Scientific Foundations of

Biochemistry in Clinical Practice

Scientific Foundations of

Biochemistry in Clinical Practice

Second edition

Edited by

David L. Williams
MA, MB, PhD, CChem, FRSC, FRCPath
Director of Pathology and Consultant Chemical Pathologist, Royal Berkshire and Battle Hospitals NHS Trust, Reading; Honorary Professor in Physiology and Biochemistry, University of Reading, UK

Vincent Marks
MA, DM, FRCP(Lond), FRCP(Ed), FRCPath, FIFST, MBAE
Professor of Clinical Biochemistry, University of Surrey; Consultant Chemical Pathologist, Royal Surrey County and St Luke's Hospital Trust, Guildford, UK

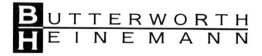

Butterworth-Heinemann Ltd
Linacre House, Jordan Hill, Oxford OX2 8DP

A member of the Reed Elsevier plc group

OXFORD LONDON BOSTON
MUNICH NEW DELHI SINGAPORE SYDNEY
TOKYO TORONTO WELLINGTON

First published 1983
Second edition 1994

To the best of the editors' and publisher's knowledge, the
information in this book is accurate and up to date at the time
of publication. However, neither the editors nor the
publisher can accept responsibility for any inaccuracy or error

British Library Cataloguing in Publication Data
A catalogue record for this book is available from the British Library

ISBN 0 7506 0167 1

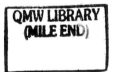
Printed in Great Britain by The Bath Press Ltd, Avon

CONTENTS

List of contributors   vii
Preface   ix
Acknowledgements   x

SECTION 1

GENERAL METABOLIC DISORDERS

1. Nutritional Disorders   1
   J. W. T. Dickerson

2. Obesity   25
   V. Marks

3. Disorders Involving Disturbance in Hydrogen Ion Concentration and Blood Gases   31
   J. F. Zilva

4. Disorders of Fluid and Electrolyte Balance   53
   G. Walters and D. St. J. O'Reilley

5. Polyuria and Disorders of Thirst   76
   D. Donaldson

6. Diabetes Mellitus   103
   M. Nattrass

7. The Clinical Biochemistry of Alcohol   121
   S. B. Rosalki

8. Psychiatric Disorders of Biochemical Origin   144
   D. Donaldson

9. The Clinical Biochemistry of Neoplasia   161
   C. R. Tillyer

SECTION 2

CLINICAL BIOCHEMISTRY IN THE CARE OF SICK PATIENTS

10. Clinical Biochemistry in Intensive and Postoperative Care   189
    A. C. Ames

11. Clinical Biochemistry and Transplantation Surgery   199
    G. Z. Maguire and A. K. Trull

12. Nutrition of the Sick Patient   218
    J. W. T. Dickerson and J. B. Morgan

SECTION 3

CLINICAL BIOCHEMISTRY OF PREGNANCY AND CHILDHOOD

13. Prenatal Screening for Neural Tube Defects and Down's Syndrome   231
    J. Wong

14. Prenatal Diagnosis of Inherited Metabolic Diseases   237
    J. B. Holton and L. Tyfield

15. Neonatal Screening for Biochemical Disorders   245
    J. B. Holton and L. Tyfield

16. Inherited and Acquired Mental Deficiency   253
    J. Stern and A. H. Wilcox

17. Neonatal and Paediatric Biochemistry   292
    V. Walker

SECTION 4

DISORDERS OF THE RENAL TRACT

18. The Chemical Analysis of Urine   317
    G. S. Challand and J. L. Jones

19. Tests of Kidney Function   325
    R. B. Payne

20. Renal Stones   338
    S. G. Hanson

SECTION 5

DISORDERS OF THE GASTROINTESTINAL TRACT

21. The Assessment of Gastrointestinal Function   347
    M. H. Z. Labib and B. J. M. Jones

22. Tests of the Functions of the Liver   383
    N. McIntyre and S. B. Rosalki

23. Clinical Diagnosis and the Acute Abdomen   399
    H. Ellis

SECTION 6

DISORDERS OF THE BLOOD CONSTITUENTS

24. Haem Synthesis and the Porphyrias   409
    G. H. Elder

25. Haemoglobinopathies   420
    D. Williamson, R. W. Carrell and H. Lehmann

26. Disorders of Iron Metabolism   446
    M. Worwood

27. Anaemias   453
    C. Barton

28. Abnormalities of the Plasma Proteins   464
    J. T. Whicher

29. Clinical Biochemistry of Blood Coagulation   495
    D. E. Austen

SECTION 7

DISORDERS OF THE NEUROMUSCULAR SYSTEM

30. Calcium Metabolism and Disorders of Bone   515
    J. A. Kanis

31. Rheumatoid Arthritis and Connective Tissue Diseases   546
    A. L. Parke

32. Clinical Biochemistry of the Central Nervous System   560
    G. B. Firth, G. N. Cowdrey and S. J. Frost

33. The Biochemistry of Coma   581
    J. de Belleroche and F. Clifford Rose

SECTION 8

DISORDERS OF THE CARDIOVASCULAR SYSTEM

34. Hypertension   585
    D. L. Williams and E. J. Burgess

35. Hyperlipidaemia   601
    A. J. Winder

36. Chest Pain   614
    V. Marks

SECTION 9

ENDOCRINE DISORDERS

37. The Hypothalamus and Pituitary and Tests of their Functions   621
    J. W. Wright

38. The Thyroid Gland and its Disorders   634
    D. L. Williams and R. Goodburn

39. Hypoglycaemia   662
    V. Marks

40. Gastrointestinal Hormones   670
    V. Marks

41. Disorders of the Adrenal Cortex   681
    P. J. Wood

42. Disorders of the Reproductive System   707
    J. W. Wright

SECTION 10

BIOCHEMICAL ASPECTS OF TOXICOLOGY AND PHARMACOLOGY

43. The Biochemistry and Toxicology of Metals
    A. P. Taylor

44. Laboratory Investigation of the Poisoned Patient
    M. J. Stewart

45. The Regulation and Monitoring of Drug Therapy
    G. Mould

Index   771

CONTRIBUTORS

Anthony C. Ames, BSc, MB, BS, FRCPath
Consultant Chemical Pathologist, Glamorgan
Health Authority, Neath General Hospital

D. E. Austen, BSc, PhD, CChem, FRSC
Clinical Scientist, Oxford Haemophilia Centre,
Churchill Hospital, Oxford

C. J. Barton, MA, MB, BChir, MSc, MRCP,
FRCPath
Consultant Haematologist, Royal Berkshire and
Battle Hospitals NHS Trust, Reading

J. de Belleroche, BA, BSc, PhD
Reader in Neurochemistry, Charing Cross and
Westminster Medical School, London

E. J. Burgess, BSc, MB, BS, PhD, CChem, MRSC,
MRCPath
Consultant Chemical Pathologist, North
Hampshire Hospital, Basingstoke

Robin Carrell, MA, PhD, FRCP, FRCPath
Professor of Haematology, University of
Cambridge

G. S. Challand, BSc, MA, PhD, MCB, CChem,
FRSC, FRCPath
Consultant Biochemist, Royal Berkshire and
Battle Hospitals NHS Trust, Reading

G. N. Cowdrey, PhD, MPhil, FIMLS
Principal Biochemist, Hurstwood Park
Neurological Centre, Haywards Heath

John W. T. Dickerson, PhD, CBiol, FIBiol, Hon
FRSH
Emeritus Professor of Human Nutrition,
University of Surrey, Guildford

David Donaldson, MB, ChB, MRCP, FRCPath
Consultant Chemical Pathologist, East Surrey
Hospital, Redhill and Crawley Hospital, West
Sussex

G. H. Elder, BA, MD, FRCP, FRCPath
Professor of Medical Biochemistry, University of
Wales College of Medicine, Cardiff

Harold Ellis, CBE, DM, MCh, FRCS
Emeritus Professor of Surgery, University of London

G. B. Firth, MSc, PhD, MRSC, CChem, MBiol,
CBiol, MCB, FRCPath
Consultant Clinical Biochemist, The Princess
Royal Hospital, Haywards Heath

S. J. Frost, BSc, MSc, MCB, MRCPath, MRSC
Principal Biochemist, The Princess Royal Hospital,
Haywards Heath

Richard Goodburn, BSc, PhD
Principal Biochemist, Ashford Hospital,
Middlesex

Sally G. Hanson, MB, BS, MRCPath
Associate Specialist in Clinical Biochemistry and
Clinical Nutrition, Royal Surrey County Hospital,
Guildford

J. B. Holton, BSc, PhD, ARCS, FRCPath
University Department of Child Health, Royal
Hospital for Sick Children, Bristol; formerly
Senior Lecturer in Clinical Chemistry, Southmead
Hospital, Bristol

Barry J. M. Jones, BSc, MD, FRCP
Consultant Gastroenterologist, Russells Hall
Hospital, Dudley

Jill Jones, BSc, PhD
Post Graduate Researcher, School of Medicine,
University of California, San Diego, USA

J. A. Kanis, MD, FRCP, FRCPath
Professor in Human Metabolism and Clinical
Biochemistry, Sheffield University Medical School

M. H. Labib, MB, ChB, MRCPath
Consultant Chemical Pathologist, Russells Hall
Hospital, Dudley

G. A. Maguire, MA, MSc, MCB, PhD, MRCPath
Top Grade Biochemist/Honorary Consultant in
Clinical Biochemistry, Addenbrooke's Hospital,
Cambridge; Associate Lecturer, University of
Cambridge

Vincent Marks, MA, DM, FRCP(London &
Edinburgh), FRCPath, FIFST, MBAE
Professor of Clinical Biochemistry, University of
Surrey; Consultant Chemical Pathologist, Royal
Surrey County and St. Luke's Hospitals Trust,
Guildford

Neil McIntyre, BSc, MD, FRCP
Professor of Medicine, Royal Free Hospital School
of Medicine, London

Graham Mould, BPharm, MSc, PhD, MRPharmS
Director, Clinical Pharmacokinetic Unit, Royal
Surrey County and St Luke's Hospitals Trust,
Guildford

Malcolm Nattrass, BSc, MB, ChB, PhD, FRCP,
FRCPath
Consultant Physician, General Hospital,
Birmingham

D. S. J. O'Reilly, MSc, MD, MRCPath
Consultant Clinical Biochemist, Glasgow Royal
Infirmary

Anne Parke, MB, BS, FRCP(C)
Associate Professor of Medicine, University of
Connecticut School of Medicine, Farmington, USA

R. B. Payne, MD, PhD, FRCPath
Consultant Chemical Pathologist, St James'
University Hospital, Leeds

S. B. Rosalki, MD, DSc, FRCP, FRCPath
Consultant in Chemical Pathology and Human
Metabolism, Royal Free Hospital and School of
Medicine, London

F. Clifford Rose, FRCP
Director, London Neurological Centre, Harley
Street, London

J. Stern, BSc, PhD, FRCPath
Top Grade Biochemist, St Helier NHS Trust,
Carshalton

M. J. Stewart, BSc, PhD, MCB, FRCPath, FIM
Consultant Scientist, Institute of Biochemistry,
Glasgow Royal Infirmary

A. P. Taylor, BSc, MSc, PhD
Top Grade Biochemist, Royal Surrey County and
St Luke's Hospitals Trust, Guildford; Senior
Research Fellow, Robens Institute of Health and
Safety, University of Surrey, Guildford,

Colin R. Tillyer, BSc, MB, BS, MRCS, PhD,
MRCPath
Consultant Chemical Pathologist, Royal Marsden
Hospital, London

Andrew Trull, PhD
Principal Clinical Biochemist, Addenbrooke's
Hospital, Cambridge

L. A. Tyfield, BSc, MSc, PhD, MRCPath
Principal Scientist, Southmead Hospital, Bristol

Valerie Walker, BSc, MD, ChB, FRCPath
Consultant Chemical Pathologist, Southampton
General Hospital; Honorary Senior Lecturer,
University of Southampton School of Medicine

Glyn Walters, MD, FRCP, LRSC, FRCPath
Emeritus Consultant in Chemical Pathology,
Bristol Royal Infirmary

J. T. Whicher, MB, BChir, MA, MSc, MRCPath
Professor of Molecular Pathology and Experimental
Cancer Research, University of Leeds

A. H. Wilcox, MA, MB, BChir, MSc, MRCPI,
MRCPath
Consultant Chemical Pathologist, The St Helier
NHS Trust, Carshalton

David L. Williams, MA, MB, PhD, CChem, FRSC,
FRCPath
Director of Pathology and Consultant Chemical
Pathologist, Royal Berkshire and Battle Hospitals
NHS Trust, Reading; Honorary Professor in
Physiology and Biochemistry, University of
Reading

D. Williamson, PhD
Senior Research Associate, Department of
Haematology, University of Cambridge

Tony Winder, MA, DM, PhD, MSc, FRCPath,
MRCP
Professor of Chemical Pathology and Human
Metabolism, Royal Free Hospital and School of
Medicine, University of London

John Wong, BAO, MA, MSc, MB, BCh, MRCPath
Consultant Chemical Pathologist, Queen Mary's
University Hospital, Roehampton

Peter J. Wood, BSc, MSc, PhD, CChem, FRSC
Consultant Biochemist, Southampton General
Hospital; Honorary Senior Lecturer, University of
Southampton School of Medicine

Mark Worwood, BSc, PhD, FRCPath
Reader in Haematology, University of Wales
College of Medicine, Cardiff

J. W. Wright, MSc, MRCPath, FRCP
Consultant in Clinical Biochemistry, St Luke's
Hospital, Guildford; Reader in Metabolic
Medicine, University of Surrey, Guildford

Joan F. Zilva, MD, BSc, FRCP, FRCPath
Professor Emeritus in Chemical Pathology,
University of London

Preface

The ten years that have elapsed since the first edition of this book have seen an ever-growing recognition of the importance of biochemistry to the practice of clinical medicine. Much of the interest and most of the media attention has been given to the elucidation of the molecular and genetic bases of disease. This has not only increased our understanding but also our ability to detect disease and do something about it before it has ravaged the body irreparably. As a result, although it is still possible to treat patients without access to a clinical biochemistry laboratory, even fewer clinicians today would be prepared to do so than in the past, unless there is absolutely no alternative.

Nevertheless, the enormous advances in technology that have taken place have made it possible to produce reliable, accurate and timely analytical data for many substances of clinical importance outside the confines of the traditional clinical laboratory. As a result there has been a tendency to forecast the demise of clinical biochemistry as a medical discipline; this view is particularly prevalent amongst third-party payers and those who know least about the complexity of the subject. On the contrary it is the very ease with which some analyses can now be conducted that makes knowledge of the factors that determine their usefulness, the order and frequency with which they are performed, and the significance of the results even more important than in the past.

Methodology, and the physical principles upon which it depends, was covered in the first volume of this series. The present volume is devoted mainly to the pathophysiological aspects of clinical biochemistry with particular emphasis on its practical application to the investigation and treatment of patients. The needs of the practising clinicians and chemical pathologists were foremost in the minds of the editors in selecting the topics to be covered and their authors, most of whom have had extensive practical, as well as academic, experience of their subject matter. The format follows closely that adopted in the first edition but all the chapters have been extensively revised by their original authors or rewritten by new ones.

Acknowledgements

The editors are greatly indebted to the authors of the constituent chapters for agreeing to contribute to this volume and for their patience during its gestation. They are also grateful for the unstinting secretarial efforts of Mrs Sheila Smith and Mrs Margaret Merry.

SECTION 1
GENERAL METABOLIC DISORDERS

1. Nutritional Disorders
J. W. T. Dickerson

Protein–energy malnutrition
  Introduction
  Protein–energy malnutrition in children
Vitamin deficiency and excess
  Introduction
  Clinical features
  Assessment of vitamin status
Trace element deficiency and excess
  Introduction
  Clinical features
  Determination of trace element status
Conclusions

PROTEIN–ENERGY MALNUTRITION

Introduction

The human body possesses considerable powers of adaptation to changes in its environment and this is nowhere more marked than in response to a decrease in nutrient availability. It is clear then that we cannot suppose that there is only one 'normal' nutritional state of the organism, and adaptation over a wide range of nutrient availability is compatible with health. Protein–energy malnutrition (PEM) represents a breakdown of adaptive mechanisms, which is manifested as clinical illness.[1] PEM is characteristically a disorder of children and as such is the most widespread and serious nutritional problem known to medical science. As we shall see, the causes are complex, with a large number of interacting factors, but the basic cause is lack of sufficient food of the right kind. PEM may, however, occur as a secondary consequence of other diseases that interfere with the ingestion of food or the absorption of nutrients, or in which there are losses by abnormal routes (i.e. fistulae) (*see* Ch. 12). The most severe form of malnutrition in adults is that which occurs in patients with cancer and is known as cancer cachexia (*see* Ch. 9). Disorders associated with obesity are discussed in the next chapter.

Protein–energy Malnutrition in Children

Classification
PEM is a term coined originally as 'protein–calorie malnutrition' to cover a spectrum of conditions ranging from marasmus at one extreme to kwashiorkor at the other. The term 'marasmus' is derived from the Greek *marasmos* meaning wasting and has been recognized for centuries as being, with gastroenteritis, a

TABLE 1.1
WELLCOME CLASSIFICATION OF INFANTILE MALNUTRITION[2]

	*Percentage of expected weight for age**	*Oedema*
Marasmus	< 60	Absent
Marasmic kwashiorkor	< 60	Present
Kwashiorkor	60–80	Present
Underweight	60–80	Absent

* Taken as the 50th percentile of the Boston standards.[3]

major cause of infant mortality. The term 'kwashiorkor' was first used by Dr Cicely Williams in 1933 to describe a condition that she recognized in the then Gold Coast. The word is taken from the *Ga* language of Ghana and literally means 'the disease the first child gets when the second is on the way'.

In marasmus the child is underweight with very little body fat and consequent loosening of the skin. There is also muscle atrophy and, depending on the chronicity of the condition, short stature. Kwashiorkor, on the other hand, is characterized by skin and hair changes, oedema, 'moon face', fatty liver, hypoalbuminaemia and psychomotor changes. The clinical manifestations of this disease differ in different parts of the world, as also does the age of development. These differences have tended to lead to some confusion in nomenclature and classification of the different forms of PEM.

A classification of PEM should be suitable for use in:

1. The international classification of diseases
2. Prevalence studies and other observations in communities
3. Clinical and research investigations.

The simplest classification is that known as the Wellcome classification (Table 1.1), which is based simply on the deficit in body weight and the presence of oedema. This classification has advantages because of its simplicity, but it cannot be applied when the age of the patient is not known and does not take into account the chronicity of the disease process.

McLaren et al.[4] introduced a simple scoring system for classifying the severe forms only (Table 1.2). This method is precise and provides a means of objectively classifying the type of patients likely to be hospitalized. It does, however, require access to laboratory facilities. Another method, introduced by Kanawati and McLaren[5], requires only the use of a stiff tape-measure and is based on the ratio of mid-arm circumference to head circumference, which is independent of age at least from 3 months to 48 months and is similar for the two sexes (Table 1.3). This method is, however, rough, unsuitable for use in individual children and is intended for use only in screening large numbers.

It seems desirable that any classification of PEM should take into account deficits in weight and height for age. One such classification is shown in Table 1.4. The diagnosis of the kind of severe PEM with which the child presents, kwashiorkor or marasmus, may change quickly for if oedema is lost a kwashiorkor child becomes a marasmic one.

Pathogenesis

Although PEM is a nutritional deficiency disease, it is doubtful if nutrition can ever be separated from the whole variety of social factors that makes up the complex environment in which children grow up. Thus, economic stringencies, overcrowding, poor hygiene, and religious and other taboos all contribute to the development of the condition. The exact form of PEM that develops depends on the age of the child, the duration of breast-feeding and also on weaning practices. Industrialization has influenced the nature of the most prevalent types of PEM in different communities. From an analysis of these factors in the Lebanon and in Jordan, McLaren[7] put forward a scheme (Fig. 1.1) to account for the pathogenesis of the extreme forms.

Classically it was held that marasmus is caused by a shortage of food, predominantly of energy, and that kwashiorkor is caused by a shortage of protein of the right kind but that the energy supply might be adequate. It has become clear that this simplistic view is a misconception, and that this has had important consequences for it has led to the idea that there is a 'protein gap', which has been described, in fact, as a 'protein fiasco'. In India, children have been described as developing either marasmus or kwashiorkor whilst consuming the same diet. It now seems clear that whether a child who is on the 'knife-edge' of good nutrition develops marasmus or kwashiorkor is determined by a number of non-dietary forces. Diet may be said to have a permissive rather than a determinative role in the human situation. This is clearly not so in animal experiments where a diet may be made determinative by eliminating other factors. A kwashiorkor-like condition can be produced in rats or pigs by feeding a diet containing a small amount of protein with excess or adequate energy. Similarly, by reducing the amount of a good diet allowed to the animals, severe stunting or a marasmic-type condition can be produced.

Prevalence

Two terms are used by epidemiologists to describe the distribution of disease in communities. They are 'incidence' and 'prevalence'. The incidence rate is the number of new cases that comes into being during a specified period in a specific group of the population. Point prevalence is the proportion of the population that has a disease at a particular instant.

All attempts to estimate the prevalence of PEM are subject to a considerable degree of uncertainty but information has been collected for a number of years by the World Health Organization (WHO) and Bengoa[8] reported data from 77 nutrition surveys in 46 developing countries, totalling nearly 200 000 children mostly under 5 years of age. Based on weight-for-height data extrapolated from these figures it was estimated that about 100 000 000 children throughout the world are suffering from moderate or severe PEM. Of these, about 31% would be found in Asia, 26% in Africa and 19% in Latin America. Mortality rates

TABLE 1.2

SIMPLE SCORING SYSTEM FOR PROTEIN–ENERGY MALNUTRITION[4]

	Points
Oedema	3
Dermatosis	2
Oedema + dermatosis	6
Hair change	1
Hepatomegaly	1
Serum albumin (g/L)	
< 10	7
10.0–14.9	6
15.0–19.9	5
20.0–24.9	4
25.0–29.9	3
30.0–34.9	2
35.0–39.9	1
> 40.0	0

Classification	Points scored
Marasmic	0–3
Marasmic kwashiorkor	4–8
Kwashiorkor	9–15

TABLE 1.3

ASSESSMENT OF MARGINAL MALNUTRITION[5]

	Mid-arm circumference/ head circumference	Percentage of weight for age
Nutritionally healthy	> 0.310	> 90
Mild–moderate PEM *	0.310–0.280	60–90
Severe PEM	< 0.250	< 60

* PEM, protein–energy malnutrition.

TABLE 1.4

CLASSIFICATION OF NUTRITIONAL STATUS IN EARLY CHILDHOOD [6][†]

Classification	Observed weight as percentage of ideal weight / length age
Overweight	> 110
Normal range	90–109
Mild PEM *	85–89
Moderate PEM	75–84
Severe PEM **	< 75

* PEM, protein–energy malnutrition.

** Marasmus (no oedema) or kwashiorkor (with oedema).

† Authors give a nomogram for rapid calculation and classification.

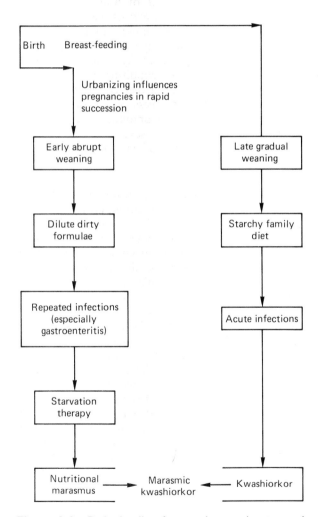

Figure 1.1 Paths leading from early weaning to nutritional marasmus and from protracted breast feeding to kwashiorkor.

for children during the first year of life and in the period 1–4 years are related to the incidence of PEM and may be used as an indirect guide in assessing nutritional status in a community.

The relative prevalence of marasmus and kwashiorkor differs in different communities. Some of the reasons for these differences have already been suggested (*see* Fig. 1.1). Of the surveys quoted by Bengoa, only 22 distinguished between the two conditions and 17 of these reported more marasmus than kwashiorkor. This is in line with present information which does suggest that marasmus is emerging as the predominant form, although it does, in fact, tend to be neglected in estimates of PEM prevalence and only kwashiorkor, which is a notifiable disease in certain areas, is reported. There is no doubt, however, that the predominant need of the world's children is for food, and not specifically for protein.

Clinical Features

Marasmus. The most striking feature of marasmus is the marked deficiency in weight and to a lesser extent in height. The marasmic infant is grossly emaciated, with an apparently large head, staring eyes and shrunken muscles under redundant folds of skin. The skin itself is thin, with no subcutaneous fat. The marasmic infant is usually irritable and fretful but may also display the features of apathy and misery that are so characteristic of kwashiorkor. Anorexia is less common in marasmus and the appetite is often good. The performance of these children in mental tests may be improved by sensory stimulation in addition to nutritional rehabilitation. However, the completeness of rehabilitation may well depend upon the age of the child, being less likely in children who have had chronic early malnutrition. Skin and hair changes may occur in marasmus but they are less common and less marked than those in kwashiorkor. Hepatomegaly is found less frequently in marasmus than in kwashiorkor.

Kwashiorkor. Oedema is the cardinal feature of kwashiorkor. The severity differs widely from one child to another and may manifest itself by puffiness around the eyes and swelling of the feet and hands, or in other cases it may be more generalized. The accumulation of fluid in the extremities may mean that severe dehydration may be present in a child with oedematous legs. Most children with kwashiorkor are underweight for their age. Marked muscle wasting may be masked by overlying well-preserved subcutaneous tissue and by oedema. Deficits in height suggest that the disease manifests itself more acutely than marasmus, although bone age and growth in length and head circumference are retarded. Some of the most striking clinical features of kwashiorkor are the skin and hair changes, though these are not present in all cases and are reversible on recovery. The skin changes include hypopigmentation and 'flaky-paint' dermatosis. In some cases the thin, shiny skin is tautly stretched on oedematous limbs or trunk; often the skin breaks down, with ulceration at the flexures in the groin and on the buttocks. The hair shows a wide range of abnormalities, especially when the disease is of long duration. Hair that is normally dark and curly becomes lighter and straighter. Dispigmented hair may alternate with darker hair according to the nutrient supply at the time when the hair was being formed; this has been described as the 'flag' sign. Hair is dry, thin and silky and is easily plucked from the scalp. In some parts of the world there is marked hepatomegaly, which is mainly due to fatty infiltration of the organ. Hepatomegaly, like the hair changes, does not occur in all cases of kwashiorkor and is therefore not diagnostic of the condition. Children with kwashiorkor are characteristically listless, apathetic, miserable and irritable. Anorexia is common and often requires intragastric tube feeding in those children where it persists. The causes of the psychological disturbances are doubtlessly complex and involve the effects of sensory deprivation. These, together with the age of the child, play an important role in determining whether the disease process is fully reversible in terms of mental function.

Marasmic Kwashiorkor. As the name implies, children are classified as having marasmic kwashiorkor when they present clinical features of both marasmus and kwashiorkor and are regarded as presenting intermediate forms of severe PEM. As shown in Table 1.1, oedema is present and body weight is less than 60% of expected standard for age. Skin and hair changes, psychological changes and a palpable fatty liver characteristic of kwashiorkor are often found in children with marasmic kwashiorkor.

Prognosis and Mortality in Severe PEM
Severe PEM is associated with infection, especially of the lower respiratory tract, and with gastroenteritis. Marked fluid and electrolyte disturbances may occur as a result of the diarrhoea, and mortality in severe PEM is high, although the rate differs in different regions. Most workers report a mortality of over 20%. A majority of deaths occur within the first few days of hospitalization. Factors that influence prognosis include infection, electrolyte and fluid imbalance, the magnitude of weight deficit, marked liver enlargement, hypothermia, hypoglycaemia, severe skin changes, xerophthalmia and evidence of disturbance in liver function. Opinions may differ as to those features that are associated with a grave prognosis but workers in Africa have reported that hypothermia with a rectal temperature of less than 35°C carries a grave prognosis. Profound hypoglycaemia is life threatening and requires immediate treatment.

Pathophysiology and Metabolic Disturbances
There is a considerable literature dealing with the pathological and biochemical changes in PEM. The brief account given in the previous edition of this book was based on a review published in 1972.[9] During the past few years there has been a complete revolution in our concepts of the mechanisms leading to the two major forms of the disease, marasmus and kwashiorkor. The following is a brief account of

recent views; a fuller account will be found elsewhere.[10]

Marasmus. In children, as in adults, a reduced food intake may be caused by one, or a number of factors—starvation, infection, malabsorption, psychiatric abnormality or neoplasia, or to an initial specific nutrient deficiency such as that of protein or zinc. Children stop growing and children (and adults) lose weight. In children, height for age and weight for age are used in the anthropometric classification of PEM (see Tables 1.1, 1.3 and 1.4).

As weight is lost, nutritional requirements fall, consequent upon the reduced lean body mass. However, there is also evidence that rather more than normal of the amino acids released from protein breakdown are used for the resynthesis of protein rather than being oxidized. Biochemical adaptation also occurs, further reducing requirements. The most important of these adaptations is a reduction in the activity of the sodium pump in cell membranes, with resultant saving in energy utilization. Further saving in energy expenditure results from a reduction in protein turnover. Furthermore, malnourished individuals reduce their spontaneous activity and there is a reduced willingness to undertake mechanical work.

Thus there are reductions in activity at different levels and these lead to physiological changes that have important consequences for treatment and rehabilitation. Changes in cardiac function put the individual at risk of cardiac failure. Reduced renal function coincident with excess body sodium and extracellular fluid can lead to acute circulatory overload and sudden death. Changes in gastric acid and digestive enzymes may result in malabsorption. Body temperature control is disturbed and the individual patient becomes poikilothermic. The inflammatory response and immunocompetence are reduced, so that infection may be difficult to recognize.

Body composition is changed (see below) and as a consequence of this and of the changes in physiological and metabolic responses, the body's reserves are depleted and its ability to respond to increased demands and environmental changes is reduced. Thus, one can visualize a number of vicious cycles developing consequent upon infections and nutritional deficiency.[10] Intestinal infections give rise to diarrhoea, which then causes deficiencies of nutrients and particularly of minerals. Skin breakdown occurs as a result of malnutrition, allowing access to bacteria. Thus, the consequences of all these changes are that the patient is anorexic and has a reduced ability to digest food and absorb nutrients. If allowed to continue, this is a self-perpetuating condition—a downwardly directed spiral with death as the inevitable result.

Treatment regimens must be aimed at breaking these vicious cycles, reversing the changes that have occurred, but working dietetically within the pathophysiological constraints of the patient's condition.

Kwashiorkor. The child with kwashiorkor has a distinctly different appearance from one with marasmus. Body fat is well preserved, the skin discoloured, the hair sparse and thin, and the liver enlarged (*see below*). The condition is very difficult to reproduce in experimental animals and preventive measures have been unsuccessful. A number of hypotheses have been proposed to account for the condition. Thus, protein deficiency, niacin deficiency, antidiuretic-hormone-like action of excess free ferritin, dysadaptation to a protein-deficient diet, hormonal dysadaptation and aflatoxicosis have all been suggested as reasons for the development of the condition in different countries. Is there a basic single nutritional/metabolic explanation—a unifying hypothesis? Golden[11,12] has suggested that kwashiorkor results from an imbalance between the production of free radicals in the patient and their safe disposal. This suggestion challenges the concept of marasmus and kwashiorkor as being at opposite ends of a spectrum of PEM. According to Golden, marasmus is caused by both energy and protein deficiency whereas kwashiorkor is the direct result of the presentation of infective and toxic agents to a body in which antioxidant and free-radical protective mechanisms are reduced by dietary deficiency of specific nutrients (vitamin E, vitamin A, carotene). In fact, Golden lists a further 10 different nutrients that may be involved: sulphur amino acids, copper, zinc, manganese, iron, selenium, riboflavin, nicotinic acid, magnesium, and thiamin. Inadequate protective pathways result in iron-catalysed chain reactions, which, in turn, lead to inadequate repair. This then leads to the characteristic clinical signs of the disease.

Thurnham[13] has reviewed the literature relating to antioxidants and pro-oxidants in malnourished populations.

Body composition. Slowing or cessation of growth in PEM is associated with a gradual increase in total body water relative to body weight. This occurs as a result of the mobilization of fat and the wasting of muscle and other tissues. Hansen et al.[14] showed that there is a direct relation between the deficit in body weight and the proportion of water in the body. The increase in total body water is due to an expansion of the volume of extracellular fluid and this is particularly marked in the presence of oedema.

A decrease in the cell mass accounts in part for the lower than normal concentration of potassium found in the body in PEM. At first the decrease in potassium is proportional to the loss in body nitrogen, but diarrhoea causes a disproportionate loss, with the result that there is a greater fall in potassium than in nitrogen in the cells. Potassium depletion plays an important part in metabolic disturbances at the cellular level, particularly in muscle, kidney and pancreas. Brain potassium is also depleted in patients with diarrhoeal losses. Studies with the whole-body counter based on determinations of the naturally occurring isotope ^{40}K have shown that, in kwashiorkor, the mean concentration of potassium in the body was 31 mM/kg and in marasmus, 39 mM/kg.[14] On recovery, values rose to 45 mM/kg (normal range 45–55 mM/kg).

In children dying of severe PEM, chemical analysis of whole bodies showed deficits of sodium, calcium and phosphorus of 7, 23 and 21% of expected values.[15] There is evidence that the cellular depletion of magnesium, like that of potassium, may be greater than that of nitrogen in muscle of children dying of PEM.

Total body protein is severely reduced in PEM and total body analysis of a limited number of cases showed deficits of 20–45% when compared with expected values. Compared with children of the same height, those with PEM had a greater deficit of total protein than of body weight. The principal loss is of non-collagen protein and on a whole-body basis, collagen is relatively little affected. However, this is probably not true of all tissues and in particular not of the skin, from which collagen is lost to a marked extent as a result of dietary deficiencies of energy or of protein.[16]

The muscle mass is greatly diminished, with degeneration and loss of fibres and shrinkage of remaining fibres.

In marasmus, body fat may be as little as 5% of the body weight (normal value, approx. 19%). Subcutaneous fat is well preserved in kwashiorkor and in this condition the liver may contain up to 50% of its wet weight as fat. Liver fat may, in fact, contribute 0.4–40% of the total body fat but there is no constant relation between the amount of fat in the liver and that in the subcutaneous tissues.

The macroscopic, yellow greasy appearance of the fatty liver of PEM is very striking. Microscopically the fat appears first in the periportal area and spreads to the central vein area of the liver lobules and distends the liver cells. The excess fat is mainly triglyceride. Liver cirrhosis does not develop as a consequence of fatty infiltration, but is more likely to be due to viral or tropical parasitic infections, alcohol or other hepatotoxins. Aflatoxin may also be a cause in some areas.

The lipid that accumulates in the liver in PEM is triglyceride and this has a similar fatty acid composition to that of adipose tissue. It seems likely that the accumulation is due to a combination of an increased flux of fatty acids from adipose tissue together with decreased hepatic synthesis of β-lipoprotein, which normally transports triglycerides from the liver. In untreated kwashiorkor the concentration of β-lipoproteins in the plasma is reduced but rises on treatment. Synthesis of the apoprotein part of the lipid-transporting mechanism seems to be particularly sensitive to dietary protein intake. The results of a study of plasma and liver lipids (Table 1.5) are in agreement with these suggestions.

Pancreatic function is abnormal in PEM and histo-

TABLE 1.5
RELATION OF SERUM LIPIDS AND LIPOPROTEINS TO FATTY LIVER IN KWASHIORKOR [17]

	Liver fat grading	Serum albumin (g/L)	Total cholesterol	β-lipoprotein cholesterol	α-lipoprotein cholesterol	Triglycerides	Total phospholipids
				mmol/L(mg/100 mL)			
A. Severe fatty liver	3–4 +	16.4	2.30 (89)	1.35 (52)	0.96 (37)	2.02 (78)	3.52 (136)
B. Mild fatty liver	0–2 +	21.4	2.69 (104)	1.79 (69)	0.88 (34)	2.67 (103)	3.47 (134)
A/B × 100		77.0	2.25 (87)	1.97 (76)	2.77 (107)	1.97 (76)	2.62 (101)
Controls			4.22 (163)	3.19 (123)	1.06 (41)	2.69 (104)	5.15 (199)

logically there is atrophy of the acinar cells though not of the islets. Exocrine function is depressed in untreated cases but responds rapidly to treatment. The endocrine function of the pancreas has attracted considerable attention and in particular that of the β cells and insulin production. Fasting plasma insulin concentrations are low in kwashiorkor and rise on recovery. Insulin response to oral glucose is low in kwashiorkor and in most marasmic children. Intravenous glucose yields a greater incidence of normal responses. When the response is impaired, the rate of return to normality is variable, with many patients taking 2–10 months after leaving hospital to recover normal responses in insulin secretion.

Disturbances in the structure and function of the gastrointestinal tract play an important role in the development of PEM and in the potential for ultimate recovery.

Macroscopically, at autopsy, the bowel appears atrophic. In the jejunum the most severe mucosal changes probably occur in kwashiorkor rather than in marasmus, but the changes range from almost normal villi to severe villous atrophy with only convolutions or ridges being seen. The crypts between the villi are not affected so severely. These changes are not specific to PEM but occur in a number of small-intestinal pathologies, notably sprue and coeliac disease. Moreover, the initial changes occur as part of the normal mucosal pattern in most tropical areas of the world. The change from the normal finger-like villi to spade villi with the occasional convolution or ridge is probably an adaptation to the 'luminal *milieu*' as distinct from atrophy of existing villi. The appearance of intestinal villi is also affected by bacterial contamination. Histologically, the epithelial cells lose their columnar shape and become cuboidal, and there is atrophy of the brush border. Paneth cells may be reduced and inflammatory cells (usually plasma cells) infiltrate the underlying lamina propria.

Electron-microscopic studies have concentrated on the appearance of lipid droplets, which were more numerous in the cells of the villous tip than in those of the crypt. The appearance was reported as being similar to that found in β-lipoprotein deficiency, in which there is a failure of chylomicron formation and accumulation of lipid droplets in the mucosal cells. Other studies on a small number of cases of severe kwashiorkor have reported no lipid in villous cells. In contrast, these workers described considerable disorganization of intracellular architecture, not only of the epithelial cells but also of endothelial cells lining the villous capillaries. They suggested that these changes could result in marked malfunction and malabsorption. They did note, however, that marked improvement occurred in a few days when rehabilitation was attempted, even in those children who subsequently died. Differences in diet prior to obtaining the samples could well account for the differences in these two reports.

Enzyme activity within the mucosal cells is reduced in PEM. The enzymes most particularly affected are the disaccharidases, peptidases, adenosine triphosphatase and alkaline phosphatase, all of which are normally located in the brush border. Of these enzymes, lactase has received the most attention and lactose intolerance is common in PEM, particularly in kwashiorkor. Although feeds containing lactose increase stool weight during the initial recovery phase, this phenomenon is often short-lived and does not require a lactose-free diet. In severe cases, sucrose and glucose intolerance also occur. Lactose intolerance may persist after recovery from PEM but the children usually tolerate milk well.

The large intestine is hypotonic, with thinning and increased vascularity of the walls. Histologically the surface epithelial cells are flattened and the mucous glands show cystic dilatation with increased numbers of inflammatory cells, particularly plasma cells, in the submucosa.

The long-term effects of PEM on the alimentary tract obviously have a bearing upon the prognosis for recovery of the child. Some workers[18] have reported that cellular improvement in the villi occurs only slowly; others reported reversion to a normal appearance within 9 months.[19] However, most of these reports have been from areas where tropical sprue is endemic and it could well be that the mucosal changes are not primarily the result of malnutrition but of some other factor that is responsible for both malnutrition and the mucosal changes. This other factor could be bacterial colonization, for Tompkins et al.[20] have shown that persistent colonization within the mucosa by enterobacteria is related to continued mucosal abnormality. Genetic differences may also play a role.

In acute PEM the mucosal atrophy of the small intestine and the exocrine pancreas, the abnormalities at subcellular level, the depression of enzyme activities, and the reported decreased concentration of conjugated bile salts in the upper jejunum all work together to reduce absorption. It would appear, however, that total mucosal function is still adequate for the absorption of the necessary nutrients to allow for rapid complete recovery of all but the most severely marasmic children. Problems arise mainly from the entry of non-absorbed residue into the lower gut, with resulting bacterial fermentation and altered osmotic pressures within the intestinal lumen, and an invasion of the upper gut by bacteria from the colon. In spite of all the apparent problems and difficulties there seems to be no evidence of any persisting malabsorption after recovery from PEM apart from a lactose intolerance, which is common in the ethnic groups amongst which PEM is common.

Protein and Amino-Acid Metabolism. Changes in body proteins occur in all forms of PEM. Those in certain tissues have already been mentioned because of their role in the pathogenesis of the disorder. Because of the ease with which they can be determined and the accessibility of the material, as well as their potential as a diagnostic tool, considerable attention has been devoted to the plasma proteins. The amount of total protein tends to be reduced in all forms of PEM but the concentrations are lowest in kwashiorkor, with the greatest reduction in the albumin fraction. In a study of malnourished and recovered children receiving high- and low-protein diets, James and Hay[21] showed that the rate of synthesis of albumin increased or decreased in response to a high- or low-protein diet, respectively. Furthermore, corresponding changes in the catabolic rate occurred after a lag period of about a week. They further showed that adaptation to a low-protein diet involved a decrease in the extravascular albumin mass with an increase in the intravascular albumin content. These observations have been confirmed in a study of experimental malnutrition.[1]

There is experimental evidence that at least two separate factors may be involved in determining whether hypoalbuminaemia appears in PEM. Thus, experiments in rats fed diets containing different concentrations of protein showed that, whilst the lower the protein concentration of the diet the greater was the extent of hypoalbuminaemia developed, dietary restriction with an increase in plasma glucocorticoid concentration and body wasting could initially delay the development of the hypoalbuminaemia. However, in the final stages of wasting that ensued a low plasma albumin could develop because of failure of the mechanisms that had earlier been able to preserve its normal concentration. It was suggested that these two separate mechanisms might have a parallel in the human situations in developing countries.

Gamma-globulin metabolism, unlike that of albumin, is unaffected by PEM and in the presence of infection the rate of synthesis is increased.[22] The concentration of transferrin in the plasma is markedly reduced in severe PEM. In a study[23] in which the serum albumin and transferrin were measured in children suffering from marasmus, kwashiorkor and marginal undernutrition it was concluded that the plasma transferrin concentration provides an index of severity in severely malnourished children. The plasma transferrin concentration showed a significant linear relation with deficits in length for age and weight for length. Moreover, in severely undernourished children who died, the plasma transferrin concentrations, in contrast to those of albumin, were lower than in those who survived.

Techniques are now available by which it is possible to measure total body protein turnover. Picou and Taylor-Roberts[24] used these techniques in malnourished children who were fed an adequate diet. They showed that at the onset of treatment the malnourished children had higher rates of protein synthesis, catabolism and turnover than recovered children. A reduction of protein intake was followed by an increase in the catabolic rate with no change in protein synthesis. These studies clearly demonstrated the adaptive mechanisms, which have been confirmed in experimental animals, by which the body conserves nitrogen in response to a dietary deficiency. It was shown that the fall in the excretion of urinary nitrogen that follows the consumption of a diet low in protein is brought about by a marked reduction in the proportion of the amino-acid flux converted to urea. Thus, when a high protein diet was fed, 23% of the amino-acid flux was converted to urea, whereas after consumption of a low-protein diet the amount converted was reduced to 2.4%.

An important aspect of this shift is the changes in the body whereby protein synthesis in certain tissues, particularly skeletal muscle, is reduced, whereas that in other tissues, such as the liver, is well maintained. It has been suggested that glucocorticoids play an important role in bringing about these tissue adaptations in protein metabolism. Confirmation of this has been obtained in an experiment in which weanling rats were given a diet containing 3.1% protein by weight and received at the same time 1.25 mg of cortisone acetate per day.[25] Under these conditions the plasma albumin concentration rose and there was a rise in the liver weight and in its protein content whereas the protein content of skeletal muscle fell. These changes in muscle and liver proteins were accompanied by changes in the corresponding free amino-acid pools, for the free amino acids of muscle generally decreased in concentration whilst those in the liver rose.

TABLE 1.6

METABOLIC RATE OF MALNOURISHED, RECOVERING, RECOVERED AND CONTROL CHILDREN EXPRESSED IN TERMS OF DIFFERENT TERMS OF REFERENCE[26]

	kJ $kg^{-1}d^{-1}$	kJ $(kg^{0.375})^{-1}d^{-1}$	kJ $100\ cm^{-1}d^{-1}$	kJ $(m^2)^{-1}d^{-1}$	kJ $(mmol\ TBK^{0.75})^{-1}d^{-1}$
Malnourished	210	315	1654	3450	17.9
Recovering	284	453	2852	5010	26.1
Recovered	251	417	2772	4827	24.2
Controls	236	409	2914	4857	22.9

Plasma Amino Acids. In untreated severe PEM the amounts of total amino acids may be reduced to half of their normal value. In kwashiorkor there is a fall of the concentrations of most of the essential amino acids, particularly the branched chain threonine and tryptophan. The concentrations of lysine and phenylalanine are less affected and the concentrations of the non-essential amino acids are fairly well maintained or even increased. The concentration of histidine is raised, probably due to decreased activity of hepatic histidinase. Another consequence of the impaired metabolism of histidine is the excretion of imidazole acrylic acid.

Urea Metabolism. In severe PEM the plasma concentration and urinary excretion of urea are reduced.

Carbohydrate Metabolism. There is general agreement that the blood glucose concentration is lower in malnourished than in recovered or normal children. The hypoglycaemia is of two types. Thus, it may be asymptomatic, noted in blood sugar determinations, or profound and almost invariably fatal. The clinical history of the children showing the profound type of hypoglycaemia frequently shows that they have been anorexic and have not fed for 12–24 h.

Glucose tolerance tests show delayed disappearance of blood glucose. Plasma insulin concentrations are low in PEM, and the insulin and glucagon response to intravenous glucose administration is impaired. The response returns to normal but only after some 2–10 months of rehabilitation. It has been suggested that the carbohydrate intolerance found in PEM predisposes the children to diabetes. The reasons for the insulin insensitivity in PEM are probably complex. The raised concentrations of cortisol and growth hormone found in the condition might play a part, for both of these hormones increase peripheral resistance to insulin. Chromium deficiency may also contribute to the condition, and potassium deficiency has been implicated because deficiency of this element results in impaired insulin release in response to glucose infusion.

There is evidence of impairment of peripheral glycolysis, which persists after recovery and which occurs at a stage of glycolysis after the phosphofructokinase step.

Gluconeogenesis is in part dependent on amino-acid availability and liver function. Tissues like the brain and erythrocytes, which usually use glucose, become dependent on hepatic gluconeogenesis in PEM and for this alanine from skeletal muscle is the principal precursor. With prolonged fasting the brain adapts to the use of ketones as fuel. It is not known to what extent this may occur in children with PEM. Hepatic glycogen concentrations are generally depressed in PEM, though there have been reports of elevated concentrations in kwashiorkor.

Energy Metabolism. The basal metabolic rate depends on the composition of the body, on cellular activity, or both. A number of bases of reference have been used in studies on children with PEM, but regardless of the reference used, the metabolic rates of malnourished children have been found to be lower than in recovering or control children (Table 1.6). Energy intake is usually the limiting factor in controlling the rate of recovery from uncomplicated PEM. With a high energy intake of the order of 490 kJ/kg per day (119 kcals/kg per day) and a moderate protein intake, rapid rates of weight gain can be achieved. It is reckoned that for each gram of tissue gain, 20 kJ (5 kcals) is required. A postprandial increase in metabolic rate is probably related to the energy cost of growth.

Thermoregulation. Rectal temperatures of 35.5°C (96°F) or less occur in patients with PEM, and in some parts of the world such low temperatures have been regarded as indicative of a poor prognosis. The degree of hypothermia is related to the severity of malnutrition. Moreover, hypothermia is more common in marasmic children, with their marked reduction in skinfold thickness, than it is in children with kwashiorkor, who have relatively well-preserved subcutaneous tissues. Another factor in the pathogenesis of hypothermia is an inadequate supply of substrates for energy production. This applies particularly to the child with marasmus. There is a marked rise in the temperature when food is provided. Hypothermia may be an indication of asymptomatic hypoglycaemia in the severely malnourished infant.

Oedema. The aetiology of oedema in kwashiorkor is complex. It cannot occur in the absence of sodium and water retention, and hypoproteinaemia is a predisposing factor. Albumin is the most important substance contributing to plasma colloidal osmotic pressure, but in studies in Uganda it has been found that the serum plasma colloidal osmotic pressure did not fall significantly until the albumin concentration fell to values of between 25.1 and 27.5 g/L. A significant correlation between the two did not appear until the plasma albumin concentration was low.[27] Increases in the concentration of globulins could account for the lag in fall of the colloidal osmotic pressure. An increased activity of arginine vasopressin (antidiuretic hormone) may also play an important role in the aetiology of oedema in kwashiorkor. It has also been suggested that increased aldosterone production is a causative factor but there is no good evidence to support this suggestion.

Diagnosis and Assessment of Severity
The diagnosis of severe PEM is usually straightforward; marasmus and kwashiorkor are easily diagnosed by the clinical features already mentioned. However, it is important that the diagnosis is correct before treatment is commenced. The identification of the child at risk of developing clinical PEM, and the detection of mild or moderate PEM and its proper assessment can make an important contribution to preventive medicine. True preventive medicine requires the identification of social, economic and other factors that predispose children to PEM. However, for the present purpose I will concentrate on those methods with which the clinical biochemist is most likely to be concerned—anthropometry and laboratory investigations. The latter fall into two groups: those used to detect malnutrition and those necessary for treatment.

Anthropometry. This is the main method by which the severity of malnutrition and the chronicity of deprivation can be assessed. It can only be used, however, if the age of the child is known, for the interpretation of the measurements depends upon reference to standards for age.

The standardization of techniques for anthropometry is of prime importance. The operator needs to be practised at the techniques so that the various measurements can be made in a strictly reproducible fashion. Moreover, s/he needs to have equipment that will enable the measurements to be made accurately and quickly. Without sound equipment and training, anthropometric measurements are likely to be of little value.

The ratio of weight to ideal weight for age is a satisfactory expression of deficit of body size. Weight for height is probably a better index of wasting than weight for age and is a measure of 'acute' marasmus.

Percentage weight for height is calculated as follows:

$$\frac{\text{Weight of child} \times 100}{\text{Weight of standard child of the same height}}$$

A deficit in height for age usually indicates that the child has suffered chronic nutritional deprivation as stunting of the skeleton takes longer to become manifest than does a deficiency in body weight.

Ideally, 'normal' reference growth data should be available for each ethnic group in order to control for the genetic contribution to growth patterns. However, the most used standards are the Harvard or Boston standards and, in the UK, those produced by Tanner and his colleagues.[3]

Fat can be conveniently assessed by making use of the fact that in man much of the total body fat, probably about 50%, is subcutaneous and the 'thickness' of this can be measured with a skinfold caliper. If convenient, the skinfold thickness at more than one site should be measured in order to allow for individual differences in the distribution of subcutaneous fat. The four sites suggested by Durnin and Womersley[28] are the biceps and triceps at the midpoint between the acromion and olecranon processes, the subscapula at the point of the shoulder blade and the suprailiac measured at the tip of the iliac crest. The sum of these skinfold thicknesses may then be used to calculate the total body fat as a percentage of the body weight, using a nomogram.[5]

Mid upper-arm circumference can be used to provide useful information about muscle mass if combined with measurement of the triceps skinfold. The measurement has an added attraction in that it requires only a steel or non-stretchable plastic tape-measure. The arm circumference represents a summation of the bone, muscle, fat and skin of the arm. What has become known as the 'mid upper-arm muscle circumference' can be calculated as follows:

$$\text{Muscle circumference} = \text{arm circumference} - (\pi \times \text{triceps skinfold}).$$

Hair Morphology. The hair root is a site of active protein synthesis throughout life. Moreover, samples are easily obtained with little or no discomfort to the subject and their examination requires only the availability of a simple microscope. Details of the method of obtaining hair samples together with interpretation guidelines were presented by Bradfield.[29] These guidelines are shown in Table 1.7. The hair root is affected differently in kwashiorkor and marasmus; this is not surprising, as hair changes are a characteristic feature of the former condition. In kwashiorkor, the number of growing roots (anagens) is significantly less than normal, and usually they show severe atrophy. The mean bulb diameter may be reduced to one-third of normal values. The number of bulbs in the resting

TABLE 1.7

SUGGESTED STANDARDS FOR THE NUTRITIONAL INTERPRETATION
OF HAIR ROOT SPECIMENS[29]

Measurement	Normal	Moderate malnutrition	Severe malnutrition
Mean bulb diameter (mm $\times 10^{-2}$)	>11	6–11	<6
Atrophy (percentage of anagen)	0–25	26–50	>50
Anagens (percentage)	>50	30–50	<30
Telogens (percentage)	<20	20–45	>45

(telogen) phase is significantly increased. In marasmus, there is almost complete lack of bulbs in the growing phase and more broken hairs are found in marasmus than in kwashiorkor. Bradfield has concluded that the method is useful for the detection of the presence of malnutrition and not for the assessment of its severity.

Plasma Albumin Concentration. Marked hypoproteinaemia, in particular hypoalbuminaemia, is a characteristic of severe kwashiorkor. There has been considerable debate as to whether this determination is a sufficiently sensitive indicator of marginal malnutrition, but Whitehead et al.[30] have shown that when the concentration reaches 30 g/L, all the metabolic changes associated with kwashiorkor develop. This information provided a basis on which to make the following interpretation guidelines: concentrations (g/L) >35, normal; 30–34, subnormal; 25–29, low; < 25, pathological.

Other Plasma Proteins. *Transferrin.* This iron-carrying globulin is much more reduced in percentage terms than albumin. However, its use as an index of malnutrition requires further investigation, for the amounts are evidently affected by iron, as well as protein status. Furthermore, more needs to be known about differences in the values in kwashiorkor compared with those in marasmus.

Thyroxine-binding prealbumin. This protein has a half-life of only 2 days, which renders it extremely sensitive to a reduced protein and energy intake of a few days' duration. It has been suggested that it declines in 3 days in response to a reduced energy intake, even when protein intake is adequate.[31] Other studies have suggested that prealbumin, whilst declining rapidly in PEM, responds equally rapidly towards normal when patients are given nutritional support (total parenteral nutrition).[32] Values of 50–100 mg/L are indicative of modest and less than 50 mg/L of severe protein depletion.

Retinol-binding protein (RBP). This transport protein has a half-life of only 12 h. Low serum RBP concentrations in Senegalese malnourished children returned to normal following nutritional support.[33] Low values in adults also returned to normal after 5 days of total parenteral nutrition.[32] Unfortunately, other factors influence serum RBP concentrations, notably liver disease, zinc deficiency and hyperthyroidism, which all decrease it. The normal range for RBP has been reported to be 30–65 mg/L[34] and 26–76 mg/L.

Plasma Amino-acid Patterns. It has been suggested that the pattern of amino acids in the plasma, which is abnormal in kwashiorkor, could be used as a means of detection of children at risk of this form of PEM.[35] Simple, semiquantitative determinations of non-essential and essential amino acids enable the calculation of a ratio:

$$\text{Ratio} = \frac{\text{glycine} + \text{serine} + \text{glutamine} + \text{taurine}}{\text{valine} + \text{leucine} + \text{isoleucine} + \text{methionine}}$$

In normal children the value of the ratio was 1.5; in subclinical malnutrition values range from 2.0 to 4.0, whilst in frank kwashiorkor they were above 3.5 with a mean value of 5.0. The main attraction of this method, which was developed in Uganda, was its sensitivity to malnutrition at an earlier stage than the plasma albumin. However, there are a number of problems with the interpretation, for the ratio very rapidly returns to normal when a good diet is given and it is clearly very sensitive to the protein content of the diet. An interpretation of the values is shown in Table 1.8.

Urinary Creatinine–Height Index. Skeletal muscle is vulnerable to malnutrition and an estimate of muscle mass would provide a useful assessment of nutritional status. Biochemical assessment is based on the fact that creatinine is a breakdown product of creatine, nearly all of which is contained in muscle. The 24-h excretion of creatinine is therefore related to the muscle mass, with 1 g of creatinine excreted being equivalent to 20 kg of muscle in children. The creatinine–height index is the ratio between creatinine excreted by the subject in 24 h divided by the daily creatinine output of the average normal child of the same height. Normal values are given in the original publication.

Values determined by this method showed a good correlation with estimates of musculature obtained

TABLE 1.8
INTERPRETATION OF FASTING SERUM AMINO ACID RATIOS IN
CHILDREN [36]

Ratio	Interpretation
< 2.0	Adequate diet
2.1–3.5	Low protein/high carbohydrate diet being eaten at insufficient amounts of protein to meet requirements; serum albumin probably decreasing, leading to subclinical kwashiorkor
> 3.5	Indicative of severe dietary deprivation and impending kwashiorkor

from the total body potassium measurements made in a whole body counter, and with estimates of musculature derived from soft tissue radiography.

Other Methods. Other methods that have been suggested as suitable for the detection of malnutrition in children include the urinary urea:creatinine ratio, the hydroxyproline–creatinine index, the urinary excretion of 3-methylhistidine, and determinations of both plasma and urinary ribonuclease. Further validation of each of these methods is required before they can be used with confidence.

Investigations During Treatment
The metabolic disturbances that occur in patients hospitalized for PEM are complex. However, a few simple determinations are all that are really necessary for their day-to-day care.

Anaemia is common and blood smears should be examined in order to determine the type that is present. The prothrombin index is also commonly depressed, particularly in septicaemic patients. Septicaemia is often associated with jaundice. The plasma bilirubin concentration should be determined in order to detect mild jaundice. Plasma electrolytes should also be determined, as a very low plasma potassium (approx. 1.5 mmol/L) is commonly seen. The low plasma urea of kwashiorkor is raised by an adequate protein intake. The plasma concentration of albumin is a sensitive guide to recovery.

Blood glucose determinations are necessary for the detection of asymptomatic hypoglycaemia though these can be done roughly with Dextrostix (Ames Company) or similar products.

Bacteriological investigations are necessary to exclude the presence of infections and the tuberculin test should always be done on admission.

Discussion of the dietary approach to the rehabilitation of children with PEM is beyond the scope of this chapter and will be found elsewhere.[10]

VITAMIN DEFICIENCY AND EXCESS

Introduction

Vitamins are organic substances that are essential to health. They cannot be made in the body, at least not in amounts sufficient to meet metabolic requirements, and must thus be supplied in the diet. With one notable exception (vitamin D, or cholecalciferol), vitamins function as cofactors for enzyme systems. Broadly speaking, the vitamins can be divided into two groups according to whether they are fat or water soluble. Ill effects from the ingestion of large quantities of water-soluble vitamins are rare and transient. In contrast, ill effects resulting from the consumption of large doses of some fat-soluble vitamins, particularly retinol (vitamin A) and cholecalciferol (vitamin D) can be serious and even fatal. As with protein and energy, the effects of deficiencies and excesses are more serious in the rapidly growing fetus and child than in adults. However, as we shall see, deficiencies of some vitamins present a public health problem in certain ethnic minority groups and amongst old people.

It is important to remember that deficiency diseases are the end-result of a series of changes (Fig. 1.2) and that they take time to develop. The fact that an individual does not show clinical evidence disease does not mean that there is no deficiency of a particular vitamin.

Biochemical indicators of circulating vitamin concentrations may yield low values, even in the absence of overt disease. There is considerable debate as to the significance of such values and they are generally said to indicate a state of 'subclinical deficiency'. There are two situations in which such deficiencies may be serious: in the sick, in whom there may be increased requirements, and in the elderly, in whom homeostatic mechanisms may be somewhat brittle.

It is also important, in this connection, to recognize that a level of deficiency which is not sufficient to produce disease may, nevertheless, result in some impairment of function. Many signs of impaired function are somewhat non-specific and only detected by experienced observers.

The situation is made more complex by interactions between certain vitamins whereby excess of one may 'protect' or 'conserve' another. In addition, blood concentrations of vitamins that circulate in the plasma bound to specific proteins may be low due to a deficiency of the binding protein. Thus, retinol circulates in the plasma bound to RBP, which forms part of the prealbumin fraction. The synthesis of RBP is dependent on the availability of zinc so that low zinc status can be responsible for a low level of retinol. Both retinol and cholecalciferol are stored in the liver, and in the case of retinol, it is clearly possible for the liver store to be adequate and yet the

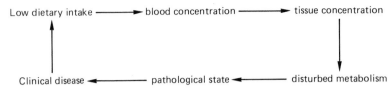

Figure 1.2 Sequence of changes leading to the development of a deficiency disease.

circulating amount, and consequently the amount reaching tissues, to be low.

Clinical Features

Vitamin A deficiency causes xerophthalmia. A mild form of this disorder, confined to the conjunctiva, is common in many countries and is not in itself serious. However, it serves as a warning for if the deficiency becomes more severe and spreads to the cornea, there is danger of corneal ulceration and a permanent defect of vision. In severe cases there is softening of the cornea, keratomalacia, which if not treated immediately leads to permanent blindness. Keratomalacia is often associated with PEM in young children. Indeed, the peak age at which blindness is most likely to occur is between 2 and 5 years, when kwashiorkor is common, but it can occur in association with marasmus in the first year of life.

Vitamin A deficiency is most prevalent in countries where rice is the dietary staple. The diet contains practically no milk or butter and very small amounts of fresh vegetables and fruit. It therefore lacks both retinol and carotenoids that can be converted into retinol in the body. Xerophthalmia and keratomalacia occur in the first year of life amongst artificially fed infants but are rare amongst the breast-fed. It is estimated that more than 10 million children develop xerophthalmia each year and of these half a million become permanently blind as the result of keratomalacia.

In experimental animals, vitamin A deficiency causes metaplasia in the cornea as well as in the respiratory and upper alimentary tracts, and in the urinary and reproductive tracts. The squamous metaplastic epithelium produces large amounts of keratin.

The WHO has given code numbers to the different forms of xerophthalmia and associated conditions (Table 1.9). One of these, night blindness (XNN) is an early symptom of vitamin A deficiency resulting from interference with the synthesis of the pigment rhodopsin, which is found in the rods of the retina. It is the aldehyde form of the vitamin (retinal) that participates in this reaction.

A number of other conditions, e.g. exposure, trauma, bacterial infection, measles and trachoma, cause corneal lesions and keratomalacia, and vitamin A deficiency must therefore be distinguished from them.

Vitamin A has been called the 'anti-infective' vitamin and there is no doubt that severe vitamin A deficiency predisposes the individual to infection. However, isolated vitamin A deficiency is a relatively rare occurrence in man and is frequently associated with some degree of PEM or mineral (iron or copper) deficiency, or both. These deficiencies themselves also affect the immune system. The major problem[38] therefore has been to try to sort out the relative contributions of each of these deficiencies on immunological function.[39]

Despite the problems, there are several reports showing that vitamin A affects the outcome of infection.[38] Thus, vitamin A deficiency when coincident with PEM results in lower levels of secretory IgA in nasal washings. In children with measles, secretory IgA and lysozyme were lower than in controls but there was no correlation between low vitamin A values and the immune factors in the tears. In a clinical study, a reduction in fatality rate from measles among Tanzanian children less than 2 years old resulted from administration of 60 mg vitamin A orally for 2 days.[40] In Indonesia, a prospective study in which a 6-monthly dose of vitamin A (60 mg) was given to preschool children resulted in a 34% lower mortality in the intervention group.[41] However, interpretation of the study is difficult, owing to lack of information about baseline mortality and specific cause of death, or about access of either the intervention or the control groups to health services.

The above studies were performed in areas where xerophthalmia is endemic and effects of vitamin A supplementation expected. Vitamin A deficiency is not endemic in Australia. It is therefore of greater interest that supplementation of Australian children with a history of frequent respiratory infections caused a 25% reduction in frequency of respiratory disease; the children received 450 mg/kg daily for 11 months.[42] In South Africa, administration of 60 mg vitamin A orally for two consecutive days to children with severe measles resulted in reduced mortality and morbidity rates.

There is some evidence that vitamin A and particularly its precursor, β-carotene, may have a protective action in relation to epithelial cancers because of their activity as antioxidants and free-radical scavengers. This has been discussed elsewhere.[43]

Populations at risk of vitamin A deficiency should be given a prophylactic oral dose of 66 000 μg vitamin A every 6 months.

Vitamin A can be toxic and both acute and chronic poisoning have been described. Acute poisonig has followed the administration of single, large doses of

TABLE 1.9
FORMS OF XEROPHTHALMIA AND ASSOCIATED CONDITIONS[37]

Code	Form and associated condition	Description
X1A	Conjunctival xerosis	Bulbar conjunctiva dry, thickened, wrinkled, and pigmented with a 'smoky' appearance
		Similar condition caused by long periods of exposure to glare, dust, and infections
		In children under 1 year, likely to be due to dietary deficiency
X1B	Conjunctival xerosis with Bitot's spots	
X2	Corneal xerosis	Cornear dry, dull, hazy and lacks lustre; insensitive to touch
X3A	Corneal xerosis with ulceration	Cornea ulceration may occur from many causes
		Erosion occurs, which in the absence of infection heals by scarring
X3B	Keratomalacia	Develops from xerosis, little chance of preventing blindness
XNN	Night blindness	An early symptom of vitamin A deficiency
Xf	Xerophthalmia fundus	Ophthalmoscopic examination shows white or yellow scattered spots along sides of blood vessels
XS	Corneal scars	White, opaque patches on the cornea; effect on vision depends on size of scar; likely to be due to vitamin A deficiency in areas where this is prevalent

about 100 000 μg to children. There are symptoms of raised intracranial pressure, with headache, vomiting and restlessness. Chronic poisoning takes several weeks or years to develop, depending on the age of the child and the dosage. Infants can become hypervitaminotic within a few weeks on 20 000 μg/day. A bizarre clinical picture is presented and vitamin A toxicity may not be suspected. The hair becomes coarse and sparse, the skin dry and rough, the lips cracked and the eyebrows denuded. Hepatosplenomegaly develops, with headache and generalized weakness. The bones also show deformities and osteoporosis.

Carotenaemia occurs in individuals who consume an abnormal quantity of carrots or carrot juice. Death may result from the following of such a fad regimen.

Vitamin D

Rickets and osteomalacia are the result in children and adults, respectively, of a deficiency of vitamin D. The child with rickets is often restless, fretful and pale, with flabby, toneless muscles. Excessive sweating of the head is common; the abdomen is distended as a result of the weak abdominal muscles. Diarrhoea is a common feature and the child is also prone to respiratory infections. Development is delayed and in severe cases growth may be severely impaired.

The bony changes are the most characteristic and easily identifiable sign of rickets. There is widening of the epiphyses where cartilage meets bone. The earliest recognizable lesion is craniotabes—small, round, unossified areas in the skull bones. Another early sign is enlargement of the epiphyses at the lower end of the radius and at the costrochondral junctions of the ribs—described as the 'rachitic rosary'. 'Bossing' of the frontal and parietal bones

may occur, with delayed closure of the anterior fontanelle. If allowed to continue the child with rickets develops deformities. These include the so-called pigeon-chest, in which there is undue prominence of the transverse depression of the chest, making breathing difficult. Kyphosis of the spine may develop in the second or third year as a result of gravitational and muscular strains, caused by sitting or crawling. There may also be enlargement of the lower ends of the femur, tibia and fibula, and when the child begins to walk the weight may cause deformities of the shafts—knock-knees (genuvalgum) or bow-legs (genuvarum). Rickets is most likely to be seen in Britain in children whose parents come from India and Pakistan.[44] Congenital rickets may occur in babies of osteomalacic mothers, usually presenting as neonatal hypocalcaemic seizures. Preterm rickets, formerly called the rickets of prematurity, is thought to be due to the very rapid linear growth of the preterm infant. This contrasts with the rapid weight gain of the low birth-weight, dysmature (light-for-dates), term infant, whose main problem is hypoglycaemia. Infantile rickets was formerly common in Britain, due to the feeding of unfortified substitutes for breast milk for some time after birth. The earliest sign is craniotabes and costrochondral beading. Toddler rickets affects mainly those aged 9 months to 3 years who have received an adequate intake of vitamin D for the first 4–6 months but whose intake then falls due to a switch from fortified to doorstep milk. Toddler rickets may be severe enough to cause pelvic contracture and genuvarum in babies already walking. Rickets is all too common amongst Asian immigrant adolescents, who are usually Muslims adhering to their religion, dress, language and dietary habits. The diet of many of these immigrants contains a large proportion of chapatis and other bread made from whole

	Osteomalacia	Osteoporosis
Clinical features		
Skeletal pain	Major complaint, usually persistent	Episodic, usually associated with fracture
Muscle weakness	Usually present, resulting in characteristic waddling gait	Absent
Fractures	Relatively uncommon, healing delayed	The usual presenting feature, heals normally
Skeletal deformity	Common, especially kyphosis	Only occurs with fracture
Biochemical features		
Plasma Ca and P	Often low	Normal
Plasma alkaline phosphatase	Often high	Normal
Plasma vitamin D	Low	Normal
Urinary calcium	Often low	Normal or high
Radiographic features		
Low bone density	Widespread	Irregular, most marked in the spine
Loss of bone detail	Characteristic	Not a feature
	Diagnostic	Absent
Biopsy		
Histological changes	Excess osteoid, normal quantity of bone	Reduced quantity of bone, fully mineralized

wheat flour. Arneil[44] points out that despite pain in limbs, awkward and deteriorating mobility, and marked genuvalgum the condition is often overlooked by teachers, nurses and doctors. Modesty and purdah play an important role in veiling the deformed limbs of pubertal Asian females.

Osteomalacia occurs in women of child-bearing age who have been depleted of calcium by repeated pregnancies. It is common amongst Muslims who practise purdah and is due to the consumption of a poor diet and the absence of exposure to sunlight. The disease is also not uncommon in non-immigrant older women in the UK and occurs particularly in those who, because of disability, cannot go out easily. Indeed, there is evidence that lack of exposure to sunlight is the main aetiological factor. Osteomalacia often coexists with osteoporosis. Distinctive features of these two conditions are shown in Table 1.10.

Osteomalacia occurs in up to 25% of subjects who have undergone gastrectomy, with signs of bone disease appearing 10–14 years after surgery. A failure to absorb vitamin D or a dietary deficiency of vitamin D and calcium have been suggested as possible reasons. Osteomalacia also commonly occurs as a consequence of chronic diseases of the digestive system such as cystic fibrosis and coeliac disease. A complex bone disease known as renal osteodystrophy occurs in patients with chronic renal failure. This disease is osteomalacia with varying degrees of osteitis fibrosa, osteoporosis, osteosclerosis and, in children, growth retardation. The disease is resistant to treatment with all but very high doses of vitamin D. Due to the renal disease there is a failure to synthesize 1,25-dihydroxycholecalciferol ($1,25(OH)_2D_3$).

Rickets and osteomalacia have been described in patients receiving long-term anticonvulsant drug therapy, particularly with phenytoin and phenobarbitone. One possible explanation is that these drugs induce hepatic microsomal enzymes, which convert 25-hydroxycholecalciferol to inactive metabolites. Another possible explanation is that the anticonvulsant drugs disturb mineral metabolism perhaps by inhibiting vitamin D function. These explanations are not mutually exclusive and evidence has been obtained in favour of both of them. Practically, it is important to note that the requirements of such patients are raised and that preventive measures against deficiency are adequate to meet this raised requirement. Children on these drugs probably require 25 μg per day, compared with 10 μg per day for children not on the drugs.

Genetically determined forms of vitamin D-resistant rickets occur. Hypophosphataemic vitamin D-resistant rickets is inherited as an X-linked dominant genetic defect, although new cases occur sporadically, presumably as new mutations. Vitamin D-dependent rickets is a rare disorder with autosomal recessive heritability.

There is a narrow gap between the nutrient requirement and the toxic dose of vitamin D. As little as five times the recommended intake, i.e. 50 μg per day, over prolonged periods can lead to hypercalcaemia and nephrocalcinosis in adults. Toxicity can occur in children from a mother mistaking her instructions in administering a concentrated vitamin D preparation. The earliest toxic symptom in children is usually loss of appetite with nausea and vomiting. Thirst and polyuria develop and constipation may alternate with diarrhoea. Pains in the head frequently occur, and the child becomes thin, irritable and depressed, and gradually stuporose. Metastatic calcification has been described in fatal cases.

The syndrome of supravalvular aortic stenosis has been presumed to be due to hypersensitivity to vitamin D. In this condition there is aortic stenosis with left ventricular hypertrophy, myocardial focal necrosis, fibrosis and calcification. Affected children have a close craniofacial similarity to those with severe idiopathic hypercalcaemia and like these may be mentally defective. Patients with this condition seldom received more than 75 μg of dietary vitamin D per day and the question arises as to whether they received too much vitamin D before birth.

There is a wide variation in the 24-h excretion of calcium between individuals in different parts of the world. In Britain the upper limit of normal is taken as 400 mg (10 mmol) for men and 300 mg (7.5 mmol) for women. Hypercalciuria on a normal diet is most commonly related to an abnormally high absorptive capacity for calcium and individuals with the condition have an increased tendency to form urinary calculi. Clearly, the enhanced absorption of calcium in idiopathic hypercalciuria could be due to stimulation of the conversion of vitamin D to its active forms. It might also be due to increased sensitivity of the intestinal mucosa to vitamin D, though it seems difficult to explain changes on this basis.

Although hypercalcaemia occurs in less than 20% of patients with sarcoidosis, hypercalciuria is found more often and evidence of hyperabsorption of calcium is an almost constant finding in the active disease. As with idiopathic hypercalciuria, there is a seasonal change in calcium absorption, and this is related to a hypersensitivity to vitamin D, which can be corrected with glucocorticoids.

Vitamin E
Primary vitamin E deficiency has been reported only in premature infants who are born with an inadequate reserve of the vitamin. If given a dietary formula with a high content of polyunsaturated fat or iron medication, they may develop a haemolytic anaemia with an associated thrombocytosis, generalized irritability and oedema. Recent interest has focused on the possible use of prophylactic vitamin E supplements in the premature infant.[46] Supplements have been suggested to be of value in the prevention of intracranial haemorrhage, bronchopulmonary dysplasia and retrolental fibroplasia, complications associated with oxygen therapy in premature infants.[47] However, the strongest evidence of benefit is in the prevention of retrolental fibroplasia, but caution is needed and the form in which vitamin E is to be given must be carefully considered.

Evidence of vitamin E deficiency has been described in patients with malabsorption of fat due to cystic fibrosis, abetalipoproteinaemia and other diseases. Red cell survival is reduced but anaemia and clinical manifestations are unusual. Vitamin E toxicity, manifested as multiple haemorrhages, has been described in a patient taking warfarin with high doses of the vitamin. Warfarin and vitamin E antagonize the action of vitamin K in provoking the clotting of blood. Vitamin E is now being taken in large doses (up to 1000 iu per day) to prevent clotting problems and also to prevent senile changes in the brain. There is no real evidence that it does either in the human. There is some evidence, however, that high doses may be beneficial in the treatment of intermittent claudication.

Vitamin K
Primary deficiency of vitamin K is rare in adults but has been seen in infants. Some cases of hypoprothrombinaemia in infants are cured by giving vitamin K.

As vitamin K is fat soluble, any disease process that interferes with the absorption of fat from the gut is likely to lead to a deficiency of the vitamin. Severe bleeding after an operation for relief of jaundice due to obstruction of the common bile duct used to be feared by surgeons. It is now customary to give vitamin K by injection before the operation in order to reduce this danger. Bleeding due to vitamin K deficiency may occur in coeliac disease and other conditions in which fats are not collectively absorbed. Vitamin K deficiency with hypoprothrombinaemia and bleeding can also follow the administration of antibiotics, which reduce the colonic flora in individuals who have been eating poorly.

Infants of mothers on hydantoin therapy should receive prophylactic vitamin K, as they appear to be particularly susceptible to the drug-induced deficiency of the vitamin.

As already indicated, warfarin antagonizes the action of vitamin K and overdosage with warfarin can be overcome by an adequate dose of phytomenadione (vitamin K_1).

Thiamin (Vitamin B_1)
Beriberi due to thiamin deficiency was formerly common amongst the rice-eating peoples of the East. Three forms of the disease occur: (i) wet beriberi characterized by oedema often associated with high-output cardiac failure; (ii) dry beriberi, a polyneuropathy, and (iii) the infantile form. Thiamin deficiency is also involved in three conditions that are not uncommon in chronic alcoholics and occur in all parts of the world. These are (i) alcoholic polyneuropathy, clinically indistinguishable from dry beriberi, (ii) a thiamin-responsive cardiomyopathy, and (iii) an encephalopathy, the Wernicke–Korsakoff syndrome.

Early symptoms and signs are common to both wet and dry beriberi. The onset is usually insidious, with anorexia and ill-defined malaise associated with weakness of the legs. Oedema of the legs and face

TABLE 1.11
PRESENTATION OF INFANTILE BERIBERI[48]

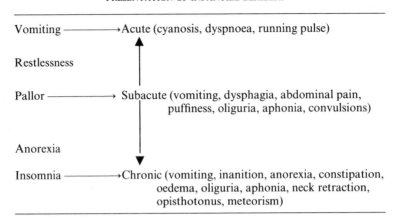

Vomiting ————→ Acute (cyanosis, dyspnoea, running pulse)

Restlessness

Pallor ————→ Subacute (vomiting, dysphagia, abdominal pain,
puffiness, oliguria, aphonia, convulsions)

Anorexia

Insomnia ————→ Chronic (vomiting, inanition, anorexia, constipation,
oedema, oliguria, aphonia, neck retraction,
opisthotonus, meteorism)

may become manifest. Tenderness of the muscles occurs on pressure and there are complaints of 'pins and needles' (paraesthesiae) and numbness of the legs. Anaesthesia of the skin, particularly over the tibiae, is common. The patients are only slightly incapacitated but at any time the disease may develop into either of the severe forms.

Oedema is the most characteristic feature of *wet beriberi* and may develop rapidly to involve legs, face, trunk and serous cavities. Palpitations are marked and there may be breathlessness; anaemia and dyspepsia are common. Often there is pain in the legs after walking, similar to that resulting from ischaemia of muscle. Neck veins become distended and show visible pulsations. High systolic and low diastolic pressures occur in the arteries. If the circulation is well maintained, the skin is warm to the touch, owing to associated vasodilation. When the heart begins to fail the skin becomes cold and cyanotic. The mind is usually clear. Sudden increase in oedema may occur, with acute circulatory failure, extreme dyspnoea and death.

The essential feature of *dry beriberi* is polyneuropathy. Early symptoms and signs are as described above. Muscles become progressively wasted and weak, and walking increasingly difficult. The thin, emaciated patient becomes progressively weaker and may succumb to an infection. The *infantile* form of *beriberi* is always a more or less acute disease due to a deficiency of thiamin in breast milk. The early signs are mild and easily missed by the mother but the disease progresses rapidly and is fatal if not treated at between 2–4 months of age. It is milder and less common after 6 months. The mothers show few signs of the disease themselves.

The clinical features are summarized in Table 1.11. Three main syndromes have been described:

1. The acute cardiac variety is of sudden onset at between 2 and 4 months of age with physical signs of acute cardiac failure and death may occur within minutes or hours.

2. Aphoria occurs between 5 and 7 months and coughing and choking suggest respiratory infection. The child emits a characteristic noiseless cry with laryngeal nerve paralysis, or oedema of the larynx.

3. The pseudomeningeal variety simulates meningitis in the older infant 8–10 months of age, with apathy, drowsiness, head retraction and signs of raised intracranial pressure.[49]

Beriberi is rare after the age of 1 year. In older children it manifests itself in a way similar to that of adults.

Alcoholics who have eaten little or no food for many weeks may develop a disorder of peripheral nerves indistinguishable from dry beriberi. More than one nerve may be involved, with the lesions being symmetrical and the nerves of the lower limbs being affected more severely than the upper limbs. Usually there is dysfunction of both sensory and motor fibres. The effects on the sensory fibres may be paraesthesiae or sometimes severe nerve pains. Motor nerve involvement manifests itself as foot drop, muscle wasting and impaired knee and ankle jerks.

Wernicke–Korsakoff syndrome is characterized by weakness of eye muscles (ophthalmoplegia), accompanied sometimes with jerky rhythmical movements of the eyes (nystagmus). If the patient can stand, he or she is unsteady (ataxic). The psychosis that is part of the syndrome is characterized by a severe defect in memory and learning. Confabulation is a characteristic feature though not always present. Memory of distant events is good but that for recent events is poor. However, the individual tends to provide a superficially convincing tale about these events rather than admit that he or she has forgotten them.

Subclinical thiamin deficiency occurs in old people and may indeed manifest itself as a cardiomyopathy. It can also be a cause of confusion in old people, particularly when there is the added stress of an infection or surgery. In the elderly, thiamin deficiency may be caused by poor dietary habits, low intake and interference with the absorption of the vitamin by antacids. The cytotoxic drug, 5-fluorouracil, causes subclinical deficiency, probably due to interference with the phosphorylation of thiamin.[50] Large doses of thiamin are diuretic. Vomiting, epigastric fullness, severe cramps and respiratory distress may also occur.

Riboflavin (Vitamin B$_2$)

Ariboflavinosis can be a cause of angular stomatitis, cheilosis and nasolabial seborrhoea in malnourished subjects. Deficiencies of the vitamin may contribute to the mouth and lip lesions found in old people. However, it seems that lesions of the mucocutaneous surfaces of the mouth are only modestly specific and do not always respond to riboflavin.[51] The anaemia that sometimes accompanies riboflavin deficiency responds more readily to iron and riboflavin than to riboflavin alone. There is some evidence that the effects of riboflavin deficiency, such as on collagen synthesis, may be complicated by induced metabolic deficiency of vitamin B$_6$.

Nicotinic Acid (Niacin) and Nicotinamide (Vitamin B$_3$)

Pellagra, the disease caused by nicotinic acid deficiency, is endemic amongst poor peasants who subsist chiefly on maize. The typical clinical features are loss of weight, increasing debility, an erythematous dermatitis, gastrointestinal disturbances, especially glossitis and diarrhoea, and mental changes. It is said to be characterized by the three Ds—dermatitis, diarrhoea and dementia. However, in mild cases, depression may be the main presenting feature, with possibly some skin changes.

The erythema has a characteristic distribution, appearing symmetrically over the parts of the body exposed to sunlight, especially the back of the hands, wrists, forearms, face and neck (Casall's collar). Diarrhoea is common but not always present; the mouth is sore and often shows angular stomatitis and cheilosis. The tongue characteristically has a 'raw beef' appearance—red, swollen and painful.

In mild cases the symptoms in the nervous system consist of weakness, tremor, anxiety, depression and irritability. In severe acute cases, delirium is common and in chronic cases dementia develops. In chronic cases there may be peripheral symptoms, with increased sensation in the feet to touch. Spasticity and exaggerated tendon reflexes occur. There may also be foot drop and the impairment of tendon reflexes. Some of these features are those of combined subacute degeneration of the cord and may be due to associated vitamin B$_{12}$ deficiency. Loss of position sense may give rise to ataxia.

Pellagra may be precipitated by the antituberculosis drug isoniazid in patients who have been given poor diets. This occurs because isoniazid acts as an antagonist to pyridoxine, which is a necessary coenzyme for the conversion of tryptophan to nicotinamide. In Western societies, pellagra is occasionally seen in alcoholics and in patients with malabsorption syndrome. It can also occur in patients receiving low-protein diets, such as those used in the treatment of chronic renal failure, when prophylactic vitamins are not also given. Patients on intermittent dialysis are particularly at risk as the vitamin supplements may be inadvertently forgotten. Pellagrous skin lesions have been described in Hartnup disease in which there is an aminoaciduria including tryptophan, and a defect of tryptophan absorption in both the renal tubules and the intestinal mucosa. The pellagrous skin rash found in this condition responds promptly to nicotinamide.

Toxic effects of 'gram doses' include pruritus, hepatotoxicity, arrhythmias, and hypotension.

Pyridoxine (Vitamin B$_6$) and Related Compounds

Dietary deficiency of pyridoxine is rare because of the wide distribution of the vitamin in food. Convulsions have occurred in infants in the USA from feeding them a formula that provided little vitamin B$_6$ due to a manufacturing error. Biochemical evidence suggesting pyridoxine deficiency has been found in patients with malabsorption and in PEM. Several drugs interact with pyridoxine and increase the requirement of the vitamin, notably isoniazid, hydrolazine, penicillin and oestrogens. A proportion of women taking oestrogen-containing oral contraceptives experience nausea, headaches and depression that are associated with abnormalities in tryptophan metabolism. The amounts of vitamin B$_6$ required to reverse these abnormalities (20–50 mg/day) are considerably higher than the recommended daily allowance (2 mg/day) and this suggests that the effects are pharmacological rather than nutritional.[52]

Convulsions cured by comparatively large doses of pyrodoxine have been described in otherwise well-nourished children. These have been attributed to a pyridoxine dependency, which appears to be an inborn error of metabolism. Rarely, a hypochromic sideroblastic anaemia occurs in adults that responds to large doses (20–100 mg/day) of pyridoxine.

Large doses of vitamin B$_6$ have been said to be of use in the treatment of a wide range of clinical conditions. The safe level for all individuals has not yet been determined.[53] Peripheral sensory neuropathy and ataxia have been reported in women taking 'gram doses'.

Cyanocobalamin (Vitamin B$_{12}$) and Related Substances

Megaloblastic anaemia due to vitamin B$_{12}$ deficiency has been described in a few very strict vegetarians (i.e. vegans), owing to the fact that this vitamin is restricted in its distribution in foods to foods of animal origin. Vitamin B$_{12}$ is stored in the liver and at birth there is sufficient of the vitamin for about 12 months. The liver of adults usually contains enough for about 5 years.

Kwashiorkor with accompanying megaloblastic

anaemia due to vitamin B_{12} deficiency has been described in children of around 13 months of age who have been reared on fad diets.

The absorption of vitamin B_{12} from the distal part of the ileum requires its conjugation with a glycoprotein secreted by the parietal cells in the stomach (Castle's intrinsic factor). Failure to produce this factor in pernicious anaemia is due to an autoimmune reaction that destroys the secretory cells of the stomach. Secretion is also reduced in atrophic gastritis, after partial gastrectomy, particularly of the Polya type and, of course, after total gastrectomy. In a variety of intestinal diseases, e.g. malabsorption syndrome, especially the blind-loop syndrome, an increased bacterial flora may reduce the absorption of vitamin B_{12}. The vitamin is also not absorbed in ilial disease. A number of drugs, e.g. β-aminosalicylic acid, biguanides, slow-release K, and colchicine, interfere specifically with the absorption of the vitamin.

The onset of symptoms in vitamin B_{12} deficiency is insidious, with a history of increasing lassitude over perhaps 14–17 months. The longest history is found in patients with neurological disease. The common symptoms are weakness, tiredness, dyspnoea on exertion, paraesthesiae and a sore tongue. With severe anaemia, evidence of cardiac failure may appear, such as oedema of the feet. Patients with pernicious anaemia are often slightly jaundiced and pyrexic, and show premature greying of the hair. The tongue is often smooth, clean and shiny.

Vitamin B_{12} plays an important role as a coenzyme in the reactions that result in the removal of cyanide from the body by its conversion to thiocyanate. Optic atrophy due to cyanide occurs in heavy smokers and is often effectively treated with hydroxycobalamine. Retrobulbar neuropathy and spinal ataxia occur together in Western Nigeria among people for whom cassava is the staple diet. The syndrome, called tropical ataxic neuropathy, appears to be caused by chronic ingestion of small amounts of cyanide from cassava. It is believed that the disease arises because the diet does not contain sufficient sulphur-containing amino acids and vitamin B_{12} to metabolize the cyanide.

Folate (Folic Acid, Folacin)

Periconceptual maternal folate deficiency may be involved in the aetiology of neural-tube defects.[54, 55] An experimental study in guinea pigs has suggested that periconceptual intakes of folic acid and vitamin C greater than those required to prevent macrocytic anaemia and scurvy, respectively, may be required to ensure a normal pregnancy outcome.[56]

Megaloblastic anaemia due to a simple dietary deficiency of folate occurs amongst poor people in the tropics and can occur in Western societies during pregnancy, owing to the increased demands for the vitamin. Absorption from the upper small intestine is often impaired in gastrointestinal diseases.

Folic acid deficiency is common in persons admit-

ted to old people's homes or psychiatric hospitals. It may cause certain types of dementia and low concentrations have been found in patients with senile dementia.[57]

Anticonvulsant and other drugs, including alcohol, reduce the blood concentrations of the vitamin but rarely cause megaloblastic anaemia. A low blood folate can also occur in patients being given intravenous amino acid solutions containing high concentrations of methionine. The reason for this is that methionine requires folate for its metabolism via the transsulphuration pathway to cysteine.

Ascorbic Acid (Vitamin C)

The diagnosis of scurvy, due to ascorbic acid deficiency, is often suggested by the gingivitis that is characteristic of the disease. The gums are spongy, swollen and red, and bleed at the lightest touch. Cutaneous bleeding also occurs, often initially on the lower thighs just above the knees. The perifollicular haemorrhages may subsequently appear on the buttocks, abdomen, legs and arms, and are often followed by petechial haemorrhages not associated with hair follicles. Corkscrew hairs may appear, particularly on the abdomen, due to a heaping up of keratin-like material on the surface and around the mouth of the follicle. Later, large cutaneous bruises (ecchymoses) can occur spontaneously on the skin. The patient will sometimes present with painful joints.

Scurvy has been produced experimentally in volunteers and these presented some additional features including ocular haemorrhages (particularly in the bulbar conjunctiva), Sjögren's syndrome, i.e. loss of secretion of salivary and lacrimal glands and swelling of the parotid glands, femoral neuropathy, oedema of the lower limbs and psychological disturbances, hypochondriasis and depression. Early signs are that the patient complains of feeling feeble and listless for some weeks. These signs precede the changes in the gums and skin. Scurvy can occur in infants from a reduction in the small amount of vitamin C present in milk. The first sign of bleeding in scorbutic infants is usually a subperiosteal haemorrhage immediately overlying one of the long bones—frequently the femur—producing the characteristic frog-like position. This gives rise to intense pain, and the infant may cry agonizingly and scream even louder when lifted.

A subclinical deficiency of ascorbic acid is common amongst the elderly and should always be suspected in old people, particularly widowers, who may not be accustomed to providing for themselves. Only a few foods are rich in the vitamin and it is easily lost during the preparation of meals. Use of the 'meals-on-wheels' service is no guarantee that provision of ascorbic acid is satisfactory.

The requirement for ascorbic acid is increased by stress and low blood concentrations occur in patients undergoing surgery. Certain drugs, notably pred-

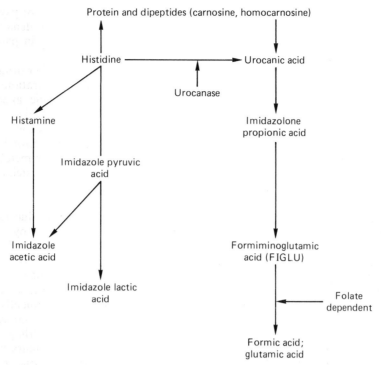

Figure 1.3 Metabolic pathways of histidine: the oxidation pathway yields formic and glutamic acids; this pathway is blocked at the urocanase step in kwashiorkor and histidinaemia; folate deficiency results in elevated excretion of FIGLU.

nisone, increase the requirement for the vitamin and may produce scurvy.

Biochemical aspects of the functions of vitamin C and the possibilities of toxicity have been discussed elsewhere.[58]

Assessment of Vitamin Status

Clinical examination, combined with a dietary history and haematological or radiological examination, depending on the nature of the vitamin, may in some cases be sufficient for the diagnosis of a vitamin deficiency. However, the early detection of vitamin deficiencies at the so-called subclinical or biochemical level relies on the determination of the amounts of the various vitamins in body fluids and tissues. The significance to be attached to low concentrations of vitamins in the body in the absence of clinical or other manifestations of deficiency depends on the age of the subject, the environment, and stresses that may be experienced. Generally speaking, low concentrations are of more potential importance in the sick, in whom they may interfere with metabolic processes involved in recovery, and in the elderly.

Biochemical methods that are used for the determination of vitamin status are shown in Table 1.12 (for a review, *see* Thurnham[77]). For some vitamins, ascorbic acid and folic acid, for example, plasma or serum concentrations can be measured. These are probably unreliable indicators of vitamin status for they change readily in response to recent intake. For other vita-

mins, niacin for example, blood concentrations are difficult to measure and status is more readily assessed from measurements of the urinary excretion of the vitamin or a metabolite, in the case of niacin, *N*-methylnicotinamide. Such determinations usually require the collection of a 24-h urine sample. Alternatively, it may be sufficient to express excretion as a ratio to creatinine. However, the excretion of creatinine is related to muscle mass, as well as to renal function, and changes with age, so that different 'normal' or reference values must be used for subjects of different ages.

Vitamins function as coenzymes at various stages in metabolic pathways. Deficiency of a vitamin will lead to a reduction in the activity of a particular enzyme and may cause both a build-up of metabolites before that point in the metabolic pathway and increased excretion of one or more metabolites. Thus, for example, folic acid is necessary for the complete conversion of histidine to formic acid and glutamic acid (Fig. 1.3), and specifically for the last stage of this pathway, that of formiminoglutamic acid (FIGLU) to formic and glutamic acids. It follows, therefore, that when a histidine load is given to a subject who is folate deficient, a greater than normal amount of the histidine will be excreted as FIGLU. The tryptophan load test for pyridoxine deficiency is based on a similar principle.

Determination of status for a number of vitamins in the B group (e.g. thiamin, riboflavin and

TABLE 1.12

BIOCHEMICAL METHODS FOR THE DETERMINATION OF VITAMIN STATUS

Vitamin	Methods	Comments	References
A	Plasma retinol and β-carotene	Normal levels of vitamin A taken as 50–100 μg/100 mL	59
	Plasma retinol-binding protein	Low concentrations alone do not indicate deficiency	
		Deficiency should be confirmed by assessment of dietary intake and measurement of dark adaptation	60
D	Plasma alkaline phosphatase	Raised concentrations of alkaline phosphatase occur in rickets and osteomalacia but are non-specific for vitamin D deficiency	
	Plasma 25-hydroxycholecalciferol	Normal values for 25-hydroxycholecalciferol vary with the method used	61
E	Plasma tocopherol	Plasma concentration varies with total plasma lipids	59
		Representative lower limits of normal taken as 5 μg/mL or 0.8 mg/g lipid	62
	Erythrocyte haemolysis	High peroxide haemolysis not specific to vitamin E deficiency	63
Thiamin	Blood pyruvate and lactate	Raised concentrations non-specific for thiamin deficiency	64
	Red-cell (or whole blood) transketolase and stimulation (TPP % value)	Red-cell transketolase and particularly raised TPP % value is most reliable index	
		Values > 15 probably indicate deficiency	65
Riboflavin	Red-cell glutathione reductase (GR) and GR stimulation ratio	Stimulation or activation ratios > 1.30 indicative of riboflavin deficiency	66
			65
	Urinary excretion of riboflavin		67
Nicotinic	Urinary excretion of N'-methyl nicotinamide (NMN)	Excretion of < 0.6 mg/6 h is subnormal; excretion of 0.2 mg or less/6 h indicative of deficiency	68
		Ratio of NMN to creatinine in 2-h urine collected between 10 a.m. and 12 a.m. similar to values obtained on 24-h urine	69
	Urinary excretion of NMN after an oral dose of nicotinamide	For load test, 50–200 mg nicotinamide given	
		Normally nourished subjects excrete 20% of dose as NMN in 24 h	
Pyridoxine	Red-cell aspartate transaminase (AST) and red-cell AST stimulation	The red-cell AST stimulation test is a convenient method of determining pyridoxine status	70
	Enzymological assay of pyridoxal phosphate with tyrosine decarboxylase	After a tryptophan load, deficient individuals excrete an increased amount of xanthurenic acid and an increased ratio of hydroxykynurenine: hydroxyanthranilate	71
			65
	Tryptophan load test		
Folate	Serum folate	Normal range 3–25 μg/L: concentrations reduced by loss of appetite; low value not sufficient to diagnose deficiency, indicates negative folate balance at time	72
	Red-cell folate	Normal range 150–600 μg/L packed cells	
		Normal range varies considerably in different laboratories	
		Low levels always indicative of folate deficiency	
		Diagnosis confirmed by satisfactory treatment with 200 μg/day	
	Histidine load test	15 g L-histidine given: folate deficiency indicated by excretion of > 18 mg formimino-glutamic acid (FIGLU) in first 8 h	73
			74
B_{12}	Serum concentration	Normal range quoted as 170–1000 μg/mL but varies with the method used	
	Methylmalonic acid (MMA) excretion	Normal range 0.2–15.3 mg MMA/24 h	75
		Level of excretion increased in B_{12} deficiency, particularly if urine is collected after giving valine or isoluecine	
		Less sensitive and less convenient than measurement B_{12}	
Ascorbic	Plasma and leucocyte ('buffy coat') concentrations	Plasma concentrations reflect recent intake but repeated values < 0.2 mg/100 mL probably indicate deficiency	76
		Leucocyte concentrations reflect tissue concentrations; values < 25 μg/10^8 cells indicate deficiency	
	Saturation test	Adequately nourished individuals excrete most of the load	
		Depleted individuals retain a proportionately greater amount	

pyridoxine) can be made by measuring the activities of enzymes in the red cell for which they act as cofactors. A more reliable index is given by the 'activation coefficient', which is the rise in enzyme activity when the vitamin is added to deficient red cells expressed as a ratio, or percentage, of that already present.

TRACE ELEMENT DEFICIENCY AND EXCESS

Introduction

Metal ions are essential for the activity of about one-third of all enzymes. These enzymes may be divided into two groups, the metallo-enzymes and the metal-ion activated enzymes. A metallo-enzyme contains the mineral as an integral part of the structure of the molecule, which does not dissociate under physiological conditions. In contrast, the metal is only loosely bound to metal-ion activated enzymes; it may be replaced by other metals, and may show some activity when removed altogether. The six most important of these metals are iron, copper, zinc, manganese, molybdenum and cobalt. Other metals present in the human body in still smaller concentrations include nickel, chromium, selenium, tin and vanadium. Other minerals known to be important in man are iodine and fluorine, and there have been suggestions that silicon may play an important role in relation to atherosclerosis. This review will be restricted to those trace minerals that are known to be involved in human disease and that are therefore of particular interest to the clinical biochemist—zinc, copper, manganese, chromium and cobalt. There have been recent reviews of these aspects of iron[78] and trace elements.[79]

Clinical Features

Zinc

A syndrome of zinc deficiency has been described in young men in Iran and Egypt. Affected patients were dwarfed and sexually retarded, and showed endocrine abnormalities that resembled hypopituitarism. Multiple deficiencies cannot be ruled out in these patients but they did respond clinically to zinc supplementation. Zinc deficiency may retard wound healing but zinc is not a panacea to aid this process. Zinc deficiency may be a cause of dermal ulcers in patients on long-term treatment with corticosteroids and play a role in delaying the healing of leg ulcers. In the latter disorder, zinc supplements are effective in promoting healing only in those patients who have a low plasma zinc. Zinc deficiency may diminish or pervert the senses of taste and smell. Zinc plays an important role in tissue growth and maternal zinc deficiency may play a role in human teratogenicity and fetal growth retardation.

Increased urinary excretion of zinc resulting in zinc depletion occurs in patients with alcoholic cirrho-

sis, and after surgery. Malabsorption syndromes, pancreatitis, diabetes and sickle-cell anaemia are associated with a depletion of body zinc and low plasma concentrations are found in women taking oral contraceptives.

Zinc deficiency occurs in patients receiving long-term parenteral nutrition if they are not being given appropriate mineral supplements. The condition presents as a red, blotchy dermatitis of the face, axillae and other parts of the body. The appearance of the skin lesions is similar to that found in the inborn error of zinc metabolism known as acrodermatitis enteropathica. This disease is inherited as an autosomal recessive characteristic and the disease presents at weaning, or earlier if the infant is not breast-fed. Severe dermatitis of the extremities is associated with severe diarrhoea and the children die in infancy unless treated. The cause of the disease is an inability to absorb zinc from the intestine but the mechanism is unknown.

Symptomless elevation of the plasma zinc concentration has been reported as a characteristic of an inherited disorder. Zinc intoxication has occurred following domestic renal haemodialysis using water stored in a galvanized tank.

Copper

Three syndromes of copper deficiency have been described in human infancy, two of them being acquired and the other an inborn error of metabolism. The first is a condition manifesting itself mainly as anaemia and found in infants maintained largely on cow's milk. The condition responds to the administration of both copper and iron. In the second syndrome, anaemia is associated with diarrhoea and skeletal rarefaction, and responds well to copper but not iron. The inborn error is known as Menkes' kinky hair syndrome. It is inherited as a sex-linked recessive disorder characterized by growth retardation, progressive mental deterioration, degeneration of aortic elastin, metaphyseal abnormalities in the skeleton with changes similar to scurvy, hypothermia, and a peculiar defect in hair keratin and pigmentation ('kinky hair'). Most of these abnormalities reflect the known activities of copper-containing enzymes. The disease is due to a failure to absorb copper from the intestine and for this reason oral copper supplements are ineffective whereas parenteral copper improves the condition.

The second inborn error of copper metabolism, that of Wilson's disease or hepatolenticular degeneration, is associated with copper excess. As in Menkes' syndrome, serum copper and caeruloplasmin concentrations are low but, in contrast, copper is absorbed and deposited in steadily increasing amounts in the tissues, particularly in the liver, brain, iris and kidneys. This steady accumulation results in toxicity, with cirrhosis of the liver, and in mental deterioration with ataxia and choreiform movements. Treatment of Wilson's disease relies on the use of chelating agents, such as penicillamine, which increases the urinary excretion of copper (and also of zinc).

Low plasma concentrations of copper may occur in malabsorption syndromes and in the nephrotic syndrome. High plasma concentrations occur in patients with certain kinds of tumour, e.g. Hodgkin's disease, and in Addison's disease. The clinical significance of these changes is not known.

Manganese

The drug hydralazine was used extensively in the treatment of hypertension. In common with a number of other drugs (including procainamide), long-continued use of hydralazine can produce a syndrome identical to idiopathic lupus erythmatosus. Patients suffering from both the drug-induced and naturally occurring syndrome have benefited from the administration of manganese salts. A link between rheumatoid arthritis and manganese metabolism has been suggested.

Manganese deficiency in animals gives rise to ataxia and convulsions. Intoxication in humans can give rise to parkinsonism, extrapyramidal syndromes, hallucinations and psychomotor instability.

Chromium

A link has now been established between chromium and glucose metabolism, with improvements in glucose tolerance being claimed in elderly people as a result of the administration of supplements of 150 μg/day of chromium chloride. The hair chromium of diabetic children is markedly reduced.

Cobalt

Cobalt is an important constituent of vitamin B_{12}. It has not been definitely established whether the metal has a role in human nutrition apart from this. However, there is a report of a single child in a cobalt-deficient area in Scotland with marked geophagia who responded to cobalt by mouth. Pharmacological doses of inorganic cobalt salts induce polycythaemia in many species, including man, and doses of 20–30 mg daily have been used with iron in the treatment of iron deficiency anaemia. However, they should not be used in this condition unless cobalt deficiency is suspected, as suppression of thyroid activity, goitre and cardiomyopathy can occur as a result of cobalt toxicity, particularly in infants. As cobalt does stimulate production of renal erythropoietin it has been used to raise the amount of haemoglobin in anaemia of chronic renal failure. An undesirable complication of such treatment is that the blood lipid concentrations are also raised.

Determination of Trace Element Status

Plasma or serum concentrations, though commonly measured, may be unreliable indices of trace-element nutriture. There has been interest in the use of hair as a biopsy material. This has obvious advantages in that the taking of the sample is non-invasive and hair contains higher concentrations of many trace elements than in plasma. Moreover, the results of hair analysis may be more informative of tissue concentrations and yield a better background of a patient's nutriture because they reflect it over a greater time-span. Futhermore, much of the developing interest in the possible role of trace elements in clinical conditions such as psychiatric disorders centres not so much on deficiency or excess of a single mineral but on the relation between different minerals, for it is known that relative excesses or deficiencies and ratios between related elements, such as copper and zinc, may be more important clinically than the absolute concentrations of either independently. Such considerations mean that more information is likely to be gained from a trace-element profile than from a single plasma determination and a profile is more easily determined on a hair sample.

CONCLUSIONS

In our present state of knowledge the limits of what may be considered 'normal' nutritional status are purely arbitrary. It is only when metabolic processes are disturbed and overt disease develops that we can refer to under- or overnutrition. Be this as it may, nutritional status is an important aspect of patient welfare. Disease may precipitate nutrient deficiencies by increasing requirements, interfering with intake, causing abnormal losses or resulting in malabsorption. Furthermore, nutritional deficiencies may have important interactions with treatment, whether by drugs, surgery or radiotherapy. Assessment and maintenance of nutritional status is therefore an important part of the holistic approach to the management of the sick.

REFERENCES

1. Waterlow J.C. (1968). Observations on the mechanism of adaptation to low protein intakes. *Lancet*, **ii**, 1091.
2. Editorial (1970). Classification of infantile malnutrition. *Lancet*, **ii**, 302.
3. Vaughan V.C., McKay R.J., Behrman R.E. eds. (1979). *Nelson Textbook of Pediatrics*, 11th edn, London: W.B. Saunders, pp. 10–16.
4. McLaren D.S., Pellett P.L., Read W.W.C. (1976). A simple scoring system for classifying the severe forms of protein–calorie malnutrition in early childhood. *Lancet*, **i**, 533.
5. Kanawati A.A., McLaren D.S. (1970). Assessment of marginal malnutrition. *Nature*, **228**, 573.
6. McLaren D.S., Read, W.W.C. (1972). Classifications of nutritional status in early childhood. *Lancet*, **ii**, 146.
7. McLaren D.S. (1966). A fresh look at protein-calorie malnutrition. *Lancet*, **ii**, 485.
8. Bengoa J.M. (1974). The problem of malnutrition. *WHO Chron.*, **28**, 3.
9. Whitehead R.G., Alleyne G.A.O. (1972). Pathophysiological factors of importance in protein-calorie malnutrition. *Br. Med. Bull.*, **28**, 72.

10. Golden M.H.N. (1988). Marasmus and kwashiorkor. In *Nutrition in the Clinical Management of Disease*, 2nd edn (Dickerson J.W.T., Lee H.A. eds.) London: Arnold, pp.88–109.

11. Golden M.H.N. (1985). The consequences of protein deficiency in man and its relationship to the features of kwashiorkor. In *Nutritional Adaptation in Man* (Blaxter K.B., Waterlow J.C. eds.) London: Libbey, pp. 169–187.

12. Golden M.H.N. (1987). Free radicals in the pathogenesis of kwashiorkor. *Proc. Nutr. Soc.*, **46**, 53.

13. Thurnham D.I. (1990). Antioxidants and pro-oxidants in malnourished populations. *Proc. Nutr. Soc.,* **49**, 247.

14. Hansen J.D.L., Brinkman G.L., Bowie M.D. (1965). Body composition in protein–calorie malnutrition. *S. Afr. Med. J.,* **39**, 491.

15. Garrow J.S., Fletcher K., Halliday D. (1965). Body composition in severe infantile malnutrition. *J. Clin. Invest.,* **44**, 417.

16. Cabak V., Dickerson J.W.T., Widdowson E.M. (1963). Response of young rats to deprivation of protein or of calories. *Br. J. Nutr.*, 17, 601.

17. Truswell A.S., Hansen J.D.L., Watson C.E., Wannenburg P. (1969). Relation of serum lipids and lipoproteins to fatty liver in kwashiorkor. *Am. J. Clin. Nutr.*, **22**, 568.

18. Cook G.C., Lee F.D. (1966). The jejunum after kwashiorkor. *Lancet*, **ii**, 1263.

19. Berkel I., Kiran O., Say B. (1970). Jejunal mucosa in infantile malnutrition. *Acta Paediatr. Scand.*, **59**, 58.

20. Tomkins A.M., Drasar B.S., James W.P.T. (1975). Bacterial colonisation of jejunal mucosa in acute tropical sprue. *Lancet*, **i**, 59.

21. James W.P.T., Hay A.M., (1968). Albumin metabolism: effect of the nutritional state and the dietary protein intake. *J. Clin. Invest.*, **47**, 1958.

22. Cohen S., Hansen J.D.L. (1962). Metabolism of albumin and α-globulin in kwashiorkor. *Clin. Sci.*, **23**, 357.

23. Reeds P.J., Laditan A.A.O. (1976). Serum albumin and transferrin in protein-energy malnutrition. *Br. J. Nutr.*, **36**, 255.

24. Picou D., Taylor-Roberts T. (1969). The measurement of total protein synthesis and catabolism and nitrogen turnover in infants in different nutritional states and receiving different amounts of dietary protein. *Clin. Sci.*, **36**, 283.

25. Lunn P.G., Whitehead R.G., Baker B.A., Austin S. (1976). The effect of cortisone acetate on the course of development of experimental protein–energy malnutrition in rats. *Br. J. Nutr.*, **36**, 537.

26. Brooke O.G., Cocks T. (1974). Resting metabolic rate in malnourished babies in relation to total body potassium. *Acta Paediatr. Scand.*, **63**, 817.

27. Coward W.A. (1975). Serum colloidal osmotic pressure in the development of kwashiorkor and in recovery: its concentrations and oedema. *Br. J. Nutr.*, **34**, 459.

28. Durnin J.V.G.A., Womersley J. (1974). Body fat assessed from total body density and its estimation from skinfold thickness: measurements on 481 men and women aged 16 to 72 years. *Br. J. Nutr.*, **32**, 77.

29. Bradfield R.B. (1972). A rapid technique for the field assessment of protein–energy malnutrition. *Am. J. Clin. Nutr.*, **25**, 720.

30. Whitehead R.G., Coward W.A., Lunn P.G. (1973). Serum-albumin concentration and the onset of kwashiorkor. *Lancet*, **i**, 63.

31. Fischer J.E. (1982). Plasma proteins as indicators of nutritional status. In *Nutritional Assessment: Recent Status and Future Directions and Prospects*, Report of Second Ross Conference on Medical Research (Levenson, S.M. ed.) Columbus, OH: Ross Laboratories, pp. 25–26.

32. Carpentier Y.A., Barthel J., Bruyns J. (1982). Plasma protein concentration in nutritional assessment. *Proc. Nutr. Soc.*, **41**, 405.

33. Ingenbleek Y., et al. (1975). Albumin/retinol binding protein (TBA/RBP) complex in assessment of malnutrition. *Clin. Chim. Acta*, **63**, 61.

34. Shetty P.S., Watrasiewiez K.E., Jang R.T., James W.P.T. (1979). Rapid-turnover transport proteins: an index of subclinical protein-energy malnutrition. *Lancet*, **ii**, 230.

35. Whitehead R.G., Dean R.F.A. (1964). Serum amino acids in kwashiorkor, I. and II. *Am. J. Clin. Nutr.*, **14**, 313; 320.

36. Alleyne G.A.O., Hay R.W., Picou D.I., Standfield J.P., Whitehead R.G. (1977). *Protein–Energy Malnutrition*, London: Arnold.

37. World Health Organization (1976). *Vitamin A Deficiency and Xerophthalmia*, Technical Report Series WHO No. 590, Geneva: WHO.

38. Tomkins A., Hussey G. (1989). Vitamin A, immunity and infection. *Nutr. Res. Rev.*, **2**, 17.

39. Tomkins A.M., Watson F. (1989). *Malnutrition and Infection: A Review*, Geneva: WHO.

40. Barclay A.J.G., Foster A., Sommer A. (1987). Vitamin A supplements and mortality related to measles: a randomised clinical trial. *Br. Med. J.*, **294**, 294.

41. Sommer A. et al. (1986). Impact of vitamin A supplementation on childhood mortality: a randomised controlled community trial. *Lancet*, **i**, 1169.

42. Pinnock C.B., Douglas R.M., Badcock N.R. (1986). Vitamin A status in children who are prone to respiratory tract infections. *Aust. Paediatr. J.*, **22**, 95.

43. Williams C.M., Dickerson J.W.T. (1990). Nutrition and cancer. *Nutr. Res. Rev.*, **3**, 75.

44. Arneil G.C. (1979). Progress in the prevention and treatment of nutritional rickets. In *The Importance of Vitamins to Human Health* (Taylor T.G. ed.) Lancaster: MTP, pp. 151–162.

45. Passmore R., Eastwood M.A. (1986). *Davidson and Passmore Human Nutrition and Dietetics*, 8th edn, Edinburgh: Churchill Livingstone, p.308.

46. Bell E.F. (1987). History of vitamin E in infant nutrition. *Am. J. Clin. Nutr.*, **46**, 183.

47. Muller D.P.R, (1987). Free radical problems of the newborn. *Proc. Nutr. Soc.*, **46**, 69.

48. Burgess C.R. (1958). Infantile beriberi. In *Nutritional Diseases* (Proceedings of a conference on beriberi, endemic goiter and hypervitaminosis A). *Fed. Proc.*, 17, No.3, Part II, Suppl 2, p.39.

49. Jelliffe D.B. (1968). *Infant Nutrition in the Subtropics*, WHO Monograph Series No. 29, 2nd edn, Geneva:WHO, p.98.

50. Aksoy M., Basu T.K., Brient J., Dickerson J.W.T. (1980). Thiamin status of patients treated with drug combinations containing 5-fluorouracil. *Eur. J. Cancer*, **16**, 1041.

51. Bates C.J. (1987). Human riboflavin requirements, and metabolic consequences of deficiency in man and animals. *World Rev. Nutr. Diet*, **50**, 215.

52. Bender D.A. (1987). Oestrogens and vitamin B6—actions and interactions. *World Rev. Nutr. Diet*, **51**, 140.

53. Gaby A.R. (1990). The safe use of vitamin B6. *J. Nutr. Med.*, **1**, 153.

54. Smithells R.W., Sheppard S., Schorah C.J. (1976). Vitamin deficiencies and neural tube defects. *Arch. Dis. Child.*, **51**, 944.

55. Laurence K.M., Jones N., Miller M.H., Tennant G.B., Campbell H. (1981). Double blind randomised controlled trial of folate treatment before conception to prevent recurrence of neural tube defects. *Br. Med. J.*, **282**, 1509.

56. Habibzadah N., Schorah C.J., Smithells R.W. (1986). The effects of maternal folic acid and vitamin C nutrition in early pregnancy on reproductive performance in the guinea-pig. *Br. J. Nutr.*, **55**, 23.

57. Thomas D.E., Chung-a-On K.O., Dickerson J.W.T., Tidmarsh S.F., Shaw D.M. (1986). Tryptophan and nutritional status of patients with senile dementia. *Psychol. Med.*, **16**, 297.

58. Dickerson J.W.T., Williams C.M. (1990). Vitamin-related disorders. In *The Metabolic and Molecular Basis of Acquired Disease*, vol. 1 (Cohen R.D., Lewis B., Alberti K.G.M.M., Denman A.M. eds.) London: Baillière Tindall, pp. 634–669.

59. Hansen L.G., Warwick W.J. (1969). A fluorometric micromethod for serum vitamins A and E. *Tech. Bull. Registr. Med. Techn.*, **39**, 70.

60. Glover J. (1973). Retinol binding proteins. *Vitam. Horm.*, **31**, 1.

61. Edelstein S., Charman M., Lawson D.E.M., Kodicek E. (1974). Competitive protein-binding assay for 25-hydroxycholecalciferol. *Clin. Sci. Mol. Med.*, **46**, 231.

62. Horwitt M.K., Harvey L.C., Dahm C.H. Jr., Searcy M.T. (1972). Relationships between tocopherol and serum lipid levels for determination of nutritional adequacy. *Ann. NY Acad. Sci.*, **203**, 223.

63. Nitowsky H.M., Tildon J.T. (1956). Some studies of tocopherol deficiency in infants and children. III. Relation of blood catalase activity and other factors to hemolysis of erythrocytes in hydrogen peroxide. *Am. J. Clin. Nutr.*, **4**, 397.

64. Dreyfus P.M. (1962). Clinical application of blood transketolase determinations. *N. Engl. J. Med.*, **267**, 596.

65. Bayoumi R., Rosalki S.B. (1976). Evaluation of methods of co-enzyme activation of erythrocyte enzymes for detection of deficiency of vitamins B_1, B_2 and B_6. *Clin. Chem.*, **22**, 327.

66. Saubelich H.E. et al. (1972). Applications of the erythrocyte glutathione reductase assay in evaluating riboflavin nutritional status in a high school student population. *Am. J. Clin. Nutr.*, **25**, 756.

67. Glatzle D., Korner W.F., Christeller S., Wiss O. (1970). Method for the detection of a biochemical riboflavin deficiency. Stimulation of $NADPH_2$-dependent glutathione reductase from human erythrocytes by FAD *in vitro*. Investigations on the vitamin B_2 status in healthy people and geriatric patients. *Int. J. Vitam. Nutr. Res.*, **40**, 166.

68. De Lange D.J., Joubert C.P. (1964). Assessment of nicotinic acid status of population groups. *Am. J. Clin. Nutr.*, **15**, 169.

69. Goldsmith G.A., Miller O.N. (1967). Niacin. In *The Vitamins* (Gyorgy P., Pearson W.N. eds.) London: Academic Press, pp. 136–167.

70. Marsh M.E., Greenberg L.D., Rhinehart J.F. (1955). The relationship between B_6 investigation and transaminase activity. *J. Nutr.*, **56**, 115.

71. Sauberlich H.E. et al. (1972). Biochemical assessment of the nutritional status of vitamin B_6 in the human. *Am. J. Clin. Nutr.*, **25**, 629.

72. Chanarin I., Kyle R., Stacey J. (1972). Experience with microbiological assay for folate using a chloramphenicol-resistant *L. asei* strain. *J. Clin. Pathol.*, **25**, 1050.

73. Tabor H., Wyngarden L. (1958). A method for the determination of formimino-glutamic acid in urine. *J. Clin Invest.*, **37**, 824.

74. Kohn J., Mollin D.L., Rosenbach L.M. (1961). Conventional voltage electrophoresis for formimino-glutamic acid determinations in folic acid deficiency. *J. Clin. Pathol.*, **14**, 345.

75. Chanarin I., England J.M., Mollin C., Perry J. (1973). Methylmelonic acid excretion studies. *Br. J. Haematol.*, **25**, 45.

76. Denson K.W., Bowers E. (1961). The determination of ascorbic acid in whole blood cells. A comparison of W.B.C., ascorbic acid and phenolic acid excretion in elderly patients. *Clin. Sci.*, **21**, 157.

77. Thurnham D.I. (1985). The interpretation of biochemical measurements of vitamin status in the elderly. In *Vitamin Deficiency in the Elderly* (Kemm J.R., Ancill R.J. eds.) Oxford: Blackwell Scientific, pp. 46–67.

78. Peters T.J., Pippard M.J. (1990). Disorders of iron metabolism. In *The Metabolic and Molecular Basis of Acquired Disease* (Cohen R.D., Lewis B., Alberti R.G.M.M., Denman A.M. eds.) London:Baillière Tindall, pp. 1870–1884.

79. Simmer K., Thompson R.P.H. (1990). Trace elements. In *The Metabolic and Molecular Basis of Acquired Disease*, vol. 1 (Cohen R.D., Lewis B., Alberti K.G.M.M., Denman A.M. eds.) London: Baillière Tindall, pp. 670–683.

2. Obesity
V. Marks

Definition
Assessment of obesity
Reason for concern
Classifications of obesity
Aetiology
    Chemical nature of food
    Appetite and gluttony
The hormonal concomitants of obesity
    Insulin
    Gut hormones
    Growth hormone
    Sympathetic nervous system
Treatment
Conclusion

Obesity is the metabolic equivalent, in clinical practice, to hypertension; it is a risk factor for a number of illnesses and is itself a consequence of many diseases, in a tiny minority of which it is the dominant or presenting feature. In most cases no pathophysiological cause can be found to explain the physical features and the decision whether to treat the obesity or not is empirical and based purely upon statistical probabilities or, more commonly, upon subjective assessment. People who are most concerned about obesity are usually those least at risk from its deleterious effects upon health.

Though often considered to be a nutritional disorder, obesity is only very rarely due to genuine overnutrition (that is, nutritional intake over and above the reference values for energy intake of normal-weight individuals of similar age, sex, size and habits). It is more often merely a physiological variant of normal body habitus of no pathological significance.

DEFINITION

Obesity can best be described as the excessive accumulation of adipose tissue, but as this is both extremely difficult to define and to measure in the living subject, it is usually defined in relation to norms established for weight in subjects of similar age, sex and height to the propositus. These norms do not necessarily coincide with values established for optimum health, especially if this is defined as the weight-for-age that is associated with maximum longevity. Weight norms have largely been derived from weight and height measurements made on people taking out life insurance. Weight is, however, at best only an approximation to the amount of fat in a person's adipose tissue, and must therefore be looked upon with circumspection as an indicator of obesity. One way of dealing with this problem has been to have three different reference ranges for weight-for-height, according to a hypothetical frame structure, namely 'light, medium and heavy'. There is little reason to believe that such a classification has any validity beyond the subjective assessment of the observer. A common, and increasingly popular, method of expressing the relation of a person's weight to height is the so-called body mass index (BMI) or Quetelet index. This is a numerical expression derived by dividing the weight in kilograms by the height in metres squared (i.e. kg/m^2). It too suffers from the disadvantage that, in any single individual, it does not distinguish a high BMI resulting from above-average muscular development from that due to adiposity. Various attempts have been made to assess the degree and extent of adiposity more objectively but with, at best, limited success.

ASSESSMENT OF OBESITY

Visual assessment of the naked individual taken in conjunction with the BMI is probably as effective as any method currently available for assessing the extent and distribution of excessive adiposity, but lacks scientific rigour. The method generally looked upon as the 'gold standard' for assessing fat stores is based upon the fact that adipose tissue has a lower density (specific gravity) than muscle and other tissues. Consequently, by weighing an individual in air and in water it is possible to calculate the extent of their adiposity, providing that certain assumptions are made. This hydrostatic method, though possible within a research setting, is clearly unsuitable for clinical use, and in any event is far from ideal. A more convenient, simple to perform (though tedious) method of measurement of adiposity is to measure skinfold thickness with calipers over a number of defined loci—often reduced to one or two, i.e. the anterolateral abdominal wall and over the triceps.

Such measurements correlate reasonably well with assessments made from hydrostatic weighing. Other methods for assessing adiposity that depend upon one or more assumptions being accepted as correct include assay of total body potassium by measurement of ^{40}K, deuterium oxide dilution, ultrasonography, total body impedance and/or conductance. None is really suitable for clinical use and unlikely therefore to replace visual assessment and measurements of skinfold thickness for clinical purposes. A recently introduced measurement based upon infrared interactants, which has found extensive application in animal husbandry, is simple to perform and requires comparatively little in the way of instrumentation. In man it can be done within the space of just a minute or two at the bedside or in the clinic but is still unproven in practice.

Most investigators have, in the past, defined individuals weighing more than 115% of the mean for their sex, age and height as obese. This would now normally be considered to be too all-inclusive and to have no pathophysiological significance. A more commonly accepted definition of obesity is a BMI of more than 30, values between 25 and 30 being considered as indicative of overweight or plumpness. There is, however, good evidence from published data on weight, height, age and sex that optimum body weight, BMI or adiposity increase linearly with increasing age up to, and including, the seventh decade of life. Whilst in subjects aged between 20 and 30 years maximum longevity is associated with an average BMI of 20, regardless of their sex, at the seventh decade of life the optimum BMI has risen to 27 or more. These conclusions, which are based on data collected from the Body Build study in which the outcome of 4.2 million persons who took out life insurance policies was analysed, are different from those usually quoted and which are based on earlier, less thoroughly researched information. As a result it is still widely believed that there is a hypothetical ideal body weight which is achieved in early adult life and should be maintained for the rest of it.

REASON FOR CONCERN

Until comparatively recently, obesity was not looked upon by either the medical community or by society as a whole as a matter for concern. Indeed, in many societies, obesity was admired both in men, as a sign of wealth and power, and in women, as one of beauty. The demonstration that obesity is associated with increased morbidity from a number of disorders, as well as increased mortality, has done a lot to change this attitude. Undoubtedly the biggest single factor, however, has been the change in the perception of beauty and the social pressures put upon people, especially women, to conform to type, which has been dictated by fashion and bolstered by commercial interests from the clothing and slimming industries. The latter, in particular, is a product and beneficiary of the very genuine medical concern for the health of the markedly obese. It has, however, exploited this to such an extent that not only do people who run a genuinely increased risk of illness from obesity buy their products, but also people (especially young women and even children) who, though only comfortably plump (that is, of near ideal body weight medically), consider themselves overweight according to current fashion and therefore unattractive. There is accumulating evidence that deliberate attempts to lose weight when it is not indicated can, and do, cause physical as well as mental damage in susceptible subjects as well as failure to thrive and even physical stunting in children.

CLASSIFICATIONS OF OBESITY

Obesity is often treated as though it were of uniform type and pathogenesis, despite the clear evidence of the observer's own eyes that it is not. Largely as a result of the efforts of a French physician, Jean Vague, it is now commonplace to distinguish between an android, or central, type of obesity and a gynaecoid, or peripheral, type. These are often referred to colloquially as 'apples' and 'pears', respectively. The two types of obesity differ in their aetiology, metabolism and clinical significance, as well as visually; even so, correct classification is not always either simple or correct. Nevertheless, most publications that purport to deal with the medical consequences of obesity do not even attempt to make a distinction between the two major phenotypic manifestations of overweight and their conclusions must therefore be viewed with circumspection.

Other classifications of obesity have been put forward, but none has found widespread acceptance. One that enjoyed considerable popularity a couple of decades ago was based upon the premise that obesity in infancy and childhood led to increased replication of adipocytes and fat-tissue hyperplasia (hence hyperplastic adiposity), while weight gain later in life was supposed to be due to increased deposition of triglyceride in pre-existing adipocytes, i.e. hypertrophic adiposity. This theory has withstood neither critical examination nor the test of time.

Other theories that have been put forward to explain obesity are based upon real or supposed aetiological factors but, apart from a few well-recognized but generally rare examples, such classifications are not warranted.

AETIOLOGY

It is surprising, but understandable, that until comparatively recently the link between food intake and obesity was not appreciated either by medical or lay people, since rarely does everyday experience reveal any clear correlation between what an individual eats, on a day-to-day basis, and his or her body mass. It was only during the early part of the twentieth century, when scientific attention was directed to the nature of obesity and the laws of thermodynamics were applied to biology, that what has come to be recognized as the 'calorie' theory of obesity was adopted as a self-evident truth.

According to this 'theory', energy derived from the absorption and conversion of food into carbon dioxide and water is expended as heat and/or physical work, any excess of intake over output being deposited as fats and any deficiency being met by temporary extraction from stores. In more prolonged periods of withdrawal from food, energy is supplied by conversion of tissue proteins into carbon dioxide, water and nitrogenous waste products. Since it first gained universal acceptance, this theory has provided the basis for all of the apparently rational treatments of obesity and has received official recognition by legal requirements that all foods claiming to be of benefit for the treatment of obesity carry the proviso 'only as part of a calorie-controlled diet'. Whilst the truth of the proposition upon which the theory is based cannot be gainsaid, the 'calorie' theory of obesity has outlived its usefulness and, by concentrating the attention of investigators almost entirely upon the energy *content* of a person's food (i.e. intake) rather than upon the interaction between it and the individual (i.e. the physiological response it evokes), it impedes progress in understanding how and why diets of comparable energy content have different propensities to foster or inhibit weight gain depending upon such variables as the size and number of meals, their timing and composition, and so on.

There are, in addition, a large number of personal factors: for example, the person's genetic make-up, exercise level, general state of health and such age- and time-related life-events as adolescence, pregnancy and the menopause. These may doom to failure any attempt to understand the pathogenesis and, consequently, the chances of introducing an effective treatment of obesity that is based wholly or largely on the supposed ability to calculate desirable energy inputs. A more fundamental and biological approach is required than has hitherto been popular amongst all but a small group of dedicated workers if any progress is to be made in this direction.

A pathoanatomical cause can be uncovered in only a tiny minority of patients with morbid obesity, i.e. those with a BMI of more than 30. In many cases no reason can be found. There is, however, a large body of evidence, from twin and adoption studies, to indicate the importance of a genetic element in the propensity to develop obesity. Contrary to expectation, there is only a very small contribution from home background and habit. Only very rarely, and then generally in very highly inbred and isolated communities and tribes, does the hereditary element manifest itself in simple Mendelian inheritance. Nevertheless, studies of obese inbred communities, and of their laboratory animal analogue, have provided pointers to possible mechanisms whereby the inherited traits might predispose to fat deposition. Such traits would appear to have survival value in peoples who, until recently, had a seasonal or even more precarious access to food. Indeed, the most clearly defined examples of hereditary obesity are found in island and other isolated communities where conditions of intermittent deprivation are most likely to have been encountered in the past.

Chemical Nature of Food

The energy yield of whole foods or of their individual constituents in the classical bomb calorimeter provides the basis of all of the food tables currently in use. However, except for elemental diets, the exact composition and energy content of a diet can only be estimated from such tables, even when allowance for wastage is made, as foods always vary to a greater or lesser extent amongst themselves. The way in which fats, proteins and carbohydrates are handled within the body varies upon circumstances. There are, how-

ever, good reasons for believing that when energy in the diet comes from fat it is more available for deposition as fat in adipocytes at lower energy cost than when it is derived from carbohydrate, protein or alcohol. In its simplest, and consequently most simplistic, form dietary fat is fattening: a proposition exactly the reverse of one that held sway less than two decades ago when energy from carbohydrate sources was thought to be particularly important in causing obesity.

Evidence that the energy value of food constituents as derived from bomb calorimetry might not be directly transferable to our understanding of human nutrition comes from a study of the polyols, sorbitol and xylitol, where, because of the interaction of these nutrients with the microflora of the gut, at least some of the 'energy' they contain is unavailable to the host. Why precisely 'calories' derived from alcohol appear not to behave in the same way as those derived from carbohydrate, for example, is not understood. It may be because alcohol increases heat loss from the body and consequently increases metabolism; it may be no more than an artefact of observation.

Appetite and Gluttony

The concept of an 'appestat' situated somewhere in the brain, most probably in the hypothalamus, which regulates the desire to eat and hence food intake, is based upon evidence derived from laboratory animals as well as from clinical observations on people with neurological lesions. Damage, or stimulation, to various well-defined nuclei within the hypothalamus can, depending upon the location, lead to changes in eating behaviour that range from a voracious (indeed insatiable) desire to eat to complete anorexia, which is capable of leading to death from starvation even in the midst of plenty. Such evidence, coupled with the argument that if food intake is sufficiently reduced, either by voluntary or involuntary means, weight loss is an invariable consequence, has favoured a behavioural approach to the aetiology of obesity at the expense of a more mechanistic or pathophysiological approach. Whilst there is no evidence that physical or anatomical lesions of the appetite centres in the brain are ever more than an extremely rare cause of obesity in man, there is intense interest in the way that neurotransmitters, of both polypeptide and simpler molecular structure, can influence appetite and hence food intake. It is, for example, unknown where lies or even what constitutes the control loop; i.e. where the sensors are which determine (once a certain, seemingly predetermined degree of adiposity has been achieved) that appetite will diminish to such an extent that dietary energy intake once again comes into equilibrium with short-term energy expenditure. The nature and mode of action of this hypothetical 'ponderostat' is as mysterious now as was the 'glucostat', which controls the concentration of glucose in the blood, before the discovery of insulin and the regulation of its secretion by the β-cells of the pancreas. It is, however, probably just as real and amenable to understanding (and eventually to modulation by pharmacological and other methods).

THE HORMONAL CONCOMITANTS OF OBESITY

The common belief amongst the lay public that most forms of obesity are a manifestation of endocrinological imbalance has its basis more in historical misconception than in verifiable evidence. There is, however, a germ of truth in it and possibly more. Space-occupying and other lesions of the hypothalamus can, and sometimes do, lead to excessive weight gain in children as well as in adults; hypothyroidism can, but rarely does, lead to moderate overweight, though only partly because of excessive deposition of fat in adipose tissue. Hypothyroidism is never a cause of gross or morbid obesity and replacement therapy with thyroxine in hypothyroid patients rarely leads to more than trivial weight loss. Hyperthyroidism, on the other hand, whether due to oversecretion of thyroid hormones by the thyroid gland or to the administration of excessive quantities of thyroxine, often does lead to a loss of adipose tissue as well as to the more serious losses of muscle and bone tissue. Ordinarily energy expenditure is compensated for, and occasionally overcompensated for, by an increase in appetite and consequently of food intake. In some cases, this can even lead to a paradoxical weight gain. Adrenocortical hyperactivity of the Cushing's variety, i.e. glucocorticoid excess, is typically associated with modest truncal obesity, the visual effect of which is accentuated by muscular wasting of the limbs. There is, in this condition as in almost all others associated with obesity, an absolute increase in the amount of insulin secreted in response to eating as well as in the basal or fasting state.

Endogenous hyperinsulinism due to insulinoma is itself a well-known but exceedingly rare cause of obesity, as is hyperinsulinism caused by functional overactivity of the β-cells that occurs in some infants whilst *in utero*. In a tiny minority—those with the so-called nesidioblastosis syndrome—excessive deposition of fat is the rule.

As all types of obesity, but especially that of the truncal variety, are associated with fasting hyperinsulinaemia and an exaggerated insulinaemic response to feeding and other insulinotropic stimuli, it seems permissible to generalize by saying that excessive insulin action on adipose tissue cells is a prerequisite for the development of obesity, but is not its immediate cause. A corollary of this is that rapid weight loss, due largely to mobilization of fatty acids from adipose tissue and their use as an energy source, is one of the earliest features of insulinoprivic diabetes.

Obesity is often associated with type 2 (non-insulin dependent) diabetes (NIDDM). This probably results from a combination of factors, not the least important of which is the close association of genes that programme for obesity with one or more of the genes that control β-cell function and particularly their ability to produce, process and secrete proinsulin and its cleavage products (insulin, C-peptide, split proinsulin and des-proinsulin). There is increasing evidence that an early and, indeed, possibly essential step in the development of NIDDM is an inability to cleave proinsulin completely into insulin, the most biologically active of the proinsulin cleavage products. The increased demand that is put upon the β-cell by peripheral insulin resistance is thought to be a non-sustainable burden upon the cell's secretory capacity and to lead to its eventual failure. In the interregnum, relatively large amounts of the proinsulin cleavage products that have some, though not all, of the properties of native insulin are secreted into the blood. They probably also exert differential effects upon the different insulin-sensitive tissues, e.g. muscle, adipose tissue, liver. Too little is known about the biological effects of the proinsulin cleavage products to say whether they are relatively more effective in suppressing lipolysis and encouraging lipogenesis in adipocytes than they are in fostering glucose uptake by muscle and hepatic cells, and how they compare with native insulin. Nevertheless, insulin resistance in obese subjects, with or without NIDDM, is confined largely, if not exclusively, to glucose uptake and/or metabolism by striated muscle and liver cells and is seemingly not involved with fatty acid uptake, release and metabolism by adipocytes.

Insulin

It is as difficult to exaggerate the importance of insulin in the pathogenesis of obesity as it is in diabetes. It is more than mere coincidence that the two conditions are so intimately connected.

Insulin is the main anabolic hormone in the body, working in conjunction with growth hormone, whose presence is necessary for its adequate and appropriate secretion. Insulin promotes protein, glycogen and triglyceride synthesis, and their incorporation into the fabric of the body. It decreases proteolysis, glycogenolysis and lipolysis, which are prerequisites for their utilization as fuels. Insulin production and secretion are promoted by the ingestion and absorption of food; its secretion is inhibited by fasting. Insulin is synergistic with growth hormone to promote protein synthesis by tissues and, in the liver, to produce insulin-like growth factor (IGF-1) and IGF-binding proteins, but antagonistic to growth hormone with regard to fat and carbohydrate metabolism. Growth hormone secretion is increased by food deprivation, which has just the opposite effect upon insulin. This combination of events serves to encourage the mobilization of fat from adipocytes and make free fatty acid available for use as a fuel. Growth hormone secretion is usually impaired in obese subjects, and partially, but not completely, restored by food deprivation. What role it has to play in the pathogenesis of obesity is still unclear.

Gut Hormones

Soon after the introduction of the immunoassay for the measurement of insulin in blood, it became apparent that obesity was the most common cause of both fasting and stimulated hyperinsulinaemia, but unlike the circumstances that obtained in patients with 'primary hyperinsulinism' due to insulin, the pancreatic β-cells of obese patients responded normally to the inhibitory effects of fasting and hypoglycaemia. They did, however, respond excessively to most β-cell stimuli, including the enteric hormones.

Gastric inhibitory polypeptide (GIP), and the more recently discovered glucagon-like peptide-1$_{(7-36)}$ amide (GLP-1$_{(7-36)}$ amide), are amongst the intestinal hormones that are believed to mediate insulin secretion in response to food. Both hormones enhance glucose uptake and its conversion into triglyceride in adipose tissue *in vitro*, and GIP activates the lipoprotein lipase of adipose tissue. This would tend to favour the efficient uptake of dietary fat by adipocytes and its storage as fat.

GIP secretion is stimulated by carbohydrates and by long-chain fatty acids. All genetically obese strains of laboratory animals so far investigated have been found to have much more GIP in their gut wall and blood than normal-weight animals of the same strain. They also show exaggerated responses to the ingestion of energy-providing nutrients. In human obesity the state is less clear. Although obese subjects generally have a higher plasma GIP than lean individuals, evidence implicating GIP in the aetiology of sporadic obesity is far from clear. In genetically obese individuals such as the Pima Indians, on the other hand, GIP concentrations in plasma are elevated and they respond excessively to feeding. In summary, GIP appears to fulfil many, if not all, of the roles expected of a hormonal mediator of an obesity gene.

Growth Hormone

Abnormalities of growth hormone secretion are almost as characteristic of obesity as those of insulin. They are similar in being at least partially reversible by diet-induced weight loss. The plasma growth-hormone response to most physiological stimuli is reduced in the obese subjects, but not by as much as in the postabsorptive phase, where the normal rise in growth hormone is almost totally abolished. The pathophysiological significance of this effect, and how it is produced, are unknown. Although it is less likely than the exaggerated insulinaemic response to stimulation by food to play a causative role in obesity, it may well have a role to play in perpetuating it. Moreover, it provides further evidence that a defect

in hypothalamic function is common in obesity, but whether as a primary or secondary event is far from clear.

Alterations in the secretion of many other hormones, of which prolactin is perhaps the most interesting, also occur in some obese subjects. Some, such as alterations that are observed in oestrogen metabolism, are secondary to the increased adipose tissue mass and an increased metabolic conversion of one steroid into another. Others, such as abnormalities of prolactin and of cortisol secretion, may have a pathogenetic role. The pathophysiological significance of these changes is, however, still poorly understood, and part of their importance lies in the diagnostic confusion they cause.

Sympathetic Nervous System

The impaired response of plasma noradrenaline and, to a lesser extent, of plasma adrenaline to hypoglycaemia in obese subjects may be either a consequence of obesity or a primary defect of pathogenetic significance. Like growth hormone and prolactin secretion the sympathetic nervous system is controlled by the hypothalamus, and is important in initiating lipolysis in adipose tissue. There is some evidence that this too may be impaired in obese subjects.

TREATMENT

There is at present no satisfactory or specific treatment for obesity, except in those rare instances where an identifiable cause can be found and rectified. Reduction of total energy intake to below the subject's energy expenditure, on the other hand, invariably produces weight loss but is extremely difficult to achieve in free-living subjects. Innumerable diets, some of them quite preposterous and antiscientific, have been said to be effective in facilitating weight loss but none has withstood either critical examination or the more practical challenge of time.

Synthetic, liquid, very low-calorie diets are effective in the short term, mainly, if not entirely, because they are easier for patients to adhere to than diets consisting of ordinary food. The 'benefits' are, however, generally short lived. Moreover, because weight loss achieved in this way is associated with loss of lean tissue as well as of fat from adipose tissue, it is of questionable value except as a short-term symptomatic treatment. Various heroic surgical manoeuvres have been tried from time to time but most have been abandoned as producing more harm than benefit in the long term. They are, at best, symptomatic treatments.

CONCLUSION

Morbid obesity is a common genetic disorder that expresses itself, like many genetic disorders, only when certain preconditions are met. In the case of obesity, the precondition is a plentiful supply of food. It is, however, unreasonable to consider morbid obesity as being of nutritional or dietary origin, as this diverts attention away from the basic, but unknown, metabolic defects that are undoubtedly responsible for it in the majority of cases.

FURTHER READING

Oomura Y., Tarui S., Inoue S., Shimazu T. eds. (1991). *Progress in Obesity Research*, Proceedings of the VIth International Congress on Obesity 1990, London: Libbey.

3. Disorders Involving Disturbances in Hydrogen Ion Concentration and Blood Gases

Joan F. Zilva

Introduction
Buffering
    The Henderson–Hasselbalch equation
    Bicarbonate buffering
    Haemoglobin and other proteins
    Phosphate buffering
Control of the components of the extracellular
    bicarbonate buffer pair
    Control of carbon dioxide by the respiratory
      centre and lungs
    Erythrocytes and the role of haemoglobin
    Control of bicarbonate by the kidneys
    Handling of bicarbonate ion by the
      gastrointestinal tract
Assessment of hydrogen ion status
    Plasma total carbon dioxide
    Measured values on arterial blood
    Derived values
Disturbances of hydrogen ion balance
    Acidosis
    Alkalosis
    Effects of salicylates
Investigation of hydrogen ion disturbances
    Interpretation of plasma (T_{CO_2})
    Anion gap
    Indications for arterial estimations

In this chapter the concentration of a substance is denoted by placing square brackets round the chemical symbol.

INTRODUCTION

Carbon dioxide (CO_2) and water are generated by complete aerobic metabolism of the hydrogen, carbon and oxygen in the skeletons of organic compounds. The CO_2 is of central importance in hydrogen ion homeostasis. Other metabolic processes release a net daily amount of about 50–100 *milli*mol of hydrogen ion (H^+) into about 15–20 L of extracellular fluid. Homeostatic mechanisms are so efficient that the normal extracellular hydrogen ion concentration $[H^+]$ is only about 40 *nano*mol/L (pH 7.4) and varies little despite changing loads during the day.

Physiological processes that generate hydrogen ions are summarized in Table 3.1. They fall into two groups.

1. *Complete metabolism of organic constituents other than carbon, hydrogen and oxygen.* The two most important metabolic processes generating hydrogen ions are conversion of amino nitrogen to urea and of sulphur in the sulphydryl (SH) groups of amino acids to sulphate. For this reason, people eating protein-rich diets, especially containing a high proportion of sulphur amino acids, pass relatively acid urine. Although such a diet may aggravate acidosis, it is unlikely to be the primary cause.

2. *Incomplete catabolism of carbon skeletons.* Oxygen is essential for complete metabolism of carbohydrate and fatty acids to CO_2 and water. The following examples of anaerobic processes generate H^+, directly or indirectly.

    (a) Incomplete metabolism of carbohydrate yields H^+ and lactate, derived from pyruvate. During strenuous exercise the rate of anaerobic muscle glycogenolysis may exceed the rate of aerobic pyruvate metabolism and lactic acid accumulates;

    (b) Incomplete metabolism of fatty and ketogenic amino acids yields ketoacids, derived from acetyl coenzyme A (Acetyl CoA). During periods of fasting the rate of ketogenesis may exceed the rate of aerobic acetyl CoA metabolism and ketoacids accumulate.

TABLE 3.1.
EXAMPLES OF PHYSIOLOGICAL PROCESSES YIELDING HYDROGEN IONS

Metabolism of Non-Carbon Groups	*Products*
Oxidation of sulphur	Sulphate^{2-} + $2H^+$ per $-SH^-$
Metabolism of nitrogen	Urea + H^+ per $-NH_3^+$
Incomplete Metabolism	
Anaerobic glucose metabolism	2 lactate$^-$ + $2H^+$ per glucose molecule
Incomplete fatty acid metabolism	Acetoacetate$^-$ + H^+ ⎱ per acetyl CoA
or	3-hydroxybutyrate$^-$ + H^+ ⎰ (or per fatty acid molecule)

No attempt has been made to balance these equations.
The production of hydrogen ions is not always a direct consequence of the reaction.
Interested readers should consult the references at the end of the chapter for more detailed information.

The rate of these two H^+ generating processes may be much increased in pathological states.

Three very simple compounds are essential for hydrogen ion homeostasis:

- *Water* is ubiquitous and incorporates hydrogen ions which have been buffered by bicarbonate in an unionized (inactive) form.
- *Carbon dioxide* is constantly produced by aerobic metabolism.
- *Bicarbonate* and hydrogen ion are produced when water and carbon dioxide combine.

Two organs are essential to coordinate the system:

- The *lungs*, controlled by the cerebral medullary respiratory centre, adjust the extracellular CO_2 concentration.
- The *kidneys*, using CO_2 and water, control the extracellular *bicarbonate* concentration.

A most important reaction affecting hydrogen ion homeostasis is the very simple, reversible one involving the three components mentioned above:

$$H^+ + HCO_3^- \overset{a}{\rightleftharpoons} H_2CO_3 \overset{b}{\rightleftharpoons} CO_2 + H_2O \quad (1).$$

Before discussing how these mechanisms work *in vivo* I shall outline some important aspects of buffer action and explain which metabolites can act as effective buffers in the body.

BUFFERING

A buffer pair is made up of a weak (little dissociated) acid and its conjugate base. If either free H^+ or free hydroxyl ions (OH^-) are added to a solution of such a pair they will be partly converted to the unionized form.

Thus, if HB denotes a weak acid and B^- its conjugate base, and if the solid arrows indicate the predominant direction of the reaction and the dotted arrows the reverse one, then

$$B^- + H^+ \rightleftharpoons HB \quad (2),$$

or

$$HB + OH^- \rightleftharpoons H_2O + B^- \quad (3).$$

Obviously the buffering capacity depends partly on the concentration of the buffer. If so much H^+ is added that its concentration exceeds that of B^-, the excess cannot be buffered. Moreover the reaction is reversible (*see* equation 2) and as $[B^-]$ falls and $[HB]$ rises the relative rate of the reverse reaction increases and buffering becomes progressively less effective. If the concentration of HB in the initial mixture is much greater than that of B^- it will be a poor buffer for even small amounts of added H^+. The nearer the ratio of $[HB]$ to $[B^-]$ is to unity, the more effective is the buffer system in minimizing changes due to the addition of either H^+ or OH^-. If $[B^-]$ is much greater than $[HB]$ it will be more efficient in buffering H^+ than OH^-.

The Henderson–Hasselbalch Equation

If the equilibrium constant, K_a, is included in equation 2 the relative concentrations of the reactants at equilibrium can be expressed as follows:

$$[B^-][H^+] = K_a[HB] \quad (4),$$

or

$$[H^+] = K_a \frac{[HB]}{[B^-]} \quad (5).$$

When $[HB] = [B^-]$, then $[HB]/[B^-] = 1$ and thus, at equilibrium, $[H^+] = K_a$. A buffer system is therefore most effective if the hydrogen ion concentration is near its equilibrium constant.

The Henderson–Hasselbalch equation uses the term pH rather then $[H^+]$. pH is log $1/[H^+]$ when $[H^+]$ is expressed as mmol/L. If pK_a is log $1/K_a$, equation 5 can be rewritten

$$pH = pK_a + \log\frac{[B^-]}{[HB]}.$$

Using the pH notation, the effectiveness of a buffer system can be predicted as follows. The antilog of 1 is 0. When $[HB]/[B^-] = 1$, $pH = pK_a$. A buffer pair is therefore most effective in maintaining a pH near its pK_a; it can be shown to have a significant action within about 1.5 pH units on either side of this. Because normal extracellular pH is about 7.4, the nearer the pK_a of a buffer is to 7.4 the more effective it will be; buffer with pK_a outside the range 5.9–8.9 will have little useful effect.

Metabolic processes generate H^+ rather than OH^- and a pK_a nearer the lower end of the range (that is, $[B^-]$ is greater than $[HB]$) is usually less physiologically disadvantageous than one at the upper limit.

The importance of buffer pairs *in vivo* should thus be considered with two factors in mind:

1. the concentration of the buffer;
2. the pK_a of the buffer.

Bicarbonate Buffering

The physiological concentration of bicarbonate of about 25 mmol/L is quantitatively adequate for buffering in plasma and interstitial fluid (which together make up the extracellular fluid) and in the glomerular filtrate. Inside cells the concentration is too low for it to have a significant function.

Bicarbonate ion (HCO_3^-) and carbonic acid (H_2CO_3) form the buffer pair for which the Henderson–Hasselbalch equation can be written:

$$pH = pK_a + \log\frac{[HCO_3^-]}{[H_2CO_3]}.$$

The concentration of H_2CO_3 cannot be measured directly, but the partial pressure of CO_2 (P_{CO_2}) can. Inspection of the important equation 1 (buffering of

H$^+$ by bicarbonate) shows that H_2CO_3 is in equilibrium with CO_2:

$$H^+ + HCO_3^- \overset{a}{\rightleftharpoons} H_2CO_3 \overset{b}{\rightleftharpoons} CO_2 + H_2O \quad (1).$$

H_2CO_3 can therefore be replaced by CO_2 in the Henderson–Hasselbalch equation:

$$pH = pK_a' + \log\frac{[HCO_3^-]}{[CO_2]},$$

where pK_a' represents the combined pK_a for reactions (a) and (b) in equation 1. This pK_a' has a value of about 6.1.

[CO_2], expressed in mmol/L, can be calculated by multiplying measured PCO_2 by the solubility coefficient for carbon dioxide. The value of this coefficient is 0.225 if PCO_2 is expressed in kilopascals (kPa) and 0.03 if it is expressed in mmHg.

Therefore if [HCO_3^-] is expressed in mmol/L and PCO_2 in kPa,

$$pH = 6.1 + \log\frac{[HCO_3^-]}{PCO_2 \times 0.225}.$$

The pK_a' of 6.1 is near the lower limit of 5.9 for an effective buffer system at pH 7.4. If 7.4 is inserted for pH in the Henderson–Hasselbalch equation, $\log[HCO_3^-]/[CO_2]$ will be $7.4 - 6.1 = 1.3$. The ratio of [HCO_3^-] to [CO_2] at pH 7.4 is therefore the antilog of 1.3, which is 20. *The concentration of base is therefore much higher than that of acid and buffering will be more effective for H$^+$ than for OH$^-$.* This is advantageous because, as already mentioned, H$^+$ rather than OH$^-$ is produced by the body. The physiological effectiveness of the system is also enhanced by dissociation of H_2CO_3 to gaseous CO_2, the level of which can be kept low by the lungs, and by the catalysis of the interconversion of carbonic acid and CO_2 by carbonate dehydratase (*see* equation 1).

The bicarbonate system is of prime physiological importance and acts in conjunction with other buffers.

Buffering by Haemoglobin and other Proteins

The complex buffering action of proteins depends on the polar groups of the constituent amino acids, the pK_a values of which are affected by neighbouring groups. No accurate figure can be given either for the concentration of the buffering groups, or for the pK_a of a protein.

Plasma proteins diffuse only slowly through capillary walls and protein concentration in interstitial fluid is very low. This contrasts with HCO_3^-, which diffuses freely and is of almost the same concentration in interstitial fluid as in plasma. Proteins are predominantly intracellular and haemoglobin is confined to erythrocytes. Proteins acting alone hardly contribute to extracellular buffering, just as bicarbonate acting alone is ineffective inside cells.

Haemoglobin

At pH 7.4, haemoglobin is a better buffer than most proteins because of the relatively high concentration of imidazole groups, with a pK_a of about 7, of the constituent histidine molecules. Although the erythrocyte haemoglobin concentration is only about 4 mmol/L (that is, 2 mmol/L in whole blood), each molecule incorporates several buffering groups. The buffering capacity is therefore higher than the concentration of the whole protein would suggest.

Haemoglobin is also a much more effective blood buffer than plasma proteins because it is enclosed, with carbonate dehydratase, in erythrocytes. It will be shown later that this enables the bicarbonate and haemoglobin buffering systems to work cooperatively.

Deoxyhaemoglobin is a better buffer than oxyhaemoglobin; conversely, hydrogen ions decrease the affinity of haemoglobin for oxygen.

Other Proteins

The total blood molar concentration of plasma proteins is lower than that of haemoglobin and their concentrations in interstitial fluid are even lower. More importantly, the buffering capacity per mole is less and they do not work cooperatively with the carbonate dehydratase system. They are therefore unimportant as extracellular buffers.

The intracellular protein concentration is much higher than that in plasma. Proteins play a relatively important part in buffering H$^+$ before it is released from cells.

Phosphate Buffering

Mono- and dihydrogen phosphate form a buffer pair with a pK_a of about 6.8:

$$pH = 6.8 + \log\frac{[HPO_4^{2-}]}{[H_2PO_4^-]}.$$

The plasma phosphate concentration is only about 2 mmol/L so that, despite the favourable pK_a, extracellular phosphate contributes little to buffering.

The glomerular filtrate concentration is almost identical with that of plasma, but during selective water reabsorption from the tubular lumen the concentration rises, reaching about 20 mmol/L in urine. Phosphate is an important buffer in distal luminal fluid and, like haemoglobin in erythrocytes, works cooperatively with the bicarbonate system.

Extracellular and urinary concentrations of all other potential buffers are very low (for example, that of urate is about 0.2 mmol/L in extracellular fluid and about 2 mmol/L in urine) and their pK_a values are more unfavourable, even at the lower and more variable pH of urine.

In summary the three important buffers are:

  (a) the *bicarbonate* system in the extracellular fluid and glomerular filtrate, which is central to hydrogen ion homeostasis and works cooperatively with
  (b) *haemoglobin* in erythrocytes and
  (c) *phosphate* in renal tubular fluid.

It will be shown later that *ammonia* in luminal fluid, although not an effective buffer, also acts cooperatively with the bicarbonate system.

CONTROL OF THE COMPONENTS OF THE EXTRACELLULAR BICARBONATE BUFFER PAIR

Carbon dioxide, the denominator in the Henderson–Hasselbalch equation, is a 'waste product' of aerobic metabolism. It reacts with water to form bicarbonate, the numerator in the same equation, and so plays an important part in controlling another potentially toxic product of metabolism, hydrogen ion.

Control of Carbon Dioxide by the Respiratory Centre and Lungs

Carbon dioxide diffuses freely from capillaries into alveolar sacs. The concentration gradient of CO_2 from the blood into these sacs is maintained by its elimination, the efficiency of removal depending mainly on the rate and depth of breathing. The capacity of normal lungs to eliminate carbon dioxide is very high. Although metabolic acidosis increases the rate of production of CO_2 as metabolically generated hydrogen ions are buffered by bicarbonate, plasma $[CO_2]$ is kept normal, or even low, by an increase in the rate and depth of breathing; it only rises if either gas diffusion across alveolar walls or lung movement is impaired. Respiratory movement is controlled by the response of the cerebral medullary respiratory centre to the pH of the blood flowing through it and, under physiological conditions, maintains arterial P_{CO_2} at about 5.3 kPa (40 mmHg)—corresponding to about 1.2 mmol/L $[CO_2]$. This residual CO_2 is of central importance in hydrogen ion homeostasis.

CO_2 combines with water to form carbonic acid, which dissociates to bicarbonate and hydrogen ions:

$$CO_2 + H_2O \xrightarrow{a} H_2CO_3 \xrightarrow{b} H^+ + HCO_3^- \quad (1).$$

The HCO_3^- generated by this reaction can only usefully buffer metabolically produced hydrogen ions if the H^+ generated in reaction (b) is removed. The pH of the system depends on the ratio of $[HCO_3^-]$ to $[CO_2]$. To minimize changes in pH the reaction should proceed rapidly to the right so that HCO_3^- is formed as $[CO_2]$ rises at the site of production of H^+ (tissues), and should reverse rapidly to convert HCO_3^- to $[CO_2]$ as the latter falls at the site of removal of CO_2 (lungs).

Two cell types (erythrocytes and renal tubular cells) not only contain high concentrations of *carbonate dehydratase*, which catalyses the reaction, but also have a means of disposing of H^+ formed in the process. HCO_3^- is therefore made available to buffer metabolically produced hydrogen ions.

Erythrocytes and the Role of Haemoglobin

Erythrocytes are of great *physiological* importance in minimizing the change in ratio of $[CO_2]$ to $[HCO_3^-]$, and therefore the change in pH, between arterial and venous blood.

Red cells produce little CO_2 because they lack aerobic pathways. As shown in Fig. 3.1 (step 1), when CO_2 diffuses from tissues cells into the extracellular fluid, the extracellular ratio of $[HCO_3^-]$ to $[CO_2]$, and therefore the pH, falls. The rising venous P_{CO_2} creates a concentration gradient between plasma and erythrocytes. CO_2 therefore diffuses into red cells (step 2) where its reaction with water is catalysed by carbonate dehydratase (step 3). Haemoglobin in venous blood has already released oxygen to tissues, and the haemoglobin, mostly in the deoxy- form, buffers H^+ produced by the reaction (step 4); this, in turn, stimulates further oxygen release from haemoglobin. The rising intracellular $[CO_2]$ and the removal of H^+ by haemoglobin keep the net reaction proceeding in a forward direction and the intracellular concentration of bicarbonate rises. Diffusion into extracellular fluid (step 5) brings the ratio of $[HCO_3^-]$ to $[CO_2]$ (and pH) towards normal; the negatively charged HCO_3^- is replaced by chloride, which diffuses from plasma along the electrochemical gradient ('chloride shift').

This process reverses in the lungs. CO_2 diffuses from plasma across alveolar walls (Fig. 3.2; step 1), creating a concentration gradient across red-cell membranes. As CO_2 leaves these cells (step 2) the carbonate dehydratase reaction reverses (step 3) and the consequent removal of H^+ from haemoglobin (step 4) is accelerated as haemoglobin takes up oxygen to form oxyhaemoglobin, a weaker buffer. Oxygenation of haemoglobin is also stimulated by the fall of $[H^+]$. Bicarbonate diffuses into erythrocytes along the concentration gradient (step 5) and chloride diffuses out along the electrochemical gradient.

Diffusion of chloride is the rate-limiting step in both these processes.

Under physiological circumstances these reactions are so effective in minimizing a change in ratio between $[HCO_3^-]$ and $[CO_2]$ that the arteriovenous pH difference is only about 0.03–0.04 units (a change of hydrogen ion concentration of 40–43 nmol/L). Haemoglobin (Hb) buffering capacity is not exceeded because it is alternately in the form HHb and HbO_2^-; HCO_3^- is alternately formed from, and broken down to, CO_2.

If CO_2 cannot be removed at a normal rate by the lungs, most of the haemoglobin may be in the form

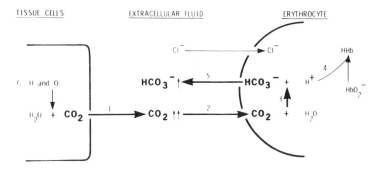

Figure 3.1 Role of haemoglobin in controlling extracellular pH during carbon dioxide release from tissues (HbO_2^- = oxyhaemoglobin, HHb = acid haemoglobin).

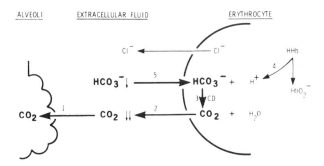

Figure 3.2 Role of haemoglobin in controlling extracellular pH during carbon dioxide removal in the lungs.

HHb and further bicarbonate generation is impaired. Thus erythrocytes can play only a minor part in correction of respiratory acidosis; this explains the limitations of the concept of 'standard' bicarbonate (see p. 40).

Control of Bicarbonate by the Kidneys

Erythrocytes are important in minimizing the arteriovenous pH difference, but have little effect on net bicarbonate balance. The kidneys are the most important organs in the control of the extracellular bicarbonate concentration.

Extracellular bicarbonate can be lost from the body by one or more of three mechanisms.

1. Bicarbonate filtered through glomeruli at the normal plasma concentration of about 25 mmol/L may not be completely reabsorbed.
2. Circulating bicarbonate may be depleted when it buffers an excess of metabolically produced hydrogen ions.
3. Bicarbonate secreted into the intestinal lumen may not be recovered completely.

The kidneys normally limit the effects of the first two abnormalities and also help to minimize that of abnormal intestinal losses.

Bicarbonate is formed within tubular cells by the carbonate dehydratase (CD) mechanism:

$$CO_2 + H_2O \xrightarrow{\text{CD}} H^+ + HCO_3^-.$$

The erythrocyte and renal tubular mechanisms differ in one important respect. The H^+ formed in red cells when CO_2 and water combine remains in the body. By contrast, that formed by the same mechanism in tubular cells can be secreted into luminal fluid and so be lost in the urine. While H^+ can continue to be secreted, HCO_3^- can continue to be formed in tubular cells and returned to the extracellular fluid; the net reaction therefore continues to the right. Secretion is an active process that can take place against a moderate hydrogen-ion concentration gradient. This gradient is maintained because the luminal cell membranes are relatively impermeable to H^+.

Tubular cells also differ from erythrocytes in producing CO_2 by aerobic metabolism. This constant CO_2 production within the cells is another factor that helps to keep the net reaction proceeding to the right. CO_2 diffuses out of the cells along a concentration gradient.

The transluminal surfaces of tubular cells are permeable to both gases and ions: by contrast, the luminal surfaces, while freely permeable to gases, are relatively impermeable to ions.

The following factors *increase* the rate of renal HCO_3^- production.

1. *A rise in extracellular or luminal $P\text{CO}_2$.* CO_2 can diffuse out of tubular cells into both luminal and extracellular fluids. An increase in CO_2 concentration in either of these fluids reduces the concentration gradient, slows diffusion out of the cells and increases intracellular $[CO_2]$. CO_2 is one of the reactants in the carbonate dehydratase reaction.

2. *A fall in extracellular $[HCO_3^-]$.* The luminal cell membranes are relatively impermeable to HCO_3^- ions,

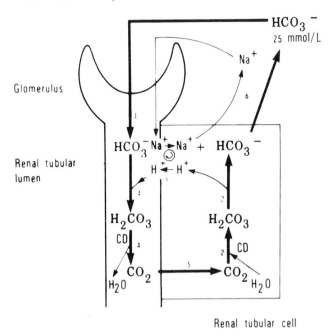

Figure 3.3 'Reabsorption' of filtered bicarbonate by the proximal renal tubular cells.

but they can diffuse through the transluminal membranes into extracellular fluid along a concentration gradient. A fall in extracellular $[HCO_3^-]$ increases the gradient and so reduces the intracellular concentration of one of the products of the carbonate dehydratase reaction. The rate of reaction is stimulated.

3. *An increased rate of secretion of H^+* into the tubular lumen increases the rate of removal of the other product of the reaction and also has a stimulatory effect.

The rate of production of HCO_3^- may be *reduced by*:

1. a fall in extracellular $P\text{CO}_2$;
2. a rise in extracellular $[HCO_3^-]$;
3. a decreased rate of secretion of H^+.

'Reabsorption' of Filtered Bicarbonate
Bicarbonate filtered through glomerular membranes (Fig. 3.3, step 1) is reclaimed by means of the carbonate dehydratase mechanism. HCO_3^- cannot be reabsorbed directly because of the relative impermeability of the luminal surfaces of tubular cell membranes to ions, but an equivalent amount to that filtered can be formed within luminal cells and returned to the extracellular fluid through the permeable transluminal membranes. This process occurs predominantly in the proximal tubules.

H^+ formed within tubular cells by the carbonate dehydratase mechanism (Fig. 3.3, step 2) is pumped into luminal fluid in exchange for the filtered cation, sodium (Na^+) (step 3). This active removal of H^+ as it

is formed inside cells continues to stimulate its production. H^+, being ionized, cannot diffuse back into the cells, but combines with the HCO_3^- that was filtered with the now reabsorbed Na^+. The cellular reaction is thus reversed in the lumen (step 4)—a process probably catalysed by carbonate dehydratase on luminal cell membranes. The CO_2 formed by this mechanism in luminal fluid can diffuse back into cells (step 5) and the intracellular reaction between CO_2 and water is stimulated. The resulting hydrogen ions are again exchanged for Na^+ in luminal fluid. Intracellular concentrations of HCO_3^- and Na^+ rise and these ions diffuse through the transluminal membranes. Each mmol of HCO_3^- filtered can combine with one mmol of H^+, and each time one mmol of H^+ is exchanged for luminal Na^+ one mmol each of HCO_3^- and Na^+ enter the extracellular fluid. Because an amount of HCO_3^- equal to that filtered can be returned to the extracellular fluid by this mechanism, bicarbonate is effectively, albeit indirectly, reabsorbed. Luminal fluid is almost bicarbonate free as it leaves the proximal tubules.

Replacement of Bicarbonate Depleted by Buffering
Bicarbonate 'reabsorption' is cyclical (*see* Fig. 3.3). It reclaims filtered bicarbonate, which would otherwise be lost, but it does not change the net amount of either bicarbonate or hydrogen ion in the body. Bicarbonate lost by extrarenal routes, such as that used during buffering or entering the gastrointestinal tract, can only be replaced if it continues to be generated in tubular cells after all filtered bicarbonate has been 'reabsorbed'. Secreted H^+ lost in the urine with anion *other than bicarbonate* enables this to happen. This should be a buffer anion, which minimizes ionization of hydrogen: if the luminal $[H^+]$ is very much higher than that in tubular cells, continuation of active secretion would need more energy than is readily available to overcome this gradient.

Urinary Phosphate and the Carbonate Dehydratase Mechanism
As filtered bicarbonate continues to be 'reabsorbed' less becomes available to buffer secreted H^+. Below pH 6.5 almost none is present. By contrast, the phosphate concentration increases because of selective water reabsorption and phosphate secretion in more distal parts of the tubules. Moreover, as the pH of the luminal fluid falls it approaches the pK_a of the phosphate pair (6.8), thus increasing the effectiveness of the buffering. As the buffering capacity of bicarbonate declines that of phosphate increases until it takes over. As in the 'reabsorption' mechanism, secreted H^+ is derived from water in the tubular cells, catalysed by carbonate dehydratase; HCO_3^- is returned to the extracellular fluid with sodium each time secreted H^+ combines with mono- to form dihydrogen phosphate (Fig. 3.4). This allows a net gain of 1 mmol of HCO_3^- per mmol H^+ buffered by phos-

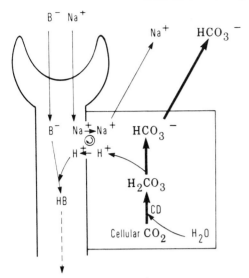

Figure 3.4 Role of filtered buffer anions in net generation of bicarbonate by renal tubular cells (B^- = non-bicarbonate buffer anion (mostly monohydrogen phosphate)).

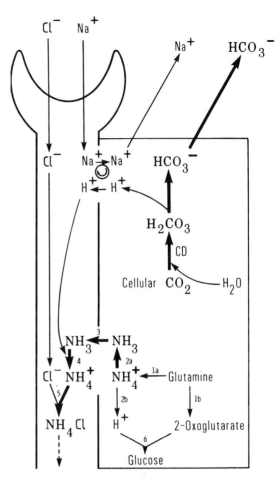

Figure 3.5 Role of urinary ammonia in net generation of bicarbonate by renal tubular cells.

phate. There is net loss of H^+ in the urine in the form of dihydrogen phosphate.

Urinary Ammonia and the Carbonate Dehydratase Mechanism

As more H^+ is secreted more monohydrogen phosphate is converted to dihydrogen phosphate until, below pH about 5.5, almost all is in this form. If tissues are generating a very large H^+ load the luminal buffering capacity may be inadequate to enable the carbonate dehydratase mechanism fully to replete extrarenal bicarbonate loss.

The more acid the urine becomes the more ammonium salts it contains. Ammonia and the ammonium ion form a buffer pair of sorts, but the pK_a of the system is about 9.2 (an effective buffering range of between pH about 8 and 11). This pair cannot act as a physiological buffer, especially in the relatively acid urine. It can, however, cooperate with the carbonate dehydratase system to replete plasma HCO_3^-.

Ammonium ion (NH_4^+) is formed in tubular cells from the two amino groups of glutamine, the two deamination steps being catalysed by glutaminase and glutamate dehydrogenase. The net effect is the production of one mmol of 2-oxoglutarate and two mmol of (NH_4^+) from one mmol of glutamine:

$$\text{Glutamine} \xrightarrow{\textit{glutaminase}} \text{Glutamate} + NH_4^+$$

$$\text{Glutamate} \xrightarrow{\substack{\textit{glutamate} \\ \textit{dehydrogenase}}} \text{2-oxoglutarate}^{2-} + NH_4^+.$$

The high pK_a of the ammonia pair indicates that most intracellular ammonium ion will not dissociate;

for example, at pH 7.2 there is 100 times as much NH_4^+ as NH_3 and at pH 7.4 the factor is 60. However, just as one member of the bicarbonate pair forms gaseous CO_2, which, unlike bicarbonate ion, can diffuse through luminal cell membranes, so ammonia can diffuse into luminal fluid while the ammonium ion cannot. If this ammonia is prevented from returning to cells more of the ammonium ion formed within cells will dissociate and its production from glutamine will continue.

Figure 3.5 shows how the cooperation between ammonium production and the carbonate dehydratase system could enable H^+ secretion into the urine and bicarbonate generation to continue. Figure 3.5 should be compared with Fig. 3.4. The action of glutaminase and glutamate dehydrogenase liberates NH_4^+ into distal tubular cells (Fig. 3.5, step 1a). This NH_4^+ is in equilibrium with a very small amount of NH_3 (step 2a). The luminal ammonia concentration is even lower than in cells and the gas diffuses along a gradient into the luminal fluid (step 3), where it combines with H^+ generated in the usual way (step 4). The luminal NH_4^+ cannot diffuse back into tubular cells. This 'trapping' of NH_3 and

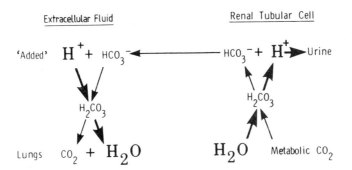

Figure 3.6 Hydrogen ion 'shuttle' between site of buffering and kidneys. (Reproduced from Mayne P.D. (1994). *Clinical Chemistry in Diagnosis and Treatment*, 6th edn, Edward Arnold).

H^+ in the lumen removes one of the products of both the glutaminase/glutamate dehydrogenase (NH_3) and the carbonate dehydratase (H^+) reactions and bicarbonate generation is accelerated. The ammonium is passed in the urine with the non-buffer anion chloride and the accompanying sodium, exchanged for secreted H^+, is returned to the extracellular fluid with bicarbonate. Chloride cannot buffer H^+ directly, as hydrochloric acid is highly ionized, but by incorporating H^+ in NH_4Cl the carbonate dehydratase system can continue to generate HCO_3^- and replete that used in buffering, even when urinary buffering capacity has been exhausted.

There is still one problem. Dissociation of NH_4^+ releases H^+ as well as NH_3 (step 2b). Unless it can be disposed of by some other route, this H^+ generated in tubular cells will use the same amount of HCO_3^- during buffering as that formed. The excretion of NH_4^+ would then have no role in hydrogen ion homeostasis. The explanation may be that in renal tubular (and hepatic) cells 2-oxoglutarate, the other product of deamination of glutamine (step 1b), can act as a substrate for gluconeogenesis and that glucose synthesis can be shown to use H^+. H^+ liberated into cells may be incorporated into glucose (step 6). The net effect would then be loss of one mmol of H^+ and gain of one mmol of HCO_3^- for each mmol of NH_3 entering the urine.

It has been claimed that, because of a lag before this mechanism becomes effective, it can only help to correct chronic acidosis.[1] However, administration of ammonium chloride acidifies the urine within a few hours.

We can now see how ingeniously the renal tubular mechanisms replete HCO_3^- used during the buffering of H^+ derived from metabolic processes. H^+ diffuses into the extracellular fluid and is incorporated locally, in an unionized form, into water; the oxygen in the water is derived from HCO_3^-. The normal respiratory centre responds to the slight rise in P_{CO_2}. The falling $[HCO_3^-]$ stimulates the renal carbonate dehydratase

mechanism and the extracellular buffering reaction is reversed, using CO_2 and water within renal tubular cells. H^+ produced here is lost in the urine incorporated in dihydrogen phosphate and, as phosphate buffering capacity falls, increasingly more is incorporated into ammonium chloride. If the addition of H^+ to extracellular fluid stops, these processes will continue only until extracellular $[HCO_3^-]$ becomes normal, when the stimulus is removed and the former steady state is reached. Urinary phosphate and ammonium are, like erythrocyte haemoglobin, acting as hydrogen ion acceptors and so allow the continued formation of HCO_3^- from CO_2.

Water carries hydrogen ions in an inert form from the site of production to a site where they can be eliminated from the body (Fig. 3.6).

Urinary Sodium and Chloride and the Carbonate Dehydratase Mechanism

Hydrogen ion secretion and therefore HCO_3^- generation in tubular cells needs sodium for exchange. Reduced availability of sodium in luminal fluid may cause acidosis and increased availability may contribute to alkalosis.

The amount of chloride filtered through glomerular membranes is an important factor affecting the amount of sodium reaching distal sites. Only the small fraction of sodium that escapes reabsorption in proximal tubules takes part in hydrogen ion exchange. Proximal reabsorption of cationic sodium depends on the availability of anion to accompany it. The two predominant filtered anions are chloride (about 100 mmol/L) and bicarbonate (about 25 mmol/L). Hypochloraemia without equivalent hyponatraemia impairs proximal tubular sodium reabsorption, allowing more to reach distal sites. Inappropriate H^+ secretion will be stimulated despite pre-existing alkalosis. This is important in determining how to treat the biochemical disturbance of pyloric stenosis.

Potassium and the Carbonate Dehydratase Mechanism

Potassium ions within renal tubular cells compete with

hydrogen ions, formed by the carbonate dehydratase mechanism, for exchange with luminal sodium ions.

An abnormally low potassium concentration in these cells favours secretion of relatively more hydrogen ions in exchange for the same amount of sodium. Increased H^+ secretion, one of the factors stimulating the carbonate dehydratase mechanism, increases return of HCO_3^- to the extracellular fluid and can cause alkalosis. By contrast, other factors stimulating the mechanism *cause* acidosis (a high extracellular P_{CO_2} or a low extracellular $[HCO_3^-]$), and the increased H^+ secretion helps to correct it; in these cases relatively more H^+ is available for exchange in cells with normal potassium concentrations and hyperkalaemia, rather than hypokalaemia, may follow the retention of potassium.

Conversely, a high intracellular potassium concentration would inhibit HCO_3^- formation and low P_{CO_2} or high $[HCO_3^-]$ tend to cause potassium depletion.

Handling of Bicarbonate by the Gastrointestinal Tract

The Gastric Mucosa

Gastric mucosal secretion of acid also depends on the carbonate dehydratase mechanism. The empty gastric cavity contains very little sodium or buffer. Hydrogen ions are secreted into it with chloride rather than, as in the renal tubular lumen in exchange for sodium. Hydrochloric acid is almost completely ionized and the pH of gastric secretion is very low: the gastric mucosa can tolerate this high degree of acidity and can maintain the large H^+ gradient between the cavity and cells. As usual, HCO_3^- is returned to the extracellular fluid each time H^+ is secreted.

The Intestinal Tract

Some bicarbonate diffuses passively into the duodenal and jejunal lumina and is probably 'reabsorbed' by an exactly analogous process to that in the kidneys (*see* Fig. 3.3).

Pancreatic cells and those lining the biliary tract actively secrete sodium bicarbonate from the extracellular fluid into the duodenal lumen, probably by the reverse process to the renal one. Each H^+ formed intracellularly exchanges with one Na^+ in the extracellular fluid instead of the lumen. It is buffered by, and so reduces the concentration of, extracellular HCO_3^-. The HCO_3^- formed within the cells with H^+ enters the biliary tract with sodium derived from that previously associated with the extracellular bicarbonate lost in the buffering.

Bicarbonate is also secreted by ileal and colonic cells, probably by the reverse mechanism of that in the gastric mucosa, with the net effect of secretion of bicarbonate in exchange for chloride. Luminal chloride exchanges for bicarbonate formed within cells; the H^+ is secreted into the extracellular fluid with the chloride, where buffering reduces plasma bicarbonate concentration, the potential anion deficit being made up by chloride. There is therefore no net movement of sodium.

The tendency to alkalosis during postprandial gastric secretion (the so-called 'alkaline tide') is normally mainly offset by bicarbonate secretion as food enters the duodenum. The rest of this bicarbonate increment is lost in the ileum and colon, together with an amount of chloride equivalent to that gained at the same site.

ASSESSMENT OF HYDROGEN ION STATUS

The bicarbonate system is central to hydrogen ion homeostasis. It will be affected if this homeostasis is disturbed in any way. The components of the system can easily be measured. Haemoglobin is important in buffering the effects of *acute* disturbances. This buffering capacity depends on both its concentration and its degree of oxygenation.

Plasma Total Carbon Dioxide

The plasma total carbon dioxide (T_{CO_2}) is made up of bicarbonate, dissolved CO_2 and carbonic acid. The following calculations show that its concentration is a very close index of that of bicarbonate.

At pH 7.4 the ratio of $[HCO_3^-]$ to the other two components is 20:1, so if the $[T_{CO_2}]$ were 21 mmol/L, 20 mmol/L of this would be accounted for by HCO_3^-. Even at a low plasma pH of 7.1 the ratio would be 10:1 and a $[T_{CO_2}]$ of 22 mmol/L would represent 20 mmol/L of HCO_3^-.

Determination of plasma T_{CO_2} concentration is the simplest, safest, most commonly performed and often the only necessary estimation of a component of the bicarbonate buffer pair. If clinical and other findings are taken into account together with a knowledge of $[T_{CO_2}]$, the state of acid–base balance usually can reliably be inferred. The estimation can be carried out on venous plasma at the same time as those of sodium, potassium, urea and, if indicated, glucose and chloride, all of which may help to elucidate the cause of an abnormal T_{CO_2}. Arterial puncture is avoided.

Simple precautions must be taken during blood collection and processing to ensure that the result truly reflects the circulating concentration. The commonest cause of an artefactually low concentration, especially in specimens from small children, is loss of CO_2 from blood into the air in the specimen tube. As CO_2 is lost, bicarbonate is converted to CO_2, which in turn, is lost into the dead space. Centrifugation may cause significant losses if there is a large space between the specimen and the stopper. Tubes should be filled nearly to the top and small specimens should be put into small tubes. Unless these criteria are fulfilled a fresh specimen should be requested, rather than a probably misleading result reported. Old and haemolysed specimens are also unsuitable because of the effect of erythrocyte metabolism.

Measured Values on Arterial Blood

There is a relatively large arteriovenous difference in P_{CO_2} and measurements other than $[T_{CO_2}]$ must be made on arterial blood. Arterial puncture is slightly more unpleasant and dangerous for the patient than venepuncture and measurement of all variables is often unnecessary. The clinician should only request or perform 'blood gas' estimations if the clinical indications are clear (*see* p. 51).

Blood should be drawn into and left in a heparinized syringe. It should be mixed by rolling the syringe gently between the hands without allowing air to enter. Results of estimations on capillary specimens are less likely to represent circulating arterial concentrations, especially if, as often in conditions in which these estimations are requested, there is peripheral vasoconstriction. If capillary puncture must be used the site should be warm and pink, and heparinized capillary tubes should be completely filled with blood and sealed. All specimens should be assayed or sent to the laboratory immediately, preferably on ice to reduce the rate of erythrocyte metabolism. Excessive amounts of heparin significantly affect results and the anticoagulant should only wet the surface of the syringe. *Plasma sodium estimation should never be performed on specimens taken into sodium heparin.* A false diagnosis of hypernatraemia is dangerous.

Measurements are made at 37°C. Corrections may be made for hypoxia and hypothermia.

The **pH** is measured by passing blood directly from the syringe or capillary tube through a glass electrode. The finding of an abnormal pH indicates a serious abnormality of hydrogen ion balance but a normal one does not exclude an abnormality. Compensatory changes may be keeping it normal.

The P_{CO_2}, a measure of respiratory disturbance, is measured by passing blood through a CO_2 electrode.

Derived Values

All values other than those already discussed are calculated automatically in modern machines from measured pH, P_{CO_2}, sometimes with haemoglobin and its degree of saturation, from the Henderson–Hasselbalch equation and haemoglobin concentration. The machines can often be programmed to suppress some or all of these derived values. This shows either lack of conviction, or commercial considerations, on the part of the manufacturers. I think it unfortunate that they are made available at all. In general those most likely to use them are those least likely to recognize their limitations. The following explanations should indicate the problems of interpreting such results.

Actual bicarbonate concentration is derived by inserting measured values of P_{CO_2} and pH into the Henderson–Hasselbalch equation for the bicarbonate pair. It is the most commonly reported of the derived values and should be a measure of the circulating arterial bicarbonate concentration. However, the cal-culation assumes that the pK_a of the bicarbonate system is constant, which is not true in all pathological states. For this reason it has been suggested that *arterial* $[T_{CO_2}]$ is a better measure of arterial bicarbonate concentration.[2] I feel that this is a purist recommendation. In my experience actual bicarbonate and venous T_{CO_2} measurements usually agree closely enough for practical purposes.

Standard bicarbonate concentration is measured *in vitro*. If whole blood taken from a patient with an abnormal P_{CO_2} is equilibrated with gas of a 'normal' P_{CO_2} of 5.3 mmol/L (40 mmHg), the bicarbonate alters, owing to the action of the erythrocytes (*see* Figs. 3.1 and 3.2). This new value is the 'standard' bicarbonate. If the circulating P_{CO_2} is high, *in vitro* correction to normal would result in a 'standard' bicarbonate concentration lower than that of the actual one; if the circulating P_{CO_2} were low the 'standard' would be higher than the actual bicarbonate. The difference should therefore indicate the *in vitro* increment or decrement in circulating bicarbonate that is due to the *erythrocyte mechanism alone*. Difficulties of interpretation are discussed on p. 46.

I have even greater reservations about the other two derived values, which seem of no more help and are more prone to error than direct measurements. *Buffer base* is said to indicate the *total* blood buffering capacity. *Base excess* or *deficit* is a hypothetical measurement of the amount of acid or base needed per litre of blood to bring all the variables to normal. These two values will not be discussed further in this chapter, but the reader may consult Astrup et al.[3] for further information.

In the following discussion changes in pH, P_{CO_2} and actual bicarbonate concentrations in each group of disturbances will be described. These changes are summarized in Table 3.2. In the last part of the chapter I shall consider which estimations give clinically useful information.

DISTURBANCES OF HYDROGEN ION BALANCE

The bicarbonate buffer pair is affected in any abnormality of hydrogen ion homeostasis and its components can easily be measured. It is therefore convenient and valid to discuss disturbances in terms of changes in this pair.

pH is determined by the ratio of $[HCO_3^-]$ to P_{CO_2}.

In so-called *metabolic* disturbances a change in the concentration of *bicarbonate* is the primary abnormality.

In so-called *respiratory* disturbances a change in P_{CO_2} is the primary abnormality.

If the concentration of the other member of the pair changes in the same direction the ratio of the two, and therefore the pH, reverts towards normal.

In *metabolic* disturbances the *compensatory* change is in P_{CO_2} and is in the same direction as the original change in (HCO_3^-).

TABLE 3.2
FINDINGS IN ARTERIAL BLOOD IN HYDROGEN ION DISTURBANCES

Type	Uncompensated			Partially compensated			Fully compensated		
	pH	P_{CO_2}	$[HCO_3^-]$	pH	P_{CO_2}	$[HCO_3^-]$	pH	P_{CO_2}	$[HCO_3^-]$
Acidosis									
Metabolic	↓↓	N	↓↓	↓	↓	↓↓	N	↓↓	↓↓
Respiratory	↓↓	↑↑	N	↓	↑↑	↑	N	↑↑	↑↑
Alkalosis				Compensation relatively ineffective					
Metabolic	↑↑	N	↑↑						
Respiratory	↑↑	↓↓	N	↑	↓↓	↓	N	↓↓	↓↓

N, normal value or range.

In *respiratory* disturbances the *compensatory* change is in $[HCO_3^-]$ in the same direction as the original change in P_{CO_2}. Compensatory changes may correct the pH partly or completely (Table 3.2) but buffering capacity remains abnormal unless the original cause is corrected.

Acidosis

Primary products of metabolism are hydrogen ions and carbon dioxide rather than hydroxyl and bicarbonate ions. This explains why acidosis is relatively common and alkalosis a rarity. Compensatory mechanisms for acidosis are more effective than those for alkalosis.

Either a fall in $[HCO_3^-]$ in metabolic acidosis, or a rise in P_{CO_2} in respiratory acidosis will cause a fall in pH:

$$pH = 6.1 + \log \frac{[HCO_3^-]}{P_{CO_2} \times 0.225}.$$

Acidosis, whether metabolic or respiratory in origin, may cause the following secondary findings:

1. *Hyperkalaemia.* Acidosis increases the ratio of $[H^+]$ to $[K^+]$, the two ions that compete in renal exchange for Na^+. In most forms of acidosis the proportion of luminal Na^+ exchanged for cellular H^+ is increased. K^+ secretion may be impaired enough to cause hyperkalaemia. Hyperkalaemia will not occur in acidosis due to intestinal loss of bicarbonate if much potassium is also lost: impairment of tubular H^+ secretion by carbonate dehydratase inhibitors or poor tubular function causes loss of *more* K^+ than usual and hypokalaemia is the rule.

2. *Osteomalacia.* An acid medium, by increasing calcium ionization, may cause bone decalcification, but only very prolonged acidosis causes overt osteomalacia with the typical clinical and radiological findings and a high plasma alkaline phosphatase activity. Despite hypercalciuria, renal calcification and calculi do not usually occur because the appropriate acidity of the urine keeps the calcium in solution. In 'classical'

renal tubular acidosis the systemic acidosis is due to an inability to secrete H^+ and calcium salts may precipitate in the relatively alkaline urine. Hypercalcaemia due to acidosis is a *very* rare complication.

Metabolic Acidosis

The primary abnormality in the bicarbonate buffer system in metabolic acidosis is a low plasma $[HCO_3^-]$; other findings in the uncompensated, partly compensated and fully compensated states are shown in Table 3.2. Stimulation of the respiratory centre by the acidosis leads to deeper than normal breathing with a consequent compensatory fall in $[CO_2]$; in severe cases this hyperventilation may be clinically evident ('Kussmaul respiration'). Compensation is impaired by any disturbance of the cerebral medullary–respiratory axis.

A primary fall in $[HCO_3^-]$ may be due to any of the following factors.

1. Use of HCO_3^- during buffering at a rate exceeding renal capacity to replace it.
2. Other extrarenal loss of HCO_3^- at a rate exceeding renal capacity to replace it.
3. Impairment of tubular mechanisms generating HCO_3^-.

Increased Use of Bicarbonate in Buffering. Production of many intermediate anionic metabolites is associated with equivalent H^+ production. Both are used during aerobic metabolism, but if one of the pathways is interrupted bicarbonate is used to buffer the unused H^+. Unless the addition of hydrogen ions is very rapid, renal tubular bicarbonate generation and hydrogen ion secretion, together with the anionic metabolite, can be increased sufficiently to prevent a significant fall in $[HCO_3^-]$. Once the rate reaches its maximum further addition of H^+ will reduce the plasma bicarbonate concentration, an equivalent amount of the retained anionic metabolite replacing the bicarbonate deficit. Although extracellular pH may be partly or completely corrected by rapid respiratory loss of CO_2, which keeps the ratio of $[HCO_3^-]$ to CO_2 normal, extracellular buffering capacity is

TABLE 3.3

EXAMPLES OF PATHOLOGICAL CONDITIONS CAUSING HYDROGEN ION OVERPRODUCTION

Conditions	Predominant anion(s)
Lactic acidosis (see Fig. 3.7)	Lactate
Ketoacidosis due to diabetes or starvation	Acetoacetate + 3-hydroxybutyrate
Long-chain ketoacidosis due to inborn errors of fatty acid metabolism	
β-ketothiolase deficiency	α-methylacetoacetate + α-methyl-3-hydroxybutyrate
Propionyl CoA carboxylase deficiency (propionic aciduria)	Propionate + associated ketoacids
Methylmalonic acidaemias	Methylmalonate + associated ketoacids
Inborn errors of branched-chain amino acid metabolism	
Maple syrup urine disease (ketoacidosis)	Branched-chain amino- and ketoacids
Isovaleric acidaemia	Isovalerate
β-methylcrotonyl CoA carboxylase deficiency (β-methylcrotonic aciduria)	β-hydroxyisovalerate + β-methylcrotonyl glycine
Glutathione synthetase deficiency (5-oxoprolinuria)	? 5-oxoproline
Administration of ammonium chloride	Chloride

reduced and, if the condition is not corrected, the pH will eventually fall.

Some of the conditions associated with such hydrogen ion overproduction are listed in Table 3.3. *Ketoacidosis* is the commonest cause in adults. *Hypoxic lactic acidosis*, although common, is usually part of a complicated picture including many other causes of acidosis.

Inborn errors should always be considered in infants when an unexpected, and authenticated, low $[T_{CO_2}]$ is found. These diseases fall into two groups: those associated with lactic acidosis due to abnormalities of carbohydrate metabolism and those with excessive production of keto- and other organic acids due to faulty fatty or amino acid metabolism.

Ketoacidosis. The acetyl group of acetyl CoA is oxidized aerobically to CO_2 and water in the tricarboxylic cycle. If its rate of production exceeds that of its removal the acetyl groups of two molecules condense to form acetoacetate, allowing coenzyme A (CoASH) to be reused for further metabolism. The net reaction is

$$2CH_3COSCoA + H_2O \rightarrow CH_3COCH_2COO^-$$
acetyl CoA   acetoacetate
$$+ H^+ + 2CoASH.$$

At first, equimolar amounts of acetoacetate and hydrogen ion are produced. Reduced NAD converts acetoacetate to 3-hydroxybutyrate; this reaction does not use the H^+ generated from acetyl CoA:

$$CH_3COCH_2COO^- + NADH + H^+ \rightarrow$$
$$CH_3CHOHCH_2COO^- + NAD^+.$$
3-hydroxybutyrate

The HCO_3^- used during buffering is thus replaced by equimolar amounts of acetoacetate and 3-hydroxybutyrate. The fall in extracellular $[HCO_3^-]$ stimulates the tubular carbonate dehydratase mechanism and, as HCO_3^- is generated, H^+ is secreted in exchange for sodium filtered with 3-hydroxybutyrate (pK_a 4.7) and acetoacetate (pK_a 3.6); these ketoacids may be detectable in the urine. Any renal impairment, whether due to an impaired glomerular filtration rate (GFR), to tubular damage or to both, will reduce the renal capacity to replace the depleted HCO_3^-.

Acetoacetate production rises if fatty acid catabolism increases relatively more than carbohydrate catabolism.

During *fasting* the plasma glucose concentration is normal or low and the availability of glucose is reduced in those cells lacking significant glycogen stores. Triglyceride catabolism in adipose tissue provides the fatty acid substrate for acetoacetate production. Ketosis may occur after only short periods of fasting and will be reversed by ingestion of carbohydrate. After prolonged starvation ketoacid production may be fast enough to swamp the homeostatic mechanisms and cause some acidosis.

In *diabetes mellitus* ketosis is also due to intracellular glucose deficiency in those cells that depend on insulin for entry of glucose, in this case despite hyperglycaemia. While production of ketoacids is only slightly increased there may be no detectable acidosis, but in full-blown ketoacidosis the plasma bicarbonate may fall to a very low concentration. Unless CO_2 can be lost through the lungs fast enough to restore the ratio to normal the pH will fall. Acidosis is aggravated if the amount of sodium filtered is so reduced by a low GFR caused by volume depletion as to limit its availability for exchange with hydrogen ion. Poor tissue perfusion, also due to volume depletion, may cause simultaneous lactic acidosis. The importance of adequate rehydration during treatment is therefore obvious.

The cause of the low $[T_{CO_2}]$ is usually evident if the plasma or blood glucose is estimated and if urine, and perhaps plasma, are tested for ketones. Knowledge of the concentration of ketones or of lactate is of academic interest, as correction of volume depletion with insulin therapy should restore both to normal. It is common to request estimations of pH, P_{CO_2} and derived values at frequent intervals, but this is only necessary if there is a superimposed respiratory condition. The effectiveness of treatment in correcting hydrogen ion balance can be monitored by measuring $[T_{CO_2}]$. In my experience overemphasis on unnecessary investigations often distracts attention from such important findings as developing hypernatraemia, which may perpetuate hyperosmolality despite control of hyperglycaemia.

Longer-chain ketoacid accumulation occurs in some inborn errors of amino- and fatty acid metabolism (Table 3.3).

Lactic Acidosis. Lactate is the product of reduction of pyruvate by reduced NAD (compare the production of 3-hydroxybutyrate from acetoacetate):

$$CH_3COCOO^- + NADH + H^+ \rightarrow$$
Pyruvate
$$CH_3CHOHCOO^- + NAD^+.$$
Lactate

Lactate and hydrogen ion production are almost always equimolar. Lactic acid may therefore accumulate when there is either overproduction or underutilization of pyruvate, or overproduction of reduced NAD.

Pyruvate is the product of anaerobic glycolysis (*see* Fig. 3.7). In the presence of oxygen it is usually metabolized to acetyl CoA and hence, in the tricarboxylic cycle, to CO_2 and water, or it may be used in the synthesis of fatty acids. Hepatic and renal cells can also use pyruvate for gluconeogenesis. Because this pathway is dependent on a supply of ATP and GTP, mostly generated by the oxygen-dependent tricarboxylic cycle, gluconeogenesis depends on the presence of oxygen. If the rate of anaerobic production of pyruvate exceeds that of utilization in oxygen-requiring pathways it is converted to lactate. Once the oxygen supply increases lactate is reconverted to pyruvate and metabolized. Metabolism of lactate, whether to glucose or to CO_2 and water, uses hydrogen ions. Liver with a normal oxygen supply uses more lactic acid, often derived from other tissues, than it produces anaerobically.

Lactic acidosis may therefore be due to any of the following factors.

1. Increased Pyruvate Production by Anaerobic Glycolysis. During strenuous *muscular exercise* pyruvate is produced faster by glycogenolysis and glycolysis in skeletal muscles than it can be metabolized aerobically,

and is converted to lactate. Once the muscles are resting the circulating lactate is reconverted to pyruvate in the liver and metabolized by aerobic pathways.

Glucose-6-phosphatase catalyses dephosphorylation of glucose-6-phosphate (G-6-P), derived from glycogenolysis and gluconeogenesis, to glucose in hepatic cells, from which glucose can enter the extracellular fluid. In *Type I glycogen storage disease* there is deficiency of the enzyme and, if glycogen breakdown is stimulated by such hormones as adrenaline or glucagon, less of the resultant G-6-P than normal can be converted to glucose and more is metabolized via pyruvate. Pyruvate may be produced fast enough to cause lactic acidosis.

Fructose, sorbitol and *xylitol* were all used in the past as energy sources during parenteral nutrition. It was found that they might precipitate lactic acidosis, especially in patients with impairment of hepatic aerobic pathways due to hypoxia. They enter hepatic cells and the glycolytic cycle at a lower extracellular concentration than glucose. The mechanism is similar to that in Type I glycogen storage disease. Glucose is the best intravenous carbohydrate source of energy

2. Reduced Pyruvate Utilization. Despite a normal rate of pyruvate production, reduced use in aerobic pathways may increase its conversion to lactate. The tricarboxylic cycle, and synthetic pathways that need ATP and/or GTP, are interdependent. Most factors impairing the tricarboxylic cycle also affect gluconeogenesis and fatty acid synthesis.

Tissue hypoxia is usually caused by poor vascular perfusion and is especially likely to be severe after cardiac arrest. Aerobic metabolism is impaired and the hypoxic liver changes from a predominantly lactic acid-consuming to a predominantly lactic acid-producing organ. This type of lactic acidosis is usually superimposed on acidosis due to renal and respiratory impairment and may sometimes accompany severe diabetic ketoacidosis.

Biguanides (metformin and phenformin) are now rarely used to treat diabetes mellitus because, by inhibiting aerobic pathways, they impair pyruvate metabolism. Diabetic patients with inadequate renal homeostatic mechanisms may develop severe lactic acidosis if treated with these drugs.

Salicylate overdosage can cause lactic acidosis, possibly because salicylates 'uncouple' oxidative phosphorylation and so impair pyruvate utilization.

Very extensive liver disease only rarely causes lactic acidosis, although hepatic gluconeogenesis accounts for most of the normal metabolism of lactate formed in other tissues such as skeletal muscle.

Pyruvate dehydrogenase catalyses conversion of pyruvate to acetyl CoA, the first step in its entry into the tricarboxylic acid cycle. Infants with genetic pyruvate dehydrogenase deficiency may present with lactic acidosis.

Primary impairment of gluconeogenesis may be due

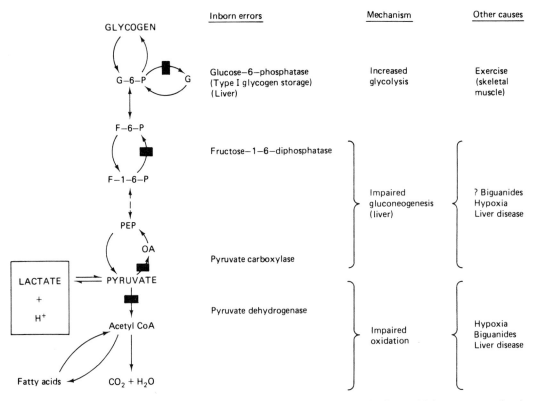

Inborn errors   Mechanism   Other causes

Figure 3.7 Schematic representation of some disturbances of pyruvate metabolism which may cause lactic acidosis (G = glucose, G-6-P = glucose-6-phosphate, F-1-6-P = fructose-1-6-diphosphate, PEP = phosphoenol pyruvate, OA = oxaloacetate).

to deficiency of one of the enzymes needed to catalyse the two irreversible steps on the glycolytic pathway. Figure 3.7 shows that gluconeogenesis can only proceed in the presence of *pyruvate carboxylase* and *fructose-1-6-dehydrogenase*. If the inborn error is associated with deficiency of either, only gluconeogenesis is affected. Pyruvate can still undergo aerobic metabolism and take part in fatty acid synthesis.

3. Increased Rate of Conversion of Pyruvate to Lactate. High concentrations of reduced NAD might be expected to increase lactate production. Mild lactic acidosis may be demonstrable after ingestion of large amounts of alcohol. Ethyl alcohol is metabolized to acetyl CoA via acetaldehyde, each step involving reduction of NAD^+, the net reaction being

$$C_2H_5OH + CoASH + 2NAD^+ \rightarrow CH_3COSCoA + 2NADH + 2H^+.$$

Possibly the lactic acidosis is due to an increased rate of conversion of pyruvate to lactate by the reduced NAD and may be aggravated if lactate utilization is impaired by liver disease. The finding is clinically unimportant. Methyl alcohol poisoning causes lactic acidosis by a similar mechanism

Other Causes of Metabolic Acidosis. *1. Ethylene Glycol and Paraldehyde Poisoning.* Ingestion of either

of these is known to cause metabolic acidosis.

Glycollate is an intermediate in ethylene glycol metabolism and its further metabolism may be rate-limiting. It is probably the anion replacing bicarbonate in the acidosis of ethylene glycol poisoning.

The cause of acidosis in paraldehyde poisoning is unknown.

2. Administration of Ammonium Chloride. During metabolism of ammonium ion to urea in the liver H^+ is generated. Ingestion of ammonium chloride in large quantities may cause acidosis, the anion replacing HCO_3^- being chloride; this is one cause of a rare hyperchloraemic acidosis (*see* Table 3.6). Ammonium chloride may be used to test the integrity of the renal carbonate dehydratase mechanism (*see* Renal tubular acidosis; p. 45).

3. Loss of Bicarbonate into the Intestinal Tract. The alkalinity of pancreatic and small-intestinal secretions is due to their high bicarbonate concentration. Usually the loss of bicarbonate into this part of the intestinal tract is balanced by generation of bicarbonate during earlier gastric acid secretion. Patients with very severe diarrhoea, or those losing a large volume through small-intestinal fistulae, may have a much increased HCO_3^- loss. As usual during extrarenal loss, the renal mechanism is stimulated by the low extracellular $[HCO_3^-]$, but if, as often happens,

TABLE 3.4

IMPAIRMENT OF RENAL TUBULAR BICARBONATE GENERATION

Cause	Mechanism
Low GFR	Carbonate dehydratase mechanism inhibited because less sodium available for exchange with hydrogen ion and less buffer available to accept hydrogen ion
Renal tubular damage	Renal tubular function impaired
Proximal renal tubular acidosis	Deficiency in proximal tubular carbonate dehydratase mechanism; bicarbonate wastage
Distal ('classical') renal tubular acidosis	Distal tubular cells abnormally permeable to hydrogen ion; distal carbonate dehydratase mechanism inhibited by H^+; inability to acidify urine
Acetazolamide	Direct inhibition of carbonate dehydratase

the fluid loss causes intravascular volume depletion the GFR may fall low enough to reduce filtration of sodium and buffer: in such cases the carbonate dehydratase system may not be able to achieve maximal generation of HCO_3^-. Replacement of intestinal loss by infusion of fluid with a low sodium concentration (for example, by dextrose saline) may cause hyponatraemia; even less sodium is then filtered, further impairing bicarbonate generation.

The clinical picture indicates the cause of the low $[T_{CO_2}]$. Volume repletion with isotonic saline maintains the GFR and prevents hyponatraemia, enabling the kidneys to replace the lost bicarbonate. Administration of bicarbonate is usually unnecessary.

Small-intestinal secretions are relatively rich in potassium. Prolonged excessive loss of these is one of the exceptions to the rule that acidosis causes hyperkalaemia.

Transplantation of the ureters into the colon or ileum, for example after total cystectomy, delivers urine into the part of the intestine where lining cells exchange luminal chloride for extracellular bicarbonate. This may cause *hyperchloraemic acidosis*. The cause should be obvious. The condition can be treated by giving sodium bicarbonate, usually orally.

Impairment of Tubular Mechanisms Generating Bicarbonate. In the two groups of acidosis already discussed renal tubular mechanisms are capable of generating bicarbonate and the urine is appropriately acid. In the group to be discussed acidosis is due to impaired hydrogen ion secretion and bicarbonate generation. The causes are listed in Table 3.4.

As already explained, a *low GFR*, by reducing the total amounts of sodium and phosphate filtered, may impair the correction of keto- or lactic acidosis, or of the acidosis due to extrarenal bicarbonate loss. A significantly reduced GFR, whether due to renal or extrarenal causes, can so impair the function of intact tubular cells that, even without further complicating factors, plasma $[T_{CO_2}]$ falls. Such a reduced GFR usually causes oliguria, with raised plasma urea and creatinine concentrations. A low GFR alone usually causes only mild acidosis. Intravascular volume

should be repleted and sodium replaced by giving the appropriate fluid, intravenously if necessary.

Renal tubular damage despite a relatively normal GFR may cause a low plasma $[T_{CO_2}]$ with normal urea and creatinine concentrations. Potassium and phosphate are also lost and the uncommon association of acidosis and hypokalaemia may provide the clue to the cause. Other evidence of tubular damage, such as glycosuria and aminoaciduria, should be sought.

Generalized renal damage, involving both glomeruli and tubules, is a much commoner cause of acidosis than are isolated glomerular or tubular dysfunction. Plasma urea and creatinine concentrations are high and there is variable hyperkalaemia. The acidosis *per se* rarely needs treating.

Renal tubular acidosis is due to failure of tubular cells to reabsorb and/or generate HCO_3^- without equivalent failure of other functions. By contrast with other causes of renal acidosis, quantitative sodium reabsorption is relatively normal. However, less hydrogen ion is secreted and so less is available for exchange, and a greater proportion of filtered sodium is reabsorbed isosmotically with chloride or in exchange for potassium. Acidosis in this group of conditions therefore has two unusual features—*hyperchloraemia* and *hypokalaemia*.

There are two forms of renal tubular acidosis. In both types the capacity to secrete ammonium in amounts appropriate to the pH of the urine is retained.

1. A defect in the *proximal tubular* carbonate dehydratase mechanism causes *impairment of bicarbonate reabsorption* and urinary bicarbonate loss is inappropriately high for the plasma level. Distal cells can still secrete H^+ and generate bicarbonate and, if plasma and therefore filtrate $[HCO_3^-]$ falls very low, little bicarbonate reaches distal tubules despite impaired proximal 'reabsorption'. The distal tubules can then function normally, the secreted H^+ mostly combining with phosphate and ammonia rather than with bicarbonate. *The ability to form an acid urine in severe systemic acidosis is retained.*

TABLE 3.5

SOME INBORN ERRORS THAT MAY CAUSE RENAL TUBULAR
ACIDOSIS

Inborn error	Tubular deposition of:
Hereditary fructose intolerance	Fructose-1-phosphate
Galactosaemia	Galactose-1-phosphate
Wilson's disease	Copper
Cystinosis	Cystine
Fabry's disease	Abnormal glycosphingolipids

2. A defect in the *distal tubule* is associated with *an inability to acidify the urine* even if there is severe systemic acidosis. In this so-called 'classical type' of renal tubular acidosis, proximal HCO_3^- reabsorption can be shown to be normal and the carbonate dehydratase mechanism is probably intact. Normal distal cell luminal membranes are poorly permeable to secreted H^+, allowing, at pH 5.4, a hydrogen ion gradient of 100 to 1 to build up between tubular and extracellular fluids: in 'classical' renal tubular acidosis the membranes may be abnormally permeable. Diffusion of secreted H^+ back into tubular cells inhibits a normal carbonate dyhydratase mechanism so that acidification of the urine with bicarbonate generation is impaired. Renal calculi or nephrocalcinosis are features of this type; the high filtered load of calcium ions common to all forms of acidosis tends to precipitate in the inappropriately alkaline urine.

Distal renal tubular acidosis may be familial or may be a transient finding in newborn infants. Both types are often secondary to damage of tubular cells caused, for example, by hypercalcaemia, ingestion of such toxins as amphotericin B or mercury, Bence–Jones proteinuria, or inborn errors causing deposition of metabolites in tubular cells, such as those listed in Table 3.5. Most of these secondary causes may, later in the course of the disease, be associated with generalized tubular damage (Fanconi syndrome).

The ability to acidify the urine may be tested by giving 0.1 mg of ammonium chloride per kg body weight orally. Normal subjects and patients with generalized renal tubular damage, or with proximal renal tubular acidosis, respond by acidifying the urine to below pH 5.2 at between 2 and 8 hours after the dose. In 'classical' renal tubular acidosis the pH remains above this level, reflecting the inability to acidify the urine in response to acidosis.

Either type of renal tubular acidosis responds to treatment with oral sodium bicarbonate and potassium supplements. Prolonged hypokalaemia, or, in the distal form, nephrocalcinosis, may cause permanent tubular damage. Early recognition and treatment are therefore important.

Acetazolamide inhibits carbonate dehydratase. Its effect is therefore similar to that of proximal renal tubular acidosis. Although large doses may cause hyperchloraemic, hypokalaemic acidosis, the small doses used to treat glaucoma rarely cause these disturbances.

Causes of acidosis that may be associated with hyperchloraemia and/or with hypokalaemia are summarized in Table 3.6.

Inborn Errors Causing Metabolic Acidosis. Many inherited metabolic disorders are associated with metabolic acidosis and these causes must be remembered if an infant presents with a low $[T_{CO_2}]$.

Acidosis associated with inborn errors may be due to:

1. Lactic acidosis due to errors of the gluconeogenic pathway or to pyruvate dehydrogenase or glucose-6-phosphatase deficiency (*see* Fig.3.7).
2. Overproduction of other intermediate metabolites with H^+ (*see* Table 3.3).
3. Renal tubular acidosis due to deposition of metabolites in renal tubular cells (*see* Table 3.5).

Respiratory Acidosis and Hypoxia

The primary abnormality in the bicarbonate buffer pair in respiratory acidosis is a high P_{CO_2}. Other findings in uncompensated, partly compensated and fully compensated states are listed in Table 3.2 (p. 41).

Compensation depends on stimulation of the renal tubular carbonate dehydratase reaction by a high P_{CO_2} (*see* p. 34). Although the capacity of normal kidneys to generate bicarbonate is very high, it takes time to produce enough to compensate fully for severe acidosis. The P_{CO_2} may stabilize at a very high level in chronic respiratory disease: the kidneys continue to generate HCO_3^- until the ratio of $[HCO_3^-]$ to P_{CO_2} is normal and a new steady state is reached with a normal blood pH and very high $[HCO_3^-]$. By contrast, a much smaller rise in P_{CO_2} in acute respiratory failure may cause severe acidosis, because it occurred too fast for enough bicarbonate to be produced to correct the ratio of HCO_3^-/P_{CO_2} and therefore the pH.

The Standard Bicarbonate in Respiratory Acidosis. Standard bicarbonate is a derived value (p. 40) and, as such, is subject to several inaccuracies. I find it much less help in assessing respiratory dysfunction than the clinical history and $[T_{CO_2}]$, occasionally together with the P_{CO_2} and pH. The result is often misinterpreted and it is important to understand the underlying concept before requesting or interpreting it.

The erythrocyte capacity to generate HCO_3^- is limited by that of haemoglobin to buffer H^+. The standard bicarbonate concentration by itself indicates the renal contribution to a rise in total bicarbonate concentration, but does not distinguish between that generated as a compensatory response to a high

TABLE 3.6

METABOLIC ACIDOSIS ASSOCIATED WITH HYPERCHLORAEMIA AND HYPOKALAEMIA

	Hyper-chloraemia	Hypo-kalaemia
Extrarenal (intestinal) loss of bicarbonate and potassium	−	+
Ureteric transplantation into the intestine	+	±
Impairment of renal tubular function:		
Generalized tubular disease	−	+
Impairment of CD mechanism only		
renal tubular acidosis	+	+
acetazolamide therapy	+	+
Administration of ammonium chloride	+	−

CD, carbonate dehydratase.

P_{CO_2} and that due to an inappropriate rise causing metabolic alkalosis. The difference between the standard and actual bicarbonate in cases of respiratory acidosis is an index of the increment in circulating bicarbonate due *only to the erythrocyte mechanism*.

Kidneys and erythrocytes both begin to generate bicarbonate as soon as the P_{CO_2} rises. In acute respiratory dysfunction a relatively high proportion (but not all) of the increase in $[HCO_3^-]$ is of red cell origin; the proportion depends on many factors, including the time since the P_{CO_2} began to rise, the haemoglobin concentration, and its degree of oxygenation and renal function. The actual bicarbonate is likely to be slightly elevated, due to contributions from erythrocytes and kidneys, but the standard bicarbonate, due to the renal contribution alone, will be less than this and, if the condition is very acute, may be within the reference limits.

Once the buffering capacity of haemoglobin is saturated, any further *in vivo* increment in bicarbonate is of renal origin. The more chronic the condition the higher the proportion of bicarbonate due to the renal contribution and the higher will be the standard bicarbonate. The only information that can be inferred is that if the actual is higher than the standard bicarbonate there is a respiratory component to the acidosis. This is likely to be obvious from the clinical picture. The finding of a high standard bicarbonate should not lead to the conclusion that there is a primary metabolic alkalosis complicating the respiratory acidosis.

Conditions Impairing Alveolar Function. Impaired alveolar function affects both oxygen and carbon dioxide transport and it is convenient to discuss these effects together.

Any of the following factors can influence gas exchange.

1. Damage to alveolar walls may impair diffusion of gases between blood and alveolar sacs.
2. Alveolar sacs may be partly or completely filled with oedema fluid.
3. Air entry to the sacs may be impaired by:
   - blockage of airways;
   - reduced depth of breathing.

The effects on arterial oxygen and carbon dioxide concentrations depend on the integrity of the blood supply to the malfunctioning alveoli.

In conditions such as *acute* and *chronic bronchitis, broncho-* and *lobar pneumonia,* and *pulmonary fibrosis, infiltration* or *collapse,* impaired function of parts of the lungs is due to more than one of the above factors.

Reduced aeration of both lungs may be due to partial blockage of the main airways, from, for example inhalation of a large foreign body or laryngeal spasm. *Chest injury, ankylosing spondylitis* or *gross obesity* may impair movement of the rib cage enough to reduce ventilation. *Cerebral medullary lesions* may impair the feedback response of the respiratory centre to a rise in P_{CO_2}, or *peripheral nerve lesions* due, for example, to poliomyelitis or peripheral neuritis may impair transmission from the cerebral medulla to the chest-wall muscles. In all these conditions the blood supply of the affected alveoli remains relatively intact.

Emphysema may produce different effects on arterial levels of oxygen and carbon dioxide because the blood supply to malfunctioning alveoli is reduced.

Pulmonary oedema impairs diffusion of oxygen more than that of carbon dioxide.

Arterial P_{CO_2} and P_{O_2} in Respiratory Dysfunction. A rise in P_{CO_2} is always associated with a fall in P_{O_2}, but a low P_{O_2} is not always accompanied by a high P_{CO_2}.

Alveolar Dysfunction with a Relatively Normal Blood Supply. Conditions with a relatively normal alveolar blood supply are more likely to cause an abnormal arterial P_{O_2} than P_{CO_2}.

The most important physiological stimulus to the respiratory centre is a fall of pH in the blood perfusing it, but hypoxia can have the same effect. If most of the alveolar walls are functionally damaged CO_2 cannot be eliminated from, nor O_2 gained by, blood perfusing them, despite the increased tidal volume due to central stimulation of respiration. However, if enough undamaged alveoli remain, increased aeration may allow them to eliminate enough CO_2 to 'compensate' for the retention in the damaged areas; it cannot, however, 'correct' the low P_{O_2} in the blood leaving the hypofunctioning sections. This contrast is due to differences in diffusibility and mode of transport of the two gases.

Dissolved carbon dioxide can diffuse from blood into alveolar air about 20 times as fast as oxygen can diffuse in the opposite direction. CO_2 diffuses more rapidly through oedema fluid. In many cases of *pulmo-*

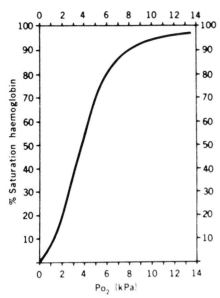

Figure 3.8 Oxygen dissociation curve of haemoglobin (pH 7.4, 37°C): haemoglobin remains over 90% saturated until the P_{O_2} falls below 8 kPa (60 mmHg); saturation falls rapidly as P_{O_2} is further reduced.

nary oedema the fall in P_{O_2} stimulates the respiratory centre, increasing the rate and depth of ventilation. Usually this increases elimination of enough CO_2 to reduce the arterial P_{CO_2} to normal or even low levels. The P_{CO_2} only rises if pulmonary oedema is very severe.

Very little blood oxygen is in simple solution. The small amount dissolved in capillary plasma diffuses into erythrocytes and equilibrates with the much larger amount in oxyhaemoglobin. At a normal P_{O_2} of about 13 kPa (100 mmHg) only about 3% of arterial haemoglobin remains unsaturated with oxygen, and even if the P_{O_2} is as low as 8 kPa (60 mmHg) only about 10% of haemoglobin is free to take up more oxygen (Fig. 3.8). Increased depth of breathing can only increase the oxygen content of arterial blood if the P_{O_2} of inspired gas is above atmospheric level. By contrast, although a little CO_2 is bound to haemoglobin as carbaminohaemoglobin, most is in simple solution and it can diffuse faster than oxygen. Normal alveoli have a very large capacity to eliminate dissoved CO_2, and increasing the ventilatory volume reduces the P_{CO_2} of blood leaving normal alveoli to abnormally low levels while hardly affecting the P_{O_2}. Thus, blood leaving malfunctioning alveoli will have a high P_{CO_2} and low P_{O_2}. As it enters the pulmonary vein this mixes with blood leaving relatively normal alveoli, which has a low P_{CO_2} and normal P_{O_2}. The outcome may be as follows:

1. *If most alveoli are functioning normally* the low P_{CO_2} in blood from them may 'overcompensate' for the high P_{CO_2} in blood from impaired areas. The normal P_{O_2} from these areas may prevent

a significant fall in P_{O_2}, but it cannot 'overcompensate'. Therefore *arterial P_{CO_2} will be low and P_{O_2} will be normal or low.*
2. *If slightly fewer alveoli are functioning normally* the arterial P_{O_2} will fall below normal. The P_{CO_2} will remain normal or low.
3. *If most alveoli are damaged* the small fraction of blood with a low P_{CO_2} will not balance that with a high P_{CO_2}. P_{O_2} *will continue to fall and the P_{CO_2} will rise.*

At a P_{O_2} below about 8 kPa (60 mmHg), haemoglobin saturation falls and the patient becomes cyanosed.

Alveolar Dysfunction with Impaired Blood Supply. If the blood supply to damaged alveoli is impaired, both arterial P_{CO_2} and P_{O_2} are relatively well preserved unless the disease is extensive.

The reduction of arterial P_{O_2} in the relatively localized pulmonary disease described above is due to mixing between blood with a low P_{O_2} and that with a normal P_{O_2}. If damaged alveoli have no blood supply arterial blood is only derived from unaffected areas and the P_{O_2} is only slightly reduced despite quite extensive lung disease. The haemoglobin oxygen dissociation curve is sigmoid. Saturation falls very little until the P_{O_2} is below about 8 kPa (see Fig. 3.8) and so cyanosis only occurs if this type of disease is very extensive. A normal respiratory centre is stimulated by the tendency of P_{O_2} to fall and the P_{CO_2} therefore falls early in this type of disease. The pink appearance of these breathless patients, usually with emphysema, has inspired the nickname 'pink puffers'. This contrasts with the less breathless 'blue bloaters' with chronic bronchitis, who are cyanosed and have a high P_{CO_2}: the 'bloating' may be due to the oedema of right heart failure and the relative absence of dyspnoea to a reduced response of the respiratory centre to *chronic* elevation of P_{CO_2} and reduction of P_{O_2}; the gradient of gas concentrations across repiratory-centre cell membranes is probably the stimulus, and a chronic steady-state allows equilibration to be achieved, so reducing the effect on the respiratory centre.

The findings in these conditions are summarized in Table 3.7.

The stimulatory effect of a low P_{O_2} must be remembered before oxygen is given to patients with chronic pulmonary dysfunction. The increase in respiratory excursion due to the low P_{O_2} may minimize the rise in P_{CO_2} and the respiratory acidosis is probably compensated for by a rise in plasma $[HCO_3^-]$. Moreover, the respiratory centre is likely to have become relatively unresponsive to the high P_{CO_2}. If the P_{O_2} is restored to normal the hypoxic respiratory drive may be reduced enough to cause dangerous acute CO_2 retention without immediate compensatory changes and the pH will fall. Haemoglobin saturation and the oxygen supply to tissues are reduced very little until the P_{O_2} is below the critical level of 8 kPa. These

TABLE 3.7
ARTERIAL BLOOD GASES IN PULMONARY DYSFUNCTION

	Blood leaving				Arterial blood			
	Dysfunctioning alveoli		Normal alveoli		Patchy disease		Extensive disease	
	P_{O_2}	P_{CO_2}	P_{O_2}	P_{CO_2}	P_{O_2}	P_{CO_2}	P_{O_2}	P_{CO_2}
Pulmonary oedema	↓	Usually N					↓	Usually N
Alveolar Blood Supply								
Normal	↓↓	↑↑	N	↓↓	↓	N or ↓	↓↓	↑
Reduced	—	—	N or ↓	↓	N or ↓	↓	↓	N or ↑

N, normal value or range.

patients should be given only enough oxygen to maintain the P_{O_2} at just above this level, ensuring continued respiratory drive with adequate tissue oxygenation.

Oxyhaemoglobin is a less effective buffer than haemoglobin. Reduction of arterial oxygenation increases haemoglobin buffering capacity and thus the ability of erythrocytes to form bicarbonate from CO_2. This slight tendency for the extracellular ratio of [HCO_3^-] to P_{CO_2} to rise in hypoxic states is relatively unimportant in offsetting the primary effects of CO_2 retention.

Conversely, buffering of H^+ by haemoglobin impairs its oxygen binding capacity and in hypoxic states the increase in carbaminohaemoglobin due a high P_{CO_2} further reduces the ability to form oxyhaemoglobin. Erythrocyte hypoxia stimulates the 'shunt' pathway by which 1:3-diphosphoglycerate, a metabolite on the glycolytic pathway, is converted to 2:3-diphosphoglycerate (2:3-DPG); 2:3-DPG, like H^+ and carbon dioxide, impairs oxygen binding by haemoglobin. This is probably an adaptive process helping to maintain release of oxygen to tissues in, for example, anaemia and chronic hypoxic states.

Alkalosis

Alkalosis is uncommon and, when it occurs, is often precipitated by the actions of the patient or the medical attendant.

Either a rise in [HCO_3^-] in metabolic alkalosis or a fall in P_{CO_2} in respiratory alkalosis will cause a rise in pH:

$$pH = 6.1 + \log \frac{[HCO_3^-]}{P_{CO_2} \times 0.225}.$$

Alkalosis, whether respiratory or metabolic in origin, may cause secondary effects that are the opposite of those due to acidosis described on p. 41.

1. *Hypokalaemia* is common in alkalosis because the reduced availability of H^+ for renal tubular exchange with sodium leads to increased urinary potassium loss. Conversely, potassium depletion causes alkalosis. It may not always be easy to distinguish cause from effect.

2. *Tetany.* Alkalosis may reduce the ionized fraction of circulating calcium enough to cause tetany. In such cases the total calcium concentration is normal.

Metabolic Alkalosis

The primary abnormality in the bicarbonate pair in metabolic alkalosis is a high plasma [HCO_3^-]. Although some compensatory CO_2 retention can be shown, this mechanism could only fully compensate severe metabolic alkalosis at the expense of serious hypoxia. Luckily the tendency of alkalosis to inhibit the respiratory centre is overridden by the consequent rise in P_{CO_2} and fall in P_{O_2}. Correction must therefore depend on inhibition of the renal carbonate dehydratase system by the high extracellular [HCO_3^-].

This inhibition slows both 'reabsorption' and net generation, and urinary bicarbonate loss may be adequate to correct the extracellular elevation. A low GFR limits the total amount that can be lost and hampers correction. An adequate GFR is an important factor in correcting either acidosis or alkalosis.

A primary rise in bicarbonate occurs in three situations.

1. *Large amounts of sodium bicarbonate* given by intravenous infusion, or even orally, may exceed the renal ability to excrete it. This is particularly likely to cause alkalosis in patients with impaired renal function.

2. *Potassium depletion.* Renal tubular generation of bicarbonate in potassium depletion is a common cause of extracellular alkalosis. The fall to normal of a high [T_{CO_2}] can be used to monitor the adequacy of potassium replacement unless there is another cause of a high extracellular bicarbonate concentration, such as chronic respiratory disease.

3. *Pyloric stenosis.* During gastric H^+ secretion,

HCO_3^- is generated. Each mmol of HCO_3^- produced by this mechanism is coupled with the loss of a mmol of chloride (Cl^-) into the gastric cavity. The sum of plasma $[HCO_3^-]$ and $[Cl^-]$ remains constant. Normally, as food passes down the intestinal tract, this gain of HCO_3^- is followed by its secretion into the duodenal cavity. If the pylorus is patent, vomiting increases loss of duodenal HCO_3^-; this counteracts the effect of its generation in the stomach and there is little disturbance of hydrogen ion balance. Obstruction between the stomach and duodenum due to pyloric stenosis reduces this loss of bicarbonate. Continuing loss of H^+ and Cl^- in the vomitus stimulates the gastric carbonate dehydratase mechanism and more bicarbonate is generated.

Only equivalent renal bicarbonate loss can prevent the development of metabolic alkalosis. Two factors may impair this correction in patients with pyloric stenosis. Firstly, volume depletion due to vomiting may reduce the GFR. Secondly, the hypochloraemia due to loss of gastric chloride reduces the chloride concentration in the glomerular filtrate. Isosmotic sodium reabsorption by the proximal tubule is impaired and more sodium is available for exchange with H^+ and K^+. The hydrogen ion secretion causes inappropriate bicarbonate 'reabsorption' and net generation, and the potassium loss aggravates that due to alkalosis: there is hypochloraemic alkalosis and hypokalaemia. This advanced state is only reached if the chloride loss and volume depletion are not corrected by infusion of saline. Once the biochemical picture is established large amounts of isosmolar saline with added potassium should be infused. Restoration of plasma $[Cl^-]$ and of the GFR enables normal kidneys to correct the alkalosis.

Respiratory Alkalosis

The primary abnormality in the bicarbonate buffer pair in respiratory alkalosis is a low PCO_2. Compensatory renal loss of and failure to generate HCO_3^- depend on inhibition of the carbonate dehydratase mechanism by the low PCO_2.

A primary fall in PCO_2 occurs if breathing is abnormally rapid or deep despite relatively normal gas transport across alveolar walls. This may occur in any of the conditions in which *oxygen exchange is impaired more than that of CO₂* (see p. 48). The slight tendency to alkalosis in such cases is less important than hypoxia.

Excessive artificial respiration is a relatively frequent cause of respiratory alkalosis in patients in intensive care units: it is difficult to judge the correct setting of the respirator by clinical observation. The alkalosis is rapidly corrected by adjusting the rate. If, as often happens, bicarbonate has, also understandably, been infused in excess, the added metabolic component increases the pH further, with severe hypokalaemia.

Hysterical overbreathing can cause respiratory alkalosis. The patient may complain of tingling in, or

spasm of, the hands because of the reduction in the ionized fraction of a normal total calcium concentration.

Raised intracranial pressure and some *brain stem lesions* may inappropriately stimulate the respiratory centre.

Salicylates and Hydrogen Ion Balance

Salicylates stimulate the respiratory centre directly and in overdose may cause respiratory alkalosis. In severe cases the 'uncoupling' effect on oxidative phosphorylation may so impair aerobic pathways that metabolic lactic acidosis develops. Both these disturbances of hydrogen ion homeostasis may contribute to low TCO_2 concentrations. The pH may be high if respiratory alkalosis is predominant, low if metabolic acidosis is predominant, or normal. Blood pH is the only measurement indicating the true state of hydrogen ion balance, but knowledge of it is unlikely to affect treatment.

INVESTIGATION OF HYDROGEN ION DISTURBANCES

It is essential to understand the mechanisms behind disorders before deciding which investigations will be useful, interpreting the results and basing the correct treatment on these results. Misunderstandings can be dangerous.

Interpretation of Plasma [TCO_2]

Estimation of plasma [TCO_2], a close reflection of bicarbonate concentration, has the advantage that it can be performed on venous blood. Plasma [HCO_3^-] *alone* tells us little about the state of hydrogen ion balance; pH depends on its ratio to PCO_2. Nevertheless, measurement of [TCO_2], together with that cheapest of all commodities, a moment's thought, often yields more reliable information than extensive investigation.

If the [TCO_2] is low the following procedure should be adopted. As soon as the diagnosis is obvious further investigation is not needed. If this result is seen early by an experienced observer, the first six steps can be accomplished without delay and this type of logical approach is likely to yield an early answer. It is rarely necessary to ask for everything at the outset.

1. *Exclude an in vitro artefactual cause* due to CO_2 loss from a specimen that has been standing overnight, or which has a large dead space above it.

2. *Estimate plasma urea and glucose* and test the urine for ketones.

3. *Reassess the clinical picture* with special reference to the presence of:
- hypotension, volume depletion or other causes of poor tissue perfusion, any of which may cause a low GFR and/or lactic acidosis;
- diarrhoea or intestinal fistulae which may lead to intestinal bicarbonate loss;
- drug history with special reference to metformin or phenformin.

In the very few cases in which the diagnosis is not yet obvious further investigation *may* be indicated.

4. *Estimate the plasma chloride concentration.* Hyperchloraemia together with a low $[TCO_2]$, without an obvious cause such as transplantation of the ureters, is most likely to be due to renal tubular acidosis. The diagnosis of distal ('classical') renal tubular acidosis may be confirmed by an ammonium chloride loading test (*see* p. 46).

5. *Estimate blood pH and PCO_2* to exclude compensated or partly compensated respiratory alkalosis.

If the acidosis is confirmed and the cause is still obscure continue as follows.

6. *Estimate lactate.* This estimation is unhelpful if tissue hypoperfusion is obvious; the acidosis in such cases is multifactorial and the underlying cause must be treated. It may help to identify rarer causes of lactic acidosis, especially in infants.

7. *Remember inborn errors in infants.* If the concentration of chloride and/or lactate is insufficient to account for all the fall in bicarbonate concentration, consider other organic acidaemias.

If the $[TCO_2]$ is high exclude hypokalaemia. Reassess the clinical picture, particularly noting if there is severe respiratory disease. Take a drug history with special reference to potassium-losing diuretics and to bicarbonate ingestion or infusion. If vomiting is severe enough to suggest pyloric stenosis estimate plasma chloride.

Anion Gap

It has been suggested that plasma chloride should always be estimated with sodium, potassium and $[TCO_2]$ and the 'anion gap' calculated. In my experience this is unnecessary if the simple procedure given above is followed. A brief explanation of the concept of the anion gap follows.

The sum of plasma cation and of plasma anion concentrations, expressed as mEq/L (numerically the same as mmol/L for univalent ions), must be equal if there is electrochemical neutrality. Sodium and potassium make the largest contributions to the cations and chloride and bicarbonate to the anions. The sum of these '*measured*' cations usually exceeds the sum of '*measured*' anions by about 15–20 mEq/L. This difference is called the 'anion gap' and is made up of

the difference between the 'unmeasured' cations such as ionized calcium and magnesium and of 'unmeasured' anions such as phosphate, urate, organic acids and plasma proteins.

A low plasma bicarbonate concentration is the hallmark of metabolic acidosis. Each mEq of bicarbonate used to buffer hydrogen ion is replaced by a mEq of the anion released with H^+. In the rare hyperchloraemic acidoses (*see* Table 3.6) this anion is chloride and the value of the 'anion gap' is therefore unchanged. In all other causes of metabolic acidosis the anion is neither chloride nor bicarbonate. The chloride concentration remains unchanged as the bicarbonate falls and the anion gap is increased. Thus the anion gap merely distinguishes between the hyperchloraemic and other acidoses.

Indications for Arterial Estimations

Estimation of arterial pH and PCO_2 is helpful in many fewer situations than usually thought.

1. If the cause of an abnormal TCO_2 is not evident, estimation of blood gases and pH may help to elucidate it.

2. If, for example, following a cardiac arrest, mixed respiratory and metabolic abnormalities of hydrogen ion homeostasis are likely to be present *and if treatment may be affected by the results*, frequent estimations may be needed to monitor control.

3. If the patient is on a respirator, frequent estimations will indicate whether adjustment is necessary.

4. If there has been an acute exacerbation of chronic respiratory disease, or if acute respiratory disease is potentially reversible, vigorous treatment, perhaps using a respirator, may tide the patient over until the condition improves. In such cases, estimation of blood gases may help. However, if there is no potential for improvement of pulmonary function the knowledge can only be of academic interest and repeated arterial puncture adds to the discomfort of the patient.

5. If arterial blood is taken for estimation of PO_2 it is sensible to estimate the other variables.

This chapter was submitted in January 1991. The author takes no responsibility for any errors due to changes in practice or theory during the intervening four years. The author also apologises if the References and Further Reading are out of date.

REFERENCES

1. Halperin M.L., Ethier J.H., Kamel K.S. (1990). The excretion of ammonium ions and acid base balance. *Clin. Biochem.* **23**, 185.
2. Kost G.J., Trent J.K.T., Saeed D. (1988). Indications for measurement of TCO_2 in arterial blood. *Clin. Chim. Acta*, **34**, 1650.

3. Astrup P., Jørgensen K., Siggaard Andersen O., Engel K. (1960). The acid–base metabolism. A new approach. *Lancet*, **i**, 1035. (This is in one of the original references explaining the concepts of the values derived from measurement of pH and P_{CO_2}.)

FURTHER READING

Jones N.L. (1990). A quantitative physicochemical approach to acid–base physiology. *Clin. Biochem.*, **23**, 189. (The author claims that it is unnecessary to invoke the Henderson–Hasselbalch equation to explain acid–base balance. Despite this difference in terminology, the philosophy is similar to that outlined in this chapter. The uselessness of the concepts of anion gap and base excess is stressed.)

McGilvery R.W. (1983). *Biochemistry: A Functional Approach*, 3rd edn., Philadelphia: W.B. Saunders. (Those interested in trying to predict disturbances producing hydrogen ions might start their search in this book, in which the author rightly stresses the importance of writing out the full stoichiometry of metabolic pathways.)

Maher E.R., Scobie J.E. (1989). Renal tubular acidosis. *Br. J. Hosp. Med.*, **42**, 116.

Diabetes Metab. Rev. (1989). **5**. (This volume contains useful reviews of all aspects of keto- and lactic acidosis.)

Scriver C.R., Beaudet, A.L., Sly, W.S., Valle D. eds. (1989). *The Metabolic Basis of Inherited Disease*, 6th edn, New York: McGraw-Hill. (This two-volume book contains several reviews of acidoses associated with inborn errors of metabolism. Volume 1 includes discussions of lactic acidosis and acidaemias due to defects in amino acid metabolism and volume 2 of renal tubular acidosis.)

The following references provide background reading on the physiology of gas exchange:

Wagner P.D. (1977). Diffusion and chemical reaction in pulmonary gas exchange. *Physiol. Rev.*, **57**, 257.

Perutz M.F. (1978). Haemoglobin structure and respiratory transport. *Sci. Am.*, **239**, 68.

4. Disorders of Fluid and Electrolyte Balance
G. Walters and D. St. J. O'Reilly

Electrolyte and water composition of the body
The renal handling of water and salt
  Factors influencing the reabsorption of water
  Factors influencing the renal tubular reabsorption of sodium
Abnormalities of the sodium and water content of the body
  Methods of assessment
  Sodium depletion
  Hypernatraemia
  Excessive water retention
  Retention of water and sodium
  Effects of hyponatraemia and their therapeutic implications
  Other guides
Potassium
  Distribution
  The renal handling of potassium and its regulation
  Hypokalaemia and potassium deficiency
  Hyperkalaemia

ELECTROLYTE AND WATER COMPOSITION OF THE BODY

On average, the total body water constitutes about 60% of the body weight in men and about 50% in women. There are very large differences between individuals, associated particularly with variations in the amount of body fat. About two-thirds of the water is in the cells and one-third outside the cells in the extracellular fluid (ECF), so that in a 70-kg man total body water is about 42 L, with 14 L of ECF and 28L of intracellular fluid. In the newborn child, total body water is 80% of body weight, 50% of this being extracellular. By the age of 12 months, total body water has fallen to the adult proportion; the ECF still constitutes slightly more than one-third of it (25% of body weight). The ECF comprises several anatomically separate compartments, namely, the blood plasma, the interstitial fluid, which lies between the cells outside the vascular compartment, the lymph, and the transcellular fluids, i.e. the small amounts of free fluid in the pleural, pericardial and peritoneal cavities, the cerebrospinal fluid, and the secretions of various glands such as the digestive secretions.

The electrolyte composition of the cells and ECF is very different, and as the transcellular fluids are secreted their composition may differ from that of the rest of the ECF. In the ECF, sodium is by far the most abundant cation whereas in the cells it is present only in about 10–20 mmol/L, the most abundant intracellular cations being potassium and magnesium; the relative amounts of the latter two vary in different tissues.

Only 93% of the plasma volume is water, the other 7% being occupied by the plasma proteins. The concentration of sodium and other ions in the plasma water will therefore be correspondingly higher than their concentration in whole plasma, e.g., the sodium concentration will be 150 mmol/L.

In the interstitial fluid the protein concentration is much lower than in plasma. As a result of a Donnan equilibrium the concentration of sodium in the interstitial fluid water will be less than in the plasma water, amounting to $0.92 \times$ concentration in plasma water.

The large differences between the sodium and potassium concentrations in the cells and the ECF are maintained by active transport of sodium out of the cell. This is mediated by a mechanism dependent on the activity of the sodium- and potassium-dependent ATPase in the cell membrane. If the rate of cell metabolism is reduced by cooling or if the cell is damaged the activity of this so-called sodium pump ceases; then sodium accumulates in the cells and potassium escapes.

The relation between the water content of the cells and the ECF is governed by differences in osmotic pressure across the cell membranes. Cell membranes are very permeable to water, and the intracellular and extracellular osmolalities must be equal; in the event of a change in one of them water will move rapidly across the cell membrane from the lower osmolality to the higher until a new equilibrium is attained. However, the cell membranes are not strictly semipermeable but are selectively permeable to solutes. Therefore the osmotic pressure across the cell membrane will be governed by the total concentration of particles to which the cell membrane is impermeable; this is sometimes known as the 'effective' osmotic pressure. Notwithstanding this, in clinical practice it is the total concentration of the osmotically active particles in the plasma water, i.e. osmolality, that is used to assess osmotic changes, and not measurements of osmotic pressure.

In the ECF, 95% of the osmolality is contributed by the electrolytes and is determined by the sodium concentration. If this changes by a large amount, say 40 mmol/L, there cannot be a compensatory change in any of the other extracellular cations because of their relatively low concentrations. Therefore, there must be a corresponding change in the total concentration of anions in order to maintain cation–anion equivalence; hence, the osmolality will change by twice the change in sodium concentration. In contrast, a large change in the most abundant anion, chloride, can be compensated for by an equal but opposite change in other anions. The sodium concentration therefore does not change and the total number of particles, and hence the osmolality, will also be unchanged. The contribution of urea and glucose to plasma osmolality is normally very small but may be large when they are pathologically raised.

The relation between the plasma and the interstitial water is dependent on other factors. The capillary wall, which separates these two compartments, is freely permeable to water and electrolytes but not to the plasma proteins. These proteins will exert an osmotic pressure across the capillary wall, known as the colloid osmotic pressure or oncotic pressure. The movement of fluid through the capillary wall is therefore dependent on the balance between the hydrostatic pressure in the capillaries forcing fluid out and the oncotic pressure drawing fluid in; these forces will be opposed by the much weaker hydrostatic and oncotic pressures of the interstitial fluid. At the arterial end of the capillary the hydrostatic pressure exceeds the sum of all the other forces so that there is a net movement of water out of the capillary. At the venous end the hydrostatic pressure is lower and the oncotic pressure is higher because of the increased protein concentration that follows the loss of protein-free fluid at the arterial end. The resultant pressure now favours the movement of fluid back into the capillary. Any fluid that does not return to the vascular compartment in this way will normally be returned via the lymphatics.

In health the plasma volume is maintained relatively constant, though small changes of about 5% do occur with alterations of posture, due to shifts of fluid into and out of the vascular compartment. After haemorrhage the capillary dynamics change so that sufficient interstitial fluid moves into the vascular compartment to restore the blood volume to normal. During this process there is also a shift of protein into the vascular compartment, thus maintaining the plasma oncotic pressure near its normal value. Restoration of the blood volume in this way will be incomplete if the ECF is diminished as a result of the loss of water and sodium.

THE RENAL HANDLING OF WATER AND SALT

In health the amount of water and electrolytes in the body is maintained within relatively narrow limits by the kidneys acting under the influence of hormones and other factors. The urine flow rate can change rapidly, e.g. during sleep after 8–10 h without drinking the urine flow rate frequently falls to less than 0.5 mL/min. This can increase more than 25-fold, to exceed 13 mL/min, within 90 min of ingesting a water load. Depending upon the solute load required to be excreted and the urine flow rate, the urine concentration can vary between 40 and 1400 mmol/kg of water, corresponding to specific gravities of 1.001–1.030. This enables the plasma osmolality to be maintained within the narrow limits of 290 ± 5 mmol/kg.

About 70% of the glomerular filtrate is reabsorbed iso-osmotically in the proximal tubule in the renal cortex. In the interstitial fluid of the medulla the concentration of sodium chloride and urea increases progressively from the corticomedullary junction to the papillary tip. As the remainder of the glomerular filtrate passes down the descending limb of Henle's loop, water is reabsorbed into the hypertonic interstitium of the medulla.

The tubular fluid therefore becomes very concentrated and may have an osmolality of 1400 mmol/kg by the time it reaches the bend of the loop of Henle. The ascending limb of the loop of Henle is impermeable to water but it actively reabsorbs chloride, sodium following passively along the electrochemical gradient thus established. The tubular fluid therefore becomes more dilute as it traverses the ascending limb, and is hypotonic to plasma when it enters the distal convoluted tubule. The thick part of the ascending limb of the loop of Henle is known as the diluting segment. Beyond it the capacity for further reabsorption of solute without water is slight, though some reabsorption of urea and electrolytes can occur in the collecting ducts, so that proper functioning of the diluting segment is necessary if the body is to excrete solute-free water. The term 'free water clearance' signifies the amount of water that is excreted in excess of that needed to carry the solute load iso-osmotically.

$$\text{Free water clearance} = V - C_{osm}$$

where V = urine flow rate; C_{osm} = osmolal clearance, i.e. $U_{osm} \times V/P_{osm}$.

The production of a concentrated urine depends on the reabsorption of water in the distal part of the convoluted tubule and the collecting tubule, which become permeable to water in the presence of the antidiuretic hormone, arginine vasopressin (AVP). Water is reabsorbed osmotically from these segments into the concentrated medulla, thereby raising the concentration of urea, etc. in the tubular fluid. The more distal part of the collecting tubule in the inner medulla is permeable to urea, which diffuses into the medullary interstitium and thus maintains its concentration.

After the reabsorption of sodium in the ascending limb of the loop of Henle, more sodium is reabsorbed in the distal convoluted tubule, under the influence of aldosterone, in exchange for potassium and hydrogen ions. The final adjustment to the amount of sodium excreted in the urine is made in the collecting ducts.

Factors Influencing the Reabsorption of Water

Physiologically a concentrated urine depends on the AVP-mediated final reabsorption of water from the collecting ducts. Excretion of a water load depends on the absence of such concentration and also on the fluid reaching the collecting ducts being hypotonic, i.e. it depends on the reabsorption of sodium chloride

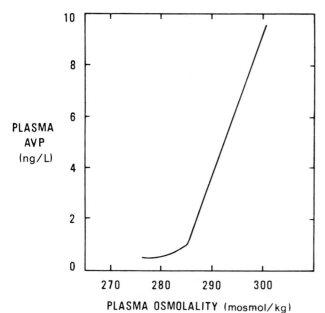

Figure 4.1 Diagrammatic representation of the relationship between plasma AVP and plasma osmolality altered by changing the sodium concentration. From the data of Robertson et al.[1]

in the ascending limb of the loop of Henle. Diuretics that prevent the reabsorption of sodium chloride in the diluting segment will therefore diminish the kidney's ability to form a dilute urine.

The elaboration of maximally concentrated urine is dependent upon AVP rendering the collecting tubules permeable to water, but the reabsorption of water through the permeable epithelium requires a hypertonic medulla. Factors that increase medullary blood flow are said to reduce the concentration of the interstitium by a wash-out effect, and therefore to diminish the maximal concentration of the urine. Diversion of blood flow to the outer cortex will have a similar effect on urine concentration as the nephrons in this part have short loops of Henle, which do not penetrate to the deepest, and therefore the most hypertonic, part of the medulla. Cortisol influences the effect of AVP; the distal part of the nephron can become maximally impermeable to water only in the presence of an adequate level of cortisol.

Factors Influencing AVP Secretion
1. Osmotic. The secretion of AVP from the posterior pituitary gland is normally regulated by changes in plasma osmolality. Physiologically, these are the result of changes in the plasma sodium concentration. It has been shown that there is a threshold of plasma osmolality, about 285 mmol/kg, below which the concentrations of AVP in plasma are too low to measure with present techniques, and above which plasma AVP increases with plasma osmolality (Fig. 4.1); a change in plasma osmolality of 3 mmol/kg, consequent on a change in the sodium concentration,

is sufficient to affect the urine concentration. The osmoreceptors are thus very sensitive, the sensitivity in any individual being indicated by the slope of the line relating osmolality to AVP concentrations in that individual.

Not all solutes have the same effect on AVP release as sodium. Increasing the plasma urea concentration does not stimulate AVP secretion unless it is done very rapidly. This is because urea readily enters the cell; it therefore does not cause an osmotic gradient across the cell membrane so that the cell volume does not change. The uptake of glucose by somatic cells is insulin-dependent. However, glucose freely enters neural cells in the absence of insulin. Therefore, in diabetes mellitus an increase in the extracellular glucose concentration will not affect the osmoreceptors directly but will draw water out of somatic cells, causing dilutional hyponatraemia. The hyponatraemia will be detected by the osmoreceptors and a decrease in the plasma AVP concentration will result. In diabetic precomatous states the development of hypovolaemia will tend to stimulate AVP secretion (*see below*).

2. Non-osmotic. AVP release is stimulated physiologically by changing from the supine to the erect posture. In pathological states its release is stimulated or inhibited by a variety of haemodynamic disturbances. These are thought to be mediated through volume (low-pressure) receptors located possibly in the left atrium, and through the high-pressure aortic and carotid baroreceptors: experimentally such responses have been abolished by interruption of the afferent pathways from the baroreceptors and left atrium.

A fall in blood volume of 10–15% in man is a powerful stimulus to AVP release, and will override the inhibition of secretion caused by a fall in plasma sodium concentration. These effects are presumably mediated through the consequent fall in the cardiac filling pressure and hence cardiac output, as impeding the venous return experimentally has similar effects, dependent on the integrity of the baroreceptors.

A rise in left atrial pressure has been shown to inhibit AVP release, and this may explain the diuresis sometimes caused by paroxysmal tachycardia. But a fall in cardiac output will stimulate AVP release through stimulation of the baroreceptors. When such opposing factors coexist, which of them predominates is variable.

There are other non-osmotic agents that appear to act directly on the brain. The infusion of noradrenaline increases water excretion, an effect that is blocked by α- but not by β-blockade. The effect is independent of haemodynamic changes and is due to suppression of AVP secretion. Conversely, isoprenaline, which has predominantly β-activity, stimulates AVP secretion.

Nausea and emesis are very potent stimuli of AVP secretion and probably account for the water-retaining syndromes observed in many clinical disorders.

Hypoglycaemia also stimulates AVP secretion via a mechanism that is not clearly understood but appears to be a direct effect of neuroglycopenia.

Plasma AVP concentrations of 0–10 ng/L generally prevail during regulation of water excretion. At the higher concentrations often seen in response to non-osmotic stimulation, vasopressin also exhibits pressor activity, stimulates glycogenolysis in the liver and increases the plasma concentrations of the clotting factor VIII.

Factors Influencing the Renal Tubular Reabsorption of Sodium

The amount of sodium presented to the renal tubules is a function of the glomerular filtration rate (GFR) and the plasma sodium concentration. Each day more than 10 times the total extracellular sodium, amounting to 24 000 mmol, is filtered and more than 99% of it is reabsorbed. During everyday activity there are fluctuations in the GFR, which do not lead to fluctuations in the amount of sodium excreted because corresponding adjustments are made to the amount of sodium reabsorbed in accordance with large or small variations in the sodium intake. Even in renal disease with a large reduction in the total GFR the individual may be able to regulate the sodium balance satisfactorily. The adjustment of tubular sodium reabsorption in accordance with fluctuations in the amount filtered is referred to as glomerulotubular balance.

The reabsorption of sodium in the distal tubule is regulated by aldosterone, secreted by the zona glomerulosa of the adrenal cortex in response to activation of the renin–angiotensin system. The major stimulus to that system is not hyponatraemia but diminished renal blood flow, such as occurs in states of hypovolaemia in which cardiac output is reduced. Expansion of the blood volume, on the other hand, inhibits the secretion of renin and hence of aldosterone. The importance of the plasma potassium concentration as a stimulus to aldosterone secretion is discussed later. Normally the distal tubule accounts for only about 8% of sodium reabsorption, compared with 70% in the proximal tubule.

It was once thought that the proximal tubular reabsorption of sodium might be regulated only by alterations in the GFR, but there is strong evidence for the existence of a 'third factor', i.e. in addition to GFR and aldosterone, which regulates sodium reabsorption in the proximal tubule. Thus, patients maintained on fixed doses of cortisol and mineralocorticoids because of Addison's disease or bilateral adrenalectomy are still able to vary their sodium excretion. Furthermore, the daily administration of a salt-retaining steroid to normal subjects induces a positive sodium balance for only a few days. Then, although the positive balance is maintained, sodium excretion in the urine rises in accordance with the dietary intake despite continuance of the mineralocorticoid.

The nature of this third factor is still uncertain.

Atrial natriuretic peptide (ANP), secreted by the cells of the right atrium in response to atrial distention and to acute and chronic sodium loading, is a prime candidate. However, renal receptors for ANP have so far been found only in the glomerulus and distal tubule but not in the proximal tubule. Early pharmacological experiments demonstrated that ANP increased the GFR and caused a prompt natriuresis. At physiological concentrations, ANP does not appear to alter the GFR and causes only a modest natriuresis. The distribution of ANP receptors so far identified in the body is very close to that of the angiotensin II receptors. At physiological concentrations, ANP antagonizes the actions of angiotensin II and also appears to inhibit aldosterone secretion directly. Thus its main influence on physiological sodium excretion may result from its modulation of the renin–angiotensin–aldosterone system. The plasma concentration of ANP is increased in conditions where there is an increase in total body sodium, such as congestive cardiac failure, chronic renal failure and Conn's syndrome. The concentrations, however, are insufficient to prevent sodium retention. The pathophysiological role of ANP in disease states is still unclear, and a disease in which disordered ANP secretion is the primary pathological disorder has not yet been described.

The possible existence of another, as yet uncharacterized, hormone that influences sodium reabsorption in the proximal tubule cannot be excluded.

ABNORMALITIES OF THE SODIUM AND WATER CONTENT OF THE BODY

Methods of Assessment

There is a tendency to consider abnormalities of sodium and water only in terms of the plasma concentration of sodium. This is of great importance because any change in osmolality resulting from a change in sodium concentration will cause water to move into or out of the cells and, if severe enough, may be fatal. However, alterations in the *total amount* of water and sodium in the ECF, which may occur without changes in plasma sodium concentration, are even more important because plasma volume contracts in parallel with the ECF volume. As the integrity of the circulation is dependent on maintenance of the blood volume, reduction in ECF volume will, if large enough, cause hypovolaemic shock. On the other hand, expansion of the ECF volume, which may also occur without alteration of sodium concentration, will lead to expansion of the plasma volume and, in some circumstances, to heart failure and acute pulmonary oedema. As the changes in the total body water and the total extracellular sodium cannot be gleaned from measurement of plasma electrolytes alone, other methods must be used.

When abnormalities occur solely during a period of observation the changes can be determined by measuring the intake and the output of water and electrolytes, and calculating the 'balance', a positive balance signifying a net gain of a substance and a negative balance signifying a net loss. This method is of great importance in clinical practice and forms the basis for formulating treatment in patients whose problems arise in hospital. However, when an electrolyte disturbance is already established by the time of admission to the hospital the most direct method of obtaining quantitative data is to measure the size of the cellular and ECF compartments, and the total body sodium, directly by means of radioisotopes or other suitable compounds.

These methods are based on the dilution principle. If an accurately known amount of a substance is introduced into a closed system in which it will mix uniformly, the volume of the system can be calculated from the dilution of the marker when mixing is complete. The favoured markers are ^3H_2O for total body water, $[^{35}S]$ sodium sulphate for ECF, and $[^{125}I]$ albumin or the dye Evans blue for plasma volume. The term 'space' is used to designate the volume of distribution of a marker, e.g. 'sulphate space'.

The 'sodium space' exceeds by about 15% the ECF volume as represented by the sulphate space, indicating that some of the sodium is in the cells. Multiplying the sodium space by the plasma sodium concentration gives the total amount of sodium with which the administered isotope has come into equilibrium. This is known as the 'exchangeable sodium'. It amounts, on average, to around 40 mmol/kg body weight, which is about 30% less than the value obtained by analysis of cadavers or by whole-body neutron activation. The reason for this is that the large amount of sodium present in bone is not exchangeable. Likewise, the exchangeable potassium can be determined. Whole-body counting of the naturally occurring isotope ^{40}K gives a value 10–15% higher than the exchangeable potassium.

Such measurements have added greatly to our knowledge of water and electrolyte metabolism, but they are unsuitable for assessing acutely ill patients because of the time required to attain equilibrium and because of the wide reference ranges.[2]

Analyses of skeletal muscle and of leucocytes have also been made, but these too do not facilitate the management of the acutely ill patient. Fortunately, in most such cases it is possible to manage the patient satisfactorily without them, by evaluating the problem from a combination of the history, which can yield very useful information on the amount of fluid lost, the physical examination, measurements of the plasma concentrations of electrolytes and urea, and a measurement reflecting total protein concentration such as plasma specific gravity or refractive index. The interpretation of these observations must be based on knowledge of the changes that are known to occur in different pathological states and of the homeostatic responses to them. It must be remembered that changes in extracellular osmolality from alteration of the sodium and glucose concentrations will result in a shift of water into or out of the cells, but that changes in plasma urea will not unless they occur very rapidly; that the loss or retention of sodium will, if the homeostatic mechanisms are intact, lead to the loss or retention of water, provided it is available; and that the homeostatic responses will be triggered by changes in concentration in some cases and by changes in volume in others.

Sodium Depletion

The normal dietary intake of sodium varies from about 50 to 150 mmol per day. There is in addition a very large turnover of digestive secretions so that the amount of sodium secreted into the digestive tract daily is five or six times the dietary intake. Secretion in the small intestine occurs through the opening of a chloride channel, sodium and water following through the paracellular spaces. Normally this is almost all reabsorbed in the small intestine, partly by an ion-exchange process at the apical brush border and partly linked to the absorption of glucose or amino acids. This mechanism, at least, is unaffected by secretion so that sodium chloride absorption is still possible during secretory diarrhoea. Excessive secretion, leading to sodium depletion if its intake is not increased, may be induced by a variety of agents. Bacterial toxins, e.g. cholera and *Escherichia coli*, become attached to specific receptors on the luminal surface and initiate a sequence of events that culminates in the opening of the anion channels. Other agents, such as inflammatory mediators, prostaglandins and neuropeptides, act via the interstitial fluid to produce the same result.

A small amount of sodium is absorbed in the colon, probably in exchange for potassium, and a very small amount of sodium is excreted in the faeces and a little in sweat. An amount equivalent to the dietary sodium is excreted in the urine. Sodium depletion is usually caused by the loss of gastrointestinal secretions or by loss through the kidney due to renal or endocrine disease. The loss of other transcellular fluids, for example cerebrospinal or pleural fluid, will, if large enough also cause sodium depletion. The normal renal mechanisms for sodium homeostasis are so efficient that a low sodium intake alone does not cause severe sodium depletion except after a prolonged period.

The composition of transcellular fluids is variable so that their loss results in the loss of various proportions of water and sodium (Table 4.1). The effect on the body fluid compartments and on the plasma sodium concentration is dependent on these proportions and on the nature of any replacement fluid that might be given.

TABLE 4.1
SOME SOURCES OF ELECTROLYTE LOSS

	Na	K	Cl
Gastric juice (acid)	70	10	125
Bile	130	4	110
Small-intestinal fluid	120	10	100
Faeces in diarrhoea	50	30	50
Rectal mucus* (villous papilloma)	100	40	100
Pleural and peritoneal fluids	as for plasma		

* Note: Although published reports emphasize the potassium loss, the sodium loss is probably of greater importance (see Fig. 4.3).

These are average values (mmol/L) but are suitable for calculating treatment in a high proportion of cases. When the losses are very large it is better to base treatment on a quantitative analysis of the fluid, since the composition of a given fluid does vary from case to case.

Sodium Depletion without Water Depletion

The sequence of events induced by sodium depletion was studied by McCance[3] by making normal subjects sweat and then replacing only the water that had been lost, so that sodium depletion without water depletion was induced. At first the plasma sodium concentration remained unchanged, but the body weight declined (Fig. 4.2) because the water ingested was excreted in the urine and a negative water balance ensued. This resulted in contraction of the ECF volume, including a reduction in plasma volume as indicated by increased concentrations of red blood cells and plasma proteins. Plasma urea concentration was also raised by the reduced renal blood flow consequent upon the contracted plasma volume. Giving water in the face of sodium loss resulted at first in excretion of dilute urine, owing to inhibition of AVP secretion, which maintained the isotonicity of the ECF at the expense of its volume.

However, after several days the weight loss ceased because water retention began and a fall in the plasma sodium concentration ensued. Presumably, release of AVP was stimulated by volume depletion, this stimulus overriding the inhibitory effect of the resultant hyponatraemia. Thus, in the later stages of sodium depletion, maintenance of plasma osmolality is sacrificed for the maintenance of plasma volume.

This experiment is sometimes inadvertently repeated in clinical practice when the loss of some secretion containing relatively large amounts of sodium is replaced by the administration of either water alone or 0.18% sodium chloride in 5% glucose, so-called fifth-normal saline, which contains only 30 mmol sodium chloride per litre. An example of this is illustrated in Fig. 4.2.

In a man aged 62, bile, lost through a T-tube after surgery for gallstones, was replaced with fifth-normal saline (see Table 4.1). After some days a dramatic fall in blood pressure occurred. Plasma

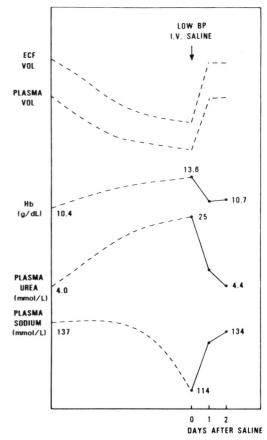

Figure 4.2 Changes in extracellular fluid (ECF) composition caused by the loss of bile and its replacement mainly with water. The numbers are the values found at the times indicated.
———— observed changes.
— — — presumed changes in accordance with McCance's observations.

urea and electrolyte concentrations at this stage are shown in the figure, together with a diagrammatic representation of the events that must have occurred before the onset of hypotension, based on the observations of McCance. Clearly, the plasma volume depletion resulting from the inadequately replaced loss of sodium had stimulated AVP release and also lowered the cardiac output to a level at which the blood pressure could not be sustained. The changes in plasma volume that had occurred are indicated by the changes in the concentrations of blood haemoglobin and plasma urea that occurred with rehydration.

The level of plasma urea found in such cases is extremely variable. It depends not only on the amount by which the GFR is reduced, but also on its duration, on the rate of protein catabolism and on increased tubular urea reabsorption, caused by reduced tubular flow rate. A rapid, large loss of circulating volume will cause a fall in blood pressure, calling for vigorous treatment, before there is time for the plasma urea to rise even though the GFR may fall to

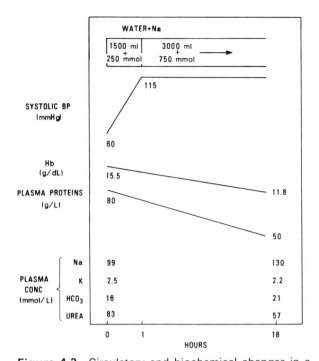

Figure 4.3 Circulatory and biochemical changes in a patient with severe sodium depletion due to the loss of mucus from a villous papilloma of the rectum.
Note the large fall in plasma urea in the first 18 h. A high urine flow rate was maintained by means of a high fluid intake, and the plasma urea returned to normal in 5 days.

TABLE 4.2

A COMPARISON OF THE CHANGES RESULTING FROM SODIUM DEPLETION (THE CASE IN FIG. 4.2) AND A CASE OF INAPPROPRIATE ANTIDIURESIS (SIAD) (THE CONCENTRATIONS ARE IN MMOL/L)

	Sodium depletion	SIAD
Plasma urea	25.0	3.0
Plasma sodium	115.0	115.0
Plasma potassium	3.8	4.0
Plasma chloride	76.0	75.0
Plasma bicarbonate	24.0	27.0
Urine sodium	2.0	80.0
Haemoconcentration	Present[1]	Absent[2]
Blood pressure	Low or tending to fall	Normal

1. Haemoconcentration may be masked by pre-existing anaemia and hypoproteinaemia.
2. Some degree of haemodilution should be present but the possibility of anaemia makes the interpretation of the haemoglobin concentration difficult.

zero. Slowly progressive changes, on the other hand, associated with maintenance of the blood pressure may cause the plasma urea to rise by 5–10 mmol/24 h to reach a level as high as 60 mmol/L, entirely due to impairment of the renal blood flow. There will be a small volume of concentrated urine containing a

large amount of urea but hardly any sodium because the fall in circulating volume resulting from sodium depletion stimulates AVP release and the sodium-retaining mechanisms. Pre-existing renal disease or the supervention of acute tubular necrosis will cause the urea to rise even faster.

The onset of hypotension in such a case is due primarily to plasma volume contraction and not to the low sodium concentration. This is illustrated by the following case (Fig. 4.3).

A woman aged 62 who presented with a detachment of the retina was found to be hypotensive with a plasma sodium concentration of 99 mmol/L resulting from sodium loss in large volumes of mucus secreted by a villous papilloma of the rectum. Resuscitation was begun immediately with intravenous isotonic saline, before the plasma electrolyte results were known. By the time they became available the blood pressure had been restored to normal by the infusion of 1.5 L of normal saline in about 1 h. The 225 mmol of sodium administered would be a small fraction of the total sodium deficit and is therefore most unlikely to have brought about resuscitation by elevating the plasma sodium concentration. The importance of volume expansion, even in patients with hyponatraemia, is further emphasized by the effect of slowing the rate of infusion too much after the initial resuscitation. As in hypovolaemic patients with normonatraemia this induces a recurrence of hypotension as the crystalloid solution equilibrates with the interstitial fluid, but the blood pressure rises again when the rate of infusion is increased to a level that ensures retention of much of the fluid in the vascular compartment.

Sodium Depletion with Water Depletion
The loss of sodium in gastrointestinal secretions or through the kidney, without water replacement, will give a different picture. The loss of any fluid with a sodium concentration approximately the same as that in plasma (Table 4.1) will obviously deplete the ECF volume without alteration of the plasma sodium concentration, apart from a tendency for it to rise slightly as a result of insensible water losses. The absence of a change in plasma sodium means that there will be no shift of water between the cells and the ECF, so that the fall in plasma volume will be unabated. Progressive contraction of the plasma volume will lead, as before, to haemoconcentration, to a rising level of plasma urea, and ultimately to hypotension. As before, the sodium-retaining mechanisms will be stimulated so that although the plasma sodium concentration is normal, sodium will disappear from the urine and the release of AVP, stimulated by contraction of the plasma volume, will produce a small volume of concentrated urine. *It cannot be stressed too strongly that a normal plasma sodium concentration does not exclude sodium depletion which*

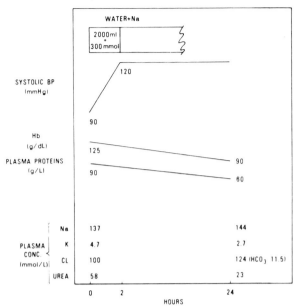

Figure 4.4 Acute hypotensive circulatory failure due to sodium depletion secondary to gastric aspiration and diarrhoea. Note the normal plasma sodium concentration. The initial contraction of the ECF volume is indicated by the fall in haemoglobin and plasma protein concentrations with treatment. The final plasma chloride concentration indicates that a mixture of chloride and bicarbonate would have been more appropriate than saline alone: this is not of great importance during rapid resuscitation, when the important point is that the fluid used should be isotonic with respect to sodium. Note how rapidly the plasma urea began to fall, a normal level being attained in 72 h.

may be so severe as to make death imminent. Such a case is illustrated in Fig. 4.4.

A different pattern develops from the loss of fluid with a much lower sodium concentration than plasma, e.g. acid gastric juice (Table 4.1). In the absence of appropriate replacement this causes the plasma sodium concentration to *rise*, thus inducing a shift of water out of the cells. Consequently, the rise in sodium concentration is minimized and the contraction of the ECF volume is less than when sodium and water are lost in equivalent amounts. But if the losses continue without replacement the changes must progress and the extracellular volume will continue to contract as the plasma sodium concentration continues to rise. It is therefore perfectly possible for circulatory failure to occur from sodium and water depletion with elevation of the plasma sodium. In practice, there is seldom more than a modest elevation of plasma sodium arising from the loss of gastric juice, probably because some replacement is usually given. The highest concentrations of plasma sodium in patients with significant sodium depletion are probably seen in infants with diarrhoea.

Some other causes of sodium depletion will be dealt with later when the problem of primary water retention is discussed.

Hypernatraemia

Water Depletion with Relatively Little Sodium Depletion

The loss of water without sodium must cause a rise in the plasma sodium concentration, and this will induce a shift of water out of the cells. The rise in sodium concentration caused by the loss of a litre of water from the ECF is greater than that caused by the loss of a litre of fluid containing 80 mmol of sodium. Therefore the former will result in a larger shift of water out of the cells to re-establish the osmotic equilibrium across the cell membrane, and hence will have the smaller residual deficit of the ECF volume. The more sodium there is in the fluid lost, the larger will be the fall in the ECF volume.

The progressive loss of water therefore leads to a rising plasma sodium concentration with minimal contraction of the ECF volume. The latter will nevertheless decline and, as in the case of sodium loss, there will ultimately be a rise in the plasma urea, though not to the same extent as in sodium depletion. As the ECF volume contracts, sodium retention will be stimulated so that the small volume of concentrated urine due to release of AVP will have a low sodium content despite the high plasma concentrations.

Conditions in which water depletion predominates are as follows.

1. *Inadequate intake.* This occurs either when fresh water is not available or when some physical disability prevents drinking. Examples are:
   (a) Carcinoma of the oesophagus.
   (b) Acutely ill elderly people living alone may be too weak to get themselves a drink; they sometimes lie undiscovered for several days after a stroke, losing extra water because of hyperventilation. It is not unusual to see patients in these categories with a plasma sodium of 150–155 mmol/L on admission to hospital.
   (c) Patients with high fever who are unable to complain of thirst, e.g. babies, or adults in coma. The development of hypernatraemia is a good indication that they are not receiving enough water.
   (d) Brain tumour or other lesions that destroy the thirst mechanism.

2. *Excessive water losses despite hypernatraemia.*
   (a) Diabetes insipidus: usually thirst ensures an adequate water intake, but when diabetes insipidus develops after a head injury the water intake will almost certainly be inadequate if the urine output is not carefully measured and the fluid balance calculated daily. A rising plasma sodium concentration in the absence of a large sodium intake should direct attention

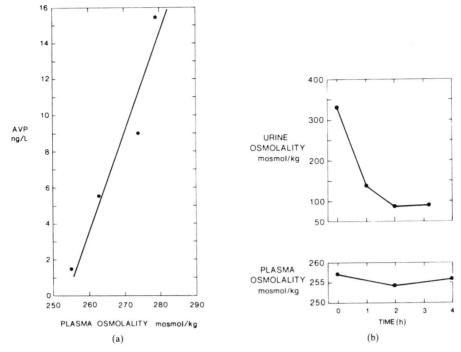

(a)   (b)

Figure 4.5   (a) Effect of an infusion of hypertonic saline on plasma osmolality and antidiuretic hormone (AVP) in a case of infectious polyneuritis with hyponatraemia. (b) Changes in urine and plasma osmolality after an oral waterload of 20 mL/kg body weight given to the same patient when the plasma sodium was 125 mmol/L. Reproduced, with permission, from Penney et al.[9]

to this diagnosis which, in these circumstances, is usually easy to confirm by measuring the urine concentration.

(b) Resetting of the osmoregulatory centre upwards. This is a rare occurrence.[4]

The plasma sodium level may be maintained anywhere between 150–170 mmol/L, and giving water fails to lower it. This is, of course, what happens in unrecognized diabetes insipidus, but the two conditions should be distinguishable by measurements of the changes in urine concentration and plasma AVP. In diabetes insipidus the urine concentration will be inappropriately low with any level of plasma sodium. With an osmoregulatory centre reset at, say, a plasma sodium level of 160 mmol/L, the urine will be dilute if the water intake is sufficient to lower the plasma sodium concentration slightly below this. But a slight rise above 160 mmol/L as a result of, say, 8 h of water deprivation, will induce a 'normal' AVP response and a rise in urine concentration, i.e. the AVP response will be similar to that in Fig. 4.1 but shifted to the right because the threshold osmolality will be high. (See also Fig. 4.5.)

(c) Osmotic diuresis: this occurs when the renal tubular fluid contains solute that cannot be reabsorbed and which therefore holds water in

the tubule. The intrarenal mechanisms are complex but lead to a large volume of urine, containing about 30 mmol/L of sodium, even if there is AVP secretion. In these circumstances the free water clearance will be negative. The plasma sodium concentration will therefore rise if the replacement of water is inadequate.

Diabetes mellitus with glycosuria is a common cause of osmotic diuresis. But the resulting tendency to hypernatraemia is opposed by the withdrawal of water from the cells by the high plasma glucose. Insulin-induced uptake of glucose by the cells will cause water to return to the cells and the plasma sodium will tend to rise further, especially if isotonic sodium solutions have been administered; this is because much of the sodium is retained while much of the water is lost in a continuing osmotic diuresis, which will persist until control of the diabetic state is re-established.

High nitrogen excretion due to high protein feeding or hypercatabolism is another cause of osmotic diuresis. Because of the limit to urine concentration a very large solute load requires a large volume of urine. The urine output may therefore appear to be 'satisfactory' even though the patient is becoming progressively water depleted (Fig. 4.6). A rising plasma

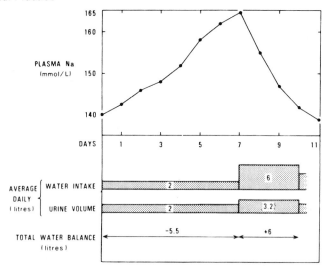

Figure 4.6 Plasma sodium concentration in a case of water depletion induced by high protein feeding. A male aged 23 with multiple injuries excreted 45–60 g urea/day when given 80 g protein/day through a nasogastric tube. Note that for the first 7 days when the sodium concentration was rising the urine output was 'good', but that on average it equalled the water intake of 2 L/day so that the patient was in negative balance by the amount of insensible loss, taken as 800 mL/day. Increasing the fluid intake to 6 L/day increased the urine output and also led to a positive balance, which corrected the abnormality in 3 days.

sodium concentration can be avoided only by ensuring an adequate water intake, making due allowance for insensible losses. It is desirable to allow an intake of about 100 ml of water for every gram of nitrogen (2 g urea) excreted.

There is clearly no sharp dividing line between the changes observed with water loss alone and those due to water loss accompanied by small amounts of sodium, the cumulative effects of which may ultimately cause acute circulatory failure. A striking example of this is provided by infants with gastroenteritis in whom circulatory failure may occur with the plasma sodium concentration as high as 160–190 mmol/L. This requires giving sodium as well as relatively more water to restore the ECF composition and its volume to normal.

Hypernatraemia Due to Excessive Sodium Intake
This sometimes arises from the administration of hypertonic sodium solutions intravenously, notably 8.4% sodium bicarbonate to correct acidosis, especially in patients with cardiac arrest. As much as one or two litres have sometimes been given, presumably due to a failure to appreciate that this solution contains 1000 mmol/L of sodium! Hypernatraemia of the order of 170 mmol/L has been reported due to hypertonic saline enemas, to the inadvertent administration of high salt-containing feeds to babies, and to the use of a salt solution as an emetic in cases of poisoning. In these the urine will be concentrated as before but with a high sodium content, because the renal tubular reabsorption of

sodium will be inhibited as a result of expansion of the ECF volume by the withdrawal of water from the cells. Withdrawal of cell water also ensures, in the absence of renal failure, a normal plasma urea. In practice, of course, the way to distinguish between hypernatraemia due to excessive sodium intake and that due to water depletion is from the history.

Effects of Hypernatraemia and their Therapeutic Implications
Patients with severe hypernatraemia are usually very ill so that clinical manifestations may be due to the primary illness. But where hypernatraemia developed acutely in babies due to the inadvertent administration of excessive amounts of salt, there was a rapid onset of confusion, followed by coma and, in some cases, death: this is attributable to cellular dehydration, especially in the brain. In the fatal cases there were striking changes in the brain, including petechial haemorrhages and subdural haemorrhage, thought to have been due to traction induced by rapid contraction of the brain volume. Although progressive water depletion ultimately proves fatal, the gradual development of a plasma sodium of 170 mmol/L in adults does not usually cause coma; some form of adaptation thus seems likely. Infants and young children with hypernatraemia due to gastroenteritis frequently exhibit fits and coma; the acute mortality rate is high and residual neurological abnormalities are common, possibly as a sequel to the anatomical lesions mentioned above. In these infants and children, fits are also associated with too rapid correction of the hypernatraemia.

The effects of acute and less acute hypernatraemia

have been studied experimentally in animals[6] and several differences between the two states have been shown. The rapid induction of hypernatraemia caused coma and death; the osmolality of the brain tissue was increased and its water content was correspondingly reduced. When hypernatraemia persisted for several days the brain osmolality again increased, but the fall in water content was less than expected from the rise in osmolality; it is suggested that in this case the increased osmolality was due to the formation and retention within the brain cells of organic molecules of relatively small molecular weight to which the name 'idiogenic osmoles' has been given, and that this is an adaptive response to prevent too much shrinkage of the brain cells.

The implications of these studies for treatment are that when hypernatraemia occurs acutely, its rapid correction by the administration of water will allow the brain volume to return to normal with benefit. But it is suggested that when hypernatraemia has been present for some days, rapid restoration of ECF tonicity will result in overhydration of the brain cells because of the intracellular idiogenic osmoles, which draw water into the cells and which dissipate only slowly. In practice it seems to take adults 24–48 h to achieve a large enough positive water balance to correct severe hypernatraemia and this does not seem to be associated with adverse effects. In infants with diarrhoea it is generally recommended that, after initial correction of any circulatory failure present with a solution of half-strength plasma or its equivalent, the hypernatraemic state should be corrected at a rate of between 1–2 mosmol/kg plasma water per hour, as these rates have been found not to induce fits. It must be emphasized, however, that a rate of 2 mosmol/kg plasma water per hour enables a plasma sodium concentration of 165 mmol/L to be corrected to 140 within 24 h, and even the slower rate allows correction of a sodium level of 155 in a little over 24 h. Slower rates of correction leave the child exposed longer to the risks of hypernatraemia and their sequelae.

Excessive Water Retention

Although sodium loss gives rise to hyponatraemia in some circumstances, hyponatraemia does not always indicate sodium loss. Conceptually, it merely indicates the presence of proportionately less sodium than water in the ECF. This may be due to the loss of sodium with the loss of relatively less water, or it may be due to the retention of water with the retention of proportionately less sodium. There are in fact many causes of water retention, in some of which retention of sodium also occurs.

It must be remembered that spurious hyponatraemia may be encountered when a blood sample is taken from a vein receiving an infusion of fluid low in sodium. Hyperlipidaemia and occasionally hyperproteinaemia in myelomatosis may also cause an

TABLE 4.3
CRITERIA FOR THE DIAGNOSIS OF THE SYNDROME OF INAPPROPRIATE ANTIDIURESIS[7]

1. Hyponatraemia with corresponding hypo-osmolality of the plasma
2. Absence of clinical evidence of fluid volume depletion
3. Concentration of the urine greater than that appropriate for the prevailing tonicity of the plasma
4. Continued renal excretion of sodium
5. Normal renal function
6. Normal adrenal cortical function

apparently low plasma sodium concentration, owing to the volume occupied by the lipoprotein or paraprotein. In such a sample a method that measures the sodium concentration in the plasma water must be used. Alternatively, an approximate value may be derived from the serum osmolality.

In order to excrete a water load efficiently the kidney must be able to elaborate dilute urine. As described above, this requires that AVP secretion be inhibited and also that the tubular fluid be dilute when it enters the collecting tubules, which is achieved by extrusion of sodium chloride in the diluting segment of the tubule. Interference with the normal inhibition of AVP secretion or with the function of the diluting segment may therefore prevent the excretion of solute-free water and hence cause hyponatraemia.

The Syndrome of Inappropriate Antidiuresis (SIAD)

To explain the water-retaining state observed in some patients with carcinoma of the bronchus, Bartter and Schwartz[7] introduced the concept of the syndrome of inappropriate secretion of antidiuretic hormone. The diagnostic criteria required to fulfil this diagnosis as outlined by Bartter and Schwartz are given in Table 4.3. Although it has been shown that ectopic secretion of AVP by tumours does occur, this is now known to be a rare cause of the water-retaining state. The plasma AVP, and in particular the AVP response to osmotic stimulation, vary from case to case (*see* Chapter 6). The term 'syndrome of inappropriate antidiuresis' (SIAD) is therefore now preferred by many. It soon became clear that this syndrome was present in patients with other forms of malignant disease such as lymphomas and carcinoma of the pancreas, and in many patients with non-malignant disease (Table 4.4). The syndrome is the most common form of euvolaemic hyponatraemia seen in clinical practice.

In this state of the plasma sodium is often less than 120 mmol/L. The expanded extracellular volume inhibits sodium-retaining mechanisms and sodium continues to be excreted in the urine. A typical set of electrolyte concentrations in this condition is shown in Table 4.2. The pattern in the SIAD differs from that of sodium depletion in that the plasma urea is normal or even low, there is abundant sodium

Trauma
Accidental and surgery

Infections
Pneumonia, peritonitis, septicaemia, urinary infections,
 tuberculosis

Pulmonary Disease
Chronic bronchitis and emphysema
Artificial ventilation

Endocrine Disorders
Hypopituitarism
Addison's disease
Hypothyroidism

CNS Disorders
Head injury
Infections
Tumours
Cerebrovascular accidents
Acute psychoses
Acute intermittent porphyria
Acute infective polyneuritis
Acute toxic polyneuritis (vincristine)

*Drugs that Interfere with the Release of AVP or Potentiate
its Action on the Renal Tubule*
Diuretics
Chlorpropamide
Vincristine, cyclophosphamide
Fluphenazine, carbamazepine, amitryptiline
Clofibrate
Thiazides
Syntocinon

in the urine if the intake is normal, there is no haemoconcentration, the blood pressure is normal and shows no tendency to fall in the upright posture, and thirst is unlikely. The acid–base state is usually normal unless other factors are present. In both cases the urine will be inappropriately concentrated for the plasma sodium concentration, though it may not exceed the concentration of plasma.

Some of the conditions listed in Table 4.4 are now considered in more detail.

After Injury or Surgery. Hyponatraemia is not uncommon within the first 2 or 3 days after surgical operations and may occur after any major injury. It has been attributed to the administration of too much hypotonic fluid and also to a shift of sodium into the cells because of damage to the cell membrane, i.e. a 'sick cell'. The latter on its own would cause water to enter the cells with sodium leaving the extracellular sodium concentration unchanged. Flear and Singh[8] attributed the hyponatraemia in the 'sick cell syndrome' to the escape from the cell of organic solutes, as yet unidentified, through a damaged cell membrane. As a result, water is drawn out of the cells and the extracellular sodium concentration falls. This ex-

planation is based on their observation that the plasma osmolality in such cases was higher than that calculated from the sodium, urea and glucose concentrations.

This sick cell syndrome may occur in any ill patient but it is very uncommon. A far more common cause of hyponatraemia, even in patients with infections, is the administration of too much water or hypotonic saline when the patient is in a water-retaining state due to AVP secretion as part of the metabolic response to injury. Such patients may, surprisingly, excrete more than 3L of urine per day if the volume of fluid given is very large. But they do not as a rule excrete the whole of the water load so that water retention gradually builds up. The duration of AVP secretion after injury varies with the severity of the injury, and sometimes it may be very prolonged. Hyponatraemia then occurs if too much water is given, but the measured plasma osmolality is not different from the calculated osmolality. As in the SIAD, overexpansion of the ECF volume causes the loss of sodium in the urine.

The mechanism that triggers such prolonged water retention is not understood, but there is evidence that in some cases at least, osmoregulation may be reset at a lower level so that AVP secretion will be switched on and off around a level of plasma sodium below the normal. This is illustrated in Fig. 4.5 above, which shows data from a case of infective polyneuritis with hyponatraemia; the plasma sodium settled at a new stable concentration of 125 mmol/L, but at this level a water load was excreted normally and the infusion of enough hypertonic saline to increase the plasma sodium concentration into the upper part of the normal range evoked a marked AVP response.

Addison's Disease. It might be thought that the inability to excrete a water load normally in Addison's disease could be adequately explained by the stimulation of AVP release by the contraction of the ECF volume resulting from sodium depletion. Correction of this abnormality by intravenous saline has been reported, but this cannot be the whole explanation because the same phenomenon occurs in hypopituitarism in which aldosterone secretion is unimpaired. A fall in the GFR, frequently indicated by a raised plasma urea concentration, would also impair water excretion by reducing delivery of fluid to the distal part of the nephron. Water handling, however, is restored to normal in both Addison's disease and hypopituitarism by cortisol. The exact nature of the abnormality is uncertain but it seems that cortisol has an effect on the collecting ducts necessary for maximal impermeability to water.

Hypothyroidism. A small proportion of patients with hypothyroidism develop hyponatraemia with the features of water retention. The mechanism is not understood but is reversed by thyroxine.

TABLE 4.5

EFFECTS OF IV HYPERTONIC SALINE (450 MMOL/L) GIVEN ON
DAYS 1 and 2 FOR WATER INTOXICATION IN A 95-YEAR-OLD
WOMAN WITH ALL THE FEATURES OF THE SIAD FOLLOWING A
FRACTURED NECK OF FEMUR

Days	1	2	3	4	5	Total
Plasma sodium (mmol/L)	111	121	134	128	123	
Sodium intake (mmol/24 h)	225	450	150	0	0	825
Sodium in urine (mmol/24 h)	*	300	150	150	120	720 +

* Not measured, but the sodium concentration in a random specimen was 80 mmol/L

Note. The data illustrate: (a) the efficacy of the treatment; (b) its safety, given normal cardiovascular and renal function; (c) the rapid recurrence of hyponatraemia when the water intake was not curtailed after the treatment.

It was quite unnecessary to give the litre of normal saline (150 mmol/L) on day 3, and the 5% dextrose in water that followed it 'to keep the drip open' was contraindicated. Unless there is a clear need for continuing i.v. therapy (which must be carefully formulated) it is best to discontinue i.v. fluids as soon as the hypertonic saline has been given.

Diuretics. It is uncommon for diuretics to cause hyponatraemia but they may do so in several ways. Those that inhibit sodium reabsorption in the diluting segment will thereby diminish the excretion of free water. Hyponatraemia may then occur, due to water retention; the plasma urea remains normal as in the SIAD, but unlike the latter hypokalaemia is often present. Recovery occurs when the diuretic is stopped, often within a few days. More rapid recovery can be achieved if necessary by giving salt with very little water (see below).

There is evidence to suggest that, in some cases at least, hyponatraemia is a consequence of severe potassium depletion, which induces a shift of sodium into the cells and possibly interferes with the regulation of AVP secretion.

A third mechanism by which diuretics may produce hyponatraemia is sometimes seen when vigorous diuretic therapy is continued after the oedema has gone. Sodium depletion and contraction of the ECF volume ensue, with malaise, weakness and a rising plasma urea in the presence of a falling plasma sodium concentration. The cautious administration of salt and water restores the ECF to normal, with a resultant fall in the plasma urea and symptomatic improvement. There is often reluctance to give salt to such patients because of the fear that it will precipitate a relapse into heart failure. But the therapeutic response can be very dramatic as in the following case:

A 52-year-old woman underwent mitral valve replacement, after which diuretics were continued for 6 weeks in the same dosage as before. She was admitted to hospital with vomiting, generalized muscle aches and weakness. Plasma sodium concentration was 120 mmol/L, potassium 2.6 mmol/L, chloride 70 mmol/L and bicarbonate 27 mmol/L; plasma urea was 52 mmol/L. There was no elevation of the jugular venous pressure and no peripheral or pulmonary oedema. In order to keep the water administration as low as possible initially, 1L of hypertonic saline containing 600 mmol sodium chloride was given intravenously over 8 h. This restored the plasma sodium to normal and only 41 mmol of sodium was excreted in the first 12 h, in contrast to the response observed in hyponatraemia due to water retention (Table 4.5). The vomiting and muscle pains had ceased by 36 h after admission and the urea was normal within a few days. There was no recurrence of heart failure.

Retention of Water and Sodium

This may be entirely iatrogenic due to the administration of so much saline that the patient is unable to excrete it as fast as it is being given, even with normal kidney function. It is particularly liable to occur in patients with acute oliguric renal failure or with chronic renal failure in which the number of functioning nephrons may be too small to handle the additional load. The plasma sodium concentration will depend on the relative amounts of salt and water that are given. If the water intake is higher than the sodium intake hyponatraemia will develop.

Hyperaldosteronism and excessive cortisol secretion are other conditions in which sodium and water retention occur, sometimes with hypernatraemia.

Fluid Retention with Oedema

Oedema occurs when the net movement of fluid out of the capillaries exceeds the capacity of the lymphatics to remove it. Apart from lymphatic obstruction the factors that promote this are increased capillary hydrostatic pressure, decreased plasma oncotic pressure, and increased capillary permeability.

A small rise in the amount of fluid in the interstitial space evokes a sharp rise in tissue hydrostatic pressure. This will increase the lymphatic drainage and oppose the flow of more fluid out of the capillaries, but above a certain level there is a dramatic fall in the pressure response to a given volume increase, and fluid then accumulates. The mechanisms of fluid retention in some cases of oedema are complex and not fully understood, especially those in which hyponatraemia is common.

Congestive Cardiac Failure. With venous congestion there is increased capillary pressure, and oedema forms. In severe cases with massive oedema, hyponatraemia develops and is a bad prognostic sign. The exchangeable sodium is grossly increased, with an increased intracellular sodium, and there is proportionally more water retention due to AVP secretion. There is usually very little sodium in the urine, owing to hyperaldosteronism. In practice a random urinary sodium concentration may be increased as a result of treatment with diuretics.

The exact mechanism of these changes is not fully understood. Non-osmotic factors, principally the reduction in cardiac output, is believed to stimulate AVP secretion via baroreceptor mechanisms. AVP secretion still responds to osmotic changes though the osmotic threshold is lowered. The reduced cardiac output also stimulates the renin–angiostension–aldosterone system, causing sodium retention. A low cardiac output will also reduce the GFR and so further impair water excretion by reducing the volume delivered to the distal tubule.

Cirrhosis of the Liver. Patients with advanced cirrhosis of the liver and portal hypertension may become oedematous and develop ascites, because of a fall in the plasma oncotic pressure due to hypoalbuminaemia. As a consequence the plasma volume is reduced. This is believed to result in the non-osmotic stimulation of AVP secretion, increased activity of the renin–angiotension–aldosterone system, and increased sympathetic nervous activity. The accompanying reduction in renal blood flow and GFR contribute to reduced water and sodium excretion. In advanced cases proportionately more water than sodium is retained, leading to hyponatraemia.

The Nephrotic Syndrome. The severe hypoalbuminaemia that results from the renal loss of albumin lowers the plasma oncotic pressure and so promotes oedema. This tends to lower the plasma volume and stimulates sodium- and water-retaining mechanisms. It should be remembered that in this condition hyponatraemia may be a spurious consequence of hyperlipoproteinaemia.

Intermittent Idiopathic Oedema. This is a distressing condition that seems to occur only in women. There is intermittent pitting oedema, and sometimes abdominal swelling, unrelated to the menstrual cycle. The mechanism is unclear and there is almost certainly more than one entity. In some patients a sudden change from supine to an upright posture precipitates a large fall in plasma volume associated with sodium retention, but this is not an invariable finding. In others, the intermittent use of diuretics, possibly to lose weight or to remove 'oedema', has been a causal factor; sodium retention and oedema recur rapidly on stopping the diuretics, and are attributed to hyperaldosteronism induced by chronic volume depletion. Permanently discontinuing the diuretics leads to recovery in most of the patients. Subclinical hypothyroidism is also associated with this form of oedema, which is relieved when therapy is instituted.

Effects of Hyponatraemia and Their Therapeutic Implications

It is a common clinical observation that, whereas

some patients with a plasma sodium concentration of 115 mmol/L due to water retention will develop the syndrome of water intoxication with anorexia, vomiting, confusion, headaches, muscle cramps, convulsions, coma, and ultimately death, others with a similar plasma sodium concentration may have none of these features. The difference is probably related to the rate of fall of sodium concentration. A large fall occurring in a few hours will induce water intoxication, whereas development over a number of days probably will not. Some adaptation therefore seems likely in the slowly developing cases.

In animals, the rapid induction of hyponatraemia was found to cause brain swelling due to an increased water content. When the sodium concentration was allowed to fall over several days there was less brain swelling, although the brain tissue osmolality was just as low because of the loss of potassium from the brain cells. Potassium is lost from the cells generally in long-standing hyponatraemia; similar adaptive changes have been observed *in vitro* with cells placed in a hypotonic solution.

These observations are relevant to treatment. If, in hyponatraemia, the brain cells in particular have adapted to the low ECF osmolality by extrusion of potassium, the rapid correction of the extracellular sodium concentration might be expected to cause cellular dehydration. If there are no symptoms or signs of water intoxication, correction may be achieved slowly by restricting the patient's water intake enough to cause a large negative balance. The total negative balance required to increase the plasma sodium concentration to 135 mmol/L is

$$\frac{(135 - \text{plasma [Na]})}{\text{Plasma [Na]}} \times \text{total body water,}$$

where total body water equals 60% or 50% of body weight (kg) in males or females, respectively. Increasing the dietary sodium or giving isotonic saline intravenously while the ECF volume is still expanded merely results in increased sodium excretion.

Signs of water intoxication are an indication for more urgent correction of hyponatraemia, which can be achieved by the intravenous infusion of *hyper*tonic saline, given over 6–8 h. The amount of sodium, in millimoles, required to raise its plasma concentration to 135 mmol/L is

$$(135 - \text{observed plasma [Na]}) \times \text{total body water.}$$

To keep the water given to a minimum, the sodium can be given as a molar solution of the chloride or, if there is an acidosis to be corrected, as a mixture of chloride and bicarbonate. This will correct the hyponatraemia and draw water out of the cells, thus transiently expanding the ECF volume still further; the excess sodium is excreted in the urine within 2–3 days and takes with it the excess water that has been withdrawn from the cells (Table 4.5). Once the plasma sodium concentration has been restored to normal or near normal in the SIAD, the improvement will only be sustained by continued water restriction.

The correction of hyponatraemia by intravenous hypertonic saline is controversial.[5] It has been reported that such treatment causes fatal pontine myelinolysis. Others have attributed fatal anatomical changes in the brain in hyponatraemia to the lack of treatment. It has been suggested that pontine myelinolysis can be avoided by giving hypertonic saline at a slow rate that increases the plasma sodium concentration by not more than 0.6 mmol/h. But water intoxication is potentially fatal and its occurrence implies the absence of the adaptive changes thought to predispose to pontine myelinolysis. The amount of sodium calculated to be necessary to restore its normal plasma concentration need not be given in a single dose; raising the plasma concentration to 125 mmol/L over about 6–8 h frequently reverses the signs of water intoxication.

Other Guides

The Anion Gap[10]

The anion gap is defined as the difference between the plasma sodium concentration (sometimes the sum of the sodium and potassium is used) and the sum of the chloride and bicarbonate; it normally falls within the range 8–15 mmol/L. Its calculation is sometimes useful diagnostically and it is useful for quality control because an error in estimating one of the components will distort the anion gap.

The sum of the cations (meq/L) equals the sum of the anions (meq/L):

$$Na - (Cl + HCO_3) = \text{proteins} + \text{unmeasured} \\ \text{anions} - (K + Ca + Mg).$$

Hence the anion gap may change because of an alteration in any of the quantities on the right-hand side of the equation.

A rise in the anion gap is the more common abnormality and is usually due to a rise in the unmeasured anions in diabetic ketoacidosis or renal failure, and, less frequently to a large salicylate overdose. A small increase may occur in alkalosis, owing to the increased anionic equivalence of the plasma proteins, and this may be combined with a further small increase due to increased protein concentration if the ECF volume is low. A much less common cause is lactic acidosis; penicillin and carbenicillin are anions in plasma and may also cause a high anion gap. Other causes that should be suspected in obscure cases include certain poisons that are metabolized to acids, such as ethylene glycol and methanol metabolized to oxalate and formate, respectively, and ethanol, which may cause lactic acidosis. A fall in the concentration of only one of the cations has too small an effect on the anion gap to be noticed.

A reduced anion gap is caused by a low plasma albumin concentration. Albumin normally contributes about 10 meq of the 15 meq or so of anions contributed by the plasma proteins. A fall in the plasma albumin to 25 g/L will therefore cause a fall of 5 meq/L in the total anions, but this is usually counterbalanced by a corresponding rise in the plasma chloride concentration, which lowers the anion gap. A low gap may also be present with a high plasma concentration of potassium, magnesium or calcium, and large amounts of lithium in cases of overdose will contribute. Recently it has been recognized that IgG has cationic properties and that high concentrations of paraproteins may result in an anion gap of only 1 or 2 meq/L, and even a negative one. Exceptionally high levels of polyclonal IgG also may cause the anion gap to be abnormally low.

Plasma and Urine Osmolality Measurements

The measurement of the osmolality of both serum and urine is widely recommended for the study of fluid balance problems, but the significance of such measurements seems often to be misunderstood and their importance grossly exaggerated. More often than not, in clinical practice, they add nothing to the information derived from other routine measurements.

In health, the plasma osmolality depends mainly on the sodium concentration, with small contributions from urea and glucose. In disease the contribution from urea or glucose is sometimes very large, but these three substances together still account for virtually the whole of the osmolality except in the comparatively few instances when substances not normally found in plasma are present, e.g. mannitol or the unidentified metabolites in the 'sick cell syndrome' (*see below*).

In *hyperosmolal states* what really matters is the *reason* for the high osmolality, because this is what determines treatment. Thus, an osmolality of say 360 mmol/kg might be due to one of the following: (i) a plasma sodium concentration of about 175 mmol/L with a slightly raised urea and a normal glucose; (ii) normal concentrations of sodium and urea, but a glucose level of 70 mmol/L; (iii) normal sodium and glucose concentrations but a urea level of 70 mmol/L. These three conditions are clearly entirely different therapeutic problems, which can only be identified by knowing the concentrations of sodium, urea and glucose. If these are known, the osmolality can be calculated: measurement of osmolality, in addition, is not helpful. There are many methods recommended for calculating the plasma osmolality.[11] The simplest is to double the plasma sodium concentration and then add the millimolar concentrations of urea and glucose if they are abnormally high.

It must be remembered that a high plasma osmolality does not necessarily indicate the need for treatment to dilute the body fluid because some substances, e.g. urea and ethanol, are distributed throughout the total body water and will not cause a change in cell size.

If there is marked elevation of only one of these

factors, serial osmolality measurements can be used *instead* of specific measurements to follow the response to treatment, but these serve no purpose if measured *as well as* the specific factor. Moreover, measuring osmolality alone may sometimes be misleading. For example, a patient with diabetic ketoacidosis resuscitated with an infusion of isotonic sodium solutions commonly sustains a rise in plasma sodium concentration as the blood glucose falls in response to insulin. The fall in plasma osmolality will then be less than the fall in the plasma glucose and could lead, mistakenly, to the administration of more insulin.

Hyperosmolality may be due to large amounts of toxic substances in the plasma, notably ethanol, methanol and ethylene glycol. Smell will direct attention to the first and, since it is usual to measure the electrolytes in coma of obscure origin, the others will be revealed by acidosis with a high anion gap.

With significant *hypo-osmolality* there must be hyponatraemia. However, the latter does not always mean hypo-osmolality because it occurs when a shift of water out of the cells is induced by high levels of some other solute, e.g. mannitol or glucose. This is the mechanism postulated in the 'sick cell syndrome'[8] in which intracellular organic metabolites that are normally confined to the cell are thought to escape into the ECF. The metabolites have not been identified and to diagnose this state it is necessary to show that the measured plasma osmolality exceeds the calculated osmolality. However, this is a very uncommon cause of hyponatraemia, most cases of which are due to the administration of too much hypotonic solution.

The value of measuring *urine osmolality* also seems to be misunderstood. It is a measure of the concentration of the urine just like specific gravity, and in normal urine there is a linear relation between the two. For most clinical purposes a very accurate assessment of urine concentration is not required, and specific gravity and osmolality give equally useful information. In the diagnosis of the SIAD or diabetes insipidus, urine specific gravity is as useful as osmolality if it is remembered that a specific gravity of 1.010 is approximately equivalent to the osmolality of normal plasma, i.e. about 290 mmol/kg.

Urine osmolality measurements are, however, essential if it is necessary to know the urine concentration when there is reason to suspect the presence in the urine of substances that increase the specific gravity more than the osmolality, e.g. glucose, very large amounts of protein, mannitol, dextran-40, or radiographic contrast media. The quantitative study of free water excretion also necessitates the measurement of plasma and urine osmolality.

Urinary Sodium Measurements

Reference has been made previously to the changes in urine sodium concentration that occur characteristically in different states. It does not follow, however, that measurements of urine sodium will necessarily contribute to the diagnosis or management of patients. Their usefulness is, in fact, very limited, and they are made far too often because their significance is misunderstood.

The question often asked when such measurements are being interpreted is what is the normal urine sodium concentration? There is no short answer to this because in health the 24-h excretion of sodium can vary from zero to several hundred millimoles according to the intake; the concentration of sodium depends also on the urine volume. In pathological states the urine sodium concentrations are always within this range and in that sense are always 'normal', but what matters is whether this is appropriate for the circumstances. For this to be determined, other information is necessary, which often but not always renders the measurement of little value.

A low urine sodium concentration of less than, say, 10 mmol/L, may, in the absence of extreme urine dilution, be due to sodium depletion. But it may also be due merely to a low sodium intake without clinically significant depletion. Moreover, such levels also occur when the exchangeable sodium is actually increased, as in heart failure and cirrhosis of the liver, owing to secondary hyperaldosteronism.

Conversely a urine sodium concentration of more than, say, 40 mmol/L in a patient with hyponatraemia might be taken to indicate a SIAD rather than sodium depletion. But additional information is necessary before this distinction can be made, because uncontrolled loss of sodium in the urine might be the cause of sodium depletion, as in Addison's disease, renal disease, diuretic therapy or osmotic diuresis.

Clearly, the urine sodium concentration cannot be interpreted on its own, but given other necessary information its measurement can on occasions be useful diagnostically. Thus, in a patient with clinical evidence of sodium depletion in whom the cause is not apparent, the urine content must be measured to determine whether this is the source of sodium loss. Likewise, in a patient acutely ill with diarrhoea and vomiting who, it is thought, might have Addison's disease, the measurement of urine sodium might enable the diagnosis to be refuted or strengthened according to whether the sodium level is very low or not.

In cases of hypernatraemia the cause should be apparent from the history, but in the absence of this, measurement of the urinary sodium will distinguish water depletion, in which it will be low, from sodium overload, in which it will be high. It follows that a low value associated with hypernatraemia should not lightly be taken to indicate that sodium retention is the cause of hypernatraemia.

The measurement of urine sodium excretion is often made ostensibly as a guide to treatment. This is useful in the relatively few patients whose kidneys cannot conserve sodium in the normal manner, as the obligatory threshold can be determined. But in most acutely ill patients the sodium that is in the urine is that which has been given in excess of the requirements, and it is misguided to measure the urinary sodium daily in order to replace it exactly in the following 24 h.

POTASSIUM

Distribution

On average, a 70-kg man will contain a little less than 4000 mmol of potassium, or 55 mmol/kg body weight, although there are very large differences between individuals. Ninety-eight per cent of this is in the cells, held in proportion to the amount of water, protein and carbohydrate; three-quarters of it is in skeletal muscle and about 7% in the bone. Naturally occurring potassium is mainly ^{39}K with a small proportion of radioactive ^{40}K, so that the total body potassium can be determined by whole-body counting of ^{40}K. The value obtained by this method is some 15% more than the exchangeable potassium measured with ^{42}K or ^{43}K. The ECF contains only 50–60 mmol in all, so that large alterations in the extracellular concentration may result from the shift of comparatively small amounts of potassium into or out of the cells. The average concentration of potassium in the cells is around 130 mmol/L, but there are large differences between different tissues.

The normal dietary intake of potassium is variable but averages about 100 mmol/day. Both meat and vegetables are rich sources so that a diet adequate in other respects is unlikely to be deficient in potassium. Most of the dietary potassium is absorbed together with the potassium in the digestive secretions, and 90% of it is excreted in the urine. About 8–10 mmol/day are excreted in the faeces, probably as a result of exchange of potassium for sodium in the colon, and there is a little lost in the sweat. The amount in both sweat and faeces is increased by aldosterone.

The Renal Handling of Potassium and its Regulation

The filtered potassium is completely, or almost completely, reabsorbed by the renal tubule, and what is excreted in the urine is added to the tubular fluid in the distal tubule in exchange for sodium. Reabsorption takes place mainly in the proximal tubule and the ascending limb of the loop of Henle, but probably continues by an active process along the whole length of the tubule, including the collecting duct. In the distal tubule, potassium enters the tubular fluid probably by passive diffusion down the electrochemical gradient created by the active reabsorption of sodium under the influence of aldosterone. Both hydrogen and potassium ions are exchanged for sodium ions at this site and the exchange process is dependent on the relative amounts of potassium and hydrogen ion in the tubular cells, as well as on the amount of sodium reaching the distal tubule. A low dietary sodium leads to a low urinary potassium, and a high sodium intake leads to a high potassium excretion, but this is not solely due to the amount of sodium available for reabsorption in the distal tubule. Although the exchange of potassium for sodium is increased by aldosterone, the effects of the hormone on sodium reabsorption and potassium excretion may be dissociated. Thus the administration of a mineralocorticoid causes sodium retention only for several days, after which sodium excretion 'escapes'. This, however, is not accompanied by a fall in potassium excretion.

The renal mechanism for regulating potassium is very responsive to changes in potassium status, and an intake as high as 200 mmol/day is easily tolerated by a corresponding increase in the urinary excretion. A low intake leads to renal conservation, though it takes a number of days to achieve maximal conservation, which, even then is not as efficient as in the case of sodium, the urine potassium seldom falling to less than 5 mmol/L.

The major factor influencing the excretion of potassium in the urine is aldosterone, which increases the exchange of potassium for sodium in the distal tubule. This is secreted not only in response to stimulation of the adrenal cortex by angiotensin II, whose activity reflects changes in sodium metabolism, but also in response to a high plasma potassium concentration. Conversely, a low plasma potassium concentration suppresses aldosterone secretion and may do so even with elevated amounts of renin.

When the potassium intake is high, the plasma concentration rises transiently during the absorptive phase, and falls in the postabsorptive phase in conjunction with a raised plasma concentration of aldosterone and increased renal excretion. Similar effects are produced by the intravenous infusion of potassium. The extent to which the plasma potassium and aldosterone rise in response to the infusion of a given amount of potassium varies with the dietary intake of potassium. On a low oral intake of 40 mmol/day, the rise of plasma potassium is higher and that of aldosterone lower than when the oral intake is 200 mmol/day. If the patient is in sodium balance, variations in the sodium intake do not affect these responses, but if the patient is sodium depleted the response to hyperkalaemia is enhanced several fold.

This interrelation between sodium and potassium intake is of great clinical importance. The administration of a high sodium intake, say 200 mmol/day, will suppress aldosterone secretion in normal subjects but not in patients with hyperaldosteronism if the potassium intake is less than the average of 80 mmol/day. But if the potassium intake is also high at 200 mmol/day, the high sodium intake will not suppress aldosterone secretion, even in a normal subject, a point of obvious importance when investigating patients for hyperaldosteronism. It is also possible for very large doses of potassium, given therapeutically, to elevate plasma concentrations and so stimulate aldosterone secretion and lead to loss of some of the potassium supplement in the urine. This, of course, also acts as a safeguard during potassium therapy provided that renal and adrenal function are normal.

The acid–base state is another important influence on the renal tubular handling of potassium. Alkalosis and acidosis, respectively, increase and decrease the intracellular potassium concentration and thus increase or decrease potassium secretion by the distal tubule.

Hypokalaemia and Potassium Deficiency

Hypokalaemia sometimes results from the transfer of a small amount of potassium from the ECF into the cells. In practice, however, it usually means potassium depletion, but the plasma concentration is not a good indication of the total body deficit. Nor does potassium depletion always cause hypokalaemia because when potassium is lost from the cells it may accumulate in the ECF if acidosis or renal failure intefere with normal renal excretion (see below). In such circumstances, rehydration of the cells or the administration of insulin and glucose rapidly causes a small shift of potassium back into the cells and the appearance of hypokalaemia.

Causes of Hypokalaemia
Starvation. This alone does not usually cause hypokalaemia as potassium is lost from the cells in proportion to the loss of protein and carbohydrate, and is excreted in the urine if there is no acidosis due to starvation. Some potassium depletion may occur if starvation is prolonged, because the kidney is unable to reduce potassium excretion to zero. Vomiting in anorexia nervosa, for example, will cause a metabolic alkalosis and thus lead to increased loss of potassium in the urine and hypokalaemia (see below).

Loss Through the Gastrointestinal Tract. All gastrointestinal secretions contain potassium and even though the concentration may not be high (see Table 4.1), the loss of such secretions is a common cause of potassium depletion; an additional factor is stimulation of aldosterone secretion as a result of sodium depletion and hence the loss of potassium in the urine. Urinary potassium loss may be further increased by alkalosis when there is loss of acid gastric juice. Plasma potassium frequently falls below 2.5 mmol/L and may be less than 2.0. Losses from the large bowel may be covered by the dietary intake until some adverse factor, such as the onset of vomiting, reduces it.

Other causes are: acute or chronic diarrhoea, including cholera and the watery diarrhoea associated with pancreatic tumours that secrete gastrin or the vasoactive intestinal polypeptide. The loss of mucus from the large bowel is another potent source of potassium loss. A villous papilloma of the rectum may secrete a litre per day or more of mucus rich in potassium and sodium (see Table 4.1). Mucus may also be lost in large amounts in ulcerative colitis and, occasionally, in carcinoma of the rectum. If the sodium intake is inadequate to replace the sodium losses hyperaldosteronism will develop and further increase the loss of potassium.

Loss Through the Kidney. *1. The metabolic response to injury.* In starvation, potassium is lost in the urine at the rate of 2.7 mmol/g nitrogen. Immediately after injury there is loss of potassium from the cells in excess of this. The amount of potassium lost in this way varies with the severity of the injury. Similar losses may occur in any acute illness, and low plasma levels will persist during convalescence unless adequate supplements are given.

2. Alkalosis. In alkalosis the hydrogen ion that is lost from the cells is replaced partly by potassium ion. The decreased amount of hydrogen ion in the renal tubular cells means that more potassium must be lost from these cells in exchange for sodium reabsorbed from the tubular filtrate; this increases the degree of hypokalaemia.

3. Diuretics. Hypokalaemia has long been recognized as a complication of treatment with diuretics, which are now so widely used to treat hypertension that their use is probably the most common cause of hypokalaemia. By causing sodium loss, diuretics stimulate aldosterone secretion and, at the same time, increase the amount of sodium at the site of aldosterone action so that potassium secretion is increased. However, the clinical significance of this change has been questioned. It has been shown that when loop diuretics and thiazides cause hypokalaemia in susceptible hypertensives, the change occurs rapidly and is maximal after only 1 week's treatment, thus rendering frequent laboratory measurements to monitor the change unnecessary. Moreover, studies of exchangeable potassium and measurements of total potassium by whole-body counting have cast doubt on the clinical importance of the hypokalaemia, as some have found that the body deficit is so small as not to be a cause for concern. Others, however, have found larger deficits on occasions and there can be little doubt that some patients on long-term diuretic therapy do acquire a sizeable potassium deficit; there are reports of some becoming so depleted that hyponatraemia developed, owing to a shift of sodium into the potassium-depleted cells, and being reversed by correcting the potassium deficit.

Notwithstanding the conclusions on the size of the potassium deficit in hypertensives, most physicians do give potassium supplements to hypertensive patients treated with diuretics. But normal plasma concentrations are restored in only a proportion of them, the others responding to the increased intake by increasing the urinary excretion. The explanation of these changes is not entirely clear. Possibly the induced sodium losses sensitize the renin–aldosterone system to the effects of potassium administration. The potassium-sparing diuretics, spironolactone, triampterene and amiloride, which block sodium/potassium exchange in the distal tubule, seem to be more effective than supplements in maintaining a normal plasma potassium. But they too do not always prevent hypokalaemia, perhaps because of incorrect dosage, and they pose a risk of hyperkalaemia.

4. Other Drugs. Carbenoxolone, a drug used in the treatment of peptic ulcer and oesophageal reflux, potentiates the action of aldosterone on the distal tubule and causes hypokalaemic alkalosis. Liquorice is another substance with similar effects due to the presence of glycyrrhizinic acid. Both of these can cause very severe symptomatic hypokalaemia.

5. Corticosteroid Excess. Aldosterone is the major factor regulating potassium excretion. Therefore hypokalaemia occurs in primary hyperaldosteronism and in secondary hyperaldosteronism due to renin-secreting tumours, Bartter's syndrome of hyperplasia of the juxtaglomerular bodies, and renal ischaemia. Excessive secretion of other mineralocorticoids such as corticosterone or deoxycorticosterone also cause hypokalaemia. Because cortisol also has some mineralocorticoid activity, hypokalaemia sometimes occurs in Cushing's syndrome and sometimes complicates the therapeutic administration of glucocorticoids.

6. Renal Disease. Potassium loss and hypokalaemia occur in several forms of renal disease. The loss may be associated with chronic parenchymal disease, particularly if there is renal ischaemia, which gives rise to secondary hyperaldosteronism, and which in turn may increase potassium loss through the remaining nephrons and will also increase loss in the faeces. The term 'potassium-losing nephritis' is sometimes used very loosely to refer to a variety of renal lesions associated with inappropriately high potassium excretion.

In acute tubular necrosis the problem is more likely to be *hyper*kalaemia, but when recovery ensues and the urine output increases, there may be uncontrolled loss of potassium in the urine. In any osmotic diuresis, the urine potassium concentration may be an 'obligatory' 20 mmol/L.

Excessive loss of potassium also occurs in renal tubular acidosis when it is the only cation available to exchange with sodium in the distal tubule, in view of the unavailability of hydrogen ion to do so. Hypokalaemia occurs frequently and may cause severe symptoms.

7. Diabetes Mellitus. Insulin promotes the cellular uptake of glucose and potassium, and the lack of it leads to the loss of potassium from the cells. Ketoacidosis also promotes the loss of potassium from the cells and interferes with potassium exchange in the distal tubule, so that a high plasma concentration is maintained. Potassium is nevertheless lost in the urine as a consequence of the osmotic diuresis, and the patient becomes potassium deficient. This becomes manifest as a low plasma potassium during treatment with insulin coupled with cellular rehydration and correction of the acidosis, all of which promote the re-entry of potassium into the cells.

8. Familial Periodic Paralysis. In this condition there are intermittent attacks of paralysis of skeletal muscle lasting up to 24 h, due to a shift of potassium into the cells. With recovery the plasma potassium returns to normal. Total body potassium between attacks has been variously reported as normal or low.

Urinary Potassium Measurements
Not uncommonly, hypokalaemia is discovered when there is no immediately obvious explanation. Loss through the kidney must then be considered, together with the possibility of chronic purgation, which the patient may not readily admit. The measurement of urinary potassium excretion may be helpful in these circumstances. The excretion of more than 25 mmol/day when the plasma potassium concentration is less than 3.0 mmol/L is presumptive evidence that the kidney is the route of loss. In cases of purgation, or of potassium deficiency from causes no longer operating, e.g. diuretic treatment or an acute illness in the recovery phase, the excretion may be down to 10 mmol/day or less. In the latter, low amounts of potassium in the urine will persist until the patient is repleted but the administration of potassium supplements to patients with Conn's syndrome will cause a dramatic rise in urinary potassium excretion before the plasma concentration approaches normal (Fig. 4.7). In alkalosis and in 'potassium-losing nephropathies' the measurement of urine potassium excretion is sometimes useful as a guide to therapy. These conditions apart, it is usually unnecessary to measure the urine potassium excretion daily in order to replace it exactly, as once repletion has been achieved the urine will contain that which is not required.

The Effects of Hypokalaemia. The membrane potential of nerve and muscle cells, and therefore their excitability, is related, among other factors, to the ratio of intracellular to extracellular potassium. Experimentally, potassium depletion with hypokalaemia has been found to cause muscular weakness, depressed tendon reflexes and loss of intestinal motility. Clinically, severe hypokalaemia has effects on skeletal muscle, cardiac muscle and possibly smooth muscle, but in general deficits of less than 300 mmol are unlikely to be manifest by clinical signs, and there is no close correlation between the level of plasma potassium and its effects. Indeed, patients with

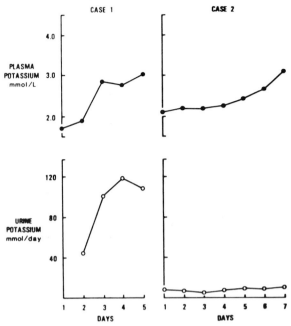

Figure 4.7 Effect of potassium supplements on plasma and urine potassium in a case of Conn's syndrome (Case 1) and one of potassium depletion due to chronic purgation (Case 2). In case 1 the supplement was 60 and 120 mmol on days 1 and 2, respectively, and thereafter was 150 mmol/day. In case 2 the supplement was 100 mmol/day throughout.

plasma concentrations as low as 1.5 mmol/L may have no symptoms whereas higher concentrations have been accompanied by flaccid quadriplegia and even respiratory paralysis, which is fortunately rare. The reason for such differences is not clear but may be due to the loss of relatively similar proportions of potassium from the intracellular and extracellular compartments, leaving the ratio little altered, or to counteracting changes in other electrolytes, e.g. magnesium or hydrogen ions.

The effect on the heart is more complex because the myocardium and the conduction system are affected differently. There is increased sensitivity to the effect of digitalis and a characteristic sequence of changes in the ECG, although this is not closely related to the plasma potassium concentration. In cases of prolonged depletion there may be morphological changes, including focal necrosis, in the myocardium.

Loss of intestinal motility is observed in experimental potassium depletion, and paralytic ileus is said to be a feature of clinical deficiency. However, there is usually a local cause for ileus and its recovery solely from correcting potassium depletion must be rare.

Chronic hypokalaemia also has adverse effects on the kidney. The ability to concentrate the urine is greatly reduced and the tubular response to AVP is impaired. Thirst and polyuria may occur, the urine volume in some patients exceeding 4 L/day. Histologically, changes are seen in the proximal convoluted tubule, but not in the collecting tubules. The former become swollen and vacuolated, but the changes have been shown by serial renal biopsies to be reversible. In long-standing depletion in animals a picture resembling chronic interstitial nephritis has been described and the possibility of this happening in man cannot be discounted.

Glucose tolerance is diminished in 50% of patients with Conn's syndrome, and reverts to normal with correction of potassium deficiency. Many publications link hypokalaemia with diminished glucose tolerance and impaired insulin release, but these are not often found in potassium deficiency.

Alkalosis associated with hypokalaemia is described in Chapter 3.

Principles of Treatment of Hypokalaemia
The total dose of potassium required to correct hypokalaemia cannot be calculated from the plasma concentration. Treatment must therefore be empirical to some extent, but clearly the rate of administration must exceed the rate of loss; the small supplements given to patients taking diuretics have no place in therapeutic regimens. [It cannot be stressed too strongly that the commercially available slow-release preparations of potassium contain only small amounts of potassium, and that as many as 10 tablets per day may provide no more than 65 mmol, which is almost always far too little for a depleted adult.]

As a general rule, when the homeostatic mechanisms are normal, therapeutic doses of potassium should be at least 100 mmol/day more than the loss. In most cases an approximate value for the latter can be derived from the data in Table 4.1, but when large volumes are lost of the fluids known to have a high potassium concentration, the fluid should be analysed. Estimation of the urinary potassium excretion is also useful in patients with severe alkalosis.

It is generally acknowledged that whenever possible potassium supplements should be given by mouth, as this is thought to be the best safeguard against overtreatment. However, it is important to establish not simply that the patient can take supplements by mouth but that he or she *will* take *enough* in this way—if not, there is no option but to give at least some of it intravenously. When the intravenous route is used there often seems to be great reluctance to give adequate amounts of potassium because of the fear of causing hyperkalaemia. The risk of this is small in depleted patients with normal homeostatic mechanisms because any elevation of plasma potassium above normal stimulates aldosterone secretion, and hence increases the urinary loss. The amount of potassium that needs to be infused to cause sustained hyperkalaemia is very large, and in severely depleted patients, with plasma concentrations below 2 mmol/L, 200–300 mmol can be infused quite safely in 12 h, preferably in glucose solutions, which will facilitate the uptake of potassium by the cells.

In the most severe cases, and especially if there is muscular paralysis, even larger amounts may be given, the infusion of up to 40 mmol/h being considered safe. During the infusion of such large amounts the ECG should be monitored continuously for large T waves, which renders unnecessary the measurement of plasma potassium every few hours.

The concentration of potassium in intravenous fluids should not usually exceed 50 mmol/L because if this solution is given too quickly it may cause severe pain along the course of the vein. Higher concentrations may be given, if infused slowly, but not through a central venous catheter because an inadvertent increase in the drip rate could be fatal.

In severe depletion the plasma potassium is likely to remain low for days after beginning treatment. Ultimately it will rise into the normal range quickly over 1 or 2 days, and to be sure of detecting this when large doses are being given it is necessary to measure the plasma concentration daily. Once a normal plasma concentration has been achieved the dose should be reduced, but not to the level of the estimated loss because this may have been underestimated—if the homeostatic mechanisms are normal it is usually better to give a little too much than to give insufficient, but, when the homeostatic mechanisms are impaired, great care is needed during potassium replacement to avoid dangerous hyperkalaemia.

Hyperkalaemia

Unlike hypokalaemia, hyperkalaemia is not related to the total amount of potassium in the body and even occurs in the presence of potassium depletion as discussed above. It may be an artefact arising *in vitro* owing to haemolysis or the breakdown of leukaemia cells during sampling. If whole blood is allowed to stand overnight before separating the plasma, levels exceeding 10 mmol/L can occur if the blood is kept at 4°C, which depresses the activity of the sodium pump. In a rare familial disorder of the red cell, rapid loss of potassium from the cell occurs even at room temperature, the plasma concentration rising to 6 mmol/L in 2 h. Such artefacts are usually identified, but lesser changes may merely obscure the presence of hypokalaemia.

Reduction in Renal Potassium Excretion
Normally, any tendency for the plasma potassium concentration to rise *in vivo* stimulates aldosterone secretion and the excess is rapidly excreted. When hyperkalaemia does develop *in vivo*, there is usually a reduced capacity for potassium excretion, which has been exceeded by the potassium intake or by the release of potassium from the cells.

The conditions that impair the renal excretion of potassium are acidosis, renal failure, mineralocorticoid deficiency, the administration of certain diuretics, and a group of conditions in which there appears to be a disorder of tubular transport, as follows.

1. Acidosis. In acidosis, potassium is displaced from the cells by hydrogen ions, and the electrochemical gradient between the cells in the distal tubule and the tubular fluid is less favourable for the excretion of potassium. The plasma potassium may be as high as 7 mmol/L even though the urine volume exceeds 2 L/day. Not all patients with acidosis show a high plasma potassium, which is often normal or even low when there is severe potassium depletion.

2. Renal Failure. In chronic renal failure, hyperkalaemia does not often present a problem until the GFR is very low, unless there is also acidosis. Adaptive changes result in the excretion of more potassium by the remaining nephrons and the excretion into the colon is also increased. Hyperkalaemia is more likely to appear in acute oliguric renal failure. This occurs in conditions in which there is also increased release of potassium from damaged tissues, viz. trauma, burns, increased catabolism, and haemorrhage into the tissues or intestine.

The plasma of stored blood contains up to 20 mmol of potassium per litre and although this seems likely to re-enter the red cells after transfusion, a proportion of the transfused cells is rapidly destroyed and the plasma potassium concentration may rise if there is renal failure. Massive blood transfusions have been reported as a cause of hyperkalaemia but this is rarely a problem if the homeostatic mechanisms are normal.

When oliguric renal failure is associated with increased tissue breakdown the plasma potassium may rise at an alarming rate, increasing from normal to 8 mmol/L in a few hours and rapidly reaching fatal levels if untreated.

3. Deficiency of Aldosterone. As in Addison's disease or as an isolated defect, this also reduces the efficiency of potassium excretion. The same effect is seen with the use of so-called potassium-sparing diuretics, amiloride, spironolactone, and triamterene, which oppose the effect of aldosterone on the sodium–potassium exchange mechanism in the distal tubule.

4. Tubular Unresponsiveness to Aldosterone (Pseudohypoaldosteronism). There have been reports of a number of cases of hyperkalaemia with acidosis in the presence of large amounts of aldosterone and renin. Many of these cases were diagnosed in infancy; renal sodium wasting was an additional feature, although this disappeared in later childhood. There was no response to exogenous mineralocorticoids and an abnormality of the aldosterone receptors in the renal tubule has been postulated. An accompanying failure of other organs to respond to mineralocorticoids has also been described.

5. Low-renin Hypoaldosteronism. This term refers to those patients in whom hyperkalaemia and acidosis are associated with a low plasma aldosterone, but also with a low plasma renin, which distinguishes the syndrome from a primary mineralocorticoid deficiency. In many of the reported cases, glomerular filtration was reduced. The low aldosterone concentration is thought to be secondary to the low renin, because salt restriction or infusion of ACTH or angiotensin have each been shown to increase aldosterone secretion, and some patients have responded to treatment with mineralocorticoids. The pathogenesis of the failure to secrete renin has not been elucidated. In a few reported cases it was shown that ECF volume and total exchangeable sodium were increased; other patients responded to treatment with thiazide diuretics. It has been postulated that there is a tubular defect that leads not only to a failure to excrete potassium but also to sodium retention. The possibility exists that this is a heterogeneous group.

6. Hyperkalaemic Periodic Paralysis. This is a condition in which a rapid shift of potassium out of the cells causes hyperkalaemia and muscular paralysis episodically. The condition is hereditary but its pathogenesis is unknown, although strenuous exercise appears to be a predisposing factor.

The Effects of Hyperkalaemia
Hyperkalaemia has effects on cardiac and skeletal muscle that depend on the plasma concentration. As this increases, cardiac conduction is depressed and arrhythmias occur. There are progressive changes in the ECG, starting with peaked T waves and culminating in ventricular fibrillation or asystole at concentrations above 11 mmol/L. In general, the earliest ECG manifestations appear with levels of about 7 mmol/L but this is inconstant and the ECG may not become abnormal until potassium concentrations exceed 9 mmol/L. A high plasma potassium also diminishes the excitability of skeletal muscle and causes weakness and even paralysis. These potentially fatal effects may be preceded by paraesthesiae but these cannot be relied upon to appear.

Principles of Treatment of Hyperkalaemia
As there may be little warning before the onset of a fatal arrhythmia, an awareness of the circumstances in which hyperkalaemia occurs is vital so that the rate of change can be assessed and corrective measures applied early. Arrhythmias can be abolished temporarily by the intravenous injection of calcium chloride, as the calcium ions block the effect of the high potassium concentration on cardiac excitability. This is a short-lived effect that does not affect the concentration of potassium but will enable procedures with more lasting effects to be instituted.

A dramatic fall in the plasma potassium can be induced by the intravenous injection of 25 g of glucose in a 50% solution together with 20 units of insulin. This causes potassium to move into the cells, and can be reinforced by creating an alkalosis with intravenous sodium bicarbonate even in non-acidotic patients. Hyponatraemia should also be corrected as this too will antagonize the effects of a high potassium.

These measures may lower the serum potassium dramatically from, say, 10 to 7 mmol/L but the fall may not be sustained for more than a few hours. It is of paramount importance, therefore, to monitor the ECG after such treatment, and if there is further deterioration despite continuing treatment some form of dialysis becomes necessary.

A slow rate of rise can be arrested by means of an ion-exchange resin administered orally together with measures to correct acidosis and cellular dehydration.

REFERENCES

1. Robertson G.L., Shelton R.L., Athar S. (1976). The osmoregulation of vasopressin. *Kidney Int.*, **10**, 25.
2. Skrabal F., Arnot R.N., Joplin G.F. (1973). Equations for the prediction of normal values for exchangeable sodium, exchangeable potassium, extracellular fluid volume, and total body water. *Br. Med. J.*, **2**, 37.
3. McCance R.A. (1936). Experimental human salt deficiency. *Lancet*, **i**, 823.
4. Thomson C.J., Freeman J., Record C.O., Baylis P.H. (1987). Hypernatraemia due to a reset osmostat for vasopressin release and thirst, complicated by nephrogenic diabetes insipidus. *Postgrad. Med. J.*, **63**, 979.
5. Ayus J.C., Krothapalli R.K., Arieff A.I. (1987). Treatment of symptomatic hyponatraemia and its relation to brain damage. *N. Engl. J. Med.*, **317**, 1190.
6. Kahn A., Brachet E., Blum D. (1979). Controlled fall in natraemia and risk of seizure in hypertonic dehydration. *Intensive Care Med.*, **5**, 27.
7. Bartter F.C., Schwartz W.B. (1967). The syndrome of inappropriate secretion of ADH. *Am. J. Med.*, **42**, 790.
8. Flear C.T.G., Singh C.M. (1973). Hyponatraemia and sick cells. *Br. J. Anaesth.*, **45**, 976.
9. Penney M.D., Murphy D., Walters G. (1979). Resetting of osmoreceptor response as cause of hyponatraemia in acute idiopathic polyneuritis. *Br. Med. J.*, **2**, 1474.
10. Emmett M., Narins R.G. (1977). Clinical use of the anion gap. *Medicine*, **56**, 38.
11. Weisberg H.F. (1975). Osmolality—calculated, 'delta' and more formulas. *Clin. Chem.*, **21**, 1182.

FURTHER READING

Baylis P.H., ed. (1989). Water and salt homeostasis in health and disease. In *Baillière's Clinical Endocrinology and Metabolism*, vol. 3, no. 2, London: Baillière Tindall.
Brenner B.M., Stein J.H., eds. (1987). *Body Fluid Homeostasis*, Edinburgh: Churchill Livingstone.
de Wardener H.E., Clarkson E.M. (1985). Concept of a natriuretic hormone. *Physiol. Rev.*, **65**, 658.
Field M., Mrinalini C.R., Chang E.B. (1989). Intestinal electrolyte transport and diarrheal disease I and II. *N. Engl. J. Med.*, **321**, 800; 879.
Rose B.D. (1989). *Clinical Physiology of Acid–Base and Electrolyte Disorders*, 3rd edn., New York: McGraw-Hill.

Schrier R.W. (1989). Pathogenesis of sodium and water retention in high-output and low-output cardiac failure, nephrotic syndrome, cirrhosis and pregnancy I and II. *N. Engl. J. Med.*, **319**, 1065; 1127.

Reference Text

Maxwell M.H., Kleeman C.R., Nairns R.G. eds. (1987). *Clinical Disorders of Fluid and Electrolyte Metabolism*, 4th edn, New York: McGraw-Hill.

5. Polyuria and Disorders of Thirst

D. Donaldson

Introduction
Basic principles of water control
  The requirement for water
  Distribution of water in the body
  Intake and output of water
  Dynamic aspects of water
  Water balance in infancy
  Homeostasis of water and sodium
Physiological control of water homeostasis
  Osmolality
  Thirst
  Water absorption
  Renal function
  Arginine vasopressin
  Consequences of imbalance of water
   homeostasis
Clinical aspects
  Primary polyuria and secondary polydipsia
  Primary polydipsia and secondary polyuria
  Miscellaneous
Laboratory investigation of polyuria and
  polydipsia
  Clinical groups
  Scheme of clinical investigation
  General principles of differential diagnosis
   and interpretation

INTRODUCTION

In clinical medicine, the symptoms of polyuria and polydipsia are commonly encountered together. Nevertheless, from the diagnostic standpoint, it is necessary to attempt to establish which of the two is the primary event, and which is the secondary consequence. It is clear, therefore, that one can at the outset divide such disorders into two groups—in one, polydipsia is primary and polyuria follows, whereas in the other, polyuria is the cause of the polydipsia. Clinically, however, both usually present simultaneously, and it is not always easy in retrospect to ascertain which came first.

The mechanisms underlying maintenance of normal hydration of the body necessarily require discussion in this context. Intake and output of water must be considered. There is, moreover, close integration between fluid intake and urinary output. The anatomical structures involved in this integration, and their normal functioning, will all be referred to in this text.

There is, for instance, continuous monitoring of the plasma osmolality by osmoreceptors in the hypothalamic area. In turn, the results of this monitoring are passed on to other areas of the brain, where physiological action is either initiated or inhibited. Elevated osmolality of the plasma, for example, causes stimulation of the thirst centre. In addition there is secretion of arginine vasopressin (AVP, previously known as antidiuretic hormone). This has, of course, been formed in the hypothalamus prior to storage in the posterior lobe of the pituitary gland. It is not fluid intake but actual excretion from the body that is determined by the AVP mechanism. This substance acts on the distal tubules and collecting ducts in the kidney, thus serving as the final control over loss of water.

A lesser monitoring role in normal circumstances is undertaken by baroreceptors located in the aortic arch, the carotid arteries and the great veins of the chest. The process of baroregulation is, however, able to promote secretion of very large amounts of AVP in circumstances where the blood pressure or blood volume has fallen precipitously.

The kidney is a vital organ in fluid balance. It is involved not only in controlling excretion of fluid from the body, but also in regulation of water intake. This is by way of the renin–angiotensin mechanism. It has been shown that angiotensin II is a potent stimulus to drinking.

Viewing these observations against the background of the biological system as a whole, it is clear that in intracellular dehydration the more important aspect is to take in water rather than merely to conserve what is already there.

The importance of each of the physiological mechanisms available for maintenance of water balance will be very apparent in the discussion on diseases involving the structures concerned. The causes of polyuria and polydipsia will be elaborated upon in turn, from both physiological and clinical aspects. Finally, those investigations that may aid in the elucidation of the clinical diagnosis will be documented and evaluated.

BASIC PRINCIPLES OF WATER CONTROL

The maintenance of water homeostasis depends essentially on a sensitive balance between the release of AVP, which controls renal output of water, and the presence of an efficient thirst mechanism, which controls input to the body.[1] It is the balance between fluid intake, AVP response to plasma osmolality, and renal response to plasma AVP that is the basis of water homeostasis. The abnormalities that may occur at any of these levels are fundamental to the disorders commonly seen in clinical practice.

In fact, both water intake and output are largely controlled by osmolality of the plasma; this in turn is largely dependent on sodium concentration. Although it is true that the sodium content largely determines the amount of water in the body of the normal individual, this is not true in pathological conditions such as hyperglycaemia, uraemia, or fol-

TABLE 5.1

DISTRIBUTION OF BODY WATER IN AVERAGE NORMAL YOUNG ADULT MALE

Source	mL/kg of body weight		% of total body water	
Intracellular	330		55.0	
Extracellular	270		45.0	
Plasma		45		7.5
Interstitial lymph		120		20.0
Dense connective tissue and cartilage		45		7.5
Inaccessible bone		45		7.5
Transcellular		15		2.5
Total Body Water	600		100.0	

From: Edelman and Leibman (1959). *Am. J. Med.*, **27**, 256.

TABLE 5.2

APPROXIMATE FLUID CONTENTS OF THE BODY COMPARTMENTS

Source	Approximate % of body weight		Approximate volume in litres	
Extracellular Fluid	20		15	
Interstitial fluid		15		12
Blood plasma		5		3
Intracellular Fluid	40		25	
Erythrocyte fluid		3		2
Non-erythrocyte fluid		37		23

lowing administration of highly osmotically active substances such as mannitol and amino acids. The mechanisms underlying osmotic diuresis in these disorders will be considered later.

The Requirement for Water

Water serves as the moisture necessary for the easy intake of nutrition to the body, and itself accounts for approximately 55–60% of the body by weight in the adult man, and 50–55% in the adult woman. There is, nevertheless, a wide range for the water content in the body—from 40% of body weight in the obese person to 70% of body weight in the lean individual. Water thus forms a large part of the body substance, both intracellularly and extracellularly (Table 5.1).

Water also acts as the medium in which metabolic reactions take place, and as the vehicle for excretion of products of metabolism, either in solution (i.e. the urine) or in the form of admixture with insoluble excretory products (i.e. the faeces). In the latter instance, water is needed for plasticity of the intestinal contents; this plasticity is essential for moulding to the continuously varying intestinal shape and pressure. Intestinal transit is thereby permitted, and hence easy expulsion of the faeces from the body follows

after a suitable interval of time, during which as much water as possible is reabsorbed. Evaporation of water from the skin surface (i.e. sweat) and from mucous membranes serves as a cooling mechanism in hot environments. The dynamic flow of water through the body in general serves to transport substances throughout the tissues, or in certain instances to convey selected compounds to parts of the body where they are required for special metabolic purposes (e.g. gastrointestinal secretions).

Distribution of Water in the Body

A 70-kg man has in his body, 40 L of water. The extracellular component is about 15 L, of which 3 L are plasma and 12 L interstitial fluid. It is increase of this latter portion that leads to clinical presentation of oedema. Intracellular fluid totals about 25 L in a 70-kg man, of which 2 L are present in the erythrocytes. The 3 L of plasma and 2 L of water in the erythrocytes totals approximately 5 L of blood (Table 5.2).

In men, body water expressed as % body wt tends to decrease slightly up to about 20 years of age. In women, however, there is a steady persistent decrease up to the menopause. This is on account of increased fat deposition—with its low water content.

Different tissues have different amounts of water—the water content, by weight, of muscle is 70%, of adipose tissue 20%, and of bone and cartilage as low as 10%.

Intake and Output of Water

The general sequence of movement of water through the body is displayed diagrammatically in Fig. 5.1. In normal circumstances, the oral route forms the only input other than the contribution from oxidation of ingested food, the latter being derived from carbohydrate, protein and fat. One gram of starch yields 0.60 g water, 1 g of protein yields 0.41 g water, and 1 g fat yields 1.07 g water. Output of water can be by several routes, i.e. urine, sweat, respiration, and faeces. In starvation, endogenous breakdown of body tissues further supplements the water supply.

Fluid Input

This is determined by the desires of the individual, other than in special circumstances where clinical requirement demands intravenous, subcutaneous, intragastric and other routes to be used. Input is influenced by thirst, by habit and also by the degree of availability of fluid. Social drinking is another aspect sometimes requiring consideration.

Fluid Output[2]

Output from the body is determined by several complex mechanisms, thus permitting release of water from the various portals of exit. There is close integration by way of feedback systems between the factors controlling intake and output, hence maintaining

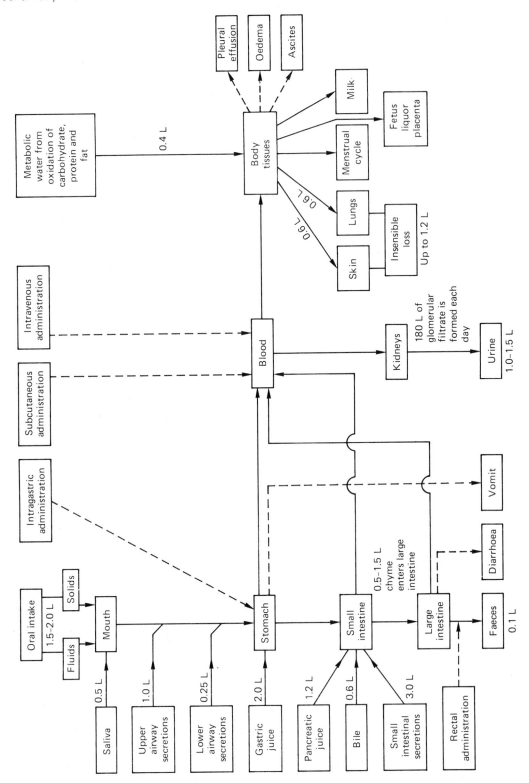

Figure 5.1 Summary of the dynamics of water in the adult human; figures represent approximate volumes in litres per 24 h.

body water at or close to the optimum concentration and amount.

Once water is within the confines of the gastrointestinal system, there are basically two ways in which it may be lost—by vomiting, or as diarrhoea. Once it has entered the tissues of the body, however, it is then involved in endogenous metabolic pathways and processes; other modes of leaving the body then become available.

In normal daily life, water is lost insensibly through the skin (600 mL/24 h) and lungs (600 mL/24 h), and is lost from the body in the urine (1500 mL/24 h). A small amount is lost in the faeces (100 mL/24 h). In pathological states, water can be sequestered in the tissues as tissue fluid (oedema, ascites, pleural effusion, etc.); this may be seen in cardiac failure, nephrotic syndrome and in hepatic disease, in addition to a large number of other clinical disorders. In females in the reproductive phase of life, a small quantity of water is lost each month in the menstrual flow and, should pregnancy occur, water will of course be incorporated into the products of conception—namely the fetus and placenta, together with the amniotic fluid. The postparturition phase is accompanied by further loss of fluid from the mother on account of lactation.

Dynamic Aspects of Water

In the normal state, the body composition of water remains fairly constant. However, in reality, there is an extraordinary degree of movement of water through the tissues. Therefore, although the quantitative composition of the organs and tissues is very constant, the flow through them is vast.

The renal system in particular displays this mobility to a remarkable degree. It is known that approximately 180 L of glomerular filtrate are formed each day. The average urine volume for an adult is of the order of 1000–1500 mL/24 h. This means that well over 99% of the fluid passing through the tubules is reabsorbed; therefore less than 1% of the glomerular filtrate becomes urine.

The gastrointestinal tract is another system of the body that shows dynamics of water flow in marked degree. In addition to orally ingested fluids, and the water content of 'solid' foods (often around 70%), both of which enter the upper end of the tract, there are many litres of gastrointestinal secretions that cascade into the system at different levels. The 24-h production of saliva is around 500 mL, gastric juice 2000 mL, pancreatic juice 1200 mL, bile 600 mL, and small-intestinal secretion 3000 mL. Almost the whole volume of these secretions, together with ingested fluid and the water content of solid foods, is absorbed in the small intestine. Only 500–1500 mL pass as chyme into the large intestine. All but 100 mL of this are reabsorbed again in the large intestine. The normal daily fluid loss via the faeces is around 100–150 mL.

With reference to the respiratory system, it is not generally appreciated that upper airway secretion (i.e. above the level of the larynx) is up to 1000 mL/24 h, most of which is reabsorbed in the gastrointestinal tract. Moreover, lower airway secretion (i.e. below the level of the larynx) is about 250 mL/24 h. Expired air also contains water vapour (up to 600 mL/24 h). The pulmonary loss, together with non-visible loss from the skin, is referred to as 'insensible loss'. In addition, the skin also produces, in certain environmental circumstances, visible sweat. Insensible loss amounts to about 1200 mL/24 h.

Water Balance in Infancy

Infants are more prone to dehydration than are adults. This is on account of their relatively greater body water content (75–80% compared with 55–60% for the adult male and 50–55% for the adult female). In addition, renal concentrating ability is poorer than in adults. Hence, in order to maintain water and electrolyte balance, intake of fluid must be sufficiently high to ensure outflow of a dilute urine. This accounts for the relatively high fluid intake requirement compared with the adult (150 mL/kg body weight per 24 h for a 1-week-old infant compared with less than 60 mL/kg per 24 h for an adult).

The premature baby is even more prone to dehydration on account of possible feeding difficulties, the even greater water content compared with that of the full-term child, the even poorer renal concentrating ability, the greater requirement for fluid than the normal full-term infant (i.e. 180 mL/kg body weight per 24 h), the increased liability to infection with consequent vomiting, diarrhoea and high respiration rate, the increased liability to diarrhoea and vomiting following on from digestive problems, and the risk of overwarming the baby.

Urine output in the normal infant of 1–3 days of age is 20 mL/24 h. At 2 weeks the urine volume is around 200 mL/24 h, and at 3 months it achieves 300 mL/24 h.

The % of body water decreases with age; by 1 year it has fallen to 60% of the total body weight.

Homeostasis of Water and Sodium

The mechanisms of homeostasis for water and sodium are interlinked, as shown in Fig. 5.2. This displays the interrelations of AVP and aldosterone. The cells of the osmoreceptor sites in the hypothalamus detect differences in osmolality between the plasma and themselves, and in turn control both AVP secretion and the sensation of thirst. AVP controls water absorption in the distal tubules and collecting ducts of the kidneys, thereby affecting urine volume. Renal blood flow is determined by several factors, and circulating volume is one. A reduced flow will lead to activation of the renin–angiotensin pathway. Aldosterone secretion controls absorption

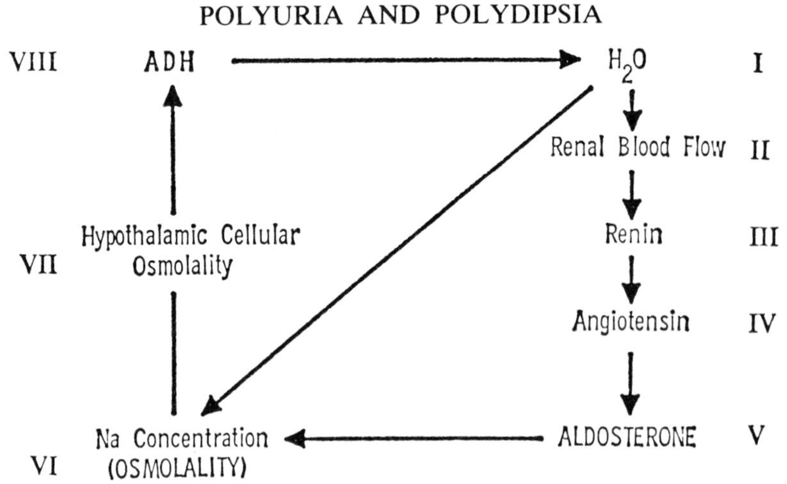

POLYURIA AND POLYDIPSIA

Figure 5.2 Simplified cycle of sodium and water homeostasis, assuming there is no influence exerted by other substances such as mannitol or amino acids, or by pathological states such as hyperglycaemia or uraemia. (Reproduced by kind permission from *Clinical Chemistry in Diagnosis and Treatment* (3rd edn, 1988), by Zilva J.F., Pannall P.R. and Mayne P.D., London: Edward Arnold.)

of sodium in the distal part of the renal tubular system. Retention of sodium leads to secretion of AVP and water retention follows, thereby restoring intravascular volume.

In essence, the extracellular sodium concentration controls AVP secretion, but the latter controls water; and water controls aldosterone secretion, which in turn controls sodium.[3] The topic of fluid and electrolyte homeostasis is covered in detail in Chapter 3; further references to the subject are also given at the end of the present chapter.[2,3,4,5,6]

PHYSIOLOGICAL CONTROL OF WATER HOMEOSTASIS

Osmolality

Accurate measurement of the freezing point of a solution (solute dissolved in water) followed by comparison of this with the freezing point of pure water enables one to make a very accurate assessment of the number of particles in that solution. These particles may be molecules, ions or molecular aggregate. Osmolality refers to the number of dissolved particles in 1 kg solvent. The usual way of determining this in the laboratory is with the aid of an osmometer. The fact that the depression of freezing point so measured is proportional to the osmolality, makes it possible to calibrate the machine to give a direct read-out in mosmol/kg. However, it should not be overlooked that the osmometer is merely a very sophisticated means of measuring the freezing point accurately.

Determination of freezing point will not provide information as to the size of the particles, nor of their shape, nor whether they are charged. It merely informs one as to how many particles there are.

When a mole (molecular weight in grams) of any solute is dissolved in 1 kg of water, the freezing point is depressed by $1.858°C$. It should be emphasized, however, that if the solute ionizes during the solution process, the ions so formed will each contribute to the freezing point depression. If, for instance, 1 mol of sodium chloride is dissolved, this will form twice as many particles (ions) when solution is complete as there were particles (molecules) in the original solute. Hence the freezing point depression will be twice that of 1 mol of urea or glucose for example, neither of which ionize on solution.

Plasma is a complex solution containing much water in which is dissolved many different types of particles. Urea and glucose are present un-ionized, but sodium chloride and potassium chloride, for instance, are ionized. In addition, plasma contains proteins; these and other large molecules contribute in only a minor way to osmolality. This is because large molecules are vastly outnumbered by the smaller ionic particles and molecules around them, which themselves contribute so much to osmolality.

Osmometry

Cooling Pure Water. The basis of laboratory determination is briefly summarized in this section. At a constant rate of cooling, pure water shows three phases on the temperature chart. The initial phase shows a straight downward slope (A in Fig. 5.3). When the temperature reaches $0°C$, the slope becomes a plateau on account of crystallization (B in Fig. 5.3), which in turn indicates that some energy has been released—in the form of heat. This temporarily nullifies the cooling process and so the actual temperature recorded remains stationary for a while. Nevertheless, when the crystallization process is complete the cooling, which continues steadily, then permits

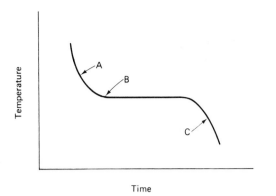

Figure 5.3 Freezing curve of a pure solvent (for explanation see text).

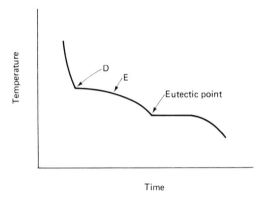

Figure 5.4 Freezing curve of a pure solution (for explanation see text).

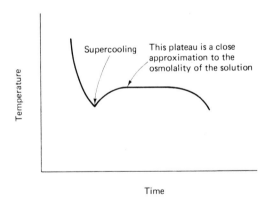

Figure 5.5 Freezing curve of plasma containing its many solutes (for explanation see text).

the temperature chart to resume its downward trend. (C in Fig. 5.3).

Cooling a Simple Solution. In the case of a solution, it is only the solvent that freezes—the solute is already 'solid'. When such a simple solution is exposed to a constant rate of cooling, freezing first occurs far away from the particles surrounded by their shells of solvent. The solvent thus commences to crystallize.

This is accompanied by a sharp decrease in the rate of cooling, on account of energy release in the form of heat (D in Fig. 5.4). The result is that the solute concentration rises as the particles are squeezed into the liquid that remains. As the concentration rises, there is in consequence even greater depression of the freezing point. A hyperbolic curve appears on the cooling chart at this point (E in Fig. 5.4).

The concentration continues to increase steadily as more and more ice is formed. Eventually the solubility limit is reached (eutectic point), and as more solvent is frozen, the solute continues to precipitate out at a steady rate.

Cooling Plasma. Different solutes have different eutectic temperatures. Therefore, the cooling curve of plasma, with its many solutes, is incredibly complex. In laboratory practice the situation is solved, however, by use of 'supercooling'. This process allows a solution to be cooled a little way below its true freezing point, without it actually freezing—this applies only if the solution is absolutely motionless. As soon as movement occurs, usually evoked by sudden vibration of a stirring rod, freezing commences and heat of crystallization is released. Freezing and thawing rapidly proceed in this blanket of slush, and the practical result is a plateau on the temperature chart. The temperature of this plateau can be used to calculate a close approximation to the osmolality of the solution (i.e. plasma) (Fig. 5.5).

Quantitative Aspects of Concentration
In the normal state, about 1000 mosmol of solute must be excreted in the urine each day. This solute is derived from breakdown of ingested nutrients, and from metabolic processes within the body. These end-products are normally excreted as a concentrated solution. Such is the concentrating ability of the renal tubular system, however, that in the normal adult, about 1 L of water is required for this purpose in each 24-h period. This concentration of approximately 1000 mosmol/kg is about three times the osmolality of normal serum. In the fasting state, the solute load requiring excretion may fall to less than half, i.e. to about 400 mosmol. Even this amount demands a urine volume of at least 400 mL for successful excretion. Extrarenal losses of water cannot be reduced to below 500 mL in 24 h.

Lesser degrees of concentrating ability are shown by the immature renal system in infancy. In addition, concentration is impaired in the renal system of elderly people, and in certain disease processes involving the kidney in adult life.

As the osmolality of serum is normally between 280 and 290 mosmol/kg, there is clearly a marked osmotic gradient between it and urine (perhaps 1000 mosmol/kg as discussed above). In fact, physiological extremes of water intake can vary the urine osmolality between 50 and almost 1500 mosmol/kg. This gradient is an expression of concentrating ability, and it diminishes with the onset of renal disease and with ageing. Eventually, in disease of the kidney, no gradient at all may exist, at which point the individual becomes unable to elevate the urine osmolality much beyond the upper limit of osmolality of normal serum. This level is around 290 mosmol/kg and equates approximately with the oft-quoted urinary specific gravity figure of 1.010. The implication behind this is that at least three times the normal volume of urine is required in order to perform excretion of the 1000 mosmol of solute by the renal system each day. The increased urine excretion that follows would lead to rapid dehydration of the body, but the onset of thirst prevents this, providing there is free availability of fluid. A mild degree of dehydration has in effect thereby stimulated the hypothalamic osmoreceptors, and polydipsia has averted further dehydration.

In the normal individual, urine achieves greater concentration overnight than during the course of the day. This ability is lost early in chronic renal disease. The consequence is the onset of nocturia, simply because the bladder cannot comfortably retain all the urine until the normal waking hour.

There are other pathological states, however, in which the osmotic load presented to the renal tubular system is greater than normal, i.e. in excess of the normal 1000 mosmol of solute per day. Diabetes mellitus is the classical example of this, in which case the urine contains large quantities of glucose, some extra electrolytes, and more water than normal.

Osmolal Clearance and Free Water Clearance

The concept of osmolal clearance and free water clearance is helpful for the understanding not only of the effect of AVP on renal tubular reabsorption of water but also of the clinical situations which can arise.

In any individual, the urine volume over 24 h is equal to the sum of osmolal clearance and free water clearance. Osmolal clearance (C_{osm}) is defined as the volume of water which is required simply to dissolve the solutes present in the urine in a solution isosmotic with plasma. If more water is present in the urine than meets this requirement, then the excess is defined as free water clearance (CH_2O). If, however, less water is present than that able to maintain the urinary solutes isosmotic with plasma, then free water clearance achieves a negative value.

During water diuresis, a high positive figure is obtained for free water clearance. In antidiuresis, however, a negative value indicates that solute-free water has been absorbed, and that the urine is more concentrated than plasma with reference to osmolality. Where there is an osmotic diuresis, there will be a rise of osmolal clearance. However, should this occur at the same time as a decrease of free water clearance, through the influence of AVP on the kidney, then total urine flow may be slightly reduced or even continue to rise—thus masking the AVP effect.

Thirst

Several physiological stimuli contribute to production of the sensation of thirst.[7] Increase in osmolality of body fluids is the main one of these.[8] It is equally effective whether there is administration of salt in excess of water, or whether there is loss of water in excess of salt; both will produce hyperosmolality. Moreover, in experimental circumstances, rapid onset of thirst occurs when hypertonic solutions of sodium chloride are administered. The high osmotic pressure thus produced in the circulation leads to withdrawal of fluid from the intracellular compartment of the body. Thirst develops, and drinking persists until the osmolality of the extracellular fluid again reverts to normal. The opposite occurs when plasma is diluted—in this case there is inhibition of thirst.

Another factor involved in thirst control is the volume of extracellular fluid. When this is decreased, there is generation of intense thirst. It is the low extracellular fluid volume, rather than lack of water itself, that is responsible. Animal experiments confirm this—deprivation of salt over a long period leads to reduction of extracellular fluid osmolality. Thirst is the consequence, and relief is obtained when the normal extracellular fluid volume is restored after giving enough sodium chloride.

In the rat, it has been found that more than 30% blood loss must occur before water intake rises above that of control animals. In man and animals, other studies with lesser degrees of blood loss have produced no consistent effects on thirst. Where drinking does ensue, however, it is found to be accompanied by elevation of plasma angiotensin II. Hence it is via activation of the renin–angiotensin system, rather than by reduced stimulation of the distension receptors in the left atrium and pulmonary veins, that thirst is so stimulated.

Extracellular and intracellular dehydration may lead to a 'dry mouth', which is relieved by drinking; but a 'dry mouth' may also be due to atropine administration. In this instance there is, of course, no change of extracellular or intracellular volume. Nevertheless drinking may occur, although it is not based on the usual sensation known as thirst. It is merely the discomfort of a dry mouth that produces drinking via a non-thirst mechanism.

Other factors influencing thirst include exposure of mucosal surfaces of the mouth, pharynx and oesophagus to water, and gastric distension, both of which temporarily reduce further intake. Changes in mood and emotion can also modify physiological stimuli controlling thirst in various ways. Lesions of certain parts of the hypothalamus may induce adipsia or hypodipsia. Moreover, electrical stimulation in the appropriate cerebral areas is known in experimental animals to arouse the sensation of thirst.

There may be a reduction in, or even absence of, thirst in the elderly, with the consequence of dehydration; however, at this time of life there may also be a lessened ability to concentrate the urine.[9] On the other hand, giving too much fluid can produce overhydration and hyponatraemia. The lowered threshold for thirst in pregnancy and during the luteal phase of the menstrual cycle may contribute to fluid retention at these times.

Temporary Relief of Thirst by Drinking
In a thirsting individual, there is prompt relief in response to the drinking of water—especially if cold. This relief occurs before water is absorbed into the circulation from the gastrointestinal tract. Thirst may return, however, after a very short while.

Entry of water to the gastrointestinal system, moreover, distends the gut, and the temporary relief of thirst may continue. In fact, distension of the stomach with a balloon can alone relieve thirst for up to 30 min.

The basis of the development of such a mechanism must surely be the prevention of overhydration, in response to thirst. It takes perhaps up to 1 h for water to be absorbed into the circulation and to reach the extracellular fluid. Should excessive drinking occur on account of thirst, there would necessarily be the danger of overdilution of body fluids.

Experimental Aspects Relating to Thirst
Experimental insertion of a balloon into the inferior vena cava of a dog has thrown more light on the thirst mechanism. If the balloon is inflated 24 h later, when the animal has fully recovered from the anaesthetic, there will be dimunution of blood return to the right atrium. Ten minutes later, drinking commences; it has been shown that the greater the fall of arterial pressure, the greater the amount of water drunk. If the balloon is left inside the inferior vena cava for several days, it can be shown that fluid intake on days when it is inflated is twice as much as on days when it is deflated.

The renin–angiotensin system has been shown to be the physiological mechanism responsible. Moreover, urine flow falls in these circumstances, and the dog, in fact, drinks itself eventually into a state of water excess.

Osmoreceptors
Early experiments yielding proof of the control of water balance by a cerebral sensory mechanism were carried out on dogs. It was suggested at that time that the cerebral receptors were stimulated by hypertonic solutions of sodium salts, sucrose and fructose flowing past them, but not by urea or D-glucose. The latter two substances equilibrate with the intracellular fluid and therefore cause no osmotic difference. However, the first three substances mentioned do not equilibrate quickly. An osmotic difference is thereby created between the interior and exterior of these cells. Dehydration of the intracellular compartment follows the passage of water from the cells towards

the newly hypertonic extracellular fluid. Hence the conclusion was that the receptors were stimulated by reduction of their own volume.

The subcellular basis of osmoreception is the presence of vesicles within neural cells of the supraoptic nuclei. They enlarge when the osmolality of extracellular fluid is less than that of intracellular fluid, and they decrease in size when the situation is reversed.

Should the concentration of osmotically active substances in the extracellular fluids rise significantly, these osmoreceptors in the supraoptic nucleus of the hypothalamus will thereby be stimulated. Neural impulses are then sent to the posterior pituitary gland where AVP is released, causing increased water absorption in the distal tubules and collecting ducts of the kidney. Osmotic stimuli are probably amongst the most important factors controlling AVP in physiological circumstances; however, a number of other factors can also influence its secretion.

Osmoregulation
Experiments involving intravenous infusion of hypertonic sodium chloride, during which plasma osmolality and AVP measurements are taken, permit the calculation of threshold values at which thirst is abolished (*see* Fig. 5.6). In normal individuals, plasma AVP is not detectable at plasma osmolality values of less than 284 mosmol/kg, and thirst is not experienced at plasma osmolality levels of less than 286 mosmol/kg. For every pmol/L rise in plasma AVP, up to a level of 6 pmol/L, the urinary osmolality value will rise by approximately 200 mosmol/kg; at this level the plasma osmolality is about 298 mosmol/kg and urinary osmolality is maximal.

Precise water homeostasis in a healthy adult is achieved largely by regulation of the balance between AVP release (which limits renal loss of water) and thirst (the process that promotes water ingestion). The principal determinant of thirst is plasma osmolality. The osmoreceptor cells that sense osmolality are located in the anterior portion of the hypothalamus; they respond to very small changes in plasma osmolality by initiating secretion of AVP and encouraging intake of water. Fluctuations of more than 2% of the basal value for plasma osmolality are rarely seen.[10–12]

The functional characteristics of the osmoreceptors governing thirst and AVP release are similar. It is likely that they exist in close proximity; however, they are occasionally involved separately in disorders of osmoregulation.

Osmoregulatory changes in pregnancy, commencing in the early stages and maintained throughout, lead to decrease in plasma osmolality by up to 10 mosmol/kg.[13] Accompanying this are reductions in the thresholds at which thirst is experienced and at which AVP release occurs; these osmotic thresholds have thereby been lowered, but by an as yet unelucidated mechanism.[14] Water homeostasis is also altered

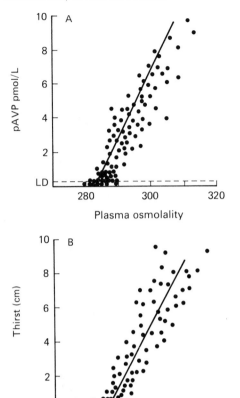

Figure 5.6 The relation between plasma osmolality (mOsm/kg) and plasma vasopressin (pAVP) in healthy man is shown in panel A, and is described by the regression line pAVP = 0.43(pOsm − 284.3), r = +0.92, p < 0.001. LD represents the limit of detection of AVP, 0.3 pmol/L (Rooke and Baylis, 1982). Panel B shows the relation between plasma osmolality and thirst and is defined by the regression line.
Thirst = 0.39 (pOsm − 285.8), r = +0.95, p < 0.001. *Modified from:* Thompson.[36]

in the elderly; they have a lessened capacity to excrete a water load.

The Renin–Angiotensin System
Renin is produced by the juxtaglomerular apparatus in the kidney. It circulates and acts on angiotensinogen in the blood to produce angiotensin I. Angiotensin-converting enzyme (ACE) then causes conversion of angiotensin I into angiotensin II. The latter in turn stimulates production of aldosterone by the adrenal cortex. In addition angiotensin II stimulates drinking and increases the blood pressure. A small portion of the angiotensin II is converted by angiotensinase A into angiotensin III, a heptapeptide; the physiological role of this compound is not yet clear.[15]

The first work claiming involvement of the renin-angiotensin system in the production of thirst was reported by Fitzsimons. Further work in the rat showed that intravenous infusion of angiotensin II produced thirst. More adventuresome application in the form of intracranial injection was found to stimulate short-term drinking even in rats that were well hydrated.

Angiotensin II, however, does not cross the blood-brain barrier, and therefore equilibrates only slowly with the interstitial fluid of brain tissue. The reason that this octapeptide can act so promptly following intravenous administration is that there are certain areas in the brain that lack this barrier. These areas are referred to as the circumventricular organs. In these areas, rapid action is likely on account of the more direct contact with blood constituents.[16]

The circulating angiotensin II is found to act at more than one such blood–brain barrier-free locus. These circumventricular organs include the area postrema, the subfornical organs, organum vasculosum and the neurohypophysis. The consequence of exposure of these areas to angiotensin II is elevation of blood pressure, secretion of AVP and ACTH, and drinking. It seems that one of the most sensitive of these areas is the subfornical organ, because the dose of angiotensin II that promotes drinking is less here than for other areas of the forebrain. Moreover, if this area is damaged selectively, intravenous angiotensin II is without any effect.

In the rat, as little as a few femtomoles of angiotensin II produces a brisk drinking response. This occurs within 1 min of injection, even if the animal is resting at the moment of the experiment. Drinking may continue up to 10 min later, and the effect is so marked that the volume imbibed in that time can reach the normal 24-h intake for the animal.

Saralasin has been shown to block the action of angiotensin II at the receptor site. Injection of this compound leads to reduction of water intake in the hour following administration, compared with the 1-h period prior to the dose.

The main site of sensitivity to angiotensin II in the brain is the subfornical organ; the vascular organ of the lamina terminalis is also responsive to it. These two sites are now recognized as the two dipsogenic areas, and are both outside the blood–brain barrier.

Angiotensin II. The molecular structure of angiotensin II is as follows:

$$\text{Asp–Arg–Val–Tyr–Ile–His–Pro–Phe}$$
$$1 \quad 2 \quad 3 \quad 4 \quad 5 \quad 6 \quad 7 \quad 8$$

It has been shown that amino acids 3–8 inclusive comprise the minimum length necessary for full biological activity. The terminal phenylalanine is essential for stimulation of the receptor site. The N-terminal aspartic acid contributes to binding and also influences duration of action. Arginine also contributes to the binding process. Amino acids 3 (valine), 5 (isoleucine), and 7 (proline), all possess side-chains that help to stabilize the secondary structure of the

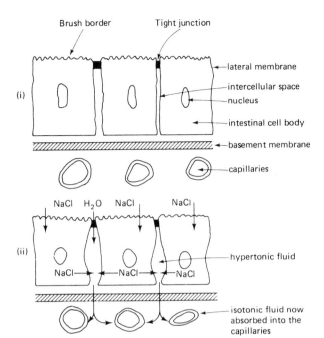

Figure 5.7 Colonic absorption of water, showing the normal sequence of events. Sodium chloride is absorbed into the intestinal cells. Following this there is transverse passage through the lateral borders of the cells, thus creating a hypertonic state. Water is now osmotically attracted into this hypertonic fluid, and thus forces itself through the tight junctions between the cells. The intercellular fluid now becomes isotonic; the elevated hydrostatic pressure thus developed aids absorption of water into the capillaries below.
Modified from: Krejs G.J., Fordtran J.A. (1978). Physiology and pathophysiology of ion and water movement in the human intestine. In *Gastrointestinal Disease; Pathophysiology, Diagnosis and Management.* (Sleisenger M.H., Fordtran J.A., eds). London: W. B. Saunders, pp. 297–330.

whole sequence. Amino acid 4 (tyrosine) and 6 (histidine) are functional groups that are essential for binding to the receptor site.

Water Absorption

Absorption of fluid by the intestinal tract is almost complete in normal circumstances. Most of this takes place in the small intestine.

Small Intestinal Absorption

Almost all of the approximately 9 L of fluid passing through the small intestine each day is absorbed there, at varying rates up to about 400 mL/h. The mechanism of absorption is very similar to that in the proximal tubules of the kidney.

Chyme leaves the stomach and enters the duodenum. It is almost isotonic with plasma at this point. Sodium, monosaccharides and amino acids in particular are actively absorbed, thus creating hypotonicity in the intestinal lumen. Water then rapidly diffuses

from this slightly hypotonic solution to the plasma. So rapid is this sequence of events that the luminal contents remain on the whole essentially isotonic, in spite of the absorption of large amounts of both solute and water.

Nevertheless, the intestinal lumen is permeable to water in both directions. In circumstances where there is high osmolality in the duodenum, water flows rapidly in the opposite direction, i.e. from the blood, to dilute this concentrated solution. Such a situation could arise where there is rapid digestion of relatively few large molecules, such as proteins and polysaccharides, to a large number of small molecules such as amino acids and monosaccharides. These small molecules will, of course, create much greater osmotic attraction for water. The result may be a marked fall of blood volume, with cardiovascular problems as the consequence.

Colonic Absorption

The main role of the colon is absorption of water and electrolytes during the onward passage of its contents. Absorption takes place throughout the whole length of the organ, although the major portion occurs on the right side.

There are a number of factors that act on the colon thereby influencing this absorption process; the concentration of sodium in the colonic fluid, togther with circulating AVP and aldosterone are three of them.

The transport of water in the intestine is a passive process, and occurs secondary to both osmotic and hydrostatic pressure gradients. These, in turn, are produced by the active transfer of solute.

Both sodium and chloride ions, for instance, are absorbed through the brush border into the columnar cells lining the intestinal tract. This is followed later by transverse passage through the lateral membranes into the hypertonic fluid lying between these cells (i.e. the intercellular space). This hypertonic fluid creates an osmotic gradient, so that water is directly attracted to it from the intestinal lumen. Water therefore forces itself between the cells through the tight junction at the distal ends of the cells, and thereby distends and dilutes the intercellular space. Elevated hydrostatic pressure has thus been created, following which the now isotonic fluid is absorbed through the basement membrane into the capillaries below. The intercellular space later becomes less tense, and the cell walls of adjacent cells return again to close proximity. The ingestion of fluids of varying tonicity can further impose osmotic gradients on this system (Fig. 5.7).

Adrenal cortical hormones influence electrolyte movement in the colon. Both the proximal and distal colon are able to absorb sodium, but only the distal portion is able to secrete potassium. This is in response to aldosterone.

AVP also has the effect of decreasing salt and water absorption in the colon in man.

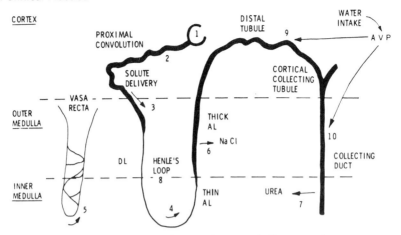

Figure 5.8 Diagram of a nephron to illustrate the factors that may influence urinary concentration. GFR (1), total solute concentration in the glomerular filtrate and proximal tubular reabsorption of sodium (2) together determine solute delivery (3) to the medullary countercurrent system. The latter's efficiency is reduced by increased flow rate through Henle's loop (4) or the vasa recta (5). Solute accumulation in the medulla depends chiefly on sodium reabsorption from the ascending limb (AL) (6) and urea absorption from the collecting duct (7). Changes in permeability of the descending limb (DL), distal tubule (9) or collecting duct (10) could affect urinary concentration. (9) and (10) are physiologically regulated by AVP, release of which is affected by water intake.
Modified from: Bissett G.W., Jones N.F. (1975). Antidiuretic hormone, in *Recent Advances in Renal Disease* (Jones N.F., ed.). *Edinburgh: Churchill Livingstone, pp. 350–416.*

Renal Function

The renal mechanisms by which urinary concentration is controlled are illustrated in Fig. 5.8.

The kidney consists basically of two parts—one is the filtration system, and the other the transport passages for the fluid so filtered. The glomerulus is the filtration unit, and there are approximately one million in each kidney. Continuous circulation of blood at the correct pressure through the glomeruli is necessary for their proper function. The filtration process takes place through the capillary network into which the afferent arteriole divides. On account of the fact that the major portion of the plasma proteins does not cross this filter, blood leaving the glomerulus via the efferent arteriole is more concentrated than that in the afferent arteriole.[17]

The composition of the fluid appearing at the commencement of the proximal tubule is almost identical with that of plasma except that it contains little if any protein, and there are no cells. Many substances in the filtrate are required by the body, and are reabsorbed readily in the tubular system. In addition there is excretion directly into the lumen of other substances not needed. As the fluid flows along the tubules, there is change not only of composition, but also of volume. The urine eventually formed collects in the bladder, which is the temporary storage organ, and from which it is voided periodically.

The membrane lining the proximal tubule and descending limb of the loop of Henle is very permeable to water, which is absorbed here in proportion to the solute that is also reabsorbed. The distal tubule and collecting ducts of the kidney are, however, controlled very differently. They are sometimes permeable to water, and sometimes not—depending on the amount of AVP in the body fluids. AVP causes increased absorption of water at these two sites.

There is control also in the distal part of this system by aldosterone and cortisone. These two hormones act on the collecting ducts to increase sodium absorption, at the same time promoting potassium loss.

Reabsorption of Water in the Proximal Tubule

Reabsorption of water in this part is a passive process along an osmotic gradient. Such a gradient is created in the proximal tubule of the kidney by active reabsorption of solutes, such as sodium and glucose. As referred to earlier, this process is similar to absorption in the small intestine. The walls of the proximal tubule are therefore freely permeable to water. As seen from Table 5.3, 140–150 L of the total 180 L filtered each day at the glomeruli are absorbed in this very vascular area; this equates with approx. 80% of the glomerular filtrate. The bloodstream carries the absorbed substances away rapidly, and distributes them as required.

Reabsorption of Water in the Loop of Henle

Of the 180 L of glomerular filtrate formed each day, approximately 35 L pass through to the descending limb of the loop of Henle. It will be seen from Table 5.3 that 75% of this is absorbed in the descending limb, thus leaving 25% to flow through the ascending limb where there is no water absorption—but where there is absorption of solute.

TABLE 5.3
RENAL BLOOD FLOW AND THE VOLUMES OF FLUID PASSING
DIFFERENT POINTS IN THE RENAL TUBULAR SYSTEM OF A
NORMAL INDIVIDUAL DURING THE COURSE OF 24 H

	mL per minute	L/24 h
Renal blood flow	1200	1800.0
Glomerular filtrate	120	180.0
Distal end of proximal tubule	24	35.0
Distal end of descending limb of the loop of Henle	6	10.0
Distal end of ascending limb of the loop of Henle	6	10.0
Urine	1	1.5

The descending limb. Isosmotic reabsorption of water in the proximal tubule means that fluid of the same osmolality as plasma enters the descending limb of the loop of Henle. This is about 280–290 mosmol/kg. By means of countercurrent multiplication, high osmolality is achieved at the distal end of the descending limb, on account of passage of sodium from the ascending to the descending limb during the onward progression of fluid. Furthermore, osmotic equilibrium is achieved between the fluid contents of the distal portion of the descending limb and the surrounding medullary tissue and blood vessels. Figure 5.9 displays the typical relationships.

The ascending limb. Osmolality of the fluid in the ascending limb is very high at the junction with the descending limb, but decreases rapidly distally. No water is absorbed in the ascending limb, but sodium absorption does occur.

Effects of AVP on the Distal Tubules and Collecting Ducts

In the distal tubules and collecting ducts of the kidney, presence of AVP is necessary for water absorption to take place. Furthermore, the renal tubule at this point must be sensitive to it, for it to work properly. Even when maximal quantities of AVP are present, a large volume passing through the distal tubules and collecting ducts will produce a water diuresis. This may occur, for example, in hyperglycaemia, uraemia or following mannitol administration. Other disorders where there is gross tissue damage may lead to protein breakdown to amino acids, and consequently to urea elevation. Osmotic diuresis and water depletion may follow. Intravenous feeding may be excessively administered, thereby leading to high production of urea from the amino acids, and hence osmotic diuresis.

AVP alters the permeability of the distal tubular system to water. Without AVP, permeability is absent, and the consequence is that hypotonic fluid leaves the renal system, and eventually a dilute urine is passed. If, however, AVP is present, there is opportunity for water to be reabsorbed as the permeability rises. Hence water passes across an osmotic gradient towards the hypertonic interstitial fluid in the medulla, and thence to the bloodstream.

This countercurrent exchange process displayed in Fig. 5.9 is seen to involve passage of water into the

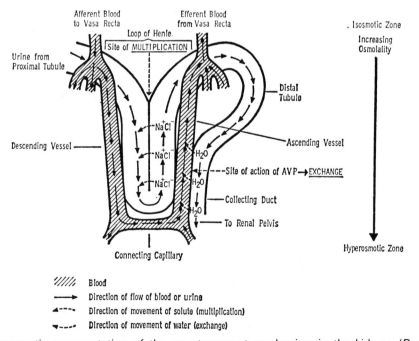

Figure 5.9 Diagrammatic representation of the countercurrent mechanism in the kidney. (Reproduced by kind permission from *Clinical Chemistry in Diagnosis and Treatment* (3rd edn, 1988), by Zilva J.F., Pannall P.R., and Mayne P.D. London: Edward Arnold.)

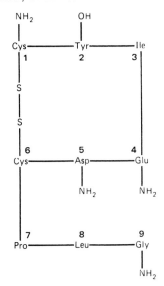

Figure 5.10 Amino acid sequence of oxytocin.

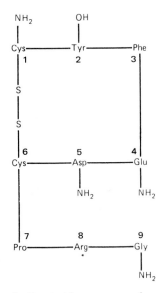

Figure 5.11 Amino acid sequence of arginine vasopressin. In lysine vasopressin, there is merely interchange of lysine with arginine (*).

ascending vasa recta along the osmotic gradient previously determined by countercurrent multiplication.

In the normal individual, AVP concentrates the urine, and in return plasma is diluted. The elderly have a reduced ability to concentrate the urine.

Arginine Vasopressin

The role of AVP is that of conservation of water. In the intact animal, however, it is clear that in intracellular dehydration, the more important aspect is to take in water, rather than only to conserve what is already there.[18]

The mechanism of increased absorption of water is by increase of pore size in the collecting ducts, sufficiently large for water, but not other solutes, to pass through.

AVP is produced by the hypothalamus and stored in the posterior pituitary gland. Its release is affected by a number of factors, and furthermore, its peripheral action can actually be impaired in certain circumstances.

Chemical Structure

There are similarities in the sequences of amino-acid residues of oxytocin, arginine vasopressin, and lysine vasopressin (Figs. 5.10 and 5.11). Lysine-vasopressin occurs in the pig and some related animals, whereas arginine vasopressin is the antidiuretic hormone in man. A number of analogues have now been prepared synthetically, and these have been used both for research and therapeutically. Both vasopressin and oxytocin have molecular weights of around 1000 Daltons.

Neurophysins

The human pituitary gland has been shown to contain at least two neurophysins, H–Np I and H–Np II, both with a molecular weight of just over 10 000 Daltons. These proteins bind vasopressin and oxytocin within the neurosecretory granules where they form in the supraoptic and paraventricular nuclei of the hypothalamus. It has been suggested that binding of neurophysins and hormones in the granules, through a weak non-covalent bond, serves as a means of decreasing the osmotic effect of the hormones.

With reference to Fig. 5.11, it is seen that the sequence of the first six amino-acid residues in the vasopressins form a ring structure. The ring is closed by means of a disulphide bond (–S–S–) between the two hemicystine (Cys) residues (amino-acid residues 1 and 6). It is known that the terminal NH_2 group of this hemicystine residue is not required for biological activity of the molecule. However, it is the means by which it binds to neurophysin, with the aid also of secondary hydrophobic bonds involving residues 2 and 3.

It seems likely that one neurophysin is associated with each hormone. Also, it is probable that the splitting of a large precursor substance gives rise to neurophysin and hormone.

Neurophysins have also been detected in tumours that have been shown to produce vasopressin, the implication of this being that both are actively produced within the neoplastic cells.

Site of Synthesis

There are neurosecretory cells in the hypothalamus— in the supraoptic nucleus and the magnocellular part of the paraventricular nucleus. These cells secrete vasopressin, oxytocin and the neurophysins. The last are the carrier proteins for the two hormones. Nerve endings of these neurosecretory cells are found in the median eminence, the infundibular stem, and the infundibular process (the neural lobe of the hypophysis).

Neurosecretion with reference to AVP is not a new concept. Indeed, the brain is now recognized to be one large neurosecretory unit, each neuron within it producing one or more neurotransmitter and/or neuromodulatory substances. These can be of many types and are largely peptide, amino acid, or amine in nature. Secretion of AVP is no longer to be regarded therefore as a strange and unique property of certain neural structures—secretion is the means by which all neurons communicate with each other, and with more distant structures of the body.

Transport and Storage

As the hormones in their neurosecretory granules, and in combination with neurophysins, travel down the axons from the hypothalamus to the pituitary gland, dissociation takes place; hence they become more concentrated.

Mechanisms Controlling AVP Secretion

Numerous neurotransmitter substances within the neurohypophysis are involved in the control of AVP release; however, the precise mechanisms are, as yet, not clearly defined.[19] Biogenic amines, amino acids and opioid peptides all play a part. These neurotransmitters are the means by which neural inputs, from both the cardiovascular system and central osmoreceptors, are relayed. Coordination of these inputs occurs within the hypothalamus, brainstem and neurohypophysis. All these inputs, positively or negatively, ultimately influence AVP release. Urinary prostaglandins show a marked increase after chronic administration of AVP.[20]

Stimulation. A multiplicity of factors is involved in release of vasopressin from its storage sites. One of the most sensitive mechanisms, and the one that is of major importance in physiological conditions, is detection of increased plasma osmolality. A very small increase of sodium is detectable by the thirst centre. In fact, a rise of as little as 2 mmol/L (i.e. approximately 1–2%) suffices to produce a marked increase in AVP output.[21]

Other factors are able to influence AVP secretion in different circumstances. Decrease of extracellular volume, hypotension, and decreased circulating volume, are three such factors. The last of these can be a very potent stimulus to AVP secretion—so potent that it can even override inhibition of AVP secretion caused by low osmolar states. Experiments in man and non-human primates reveal that a deficit of approximately 10% of the blood volume must occur before elevation of plasma AVP becomes detectable. There is evidence which implicates receptors in the region of the carotid bifurcation and in the left atrium in this process; this was referred to earlier.

Increase of AVP is noted in response to muscle pain, during emotional and mental stress, and in nausea and vomiting. All can be associated with antidiuresis. Physiological studies reveal diurnal variation, i.e. AVP secretion is increased at night, during exercise, and in the erect posture.

The nicotine test for stimulating AVP has been in use for many years, and in smokers, maximal stimulation of AVP occurs immediately after smoking. Many other drugs have now been implicated as interfering with AVP mechanisms, and the list is a growing one. Drugs and pharmacological agents that have been reported to stimulate AVP release include acetylcholine, barbiturates, bradykinin, chlorpropamide, cinchoninic acid, chlorthalidone, clofibrate, ether, ferritin, hydrochlorothiazide, methylclothiazide, morphine, nicotine, and polythiazide.[22] Carbamazepine and thioridazine may also stimulate hypo-osmolar states, but in the former instance there is some controversy regarding the mechanism of action. It is possible that there is potentiation of the action of AVP on the renal tubular system, or perhaps there is increased secretion from the posterior pituitary gland, or there may be a combination of both. However, the hypo-osmolar state reverts to normal on cessation of the drug. Chlorpropamide also potentiates the peripheral action of AVP on the renal tubule (Table 5.4).

Inhibition. Inhibition of AVP release occurs in hypo-osmolar states, elevation of extracellular fluid volume and also during exposure to ethyl alcohol. Although the effect with alcohol is weak, a marked diuresis usually follows ingestion of large quantities.

Inhibition of the peripheral action of AVP occurs in hypercalcaemia, hypokalaemia, and in states of prolonged overhydration. The peripheral action of AVP on the renal tubule is inhibited also by lithium carbonate and by demeclocycline, both of which have been used therapeutically in the syndrome of inappropriate diuresis (SIAD). The causes of this syndrome are outlined in Table 5.4. Aspects of drug-induced diabetes insipidus are recorded in Table 5.5; and a list of drugs with antidiuretic properties in Table 5.6.

Molecular Action on Distal Tubules and Collecting Ducts

AVP has been shown to act on certain receptive structures in the renal system, when it is present in the link peritubular fluid. It has no effect, however, when introduced directly into the tubular lumen.

The clinical effect of AVP may be detected as soon as 2–4 min following intravenous injection. It probably binds to receptor cells by means of covalent linkages between its own disulphide bridges (involving the cystine residues of the molecule) and sulphydryl radicals on the cell surface.

In common with many other hormones, AVP acts by way of the cyclic AMP system. Having combined with the receptor site, it then activates membrane-bound adenylate cyclase, which promptly converts ATP into adenosine 3′, 5′-monophosphate (cyclic AMP, cAMP), and pyrophosphate. In turn, cAMP is

TABLE 5.4

CAUSES OF THE SYNDROME OF INAPPROPRIATE ANTIDIURESIS
(SIAD)

1. *Tumours* (presumed ectopic production of AVP)
   Carcinoma of lung (especially oat-cell tumours)
   Carcinoma of pancreas
   Carcinoma of duodenum
   Carcinoma of suprarenal gland
   Carcinoma of prostate
   Carcinoma of ureter
   Thymoma
2. *SIAD from Probable Neurohypophyseal Dysfunction*
   Meningitis (pyogenic and tuberculous)
   Encephalitis
   Brain abscess
   Cerebral tumours
   Subarachnoid haemorrhage
   Subdural haematoma
   Head injury
   Cerebrovascular disease
   Central pontine myelinolysis
   Guillain–Barré syndrome
   Acute intermittent porphyria
   Systemic lupus erythematosus with focal cerebro-
   vascular disease
3. *Thoracic Disease*
   Pulmonary tuberculosis
   Pneumonia—bacterial, viral and fungal
   Cardiac surgery
   ? Positive pressure ventilation
4. *Endocrine Disorders*
   Addison's disease
   Myxoedema
   Hypopituitarism
5. *Drugs*
   Chlorpropamide
   Thiazide diuretics
   Carbamazepine
   Vincristine
   Cyclophosphamide
   Clofibrate*
   Metformin*
6. *Miscellaneous Conditions* (cause unknown)
   Hodgkin's disease
   Acute myeloid leukaemia
7. *SIAD Associated with Non-osmotic 'Physiological' Stimuli*
   Hypovolaemia
   Hypotension
   Pain
   Surgery
   Trauma
8. *Oedematous States in which SIAD may play a part*
   Congestive cardiac failure
   Hepatic cirrhosis with ascites
   Nephrotic syndrome

*These drugs have been shown to have actions that could lead to SIAD but the syndrome has yet to be described in patients receiving them.

From: Bisset G.W., Jones N.F. (1975). Antidiuretic hormone. In *Recent Advances in Renal Disease* (Jones N.F., ed.), Edinburgh: Churchill Livingstone.

TABLE 5.5

PHARMACOLOGICALLY INDUCED DIABETES INSIPIDUS

Posterior Pituitary Gland
Suppression of AVP release
  Phenytoin sodium

Renal Tubules
Interference with AVP action
  Lithium carbonate
  Demethylchlortetracycline
  Methoxyfluorane

TABLE 5.6

DRUGS POSSESSING ANTIDIURETIC PROPERTIES

Stimulation of AVP Secretion
Narcotics
  Morphine, other opiates
Hypnotics
  Barbiturates
Oral hypoglycaemics
  Chlorpropamide, tolbutamide
Anticonvulsants
  Carbamazepine
Antineoplastics
  Cyclophosphamide, vinblastine, vincristine
Antidepressants
  Amitryptiline
Miscellaneous
  Clofibrate, isoprenaline, nicotine derivatives

Potentiation of Action of AVP
Oral hypoglycaemics
  Chlorpropamide
Analgesics
  Paracetamol
Anti-inflammatory compound
  Indomethacin

Modified from Walmsley and Guerin.[39]

the active component that induces membrane permeability for water. Excess cAMP is, however, converted into adenosine 5'-monophosphate (5'-AMP) by means of the enzyme phosphodiesterase (Fig. 5.12). It is possible to inhibit phosphodiesterase by theophylline and other related xanthines, thereby prolonging the cellular action of cAMP.

Consequences of Imbalance of Water Homeostasis

Excessive Water Intake

Where there is a high water-load, dilution of the extracellular fluid occurs. In consequence there is a fall of osmolality and this leads to inhibition of AVP release. As the distal tubules and collecting ducts are not now permeable to water, countercurrent multiplication must necessarily occur without countercurrent exchange (*see* Fig. 5.9). A dilute urine is thereby produced. The increase of blood volume on account of the excessive water intake causes the renal blood

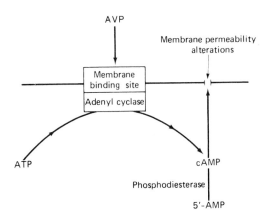

Figure 5.12 Molecular action of AVP. AVP binds with the membrane binding site, and this leads directly to activation of adenyl cyclase. This in turn converts ATP into cAMP, which mediates membrane permeability changes. Phosphodiesterase is required for conversion of cAMP into 5'-AMP.

flow to increase, thereby causing some dilution of the normally high osmolality in the medullary region (distal portion of the descending limb of the loop of Henle). This solute is then absorbed into the circulating blood and compensates for the decreased osmolality caused by drinking.

Therefore, at the same time as extra water is lost in the urine, more solute is absorbed into the circulation to compensate for the decreased osmolality of the extracellular fluid caused by the initial high water intake.

Decreased Water Intake

Decreased water intake leads to increased osmolality of the plasma, and decreased volume of the extracellular fluid. Both factors lead to AVP production. Countercurrent exchange is thereby permitted in the distal tubules and collecting ducts of the kidney. The reduced blood volume leads to diminished flow through the vasa recta, and hence permits high medullary tonicity to develop through the process of countercurrent multiplication. The consequence is reduced urine volume and absorption of the water back into the circulation, thereby again tending to increase blood volume.

Osmotic Diuresis

Proximal tubular absorption of water is a passive process. It occurs along an osmotic gradient created by solute absorption; sodium is the main contributor to this. If, however, solute is present in the glomerular filtrate, in such a high amount that it cannot be fully absorbed (e.g. glucose in diabetes mellitus), or not as fully absorbed as usual (e.g. urea in chronic renal failure), then the osmotic effect all the way down the renal tubular system will cause increased water excretion.

Furthermore, if a pharmacological agent such as

mannitol is administered, this is passed freely into the glomerular filtrate. Mannitol cannot significantly be reabsorbed actively or passively in the proximal tubule, and hence its osmotic effect causes retention of a greater amount of water than normal in the lumen. The fluid in the tubule is still isosmotic with plasma, however, largely on account of the presence of mannitol, but with a small contribution from sodium. This high volume proceeds along the whole length of the tubular system. It flows through the distal tubules and collecting ducts in greater amounts than can be absorbed there, thus causing a diuresis.

CLINICAL ASPECTS

The preceding account, including discussion on the physiological background, has been provided with the purpose of bringing into perspective each of the clinical disorders to be documented in this section. It has been seen that mechanisms responsible for maintaining water homeostasis involve a sequence of biochemical and physiological pathways utilizing feedback processes. Abnormalities may occur at any point along the line. Polyuria, polydipsia, adipsia, hypodipsia, and the SIAD all occur.[23] Reference to each of these will be made; the less common disorders are not only interesting, but study of them further aids the more complete understanding of normal homeostasis.

Polydipsia can, of course, occur apart from polyuria (often defined as a 24-h urinary output in excess of 2 L, or of 30 mL/kg in 24 h). Satisfaction of thirst may not produce polyuria if dehydration is sufficiently gross initially. Moreover, polyuria may exist in the absence of polydipsia. This can be seen, for instance, in a patient overenthusiastically transfused with intravenous fluid. He may develop polyuria, but his own desire to drink may be suppressed.

However, there are other disorders in which there is both polyuria and polydipsia. There is more than one way in which these conditions may be classified. There is the basic physiological approach, as taken in this text already, in which each of the processes in the circuit is discussed in turn. In some cases, clinical disorders are found to have only one fault in the whole urinary concentrating mechanism, and hence fit this classification neatly. However, many conditions show more than one abnormality, and hence the alternative approach is a more clinical classification. This has merit on account of the fact that it partially overcomes the problem to which reference has just been made. The latter classification, therefore, is the one that will be used in this section. Each disorder will be elaborated upon in turn, and opportunity will be taken to draw attention, where required, to the faulty biochemical and/or physiological mechanism(s) responsible.

Primary Polyuria and Secondary Polydipsia

The normal urinary volume of an adult is approximately 1–2 L/24 h, depending on fluid intake, environmental temperature and other factors. Should the volume exceed 2 L/24 h (or 30 mL/kg in 24 h), then this would generally be regarded as being polyuria; it could, of course, be physiological or pathological, and in either case might be temporary or long-standing. Measurement of urinary osmolality permits further subdivision of polyuria; if the osmolality is less than 200 mosmol/kg, then this is compatible with 'water diuresis', whereas if the osmolality is around 300 mosmol/kg, then this equates with 'solute diuresis'.

Water diuresis means water loss in excess of solute, and would imply an appropriate, or possibly inappropriate, response involving the AVP–renal tubular axis, or perhaps defective ability of AVP to act distally, i.e. at the level of the distal tubules and/or collecting ducts. Solute diuresis means solute loss as well as loss of water, with osmolality similar to that of serum; this would most likely imply that there was loss of sodium, urea or glucose, in addition to water.

Diabetes Mellitus

Diabetes mellitus is the foremost example of obligatory excretion of a solute load. The glucose content of the proximal tubular fluid exceeds the capacity of the cells to reabsorb it. Osmotic retention of water in the tubular lumen occurs; the high osmotic pressure overrides the capacity of the AVP mechanism more distally to absorb water. Glucose appears in the urine, together with extra sodium, chloride, and water. Dehydration follows the polyuria, and thirst is the consequence. Glycosuria is, of course, a feature not only of diabetes mellitus, but also of non-ketotic hyperosmolar coma. Both disorders will lead to osmotic diuresis.

Renal Disorders

The nephron is the basic unit of the kidney, and comprises the glomerulus and renal tubule. Disease processes responsible for chronic renal failure may not only involve different parts of the nephron, but may involve different nephrons in varying degree. Glomerular involvement restricts the filtration process. On account of continued protein catabolism, however, retention of urea occurs. Nevertheless, some nephrons may not be damaged at all, and as the plasma urea concentration rises, so does the amount of urea filtered by them into their proximal tubules. Osmotic imbalance is created, and hence retention of water in the tubular system results, with polyuria as the clinical outcome. In addition, some nephrons may display essentially tubular damage, rather than glomerular pathology; these tubules may reabsorb poorly and will also contribute to the osmotic diuresis referred to above.

Late chronic renal failure. In late chronic renal failure, there is reduced ability to conserve sodium. However, if dietary intake of sodium is normal, then no serious consequences ensue, but if there is persistent urinary sodium loss concurrent with restriction of intake, then reduction of extracellular fluid volume could occur. This event would secondarily lead to reduction of the glomerular filtration rate, and uraemia may be exacerbated.

Medullary cystic disease. Medullary cystic disease of the kidney also leads to urinary loss of sodium. However, in this disorder the sodium wasting is noted to occur, even in the presence of normal dietary intake. It is clear then, in this instance, that dietary supplements of sodium chloride should be taken.

Persistent obstruction of the genito-urinary tract. Persistent obstruction of the genito-urinary tract with progressive renal failure may present with polyuria. In the literature there are a number of reports in which such individuals, having been relieved of their obstruction, obtain alleviation not only of their renal insufficiency but also of their polyuria.

It is likely that there is a defect in the permeability of the collecting ducts to water, thereby simulating nephrogenic diabetes insipidus.

In patients with this disorder it has been found that relief of the polyuria and renal failure rapidly follows removal of the obstruction. The implication is that no organic damage has occurred, and that merely temporary functional changes are involved. Renal biopsies confirm that glomeruli and tubular epithelial cells are of normal appearance in these patients.

Relief of genito-urinary tract obstruction. Massive polyuria is well recognized following relief of obstruction in the genito-urinary tract.[24] The tubular damage that is present leads to defective sodium reabsorption. It is only when the obstruction has been relieved, however, that the glomerular filtrate, with its contained sodium, is permitted to test the absorptive capacity of the proximal tubule. Loss of salt and water occurs, and there is acute reduction of the extracellular fluid volume. Nevertheless, the tubular function usually recovers within a few days, and sodium absorption recommences.[22] The polyuria is therefore of short duration.

Renal transplantation. Following renal transplantation there is polyuria in some patients.[25] It is recognized that there are several possible causes of this, including fluid overload; osmotic diuresis related to retention of metabolites on account of uraemia; elevated blood glucose also giving rise to osmotic diuresis; moderate intraoperative tubular damage; and retention of preoperatively administered diuretics (e.g. frusemide).

Renal tubular dysfunction. Tubular dysfunction impairs the normal renal concentration and reabsorption processes. Amongst many functions, the countercurrent mechanisms will be disturbed, together with failure of sodium reabsorption in the proximal tubule. The latter is the essential cause of impaired water reabsorption at that level. Sodium and water are therefore lost in the urine. Nevertheless, depletion of body sodium is not likely to be great if the dietary sodium is adequate.

Predominantly tubular damage is present in the recovery phase of acute oliguric renal failure, which may in turn be due to prolonged untreated shock, or to exposure of the proximal tubule cells to toxic agents such as carbon tetrachloride. More slowly evolving disorders such as hypercalcaemia, hypokalaemia, and heavy-metal poisoning, will produce progressive damage to the tubules.

Oral ingestion of a soluble salt of mercury, for instance, leads to severe acute local inflammation at all points of contact. There is rapid onset of oral, pharyngeal, laryngeal and abdominal pain, together with nausea and vomiting within a few minutes. The mercury is absorbed into the body, and is excreted through the kidney where it is concentrated; it quickly damages the renal tubules. The consequence is a rapid onset of diuresis within 3 h of ingestion. Very soon, however, there is vomiting and dehydration, which leads to shock. In association with the progressive tubular damage, anuria and renal failure follow. Furthermore, mercury salts cause severe enteritis, with the onset of diarrhoea containing much blood. Uraemia is the usual cause of death.

Nephrogenic Diabetes Insipidus
This is caused by insensitivity of the distal tubules and collecting ducts of the kidney to AVP. It may be hereditary or acquired. Moreover, concentration of urine cannot be achieved following exposure to exogenously administered AVP; this is totally unlike the dramatic effect normally obtained in diabetes insipidus of cranial origin.

Familial nephrogenic diabetes insipidus is a very rare disorder. It is due to insensitivity of the renal tubules to AVP. Elevated concentrations of AVP have been shown in serum and urine of such patients. The biochemical basis is unknown, but two patients have been described in whom infusion of AVP did not lead to the normal rise of urinary cAMP. Moreover, cAMP injections in children with the disorder failed to cause the usual antidiuresis.

Acquired nephrogenic diabetes insipidus has a wide spectrum of causes ranging from naturally occurring diseases to administration of drugs. Renal disorders such as glomerulonephritis and pyelonephritis may cause it, as well as hydronephrosis, polyarteritis nodosa, amyloidosis, and infiltration of the kidney with myeloma tissue. Severe hypokalaemia renders the renal tubules unresponsive to AVP, and pathologically there is noted to be vacuolation of the renal

tubular cells. Hypercalcaemia leads to deposition of calcium in the renal tubular cells. Lithium carbonate therapy may also inhibit effective action of AVP on the renal tubules, thus producing a nephrogenic diabetes insipidus. Demeclocycline and methoxyflurane also interfere with the action of AVP.

Pharmacological agents probably interfere at two biochemical sites, namely with the normal ability of AVP to activate adenyl cyclase-mediated cAMP, and also with the initiation of reactions leading up to increased water permeability of the epithelial cells in the distal tubule and collecting ducts.

Hypercalcaemia. Hypercalcaemia is a particularly important cause clinically of nephrogenic diabetes insipidus. There is often loss of ability of the kidney to concentrate urine, prior to any structural damage being detectable microscopically. Later, calcification of the renal tubules can further add to the problems by causing inability to absorb water in sufficient amounts. Polyuria is the outcome, and polydipsia follows.

Lithium salts. Lithium carbonate therapy has been used in the treatment of manic depressive psychosis for a number of years. It is particularly efficacious in alleviating the manic phase. In addition, the drug has also been used in other disorders—carcinoma of the thyroid gland, thyrotoxicosis, Parkinson's disease, and inappropriate antidiuresis.

Over the years there have been reports of severe lithium intoxication leading to renal failure. Nevertheless, if serum concentrations of the drug are monitored regularly, this complication should not arise. However, experiments in animals, and observations in man, have both revealed the possibility of histological changes in the kidney following lithium exposure.

Early conclusions from the available evidence suggested that no serious side-effects would arise if the serum lithium concentration was maintained within the therapeutic range; this seems to be no longer true. It has been reported that a high proportion of patients taking oral lithium carbonate develop impairment of urinary concentration, even when serum lithium concentrations are within the therapeutic range.

Theoretically, several possible mechanisms underlying this syndrome have been considered. They include nephrogenic diabetes insipidus, cranial diabetes insipidus, and primary polydipsia.

In a series of 48 lithium-treated patients, 17 developed a urinary concentrating defect with serum lithium concentrations in the therapeutic range. Of these, 10 had nephrogenic diabetes insipidus, one had cranial diabetes insipidus, and the remainder could not be classified. There was no evidence of primary polydipsia in any of them. However, a recent study suggests that primary thirst may play a role in the expression of lithium-induced polyuria.[26]

Experiments on rats have revealed that the nephrogenic diabetes insipidus syndrome is associated with a defect in the renal production of cAMP in response to vasopressin.

In summary, therefore, lithium leads to inhibition of action of AVP on the renal tubules.

Sepsis. In patients with severe sepsis, inappropriate polyuria has been described on many occasions.[27] It can lead to severe hypovolaemia and hypotension. Physiological studies have revealed neither abnormalities of glomerular filtration rate, nor of renal blood flow. Giving such patients vasopressin injections has not prevented the polyuria. It seems, therefore, that diminished release of endogenous AVP is not the cause of this disorder. The basis is likely to be that of the effect of a toxin or of a toxic metabolic breakdown product, leading secondarily to impairment of sodium and water conservation. Another possibility was that the polyuria could represent self-protection, in the sense that there is requirement for the renal system to excrete an unidentified septic metabolite.[27]

Two patients with Gram-negative pneumonia have been documented in which hypotension was treated with intravenous dopamine hydrochloride.[28] Both patients developed polyuria with excessive loss of sodium in the urine. Dopamine hydrochloride normally has the advantage over adrenaline in that it produces increased cerebral, renal and mesenteric blood flow. However, in these two individuals it is possible that the dopamine may have enhanced the hypotension by increasing the diuresis, thereby leading to hypovolaemia. It was suggested that the Gram-negative infection might have played a significant part by enhancing the effect of the drug on the vasculature of the renal system.

Cranial Diabetes Insipidus

The pathological causes of cranial diabetes insipidus can be further subdivided according to the site of the lesion. This may be in the hypothalamus,[30] in the hypothalamo–hypophyseal tract, or in the posterior lobe of the pituitary gland.

In order for disease to be expressed clinically, there must be destruction of at least 80% of the AVP-producing neurons. It is usual for the thirst mechanism to be retained, although it is possible for there to be either excessive thirst, or even hypodipsia.

In many cases the cause of the condition is idiopathic (although up to 30% have detectable antibodies to the AVP-producing cells), but primary and secondary tumours feature prominently. Craniopharyngiomas, benign and malignant pituitary tumours, and other tumours adjacent to the pituitary gland (e.g. meningiomas) may all be responsible. Metastatic deposits from bronchial and breast tumours sometimes cause diabetes insipidus. Trauma in that region, such as may occur in head injuries, or following surgical intervention, can be the basis of destruction of the AVP-producing and releasing mechanisms; the

diabetes insipidus in such cases may be temporary or lifelong. Occasionally diabetes insipidus follows a childhood exanthem, and very rarely the disorder may be congenital or hereditary. Familial cranial diabetes insipidus is rare; one very rare variant of this is the DIDMOAD (Wolfram) syndrome, comprising Diabetes Insipidus, Diabetes Mellitus, Optic Atrophy and Deafness. Chronic granulomatous lesions that may cause it include eosinophilic granuloma, Hand–Schüller–Christian disease, sarcoidosis, syphilis (gumma), and tuberculosis (tuberculoma). Diabetes insipidus is sometimes seen to complicate basal meningitis.

Sheehan's syndrome is caused by infarction of the pituitary gland following post-partum haemorrhage; it is rare in communities with high standards of obstetric care. Pregnancy can worsen existing diabetes insipidus, but the condition can sometimes develop during pregnancy.

The symptoms are less severe if the anterior pituitary gland is also involved in the disease process, as cortisol also plays a part in normal water excretion. Conversely, partial diabetes insipidus may be worsened in the presence of exogenous ACTH or adrenal glucocorticoids. Reference to Table 5.3 indicates that in the normal individual, of every 6 mL of tubular filtrate emerging from the distal end of the ascending limb of the loop of Henle, 5 mL are reabsorbed through the AVP mechanism, and hence only 1 mL becomes urine. In the absence of AVP it is clear that the whole 6 mL entering the distal tubule is likely to become urine. Typically, therefore, the urine volume in diabetes insipidus is up to six times the normal volume, i.e. instead of 1000–1500 mL/24 h, there may be 6000–9000 mL/24 h, and it is of low osmolality.

In cases where the dipsogenic areas of the hypothalamus are involved, thirst will not be a feature. The osmostat mechanism is set much higher than normal and hence polyuria occurs alone. This group of disorders is discussed separately on p. 96 under the heading of 'Hypodipsia and Adipsia'. In all other instances, however, the usual primary polyuria and secondary polydipsia is characteristic.

Osmotic Diuresis

A number of reports have indicated that blood urea levels may be elevated when babies are fed with overstrength cows' milk. The higher the blood urea, the more likely it is that overstrength feeds are being given. Dehydration is caused by osmotic diuresis.

Another clinical cause is intravenous feeding; excessive administration leads to high production of urea from the contained amino acids. Again osmotic diuresis may follow.

Moreover, excessive protein feeds given orally, or via a tube directly into the stomach, can also lead to osmotic diuresis, and elevated blood urea. It is not always apparent that the diuresis has a nutritional basis in this case, as the medical practitioner may not be directly supervising the feeding process. In any case of unexplained diuresis, enquiry should always be made concerning not only the mode of feeding, but also the quantities being given.

Diuretic drugs decrease sodium absorption by the renal tubular system, thus causing natriuresis; this leads to an osmotic (sodium) diuresis, with body depletion of both sodium and water. Usually normonatraemia is maintained, but sometimes hyponatraemia occurs. There are, however, other clinical situations in which there is sodium loss, e.g. Addison's disease (in which the basis of the natriuresis is diminished absorption of sodium in the distal renal tubules and collecting ducts as a result of deficiency of adrenocortical hormones), renal salt-losing disease, renal tubular acidosis, and cases of high dietary intake of sodium.

Therapeutically used osmotic diuretics include mannitol, trometamol and urea. All of them reduce the water content of the body, and some are used to reduce or prevent cerebral oedema.

In addition, excessive radiation of radiosensitive tumours has been observed to produce an osmotic diuresis associated with massive increases in the concentration of circulating uric acid.

Mannitol. Mannitol is a hexahydric alcohol related to mannose. It does not possess significant energy value, but can be given intravenously for the purpose of producing osmotic diuresis in certain patients with oedema and ascites, and also in some cases of oliguria and anuria. In addition it can be used to initiate diuresis in patients who have had self-administered drug overdoses.

It is reported that doses of mannitol in excess of that normally recommended may cause symptoms of water intoxication. Even normal doses of mannitol may cause the patient to complain of thirst. Moreover, on account of its high osmotic effect, should the mannitol become extravasated, local oedema will develop, followed occasionally by thrombophlebitis.

Trometamol. Trometamol is an organic amine base that causes osmotic diuresis following intravenous infusion. It penetrates into intracellular compartments and has been used as an osmotic diuretic.

Urea. Urea is an osmotic diuretic that is sometimes used to reduce intracranial pressure due to cerebral oedema.

Iatrogenic Polyuria

Excessive volumes of intravenous fluid can overload a patient's circulation, with polyuria as the outcome. Should the fluid given be of low sodium content, then dilutional hyponatraemia might also result. If the infusion had closely followed a surgical procedure, then the stress response of release of AVP in this state could limit ability to dilute the urine, at the same time increasing the likelihood of water retention. The probability of water retention, with the

danger of water intoxication, could be compounded yet further by the presence of drugs that have antidiuretic effects (*see* Table 5.6).

Alternatively, excessive dosage with diuretic compounds can release sodium (and water, too) from the body in vast amounts; if in such circumstances the individual is unable to respond in the normal way by drinking more fluid (e.g. because of coma, stupor, serious illness, weakness, old age, infancy, and lack of proper care, attention and observation), then severe dehydration of rapid onset would result in circulatory collapse.

Polyuria is occasionally encountered on a temporary basis in test circumstances, when a patient is asked to drink copiously. The large volume of urine that follows, will, of course, be recorded in the patient's notes. This must not, however, be misinterpreted as representing his or her normal daily output—but should be recognized as the temporary iatrogenically produced volume that it is.

In addition, medical advice to a patient to increase fluid intake over a long period can sometimes, in an obsessive personality, be taken to extreme lengths, with gross polyuria as the outcome (*see* Psychogenic polydipsia *below*).[31]

Primary Polydipsia and Secondary Polyuria

There are a number of disorders in which polydipsia precedes the polyuria. Conditions of stress involving psychiatric or psychological mechanisms may be the fundamental basis in some cases. In other instances the osmotic threshold for thirst onset may be unusually low; sometimes, the plasma osmolality at which thirst is no longer appreciated may be even lower than that at which secretion of AVP ceases. Such patients continue, therefore, to feel thirsty and to drink at plasma osmolality values below those that stimulate AVP secretion.

Psychogenic Polydipsia

A number of psychiatric disorders can lead to this state of polydipsia, which may itself range from mild to utmost severity. These individuals may have a severe psychosis (e.g. schizophrenia), or they may indeed appear to be relatively normal people, merely presenting with complaints of thirst and polyuria. If the condition is sufficiently severe, water intoxication may occur. Chronic ingestion of large volumes of water can impair the renal concentrating mechanism, and sometimes there is difficulty in differentiating this condition from true diabetes insipidus. Those who are severely mentally impaired may well present with polydipsia, drinking any fluid that is freely available, including flowerpot water, puddles and even from the toilet, etc. Psychogenic polydipsia is occasionally seen between the ages of 3 and 4 years. Lack of water requirement during the night is a feature, compared with the desperate need for it in cranial diabetes insipidus.

There is ingestion of a larger amount of water

than the renal system is able to excrete. The normal kidney cannot excrete more than just over 1 L/h. The consequence is that the extracellular volume expands, and dilutional hyponatraemia occurs. The renin–angiotensin system is inhibited by the overloaded circulation; hence there is renal wasting of sodium. The specific gravity and osmolality of the urine are very low, perhaps as low as sp.gr. 1.001. However, the first urine sample in the morning may be of higher osmolality than samples throughout the rest of the day, on account of possible reduction of drinking during the night hours.

Compulsive Water Drinking

Both psychogenic polydipsia and compulsive water drinking may occur in patients with a psychiatric disorder. In compulsive water drinking, however, there seems to be a primary abnormality in the thirst mechanism. Sometimes, patients may have received phenothiazine treatment for psychiatric illness; these drugs do possess anticholinergic properties and may lead to a sensation of dryness of the mouth, with the consequence that fluid intake rises in an attempt to quench the thirst. Head injuries may be followed by temporary or lifelong cranial diabetes insipidus; however, hypodipsia and compulsive water drinking have both been recognized in patients with cranial diabetes insipidus due to head injuries where the thirst centre has also been damaged.

Hypokalaemia

It is well recognized that there is an association between hypokalaemia and polyuria.[32] It is now established that in potassium depletion, two possible mechanisms could influence water homeostasis, one being central and the other renal. The central process involves stimulation of the thirst centre, thus leading to polydipsia, which in turn will account for some of the polyuria observed in hypokalaemia. However, potassium deficiency also leads to an effect on the kidney, thereby diminishing ability of the renal tubule to achieve maximal urinary concentration. The latter process is not dependent on the former.

Experiments in rats have been largely used to determine the physiological details of the effects of hypokalaemia on water balance. Incontrovertible evidence that potassium depletion could be associated with polyuria and polydipsia via impaired maximal urinary concentration had been well established, but it was only realized later that perhaps the more important effect was stimulation of the thirst centre.

Polyuria and polydipsia may therefore be caused by chronic hypokalaemia from any cause. Firstly, there is resistance to the normal action of AVP at renal level, and secondly the hypokalaemia leads to diminished renal medullary tonicity. Thirdly there may be stimulation of the thirst mechanism.

Renin-secreting Wilms' Tumour

Plasma angiotensin II, a potent stimulus to the thirst mechanism, although unable to cross the blood–brain barrier, is able to act directly and promptly on the dipsogenic centre because it is a circumventricular organ, i.e. there is no blood–brain barrier at that location. What is true for physiological levels is especially true for pathologically high amounts of angiotensin II, e.g. caused by a renin-secreting tumour; in such a situation, profound thirst would be expected.[33]

Miscellaneous

Hypodipsia and Adipsia

A number of patients have been described with hypodipsia and hypernatraemia, in the presence of hypothalamic and suprasellar damage.[34] Autopsy studies have revealed a variety of pathological lesions. The mechanism is likely to be that damage to the thirst centre causes disordered secretion of AVP through uncoupling of the osmoreception–AVP release system. The consequence is that plasma osmolality may become grossly elevated largely because of hypernatraemia. Sodium retention would be expected, on account of low glomerular filtration rate, and secondary hyperaldosteronism.

Clinically, these patients show personality change, drowsiness, impaired concentration and memory, lethargy, apathy, confusion, weakness and low labile blood pressure, but do not show obvious dehydration or polyuria. The urine osmolality is inappropriately low in spite of marked elevation of plasma osmolality. Moreover, on rehydration, plasma electrolyte abnormalities may return to normal, but an abnormal plasma/urine osmolality ratio persists. Typically the plasma sodium achieves 150–160 mmol/L or more, and the plasma osmolality 310 mosmol/kg or more. The urine osmolality is often less than 200 mosmol/kg. Plasma volume was reduced in several patients in whom it was studied. In one patient extracellular fluid volume was also decreased.

A typical feature is that these patients do not complain of thirst, although some confess to the sensation of dryness of the mouth. It is clear therefore that unless special questions are directed to the possible absence of thirst, the patient will not volunteer it. Thirst may not be totally absent, and it may be that drinking only occurs when the serum sodium is sufficiently high to activate the osmoreceptors—as though the 'osmostat' has been set at a biologically unacceptable high level.

In these patients, rehydration sufficient to bring the serum sodium to within the normal range may not decrease the osmolality proportionally—it is considered that the high plasma osmolality is due to increased total solute. Moreover, overhydration leaves the urine osmolality inappropriately high; there thus seems to be a failure to detect and respond appropriately to the plasma osmolality. In some patients it was noticed that full rehydration did not produce a urine osmolality as low as is generally seen in classical diabetes insipidus.

A multitude of pathological lesions has been noted as being the basis of the disorder. They include granulomas (e.g. eosinophilic granuloma), secondary carcinomatous deposits (e.g. from the bronchus), meningioma, craniopharygioma, and germinoma. Lesions in one patient were found in the area of the pituitary stalk, infundibulum of the third ventricle, hypothalamus, mammillary bodies, mammillothalamic tracts, and specifically not in the supraoptic and paraventricular nuclei which remained intact. In other patients, the supraoptic and paraventricular nuclei have been infiltrated by tumour. The disorder is therefore a subdivision of diabetes insipidus—but specifically of hypothalamic origin; moreover, it is even restricted to the dipsogenic areas of the hypothalamus.

Syndrome of Inappropriate Antidiuresis

There is a large number of diseases in which the complication of the SIAD may occur. The excessive secretion of AVP leads to reduced serum osmolality and hyponatraemia. The urine osmolality is inappropriately higher than the plasma reading. This is due to persistent sodium loss on account of inhibition of the renin–angiotensin mechanism, which in turn is due to the overloaded circulation. Peripheral oedema is not a feature of the disorder.

Urine osmolality is not low, on account of the unimpaired action of AVP on the distal tubules and collecting ducts of the kidney. In normal circumstances, of course, the feedback system tends to control AVP production according to requirements. A low plasma osmolality would therefore normally lead to reduction of AVP secretion. Where AVP is autonomously produced, however, or persistently stimulated by some abnormal mechanism, no such feedback occurs.

The full syndrome is not difficult to diagnose. There may be more difficulty, however, in the case of the incomplete disorder. In these cases the blood shows no changes of sodium or osmolality until a stress test in the form of a water load is applied. If the patient has more circulating AVP than normal, there will be delayed excretion in response. Moreover, the plasma will become hypotonic at this time.

There are now many recognized causes of this syndrome (*see* Table 5.4); among these nausea and vomiting are recognized to be potent stimuli for AVP release and may be important in some cases of inappropriate antidiuresis associated with some drugs, certain clinical disorders and postoperatively. Insulin-induced hypoglycaemia produces a three- to fourfold rise in plasma AVP and could play a part in some cases. It is well known, for instance, that many malignant tumours are able to synthesize and secrete polypeptide substances, including AVP. Moreover, neurophysins have also been detected in tumour tissue.

In other disorders producing the SIAD, the AVP originates from its normal site in the hypothalamus. Excessive amounts occur either because of cellular damage in the hypothalamus, or on account of unusual stimulation.

The occurrence of SIAD in respiratory disease has produced more than one theory as to its origin. Reduced filling of the left atrium has been suggested as being the stimulus to AVP production in inflammatory lung disease. However, extraction of the lung in one patient with pulmonary tuberculosis yielded a large amount of AVP, although no conclusion could be drawn as to whether this was locally produced, or whether it was secreted in the normal way and merely trapped there.

There have also been reports of patients who developed water intoxication following oxytocin infusion, given for the induction of labour or abortion. Indeed fatalities have been recorded. The mechanism is presumably that of the antidiuretic effect of oxytocin, in combination with the large volumes of water in which it is administered.[35]

Drugs that promote the action of AVP could do so in several theoretical ways. They could stimulate AVP release, prolong the half-life of the hormone, enhance its action on the kidney, or perhaps the drug itself could have an antidiuretic effect by some other means. Some of the drugs responsible are listed in Tables 5.4 and 5.5.

LABORATORY INVESTIGATION OF POLYURIA AND POLYDIPSIA

When one considers the laboratory investigation of polyuria and polydipsia, it is clear that the clinical disorders discussed in the previous section fall into three groups.

Clinical Groups

Group 1

It is recognized that in certain diseases, polyuria and polydipsia occur as late complications. There is no surprise at the onset of diuresis when a patient enters the recovery phase of acute oliguric renal failure. Diuresis is anticipated, its cause is known, the patient is already in hospital, and laboratory investigations are orientated towards management, rather than establishing the diagnosis. Similarly, the possible polyuric and polydipsic complications of other renal disorders such as known chronic renal failure, medullary cystic disease, persistent obstruction of the genito-urinary tract, relief of genito-urinary obstruction, and renal transplantation are well documented. Nephrogenic diabetes insipidus caused by severe sepsis is referred to in the previous section, and its possibility should be kept in mind. The cause of polyuria will be obvious if a patient is receiving osmotic diuretics such as mannitol or urea. It may not be so apparent if the diuresis is caused by the feeding of overstrength cows' milk to babies, or by excessive protein feeds in adults. This applies, whether the agent is orally self-administered, or given via a tube directly into the stomach. In these circumstances, enquiry will be necessary regarding the mode of feeding, how much is being given at each feed, and how often.

Group 2

The clinical presentation of diabetes mellitus, chronic renal failure, hypercalcaemia and hypokalaemia is often with polyuria and polydipsia, in association with other complaints. If the patient does not directly admit to polyuria, routine questioning with reference to the urinary system should establish it. The laboratory investigations required here are simple and routine.

Urine glucose, blood glucose, serum urea and creatinine, urine protein and microscopy, serum calcium and serum potassium are usually sufficient initially to confirm, or exclude, any of these disorders. Should any prove abnormal, it will be necessary to pursue each in the conventional way.

It is also necessary to exclude the possibility of iatrogenic polyuria and polydipsia, and self-medication. The patient should be questioned about the taking of drugs such as diuretics, hypnotics and opiates, and also about alcohol consumption.

Group 3

More discussion is necessary about individuals belonging to the third group. These patients may present with polyuria and polydipsia, but none of the obvious causes listed under groups 1 and 2 can be established. Group 3 comprises psychogenic polydipsia, cranial diabetes insipidus, and nephrogenic diabetes insipidus.

Before proceeding to detailed investigations, iatrogenic polydipsia must also be considered and excluded. The patient should be questioned about excessive fluid intake, either taken voluntarily or on the advice of a physician, perhaps received a long time ago. This may have been suggested initially, for example, following the finding of cystine stones in the renal tract.

In the history taking, some care does need to be observed in positively establishing polyuria and polydipsia. It is not always volunteered or divulged on direct questioning. Occasionally it is found that excessive requirement for fluid has become so much a way of life, that it is now accepted as normal. The nocturnal ritual of placing a large jug of water on the bedside table, and the daily ritual of taking a bottle of dilute orange squash to work, can easily be missed. Very detailed enquiry about daily habits is essential when there is suspicion of disease involving the hypothalamic–pituitary area.

The chance observation that a 24-h urine volume recorded on a laboratory form is well above the normal range can be an important pointer to polyuria, particularly if seen on more than one occasion.

The adipsia or hypodipsia of hypothalamic disease involving the dipsogenic centre(s) needs special mention. These patients do not complain of lack of thirst. They just do not drink, as their physiological mechanisms fail to recognize thirst any longer as being a normal requirement, until the serum sodium is grossly elevated. At this high level the patients may drink, but cessation will soon occur so that the serum sodium and osmolality do not fall below the new level determined by the elevated osmostat mechanism.

It is important for the physician to interpret correctly the patient's own history and not to misinterpret as polyuria what is really frequency of micturition associated with a urinary tract infection. Furthermore, attention focused on the urinary system may cause the patient to misrepresent the symptoms. The patient may think he or she is passing a large volume of urine, and yet all laboratory tests, and detailed history, may be unable to confirm it. Special enquiry regarding drug therapy is important; it may be that anticholinergic compounds or tricyclic antidepressants are being taken, in which case a dry mouth and 'thirst' may be the outcome.

Scheme of Clinical Investigation

This scheme is suggested to serve as a framework for biochemical investigation of patients with polyuria and polydipsia. It is easily modifiable to suit special circumstances and requirements. Reference to discussion in the previous section on the clinical grouping system is necessary before proceeding.[36]

Patient Preparation and Procedure for Water Deprivation Test and Desmopressin Acetate Response Test (Fig. 5.13)

1. *Exclude* patients belonging to Group 1. Their future investigations are directed towards management rather than diagnosis of the polyuric state.

2. *Exclude* patients belonging to Group 2 by ascertaining urine glucose, blood glucose, serum urea, serum creatinine, urine protein, urine microscopy, serum calcium, and serum potassium. Ask regarding diuretics, hypnotics, opiates, and alcohol.

3. Patients of *Group 3* are now left by exclusion. Observe the patient for 1 day. Put on a fluid intake and output chart. Collect all urine samples passed, and measure the volumes and osmolalities of each. If many are presented, then a small random selection only need be analysed. Calculate the total 24-h urine volume.

4. The *water deprivation test* now follows.[37] Smoking is forbidden to the patient throughout the whole procedure. Weigh the patient initially. Permit a light breakfast and normal fluid intake on the morning of the test. During the test, exclude all access to fluid for 8 h, but be prepared to stop test if body weight falls by greater than 3%, or if the patient begins to feel unwell and looks dehydrated. Collect all urine samples passed and measure volumes and osmolality. Collect serum samples 2-hourly, and measure the osmolality of each.

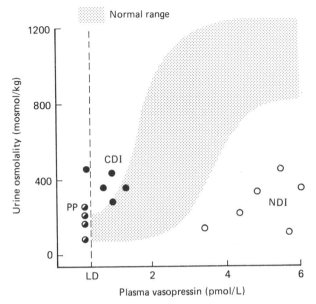

Figure 5.13 Typical results of plasma vasopressin and urine osmolality following fluid deprivation in patients with cranial diabetes insipidus (CDI) (●), primary polydipsia (PP) (◑) and nephrogenic diabetes insipidus (NDI) (○). Stippled area shows the range of the normal response; LD is the limit of detection of the vasopressin assay. Patients with partial CDI may have relatively concentrated urine for the low plasma vasopressin; those with NDI are differentiated by the low urine osmolality with respect to plasma vasopressin.
From: Baylis P.H. (1989). Vasopressin: physiology and diabetes insipidus. *Med. Int.*, **63**, 2616, with permission.

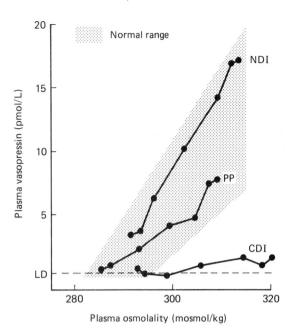

Figure 5.14 Typical plasma vasopressin responses to infusion of hypertonic saline in patients who have cranial diabetes insipidus (CDI), primary polydipsia (PP) and nephrogenic diabetes insipidus (NDI). Stippled area shows the range of the normal response; LD is the limit of detection of the vasopressin assay. Note basal CDI results are in normal range, but with osmotic stimulation plasma vasopressin is subnormal.
Source: as Figure 5.13.

5. At the end of the 8-h period of water deprivation, do the *desmopressin acetate response* test[38] using the synthetic vasopressin substance desmopressin, desaminocys[1]-D arg[8]-vasopressin (DDAVP). DDAVP (2 μg) is given intramuscularly. Again collect all urine samples passed over the next 16 h, i.e. up to the end of the whole 24-h period from the commencement of the water deprivation procedure. Measure each urine volume and osmolality. Collect three or four serum samples over this period for osmolality determinations. During the DDAVP test, food is given as normal. This is the end of the test.

6. *Interpretation* of this scheme is given on p. 100.

Nicotine Test
Maximal stimulation of AVP occurs immediately after smoking. For many years the smoking of one to three cigarettes rapidly with deep inhalation, or the intravenous nicotine test, was used to test the capacity of the hypothalamopituitary area to secrete AVP.

Intravenous nicotine in sufficient dose leads to an antidiuretic response in the normal person within 30 min of administration. There is decrease of urine flow, together with reduction of free water clearance. The urine concentrations of solutes increase. This response is absent in the patient with cranial diabetes insipidus.

The test is time consuming, not entirely reliable, and moreover, patients may suffer toxic effects such as nausea, vomiting and vertigo. There seems little merit in doing this test now that osmolality is so easily and quickly measured. Nevertheless, knowledge of the principle of it serves as a reminder that patients must not be permitted to smoke before or during investigations of polyuria and polydipsia.

Intravenous Hypertonic Saline Test (Fig. 5.14)
This test was used for many years for testing the hypothalamopituitary capacity to secrete AVP. A 3% infusion of saline (10 mL/kg) was given over 45 min. The normal antidiuretic response, seen within 60 min of infusion, does not occur with cranial diabetes insipidus.

This test is clinically time consuming, and is reported to be not always in agreement with the nicotine test. Now that osmolality tests on the urine and serum are so easily available, this test would seem to have little value in clinical diagnosis, apart from the rare requirement to calculate the threshold of AVP release, by plotting serum osmolality in mosmol/kg against plasma AVP in pmol/L.

Urinary Arginine Vasopressin Test

Urinary AVP is measured by radioimmunoassay. It is rarely required, however, as osmolality tests nearly always provide the diagnosis, are so easy, and are much less expensive.

Urine levels are dependent on the clinical state of the patient, and certain drugs already referred to will influence the value obtained.[39] The clinical state at the time of collection is important, as secretion depends on plasma osmolality and volume.

Special requirements for collection of urine need to be observed. The local laboratory will need to be consulted. In general, however, about 15 mL should suffice, as long as it is collected into a plastic container, and made acid with 1 mL of 1 M HCl per 5 mL urine immediately it has been passed. The urine and acid must be mixed well, and then stored at $-20°C$.

Plasma Arginine Vasopressin

Progress in the measurement of plasma AVP has been made in recent years; not only have the extraction procedures to remove AVP from plasma been improved, but also it is now possible to produce sensitive antibodies to the hormone. Incorporation of these newer plasma AVP assays into the water deprivation and hypertonic saline infusion tests can sometimes improve diagnostic potential in helping to differentiate cranial diabetes insipidus, nephrogenic diabetes insipidus and psychogenic polydipsia.

General Principles of Differential Diagnosis and Interpretation

Plasma AVP, plasma osmolality and urine osmolality are theoretically the three most important factors in understanding the differential diagnosis of psychogenic polydipsia, cranial diabetes insipidus, and nephrogenic diabetes insipidus. Plasma AVP is not readily available as a routine test, but the osmolality determinations are.

The Normal Individual

The normal serum osmolality is between 280 and 290 mosmol/kg. It does not matter whether serum or plasma is used for the determination of osmolality, as the figures obtained are virtually identical.

Overnight deprivation of fluid may possibly elevate serum osmolality to 295 mosmol/kg, and urine osmolality to more than 1000 mosmol/kg. The first urine specimen after sleep is likely to be the most concentrated of the whole day.

Intramuscular DDAVP administration following overnight deprivation of water cannot lead to greater osmolality of urine; the endogenous AVP is already being secreted maximally, and exerting its full effect.

Psychogenic Polydipsia

This is characterized by appropriately low plasma and urine osmolalities in the presence of low plasma AVP. In this disorder there is normally fluid intake in excess of the capacity of the renal system to excrete it. The tendency is therefore, for serum sodium and osmolality to be towards, at, or below the lower limit of the normal range for the laboratory concerned. Serum osmolality may even be below 255 mosmol/kg and urine osmolality less than 50 mosmol/kg. If it is possible to collect all samples of urine passed, it is likely that the early morning one will have an osmolality greater than those during the remainder of the day. This is on account of the reduced or absent fluid input during sleep. Urine volume and fluid input should both be measured over 24 h, if possible, but in a severely psychiatrically disturbed patient this may not prove feasible.

Deprivation of fluid intake may lead to elevation of serum osmolality to the upper end of the normal range, around 290 mosmol/kg. Urine osmolality may rise to the same level or greater, depending on the severity of the condition initially. It is not likely, however, to rise as much as in the normal person, but it may reach 600 mosmol/kg.

Intramuscular injection of DDAVP following water deprivation causes water absorption in the distal tubules and collecting ducts of the kidney. There could be, in consequence, a decrease of serum osmolality to perhaps 255 mosmol/kg, as drinking may not be inhibited. Urine osmolality, however, may not change much from the elevated level achieved following fluid deprivation; it may rise to 750 mosmol/kg. If the condition is severe, it may be that urine osmolality remains low after fluid deprivation. Hence there will be opportunity for elevation of it following the intramuscular DDAVP injection, perhaps to 500 mosmol/kg.

Exposure to DDAVP can be dangerous sometimes in psychogenic polydipsia, as the patient may suffer from overhydration some hours afterwards if fluid intake is not curtailed.

Cranial Diabetes Insipidus

This is characterized by low or absent plasma AVP in the presence of high plasma osmolality. The disorder is normally accompanied by urine output being in excess of the capacity of the individual to counteract it by drinking. The tendency, therefore, is for serum sodium and osmolality to be near, at, or above the upper limit of the reference range. Urine osmolality of all separate specimens passed throughout the course of the day tends to show a fixed low level. The early morning sample does not have a higher osmolality than the others; this is unlike psychogenic polydipsia. Urine volumes over 24-h periods should be recorded, and a fluid intake/output chart commenced.

Water deprivation causes the serum osmolality to increase beyond 295 mosmol/kg, perhaps even to 305 mosmol/kg. Nevertheless, urine osmolalities remain at the same low level as found initially, maybe around 150 mosmol/kg. Abundant urine continues to be passed. In milder degrees of the illness, the urine can be concentrated to some degree, and the osmolality rises towards or even surpasses that of serum; it may reach 400 mosmol/kg.

Deprivation of fluids in cranial diabetes insipidus may indeed be dangerous if overdone. The patient may become dehydrated rapidly, and may appear sunken eyed, grey and lethargic. Water is relatively heavy and, therefore, loss of much urine in the absence of intake will lead to weight reduction. Great care should be exercised in supervising this test. It should be stopped as soon as sufficient information has been gained and immediately that there is any cause for concern regarding the patient's well-being, as vasomotor collapse is possible in severe dehydration. Hourly weighing of the patient will alert the clinician to consider ending the test should the body weight fall by greater than 3%. The test must therefore only be done by day when there is strict supervision by experienced staff.

Accurately timed 1- or 2-h volumes of urine may also be collected for determination of AVP both before and after fluid deprivation, for as long as can safely be maintained. Special requirements for the collection and storage of the urine are quoted in the section entitled 'Urinary Arginine Vasopressin Test' above.

Administration of intramuscular DDAVP leads to a very dramatic fall of urine output, the appearance of the urine changes from colourless to yellow, the osmolality rises, and the patient not only begins to feel improved but also looks better. Urine osmolality may reach 800 mosmol/kg in mild cases, and around 450 mosmol/kg when the disorder is more severe.

Nephrogenic Diabetes Insipidus
Patients with this disorder are found to have an appropriately high plasma AVP in the presence of a low urine osmolality.

Findings of the water deprivation test in this disorder are similar to those in cranial diabetes insipidus. Fluid intake and output should be recorded over 24-h periods.

Administration of DDAVP intramuscularly to a patient with nephrogenic diabetes insipidus is without effect on urine output, and the osmolalities do not change from the initial values.

Hypodipsia and Adipsia
Biochemical features include high serum sodium, perhaps between 150 and 160 mmol/L but maybe more. In spite of this, thirst is significantly absent as the 'osmostat' is elevated. Serum osmolality is usually in excess of 310 mosmol/kg. The urine osmolality is inappropriately low, and may be less than 200 mosmol/kg. On rehydration, the serum electrolytes may return to normal, but there may be persistence of an abnormal plasma/urine osmolality ratio.

Syndrome of Inappropriate Antidiuresis
Biochemical findings include reduced serum sodium

and osmolality. The serum sodium may be down to 120 mmol/L and the osmolality around 240 mosmol/kg. Urine osmolality is inappropriately higher than plasma osmolality, and this is due to the loss of sodium. This occurs on account of the overloaded circulation producing inhibition of the renin–angiotensin mechanism, and because of the persistent excessive activity of AVP on the renal tubules and collecting ducts.

The incomplete disorder, however, may require a stress test in the form of a water-load. In this case delayed excretion of the water occurs on account of the elevated AVP activity. At the same time, the plasma will become hypotonic.

REFERENCES

1. Andersson B. (1978). Regulation of water intake. *Physiol. Rev.*, **58**, 582.
2. Zilva J.F., Pannall P.R., Mayne P.D. (1988). The kidney: renal calculi. In *Clinical Chemistry in Diagnosis and Treatment*, London: Edward Arnold, pp. 1–24.
3. Zilva J.F., Pannall P.R., Mayne P.D. (1988). Sodium and water metabolism. In *Clinical Chemistry in Diagnosis and Treatment*, London: Edward Arnold, pp. 25–55.
4. Guyton A.C. (1991). Renal and associated mechanisms for controlling extracellular fluid osmolality and sodium concentration. In *Textbook of Medical Physiology*, Philadelphia: W.B. Saunders, pp. 308–319.
5. Foote J.W. (1990). Hyponatraemia: diagnosis and management. *Hosp. Update* (March), 248.
6. Paterson K.R. (1990). Hyponatraemia. *Prescribers J.*, **30**, 28.
7. Ramsay D.J. (1989). The importance of thirst in maintenance of fluid balance. In *Baillière's Clinical Endocrinology and Metabolism*, vol. 3, no. 2 (Baylis P.H. ed.) London: Baillière Tindall, pp. 371–392.
8. Thompson C.J., Baylis P.H. (1988). Osmoregulation of thirst, *J.Endocrinol.*, **117**, 155.
9. Rolls B.J., Phillips P.A. (1990). Aging and disturbances of thirst and fluid balance. *Nutr. Rev.*, **48**, 137.
10. Baylis P.H. (1989). Regulation of vasopressin secretion. In *Baillière's Clinical Endocrinology and Metabolism*, vol. 3, no. 2 (Baylis P.H. ed.) London: Baillière Tindall, pp. 313–330.
11. Baylis P.H., Thompson C.J. (1988). Osmoregulation of vasopressin secretion and thirst in health and disease. *Clin. Endocrinol.*, **29**, 549.
12. Baylis P.H. (1989). Vasopressin: physiology and diabetes insipidus. *Med. Int.*, **63**, 2616.
13. Davison J.M., Lindheimer M.D. (1989). Volume homeostasis and osmoregulation in human pregnancy. In *Baillière's Clinical Endocrinology and Metabolism*, vol. 3, no. 2 (Baylis P.H. ed.) London: Baillière Tindall, pp. 451–472.
14. Lindheimer M.D., Barron W.M., Davison J.M. (1989). Osmoregulation of thirst and vasopressin release in pregnancy. *Am. J. Physiol.*, **257** (Renal Fluid Electrolyte Physiol. 26), F159.
15. Mitchell K.D., Navar L.G. (1989). The renin–angiotensin–aldosterone system in volume control. In *Baillière's Clinical Endocrinology and Metabolism*, vol. 3, no. 2 (Baylis P.H. ed.) London: Baillière Tindall,

pp. 393–430.

16. Weindl A. (1973). Neuroendocrine aspects of circumventricular organs. In *Frontiers in Neuroendocrinology* (Ganong W.F., Martini L. eds.) New York: Oxford University Press.

17. Guyton A.C. (1991). Renal disease, diuresis and micturition. In *Textbook of Medical Physiology*, Philadelphia: W.B. Saunders, pp. 344–354.

18. Vokes T.J., Robertson G.L. (1988). Disorders of antidiuretic hormone. In *Diagnostic Evaluation of Endocrine Disorders I, Endocrinology and Metabolism Clinics of North America*, **17**, no. 2, Philadelphia: W. B. Saunders, p. 281.

19. Chowdrey H.S., Lightman S.L. (1989). Neuroendocrine control of blood tonicity and volume. In *Baillière's Clinical Endocrinology and Metabolism*, vol. 3, no. 2 (Baylis P.H. ed.) London: Baillière Tindall, pp. 229–247.

20. Bankir L., Bouby N., Trin-Trang-Tan M-M. (1989). The role of the kidney in the maintenance of water balance. In *Baillière's Clinical Endocrinology and Metabolism*, vol. 3, no. 2 (Baylis P.H. ed.) London: Baillière Tindall, pp. 249–311.

21. Guyton A.C. (1991). The pituitary hormones and their control by the hypothalamus. In *Textbook of Medical Physiology*, Philadelphia: London: W.B. Saunders pp. 819–829.

22. Andreoli T.E. (1988). Disorders of fluid volume, electrolyte and acid–base balance. In *Cecil Textbook of Medicine* (Wyngaarden J.B., Smith L.H. eds.) Philadelphia: W.B. Saunders, pp. 528–558.

23. Robertson G.L. (1988). Differential diagnosis of polyuria. *Annu. Rev. Med.*, **39**, 425–442.

24. Nagar D., Ferris F.Z., Schlacht R.A. (1976). Obstructive polyuric renal failure following renal transplantation. *Am. J. Med.*, **60**, 702.

25. Husberg B., Hellsten S., Bergentz S., Hansen T., Moller-Jensen K. (1977). Massive diuresis after renal transplantation due to retention of furosemide. *Transplantation*, **23**, 101.

26. Penney M.D., Hampton D. (1990). The effect of lithium therapy on arginine vasopressin secretion and thirst in man. *Clin. Biochem.*, **23**, 233.

27. Cortez A., Zito J., Lucas C.E., Gerrick S.J. (1977). Mechanism of inappropriate polyuria in septic patients. *Arch. Surg.*, **112**, 471.

28. Flis R.S., Scoblionco D.P., Basti C.P., Popovtzer M.M. (1977). Dopamine-related polyuria in patients with Gram-negative infections. *Arch. Intern. Med.*, **137**, 1547.

29. Walmsley R.N., Guerin M.D. (1984). Renal disease. In *Disorders of Fluid and Electrolyte Balance*, Bristol: John Wright, pp. 202–205.

30. Page S.R., Nussey S.S., Jenkins J.S., Wilson S.G., Johnson D.A. (1989). Hypothalamic disease in association with dysgenesis of the corpus callosum. *Postgrad. Med. J.*, **65**, 163.

31. Berry E.M., Halon D., Fainaru M. (1977). Iatrogenic polydipsia. *Lancet*, **ii**, 937.

32. Berl T., Linas S.L., Aisenbrey G.A., Anderson R.J. (1977). On the mechanism of polyuria in potassium depletion—the role of polydipsia. *J. Clin. Invest.*, **60**, 620.

33. Sheth K.J., Tang T.T., Blaedel M.E., Good T.A., (1978). Polydipsia, polyuria and hypertension associated with renin-secreting Wilms' tumour. *J. Paediatr.*, **92**, 921.

34. Lascelles P.T., Lewis P.D. (1972). Hypodipsia and hypernatraemia associated with hypothalamic and suprasellar lesions. *Brain*, **95**, 249.

35. Morgan D.B., Kirwan N.A., Hancock K.W., Robinson D., Ahmad S. (1977). Water intoxication and oxytocin infusion. *Br. J. Obstet. Gynaecol.*, **84**, 6.

36. Thompson C.J. (1989). Polyuric states in man. In *Baillière's Clinical Endocrinology and Metabolism*, vol. 3, no. 2 (Baylis P.H. ed.) London: Baillière Tindall, pp. 473–497.

37. Lascelles P.T., Donaldson D. (1989). Water deprivation test. In *Diagnostic Function Tests in Chemical Pathology*, Dordrecht: Kluwer Academic, pp. 160–162.

38. Lascelles P.T., Donaldson D. (1989). Desmopressin acetate response test. In *Diagnostic Function Tests in Chemical Pathology*, Dordrecht: Kluwer Academic, pp. 37–38.

39. Walmsley R.M., Guerin M.D. (1984). Drugs affecting water and electrolyte homeostasis. In *Disorders of Fluid and Electrolyte Balance*, Bristol: John Wright, pp. 256–264.

6. Diabetes Mellitus

M. Nattrass

Glucose metabolism
Fat metabolism
Insulin
Aetiology of diabetes
    Type 1 diabetes
    Type 2 diabetes
Pathogenesis
    Insulin resistance
Diagnosis
    Blood glucose estimation
    The patient
    The diagnosis of diabetes and impaired
      glucose tolerance
Treatment
    Diet
    Oral hypoglycaemic agents
    Insulin
    Monitoring treatment
Hyperglycaemic emergencies
    Diabetic ketoacidosis
    Hyperglycaemic non-ketotic diabetic coma
    Lactic acidosis
Hypoglycaemia
Long-term complications of diabetes
    Diabetic neuropathy
    Diabetic retinopathy
    Diabetic nephropathy
    Macrovascular disease
    Protein glycosylation

GLUCOSE METABOLISM

Few biochemical measurements have attracted as much interest as blood glucose. In part this is because it is not only a disease marker but a reflection of biological function. With blood glucose measurement goes the feeling that the very biological support of life itself is being examined.

Of course, it is necessary to be reminded of first principles—that blood glucose simply reflects rates of production and utilization. This 'bath-tub principle' has assumed increasing importance in recent years with the concept that insulin resistance affects hepatic glucose output and peripheral glucose utilization.

The liver is the major source of glucose production in normal man in the postabsorptive state. After an overnight fast, glucose production rates are around $12\,\mu$mol/kg per min (2 mg/kg per min), of which approximately 75% comes from hepatic glycogen breakdown with the remaining 25% from gluconeogenesis. Glycogen stores in the liver amount to only about 120 g and with prolongation of fasting there comes increasing dependence upon hepatic gluconeogenesis.

Glycogen breakdown is regulated by phosphorylase, one of the many enzymes now known to exist in active and inactive forms where interconversion depends upon phosphorylation/dephosphorylation reactions. The active form, glycogen phosphorylase **a** is phosphorylated and the inactive form **b** dephosphorylated. Phosphorylase **b** kinase converts the enzyme to the active form and itself is activated by phosphorylation. Breakdown of glycogen into glucose 6-phosphate is followed by conversion into glucose by glucose 6-phosphatase, the enzyme of importance in type I glycogen storage disease (von Gierke's disease).

Gluconeogenesis is an altogether more complex process. The major gluconeogenic precursors are lactate, pyruvate, glycerol and alanine. Normal values after an overnight fast are given in Table 6.1. The

TABLE 6.1
POSTABSORPTIVE CONCENTRATIONS OF INTERMEDIARY
METABOLITES IN WHOLE BLOOD IN NORMAL MAN

Metabolite	Concentration range (mmol/L)
Lactate	0.31–1.09
Pyruvate	0.03–1.00
Alanine	0.14–0.45
Glycerol	0.02–0.13
Non-esterified fatty acids	0.33–0.89
3-hydroxybutyrate	0.01–0.28
Acetoacetate	0.01–0.10

source of these gluconeogenic precursors is carbohydrate metabolism in peripheral tissues. Most tissues release lactate and pyruvate from partial oxidation of glucose. Erythrocytes do not possess Krebs cycle enzymes and can therefore metabolize glucose only to lactate and pyruvate. Alanine serves the dual purpose of transporting both a carbohydrate skeleton and nitrogen from muscle to liver. It is now well recognized that the carbohydrate skeleton of alanine is derived from pyruvate,[1] and hence from glucose, and should rightly be included in present-day concepts of the Cori cycle. Glycerol release from fat cells comes from stored triglyceride and hence the carbon skeleton originates in, and can be converted back to, glucose. Fatty acids may be re-esterified in the fat cell but this tissue is devoid of α-glycerokinase required for re-esterification of glycerol and thus release serves as a marker of lipolysis. Uptake by the liver feeds glycerol into gluconeogenesis at the level of triose phosphate.

Postprandially the liver receives a large quantity of glucose from the gut. From being active in glucose production, glycogen breakdown and gluconeogenesis must now be halted and stores of glycogen replaced.[2] The liver is extraordinarily effective in removing glucose from the portal circulation. A meal containing 1.1 mol (200 g) of carbohydrate, which is 10 times the size of the total body pool of glucose, will raise the peripheral blood glucose concentration by only 2–3 mmol/L (36–54 mg/100 mL). In part this is due to increased peripheral disposal of glucose but the liver makes a substantial contribution to curtailing an excessive rise in glucose by removing 50% of it during the first pass. Clearly, with the limitation in glycogen stores not all of the hepatic uptake of glucose is stored as carbohydrate. A small amount only is metabolized within the liver but a substantial proportion is converted into fatty acids, which leave the liver as triglyceride.

In peripheral tissues, glucose uptake is predominantly mediated by prevailing glucose concentration. In some important tissues, such as brain, nerve, and retina (as well as liver), this process governs glucose uptake over the range of glucose concentrations. In others, such as muscle and fat tissue, non-basal glucose uptake is insulin dependent. Available glucose repletes glycogen stores, particularly of muscle but also other tissues, and supplies energy for the tissues. Glycolysis and Krebs cycle activity are important for this latter process. There is an important difference between these two pathways contributing to glucose oxidation. Glycolysis is anaerobic and takes place in the cytosol while Krebs cycle activity is aerobic and located in the mitochondria. The link between the two is pyruvate conversion to acetyl CoA regulated by the important enzyme pyruvate dehydrogenase. Entry into the Krebs cycle carries the penalty of no return. Until pyruvate becomes acetyl CoA there exists the possibility of recycling to glucose and carbohydrate stores. Entry into the Krebs cycle results in net loss to the organism of these stores—a biochemical disaster to man with limited availabilty of food or an evolutionary quirk to benefit the sugar-guzzling West.

FAT METABOLISM

Fat metabolism is of equal importance in diabetes as carbohydrate metabolism. Diabetic ketoacidosis still claims lives, while macrovascular disease is the single largest cause of death in the diabetic population. Fat storage, as triglyceride in the adipocyte, relies upon the transport to peripheral tissue of fatty acids synthesized in the liver. Although this transfer is made as triglyceride, the fatty acids are released at the fat cell by lipoprotein lipase. After entry into the cell, esterification is with α-glycerophosphate derived from glucose through partial glycolysis.

Breakdown of triglyceride, controlled by a second lipase enzyme—hormone-sensitive lipase—results in the release of glycerol and partial release of non-esterified fatty acids (NEFA). Some NEFA may be re-esterified intracellularly without release. While glycerol is taken up by the liver for gluconeogenesis,

NEFA is similarly transported to the liver for hepatic uptake and either re-esterification or degradation. For degradation, NEFA enter the mitochondrion utilizing the two carnitine acyl transferase enzymes.[3] β-Oxidation results in the generation of acetyl CoA, which may enter the Krebs cycle or lead to formation of the ketone bodies. Acetoacetate and 3-hydroxybutyrate are present in normal subjects (Table 6.1), while acetone may be easily detectable on the breath of a patient with diabetic ketoacidosis. The liver is the only site in man for the production of ketone bodies, although peripheral utilization (particularly by muscle) is the degradative pathway for acetoacetate and 3-hydroxybutyrate. All three ketone bodies may be excreted in urine; acetone may also be excreted in breath.

INSULIN

The complex interlinking of different facets of metabolism requiring rapid adaptation to changes in environment, particularly the change from the fasted to the fed state, necessitates a prompt and clear signal. This signal is provided by insulin.

Insulin is a polypeptide of 39 amino acids arranged as an A- and B-chain joined by disulphide bridges. The double-chain structure results from its origin as proinsulin[4] when a peptide length joins the end of the A-chain to the B-chain (Fig. 6.1). This connecting peptide chain, C-peptide, is secreted in equimolar amounts with insulin, appears to be inert, and in contrast to insulin is excreted virtually unchanged in urine. In recent years it has served as a useful marker of endogenous insulin secretion, allowing assessment when circulating insulin antibodies result from exogenous insulin administration.[5] As with other hormones, proinsulin is preceded in the cell by preproinsulin.

Release of insulin from the β-cell of the islets of Langerhans is occasioned by a stimulus that may take many forms. In real life it is most often a mixed

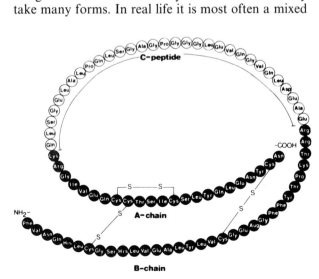

Figure 6.1 Structure of proinsulin.

meal and the summation of the constituent parts of the stimulus—glucose, amino acids, gut hormones and a neural component. The rapid rise in insulin that follows this stimulus inhibits hepatic output of glucose by inhibition of phosphorylase and stimulation of glycogen synthase, and by diverting gluconeogenesis to glycogen storage in the initial phase.

Insulin is not required for hepatic uptake of glucose but is essential for peripheral uptake by the metabolically active tissues, skeletal muscle and adipocytes.

Insulin exerts effects upon both lipid storage and breakdown. Lipoprotein lipase at the capillary endothelium is stimulated by insulin to release fatty acids. With simultaneous stimulation of glucose uptake into the fat cell, α-glycerophosphate is made available for esterification. Hormone-sensitive lipase is inhibited by an increase in circulating insulin concentrations.

The means by which insulin in the circulation achieves these considerable metabolic effects is only partly understood. The first action of insulin is binding to its receptor on the cell surface (Fig. 6.2). The receptor is composed of α and β subunits arranged across the cell membrane.[6] Binding of insulin to its receptor is followed by internalization of the hormone–receptor complex. Dissociation leads to a return of receptors to the cell membrane and probable degradation of insulin. The initial stages of hormone–receptor binding are now much better understood: they involve autophosphorylation of the receptor through tyrosyl kinase activity; subsequent steps, which involve amplification of the signal, await elucidation.

There are important conceptual considerations in the simple if extensive role of insulin in metabolism. Firstly, there is the sensible logic of insulin as the prime anabolic hormone of adult life. The major role of insulin is clearance (storage) in times of plenty, when insulin concentrations are high, to reduce wastage by stopping glucose production in the liver at this time when the substrate is abundantly available. Equally important is that the reduction in circulating insulin with change from the fed to the fasted state results in release of inhibition and the discontinuation of stimulation—which effects allow substrates to

become available for the postabsorptive state. This concept, that a decreased insulin signal is important in its own right and as an active process, contributes to the approach to insulin treatment in diabetic patients. Thirdly, it should be realized that the effects of insulin upon different metabolic pathways are hierarchical in insulin concentration. Stimulation of glucose uptake into peripheral tissues requires an insulin concentration of around 100 mU/L, while at the other extreme inhibition of lipolysis occurs with small (less than 10 mU/L) changes in insulin from basal. Between these two lies inhibition of hepatic glucose output.[7]

AETIOLOGY OF DIABETES

Current classifications of diabetes recognize two main types.[8] In a clinical classification (Table 6.2), these

TABLE 6.2
CLINICAL CLASSIFICATION OF DIABETES

Diabetes mellitus:
  Insulin-dependent
  Non-insulin dependent

  Associated with other conditions and syndromes:
    pancreatic disease, endocrine disease, drug or chemical
    induced, insulin receptor abnormalities, genetic
    syndromes, etc.
  Malnutrition-related diabetes
Impaired glucose tolerance
Gestational diabetes

Modified from World Health Organization protocol.[8]

are insulin-dependent (IDDM) and non-insulin dependent (NIDDM), while an aetiological classification describes type 1 and type 2 diabetes mellitus. There is a tendency to use the two classifications interchangeably, with type 1 equated with IDDM and type 2 with NIDDM; this is not entirely correct. The division of diabetes into these two broad categories does not preclude the association of diabetes with other primary diseases and follows a certain logic. IDDM, formerly juvenile-onset or ketosis-prone diabetes, has a younger age of onset and a dependence upon insulin; the opposite is true for NIDDM, formerly called maturity-onset diabetes. As well as the clinical presentation, the aetiology and pathogenesis of the two types of diabetes are distinct.

Type 1 Diabetes

Type 1 diabetes is associated with a particular genetic make-up.[9] The human leucocyte antigens (HLA) DR3 and DR4 occur more commonly in patients with this condition, with a corresponding decrease in HLA-DR2. These observations were preceded by the association of type 1 diabetes with certain of the A and B antigens but it is now recognized that these

Insulin binding

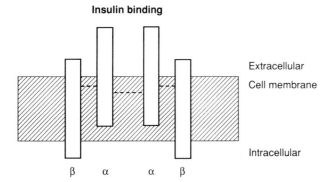

Extracellular

Cell membrane

Intracellular

β   α   α   β

Figure 6.2 Structure of the insulin receptor.

antigens are in linkage disequilibrium with the DR antigens, i.e. a particular antigen is associated with HLA-DR3. Recent work has concentrated on an examination of the DR antigens, with studies of the Dr, Dp, Dq regions. It should be stressed that considerable genetic heterogeneity can be found in type 1 diabetes if we abandon parochial concepts and consider differences in racial origin. The finding of an association with a particular antigen allows a calculation of relative risk for the holder of developing diabetes. HLA-DR3 and -DR4 are, however, preponderant in the normal population, many of whom never develop diabetes. Indeed, while much attention has focused on the positive association as conferring susceptibility, the negative association resulting in protection has received much less consideration.

The fact that the HLA associated with increased risk of type 1 diabetes are common in the non-diabetic population has led to a search for an environmental interaction. The idea of an infective agent has some attraction in view of the HLA association with the immunological response. Viral agents have for many years been considered a likely environmental factor. Much of the evidence is circumstantial. There is an increased incidence of diabetes at certain ages and a seasonal variation, both of which have been likened to patterns of infective diseases. This evidence dates from a time when the onset of this type of diabetes was considered sudden, measurable in days or weeks, although it is now recognized that the prediagnostic delay may be up to 2 years. Certain viruses can clearly be associated with diabetes. Thus, in congenital rubella there is a marked increase in diabetes over expected rates. Less firm evidence comes from data on viral antibodies, particularly to Coxsackie B4, which occur more often in newly diagnosed diabetic children than in controls. Again, with recognition of a slower rate of onset, it is less clear whether this infection could instigate diabetes or simply unmask it. Finally, it is possible to induce diabetes in laboratory animals with a variety of viruses, such as cytomegalovirus and Venezuelan equine virus.

Chemical toxins to the β-cell have also been sought. Alloxan and streptozotocin are toxic to the β-cell and are used to produce diabetes in animals. Similar chemical compounds may exist in a normal diet, although the potential for identification must be remote.

It is clear, however, that some genetic–environmental interaction requires a third component for expression of the disease. This is provided by the finding of autoantibodies to islet cells in the serum of newly diagnosed, type 1 diabetics. Whether these arise spontaneously or result from subclinical β-cell damage remains unresolved,[10] although the current generation of medical students are firm in their assurance of type 1 diabetes as an autoimmune disease!

Type 2 Diabetes

Less (or even less) is known of the aetiology of type 2 diabetes (Table 6.3). Studies in identical twins[11] have indicated a strong genetic predisposition. In identical twins with type 2 diabetes, concordance rates approach 100%, in contrast to the 50% concordance in type 1 diabetes. The nature of the genetic predisposition remains unknown, although the majority of evidence excludes an HLA association. The environmental factor also defies elucidation. It is generally thought that obesity is the main identified environmental factor. Evidence to support this may be quoted: a fall in the incidence with calorie restriction; the association with diabetes seen in every diabetic clinic; and the correction of diabetes by weight loss. All this is less convincing than at first sight and there remains the nagging doubt of no association with obesity in twin studies, and the extraordinary number of people who can achieve over 200% ideal body weight without developing diabetes.

PATHOGENESIS

The pathogenesis of type 1 diabetes results from insulin deficiency. It is probably necessary to loss 90% of functioning β-cells for diabetes to result from insulin deficiency. This having been achieved the deranged metabolism is entirely predictable from a knowledge of the action of insulin. Increased glucose production from unrestrained hepatic glucose output, and decreased uptake of glucose into peripheral insulin-sensitive tissues, both contribute to a rise in blood glucose concentration. Simultaneously a lack of inhibition upon lipolysis leads to increased release of NEFA, hepatic uptake, and hepatic ketogenesis. It is less clear, although likely, that peripheral uptake of ketone bodies may also be impaired. In view of the sensitivity of lipolysis to inhibition by insulin, ketone bodies are a marker of insulin deficiency.

In type 2 diabetes the pathogenesis is more complex and less certain. In this disease the debate has revolved around insulin deficiency or insulin resistance as the cause. The roots of the discussion lie in studies made shortly after the insulin assay was introduced and the issues are most pointed in relation to the group of patients that has both obesity and NIDDM. If glucose tolerance tests are made in lean subjects, obese, non-diabetic subjects and obese diabetic patients, the obese non-diabetics will be found to have a considerably greater insulin response than the lean controls. Provided the obese diabetic group can be matched for blood glucose concentrations during the test, their insulin response will be intermediate between the other two groups. Thus, for a similar blood glucose concentration, the higher insulin response of obese diabetics than lean normals indicates an element of insulin resistance, while the lesser insulin response than that of obese non-diabetics indicates an element of insulin deficiency.

TABLE 6.3
AETIOLOGICAL CLASSIFICATION OF DIABETES

	Type 1	*Type 2*
Genetic susceptibility	HLA linked	Present—not identified
Environmental factors	Viruses	Obesity
	Chemical toxins	
Immunological factors	Islet-cell antibodies	Absent

Insulin Resistance

The idea that a diabetic subject may have a 'normal' or even raised plasma insulin and yet still be hyperglycaemic has led to the concept of insulin resistance. This is an important area, which has received much attention in recent years.

Theoretical Concepts in Insulin Resistance

If a process sensitive to insulin is considered, for example glucose uptake into cells, it can be argued that there are two ways in which it can go wrong (Fig. 6.3). Firstly, it may be possible to stimulate glucose uptake to a maximal rate but greater than normal insulin concentrations are required—a right shift in the dose–response curve. Secondly, there may be a normal response to insulin but only up to a submaximal (say 80%) rate. The third possibility in practice is a mixture of the two, i.e. a right shift of the dose–response curve achieving only a submaximal response.[12]

Methods of Studying Insulin Resistance

A number of techniques exist for studying insulin resistance. In the 1930s, Himsworth and Kerr identified two types of diabetics, denoting them insulin sensitive or insulin insensitive in their responses to combined glucose and insulin administration.[13] Reaven devised a quadruple infusion test of fixed doses of insulin and glucose, combined with adrenaline to inhibit endogenous insulin and propranolol to block side-effects of adrenaline.[14] The test results show insulin resistance when, for matched insulin levels, steady-state plasma glucose concentrations are higher in a particular group. Modifications of this technique have been devised whereby somatostatin replaces adrenaline and propranolol.

The most common method used to study insulin resistance is the euglycaemic clamp.[15] After an overnight fast, glucose and insulin are infused into a patient at varying doses. Glucose infusion is adjusted to maintain euglycaemia, while a dose of insulin is used that will produce a required circulating concentration. This may be 50, 100, 1000, or even 10 000 mU/L. If the procedure is combined with isotopic glucose infusion, the effect of different insulin concentrations upon glucose turnover can be studied. This allows the construction of dose–response curves for insulin upon hepatic glucose output or peripheral glucose utilization.

Causes of Insulin Resistance

These are:

1. Abnormal β-cell secretion (pseudo-insulin resistance):
(a) familial hyperproinsulinaemia;
(b) mutant insulin.

2. Circulating insulin antagonists;
(a) hormonal—catecholamines, glucagon, cortisol growth hormone, thyroxine, oestrogens, prolactin, AVP;
(b) metabolites—non-esterified fatty acids, ketone bodies, hydrogen ion;
(c) immunological—anti-insulin antibodies, anti-insulin receptor antibodies.

3. Changes in insulin receptors:
(a) decreased number;
(b) altered affinity.

4. Postbinding impairment.
These resistant factors are next considered in more detail.

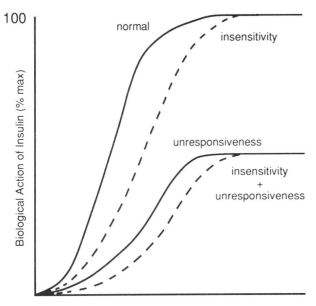

Figure 6.3 Theoretical patterns of insulin resistance (adapted from Kahn).[12]

TABLE 6.4
METABOLIC EFFECTS OF COUNTERREGULATORY HORMONES

	Glucagon	Catecholamines	Growth hormone	Cortisol
Glycogen breakdown	+ + +	+ + +	+	+
Gluconeogenesis	+ +	+	+	+
Peripheral glucose uptake	0	−	−	−
Lipolysis	0	+ + +	+	+
Ketogenesis	+ +	+	+	+

Pseudo-Insulin Resistance. Apparent insulin resistance arises when endogenous insulin as measured by radioimmunoassay is elevated but there is a normal response to exogenous insulin. In familial hyperproinsulinaemia,[16] radioimmunoassay insulin is elevated, owing to the measurement of large amounts of proinsulin. Initially it was thought that this disorder resulted from an inability to cleave proinsulin in its processing within the β-cell but careful sequencing of the proinsulin from these patients has revealed a single substitution in the B chain of arginine by histidine. Quite why this should result in failed cleavage is not clear. The second abnormality in this category is the presence of a mutant insulin with reduced biological acivity. The best defined of these occurs with a B24 substitution of phenylalanine.[17] The active site of insulin includes the area around B24 and this substitution robs the insulin molecule of most of its activity. As with familial hyperproinsulinaemia, response to exogenous insulin is normal.

True Insulin Resistance. It is widely recognized that a number of hormones have antagonistic actions to insulin in many facets of metabolism (Table 6.4). Indeed these catabolic hormones are often grouped together as gluco-counterregulatory hormones. Of greatest importance are the catecholamines and glucagon. Catecholamines inhibit insulin secretion but, independent of this effect, increase hepatic glucose output through stimulation of glycogen breakdown and are potent stimulators of lipolysis. Increased release of NEFA results in catecholamines being indirectly ketogenic. Glucagon similarly stimulates glycogen breakdown in liver, although it is without effect at physiological concentrations on lipolysis. Within the liver, glucagon is directly ketogenic.

Often grouped with catecholamines and glucagon are cortisol and growth hormone. Although rising promptly in response to hypoglycaemia, their metabolic effects take some time to become apparent. Chronic overproduction of any of these hormones, as in phaeochromocytoma, glucagonoma, Cushing's syndrome or acromegaly, results in insulin resistance. In general it can be assumed that diabetes or impaired glucose tolerance accompany these syndromes when insulin secretion is unable to rise to levels sufficient to obviate their effects. Of more general interest is the response to these hormones in stress. The acute stress of injury or infection is widely recognized to result in glucose intolerance, following elevations of one or more of the catabolic hormones. Perhaps the most common example is with myocardial infarction and the massive surge of catecholamines that follows. In the severely shocked patient, other hormones not normally thought of as catabolic display anti-insulin effects, such as the glycogen breakdown that follows release of vasopressin in shock. The minor degrees of insulin resistance that can be identified in the presence of elevated thyroxine, prolactin, or other hormone are of doubtful importance.

In addition to hormonal antagonism, certain metabolites can result in an impairment of insulin action. In general terms this impairment is less than traditional belief would have it. In diabetic ketoacidosis with elevated hydrogen ion, NEFA, and ketone bodies, all of which result in insulin resistance, the effect upon a response to administered insulin is only modest impairment.

The role of NEFA in insulin resistance merits further discussion. Since Randle and his colleagues[18] proposed a glucose/fatty acid cycle on the basis of their experiments in the perfused rat heart the precise role of this cycle has eluded definition. In brief, they found that in the presence of elevated NEFA concentrations, glucose utilization by heart muscle was decreased. Conversely, when glucose utilization was enhanced by perfusing with glucose and insulin, fatty acid oxidation was inhibited. Newsholme[19] has stressed the precision with which the cycle could be controlled in the human animal. Falling insulin concentrations allow NEFA mobilization, which impairs glucose utilization and thus spares glucose; should glucose begin to rise, stimulation of insulin secretion inhibits lipolysis. An additional safety feature of the cycle is that NEFA stimulate insulin secretion and a rise to toxic concentrations of NEFA is therefore prevented. Recent interest in this cycle has focused on the role of NEFA in insulin resistance. It has become apparent that when insulin resistance is present it cannot only affect glucose metabolism. Many groups have demonstrated insulin resistance in fat metabolism (equated with a right shift in the dose–response curve for insulin vs. NEFA and glycerol) accompanying resistance in carbohydrate metabolism. Could the elevated NEFA observed be the cause of insulin resistance in glucose metabolism? That question is currently unanswered.

The Kahn model of insulin resistance[12] originally proposed that a right shift of the dose–response relation (insulin insensitivity) was analogous with a pure receptor defect, while a failure to realize a maximal response (insulin unresponsiveness) was a feature of a postreceptor defect. Simply argued, only the most severe loss of insulin receptors (more than 90%) would become response-limiting. In all other conditions, enough receptors could be recruited, given a sufficiently high dose of insulin, that a maximal response could be achieved. On the other hand, if the rate-limiting step was a postreceptor defect, then no matter how high the insulin concentration this would remain rate-limiting. Such a distinction is of little value in practice and probably also in theory. It was originally presented when insulin receptors were expected by some to answer many questions in diabetes. Time has shown that they have been of immense interest and stimulus to basic research and distinctly disappointing in clinical or metabolic medicine.

The original distinction, that insulin resistance could arise through receptor binding or postbinding events, was useful. Reduced number or altered affinity of receptors could impair the biological response to insulin. In practice, pure receptor defects, if they exist at all, are rare and occur in the unusual syndromes. Similarly, a pure postreceptor defect is unknown and probably impossible, as it would alter circulating glucose and insulin concentration and hence insulin receptors.[20]

These considerations are of more than theoretical concern in the common diseases of obesity and NIDDM. A feature of both is a blood glucose concentration inappropriately high for the prevailing insulin concentration. Furthermore, by using the techniques described above it can be shown that the biological activity of insulin is impaired. The process that has received the most attention is glucose uptake into peripheral tissues and it is clear that, in both conditions, this is markedly reduced compared with controls when examined at similar insulin concentrations. The use of pharmacological concentrations of insulin (between 1000 and 10 000 mU/L) fails to achieve a maximal response in most patients. Hepatic glucose output can also be shown to be insensitive to insulin, although in the majority of reports the defect is of the type where a maximal response can be achieved but fractions of this maximal response require higher insulin concentrations than controls—a right shift in the dose–response curve. Recent work has attempted to study fat metabolism in these states and accruing evidence indicates that this too displays insulin resistance.

Thus, in NIDDM, insulin resistance and reduced insulin secretion can both be demonstrated. Whether one is a consequence of the other, and if so which is the primary defect, is not clear. Longitudinal studies in man are notoriously difficult to perform, especially when there is little indication which subjects will eventually develop diabetes. Studies at diagnosis and subsequently in the course of the disease may start too late, although the natural history of the disorder may suggest that the progression of treatment with time—diet to tablets to insulin—indicates a progression to hypoinsulinaemia. It is tempting to draw the parallel with the rhesus monkey (*Macaca mulatta*), in which years of insulin resistance precede the onset of diabetes and insulinopenia.[21]

DIAGNOSIS

Despite the varied aetiology and pathogenesis of diabetes mellitus, whether it be type 1 or 2, associated with a disease such as dystrophia myotonica, or part of a rare and unusual syndrome such as leprechaunism, the unifying feature is a raised blood glucose. In the general population the distribution of blood glucose concentration is not bimodal but a continuum skewed to the right, and it should be recognized that the cut-off point below which blood glucose is considered normal and above which it is considered to indicate diabetes is somewhat arbitrary. This was certainly true of earlier diagnostic criteria but more recent criteria are more surely grounded on evidence from long-term epidemiological findings. The crucial question is of defining the blood glucose concentration above which the full-blown clinical syndrome of diabetes, i.e. with its complications, becomes a possibility and below which such events do not occur or are exceedingly unusual. A number of population studies indicate that this cut-off is around 10–12 mmol/L. More precisely, the risk of microvascular complications becomes increased above a capillary blood glucose concentration 2 h after 75 g glucose orally of 11.1 mmol/L (200 mg/100 mL). As discussed below, there are major differences between the specific complications of diabetes—retinopathy, nephropathy, and neuropathy—and the nonspecific macrovascular disease. These differences persist in risk relation (or association) with blood glucose concentration. It is more likely that this relation of macrovascular disease with blood glucose exhibits no particular cut-off point but increases gradually with the concentration. In defining new diagnostic criteria for diabetes, some of these problems were answered by the introduction of an intermediate category between normal and diabetic, called impaired glucose tolerance. Patients in this category have an incidence of atherosclerosis intermediate between normals and the high prevalence of the diabetic population. One other feature marks this group and that is a greater than normal tendency for progression to diabetes with time.

Blood Glucose Estimation

The sample

Certain methodological considerations must be allowed in order to give precision to diagnosis and, more importantly, to our thinking. Venous and capillary blood samples are most commonly used for blood glucose estimation. Ideally one would argue in favour of arterial blood but the acceptability of arteriopuncture is likely to be poor. Arterial and venous blood give similar results for blood glucose measurement in the postabsorptive state. After feeding or oral glucose ingestion, values diverge because of peripheral tissue uptake of glucose. The degree of difference will depend on the arterial glucose concentration, the insulin concentration, and the degree of insulin resistance in peripheral tissue. This changing difference disallows a precisely applicable comparison. Capillary blood will therefore give higher blood glucose values than venous blood, by a factor of 10% for practical purposes.

Whole blood or plasma

Glucose enters erythrocytes with the aim of providing energy. At entry it is immediately phosphorylated and, to all intents and purposes, does not exist as free glucose. The net effect of measuring whole-blood glucose is therefore to measure plasma glucose diluted with intracellular water. One important factor that will contribute to the difference is the number of red cells, which confounds a precise relation of whole-blood and plasma glucose. Again a useful working rule is that the plasma value is 10% higher than that of whole blood.

Methods of blood glucose measurement

It is tempting to imagine that specific enzymatic blood glucose methods, e.g. hexokinase or glucose oxidase, are now so widely used that others can be forgotten. On a world-wide scale this cannot be considered correct. The number of 'historical' methods for measuring reducing substances, sugar, or glucose are so numerous that detailed discussion is impossible. Suffice it to say that the user has a responsibility to know the limitations of a method, particularly its specificity, precision and accuracy, if rational interpretation of the result is to be obtained. This responsibility lies no less squarely on the shoulders of the user of specific glucose methods. The diagnostic criteria for diabetes mellitus are based on specific methods of measurement for blood glucose.

The Patient

The state of the patient and knowledge of drugs administered are important in interpretation of blood glucose measurements. Disturbed carbohydrate metabolism is an accompanying feature of major illness, as reflected in the number of patients with elevated glucose concentration seen in an intensive or coronary-care unit. A number of drugs can result in a high measurement, either through interference in a method or by altering glucose homeostasis in the patient. The most commonly encountered in the latter category are thiazide diuretics and corticosteroids.

The relationship of the diagnosis of diabetes with glucose intolerance during severe illness or from thiazide or corticosteroid administration is an uneasy one. After open-heart surgery, for example, insulin may be necessary to control blood glucose concentration, although whether subsequently the patient will have diabetes is uncertain. Debating the niceties of this point is of little value to the patient, who should be treated as if having diabetes. Better that the debate should continue after recovery than that the metabolic derangement be the final blow which tips the scales against it.

Many patients with diabetes are diagnosed after the introduction of thiazides. Whether this is the final overdemand on an already compromised metabolism, or whether it simply reveals the diagnosis, is unclear.

Pregnancy is a special case. Not only is carbohydrate metabolism altered by this physiological state but there is clearly a type of diabetes associated with it, which remits after delivery—gestational diabetes. The rate of development of NIDDM in later life (60–80% before age 60) would suggest a predisposition to diabetes, temporarily unmasked by pregnancy and becoming manifest later. This brief reference to pregnancy is a reminder that, in contrast to the obsolete terms prediabetes, chemical diabetes, and latent diabetes, the only remaining definition with specific value is that of potential diabetes, as in a collection of risk factors which increases the chance of diabetes developing in pregnancy and therefore gives direction to screening for diabetes.

The Diagnosis of Diabetes and Impaired Glucose Tolerance

Approximately 80% of diabetic patients are diagnosed by random blood glucose measurement. The relation to a recent meal is of some importance but in a negative rather than a positive manner. In other words it does not matter how near to a recent meal the sample is taken, but it does matter if the patient has fasted. The obsession of non-specialists and general practitioners with measuring fasting blood glucose is both pointless and erroneous. In the presence of symptoms, a random venous plasma glucose of more than 11.1 mmol/L (200 mg/100 mL) is diagnostic of diabetes. The diagnosis of diabetes has such ramifications throughout everyday life that the World Health Organization (WHO) advice[8] that diagnosis should not be based on one abnormal blood-glucose result is sensible. How often this is followed in practice is debatable. The WHO reliance on symptoms, as any practising diabetologist will indicate, is the opposite of sensible because many patients have symptoms only in retrospect.

Only when random blood-glucose results are

equivocal is a glucose tolerance test indicated. This is done under specific conditions (Table 6.5). After a fasting sample, 75 g anhydrous glucose diluted with water are drunk. This solution should not be too concentrated, as excessive hyperosmolarity may lead to vomiting and even without vomiting to poor absorption. There is no justification for taking half-hourly samples for 2 h. Diagnosis is based on the fasting and 2-h blood, with a sample taken at 1 h providing additional confirmation and sometimes of use in identifying a pattern found in some non-diabetic conditions. Nor is there any justification for proceeding to a glucose tolerance test when the fasting blood glucose is unequivocally raised.

Interpretation

Specific criteria are laid down for interpretation (Table 6.6). Three specific states are recognized: normal, impaired glucose tolerance and diabetes mellitus. It does not take a mathematical genius to realize that with three levels for two measurements there are nine possible combinations of result for fasting and 2-h measurements.[22] The interpretation of the six non-diagnostic combinations is not the responsibility of the laboratory but of the clinician in the light of the clinical presentation.

Measurement of glycosylated proteins is not included in the diagnostic criteria. If normal or unequivocally raised, a measurement may provide useful confirmatory evidence but poor discrimination of impaired glucose tolerance.[22]

TREATMENT

For appropriate treatment of diabetes it must be decided whether the patient is likely to have the insulin-dependent or non-insulin dependent disease. The majority of symptoms experienced by a newly diagnosed diabetic do not help in this decision. Indeed, it is rather easier to point to factors that do *not* discriminate than to list helpful findings. The intensity of symptoms, polyuria and polydipsia in particular, reflect the degree and duration of hyperglycaemia, which in turn is partly determined by previous fluid intake in response to thirst. Thus, quenching

TABLE 6.5
PROCEDURE FOR AN ORAL GLUCOSE TOLERANCE TEST

1. Ensure preceding diet of > 150 g carbohydrate for 3 days prior to test
2. Fast patient for 10–14 h before test
3. After fasting glucose, give 75 g anhydrous glucose in 300 mL (flavoured) water drunk over 5 min
4. Patient should sit quietly and not smoke
5. Second blood sample at 2 h
6. Urine samples should be collected at 0 and 2 h for detection of renal glycosuria with a normal oral glucose tolerance test

of thirst produced at a blood glucose of 15 mmol/L by the readily available cans of refined sugar may lift the blood glucose to 30 mmol/L but will not alter the type of diabetes. In the presentation the physician pays most attention to a history of weight loss. Some of the lost weight will be fluid, some protein, and the remainder fat. As discussed elsewhere in this chapter, lipolysis is exquisitely sensitive to inhibition by insulin and fat breakdown indicates severe insulinopenia. Fat breakdown is confirmed by the finding of urinary or plasma ketone bodies. A common misapprehension in this situation is that ketonuria may be the result of simultaneous fasting. An example is the newly diagnosed diabetic presenting with weight loss where oral intake has been poor. The accepted normal physiology of fasting shows ketone body production increasing in response to declining glucose and insulin concentrations. This is not so in our diabetic, who will have a blood glucose of sufficient concentration to stimulate insulin secretion. That this has not occurred, even to the extent of producing small amounts of insulin sufficient to inhibit lipolysis, must inevitably lead to the conclusion of severe insulin deficiency, and in treatment terms, insulin dependence.

The conclusion that the patient is non-insulin dependent is arrived at by exclusion—that is he/she is not insulin dependent—although other details of the patient inevitably play a part, especially age and size. Non-insulin dependent diabetic patients will be treated with a diet, or with diet plus tablets, or with diet plus insulin. It is important to understand that treatment with insulin because of persistent hyperglycaemia on diet and tablets does not change a non-insulin dependent diabetic into an insulin-dependent one but rather he or she is an insulin-treated, non-insulin dependent diabetic patient. As the reader may imagine, such precision of language beloved of expert committees does not get much day-to-day usage!

Diet

Dietary treatment of diabetes has followed dietary fashion in the general population. For many years the basis of the diabetic patient's diet was carbohydrate restriction. This originated in the pre-insulin days when strict carbohydrate restriction (or perhaps exclusion) could prolong the life of the insulin-dependent patient by a few months. With treatment came some degree of relaxation of carbohydrate intake but restriction remained a dietary bulwark. This led to the unhappy situation where atheroma was the major cause of mortality in diabetic patients yet they were being prescribed a diet restricted in carbohydrate, (financially) restricted in protein, and consequently a greater percentage of their calories came from fat. This situation was reversed when many groups showed that diabetics could eat more carbohydrate without a deleterious effect upon diabetic control.

TABLE 6.6
INTERPRETATION OF THE ORAL GLUCOSE TOLERANCE TEST

Diagnostic interpretation sample	Venous whole blood (mmol/L)	Capillary whole blood (mmol/L)	Venous plasma (mmol/L)	Capillary plasma (mmol/L)
Diabetes				
Fasting glucose	⩾6.7 (120 mg/100 mL)	⩾6.7 (120. mg/100 mL)	⩾7.8 (140 mg/100 mL)	⩾7.8 (140 mg/100 mL)
2-h sample	⩾10.0 (180 mg/100 mL	⩾11.1 (200 mg/100 mL)	⩾11.1 (200 mg/100 mL)	⩾12.2 (220 mg/100 mL)
Impaired Glucose Tolerance				
Fasting glucose	<6.7 (120 mg/100 mL)	<6.7 (120 mg/100 mL)	<7.8 (140 mg/100 mL)	<7.8 (140 mg/100 mL)
2-h sample	6.7–10.0 (120–180 mg/100 mL)	7.8–11.1 (140–200 mg/100 mL)	7.8–11.1 (140–200 mg/100 mL)	8.9–12.2 (160–220 mg/100 mL)

Certain commonsense considerations were evident—the extra carbohydrate should not be taken as a refined sugar but complex carbohydrate was acceptable. Thus the diabetic's diet is now designed to reduce fat intake by supplying 40–60% of the calories from carbohydrate. In practice the higher figure is quite difficult to attain with the carbohydrate supplied as complex carbohydrate/high fibre.

Oral Hypoglycaemic Agents

There are two groups of oral hypoglycaemic agents used in the treatment of NIDDM.

The first group, the sulphonylureas, contains many drugs with similar action. Initially, blood glucose is lowered by an increase in circulating insulin concentration. Thus efficacy depends upon the patient's pancreas being able to produce more insulin. After a few months, however, the improvement in blood glucose concentration is maintained despite circulating insulin concentrations returning to pre-treatment levels. This ability to improve the circulating efficiency of insulin has been termed an extrapancreatic effect. The precise nature of this effect has proved elusive. Various suggestions have been put forward, including reduced hepatic extraction of insulin, but recent attention has focused upon an improvement in postreceptor binding effects of insulin, that is, a reduction in insulin resistance. It is of interest that this extrapancreatic effect is non-specific. Similar results can be obtained with diet-only treatment when, with weight loss, improved blood glucose concentrations are maintained by a reduced concentration of circulating insulin.

The second group of oral hypoglycaemic agents contains only one drug available in the UK. Metformin is a biguanide of the family that also contains phenformin and buformin. Biguanides lower the blood glucose concentration by reducing intestinal absorption of glucose, inhibiting hepatic gluconeogenesis, and promoting peripheral glucose uptake. While not acting through insulin secretion, they need the permissive effect of circulating insulin concentrations. The lower blood glucose produced by a direct effect upon metabolism results in lower insulin concentrations, which is an advantage in the treatment of patients with NIDDM who are obese and hence have hyperinsulinaemia. The biguanides have unwanted metabolic side-effects, although metformin produces fewer than the others. Indeed phenformin was withdrawn from the UK market because of its propensity for producing lactic acidosis. Metformin rarely produces lactic acidosis and most reports are of patients with associated renal impairment. The significance of the lesser metabolic abnormalities, hyperlactataemia, hyperalaninaemia and hyperketonaemia, are uncertain.[23]

Insulin

The actions of insulin to reduce blood glucose concentration are detailed elsewhere in this chapter. In a patient with insulin deficiency it is extremely difficult to achieve the minute-by-minute regulation of blood glucose concentration that is found in the normal subject. In part this is because of the limitations of insulin preparations but it is also due to attitudes to insulin injections and the practical limitation that exogenous insulin is delivered into the peripheral circulation rather than the more physiologically important portal circulation.

The many insulin preparations available fall into three broad categories—quick, intermediate, and long acting. Intermediate and long-acting insulins are manufactured by addition of agents that retard absorption to quick-acting insulin. Protophane and zinc are the major complexing agents. Therapeutic insulins also divide according to species. Beef, pork and human insulins are available. Human insulin is manufactured by genetically programmed bacteria or yeasts.

If normal physiology is considered it is apparent

that the amounts of circulating insulin have two components—an overnight basal secretion and meal- and snack-stimulated peaks. In recent years, attempts have been made to mimic this normal pattern in the diabetic by given one intermediate-acting insulin late at night to provide the counterpart of the basal, overnight insulin, and then three injections of quick-acting insulin immediately before the main meals. Acceptance of such a regimen has been enhanced by the replacement of the conventional insulin syringe with pen injection devices with insulin cartridges.

Monitoring Treatment

Control of diabetes is held to be important in the prevention of its long-term complications.[24] The evidence that this is so comes from three sources. Firstly, retrospective studies of human diabetics indicate that fewer complications occur in groups of patients who are well controlled. There are many such studies in the literature yet there is a serious flaw underlying the results. It takes upward of 10 years from the onset (but not necessarily the diagnosis) of diabetes to develop long-term diabetic complications. Assessing the level of control over 10 years is fraught with difficulties, especially as most of the studies preceded the advent of glycosylated protein assays. The majority of studies, therefore, are based upon random blood-glucose measurement at clinic attendance, and/or the clinicians' attempts to grade control from home and hospital urine tests. In addition to this problem, the design (or more strictly, lack of design) of these studies fails to answer the problem of whether all participants have diabetes of a similar tendency to develop complications—in other words, whether diabetes that is easy to control is also less likely to result in complications.

Animal experiments also give evidence for a relation between control and complications. Small animals can be made diabetic by injecting alloxan or streptozotocin and allocated to two levels of diabetic control. Complications develop more rapidly in the poorly controlled group. This type of diabetes, however, lacks the genetic component of human diabetes.

Prospective studies of this relation have proved more difficult. Where they have been made, the weight of evidence supports the view that the better the diabetic control, the less likely that complications will develop. Unfortunately, achieving and maintaining two levels of diabetic control is difficult without relegating one group of patients to 'poor' control for 10 + years—an idea that most physicians and ethical committees would rebel against. Not surprisingly, the studies have left some room for doubt but most physicians would agree that control plays some, if not the total, part in preventing complications. Thus the working hypothesis for the management of the diabetic patient is to obtain the best degree of diabetic control as is possible without unacceptable disruption of the patient's life.

It is important to have a realistic concept of good diabetic control. In theory, good control would be equivalent to euglycaemia but this may only be realistic for patients on diet only, for some on oral agents, and for hardly anyone on insulin. For reasons outlined elsewhere, the achievement and maintenance of normoglycaemia in patients using insulin is very difficult with the exception of those in the 'honeymoon' period—the period of some 6 months after the introduction of insulin therapy—and of women during pregnancy. To be realistic, therefore, acceptable levels of control have been defined (Table 6.7).[25]

Glycosylated Proteins

Achieving the best possible diabetic control necessitates a reliable assessment of that control. In the clinic this has been provided in recent years by measurement of the glycosylated proteins haemoglobin A_1 (HbA_1) or fructosamine. Such measurement gives objective evidence of diabetic control in the weeks preceding clinic attendance.

Posttranslational glycosylation of protein depends upon the degree of glycaemia that the protein is exposed to during its lifetime. HbA_1 reflects diabetic control over the preceding 4–6 weeks, while fructosamine gives an assessment of control in the preceding 1–3 weeks. Of the minor glycosylated products of HbA the largest contribution is from HbA_{1c}. Methods for measuring HbA_{1c}, however, are less amenable to use in a diabetic clinic which generates a large number of samples than those that measure total HbA_1.[26] Some confounding conditions that affect the turnover rate of the protein lead to aberrant results. Non-enzymic glycosylation of the ε-amino

TABLE 6.7
ACCEPTABLE LEVELS OF DIABETIC CONTROL

	Good	Acceptable	Poor
Blood glucose			
Fasting	4.4–6.7 mmol/L (80–120 mg/100 mL)	< 7.8 mmol/L (140 mg/100 mL)	< 7.8 mmol/L (140 mg/100 mL)
Postprandial	4.4–8.9 mmol/L (80–160 mg/100 mL)	< 10 mmol/L (180 mg/100 mL)	< 10 mmol/L (180 mg/100 mL)
HbA₁	< mean ± 2 SD	< mean ± 4 SD	> mean ± 4 SD

groups of lysine residues of albumin produces a product christened 'fructosamine'. Measurement of this protein has a number of advantages over HbA_1 in that it can be readily automated, is cheap by comparison, and has good analytical precision. As glycosylation of albumin contributes approx. 80% to the final result, physiological or pathological conditions that reduce the serum albumin concentration may modify the result obtained and it has been suggested that the result should be corrected for the serum albumin. Due to the more recent introduction of the assay, it is less well investigated in clinical use.[27]

Home Monitoring

An equally impressive revolution in monitoring in recent years has been the introduction of home blood-glucose monitoring. Reagent strips for the measurement of blood glucose were available in the 1960s but it was not until the work of Sonksen and Tattersall and their colleagues in the 1970s that the full potential for use by patients was revealed.[28,29] Most of the strips are based upon immobilized glucose oxidase with a colour end-point proportional to the substrate concentration. Such is the ease with which blood glucose can be measured using reagent strips that their use has spread from home to health centre, outpatient clinic, casualty department, ward or laboratory. While their use is convenient and cheap, reservations remain about reliability and the appropriateness of using extralaboratory measurements.[30]

The ability to measure blood glucose at home has revolutionized the life of many diabetics, particularly those patients on insulin who can derive reassurance and information for changes in their insulin regimen. For non-insulin dependent diabetics, home blood-glucose measurement is more a record-keeping exercise than a means for modifying treatment. Records in both groups of patients should be read in the light of objective assessment of control, that is glycosylated protein. It is surprising how often major discrepancies between the two methods of assessing control are found.

In the clinic, other aspects of monitoring deserve attention. Microalbuminuria and Albustix-positive proteinuria require documentation, as does 24-h quantitative excretion of the latter. Lipids are also an important part of monitoring.

HYPERGLYCAEMIC EMERGENCIES

Hyperglycaemia with dehydration and with or without acidosis is a medical emergency. Diabetic ketoacidosis is the most common form, while the more unusual hypersosmolar non-ketotic diabetic coma and lactic acidosis carry a high mortality.

Diabetic Ketoacidosis

Diabetic ketoacidosis is a risk throughout the life of the insulin-dependent diabetic from diagnosis to old age. It is defined as severe, uncontrolled diabetes requiring emergency treatment with intravenous fluids and insulin and presenting with a total ketone body concentration of more than 5 mmol/L. As ketone bodies are rarely measured anything but retrospectively, the diagnosis is based on clinical presentation, dehydration and acidosis. There is no level of blood glucose in the definition for the very good reason that while usually presenting with hyperglycaemia, diabetic ketoacidosis may present with only minor elevation of blood glucose or even euglycaemia.

Pathogenesis

The metabolic abnormalities result from a relative insulin lack with excess catabolic hormone secretion. Some insulin can be detected in the blood of patients with diabetic ketoacidosis but it is clearly insufficient to counteract the catabolic response associated with infection, thrombotic episodes (including myocardial infarction), and trauma. Often the relative insulin lack is compounded by inappropriate advice or action resulting in a reduced insulin dose during intercurrent illness. The end-result of relative insulinopenia and catabolic hormone excess is to increase glucose production and decrease utilization; promote fat breakdown and reduce storage; promote intrahepatic ketogenesis and reduce peripheral ketone-body utilization. The concentrations of blood glucose and ketone bodies rise. Above the renal threshold for glucose (about 10 mmol/L (180 mg/100 mL)) glycosuria occurs. Initially fluid loss can be counteracted by oral intake but as blood glucose continues to rise fluid and electrolyte loss is increased. At this stage, fluid loss cannot be obviated by oral intake. Ketone bodies, initially buffered by normal systems, gradually exceed this capacity; pH and bicarbonate fall, stimulating respiration, and Pa_{CO_2} also falls. The acidosis is accompanied by deep, rapid ventilation (Kussmaul respiration), nausea and vomiting, which combine to increase fluid and electrolyte loss.

Diagnosis

The patient presents with a history of thirst, polyuria, nausea and vomiting, and on examination is dehydrated, with Kussmaul respiration. Diabetic coma is a misnomer for this condition because only about 25% of patients are comatose. On urine testing, glycosuria and ketonuria are present and the diagnosis should be rapidly confirmed by measurement of blood glucose and gases. Baseline measurements of electrolyte concentrations are mandatory because they will govern the electrolyte administration in the early stages of treatment.

Treatment

The principles of treatment are rehydration, electrolyte replacement and insulin.

Rehydration is usually undertaken with saline (150

mmol/L (0.9%)) and, except in the elderly or where heart disease is present, the rate of infusion is rapid. In the first 3 h, 3 L can be given, followed by a further 3 L in the next 10 h. The rate may need adjustment in the light of urine output. The urine loss may be great, owing to the osmotic effect of glycosuria, but oliguria and occasionally anuria may be present if the patient has prolonged hypotension or severe dehydration. The strength of saline may be changed if the plasma sodium exceeds about 150 mmol/L. Plasma sodium at presentation may be low, normal or high, depending upon the relative losses of sodium or water. Grossly lipaemic serum may also be apparent at presentation, leading to pseudohyponatraemia with some methods of measuring sodium. In this instance, the plasma sodium may apparently rise rapidly with rehydration and clearance of the lipaemia with insulin. When alternative saline solutions are available, 75 mmol/L (0.45%) or even 30 mmol/L (0.18%) may be used. Both carry the risk of causing haemolysis if too much (more than 2 L) is infused.

It is of paramount importance to avoid hypokalaemia or hyperkalaemia during treatment, as both may cause cardiac arrhythmias with fatal consequences. As with sodium, potassium may be low, normal, or high at presentation. During treatment the main risk is from hypokalaemia. Plasma potassium will fall with rehydration and this is exaggerated if alkali is used. In addition, insulin administration results in potassium uptake into cells, so increasing the likelihood of hypokalaemia. Overenthusiastic replacement of potassium carries cardiac risk and thus the physician treads a narrow line when prescribing potassium replacement. Clearly the laboratory has a role in providing information for appropriate infusion concentrations.

Insulin is given in small but frequent amounts[31] with the aim of achieving a circulating concentration that will inhibit hepatic glucose output and promote glucose utilization, so leading to a fall in blood glucose, and that will inhibit lipolysis, leading to a fall in hepatic ketogenesis and thus correction of the acidosis. An intravenous infusion of 6 units/h is a widely used regimen, although intramuscular insulin (20 units at diagnosis followed by 6 units hourly) works just as well. Rapid-acting insulin is always used and the subcutaneous route is avoided because of the danger of poor perfusion and absorption.

There are a couple of controversial areas during treatment. The first concerns the use of alkali. In theory, severe acidosis may impair myocardial contractility and diminish the glycolytic rate. Partial correction of the acidosis with sodium bicarbonate (150 mmol given over half an hour) is not without risk, however, through accentuating potassium loss in the urine.

Linked to the use of alkali is a second area of concern. At presentation, the amount of 2:3 disphosphoglycerate (DPG) is low, with consequences for peripheral oxygen delivery. Administration of phosphate will raise the 2:3 DPG levels, with theoretical benefit. The major problem with giving phosphate is that it needs to be done as a potassium salt. The amount of potassium required, however, far exceeds the amount of phosphate and some juggling of potassium additives is needed. This complicates the regimen and most physicians agree that the potential for error outweighs the potential benefit. Interestingly, the effect upon the oxyhaemoglobin dissociation curve of low 2:3 DPG levels is offset somewhat by an opposite shift due to acidosis. This benefit is lost if the acidosis is modified rapidly by alkali administration.[32]

Treatment is modified when the blood glucose falls to about 14 mmol/L (250 mg/100 mL). Fluid is changed to a glucose solution (5 or 10% dextrose) and the amount of insulin is reduced. Infusion of potassium is continued as appropriate. This glucose/insulin/potassium infusion can be maintained until the patient resumes oral intake.

The role of the laboratory in the management of diabetic ketoacidosis is of obvious importance. In any series reporting patients with diabetic ketoacidosis, approaching half of the deaths occur during treatment and often without obvious pathology at autopsy. Careful monitoring reduces such unexplained mortality and contributes to better survival in the remaining patients with severe associated illness. At diagnosis of ketoacidosis the laboratory contributes to an assessment of the severity with glucose, electrolyte, and acid–base measurements. During treatment, 4-hourly electrolyte measurement is necessary and occasionally potassium may require more frequent estimation. Inevitably, junior doctors inexperienced in ketoacidosis management will place greater demands upon the laboratory. Thus it should be; experience shows a mortality of 6% in centres with a major interest in the condition compared with 12–15% in less experienced centres.

Hyperglycaemic Non-ketotic Diabetic Coma

A less common form of 'diabetic coma' is the hyperglycaemic non-ketotic. The aetiology and pathogenesis of the condition are not clear and suggestions only may be derived from the clinical presentation and outcome of management. Thus the presentation is often preceded by ingestion of refined carbohydrate drinks in an attempt to assuage the thirst of diabetes. Two groups are particular prone to this condition—the elderly and patients of Afro-Caribbean origin. Once the acute condition has been successfully treated, patients may be treated by diet with or without oral hypoglycaemic agents. Thus the suggestion has been made that patients presenting with hyperglycaemic non-ketotic coma have sufficient insulin circulating to inhibit lipolysis and ketogenesis but insufficient to stimulate glucose uptake into cells.

The condition is diagnosed when hyperglycaemia

is accompanied by a plasma osmolaelity of more than 340 mmol/kg with no significant degree of metabolic acidosis. Some degree of ketonuria may be present.

The management of hyperglycaemic non-ketotic coma is similar to that for ketoacidosis; rehydration, insulin, and electrolytes and the demands upon monitoring are therefore identical. It is worth bearing in mind that, although less common than diabetic ketoacidosis, the mortality is higher (approx. 33%).

Lactic Acidosis

Lactic acidosis is a rare accompaniment of diabetes. Diabetics are not immune from lactic acidosis resulting from hypovolaemic or septicaemic shock, and they have the additional risk of lactic acidosis associated with diabetes *per se*, or with biguanide treatment of diabetes. Quite why diabetes should carry a risk for lactic acidosis is not clear, although pyruvate dehydrogenase is modified by insulin and nutritional status. Lactic acidosis was a real risk with the biguanides phenformin and buformin but is considerably less of a risk with metformin.[23] Indeed, in the majority of reported cases of metformin-associated lactic acidosis, contraindications to use of the drug were present in the patients. The precise mechanism of action of biguanides is not understood but administration results in small increases in lactate and other gluconeogenic precursors in otherwise healthy diabetics.

HYPOGLYCAEMIA

The definition of hypoglycaemia in non-diabetic subjects persists into diabetes—a blood glucose concentration of less than 2.2 mmol/L. Such a figure is of use only as an *aide-mémoire* and has no value as a precise definition of hypoglycaemia. It is not even clear, in the diabetic patient, whether the absolute blood glucose concentration is the trigger for either neuroglycopenia or the hormonal counter-regulatory response. A number of diabetic patients will claim experience of hypoglycaemic symptoms when they are normoglycaemic or even hyperglycaemic. A potential explanation of this may lie in *rate of fall* of blood glucose as a trigger to hypoglycaemic symptoms in addition to absolute concentration.

Hypoglycaemia triggers the symptoms of neuroglycopenia and the counter-regulatory response, which is itself a source of adrenergic symptoms and signs. Neuroglycopenia results in altered sensory perception, particularly perioral tinglings, light-headedness, and confusion progressing to convulsions and coma. As the brain is dependent upon glucose as a substrate, these sequelae are predictable and it is important to recognize that diabetic hypoglycaemia is always accompanied by hyperinsulinism such that other potential substrates for brain metabolism, for example NEFA and total ketone bodies, are unavailable through suppression of lipolysis and ketogenesis.

This situation exists until the counter-regulatory response is established.

The ability of insulin to induce hypoglycaemia has been well used in medicine in the investigation of pituitary disease. Hypoglycaemia triggers the release of growth hormone and ACTH and hence cortisol, all of which have actions upon metabolism antagonistic to insulin. These effects, although well recognized, are of minor importance in the correction of acute hypoglycaemia. In this situation it is the catecholamines and glucagon that are of major import. Both raise blood glucose by mobilizing the glycogen stores of the liver, while adrenaline and noradrenaline are potent stimulators of lipolysis and glucagon plays a role in ketogenesis.

Precipitating factors in hypoglycaemia are many and varied, although the most common are missed meals and unplanned exercise. Both of these result in inappropriately high insulin concentrations for the prevailing blood glucose concentration in an insulin-dependent diabetic patient. Mild hypoglycaemic symptoms occur commonly in patients on sulphonylureas, but severe hypoglycaemia is unusual. In all respects, hypoglycaemia in the non-insulin dependent diabetic is identical to that of the insulin-dependent diabetic, although it is worth drawing attention to the presentation of severe hypoglycaemia in elderly patients with NIDDM as a hemiplegia or other neurological deficit. This diagnosis should not be missed.

Treatment

The suspicion of hypoglycaemia demands treatment without waiting for confirmation of the diagnosis. It is nevertheless necessary to obtain a sample for subsequent measurement of blood glucose, as treatment may result in recovery in normoglycaemic conditions, and conversely may not result in immediate recovery in a patient where hypoglycaemia has been severe and prolonged even with the restoration of normoglycaemia. Measurement of insulin concentrations in diabetic hypoglycaemia is of no interest or importance.

Treatment is with intravenous glucose. Traditionally, 40 ml of 50% dextrose are given, although this is something of an 'overkill'. It can be difficult to inject this viscous fluid into a confused patient and extravasation can have severe consequences to surrounding tissues, leading to sloughing. For this reason, glucagon, 1 mg intramuscular or subcutaneously, may be preferred. It should be noted that the hyperglycaemic response to glucagon is of the order of 1–2 mmol/L (18–36 mg/100 mL) and thus it may be insufficient to produce normoglycaemia. Nevertheless, it is usually enough to awaken a patient sufficiently for oral glucose to be given.

Sulphonylurea-induced hypoglycaemia may be more problematical in treatment. Patients with NIDDM are capable of insulin secretion yet they also receive either glucose or glucagon as treatment. As both are potent secretagogues of insulin, hyperinsulinism may be enhanced and protracted. For this reason these patients must be admitted to hospital and receive careful monitoring of blood glucose during the customary treatment with an intravenous glucose infusion.

LONG-TERM COMPLICATIONS OF DIABETES

The long-term complications of diabetes are divided into those arising from disease of small blood vessels, retinopathy and nephropathy, and those from disease of large arteries, collectively called macrovascular disease. Diabetic neuropathy sits uneasily in this classification, with uncertainty surrounding its derivation from microvascular disease and increasing evidence of a biochemical pathogenesis.

Diabetic Neuropathy

A useful clinical classification of diabetic neuropathy is:

1. Distal symmetrical sensory polyneuropathy.
2. Proximal painful neuropathy.
3. Isolated nerve palsies.
4. Autonomic neuropathy.

This also provides some suggestion of a multifactorial causation. Thus, isolated nerve palsies may be predicted to improve with time, proximal neuropathy may remit with improved diabetic control, while distal symmetrical polyneuropathy, and particularly autonomic neuropathy, appear to run a course independent of attempts at intervention. The time-course of improvement of isolated nerve palsies corresponds to the recanalization of blood supply, which might be expected if the original sudden onset had been due to thrombosis of a small vessel supplying the nerve. Such small-vessel disease has also been suggested as causal in all types of diabetic neuropathy, although support for this view has waned in recent years with increasing evidence of a biochemical causation.

It is of some interest that tissues damaged in long-term diabetic patients are those where insulin is *not* required for glucose entry. This is particularly true of peripheral nerve. Thus, high blood-glucose concentrations are reflected in high intracellular concentrations of glucose, which in nerve are not rate-promoting for glycolysis. Instead a second pathway for glucose disposal is activated, the polyol pathway (Fig. 6.4). In this pathway, glucose is converted to sorbitol by aldose reductase and then to fructose by *sorbitol* dehydrogenase. This latter enzyme is rate-limiting in the pathway and consequently there is an accumulation of sorbitol. Sorbitol does not diffuse readily across cell membranes and intracellular accumulation leads to an osmotic effect with subsequent cell damage. It has been shown in human and experimental diabetes that the amounts of glucose, sorbitol and fructose are raised in nerve, supporting this hypoth-

Aldose reductase

$$Glucose + NADPH + H^+ \rightleftharpoons Sorbitol + NADP^+$$

Sorbitol dehydrogenase

$$Sorbitol + NAD^+ \rightleftharpoons Fructose + NADH + H^+$$

Figure 6.4 Sorbitol pathway.

esis, although reciprocal changes in myo-inositol concentrations are thought by some to be of primary importance. The 'polyol pathway' hypothesis has led to clinical trials with aldose reductase inhibitors in an attempt to reverse diabetic neuropathy. Results have been disappointing, perhaps because clinical diabetic neuropathy is too late a stage for reversibility to be found. Alternatively, perhaps sorbitol is of no causal import or inhibition of aldose reductase is not achieved.

Diabetic Retinopathy

The pathogenesis of diabetic retinopathy is full of uncertainty. It is clear that the diabetic retina shows abnormalities of blood flow, although the precise role for these abnormalities remains in doubt. Similarly, a variety of abnormalities in rheology and coagulation can be demonstrated in patients with diabetic retinopathy. Viscosity is increased, platelet sensitivity is increased, and the levels of β-thromboglobulin and factor VIII are raised. However, changes in blood rheology and coagulation are common in diabetics both with and without retinopathy. Some changes are clearly related to diabetic control, and it is difficult to guess whether the changes are, themselves, secondary to the presence of the diabetic complication. Fortunately, with greater (but not total) certainty there remain a number of studies implicating diabetic control in the progression of retinopathy and, in the absence of a clearer pathogenesis, work aimed at improving control is worthwhile.

Diabetic Nephropathy

It will come as no surprise that the pathogenesis of diabetic nephropathy, the second microvascular complication of diabetes, is only marginally clearer than that outlined above for retinopathy. The kidney has the advantage (for the investigator if not the patient) that it is readily accessible to the biopsy needle, tissue can be inspected, and a positive abnormality identified. This abnormality is thickening of basement membrane. Glomerular basement membrane is composed of collagen and non-collagenous and carbohydrate mixtures. The type IV collagen contains significant amounts of proline, hydroxyproline, hydroxylysine and glycine. The non-collagenous content includes glycosaminoglycan, proteoglycans and laminin. About 10% of glomerular basement membrane is carbohydrate, including glucose, galactose, mannose and glucoronic acid. Glucose/galactose disaccharides are linked to hydroxylysine in the peptide chain. Other combinations are linked to the chain either by disulphide bonds through serine or by glycosylamine bonds through asparagine.

The development of diabetic nephropathy follows a typical route. After a number of years of diabetes, and usually with the other microvascular complication of retinopathy already evident, a patient will develop initially slight and intermittent proteinuria (Albustix positive). After a variable length of time this proteinuria becomes both heavy and constant, and some time later the signs of declining renal function will become evident in the blood. Once creatinine concentrations begin to rise they do so inexorably. Indeed, once this stage has been reached a plot of time vs. the reciprocal of the creatinine concentration can be extrapolated to date the occurrence of creatinine concentration at which death will result.

In recent years, attention has been drawn to the pre-(Albustix positive) proteinuria phase. With more sensitive techniques for detecting proteinuria, albumin may be found in normal people, in diabetics without renal damage and, importantly, in diabetics with renal damage but who do not yet have Albustix-positive proteinuria. This degree of proteinuria has been termed, somewhat inaccurately, microalbuminuria. The rather extravagant claim has been entered that renal damage is, at this stage, reversible—the amount of microalbuminuria declining with improved control, control of blood pressure, and low-protein intakes—and consequently some knowledge of the estimation and application of microalbuminuria is necessary.

Microalbuminuria

Who should be screened for microalbuminuria? As it is an early marker of tissue damage, and unless we can identify a group of diabetic patients not at risk of complications, the answer must be *all*. How often they should be screened is difficult; annually while negative—then more often when microalbuminuria is detected. Various protocols exist for re-testing positive patients but all depend upon the degree of intervention employed and the number of patients seen.

How should patients be screened? This question has attracted considerable attention and produced a variety of possible answers. Twenty-four hour collections of urine are notoriously unreliable and generally involve the patient in two trips to hospital, to collect and deliver the container. Timed overnight collections probably increase reliability but are of equal inconvenience. Given these considerations, attempts to find a suitable means of expressing results in a spot sample have been devised, e.g. albumin:creatinine ratio. Perhaps the best solution is screening by spot sample but follow-up of positives with a timed overnight sample.

Which factors affect albumin excretion? Microalbuminuria may be detected in diabetic patients without early nephropathy at times of poor diabetic control and after exercise. In addition, the numerous causes of heavy proteinuria will also be detected—urinary tract infections, heart failure, etc. Nevertheless, it is often clear when faced with the patient that microalbuminuria reflects diabetic kidney damage, alerting the physician to the potential risk and opportunity for intervention.

Macrovascular Disease

Macrovascular disease (atheroma) is the major cause of mortality in patients with diabetes. It is the only 'diabetic complication' that also occurs in non-diabetics, although with subtle differences—it occurs at an earlier age, is more extensive and, when peripheral, tends to be more distal than the proximal disease of the non-diabetic. It differs from microvascular disease and neuropathy by being unrelated to diabetic control. Thus, the involvement of factors other than blood glucose occupies the mind. These risk factors are identical to those in the population as a whole: smoking, hypertension, family history, and lipids. Lipids have evoked a love–hate relationship with diabetologists: some measure them and focus on the results while others can barely cope with the volume of other factors in diabetes. The latter have also been put off by the relation between diabetic control and plasma lipids. It is clear that some lipid abnormalities can be corrected by instigation of euglycaemia. This is such a difficult goal to achieve, however, that more and more diabetologists are turning to simultaneous treatment of blood glucose and raised lipids.

Protein Glycosylation

Is protein glycosylation a factor in the development of diabetic complications? Post-translational glycosylation of a number of proteins is well recognized. Glucose condenses non-enzymatically with free amino groups either at the N-terminal or ε-amino groups of lysine residues. The Schiff base that is formed undergoes an Amadori rearrangement forming a stable ketoamine linkage (Fig. 6.5). Glycosylation of haemoglobin has been studied extensively and has entered laboratory use as a long-term marker of diabetic control. The amount of glycosylated protein formed reflects the prevailing degree of glycaemia with length of exposure. In turn, length of exposure is a function of protein turnover rates. Proteins that may be glycosylated include lens proteins, albumin and collagen. Collagen and advanced glycosylation end-products form cross-links that disturb the function of the protein—for example, glycosylated

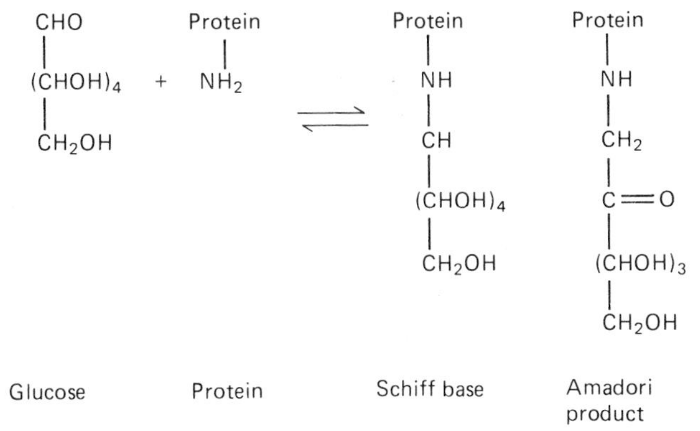

Figure 6.5 Glycosylation of proteins.

basement membrane is more resistant to enzymic digestion than when not glycosylated.

It remains to be seen to what degree the long-term complications of diabetes can be explained by glycosylation of protein. The scope certainly exists for linking microangiopathy and glycosylated basement membrane, cataract and glycosylated lens protein, and atheroma and glycosylated arterial collagen and low-density lipoprotein. It is to be hoped that the next few years will see resolution of this debate.

REFERENCES

1. Chang T.W., Goldberg A.L. (1978). The origin of alanine produced in skeletal muscle. *J. Biol. Chem.*, **253**, 3677.
2. Hers H.G. (1974). The control of glycogen metabolism in the liver. *Annu. Rev. Biochem.*, **45**, 167.
3. McGarry J.D., Woeltje K.F., Kuwajima M., Foster D.W. (1989). Regulation of ketogenesis and the renaissance of carnitine palmitoyltransferase. *Diabetes/Metab. Rev.*, **5**, 271.
4. Steiner D.F., Oyer P.E. (1967). The biosynthesis of insulin and a probable precursor of insulin by a human islet cell adenoma. *Proc. Natl. Acad. Sci. (USA)*, **57**, 473.
5. Rubenstein A.H., Clark J.L., Melani F., Steiner D.F. (1969). Secretion of pro-insulin C-peptide by pancreatic β cells and its circulation in blood. *Nature*, **224**, 697.
6. Czech M.P. (1981). Structure and function of the insulin receptor. *Am. J. Med.*, **70**, 142.
7. Alberti K.G.M.M., Nattrass M. (1978). Severe diabetic ketoacidosis. *Med. Clin. North. Am.*, **61**, 799.
8. World Health Organization (1985). *Diabetes Mellitus: Report of a World Health Organization Expert Committee*, WHO Technical Report Series 727, Geneva: WHO.
9. Hitman G.A., Niven M.J. (1983). Genes and diabetes mellitus. *Br. Med. Bull.*, **45**: 191.
10. Bottazzo G.F. (1986). Death of a beta cell—homicide or suicide? *Diabetic Med*, **3**, 119.
11. Barnett A.H., Eff C., Leslie R.G.D., Pyke D.A. (1981). Diabetes in identical twins: a study of 200 pairs. *Diabetologia*, **20**, 87.
12. Kahn C.R. (1978). Insulin resistance, insulin sensitivity and insulin responsiveness: a necessary distinction. *Metabolism*, **27** (suppl. 2), 1893.
13. Himsworth H.P., Kerr R.B. (1939). Insulin-sensitive and insulin-insensitive types of diabetes mellitus. *Clin. Sci.*, **4**, 119.
14. Reaven G.M. (1983). Insulin resistance in non-insulin-dependent diabets. Does it exist and can it be measured? *Am. J. Med.*, **74**, 3.
15. DeFronzo R.A., Tobin J.D., Andres R. (1979). Glucose clamp technique: a method for quantifying insulin secretion and resistance. *Am. J. Physiol.*, **237**, E214.
16. Gabbay K.H., De Luca K., Fisher J.N., Mako M.E., Rubenstein A.H. (1976). Familial hyperproinsulinaemia: an autosomal dominant defect. *N. Engl. J. Med.*, **294**, 911.
17. Kwok S.C.M., Steiner D.F., Rubenstein A.H., Tager H.S. (1983). Identification of a point mutation in the human insulin gene giving rise to structurally abnormal insulin (insulin Chicago). *Diabetes*, **32**, 872.
18. Randle P.J., Garland P.B., Hales C.N., Newsholme E.A. (1963). The glucose fatty acid cycle: its role in insulin sensitivity and the metabolic disturbances of diabetes mellitus. *Lancet*, **i**, 785.
19. Newsholme E.A. (1976). Carbohydrate metabolism *in vivo*: regulation of the blood glucose level. *Clin. Endocrinol. Metab.*, **5**, 543.
20. Soll A.H., Kahn C.R., Neville D.M., Roth J. (1975). Insulin receptor deficiency in genetic and acquired obesity. *J. Clin. Invest.*, **56**, 769.
21. Hansen B.C., Bodkin N.L. (1986). Heterogeneity of insulin responses: phases leading to type 2 (non-insulin-dependent) diabetes mellitus in the rhesus monkey. *Diabetologia*, **29**, 713.
22. Allbutt E.C., Nattrass M., Northam B.E. (1985). Glucose tolerance test and glycosylated haemoglobin measurement for diagnosis of diabetes mellitus—an assessment of the criteria of the WHO Expert Committee on Diabetes Mellitus 1980. *Ann. Clin. Biochem.*, **22**, 67.
23. Bailey C.J., Nattrass M. (1988). Treatment—metformin. *Clin. Endocrinol. Metab.*, **2**, 455.
24. Singh B.M., Nattrass M. (1990). Diabetes mellitus and the control of hyperglycaemia. In *New Antidiabetic Drugs* (Bailey C.J., Flatt P.R. eds.) London: Smith-Gordon, pp. 1–18.
25. Alberti K.G.M.M., Gries F.A. (1988). Management of non-insulin-dependent diabetes mellitus in Europe: a consensus view. *Diabetic Med.*, **5**, 275.
26. Lester E. (1985). The clinical value of glycated haemoglobin and glycated plasma proteins. *Ann. Clin. Biochem.*, **26**, 213.
27. Hill R.P., Hindle E.J., Howey J.E.A., Lemon M., Lloyd D.R. (1990). Recommendations for adopting standard conditions and analytical procedures in the measurement of serum fructosamine concentration. *Ann. Clin. Biochem.*, **27**, 413.
28. Sonksen P.H., Judd S.L., Lowy C. (1978). Home monitoring of blood glucose. *Lancet*, **i**, 729.
29. Walford S., Gale E.A.M., Allison S.R., Tattersall R.B. (1978). Self-monitoring of blood glucose: improvement of diabetic control. *Lancet*, **i**, 732.
30. Price C.P., Burrin J.M., Nattrass M. (1988). Extra laboratory blood glucose measurement: a policy statement. *Diabetic Med.*, **5**, 705.
31. Alberti K.G.M.M. (1977). Low dose insulin in the

treatment of diabetic ketoacidosis. *Arch. Intern. Med.,* **137**, 1367.

32. Hale P.J., Crase J., Nattrass M. (1984). Metabolic effects of bicarbonate in the treatment of diabetic ketoacidosis. *Br. Med. J.,* **285**, 1035.

33. Brownlee M., Cerami A., Vlassava H. (1988). Advanced glycosylation end-products in tissue and the biochemical basis of diabetic complications. *N. Engl. J. Med.,* **318**, 1317.

7. The Clinical Biochemistry of Alcohol

S.B. Rosalki

Introduction
  Definitions
  Metabolism of alcohol
Acute alcoholic intoxication
  Clinical features
  Biochemical confirmation
  Biochemical changes
  Biochemical changes accompanying
    alcohol withdrawal
Biochemical factors relevant to predisposition
    to excess alcohol intake and to alcoholic
    organ damage
  Genetic factors
  Trait markers
  Biochemical abnormalities that may
    predispose to alcoholic brain damage
  Biochemical mechanisms that may
    encourage or perpetuate excessive
    drinking
Biochemical changes that assist in identifying
    excess alcohol consumption
  Identification of recent alcohol intake
  Identification of chronic excess alcohol
    intake
Overview of the laboratory identification of
    alcohol excess
Clinical consultation, questionnaires and their
    relation to biochemical abnormalities
Complications of alcoholism
  Pancreatitis
  Alcoholic myopathy
  Cardiomyopathy
  Vitamin deficiency
  Alcoholic bone disease
  Alcoholic ketoacidosis
Conclusion

INTRODUCTION

At least 6% of adult males and 1% of adult females in the UK are estimated to consume excessive quantities of alcohol (ethanol).[1] Alcohol excess may give rise to acute effects (particularly intoxication), metabolic changes and chronic organ injury. Biochemical investigation can make a major contribution to their recognition and management.

This chapter will review:

1. The metabolism of alcohol.
2. The biochemical recognition and concomitants of acute alcoholic intoxication.
3. Biochemical factors possibly relevant to predisposition to excess alcohol intake.
4. Biochemical changes indicative of such predisposition ('trait' markers).
5. Biochemical abnormalities resulting from the metabolic and organ-injury effects of chronic excess alcohol intake, especially those abnormalities of value for the identification of such intake ('state' markers).

Where appropriate, relevant clinical features will also be considered.

Definitions

The following terms will be used in this chapter.

- **Excess alcohol consumption** (synonyms: 'heavy drinking'; 'alcohol abuse') may be considered as regular alcohol intake at levels at which there is a high risk of harm, particularly from organ injury. Where such intake is accompanied by actual harm, the terms *'harmful drinking'*, *'problem drinking'* or *'alcoholism'* may be used.
- **Alcoholism** (synonym: 'chronic alcoholism') has been defined as the repeated ingestion of alcohol, resulting in dependency, disease or other harm.[2]
- **Dependency** (synonym: 'alcohol dependency syndrome') is characterized by drink-orientated behaviour, tolerance to the cerebral effects of alcohol, continued drinking despite harm, and withdrawal symptoms with abstinence.

Though some harm may result at lower intakes (e.g. in hypertension or pregnancy) and many individuals will be unaffected at higher levels of consumption, there is a high risk of harm from alcohol intakes greater than 50 units (approx. 400 g alcohol) per week or 7 units (approx. 60 g) per day for males, and 35 units (280 g) per week or 5 units (40 g) per day for females.[3] One unit (approx. 8 g of ethanol) represents half a pint (284 mL) of average-strength (3.5% alcohol by volume) beer, one single measure (24 mL) of spirits (40% alcohol by volume), one glass (2 fl oz, approx. 57 mL) of sherry or similar fortified wine (approx. 20% alcohol by volume), or one glass (4 fl oz, 114 mL) of wine (approx. 11% alcohol by volume).

Metabolism of Alcohol[4,5]

1. Absorption and Excretion

After ingestion, alcohol is rapidly absorbed by diffusion, principally from the upper small intestine but with minor gastric absorption. A small amount of oxidation may occur within the stomach by gastric alcohol dehydrogenase ('first-pass metabolism'), particularly in the postprandial state in males.[6] After absorption, alcohol reaches the systemic circulation via the liver and is distributed throughout the body water, peak blood concentrations generally being reached within 1 h in fasting subjects. Small amounts of alcohol are excreted in the urine, breath, sweat and saliva.

2. Oxidation

Ninety per cent of absorbed ethanol is metabolized in the liver. The first step is oxidation to acetaldehyde; this can be catalysed by at least three different enzyme systems—alcohol dehydrogenase, catalase and microsomal ethanol-oxidizing enzyme.

Alcohol dehydrogenase normally accounts for 80% of hepatic ethanol oxidation. The enzyme is cytosolic and requires nicotinamide adenine dinucleotide (NAD) as cofactor. During ethanol oxidation, NAD is converted to its reduced form, NADH. Catalase, in peroxisomes and mitochondria, acting together with hydrogen peroxide produced by various oxidase enzymes (e.g. xanthine oxidase) accounts for less than 10% of ethanol oxidation. Microsomal oxidation activity accounts for up to 20% of ethanol oxidation in the normal subject. It uses reduced nicotinamide adenine dinucleotide phosphate (NADPH) as coenzyme, which is concomitantly oxidized to NADP during ethanol oxidation. Both catalase and microsomal ethanol oxidase have Michaelis constants (K_m) for ethanol of approx. 10 mmol/L and are principally active in ethanol oxidation when plasma ethanol concentrations exceed 20 mmol/L. In chronic alcoholics the contribution of microsomal ethanol oxidase to ethanol oxidation may double and there is an associated increase in activity of other microsomal enzyme systems.

The second step in metabolism of alcohol is the conversion of acetaldehyde to acetate by aldehyde dehyrogenase. Again, 90% of this oxidation takes place in the liver. Aldehyde dehydrogenase also uses NAD as cofactor; it is located both in the liver cytosol and mitochondria. It appears probable that the mitochondrial enzyme, which has the higher affinity (lower K_m) for acetaldehyde, is the more active in acetaldehyde oxidation. Approximately 5% of acetaldehyde produced in the liver is released into the blood. NADH formed by the action of alcohol dehydrogenase and aldehyde dehydrogenase during ethanol oxidation is oxidized by coupling to oxidative phosphorylation, with the formation and shuttling of reduced substrates from the cytosol into the mitochondria for oxidation. Acetate is released into the circulation and oxidized to carbon dioxide and water in tissue mitochondria. Availability of NAD limits the oxidation of ethanol and acetaldehyde, and acetaldehyde will accumulate if the NAD concentration is inadequate.

3. Metabolic Effects of Oxidation

The action of alcohol and aldehyde dehydrogenases in the oxidation of ethanol results in a relative increase in NADH compared with NAD. The resulting altered redox state reduces hepatic gluconeogenesis, fatty acid oxidation and protein synthesis. It increases lactate formation, triglyceride and lipoprotein synthesis, ketone-body formation and porphyrin synthesis. As a consequence of the effect on lipid metabolism, fat accumulates in the liver. Lactate competing with the excretion of urate in the distal renal tubule promotes urate retention.

Enhancement of microsomal enzyme activity from chronic alcohol excess gives rise to increased rates of ethanol oxidation and drug metabolism. Synthesis of cholesterol and lipoprotein (especially very low-density lipoprotein, VLDL) may also be stimulated. These effects are seen in recently drinking alcoholics, provided that hepatic damage is not so severe as to impair microsomal function. Simultaneous ingestion of alcohol and a drug (or drugs) will reduce drug metabolism.

4. Mechanisms of Cell Damage from Alcohol

Acetaldehyde formed by the enzymic oxidation of alcohol in the liver is thought to play a major role in the development of cell damage from alcohol, particularly in relation to alcoholic liver-cell injury.[7] Acetaldehyde may combine covalently with cell membrane proteins causing membrane damage and creating neo-antigens that activate cytotoxic lymphocytes. It may also damage hepatic microtubules by interfering with the secretion of liver proteins and promoting collagen formation.

A reduction of liver total and cytosolic aldehyde dehydrogenase is an acquired abnormality in alcoholics. Acetaldehyde is also thought to damage hepatic mitochondria. The reduced level of (mainly mitochondrial) aldehyde dehydrogenase would further impair the oxidation of acetaldehyde, with more accumulating and a vicious circle of liver damage.

Recently, attention has focused on possible hepatotoxicity and non-hepatic cell injury from the superoxide ion formed during the oxidation of acetaldehyde to acetate. The ion may damage membrane lipid, with the production of toxic metabolites from lipid peroxidation. Free-radical scavenging by the enzyme superoxide dismutase and removal of organic peroxides by combination with glutathione and the action of glutathione peroxidase, a selenium metalloenzyme, normally protect from such damage. Impairment of this protective function is suggested by the finding of reduced glutathione in the liver and low selenium concentrations in plasma in alcoholics, with increased lipoperoxides in both liver and plasma. Vitamin E, a recognized free-radical scavenger, also has lowered plasma concentration.[8]

Damage to extrahepatic tissues may be a consequence of the ability of tissue macrophages to metabolize ethanol, with damage mediated by acetaldehyde, free-radical formation, or neo-antigen formation as in the liver. Serum proteins may also be modified by circulating acetaldehyde to produce cytotoxic complexes.[9]

A proposed novel mechanism of organ damage is from fatty-acid ethyl esters formed by non-oxidative ethanol metabolism.[10] Brain, pancreas and heart (all organs particularly sensitive to alcoholic injury) have high synthetic activity for fatty-acid ethyl esters, and it is suggested that these esters may bind to mitochondria and be hydrolysed to free fatty acids, which then give rise to uncoupling of oxidative phosphorylation and impaired mitochondrial function.

ACUTE ALCOHOLIC INTOXICATION

Clinical Features

The clinical features of acute alcoholic intoxication are well known (Table 7.1). Early features include disinhibition, impaired coordination, dizziness and slurred speech. These first become evident at blood alcohol concentrations above 50 mg/dL (11 mmol/L), are generally obvious at 100 mg/dL (22 mmol/L), and almost invariable above 150 mg/dL (33 mmol/L). However, intoxication may become manifest at lower levels in those unused to drinking, in the young, and whilst the blood alcohol is rising; and at higher concentrations in those who regularly drink large amounts of alcohol. In consequence, the clinical recognition of intoxication may show an error rate of at least 12%, even among those very familiar with its clinical manifestations.[11]

At a blood alcohol above 200 mg/dL (43 mmol/L) consciousness is generally impaired, and above 300 mg/dL (65 mmol/L) there is coma. Above this, there is a danger of death, especially from respiratory failure, the median lethal level being 400–500 mg/dL (87–109 mmol/L), though survival has been been recorded up to a value as high as 1500 mg/dL (326 mmol/L).[12] After drinking and absorption of alcohol have ceased, blood alcohol concentrations may be expected to fall by an average of about 15 mg/dL an hour (range 10–25).

Biochemical Confirmation[13]

Biochemical confirmation of intoxication is required to prevent clinical misdiagnosis. It is used to confirm

TABLE 7.1
CLINICAL FEATURES OF ACUTE ALCOHOLIC INTOXICATION

Blood ethanol		
mg/dL	mmol/L	Typical effect
20	4	Euphoria
40	9	Disinhibited
60	13	Impaired judgement
80	17	Impaired coordination
100	22	Impaired control
150	33	Drowsiness, amnesia
300	65	Stupor, coma
500	109	Coma, death

that significant amounts of alcohol have been ingested, and that the symptomatology is appropriate to the observed alcohol values.

Alcohol ingestion is confirmed by ethanol measurement in blood, breath, saliva or urine.[13–15] Blood alcohol is usually measured by enzymatic (alcohol dehydrogenase) spectrophotometry or by gas chromatography. Blood samples are best stored in well-sealed, refrigerated tubes with added sodium fluoride (10 mg/mL of blood) and anticoagulant (potassium oxalate, 3 mg/mL), and will then show no change of ethanol content for at least 2 weeks. Ethanol concentration is, on average, 18% higher in plasma than in red cells and the concentration in serum or plasma is correspondingly higher than that of whole blood.

Urine with merthiolate added to prevent bacterial growth and stored at 4°C may also be used for ethanol determination, generally by gas chromatography. Urine alcohol concentrations are generally some 33% higher than the corresponding blood concentrations. Difficulty or delay in obtaining urine samples generally renders blood alcohol analysis preferable.

Breath ethanol analysis by gas chromatography, infrared spectroscopy (e.g. the 'Intoximeter', Lion Laboratories Ltd, Barry, UK), or fuel cell ('Alcolmeter', Lion Laboratories) is also used to confirm intoxication, especially for forensic purposes; fuel-cell instruments, because of their small size, may conveniently be used in the accident and emergency department for breath sampling, even in unconscious subjects.[18] A blood:breath ratio of 2300:1 is generally assumed.

Salivary alcohol concentrations[17] correlate well with, but are marginally higher than, those of blood. Dipsticks using immobilized enzyme (alcohol dehydrogenase or oxidase) and colour reagent have been suggested as suitable for the rapid, quantitative or semiquantitative measurement of salivary (or urinary) alcohol.

Where measurement of ethanol is not readily available, an indirect indication of ethanol intake and blood alcohol may be obtained by measurement of plasma osmolality (reference range, 285–295 mmol/L) by freezing-point depression, and the finding of an unexpectedly high plasma osmolality (above 320 mosmol/kg) and an increased osmolal gap from the osmolal effects of alcohol in the blood.

The addition of ethanol to plasma at a concentration of 100 mg/dL (22 mmol/L) increases plasma osmolality by some 20 mosmol/kg. Similarly, a blood alcohol of 150 mg/dL (33 mmol/L) following oral intake by healthy subjects raises plasma osmolality by some 30 mosmol/kg. The serum osmolality on admission to hospital in injured patients correlated well with recent alcohol intake, with osmolality above 320 mosmol/kg associated with a blood alcohol above 50 mg/dL (11 mmol/L) in some 90% of patients.[18] No patient with a blood alcohol above 150 mg/dL (33 mmol/L) had an osmolality below 340 mosmol/kg. In these patients, however, a 50 mg/dL (11 mmol/L) increase in blood alcohol increased the serum osmolality by approximately 20 mosmol/kg—the enhanced effect possibly being a consequence of accompanying dehydration.

An increased osmolal gap, i.e. in the difference between determined and calculated osmolality, may also suggest an increased blood alcohol. The formula calculated osmolality = 1.86 [sodium] + [glucose] + [urea] + 9 (all concentration values in mmol/L) is useful and yields a reference limit for the osmolal gap of 15 mmol/L.[19] Again, in emergency-room patients, a near 90% agreement between an increased osmolal gap and increased blood ethanol has been observed. Similarly, a correlation with measured alcohol of 0.99 has been found after alcohol ingestion. However, calculated osmolality may be 'underestimated' and ethanol concentration overestimated by this formula. This may be due to the behaviour of ethanol in plasma not conforming to that expected of an 'ideal' solution, either because the addition of ethanol alters the degree of dissociation of sodium chloride, or because of the presence of other osmotically active components of alcoholic drinks. Additionally, concomitant lactic acidosis or alcoholic ketoacidosis may contribute to the osmolal gap. Multiplication of the osmolal gap by 0.83 more closely correlates with the blood alcohol than does the gap value alone.[20]

Biochemical Changes[21,22]

A variety of biochemical changes accompany acute alcoholic intoxication. They include changes in water, electrolyte, acid–base, metabolite and endocrine status.

Intoxication is accompanied by an initial diuresis due to inhibition of vasopressin release, especially while the blood alcohol is rising. This is followed by water retention when the blood alcohol falls. There is accompanying sodium retention, together with potassium and chloride retention during both periods, but plasma concentrations are virtually unchanged. As the blood alcohol falls there may also be increased urinary excretion of zinc, calcium and magnesium.

Ingestion of large amounts of ethanol may lower blood pH and bicarbonate, and increase blood lactate and ketone bodies. Acidosis, either respiratory or metabolic, results from decreased ventilation owing to depression of the central nervous system, and hydrogen ion production from ethanol oxidation and increased ketone body (especially 3-hydroxybutyrate) formation from fatty-acid oxidation. Glucose concentrations may fall as a result of diminished hepatic gluconeogenesis. There may also be increased release of catecholamines, aldosterone, cortisol and renin, possibly as a direct effect of ethanol, from stress, or from altered redox state.

Diuresis and dehydration from intoxication may contribute to hangover, hypoglycaemia to confusion or even coma, and catecholamine release to cerebral effects. It is especially important to measure the blood glucose in suspected alcohol intoxication because of the dangers of unrecognized neuroglycopenia.

Two principal mechanisms have been postulated for the cerebral effects of acute alcohol ingestion.[23,24] The first is an anaesthetic-like effect of alcohol acting on neural membranes, either by increasing membrane fluidity with an accompanying decreased sodium entry into the cell, or by decreased sodium/potassium ATPase activity with loss of cell potassium. Both of these alter neurone polarization and impulse transmission. The second possible mechanism is altered activity of cerebral neurotransmitters, particularly from the release of brain catecholamines.

Biochemical Changes Accompanying Alcohol Withdrawal[21,22]

Recovery from intoxication may be followed by the alcohol withdrawal syndrome in those dependent on alcohol. Clinical features include mild, early tremulousness (the 'shakes'), hallucinosis ('the horrors'), and sometimes fits. Occasionally the severe features of delirium tremens, the DTs, may develop, with agitation, impaired consciousness and hallucinations.

The alcohol withdrawal syndrome has characteristic biochemical concomitants, generally with respiratory alkalosis, but with a metabolic contribution to alkalosis from low potassium or vomiting. Low plasma electrolytes, with increased urinary loss (especially of potassium, magnesium, calcium and zinc), increased plasma catecholamines, and hypoglycaemia may all be present. The low magnesim and calcium (possibly a consequence of diminished parathyroid secretion or responsiveness) are thought to contribute to the likelihood of tremor and convulsions, the altered catecholamines to agitation and sympathetic overactivity, and the hypoglycaemia to confusion. Treatment with glucose infusions may promote a fall in plasma phosphate, leading to muscle weakness and respiratory failure.

It has been suggested that profound alteration in neurotransmitters takes place in the brain,[23,24] with increased catecholamines, decreased 5-hydroxytryptamine, decreased γ-aminobutyrate and increased cyclic nucleotides, cyclic adenosine monophosphate and cyclic guanosine monophosphate. All these would contribute to the profound psychiatric disturbance.

BIOCHEMICAL FACTORS RELEVANT TO PREDISPOSITION TO EXCESS ALCOHOL INTAKE AND TO ALCOHOLIC ORGAN DAMAGE[25]

It is generally considered that genetic or environmental influences, possibly biochemically mediated, may predispose to or encourage excess drinking, and that biochemical factors may serve to perpetuate this by promoting dependency on alcohol.

Genetic Factors[26,27]

Numerous family and twin studies have suggested a significant genetic component related to excess alcohol consumption. Thus, this is far more frequent in sons of alcoholics than in the sons of non-alcoholics, even if they were separated from their biological parents in infancy. Additionally, concordance to excess alcohol consumption is twice as frequent in monozygotic as dizygotic twins, even when reared apart. Furthermore, ethanol elimination rates show wide person-to-person variation; twin studies indicate that 50% of this is genetic in origin. These observations have focused attention on the genetics of the enzymes involved in the hepatic metabolism of alcohol, particularly on the alcohol and aldehyde dehydrogenases.

Alcohol and Aldehyde Dehydrogenase Polymorphism[28,29]

Alcohol dehydrogenase is a dimeric enzyme coded at five gene loci. Three of these, *ADH1*, *ADH2* and *ADH3* on chromosome 4, are important in ethanol metabolism and respectively code for α-, β- and γ-polypeptides, which combine as homo- or heterodimers to yield active enzyme. Allelic polymorphism at the *ADH2* locus yields three types of β-polypeptide. The usual form is described as β_1. A β_2 or 'atypical' variant is found in 5–10% of white Europeans but in 85% of mongoloid orientals, and a β_3 or Indianapolis variant is found in about 25% of Afro-Americans. Polymorphism also occurs at the *ADH3* locus, giving two forms of γ-polypeptides, γ_1 or γ_2, which occur with near equal frequency in Europeans. The γ_1 form is more common in mongoloids. The polymorphic variants of *ADH2* and *ADH3* result from single amino-acid substitutions and may be identified by examination of liver tissue or of DNA extracted from peripheral blood. The polymorphic forms differ in their enzyme kinetic constants and this is thought to account for interindividual differences in ethanol elimination rates.

Attempts to correlate *ADH2* and *ADH3* polymorphism with alcoholism have failed to show any relations. Coutelle and colleagues in France[30,31] found the atypical, β_2-polypeptide forms virtually absent in alcoholics, so *ADH2* polymorphism cannot predispose to alcoholism, though the low frequency of the β_2 variant at less than 1% compared with an anticipated 5–10% might suggest a protective role. The γ_1 and γ_2 polypeptides show similar frequencies in alcoholic cirrhosis and non-alcoholic controls, and similar frequencies in alcoholic and non-alcoholic caucasoid populations. Thus, polymorphism at the *ADH3* locus also does not predispose to alcoholism nor presumably to alcoholic liver disease.

Aldehyde dehydrogenase polymorphism does, however, appear to have a more important role in relation to alcoholism. Two gene loci code for the principal forms of this tetrameric enzyme. The first, on chromosome 12, codes for the mitochondrial form of aldehyde dehydrogenase, here designated ALDH-2 or E-2, and believed to be the principal form responsible for acetaldehyde oxidation. A second locus on chromosome 9 codes for ALDH-1 (or E-1), the cytoplasmic form. Polymorphism occurs at the mitochondrial *ALDH2* locus and results in the formation of catalytically inactive 'unusual' enzyme (ALDH-2¹) instead of the usual active form (ALDH-2²). This is found in 50% of mongoloid orientals but is not generally seen in caucasoids. This inactive 'oriental' variant of aldehyde dehydrogenase cannot oxidize acetaldehyde formed after ethanol ingestion, which accumulates in the circulation and may give rise to skin flushing, nausea and tachycardia.

It can readily be understood that these unpleasant effects of alcohol ingestion in orientals with ALDH-2 deficiency would discourage drinking. This indeed is so. Workers in Japan found ALDH-2 deficiency (though designated ALDH-1 in their nomenclature) in 41% of 105 healthy subjects, but in only 2% of 175 alcoholics.[32] It is clearly protective against alcoholism.

Trait Markers

Attempts have been made to identify biochemical markers *other* than ethanol-metabolizing enzymes that may indicate predisposition to alcoholism. Such 'trait' or 'vulnerability' markers would be expected with greater frequency in so-called type 2 than in type 1 alcoholics.[33] Type 2 or 'male-limited' alcoholism, found in young adult males, is severe, largely environment-independent and has a marked genetic component, whereas type-1 or 'milieu-limited' alcoholism is milder, found in middle age in both sexes, environment-sensitive and only mildly influenced by genetic factors. Trait markers should thus be more frequent in alcoholics with a positive family history than in those whose family history is negative; should be expected to be present in non-alcoholic relatives of alcoholics; should persist in alcoholics, even when abstinent; and ideally should be shown to precede the development of alcoholism.

A number of substances have been studied and suggested as possible trait markers for alcoholism because they fulfil some, or most, of the above criteria (Table 7.2). These include low platelet monoamine oxidase;[34] increased plasma salsolinol;[35] the response of blood acetaldehyde,[36] plasma cortisol and corticotrophin (ACTH),[37] and platelet monoamine oxidase[38] to ethanol challenge; and increased platelet 5-hydroxytryptamine uptake and decreased adenylate cyclase after nucleotide stimulation.[38]

The marker that seems most closely to correlate with susceptibility to alcohol is platelet monoamine oxidase.[39] This enzyme catalyses the oxidation of various neurotransmitter amines, including noradrenaline, dopamine and 5-hydroxytryptamine, which when present in excess in the brain might be associated with alcohol-seeking behaviour and which

TABLE 7.2
POSSIBLE TRAIT MARKERS FOR ALCOHOLISM

Enhanced
Blood acetaldehyde increase after ethanol
Plasma salsolinol
Inhibition of platelet monoamine oxidase by ethanol

Decreased
Platelet monoamine oxidase
Plasma cortisol and ACTH response after ethanol
Platelet adenylate cyclase after nucleotide stimulation

can combine with ethanol-derived acetaldehyde to yield products with addictive properties. The type B monoamine oxidase isoenzyme is reduced in the platelets, particularly of type 2 alcoholics; remains low after years of abstinence; is low in the non-alcoholic relatives of alcoholics; and shows increased inhibition by alcohol in at least 70% of alcoholics. It would thus seem to act as a definite marker of vulnerability.

Most recently, studies of the dopamine D_2 receptor gene in brain have revealed a restriction fragment length polymorphism, with an A-1 allele detectable in 69% of alcoholics but only 20% of non-alcoholics.[40] If confirmed, and if identified in peripheral blood DNA, this too might prove a helpful trait marker.

Biochemical Abnormalities that may Predispose to Alcoholic Brain Damage

One of the most feared cerebral complications of alcoholism is Wernicke's encephalopathy, found in at least 2% of alcoholics. It is characterized clinically by paralysis of eye movement, ataxia, polyneuropathy and mental confusion, and pathologically by loss of midbrain neurons. It is associated with lack of thiamin (vitamin B_1) as a consequence of impaired intake, absorption or utilization of that vitamin or from an increased requirement for it. Vitamin B_1 acts as a coenzyme for three important enzymes: pyruvate dehydrogenase, α-oxoglutarate dehydrogenase and transketolase. Decreased activity of these enzymes in the brain, possibly from the effects of cytotoxic free radicals or the formation of acetaldehyde–apoenzyme adducts, may result in metabolic disturbances that account for the cerebral symptoms.

A variant transketolase with a reduced affinity (high K_m) for the coenzyme has been observed in cultured skin fibroblasts from patients with Wernicke's encephalopathy, with abnormally high levels of vitamin B_1 required for its full activity.[41] It has thus been postulated that genetic variation in transketolase may result in a population particularly at risk of Wernicke's encephalopathy from alcohol. This suggestion has not been fully confirmed,[42] though heterogeneity of erythrocyte transketolase in healthy subjects, with differing kinetics of individual transketolase fractions, has been demonstrated. A particular pattern of erythrocyte transketolase isoenzymes has also been reported in association with Wernicke's encephalopathy, though it was unassociated with altered K_m values.

The finding of chromatographically separable high- and low-affinity transketolases concurrently in the same alcoholic individuals, and the lack of reproducibility of isoenzyme patterns on isoelectric focusing, have led to the suggestion that the enzyme variant with reduced affinity and the enzyme's overall heterogeneity may result from *in vivo* damage or *in vitro* breakdown. However, the possibility of real genetic variation from pretranscriptional rather than post-translational change is not excluded.

Biochemical Mechanisms that may Encourage or Perpetuate Excessive Drinking[43]

A major feature of alcoholism is the alcohol dependency syndrome, characterized, as outlined above, by drink-orientated behaviour, craving for alcohol, tolerance to the cerebral effects of alcohol, continued drinking despite harm, and withdrawal symptoms with abstinence. All these are behavioural changes that must be assumed to be a consequence of altered cerebral metabolism. Various mechanisms could explain such metabolic alterations. The proposed explanations mostly assume that the acetaldehyde generated by hepatic oxidation of alcohol and released into the plasma alters brain function. The activity of alcohol dehydrogenase and concentrations of acetaldehyde are low in brain tissue, so that substantial local formation of acetaldehyde is unlikely. Acetaldehyde might compete with the aldehyde derivatives of monoamines, e.g. dopamine, noradrenaline and serotonin (5-hydroxytryptamine) as substrate for oxidation enzymes. The consequent impairment of monoamine aldehyde oxidation could result in the accumulation of these or their psychoactive metabolites. Monoamines can also condense with acetaldehyde or with their own monoamine aldehydes to form isoquinolines. Tryptophan derivatives such as 5-hydroxytryptamine may condense with acetaldehyde to form β-carbolines. Both isoquinolines and β-carbolines are psychoactive compounds that may show opiate-like properties and thus predispose to addiction. Acetaldehyde may also interfere with the action of the coenzyme pyridoxal phosphate (vitamin B_6). This vitamin is a cofactor for enzymes responsible for the synthesis of the neurotransmitters γ-aminobutyrate, 5-hydroxytryptamine and adrenaline.

BIOCHEMICAL CHANGES THAT ASSIST IN IDENTIFYING EXCESS ALCOHOL CONSUMPTION[44]

Those who regularly consume harmful quantities of alcohol are generally reluctant to admit the extent of their drinking. Although various clinical features may alert the physician to the possibility that a patient is

TABLE 7.3
SOME EARLY PHYSICAL SIGNS OF ALCOHOLISM

General	Unkempt, overfamiliar, smell of alcohol
Voice	Hoarse
Face	Bloated, flushed, bloodshot eyes
Skin	Bruising, dilated blood vessels
Hands	Red palms, tremor, rapid pulse
Trunk	Obese, pot-belly, male breast enlargement

TABLE 7.4
CLINICAL FEATURES OF ALCOHOLISM

At-risk Factors Present
Occupation, family history, etc.
Social Difficulties
Marital, family, work
Law contravention (assault, drunkenness, etc.)
Accidents (work, traffic)
Psychiatric Disturbance
Anxiety, depression, etc.
Symptoms of Addiction
Craving, withdrawal symptoms (fits, hallucinations, amnesia)

TABLE 7.5
CLINICAL FEATURES OF DISEASE COMPLICATIONS OF ALCOHOLISM

Hepatic/Gastrointestinal/Pancreatic
Pain, nausea, vomiting, diarrhoea, bleeding, hepatomegaly, jaundice
Neuropsychiatric
Poor concentration and memory, insomnia, blackouts, sweating, numbness, tingling
Cardiovascular
Palpitations, dyspnoea, raised blood pressure
Musculoskeletal
Pain, weakness, fractures, gout
Endocrine/Metabolic/Reproductive
Obesity, breast swelling, glycosuria, impotence, infertility, fetal abnormality
Immunological/Neoplastic
Chest infections, upper gastrointestinal cancer

drinking excessively (Tables 7.3, 7.4 and 7.5), they may not be recognized or may be misinterpreted. The clinical recognition of the alcoholic, therefore, remains difficult. Biochemical changes can provide objective evidence of chronic alcohol excess and demonstrate recent intake. Laboratory tests can facilitate the recognition of chronic excessive drinking, even when this is denied, and before the stage at which dependency or irreversible organ damage is reached. They can be used to monitor the progress and treatment of the alcoholic, and can identify hepatic and non-hepatic complications. Laboratory tests can be used both to confirm a clinical suspicion or diagnosis

of alcoholism or heavy drinking, and to screen populations at high risk or otherwise. Biochemical changes that assist in the identification of excess alcohol consumption are referred to as 'state markers'. Tests can be divided into those designed to identify recent alcohol intake by measurement of alcohol or its metabolites, and those responsive mainly to chronic excess and which identify the effects of alcohol on metabolic processes or organ damage from alcohol.

Identification of Recent Alcohol Intake

The demonstration of recent drinking, particularly when denied, may draw attention to possible chronic alcohol excess. Measurement of ethanol concentrations in breath and body fluids has been used to confirm suspicion of excess drinking and to identify drinking in selected population groups. In alcoholic patients, alcohol measurement in breath, blood, urine or sweat can be used to monitor compliance with treatment.

Alcohol Measurement for Confirmation of Alcoholism
Two groups of patients have been particularly studied: those attending liver-disease clinics and those attending alcohol treatment centres.

Liver-Disease Clinics. Random alcohol determinations are of only limited diagnostic value in patients attending clinics for liver disease. With repeated testing, up to 50% of heavy drinkers attending morning clinics may be found to have ethanol in their blood. Measurements made in the afternoon are less sensitive, with only 16% of alcoholics attending an afternoon clinic showing increased blood ethanol concentrations, and 8% of control 'social drinkers' also showing alcohol in their blood.[45]

Alcohol measurement seems most valuable for monitoring claimed abstinence in known alcoholics. In one study, 50% of daily urine samples screened for alcohol from patients with alcoholic liver disease contained alcohol, yet 50% of these patients emphatically denied alcohol ingestion.[46]

Alcohol Treatment Centres. About 35–50% of patients attending specialist clinics for problem drinkers or admitted to alcohol treatment centres have measurable concentrations of alcohol in their blood at initial examination.

Alcohol Measurement for Identification of Excessive Drinking in Selected Population Groups

Health Surveys. Thirty-six (11%) of 327 males taking part in a health survey in Uppsala, Sweden, were found to have alcohol in their urine on the day of screening.[47] One-third of the men showed additional evidence of chronic excess alcohol intake, while the remaining two-thirds were considered casual drinkers.

General Practice Surveys. Breath alcohol concentrations measured in 1000 randomly selected patients attending general practitioners' surgeries were positive in 3.5%, although in a significant proportion of these the measurement was at the lower limit of sensitivity of the detection instrument.[48] Just under half of the patients with a positive breath-alcohol reading were thought to be problem drinkers, giving a true positive rate of only 50%, and of these one-third were known to the general practitioners. In relation to the likely number of problem drinkers in the practice population, the sensitivity of random breath-alcohol measurement as a test for problem drinking would lie between 20 and 40%.

Accident and Emergency Departments. Blood alcohol concentrations have been measured in patients attending accident and casualty departments with head and other injuries; some 50% were found to have raised values, usually in the region of 100–300 mg/dL (22–65 mmol/L). Similarly, 40% of patients attending an accident and emergency service during the evening hours had positive breath-alcohol readings, one-third of these corresponding to a blood alcohol greater than 80 mg/dL (17 mmol/L).[49]

Alcohol measurements in accident and emergency departments may grossly underestimate the frequency of chronic alcohol abuse. In patients attending such a department, randomly screened by questionnaire for problem drinking, measurement of breath alcohol showed a diagnostic sensitivity of only 22%.[50] Almost 80% of positive breath tests were thought to represent casual drinking only.

Up to one-third of drivers involved in road traffic accidents and with blood alcohol concentrations exceeding 80 mg/dL (11 mmol/L) have been found to show additional biochemical changes suggestive of chronic alcohol abuse.

Acute Medical Emergencies. In a Glasgow study, 35 (7.3%) of 482 female patients consecutively admitted to acute medical beds had alcohol in their blood.[51] In 21 patients (4.3%), values exceeded 80 mg/dL (17 mmol/L).

Significance of Ethanol Increase in Body Fluids
Various studies indicate that even at high blood ethanol concentrations (greater than 80 mg/dL, 17 mmol/L) alcohol ingestion may remain unrecognized clinically in approximately 20% of subjects. In the absence of alcohol measurement, lesser degrees of ingestion would be unnoticed. Whilst moderately elevated blood alcohol concentrations may be found in casual as well as habitual drinkers, detection of higher values may be suggestive of chronic alcohol abuse. Thus, a blood alcohol above 100 mg/dL (22 mmol/L) at routine medical examination, above 150 mg/dL (33 mmol/L) without intoxication or above 300 mg/dL (66 mmol/L) at any time should be regarded as highly suggestive of alcoholism.

Blood alcohol measurement is useful for *confirmation* of alcoholism, as abnormal levels will be detected in up to 50% of known alcoholics. Measurements made on morning samples are more frequently abnormal than those on afternoon samples. On the other hand, blood alcohol measurement is of less value for *detection* of alcoholism, as most alcoholics with raised values admit to heavy drinking. When used to screen for alcoholism an abnormal ethanol concentration is to be anticipated in only 20–50% of alcoholics, whereas 50–70% of positive screenings result from casual drinking unassociated with alcoholism.

Random alcohol measurements are best employed for monitoring abstinence in known alcoholics.

Identification of Chronic Excess Alcohol Intake

The profound metabolic and toxic effect of alcohol on the liver is reflected in biochemical disturbances, which, although not specific for alcohol excess, are nevertheless valuable for its identification. In general, abnormalities of these 'state markers' are more frequent and severe in alcoholics, i.e. those in whom alcohol excess has resulted in harm. Sensitivity is lower in those merely drinking at high-risk levels. The demonstration of increased activity of plasma enzymes of hepatic origin, particularly of the enzyme γ-glutamyltransferase, has proved especially useful in the identification of chronic drinking. As these enzyme measurements are generally made as part of a 'liver function test', changes in plasma protein and bilirubin concentrations may be concomitantly, though less frequently, observed. Plasma urate and lipids, determined routinely in most clinical biochemistry laboratories, may also show alterations that may assist in the recognition of alcohol excess, and a host of more specialized investigations may show changes valuable for this purpose. Of these, measurement of the serum concentration of desialylated forms of the liver-produced protein transferrin appears the most promising. Changes in each of these state markers are considered below. Toxic effects of alcohol on other tissues, for example the bone marrow, also produce alterations, such as macrocytosis, that are also helpful in detecting alcohol abuse.

Abnormalities of Plasma Enzymes of Hepatic Origin and of Plasma Bilirubin

Plasma γ-Glutamyltransferase. It is now more than 20 years since I first demonstrated the special sensitivity of measurement of the plasma γ-glutamyltransferase (GGT, formerly known as γ-glutamyl transpeptidase) to alcohol excess.[52,53] This sensitivity has been repeatedly confirmed, and this remains the most valuable of all single biochemical measures for the detection of chronic excess alcohol intake. The enzyme originates from the liver, where alcohol induces its synthesis. This is an early effect of alcohol, which precedes abnormality of conventional liver function tests and may occur independently of abnormal liver histology, though cholestasis and hepatocellular damage may contribute to enzyme elevation when liver disease is established. The enzyme is stable for several months in frozen plasma samples and its activity can be inexpensively, simply and rapidly determined in the laboratory using automated procedures.

Increased plasma GGT activity is found in approx. 70% of alcoholics. This high prevalence occurs in both inpatients and outpatients, even in the absence of clinical evidence of hepatic disease, and independent of alcohol intake in the period immediately before testing.

In general, GGT values are on average two to three times higher than the upper reference limit in hospitalized alcoholics and one-and-a-half times higher in alcoholic outpatients. However, values up to five times that limit are frequent in both groups, and levels up to 60 times the limit have been observed in alcoholics recently drinking. Higher values at equivalent levels of consumption have been observed in Asian Indians when compared to white Europeans.

The frequency of a raised plasma GGT is largely independent of the degree of liver damage, although increased plasma GGT activity is found in less than 30% of alcoholics with normal liver histology who have not recently been drinking. However, activities of plasma GGT correlate with the degree of hepatic inflammation and necrosis found histologically, so that the highest plasma values are found in patients with severe liver disease and profound hepatic inflammatory change.

The frequency of raised plasma GGT in alcoholics is greater with regular daily drinking than with bout drinking and increases with the duration of drinking before sampling. The frequency falls in patients with advanced cirrhosis and a drinking history of more than 20 years. Possible explanations for this include: a reduction in the number of enzyme-producing liver cells; the selective survival of alcohol-resistant individuals characterized by normal enzyme levels; or nutritional deficiencies, particularly of vitamins and minerals, which may interfere with enzyme production.

Acute alcohol excess (a 'binge') does not produce significant elevation of plasma GGT activity in normal subjects, and intakes of up to 2 g alcohol per kg body weight generally produce less than 10% change. Abnormal plasma GGT concentrations may, however, result from acute alcohol intake in patients with pre-existing liver disease. A doubling of baseline levels with an increase to pathological values 24 h after challenge with 1 g alcohol per kg body weight has been observed in abstaining moderate drinkers with a normal plasma GGT, and was suggested as useful for differentiating these from non-drinkers.[54]

In previous non-drinkers, a minimum of 5 weeks' daily drinking in excess of 60 g/day seems to be required before plasma GGT activity becomes pathologically raised.

In the general population, a progressive increase in plasma GGT is found with increasing levels of alcohol consumption, with higher values in males than females. An elevated plasma GGT is found in 20% of men and 15% of women who admit regularly daily intakes of between 30–40 g, and in 40–50% of men and 30% of women drinking 60 g or more daily. This lower frequency in high-risk subjects compared with alcoholic patients may reflect the generally higher alcohol intakes of the alcoholics or organ damage resulting therefrom. Where determination of GGT is used to screen a predominantly healthy population for excessive drinking, fewer than 10–20% of subjects not drinking excessively will show a raised activity, whereas at least 50–75% of the abnormal values encountered result from alcohol excess.

Progressive reduction in plasma GGT activity occurs in drinkers who abstain. Values generally show a 50% reduction within 2 weeks (mean 10 days) and near normal values are attained within 5 weeks. More persistent elevation may be observed in patients with alcoholic liver cirrhosis. The fall in the plasma GGT is generally exponential. Serial measurements of plasma GGT activity are of value in monitoring the known alcoholic, as renewed drinking will result in a rapid return of plasma GGT activity to abnormal values.

In some patients, especially those in whom initial values for plasma GGT are less than five times the upper reference limit, the fall in activity with abstinence may be delayed. Sometimes plasma GGT activity transiently increases in patients admitted to hospital; the reason for this is unknown.

Increased plasma GGT activity is not specific for alcohol excess, as elevation may result from biliary stasis or hepatocellular injury from any cause, and may also occur in patients on long-term treatment with enzyme-inducing drugs such as phenobarbitone and phenytoin.[55] Increased activity may also be found with hepatic steatosis accompanying obesity, with raised values in approximately 8% of men with a body mass index (weight in kg divided by the square of the height in metres) above the upper reference limit (25).[56] However, a raised GGT without obvious cause should always suggest the possibility of excess drinking, particularly if other evidence of liver disorder is lacking. A rapid fall in plasma GGT with abstinence indicates that the initial elevation was probably due to alcohol excess.

Isoforms of plasma GGT have been studied in alcoholics, but this adds little to specificity. In normal plasma, two or sometimes three GGT isoforms are demonstrable by electrophoresis. The most anodal isoenzyme is the principal one in only 20% of healthy subjects, but is the principal fraction in 80% of alcoholic patients. However, a similar incidence of abnormality is observed in patients with non-alcoholic liver disease.[57] A more cathodal GGT isoform (sometimes designated GGT-4) is also increased in 60–80% of alcoholics and in less than 10% of non-drinking controls, but this abnormality may also be found in non-alcoholic (especially cholestatic or neoplastic) liver disease.[58]

Plasma GGT activity normally declines during pregnancy. A similar fall in plasma GGT to normal with advancing pregnancy has been observed in heavy drinkers who continue to drink. The recognition of excess alcohol intake in pregnancy is of particular importance because of the danger to the developing fetus. Measurement of plasma GGT activity is only useful for this purpose if made in the first trimester. Increased GGT activity from alcohol during pregnancy has been found to be a useful predictor of fetal alcohol effects,[59] and values above the reference range in the newborn have been observed in association with the fetal alcohol syndrome.[60]

Determination of plasma GGT activity may be usefully combined with measurement of the erythrocyte mean corpuscular volume (MCV), which is readily made with modern automated cell counters. Chronic alcohol consumption damages the developing red cell and increases the erythrocyte volume (macrocytosis).

In population studies there is a good correlation between MCV and alcohol intake, an increase of approx. 1.7 fL accompanying each 10-g increment in daily ethanol consumption. Macrocytosis is seen in approx. 20% of men and women drinking at high-risk levels, and in 35% of men with daily intakes above 70 g.

The prevalence of macrocytosis in alcoholics (50–60% in both males and females) is lower than that of a raised plasma GGT; the degree of abnormality is smaller, and the response to abstinence slower, it taking about 2–3 months for the MCV to return to normal after cessation of drinking. Nevertheless, some patients with normal plasma GGT activity may show an increased MCV, so that combining these measurement increases sensitivity and, if both are abnormal, specificity also. Many disorders other than alcoholism also increase the erythrocyte MCV, although alcohol excess is now the most frequent cause of an isolated increase in MCV.

Plasma Transaminases and Alkaline Phosphatase. These enzymes are widely measured in hospital inpatients, and outpatients, and in general screening as part of liver function testing. Abnormality may draw attention to liver disorder, of which alcohol excess is a major cause. Plasma aspartate transaminase (AST) and alanine transaminase (ALT) may increase as a consequence of hepatocellular injury, and plasma alkaline phosphatase (ALP) activity is increased in cholestasis, both of which may be found in alcoholic liver disorder.

Relation of Enzyme Changes to Degree of Liver Damage. The changes that occur in these plasma enzymes in alcoholic patients are most conveniently considered in relation to the degree of hepatic injury seen histologically. The clinical and histological features of each stage are summarized in Table 7.6, and enzyme changes in Table 7.7. Concomitant changes in bilirubin will also be indicated, below, because of the invariable inclusion of bilirubin in liver function testing.

Steatosis (Synonym: Fatty Liver). This is the first stage of histologically identifiable hepatic injury from alcohol. It may be the sole histological abnormality in about 60% of patients with minimal clinical liver disease. Steatosis may be accompanied by a mildly raised plasma AST and ALT; on average, the frequency of this elevation is approx. 40 and 20%, respectively. Both transaminase values generally remain below four times the upper reference limit, with AST averaging twice this limit and characteristically higher than ALT (*see below*). Enzyme activity falls by approximately 50% within 1 week of abstinence. Cholestasis from steatosis gives mild hyperbilirubinaemia (less than twice the upper reference limit) and an increased plasma ALP in 10% of patients. ALP values remain below one-and-a-half times the upper reference limit. The α_1-isoenzyme of ALP ('biliary' or high molecular-mass ALP) may be increased in plasma, even when the total ALP is within normal limits. It has been claimed that increases in plasma values of the α_1-isoenzyme are found in 60% of alcoholics, and are a more sensitive indicator than raised plasma GGT,[61] but in my experience this is definitely not so, and this isoenzyme is found in the plasma of only 20% of alcoholics overall, with a similar percentage in patients with steatosis only.

Alcoholic Hepatitis (Synonyms: Alcoholic Steatonecrosis. Sclerosing Hyaline Necrosis). This condition may follow a severe drinking bout in the precirrhotic alcoholic and is thought to develop in approx. 30% of alcoholics. The biochemical features are those of hepatocellular injury and biliary obstruction, with hyperbilirubinaemia in up to 90% of patients, and serum bilirubin concentrations up to 10 times the upper refernce limit in severe cases. Plasma AST values are raised in approx. 70% and ALT in 50% of

TABLE 7.6
HEPATIC EFFECTS OF ALCOHOL

	Clinical	*Pathological*
Steatosis	Hepatomegaly, tender liver	Fat infiltration
Alcoholic hepatitis	Anorexia, fever, pain, hepatomegaly ± jaundice	Cell necrosis, polymorph infiltration, alcoholic hyaline
Cirrhosis	Hepatomegaly, bleeding, jaundice, ascites, encephalopathy	Fibrosis, regeneration nodules

TABLE 7.7

	GGT	*AST*	*ALT*	*ALP*
Steatosis	75	40	20	10
Alcoholic hepatitis	80	70	50	40
Cirrhosis (anicteric)	75	70	50	50

GGT, γ-glutamyltransferase; AST, aspartate transaminase; ALT, alanine transaminase; ALP, alkaline phosphatase.

patients. The plasma AST is higher, but both AST and ALT are below five times the upper reference limit. The plasma ALP is raised in about 40% of patients; amounts are generally below two-and-a-half times the upper reference limit, although higher concentrations are occasionally found in patients who are deeply jaundiced.

Alcoholic Cirrhosis. Approx. 10% of chronic alcoholics with a history of 10 or more years' alcoholic excess show histological evidence of cirrhosis. The biochemical changes are predominantly those of chronic hepatocellular dysfunction. Plasma bilirubin is mildly increased, below five times the upper reference limit, in approx. 60% of patients.

Plasma AST is raised in two-thirds to three-quarters of cirrhotic patients; the plasma ALT is increased in 50%. Transaminase usually remains below five times the upper reference limit, but AST activity is substantially higher than ALT.

Plasma ALT activity is elevated in about 50% of patients overall, but in 75% with jaundice. Amounts are usually below two-and-a-half times the upper reference limit.

Effect of Acute Ethanol Intake on Plasma Transaminase and Alkaline Phosphatase. Acute alcohol intakes of 0.5–2.0 g/kg body weight have little effect on plasma transaminase or ALP values in healthy subjects. Similarly, alcohol intakes of 0.8 g/kg body weight have no significant effect on these enzymes in alcoholic patients, although intakes of 1.5–2.0 g/kg body weight may cause transient increases. Acute alcohol intakes of 3–4 g/kg body weight or more prolonged daily intakes of 1–2 g/kg body weight can lead to a doubling of the basal plasma AST within 24 h in healthy volunteers, and may occasionally result in a more significant elevation.

Transaminase and ALP compared with GGT. The frequency of a raised plasma transaminase and ALP in patients with alcoholic liver disease is substantially less than that of an increased plasma GGT, particularly in early disease. However, as estimations of plasma AST and ALP are routinely included in liver function tests they remain of value for identifying excess drinking

and the development of alcohol-related liver disease.

Enzyme Ratios. The relative insensitivity of plasma ALT and ALP when compared with plasma AST and GGT, respectively, facilitates the differentiation of alcoholic liver disease from other varieties of liver damage associated with enzyme changes.

AST:ALT Ratio. When the plasma AST is moderately raised (less than eight times the upper reference limit), AST:ALT ratios greater than 1 are found in 70–80% of patients with alcoholic steatosis, hepatitis and cirrhosis. This may assist in differentiating such AST elevation from that occurring in acute hepatitis, chronic active or chronic persistent hepatitis, obstructive jaundice and primary biliary cirrhosis, in which ALT values are greater than AST. AST:ALT ratios above 2 have been reported in approx. 70% of patients with alcoholic hepatitis or active alcoholic cirrhosis, but in only 30% of patients with non-alcohol related chronic liver disease.[62]

Mitochondrial AST. A disproportionate increase in the mitochondrial isoenzyme of AST is found in the plasma of heavy drinkers, reflecting the specific tendency of alcohol to cause mitochondrial damage. In one study, mean activity of the plasma mitochondrial AST isoenzyme was four times the upper reference limit, although total AST activity was only one-and-a-half times greater than the upper reference limit.[63] The mitochondrial isoenzyme may constitute 20% of total plasma AST activity, a higher proportion than in patients with hepatitis or cirrhosis unrelated to alcohol. More modest elevation, detected by a sensitive immunological method, has been found in over 90% of alcoholics, preceding clinical or other biochemical evidence in liver damage.[64] However, such frequencies have been observed almost exclusively in alcoholics admitted to liver units, and even in these GGT has shown comparable sensitivity, though more false positives in non-alcoholic liver disease. In an unselected population attending a centre for preventive medicine,[65] and in general practitioner outpatient surgeries,[66] neither the determination of mitochondrial AST alone, nor its percentage (ratio) compared with total AST have proved of value for the detection of alcohol consumption in excess of 80 g/day. In these groups, diagnostic sensitivities of less than 30% have been reported, markedly lower than those of concomitantly measured GGT, and accompanied by lower specificity also.

GGT:ALP Ratio. The plasma GGT:ALP ratio may also be used to differentiate alcohol-related from unrelated liver disease. Enzyme activity ratios are critically dependent on methodology. Transaminase determinations are well standardized and the ratios are widely applicable, but this does not apply to measurements of plasma GGT and ALP. It is preferable, therefore, to express these enzymes in terms of their respective upper reference limits. If this is done, the GGT:ALP ratio, which is useful in differential diagnosis, appears to be approx. 4:1. Some 80% of patients with alcohol-related liver disease exhibit a ratio above this figure.

Plasma Glutamate Dehydrogenase. Glutamate dehydrogenase (GDH) is a mitochondrial enzyme that is released into the circulation following hepatic mitochondrial damage by alcohol. Its activity may also be induced by ethanol. Plasma GDH activity is increased in 50–60% of heavy drinkers, with values averaging about twice the upper reference limit and almost all below five times this upper limit. It was claimed that the plasma GDH correlated well with the presence and histological severity of alcoholic hepatitis,[67] but this observation has not been confirmed; indeed plasma GDH activities show no relation to the histological degree of liver damage.

Increased plasma GDH activity in the alcoholic falls by 50% within 48 h of alcohol withdrawal. This rapid fall may be useful in confirming a suspicion of increased alcohol intake, but limits the value of this enzyme for screening. Methods for measuring GDH are also not entirely satisfactory, which limits its routine use.

β-Hexosaminidase. The lysosomal enzyme β-hexosaminidase (N-acetyl-β-D-glucosaminidase) has been measured in plasma for the detection of alcoholism and heavy drinking.[68] Initial studies in alcoholics admitted to hospital for detoxication and in drunken arrestees drinking more than 60 g of ethanol (averaging 270 g) daily over the preceding month indicated abnormalities (mean 2.5-fold increase) in 85–95%, with more marked sensitivity than for GGT but similar specificity. Later studies have, however, found sensitivities close to 70%, virtually identical to that of concomitantly measured GGT.[69]

In alcoholics, β-hexosaminidase activities fall rapidly towards normal within 7–10 days of abstinence. In healthy volunteers, a minor increase has been observed after 60 g of alcohol daily for 10 days. Other causes of increase include non-alcoholic liver disease, diabetes, hyperthyroidism and pregnancy. Serum β-hexosaminidase is not measured routinely in clinical laboratories, and further studies would need to demonstrate a significantly better diagnostic performance than with GGT before its use in screening for alcohol abuse could be recommended.

Anormalities Resulting Principally from the Metabolic Effects of Alcohol on the Liver

Frequently Measured Metabolities.
1. Plasma Protein Abnormalities. As the majority of the plasma proteins are synthesized in the liver, it is not surprising that their concentrations may be altered by alcohol excess.

Reduced plasma albumin concentration is uncommon in alcoholic patients in the absence of cirrhosis. Approx. 50% of alcoholics with cirrhosis develop hypoalbuminaemia as a non-specific abnormality. Other non-specific protein changes include depression of plasma prealbumin, orosomucoid, haptoglobin and transferrin concentrations and increased plasma concentrations of α_2-macroglobulin, caeruloplasmin and immunoglobulins A, G and M. Concentrations of plasma orosomucoid and other acute-phase proteins, e.g. α_1-antitrypsin and C-reactive protein, may be increased, and concentrations of transferrin decreased in the early stage of liver damage, but the plasma orosomucoid concentration falls as cirrhosis develops. Increased plasma concentrations of the collagen precursor procollagen III peptide[70] and of the protein laminin[71] may accompany the fibrosis of cirrhosis. The serum concentrations of both these correlate well with the extent of fibrosis and can be used to monitor its development and progression.

Patients with alcoholic cirrhosis may show marked elevation of plasma IgA concentrations, averaging three times the upper reference limit. This is found in about 60% of cirrhotic alcoholics. Plasma IgA concentrations may remain raised for many months after withdrawal from alcohol. In alcoholics without cirrhosis, a raised IgA is infrequent, being found in less than 30% of patients, and with levels remaining below twice the upper reference limit.

An increased plasma IgA with a reduced plasma transferrin concentration is particularly characteristic of alcoholic cirrhosis. It is found in two-thirds of alcoholics with cirrhosis but also in one-third of precirrhotic alcoholics or heavy drinkers. The combination of a modest elevation of plasma AST activity, greater than that of ALT, and a marked increase in plasma IgA concentration is also a feature of alcoholic cirrhosis. Such findings in a patient with suspect liver disorder may serve to identify alcoholism as its cause.

2. Lipid Abnormalities. Alcohol excess produces changes that predominantly affect the triglyceride (VLDL) and high-density lipoprotein (HDL) fractions.[72] The regular daily intake of more than 60 g of ethanol by healthy volunteers will rapidly produce increasing amounts of triglycerides, HDL–cholesterol and apolipoprotein A. Triglycerides start to rise within 1 week and HDL within 3–5 weeks. Single, acute intakes of 3 g ethanol/kg body weight may also produce a statistically significant increase in triglycerides within 3–10 days, and lesser intakes (1 g/kg) may increase HDL–cholesterol.

In population studies, triglycerides, HDL–cholesterol and apolipoprotein A all correlate significantly with alcohol intake. Hypertriglyceridaemia is found in some 14% of men and 7% of women drinking 'high-risk' amounts, and in 20% of men and 10% of women who regularly consume nine or more drinks (about 70 g alcohol) a day.

Hypertriglyceridaemia and/or raised HDL may be

found in some 60% of recently drinking alcoholic patients with minimal liver disease. Within the VLDL fraction there is an increase in apolipoprotein C_{III} and a decrease of C_{II}. For HDL, it is the HDL-3 fraction that is particularly increased, with raised concentrations of apolipoprotein A_1 and A_2. Apolipoprotein A_2 is more frequently increased than A_1, and A_2 is the most sensitive of all lipoproteins to alcohol excess. With the development of liver disease, the incidence of these changes falls so that overall only 30% of alcoholics show plasma lipid abnormalities. Liver disease impairs synthesis of triglycerides, lipoprotein A_1 and lecithin–cholesterol acyltransferase, and increases catabolism of HDL.

Generally, the hypertriglyceridaemia and the increases in HDL–cholesterol in the alcoholic are modest, with lipid concentrations below twice the upper reference limit. Considerably higher concentrations are found, however, in patients with pre-existing non-alcoholic lipid disorders, which alcohol may exacerbate. In the cirrhotic, concentrations of triglycerides and HDL may remain normal despite continual alcohol abuse. With abstinence, the elevation of triglycerides falls to normal within 1–2 weeks, though it may increase again within a few hours of relapse. HDL concentrations also usually return to normal within 1–2 weeks.

It has been suggested that low amounts (less than 2 units) of daily alcohol consumption may protect from death from coronary arterial disease,[73] and that this may, in part, be a consequence of the raised plasma HDL (especially HDL-2) and apolipoprotein A_1, both of which are antiatherogenic. Alcohol may also decrease the plasma concentration of the atherogenic and thrombotic lipoprotein (a)[74] and this too may be beneficial.

The aetiology of alcohol-induced hyperlipidaemia is multifactorial. Reduced oxidation of free fatty acids secondary to the altered redox state that follows alcohol ingestion is thought to stimulate the synthesis of triglycerides and VLDL. Reduced hepatic and plasma lipoprotein lipase activity may impair triglyceride clearance. The increase in plasma HDL could reflect increased hepatic microsomal activity from the enzyme-inducing effect of alcohol.

Lipid abnormalities are short-lived, show only a moderate frequency of elevation in alcoholics, which falls as liver disease progresses, and are non-specific, with triglycerides being raised in both primary (familial) hyperlipidaemia and other secondary hyperlipidaemias (e.g. from obesity, diabetes or drug therapy). All these features detract from the value of lipid abnormalities in detecting alcoholism. However, measurements of triglycerides are readily made and routinely done for the investigation of suspect hyperlipidaemia. Also, measurements of HDL–cholesterol and apolipoprotein A are increasingly used to assess risk of coronary arterial disease. As alcohol ingestion is one of the most frequent causes of secondary hyperlipidaemia, alcohol excess should be suspected whenever lipid abnormality (especially raised triglycerides) is found on medical examination. The combination of lipid abnormality with other biochemical disturbances, e.g. enzyme changes or hyperuricaemia, increases the likelihood of alcohol excess, and the inclusion of lipid tests may improve the diagnostic performance of test combinations for diagnosing alcoholism.

Plasma Urate.[44] In population studies, blood uric acid concentrations have been shown to rise progressively with increasing amounts of ethanol consumption. Hyperuricaemia is found in approx. 30% of men drinking at high-risk levels and 40% of those who consume 70 g or more of ethanol per day. A much lower frequency is observed in women.

Raised plasma uric acid concentrations are found in approx. 40–50% of male and 25% of female alcoholics on admission to hospital. After abstinence, these may fall rapidly or persist for several weeks. Sometimes a temporary increase in hyperuricaemia is observed, possibly from altered nutrition. Because of this inconsistent relation to current drinking, measurement of the plasma uric acid is of little value for monitoring drinking behaviour in the short term. Measurement of plasma uric acid concentration is of some value for detecting alcohol abuse. In combination with other biochemical changes (e.g. increased plasma enzymes and lipids), hyperuricaemia may be very suggestive of alcohol excess, and it is a frequent constituent of test combinations used for its identification. It should be remembered, however, that the plasma uric acid may vary with age, sex and weight, and that hyperuricaemia may result from renal disease, gout or from drug ingestion.

Several mechanisms contribute to hyperuricaemia in heavy drinkers. Alcohol ingestion may increase urate synthesis, lactate produced in excess as a consequence of the altered redox state resulting from alcohol oxidation may compete with uric acid for renal tubular excretion, and beer drinking may contribute to hyperuricaemia through its purine content.

Less Frequently Measured Metabolites and Markers.
1. *Serum Isotransferrins.* Transferrin is an iron-binding glycoprotein synthesized and metabolized in the liver. Transferrin in the plasma transports iron, mainly in the di-ferric form, utilizing its two iron-binding sites per molecule. Several genetic variants of the protein have been reported. In Europeans, the C variant is the major phenotype, and B and D variants are occasionally observed. The carbohydrate portion of transferrin has two branched side-chains, one showing up to three and the other up to four branches. These branches each terminate in charged sialic-acid residues and the serum transferrins are named according to the number of their sialic acid groups. The separate forms (isoforms) can be resolved by isoelectric focusing, the principal form in serum being tetrasialotransferrin of isoelectric point (pI) approx. 5.4.

Small amounts of more sialylated anodal transferrins with lower pI (pentasialo-, pI 5.3; hexasialo-, pI 5.2) and less sialylated cathodal forms with higher pI (trisialo-, pI 5.6; disialo-, pI 5.7; monosialo-, pI 5.8 and asialo-, pI 5.9) may also be present.

In 1979, Stibler and coworkers, using isoelectric focusing and immunofixation to detect serum transferrin, demonstrated qualitatively a marked selective increase in alcoholics of a so-called microheterogeneous component (isoform) of pI 5.7 (i.e. disialotransferrin).[75] This was found in 81% of alcoholics drinking in excess of 60 g of alcohol daily but only 1% of non-drinking healthy controls, and in none of patients with non-alcoholic liver disease. It was not found in healthy volunteers after a large single intake of 1.8 g alcohol/kg body weight, but appeared after 0.6 g/kg taken for 7 days. The measurement thus seemed to have considerable promise as a sensitive and specific marker of alcoholism.

Subsequent studies were carried out to confirm these results, but not all were successful, possibly because of the inherent technical difficulties or because of failure to saturate the serum samples with iron before separation, a procedure essential for reproducible results. Many of the more successful confirmatory studies have modified the procedure by the use of densitometry to provide a quantitative measure of the fraction at pI 5.7, its increase being expressed as a ratio or percentage of total transferrin (normally less than 3%)[76] or of the fraction at pI 5.4 (the so-called transferrin index, normally less than 7%).[77] Scrupulous technique is essential for measurement of these low relative values.

Most (but not all) workers using isoelectric focusing have been able to confirm 80–90% sensitivity and greater than 90% specificity for the measurement in alcoholics. In comparison with GGT determination the procedure has generally shown slightly greater sensitivity in alcoholics, slightly greater specificity in healthy controls, but far better specificity in non-alcoholic liver disease. The mechanism of the serum desialotransferrin increase in alcoholism is uncertain, impaired hepatocyte uptake from alcohol-mediated membrane dysfunction being the most favoured.

As an alternative to the difficult isoelectric focusing, chromatographic methods were developed.[78] These have used anion-exchange chromatography to separate and pH-controlled buffer to elute the fraction at pI 5.7 (disialotransferrin) and the higher pI fractions, together known as desialylated or carbohydrate-deficient transferrin (CDT). Transferrin is then measured in the eluates by radioimmunoassay.

Reagents for this assay have been prepared commercially and distributed for examination to several international groups. Most have found sensitivities and specificities for alcoholism similar to those in the original electrophoretic study. My team found an increased CDT concentration in the serum of 15 out of 20 alcoholics drinking more than 60 g of alcohol daily, and in 4 out of 73 non-drinking healthy controls. In both groups these proportions were identical to those observed with concomitantly measured GGT. However (as expected), an increase in GGT was observed in 21 out of 26 patients with non-alcohol liver disease whereas CDT was abnormal in only five.

My studies also showed a marked sex difference in CDT concentrations in healthy subjects, with higher values in women. Others have since reported minor sex differences, and also a slight increase with age in men. The rare phenotypes may also show altered CDT values; higher with the D and lower with the B variant. No major difference was observed, however, in the frequency of increased serum CDT concentrations in alcoholics between Puerto Ricans, blacks and whites in an American study.[79]

In non-alcoholic liver disease, instead of the complete lack of a raised CDT originally noticed, it has now been recognized that patients with autoimmune disease and particularly primary biliary cirrhosis may show abnormality. Up to one-third of those with this cirrhosis may show increased concentrations. I have found subnormal concentrations in 'social drinkers' with multiple myeloma, but the paraprotein might well interfere with the column binding of transferrin in the assay.

The column method (CDT) and isoelectric focusing of disialotransferrin have been directly compared in alcoholics and controls, excellent correlation being obtained between CDT and the 'transferrin index', though the index showed greater sensitivity to alcoholism in patients drinking more than 40 g of alcohol a day.[80] This good correlation is relevant to the outcome of more recent studies using isoelectric focusing, one of which has suggested its insensitivity in detecting alcohol abuse in young adult alcoholics, with less than 20% showing abnormal levels of disialotransferrin.[81] A similar low frequency of abnormality (22%) has also been found for CDT in a study of male student heavy drinkers of mean age 22 years consuming more than 27 g of alcohol daily.[82] A particularly important study, carried out in France, has examined the ability of the 'transferrin index' (the method previously correlated with the chromatographic procedure) to identify alcohol consumption in excess of 80 g/day in a general practice outpatient population.[83] It showed a sensitivity of only 45%, less than that of GGT (52%), though specificity was higher (98% vs. 80%). Some drinkers had a normal transferrin index with a normal GGT and vice versa. The raised mean disialotransferrin activities observed in house painters suggest that organic solvent inhalation might also be a source of abnormality.[84]

The manufacturers (Pharmacia, Sweden) of the original, commercially produced procedure for CDT measurement, which used pH-controlled elution from an anion-exchange column, have discontinued its production because of problems in obtaining stable buffer pH. They have substituted a procedure in which CDT is instead eluted with buffer of defined ionic strength. This has been claimed to give sensitivity and specificity for alcoholism virtually identical to the original method. It should, however, be noted that this technique measures only a part of the fraction at pI 5.7 together with higher pI fractions, and the reference range for CDT concentration is correspondingly reduced, with an upper reference limit one-quarter of that of its predecessor (about 20 mg/L compared with the previous 80 mg/L). As with the earlier column CDT method, the newer technique is demanding, being non-automated and requiring duplicate analyses. The determination time is long (at least 2 h), and the procedure requires radioisotopes and suitable counting apparatus. Though details of the diagnostic performance of this new procedure are still scanty, a preliminary study has reported a sensitivity of only 42% in recently drinking alcoholics with biopsy-confirmed fatty liver, increasing to only 63% with biopsy-confirmed cirrhosis.[85] Furthermore, false positives were observed in 10% of non-alcohol abusing controls and 16% of patients with non-alcoholic liver disease.

In summary, it would appear that measurement of disialotransferrin by one or other of its various methods has good sensitivity (about 80%) to alcoholism but has much less value for the identification of high-risk alcohol consumption in the general population. Its only clear advantage over measurement of GGT is its greater specificity in non-alcoholic liver disease, but its value is offset by technical difficulties. Further evaluation is obviously needed, and such studies are currently in progress in my laboratory and elsewhere. At this time, its principal role in the identification of alcohol abuse would seem to be as an adjunct to GGT determination, assisting in the interpretation of a raised serum GGT.

2. Abnormalities Resulting from Hepatic Enzyme Induction.[44]

Ethanol induces the synthesis of hepatic microsomal enzymes. This has a number of metabolic consequences including increased hepatic clearance of orally administered drugs, and enhanced urinary excretion of D-glucaric acid, a metabolite of the hepatic glucuronic-acid pathway. These changes can occur at a time when the liver appears normal on light microscopy.

(a) *Drug clearance*: measurement of the clearance of radiolabelled aminopyrine is a convenient, non-invasive means of assessing enzyme induction. However, only one-third of non-cirrhotic alcoholic patients show increased clearances. This low proportion may reflect the inhibiting effect of acute alcohol ingestion on drug clearance.

Hepatocellular damage may also impair drug excretory mechanisms; thus 75% of alcoholic cirrhotic patients have diminished clearances. Diminished clearance is non-specific, and is also found in non-alcoholic cirrhosis.

(b) *Urinary D-glucaric acid excretion*: enzyme-including agents, including ethanol, are known to increase the urinary excretion of glucuronic acid metabolites, especially D-glucaric acid. Increased urinary excretion of glucaric acid is found in 60–90% of alcoholics attending alcohol treatment centres and drinking heavily up to the time of admission. Urinary excretion of D-glucaric acid excretion returns to normal within about 8 days of alcohol withdrawal. There is correlation between this excretion and serum GGT activity, and the increase occurs independently of liver damage, suggesting that enzyme induction is responsible for the elevation.

Glucaric acid can be determined in 24-h urine collections or in random morning specimens, and can be related to the urine creatinine concentration. Unfortunately, the greatest frequency of abnormality is detected with methods too complex for routine laboratory use. Increased urinary excretion of D-glucaric acid is also found in patients with alcohol unrelated liver disease and in those exposed to other enzyme-inducing drugs; thus it is not specific for detecting alcohol abuse. In addition, the increase that follows alcohol consumption is only transitory and easily missed.

3. Plasma α-Amino-n-Butyric Acid:Leucine (A:L) Ratio.[44]

Following the observation that plasma concentrations of α-aminobutyric acid are elevated and concentrations of branched-chain amino acids such as leucine are depressed in animals fed alcohol, Shaw and coworkers reported an elevated A:L ratio in approx. 80% of recently drinking alcoholics on admission to hospital.[86] The changes were independent of nutritional status as well as biochemical or morphological evidence of liver damage. After 1 week of abstinence, the frequency of abnormality fell to 54%. Patients with non-alcoholic liver disease did not show raised A:L ratios.

Others, however, have shown that the A:L ratio is both insensitive and non-specific for alcoholism, and that abnormal values reflect the presence of liver damage irrespective of cause. The measurement of the A:L ratio cannot be recommended for identifying alcoholic patients, because of its poor sensitivity, poor specificity and the methodological complexities involved.

4. Erythrocyte Superoxide Dismutase.[44]

An increased concentration of the erythrocyte enzyme, cuprozinc superoxide dismutase determined by radioimmunoassay was reported in 1979 in 68% of a small series of black alcoholics. Increased activities were not found in the erythrocytes of white alcoholics. It was suggested that the superoxide radical resulting from the oxidation of acetaldehyde formed from ethanol induces the synthesis of the enzyme.

Subsequent reports on white alcoholics have related increased activity of the enzyme to the presence and severity of accompanying liver disease, normal values being found in its absence.[87] A modest elevation has been observed in non-alcoholic liver disease. The concentrations of erythrocyte superoxide dismutase in recently drinking alcoholics cluster in two groups, above and below the normal range.[88] Both groups show normalization of enzyme values after 1 week of abstinence from alcohol. Clustering might reflect differing drinking patterns immediately before admission to hospital or varying degrees of liver involvement. It could also result from induction by superoxide radicals, resulting in increased concentrations, or from a direct toxic action of ethanol on the erythrocyte enzyme, resulting in decrease.

Though it was initially thought that measuring the concentration of erythrocyte superoxide dismutase might prove useful for the identification of alcoholism, demonstrations of the inconstancy of its elevation, and its general relation to liver disease now indicate that it is not valuable for this purpose.

5. *Minor Haemoglobins and Acetaldehyde–Protein Adducts.* Erythrocyte haemolysates from alcoholics reportedly show an increased concentration of minor haemoglobin fractions, which migrate rapidly on cation-exchange resin chromatography. One of these fractions was found in 8 out of 10 alcoholics, and believed to be a consequence of adduct formation between haemoglobin and circulating acetaldehyde. The erythrocyte synthesizes 5-deoxy-D-xylose-1-phosphate from acetaldehyde and dihydroacetone phosphate, and it is this compound that is thought to form a stable adduct with haemoglobin, its concentration reflecting the long-term ('integrated') blood acetaldehyde level.

Not all workers have been able to identify abnormal haemoglobin fractions in the blood of alcoholics, but significant differences in their mean concentration in recently drinking alcoholics compared with non-alcoholic controls have been measured using sensitive chromatographic and immunological techniques.[89] Values return to normal after 24–48h of abstinence.

The measurement of haemoglobin adducts with acetaldehyde has been suggested as a marker of potential value in screening for alcoholism. However, as levels in alcoholics appear to overlap substantially with those in non-alcoholics, it does not seem to be useful for this purpose.

Acetaldehyde may also form adducts with other proteins. Adducts with myoglobin and with haemocyanin have both been detected by immunoassay in the serum of alcoholics, and at a higher mean concentration than in controls. In a preliminary study, assay of the myoglobin adducts had better diagnostic accuracy, with a sensitivity of 71% and a specificity of 91%.[90] Its further evaluation is awaited.

6. *Plasma Acetate.*[91] The oxidation of ethanol and formed acetaldehyde yields acetate; the plasma acetate is consequently increased after alcohol ingestion. The altered redox state resulting from ethanol oxidation also inhibits the further oxidation of acetate.

Plasma acetate after alcohol ingestion is higher in alcoholics than in non-alcoholics, possibly because of an increased rate of ethanol elimination in alcoholics. In both groups, increased plasma acetate concentrations are found within 1h of alcohol intake. Measurement of the plasma acetate concentration has been used to identify alcoholics but its sensitivity is poor, with less than 65% of alcoholics and heavy drinkers showing increased values. Raised concentrations are also found in non-alcoholics receiving steroid therapy.

A raised acetate in the blood of alcoholics is found only after recent alcohol intake and as long as the blood alcohol is also raised. This limits its value as a marker for alcoholism, though it may be useful in the detection of chronic heavy drinking in recently drinking subjects involved in accidents or road traffic offences.[92]

7. *Urinary Salsolinol.* Salsolinol (dihydroxy methyl tetrahydroisoquinoline) is a condensation product of acetaldehyde and dopamine. An increased salsolinol concentration has been observed in the urine of male, long-term, moderate drinkers, and in 50% of alcoholics.[93] Levels return to normal within 2–3 days of abstinence. Urinary salsolinol concentrations are also increased after acute alcohol intake in healthy subjects (orientals) with deficient hepatic mitochondrial aldehyde dehydrogenase (i.e of ALDH-2² phenotype), as a consequence of the high serum acetaldehyde concentrations after alcohol in these subjects. The urinary and plasma salsolinol concentrations are strongly correlated.

Limited sensitivity and a complex method detract from measurement of salsolinol as a marker of alcoholism. A further difficulty is that salsolinol has been identified as a constituent of various foodstuffs (e.g. chocolate, bananas) and alcoholic beverages, and this may cause problems in interpretation.

8. *Urinary Dolichols.* Dolichols are long-chain polyprenols containing an α-saturated isoprene unit. They act as glycosyl carriers and are cell-membrane constituents. Ethanol is thought to interfere with their further metabolism, as both are oxidized by alcohol dehydrogenase, though it may also increase their synthesis or impair their uptake into membranes.[94]

Urinary dolichols are increased in approx. 60% of severe alcoholics. This does not, however, appear to be a useful marker of alcoholism, because of limited sensitivity, rapid disappearance with abstinence and poor specificity, increased concentrations being found also in infections, pregnancy and with neoplasia. Determining dolichols is methodologically complex.

Biochemical Abnormalities Independent of the Hepatic Effects of Alcohol. 1. *Erythrocyte δ-Aminolaevulinic Acid Dehydratase (DALD)*.[44] Erythrocyte DALD catalyses the formation of porphobilinogen from α-aminolaevulinic acid in the pathway of porphyrin biosynthesis. In intoxicated men attending a casualty department, a highly significant correlation between DALD activity and blood ethanol concentration was found, with a significant depression of enzyme activity at a mean blood ethanol concentration of just over 200 mg/dL (44 mmol/L). Acute ethanol administration to healthy volunteers also results in rapid depression of erythrocyte DALD, lowest activities being found at 2 h and coinciding with peak blood ethanol concentrations of 150 mg/dL (33 mmol/L). Values had returned to normal at 10 h, by which time ethanol had disappeared from the blood.

Reduced activity of erythrocyte DALD has been reported in over 90% of alcoholics examined within 48 h of admission to hospital, activities returning to normal within 1 week of abstinence. However, in chronic alcoholics attending a liver disease clinic, only 38% showed depression of erythrocyte DALD, as did 9% with non-alcoholic liver disease.

Erythrocyte DALD is a labile enzyme, so that blood samples must be processed immediately. The method is inconvenient and enzyme activity may also be depressed by environmental toxins such as lead. Because of methodological complexity the test has found little application in the diagnostic laboratory for detection of alcoholism, despite apparently good sensitivity and specificity. The reduced activity from intoxication in the absence of chronic alcohol excess is also a disadvantage.

Test Combination.[44,95] Combining the results of several tests in alcoholics and heavy drinkers may yield a greater frequency of abnormality than when each test is used individually. Thus, in my study of 110 alcoholics, abnormal plasma GGT activities and/or erythrocyte MCV were found in 85% of patients, compared with 75% for GGT alone, and 50% for MCV alone.

In addition to increasing the sensitivity, tests in combination can increase diagnostic specificity: combinations of particular importance include raised plasma GGT activity with hypertriglyceridaemia and hyperuricaemia; increased plasma AST:ALT ratios, especially with IgA elevation; increased plasma GGT:ALP ratios and raised plasma GGT:urea ratios.

More sophisticated, mathematical treatment of results from multiple laboratory tests has also been used to identify heavy drinking and to distinguish alcoholic from non-alcoholic liver disease. Discriminant function analysis uses data from defined disease groups to allocate weightings for test results that produce a discriminant which minimizes within-group differences and maximizes between-group differences. Using such analysis with large numbers of test variables (up to 33 in some cases) near 100% sensitivities and specificities have been reported for discrimination between subjects drinking at high compared to low levels of risk, between alcoholics and patients with alcohol-unrelated disease, and between alcoholic and non-alcoholic liver disease.[96,97] The examination of large numbers of variables and their discriminant analysis would be impractical for most laboratories; fortunately, on using only three (best) variables in combination (GGT, MCV and ALP), sensitivities and specificities of more than 80% are found for discrimination between each of the three categories mentioned in the previous sentence.

OVERVIEW OF THE LABORATORY IDENTIFICATION OF ALCOHOL EXCESS

Of the various laboratory tests (Table 7.8), measuring plasma γ-glutamyltransferase activity combines the greatest convenience and sensitivity and is the most valuable individual procedure. Its diagnostic value is enhanced by its combination with other simple biochemical measurements routinely made by the diagnostic laboratory, particularly the plasma enzymes normally included in liver function tests, and the determination of uric acid and triglycerides. Measurements of ethanol in breath and erythrocyte MCV are simple tests that are also helpful. Test combinations enhance both sensitivity and specificity, and identify more alcoholics than single procedures. Their accuracy is greater than 80%. With the exception of the serum isotransferrin, more complex and exotic measurements seem, currently, to add little to diagnostic ability. The value of measuring isotransferrin (diasialotransferrin or CDT) is still under review. Its diagnostic sensitivity is similar to that of GGT, and its specificity with regard to non-alcoholic liver disease is superior. Analytical complexity is a distinct disadvantage.

CLINICAL CONSULTATION, QUESTIONNAIRES AND THEIR RELATION TO BIOCHEMICAL ABNORMALITIES

Biochemical tests for the identification of excess alcohol intake or the confirmation of alcoholism are not done in isolation but as part of a diagnostic process that may include clinical consultation and/or patients' responses to questionnaires. It is relevant, therefore, to consider the relation of biochemical abnormalities to these responses and their relative contributions to diagnosis.[98]

For the individual patient it is the consultation (history and clinical examination) that generally provides the initial diagnosis. This can identify more than 80% of alcohol abusers, most of whom (up to 90%) will also show some abnormality on biochemical testing, particularly when simple test combinations are used. Accuracy in consultation does, however, depend on the skill and experience of

TABLE 7.8

APPROXIMATE FREQUENCY OF SOME BIOCHEMICAL TEST ABNORMALITIES IN ALCOHOLICS

Enzymes	GGT (< 75%)
	AST (< 70%); GDH (< 70%); β-hexosaminidase (< 80%)
	DALD (> 40%); superoxide dismutase (< 70%)
Metabolites	Urate (< 40%); triglycerides (< 30%); apolipoprotein A_2 (< 80%)
	A : L (< 70%); D-glucarate (> 60%)
	Acetate (< 70%); salsolinol (< 50%); dolichols (< 60%)
Proteins	IgA (< 60%)
	Isotransferrins (< 80%)
	Haemoglobin adducts (< 80%)
Ethanol	Blood / urine / breath (< 50%)

GGT, γ-glutamyltransferase; AST, aspartate transaminase; GDH, glutamate dehydrogenase; DALD, δ-aminolaevulinic acid dehydratase; A : L, α-amino-n-butyric acid : leucine.

the physician, particularly in history taking, as physical signs may be few. In addition to being labour-intensive, consultation can also be very time-consuming and so is unsuited to screening for alcoholism.

Questionnaires are frequently used in the investigation of excessive alcohol consumption. They have the advantages of speed, convenience, simplicity and low cost, and can be self-administered and computer-administered. They do, however, rely on the patient's memory and are susceptible to deliberate concealment. Three types of questionnaire are in general use—those designed to evaluate (i) the frequency and amount of recent alcohol consumption (quantity/frequency questionnaire); (ii) attitudes to alcohol (e.g. the CAGE questionnaire, CAGE being an acronym derived from the four questions asked therein); (iii) problems resulting from alcohol excess (e.g. the brief Michigan Alcoholism Screening Test (MAST) questionnaire); or a combination of these (e.g. the Health Survey Questionnaire (HSQ).

Questionnaires identify a similar frequency to that of consultation—up to 80% of alcohol abusers. The most sensitive are those designed to detect excess consumption (quantity/frequency questionnaires). These are particularly suitable for population screening, where biochemical tests are much less sensitive (approx. 50% sensitivity with individual tests, increasing with test combinations). The CAGE and brief MAST tests are, in general, less sensitive, but identify those whose drinking has caused harm; at this stage, simple test combinations may indicate a near-identical frequency of abnormality.

Overall, therefore the sensitivities of consultations, questionnaire and biochemical investigations may be comparable, though the last are the least sensitive in some, perhaps most, clinical settings. However, it must be admitted that the various published studies do not show unanimity in their conclusions. One major study of over 2000 outpatients, and with diagnosis based on patients' records, reported that laboratory tests had better sensitivity in detecting alcohol abuse than either consultation or questionnaire.[99] Most agree that biochemical markers may reveal unexpected alcohol excess, undoubtedly complement and confirm clinical and questionnaire-based diagnoses, and are of particular value when memory is poor or there is any attempt at concealment, and for monitoring abstinence programmes.

COMPLICATIONS OF ALCOHOLISM

In addition to the hepatic, neurological and metabolic complications of alcoholism previously discussed, important consequences of alcohol abuse include disease of the pancreas, skeletal and cardiac muscle, vitamin (especially vitamin B_1) deficiency and bone disease. The biochemical changes that accompany these disorders are helpful in the confirmation of diagnosis, and may also first draw attention to alcohol abuse. They are considered below. Alcohol excess may also profoundly affect the endocrine system[100,101] and porphyrin[102] metabolism, but such effects have been extensively reviewed elsewhere, and will not be further discussed.

Pancreatitis[13]

Alcoholism is responsible for more than 10% of acute and more than 50% of chronic pancreatitis. Acute pancreatitis is characterized clinically by upper abdominal pain radiating through to the back, accompanied by vomiting and abdominal tenderness and usually preceded by an alcoholic debauch. Rarely the condition may be subclinical. Acute pancreatitis may be confirmed by the demonstration of transiently increased activity of enzymes of pancreatic origin in plasma, particularly amylase and lipase. The activity of these enzymes is raised in more than 90% of patients with acute pancreatitis, with values generally above five times the upper reference limit. In alcoholics without symptoms of pancreatic disease these enzymes are generally normal, with occasional (10–20%) borderline elevation.

Chronic pancreatitis may present with chronic and intermittent abdominal pain, steatorrhoea, jaundice or diabetes. It may result in reduced output of trypsin, lipase and amylase in duodenal juice in response to hormonal (pancreozymin) stimulation of the pancreas, or a reduced duodenal trypsin response to an oral test meal (Lundh test). Faecal enzyme activity (chymotrypsin and trypsin) may also be low. Faecal fat excretion may be increased and glucose tolerance impaired. The demonstration of reduced enzymes of pancreatic origin (pancreatic isoamylase, immunoreactive trypsin) in plasma provides a convenient way of screening for pancreatic exocrine insufficiency, with a sensitivity of about 70% and a specificity of approx. 90%. Pancreatic isoamylase activity in plasma is reduced in about 20% of alcoholics without clinical evidence of pancreatic deficiency, sometimes with an increase of the salivary fraction so that total amylase remains within normal limits. Reduction in plasma pancreatic isoamylase in the actively drinking, symptomless alcoholic may be transient, reverting rapidly to normal with abstinence. For confirmation of chronic pancreatic exocrine insufficiency, therefore, low plasma enzymes should be demonstrated during abstinence.

Alcoholic Myopathy[103,104]

Chronic alcoholism may result in myopathic changes in skeletal muscle. Acute myopathy (rhabdomyolysis) may follow recent alcohol excess. The muscles are painful and tender, and there may be myoglobinuria. The condition is rare, being found in less than 1% of hospitalized alcoholics. Histologically, there is muscle cell destruction, particularly of type I (slow twitch, aerobic glycolytic) fibres. Glycolytic and oxidative enzymes in muscle are reduced. The plasma creatine kinase is raised in more than 80% of such patients, with enzyme levels averaging four times the upper reference limit, though much higher activities are sometimes encountered.

Chronic myopathic changes with atrophy of type 2b (fast twitch, anaerobic glycolytic) fibres is found in some two-thirds of alcoholics. It may be accompanied clinically by muscle weakness and wasting. Enzymes of calcium transport and glycolytic enzymes are reduced in muscle. Plasma α-tocopherol (vitamin E) concentrations are subnormal, and enhanced free-radical activity in muscle has been postulated as an aetiological factor.

Carnosine is normally present at high concentration in muscle, especially in type 2 fibres, and has antioxidant activity. Studies of carnosinase activity in plasma in chronic alcoholic myopathy have shown reduced levels, correlating with the severity of muscle atrophy. Values increase with abstinence, paralleled by improvement of the myopathy.

A raised plasma creatine kinase is found in up to 60% of patients with symptoms of chronic myopathy, with enzyme levels averaging twice the upper reference limit. In alcoholics without clinical evidence of muscle disorder, a modest elevation of creatine kinase with enzyme values below twice the upper reference limit is found in some 20%. Assay for creatine kinase isoenzymes shows the enzyme to be the MM form originating from muscle.

Cardiomyopathy[105]

1–2% of alcoholics may show clinical cardiomyopathy, the haemodynamic test of cardiac function may be abnormal in 30–40% and 90% show myofibrillar degeneration and interstitial fibrosis of cardiac muscle at autopsy. These changes are thought to be due to the cardiotoxic action of acetaldehyde, particularly on mitochondria, with reduction of mitochondrial oxidative enzyme activity. Despite the high frequency of cardiac involvement, enzymes of cardiac origin (creatine kinase MB isoenzyme and lactate dehydrogenase LD-1 isoenzyme) are not generally demonstrable in increased amounts in plasma. This suggests that alcohol-related cardiac injury is generally unaccompanied by significant necrosis of myocardial cells, and is in conformity with the usual histological findings.

Vitamin Deficiency[106]

Alcoholism is a major cause of vitamin deficiency, which results from impaired intake, absorption or utilization, or increased demand. Deficiency of all the major vitamins has been observed, though vitamin B_1 deficiency is the most familiar because of its association with neurological or, rarely, cardiac symptoms. For the detection of vitamin B_1 deficiency, measurement of erythrocyte transketolase and its increased activity following the addition *in vitro* of its cofactor thiamine pyrophosphate (TPP effect) has been widely used. Deficiency results in reduced transketolase activity and undersaturation of the erythrocyte enzyme with cofactor, so that there is an enhanced increase in transketolose activity on adding vitamin B_1. These changes are demonstrable in some 40% of symptomless alcoholics.

Alcoholic Bone Disease[101,107]

Chronic alcohol excess is an important cause of metabolic bone disease, particularly osteoporosis. Studies of bone density by radiography or dual-photon absorptiometry indicate bone loss (osteopenia) in approx. 30% of non-cirrhotic, middle-aged alcoholics. This is generally subclinical, though an increased tendency for spontaneous fractures, and occasionally bone pain, has been observed. The bone changes have a multifactorial origin. Inadequate dietary intake of calcium, protein and vitamin D, or their impaired absorption because of enterocyte damage from alcohol or, occasionally, chronic pancreatitis may be relevant, as may altered metabolism of vitamin D or parathyroid hormone (PTH) through liver injury. Increased cortisol in response to alcohol may also act on bone to produce osteopenia. Most recent studies suggest that a direct toxic action of ethanol on bone with inhibition of osteoblast activity is the main factor.

Biochemical findings are inconsistent. In the noncirrhotic alcoholic, plasma calcium, inorganic phosphate and magnesium are within the reference range, though a slight increase in mean total calcium and ionized calcium has been reported. The amounts of plasma 25-hydroxy vitamin D are normal or low, though high values of 1:25-dihydroxy vitamin D have also been observed. The levels of PTH remain normal or are increased. Osteocalcin concentrations (which generally reflect osteoblast activity) have variously been reported as increased or reduced.

To account for some of these biochemical changes it has been suggested that dietary deficiency of vitamin D and low dietary calcium by reducing calcium absorption would tend to lower the plasma calcium. There would then be a compensatory increase in PTH. Hepatic degradation of PTH by an alcohol-affected liver might also be impaired. PTH would then act on bone to promote resorption, and stimulate renal synthesis of 1:25-dihydroxy vitamin D, resulting in an increase of plasma ionized calcium and release of osteocalcin from osteoblasts. The inconsistencies in observed plasma biochemical values may result from variation in the extent of alcohol intake and of the consequent liver damage and bone changes. Drinking shortly before sampling may also be relevant, as acute alcoholic intoxication has been found to result in transient decreases of osteocalcin and PTH.

Alcoholic Ketoacidosis[13]

This disorder is found especially in female alcoholics presenting with anorexia, abdominal pain, vomiting and dehydration following recent alcohol abuse. In its florid form, mental confusion and air-hunger may be present. Frequently, onset is preceded by starvation, and alcohol is low or absent in the blood by the time of presentation. It may account for up to 20% of hospital admissions with ketoacidosis.

Arterial pH and the plasma bicarbonate concentration are lowered, and the 'anion gap' is increased due to raised levels of 3-hydroxybutyrate in the plasma, with a lesser elevation of acetoacetate. This elevation may be overlooked if the plasma ketones are assessed by the nitroprusside reaction (Acetest or Ketostix, Ames), which is relatively insensitive to 3-hydroxbutyrate compared with its sensitivity to acetone. The plasma lactate is generally also raised; plasma glucose remains normal or minimally elevated; plasma insulin is normal or near normal. The plasma phosphate may be lowered and such lowering may be accompanied by red cell haemolysis.

Alcoholic ketoacidosis is thought to result from the ketogenic effect of acute starvation combined with that of alcohol secondary to the increased NADH:NAD ratio from alcohol oxidation by alcohol dehydrogenase.

CONCLUSION

The clinical presentations of alcohol abuse are so varied that it is important to consider alcoholism as a possible aetiological agent in a variety of organ and metabolic disorders. Indeed, no organ or major metabolic pathway is unaffected by alcohol excess.

This chapter has highlighted selected aspects of the metabolism of alcohol, the origins of alcoholism, the acute and chronic effects of alcohol abuse, and the identification of alcohol excess. It is hoped that it will provide a framework to assist the clinical biochemist to understand, to identify and to manage the biochemical consequences of alcohol excess.

REFERENCES

1. Dunbar G.C., Morgan D.D.V. (1987). The changing pattern of alcohol consumption in England and Wales 1978–1985. *Br. Med. J.*, **295**, 807.
2. Paton A., Saunders J.B. (1981). ABC of alcohol: definitions. *Br. Med. J.*, **281**, 1248.
3. Royal College of Physicians (1987). *The Medical Consequences of Alcohol Abuse: A Great and Growing Evil*, London: Tavistock Publications.
4. Lieber C.S. (1977). Metabolism of ethanol. In *Metabolic Aspects of Alcohol* (Lieber C.S. ed.) Lancaster: MTP Press, pp. 1–29.
5. Lieber C.S., de Carli L.M. (1977). Metabolic effects of alcohol on the liver. In *Metabolic Aspects of Alcohol* (Lieber C.S. ed.) Lancaster: MTP Press, pp. 31–79.
6. Frezza M., di Padova C., Pozzato G., Terpin M., Baraona E., Lieber C.S. (1990). High blood alcohol levels in women. The role of decreased gastric alcohol dehydrogenase activity and first pass metabolism. *N. Engl. J. Med.*, **322**, 95.
7. Jenkins W. (1984). Liver disorders in alcoholism. In *Clinical Biochemistry of Alcoholism* (Rosalki S.B. ed.) Edinburgh: Churchill Livingstone, pp. 258–270.
8. Tanner A.R., Bantock I., Hinks L., Lloyd B., Turner N.R., Wright R. (1986). Depressed selenium and vitamin E levels in an alcoholic population. *Dig. Dis. Sci.* **31**, 1307.
9. Wickramasinghe S.N., Marjot D.H., Rosalki S.B., Fink R.S. (1989). Correlations between serum proteins modified by acetaldehyde and biochemical variables in heavy drinkers. *J. Clin. Pathol.*, **42**, 295.
10. Laposata E.A., Lange L.G. (1986). Presence of nonoxidative ethanol metabolism in human organs commonly damaged by ethanol abuse. *Science*, **231**, 497.
11. Rutherford W.H. (1977). Diagnosis of alcohol ingestion in mild head injuries. *Lancet*, **i**, 1021.
12. Johnson R.A., Noll E.C., Rodney W.M. (1982). Survival after a serum ethanol concentration of 1 1/2%. *Lancet*, **ii**, 1394.
13. Fink R., Rosalki S.B. (1978). Clinical biochemistry of alcoholism. *Clin. Endocrinol. Metab.*, **7**, 297.

14. Denney R.C. (1984). Measuring alcohol. In *Clinical Biochemistry of Alcoholism* (Rosalki S.B. ed.) Edinburgh: Churchill Livingstone, pp. 51–64.
15. Wright J.W. (1991). Alcohol and the laboratory in the United Kingdom. *Ann. Clin. Biochem.*, **28**, 212.
16. Falkensson M., Jones W., Sorbo B. (1989). Bedside diagnosis of alcohol intoxication with a pocket-size breath-alcohol device. Sampling from unconscious subjects and specificity for ethanol. *Clin. Chem.* **35**, 918.
17. McColl K., Whiting B., Moore M.R., Goldberg A. (1979). Correlation of ethanol concentration in blood and saliva. *Clin. Sci.* **56**, 283.
18. Champion H.R., et al. (1975). Alcohol intoxication and serum osmolarity. *Lancet*, **i**, 1402.
19. Dorwort W.V., Chalmers L. (1975). Comparison of methods for calculating serum osmolality from chemical concentrations and the prognostic value of such calculations. *Clin. Chem.*, **21**, 190.
20. Geller R.J., Spyker D.A., Herold D.A., Bruns D.E. (1986). Serum osmolal gap and ethanol concentration: a simple and accurate formula. *Clin. Toxicol.*, **24**, 77.
21. Badawy A. (1984). Alcohol intoxication and withdrawal. In *Clinical Biochemistry of Alcoholism* (Rosalki S.B. ed.) Edinburgh: Churchill Livingstone, pp. 95–116.
22. McIntyre N. (1984). The effects of alcohol on water, electrolytes and minerals. In *Clinical Biochemistry of Alcoholism* (Rosalki S.B. ed.) Edinburgh: Churchill Livingstone, pp. 117–134.
23. Littleton J. (1978). Alcohol and neurotransmitters. *Clin. Endocrinol. Metab.*, **7**, 369.
24. Noble E.P., Tewari S. (1977). Metabolic aspects of alcoholism in the brain. In *Metabolic Aspects of Alcoholism* (Lieber C.S. ed.) Lancaster: MTP Press, pp. 149–185.
25. Schuckit M.A. (1984). Biochemical markers of a predisposition to alcoholism. In *Clinical Biochemistry of Alcoholism* (Rosalki S.B. ed.) Edinburgh: Churchill Livingstone, pp. 20–50.
26. Saunders J.B., Williams R. (1983). The genetics of alcoholism. Is there an inherited susceptibility to alcohol related problems? *Alcohol Alcoholism*, **18**, 189.
27. Marshall E.J., Murray R.M. (1991). The familial transmission of alcoholism. *Br. Med. J.*, **303**, 72.
28. Hittle J.B., Crabb D.W. (1988). The molecular biology of alcohol dehydrogenase; implications for the control of alcohol metabolism. *J. Lab. Clin. Med.*, **112**, 7.
29. Ehrig T., Bosron W.F., Li T-K. (1990). Alcohol and aldehyde dehydrogenase. *Alcohol Alcoholism*, **25**, 105.
30. Coutelle C., et al. (1989). Distribution of β and γ isoenzymes of hepatic alcohol dehydrogenase (ADH) in France. *Alcohol Alcoholism*, **241**, 369.
31. Couzigou P., et al. (1989). Comparative genetic polymorphism of alcohol dehydrogenase (ADH) at the *ADH-3* locus in alcoholic cirrhosis and controls in France. *Alcohol Alcoholism*, **24**, 370.
32. Harada S. (1989). Polymorphism of aldehyde dehydrogenase and its application to alcoholism. *Electrophoresis*, **10**, 652.
33. Cloninger C.R. (1987). Neurogenetic adaptive mechanisms in alcoholism. *Science*, **236**, 410.
34. Major L.F., Murphy D. (1978). Platelet and plasma amine oxidase activity in alcoholic individuals. *Br. J. Psychiatry*, **132**, 548.
35. Faraj B.A., Camp V.M., Davis D.C., Lenton J.D., Kutner M. (1989). Elevation of plasma salsalinol sulfate in chronic alcoholics as compared to non alcoholics. *Alcoholism: Clin. Exp. Res.*, **13**, 155.
36. Schuckit M.A., Rayses V. (1979). Ethanol ingestion: differences in blood acetaldehyde concentrations in relatives of alcoholics and controls. *Science*, **203**, 54.
37. Schuckit M.A., Risch S.C., Gold E.O. (1988). Alcohol consumption, ACTH level and family history of alcoholism. *Am. J. Psychiatry*, **145**, 1391.
38. Tabakoff B., et al. (1988). Differences in platelet enzyme activity between alcoholics and non-alcoholics. *N. Engl. J. Med.*, **318**, 134.
39. Whitfield J.B. (1990). Biochemical markers and susceptibility to alcohol dependence. *Clin. Biochem. Rev.*, **11**, 10.
40. Blum K., et al. (1990). Allelic association of human dopamine D_2 receptor gene in alcoholism. *J.A.M.A.*, **263**, 2055.
41. Blass J.P., Gibson G.E. (1977). Abnormality of a thiamine-requiring enzyme in Wernicke–Korsakoff syndrome. *N. Engl. J. Med.*, **297**, 1367.
42. Pratt O.E., Jeyasingham M., Shaw G.K., Thomson A.D. (1985). Transketolase variant enzymes and brain damage. *Alcohol Alcoholism*, **200**, 223.
43. Rosalki S.B. (1984). Alcoholism—an overview. In *Clinical Biochemistry of Alcoholism* (Rosalki S.B. ed.) Edinburgh: Churchill Livingstone, pp. 3–19.
44. Rosalki S.B. (1984). Identifying the alcoholic. In *Clinical Biochemistry of Alcoholism* (Rosalki S.B. ed.) Edinburgh: Churchill Livingstone, pp. 65–92.
45. Hamlyn A.N., Hopper J.C., Skillen A.W. (1979). Assessment of erythrocyte γ-aminolaevulinate dehydratase for outpatient detection of alcoholic liver disease: comparison with γ-glutamyltransferase and casual blood ethanol. *Clin. Chim. Acta*, **95**, 453.
46. Orrego H., Blendis L.M., Blake J.E., Kapur B.M., Israel Y. (1979). Reliability of assessment of alcohol intake based on personal interviews in a liver clinic. *Lancet*, **ii**, 1354.
47. Waern U., Boberg J., Hellsing K. (1979). Evaluation of indices of alcohol intake in a population of 60 year old men in Uppsala, Sweden. *Acta Med. Scand.*, **205**, 353.
48. Wiseman S.M., Tomson P.V., Barnett J.M., Jenkins M., Wilton J. (1982). Use of an alcolmeter to detect problem drinkers. *Br. Med. J.*, **285**, 1089.
49. Holt S., et al. (1980). Alcohol and the emergency service patient. *Br. Med. J.*, **281**, 638.
50. Redmond A.D., Richards S., Plunkett P.K. (1987). The significance of random breath alcohol sampling in the accident and emergency department. *Alcohol Alcoholism*, **22**, 341.
51. Northcote R.J., Martin B.J., Saillion H., Reilly D.T. (1983). Changing pattern of alcohol abuse in female acute medical admissions. *Br. Med. J.*, **286**, 1702.
52. Rosalki S.B., Rau D., Lehmann D., Prentice M. (1970). Determination of serum γ-glutamyl transpeptidase and its clinical applications. *Ann. Clin. Biochem.*, **7**, 143.
53. Rosalki S.B., Rau D. (1972). Serum γ-glutamyltranspeptidase activity in alcoholism. *Clin. Chim. Acta*, **39**, 41.
54. Nemesanszky E., Lott J.A., Arato M. (1988). Changes in serum enzymes in moderate drinkers after an alcohol challenge. *Clin. Chem.*, **3**, 525.
55. Rosalki S.B. (1975). Gamma-glutamyl transpeptidase. In *Advances in Clinical Chemistry 17* (Bodansky O.,

Latner A.L. eds.) New York Academic Press, pp. 53–107.

56. Robinson D., Whitehead T.P. (1989). Effect of body mass and other factors on serum liver enzyme levels in men attending for well-population screening. *Ann. Clin. Biochem.*, **26**, 393.

57. Rosalki S.B. (1982). γ-Glutamyltransferase isoenzymes in health and disease using a new fluorescence procedure. In *Gammaglutamyltransferases Advances in Biochemical Pharmacology* (3rd series) (Siest G., Heusghem C. eds.) Paris: Masson, pp. 147–159.

58. Tamaro G., Grossi F., Mangiorotti M., Buttolo R., Madonutti G.B., Parco S. (1989). Danno da alcool e parametri di screening: nostra esperienza sull 'uso della banda di iso-GGT 4. *Clin. Lab.*, **13**, 51.

59. Ylikorkala O., Stenman U-H., Halmesmaki E. (1987). γ-glutamyl transferase and mean cell volume reveal maternal alcohol abuse and fetal alcohol effects. *Am. J. Obstet. Gynecol.*, **157**, 344.

60. Le Roux P., Le Luyer B., Goulle J.P., Chabrolle J.P. (1987). Alcoolisme foetal. Un marqueur biologique, la gamma-glutamyl-transferase. *Presse Med.*, **16**, 444.

61. Brohult J., Fridell E., Sunblad L. (1977). Studies in alkaline phosphatase isoenzymes, relation to γ-glutamyltransferase and lactate dehydrogenase isoenzymes. *Clin. Chim. Acta*, **76**, 205.

62. Cohen J.A., Kaplan M.M. (1979). The SGOT/SGPT ratio—an indicator of alcoholic liver disease. *Dig. Dis. Sci.*, **24**, 835.

63. Ishii H., Okuno F., Shigeta Y., Tsuchuja M. (1979). Enhanced serum glutamic oxaloacetic transaminase activity of mitochondrial origin in chronic alcoholism. In *Currents in Alcoholism V* (Galanter M. ed.) New York: Grune & Stratton, pp. 101–108.

64. Nalpas B. *et al* (1984). Serum activity of mitochondrial aspartate aminotransferase: a sensitive marker of alcoholism with or without alcoholic hepatitis. *Hepatology*, **4**, 893.

65. Schiele F., Artur Y., Varasteh A., Wellman M., Siest G. (1989). Serum mitochondrial aspartate aminotransferase activity: not useful as a marker of excessive alcohol consumption in an unselected population. *Clin. Chem.* **35**, 926.

66. Nalpas B., et al. (1989). Evaluation of mAST/tAST ratio as a marker of alcohol misuse in a non-selected population. *Alcohol Alcoholism*, **24**, 415.

67. Van Waes L., Lieber S. (1977). Glutamate dehydrogenase: a reliable marker of liver cell necrosis in the alcoholic. *Br. Med. J.*, **2**, 1508.

68. Hultberg B., Isaksson A., Tiderstrom G. (1980). β-Hexosaminidase, leucine aminopeptidase, cystidyl aminopeptidase, hepatic enzymes and bilirubin in serum of chronic alcoholics with acute ethanol intoxication. *Clin. Chim. Acta*, **105**, 317.

69. Karkkainen P. (1990). Serum and urinary β-hexosaminidase as a marker of heavy drinking. *Alcohol Alcoholism*, **25**, 365.

70. Torres-Salinas M., et al. (1986). Serum procollagen type III peptides as a marker of hepatitis. *Gastroenterology*. **90**, 1241.

71. van Zanten R.A.A., van Leuwen R.E., Wilson J.H.P. (1988). Serum procollagen III N-terminal peptide and laminin P, fragment concentrations in alcoholic liver disease and primary biliary cirrhosis. *Clin. Chim Acta*, **177**, 141.

72. Cramp D.G. (1984). Lipid abnormalities in alcoholism. In *Clinical Biochemistry of Alcoholism* (Rosalki S.B. ed.) Edinburgh: Churchill Livingstone, pp. 149–160.

73. Rimm E.B., et al. (1991). Prospective study of alcohol consumption and risk of coronary disease in men. *Lancet*, **338**, 464.

74. Marth E., Cazzolato G., Bittolo B.G., Avogaro P. (1982). Serum concentrations of Lp(a) and other lipoprotein parameters in heavy alcohol consumers. *Ann. Nutr. Metab.* **26**, 56.

75. Stibler H., Borg S., Allgulander C. (1979). Clinical significance of abnormal heterogeneity of transferrin in relation to alcohol consumption. *Acta Med. Scand.*, **206**, 275.

76. Vesterberg O., Petren S., Schmidt D. (1984). Increased concentrations of a transferrin variant after alcohol abuse. *Clin. Chim. Acta*, **141**, 33.

77. Schellenberg F., Weill J. (1987). Serum desialotransferrin in the detection of alcohol abuse. *Alcohol Alcoholism*, suppl. 1, 625.

78. Stibler H., Borg S., Joustra M. (1986). Micro anion-exchange chromatography of carbohydrate deficient transferrin in serum in relation to alcohol consumption (Swedish Patent 8400587–5). *Alcoholism: Clin. Exp. Res.*, **10**, 535.

79. Behrens V.J., Worner T.M., Braley L.F., Schaffner F., Lieber C.S. (1988). Carbohydrate deficient transferrin: a marker for chronic alcohol consumption in different ethnic populations. *Alcoholism: Clin. Exp. Res.*, **12**, 427.

80. Schellenberg F., Benard J.Y., LeGoff A.M., Bourdin C., Weill J. (1989). Evaluation of carbohydrate-deficient transferrin compared with TF index and other markers of alcohol abuse. *Alcoholism: Clin. Exp. Res.*, **13**, 605.

81. Chan A.W.K., et al. (1989). Transferrin and mitochondrial aspartate aminotransferase in young adult alcoholics. *Drug Alcohol Depend.*, **23**, 13.

82. Nystrom M., Perasalo J., Salaspuro M. (1991). Carbohydrate-deficient transferrin (CDT) in serum as an indicator of heavy drinking in young university students. *Alcohol Alcoholism*, **26**, 255.

83. Poupon R.E., Schellenberg F., Nalpas B., Weill J. (1989). Assessment of the transferrin index in screening heavy drinkers from a general practice. *Alcoholism: Clin. Exp. Res.*, **13**, 549.

84. Petren S., Vesterberg O. (1989). Separation of different forms of transferrin by isoelectric focussing to detect effects on the liver caused by xenobiotics. *Electrophoresis*, **10**, 600.

85. Bell H., Raknerud N., Tallaksen C., Orjasaeter H., Hung E. (1991). Carbohydrate deficient transferrin (CDT) in serum in patients with chronic liver disease: a preliminary report. *Alcohol Alcoholism*, **26**, 236.

86. Shaw S., Stimmel B., Lieber C.S. (1976). Plasma alpha-amino-n-butyric acid to leucine ratio: an experimental marker of alcoholism. *Science*, **194**, 1057.

87. Ledig M., Doffoel M., Doffoel S., Kopp P., Bockel R., Mandel P. (1988). Blood cell superoxide dismutase and enolase activities as markers of alcoholism and nonalcoholic liver diseases. *Alcohol*, **5**, 387.

88. Rooprai K.H., Pratt O.E., Shaw G.K., Thomson A.D. (1989). Superoxide dismutase in the erythrocytes of acute alcoholics during detoxification. *Alcohol Alcoholism*, **24**, 503.

89. Peterson C.M., Polizzi CM. (1987). Improved method for acetaldehyde in plasma and in hemoglobin-associ-

ated acetaldehyde: results in teetotalers and alcoholics reporting for treatment. *Alcohol*, **4**, 477.

90. Lin R.C., Lumeng L., Shahidi S., Kelly T., Pound D.C. (1990). Protein–acetaldehyde adducts in serum of alcoholic patients. *Alcoholism: Clin. Exp. Res.*, **14**, 438.

91. Korri U.M., Nuutinen H., Salaspuro M. (1985). Increased blood acetate: a new laboratory marker of alcoholism and heavy drinking. *Alcoholism: Clin. Exp. Res.*, **9**, 468.

92. Roine R.P., Korri U-M., Ylikahri R., Penttila A., Kikkareinin J., Salaspuro M. (1988). Increased serum acetate as a marker of problem drinking among drunken drivers. *Alcohol Alcoholism*, **23**, 123.

93. Collins M.A., Nijim W.P., Borge G.F., Teas G., Goldfarb C. (1979). Dopamine-related tetrahydroisoquinolines: significant urinary excretion by alcoholics after alcohol consumption. *Science*, **206**, 1184.

94. Roine R.P., Turpeinen U., Ylikahri R., Salaspuro M. (1987). Urinary dolichol—a new marker of alcoholism. *Alcoholism: Clin. Exp. Res.*, **11**, 525.

95. Stamm D., Hansert E., Feuerlein W. (1984). Detection and exclusion of alcoholism in men on the basis of clinical laboratory findings. *J. Clin. Chem. Clin. Biochem.*, **22**, 79.

96. Hillers V.N., Alldredge J.R., Massey L.K. (1986). Determination of habitual alcohol intake from a panel of blood chemistries. *Alcohol Alcoholism*, **21**, 199.

97. Ryback R.S., Eckardt M.J., Felsher B., Rawlings B.R. (1982). Biochemical and haematological correlation of alcoholism and liver disease. *J.A.M.A.*, **248**, 2261.

98. Levine J. (1990). The relative value of consultation, questionnaires and laboratory investigation in the identification of excessive alcohol consumption. *Alcohol Alcoholism*, **25**, 539.

99. Persson J., Magnusson P.H. (1988). Comparison between different methods of detecting patients with excessive consumption of alcohol. *Acta Med. Scand.*, **223**, 101.

100. Wright J. (1978). Endocrine effects of alcohol. *Clin. Endocrinol. Metab.*, **7**, 351.

101. Fink R. (1984). The effects of alcohol on endocrine function. In *Clinical Biochemistry of Alcoholism* (Rosalki S.B., ed.) Edinburgh: Churchill Livingstone, pp. 271–288.

102. Moore M.R., McColl K.E.L., Goldberg A. (1984). The effects of alcohol on porphyrin biosynthesis and metabolism. In *Clinical Biochemistry of Alcoholism* (Rosalki S.B. ed.) Edinburgh: Churchill Livingstone, pp. 161–187.

103. Preedy V.R., Peters T.J. (1990). Alcohol and skeletal muscle disease. *Alcohol Alcoholism*, **25**, 177.

104. Peters T. (1991). Alcoholic muscle disease. *J. R. Soc. Med.*, **84**, 506.

105. Fink R., Rosalki S.B. (1979). Observations on the incidence of alcoholic cardiomyopathy. *Br. J. Alcohol Alcoholism*, **14**, 245.

106. Ryle P.R., Thomson A.D. (1984). Nutrition and vitamins in alcoholism. In *Clinical Biochemistry of Alcoholism* (Rosalki S.B. ed.) Edinburgh: Churchill Livingstone, pp. 188–224.

107. Feitelberg S., Epstein S., Ismail F., d'Amanda C. (1987). Deranged bone mineral metabolism in chronic alcoholism. *Metabolism.*, **36**, 322.

8. Psychiatric Disorders of Biochemical Origin

D. Donaldson

Introduction
   Historical context
   Biological disorders with a psychiatric
     component
   Psychiatric disorders with a biochemical
     basis
The complexity of the central nervous system
   Cellular organization
   Oxygen consumption
   Energy requirement
   Neuroregulation
   Neurotransmitter involvement in disease
     states
Neurotransmitters and psychiatric disorders
   Schizophrenia
   Depression
   Mania and hypomania
   Anxiety
   Alzheimer's disease
Neuroendocrinological aspects of psychiatric
    disorders
   Puerperal psychosis
   Depression
   Mania and hypomania
   Stress
Psychiatric disorders and clinical chemistry
   Endocrine disorders
   Metabolic encephalopathies
   Electrolyte and water disorders
   Vitamin disorders
   Mineral disorders
   Inherited metabolic disorders
Psychiatric side-effects of drug therapy
Munchausen's syndrome and other factitious
    illnesses
   Laboratory investigations
Laboratory investigations of psychiatric
    disorders
Conclusions

INTRODUCTION

Every illness, whether basically psychiatric or biological, possesses an emotional aspect as at least part of its clinical presentation. The emotional aspect could, however, comprise the major component of the disorder where there is essentially a psychosocial, family or personality problem; in particular, the illness might be reactive to certain events or to a situation. On the other hand, the emotional aspect could be a reaction to any illness, which might itself be predominantly biological (e.g. depression and/or anxiety following a myocardial infarction), although another possibility is that there might be close and intergral involvement between the mental state and basic biological processes (e.g. depression or confusion as an accompaniment of the hypercalcaemia of primary hyperparathyroidism). In yet other instances the mental features could be secondary to a microbiological infection (e.g. lethargy as the one and only complaint of a patient with an 'almost subclinical' episode of viral hepatitis) or could be attributed to the side-effects of a pharmacological agent, being either prescribed as therapy (e.g. memory impairment and confusion following bedtime dosage with the short-acting benzodiazepine, triazolam) or taken for some other reason (e.g. decreased alertness in an elderly patient due to electrolyte changes caused by the taking of laxatives and/or, perhaps, a diuretic)—of which the doctor may or may not be aware. Finally, it must never be dismissed from mind that anyone, even with a long-standing psychiatric history, may well develop a biological illness (with all its sequelae) or, indeed, an additional and unrelated psychological problem of another aetiology.

The mental contribution to the presentation of an illness as a whole may range from being trivial to substantial and might even vary in degree at different times as the symptoms unfold; moreover, it could even be manifest long before the physical expression of a biological basis becomes clinically recognized.

Historical Context

The concept that chemical disorders might underlie disturbances of the mind is not new. In ancient Greece the Hippocratic school believed that such clinical presentations might be caused by abnormalities in the humors of the brain and/or composition of the blood. Nevertheless, it was to wait until 1884 for the founder of modern neurochemistry, J. W. L. Thudichum, so eloquently to express his thoughts and visions as follows:[1]

> Many forms of insanity are unquestionably the external manifestations of the effects upon the brain-substance of poisons fermented within the body, just as the mental aberrations accompanying chronic alcoholic intoxication are the accumulated effects of a relatively simple poison fermented out of the body. These poisons we shall, I have no doubt, be able to isolate after we know the normal chemistry to its uttermost detail. And then will come in their turn the crowning discoveries to which all our efforts must ultimately be directed, namely, the discoveries of the antidotes to the poisons, and to the fermenting causes and processes which produce them.

Biological Disorders with a Psychiatric Component

The biological presentations of the disorders of clinical medicine have, over the years, been well documented, but there has been noticeably less emphasis on their emotional and/or psychiatric aspects; the reasons for this are many but must, surely, include recognition that these presentations are often dominated by the more obvious and, sometimes, more urgent biological events—which override the mental aspects. Sometimes, the psychological and biological components have a different time-scale, one having begun at an earlier or later stage of the illness than the other, thus making it difficult to associate the two with any surety. In other instances the mental symptoms are so minor that, unless they are specifically probed, the patients may not even think to mention them. A multitude of minor complaints, each individual one seemingly so trivial, may collectively cause distress to a significant degree. Some may have important diagnostic potential; nevertheless, the patient may be wary of 'being seen too readily to complain of trivia' for fear of being regarded as neurotic; hence, important clinical data may never come to light. Not only may such patients wrongly regard themselves as being neurotic, but this view may be enhanced and seemingly proven by the similarly erroneous views held by close family members, friends, acquaintances and even the medical practitioner.

The precise mode of presentation of any illness is the result of interaction between an individual and the environment; one must, in consequence, be aware of the possible combinations of any or all of the factors so far mentioned as contributing to the construction of the clinical state. All the common psychiatric symptoms (e.g. anxiety, depression, phobias, obsessions/compulsions, paranoid feelings), together with the simple emotional disorders (e.g. feeling irritable, afraid, tired, unhappy), can be either 'primary' or have a 'secondary' cause—of physical, chemical, biological, psychological or sociological origin. It is those disorders which are secondary to chemical changes that will mainly be elaborated upon in this review (e.g. the depression that may precede or accompany Addison's disease, the anxiety that can be associated with a phaeochromocytoma, and the confusion and aggression that may herald an insulinoma).

Psychiatric Disorders with a Biochemical Basis

Psychiatric disorders of biochemical origin may be prime examples of seeing a psychiatric presentation in wrong perspective. In turn, this is basically related to the variations in viewpoint of medical practitioners skilled in different disciplines. What may at first seem to be the obvious diagnosis may, quite suddenly, be revealed as being incorrect, particularly when new information has come to light or after reflection on the clinical data at hand. The importance of this is well illustrated by depression, previously attributed to some other cause, which quite suddenly becomes a very different situation when the hypercalcaemia of primary hyperparathyroidism is firmly established;

the treatment and management would then be reorientated towards partial parathyroidectomy rather than to the prescribing of pharmacological agents and, perhaps, electroconvulsive therapy. It is worth drawing attention at this point to the fact that even a number of the standard textbooks of psychiatry do not place sufficient emphasis on the chemical aspects of psychiatric disorders.

Those psychiatric disorders secondary to physical causes (e.g. a cerebral space-occupying lesion), as opposed to those with a chemical basis (e.g. of biochemical, pharmacological and toxicological origin), will receive only brief mention here. The more formal and florid psychiatric presentations, however, such as schizophrenia and endogenous depression, will also be discussed; these conditions form entities of their own, but are, nevertheless, rather more 'primary' than the main body of disorders (secondary to biochemical disturbances) to which the reader's attention is particularly directed in the section on 'Psychiatric disorders and clinical chemistry'.

THE COMPLEXITY OF THE CENTRAL NERVOUS SYSTEM

There should be no surprise at finding that the biochemistry, physiology and pathology of the brain are less completely understood than for any other organ; this becomes clear when one considers just four aspects of cerebral structure and function:

1. The anatomical intricacies of neuronal connections.
2. The high oxygen consumption of cerebral metabolic processes.
3. The constant requirement for energy which is almost entirely from glucose.
4. The complexities of neurotransmission.

The brain is, in essence, a large neuroendocrine organ, made up of vast numbers of neurons and synapses, each one being involved in reception (at neurotransmitter receptor sites), processing (the chemical processes taking place within the neuronal axon) and transmission (via the neurotransmitter molecules, receptors and re-uptake mechanisms) of information at each synaptic cleft.

Cellular Organization

At cell level there is great complexity; there are approximately 10 thousand million neurons in both the cerebral cortex and the cerebellum. In addition, each of these cells makes many connections, with there being up to 60 000 synaptic points on a single cortical neuron, although not all are from different sources.[2] These synaptic points, moreover, can be situated on the cell body of the receiving neuron, on the axon, on the trunk of the dendrites or on the spines which project from them.[3] Furthermore, there are electron-microscopic differences: excitatory synapses usually have round vesicles and a dense, continuous, postsynaptic membrane, whereas inhibitory synapses are characterized by flattened synaptic vesicles and discontinuity of the postsynaptic membrane density.

Oxygen Consumption

At physiological level, the brain proves to be the most active energy consumer of all the organs of the body; in keeping with this is its rich blood supply and high oxygen uptake. The adult human brain represents, in fact, just 2% of the total body weight (more in babies), but its high oxygen utilization of 50 ml/min equates with 20% of the body's resting oxygen needs.[3] The maximal oxygen consumption by the brain occurs at around 6 years of age. This ravenous requirement for oxygen is probably essential for maintenance of the ionic gradients across neuronal membranes, on which depend conduction of neural impulses in the many billions of neurons; glucose supplies the energy for these processes. The rate of brain metabolism is much the same both during the day and by night, although there is, perhaps, a slight increase during the rapid eye movement phase of sleep. If the supply of oxygenated blood to the brain ceases, then consciousness is lost within a period of as little as 10 s; a similar effect would follow the onset of severe hypoglycaemia of any cause.

Energy Requirement

The constant requirement for energy by the brain is approximately 1700 KJ/day; this represents approximately 20% of the total energy needs of a normal resting adult. The source of energy is almost entirely glucose, although the ketones 3-hydroxybutyrate and acetoacetate can also be utilized in small amounts; glycogen, too, is present in the brain, but the content of merely 0.1% is insufficient for it to be an important source of energy. There is heavy reliance on the glucose present in the extracellular fluid, because the brain is neither able to store nor synthesize glucose; moreover, the entry of glucose to the brain is not under hormonal control. It is the conversion of approximately 120 g of glucose each day to carbon dioxide, water and energy that supplies this high energy need. The consequence is that significant hypoglycaemia drastically impairs neuronal function; marked hyperglycaemia also disrupts cerebral function, but in other ways.

Neuroregulation

In the central nervous system (CNS), transfer of information from one neuron to another occurs by way of the release of one or more substances from the first neuron, which bind and act at specific receptor sites on the second neuron.[3] This binding, in turn, promotes a sequence of biochemical effects in the second neuron, with consequent physical changes. There are four groups of neuroregulators.[4]

1. *Neurotransmitters*, e.g. the 'classic' transmitter compounds, which include acetylcholine, noradrenaline, dopamine, and serotonin (5-hydroxytryptamine, 5-HT), together with the excitatory amino acids (e.g. glutamic and aspartic acids), and the inhibitory, amino acid-based transmitters such as γ-aminobutyric acid (GABA) and glycine. These compounds all produce shortlasting, rapid onset, postsynaptic effects (e.g. depolarization close to the point at which they are released).

2. *Neuromodulators*, e.g. endorphins, substance P and somatostatin. They modify, either by enhancing or lessening, the response to a neurotransmitter; they also act close to the point of their release, but do not actually precipitate depolarization.

3. *Neurohormones*, e.g. vasopressin and angiotensin II. They are released into the bloodstream; unlike neurotransmitters and neuromodulators, they act remotely on receptors somewhere else in the body. Their effects are, therefore, of later onset, of longer duration and far distant.

4. *Neuromediators*, e.g. adenosine 3', 5'-monophosphate (cyclic AMP, cAMP) and guanosine 3', 5'-monophosphate (cyclic GMP, cGMP). These compounds act as second messengers at specific sites of synaptic transmission, participating in elicitation of the postsynaptic response to a neurotransmitter.

For further information about these vital substances, readers are referred to the very extensive literature that has accumulated on them.

Neurotransmitter Involvement in Disease States[5]

Several groups of clinical disorders, e.g. those of movement, mood and intellect, possess important underlying neurotransmitter involvements of varying degree and at different locations within the CNS. Neurotransmitter abnormalities are implicated in disorders of movement (e.g. Parkinson's disease, Huntington's disease, motor neuron disease), disorders of mood (e.g. unipolar depression, manic–depressive illness, anxiety) and diseases involving the intellect (e.g. Alzheimer's disease, Jakob–Creutzfeldt disease, Hallervorden–Spatz disease, Lewy body dementia, Wernicke's encephalopathy, Korsakoff's psychosis, schizophrenia). In addition, neurotransmitter involvement has been implicated in many other disorders, such as coma, head injury, cerebral infarction, epilepsy, alcoholism and the mental retardation states of metabolic origin seen particularly in childhood.

NEUROTRANSMITTERS AND PSYCHIATRIC DISORDERS

The psychiatric disorders included in this section will be dealt with primarily from the angle of their neurotransmitter involvements; any other biochemical, physiological, clinical and genetic abnormalities will either not be included or only cursorily documented.

Schizophrenia[5,6]

In developed countries, schizophrenia occurs in approximately 1% of the adult population at some point during their lives. It comprises a group of psychoses with either 'positive' or 'negative' symptoms. Positive symptoms consist of hallucinations, delusions and disorders of thought; negative symptoms include emotional flattening, lack of volition and a decrease in motor activity. The two syndromes alluded to above are called type 1 and type 2 schizophrenia, respectively; it is the former which is likely to be associated with hyperactivity of the dopaminergic system centrally.

Dopamine

Administration of amphetamines and amphetamine-like drugs increases dopamine release in normal volunteers; in parallel with this enhanced dopaminergic neurotransmission, there is intensification of the positive symptoms of the disorder in a patient with schizophrenia. On the other hand, neuroleptic drugs effectively cause dopamine receptor blockade by occupying the dopamine receptors, thus blocking the effect of dopamine on postsynaptic structures; in parallel with this reduced dopaminergic neurotransmission there is amelioration of the positive symptoms of schizophrenia. To be more precise, the antipsychotic potency of such drugs parallels blocking activity involving the D_2, rather than the D_1, receptor. The highly selective D_2-receptor antagonists, sulpiride and remoxapride (both being substituted benzamide compounds), are just two of the antipsychotic drugs used in the treatment of schizophrenia. Clozapine, too, sometimes successful in the therapy of severe and intractable schizophrenia, causes blockade of the D_2 receptors—but is of weaker action than other neuroleptic agents in not causing elevation of serum prolactin; however, successful therapeutic effect may be based on antagonism of both D_2 and $5HT_2$ receptors. The earlier finding of an elevated number of D_2-binding sites in post-mortem brain tissue of patients with schizophrenia might be simply a compensatory response to the effect of antipsychotic drugs over a long period of time, rather than being due to the disease itself.

Moreover, the findings are not fully supported by recent studies of positron emission tomography scanning in patients who had not received such drug treatment.

Other Neurotransmitters

There is evidence to suggest that abnormalities of both catecholamine and glutamate metabolism or neurotransmitter function may be involved in the aetiology and/or manifestations of schizophrenia.

Depression[5,7]

Depression, characterized by a pathological lowering of mood of more severe degree and of longer duration than those swings that occur in normal circumstances, is traditionally regarded as either reactive to life-events or endogenous; stress may be a precipitating factor in either case. In equilibrium with the change of mood there are biological accompaniments such as disturbance of sleep pattern with a tendency to early morning wakening, loss of appetite, loss of weight and a lessening or loss of libido.

Many neurochemical findings are coming to light implicating a biological basis for the 'functional disorders' (depression and anxiety), at least for certain subtypes. Abnormalities of monoamine function have been recognized in depression for many years, not only involving noradrenaline but also dopamine and 5-HT. Other evidence along these lines will now be briefly documented.

Catecholamines

Amphetamine administration has long been known to elevate mood; this is known to be accompanied by increased activity of noradrenergic and dopaminergic neurons. However, the introduction of reserpine, used in therapy of hypertension in the early 1950s, revealed that some patients so treated developed depression; it was found that the drug depleted neuronal stores of monoamines. Hence, it was surmised that those patients suffering from endogenous depression might, perhaps, be unable to produce naturally sufficient monoamines for neuronal transmission. In keeping with the 'noradrenergic hypothesis' was the later observation that antidepressant drugs could potentiate monoamine neurotransmission, increasing either noradrenaline or 5-HT at aminergic synapses. Moreover, tricyclic antidepressants were found to inhibit the reuptake mechanisms for noradrenaline and 5-HT, thereby increasing synaptic concentrations of these amines; monoamine oxidase inhibitor (MAOI) drugs were found to do likewise. In excess of 100 drugs, many of them structurally different from tricyclic compounds and MAOIs, have now been used in the treatment of depression, each one of which produces an increased amount of available noradrenaline and/or 5-HT at the synaptic cleft.

Depression may be a feature in up to 50% of patients with neurodegenerative disorders such as Parkinson's disease and Alzheimer's disease. The neuronal loss in the locus ceruleus, typical of Alzheimer's disease, is greatest in those patients who have depression and they also have lower concentrations of noradrenaline than do those who lack depressive features. Approximately 50% of patients with Alzheimer's disease have less noradrenaline than normal in the majority of cortical and subcortical areas of the brain that have been examined to date.

All these facts seem, at first reading, to fit neatly into this hypothesis; however, from later findings it becomes clear that some reappraisal and modifications are necessary. The increased amounts of monoamine transmitters at the synapses, although quickly produced in response to antidepressant therapy, is in contrast with the much slower clinical recovery of the patient from depression, which takes about 2 weeks to begin and which may only be maximal several weeks later. Moreover, should acute depletion of either noradrenaline and/or 5-HT occur experimentally in a normal individual then depression does not, in the short term, occur.

Other Neurotransmitters

There is evidence to suggest that abnormalities of acetylcholine, 5-HT and dopamine are involved, probably causally, in some or all patients with depressive illness.

Mania and Hypomania[6]

Mania or hypomania comprises one phase of manic–depressive psychosis (bipolar manic–depression). Clinical presentation may take the form of irritability, restlessness, elation, euphoria, increased talkativeness at rapid rate, increased energy, increased appetite for food, overactivity, hostility, aggressiveness, delusions of grandeur, an inflated self-esteem, loss of insight, easy distractability, a decreased need for sleep and social and sexual disinhibition; there may, in addition, be revealed 'flights of ideas' and a subjective feeling of 'racing of thoughts'. Furthermore, the patient may be found to be extravagantly spending money and to be becoming involved in financially unsound business schemes. Like unipolar depression, hypomania is associated with abnormalities of the catecholamines and other neurotransmitters.

Anxiety[6,8]

The clinical expression of anxiety, in its different forms, includes both psychological and biological symptoms. From the psychological aspect there may be fear, irritability and restlessness, together with excessive sensitivity to noise, impairment of concentration and sleep disturbance. The biological accompaniments of anxiety comprise the consequences of autonomic overactivity, skeletal muscle tension and the effects of hyperventilation. Autonomic overactivity leads to palpitations and sweating, dryness of the mouth, diarrhoea, frequency of micturition and, sexually, to impotence or frigidity; muscular tension can cause headache and pain in the neck and in the back. Hyperventilation can cause the patient to feel dizzy or faint, with paraesthesiae and palpita-

tions. Similar symptoms, presenting suddenly, in marked degree and perhaps of unexpected onset, are referred to as 'panic attacks'; symptoms comprise combinations of the following: palpitations, breathlessness, sweating, trembling, a feeling of dizziness or faintness, paraesthesiae or numbness, flushing and nausea, together with depersonalization and a fear of impending death.

Evidence is accumulating for there being a biological basis to anxiety, as there also is for the other 'functional disorder', i.e. depression. As with the more severe or psychotic illnesses referred to above, there is evidence of a role for catecholamine, 5-HT and GABA neurotransmitter dysfunction in the pathogenesis of anxiety states.

GABA

GABA is of particular interest. The $GABA_A$ receptor possesses a chloride channel complex; it has at least four separate binding sites, one of which binds benzodiazepine drugs, anxiolytic compounds and β-carbolines. Benzodiazepine binding occurs to high degree in the cerebral cortex and amygdala; in some way it seems to unmask GABA receptors in many areas of the brain, thereby permitting enhanced GABA binding, with the consequence of optimal GABAergic neuronal activity, i.e. inhibitory in function.

Endogenous anxiolytics and, perhaps, anxiogenic molecules, too, may both exist *in vivo*; it is possible that a 104 amino-acid peptide, called diazepam-binding inhibitor, which can markedly reduce the duration of opening of ion channels, is a candidate.

Alzheimer's Disease[5]

Alzheimer's disease is characterized by the onset in middle age of a slowly progressive dementia; there is loss of memory for past events, inability to lay down new memories and impairment of intellect—all leading to a lessened capacity for dealing with the tasks and problems of daily living. It is the most common cause of both presenile and senile dementia. Alzheimer's disease is not the non-specific degenerative disorder of the CNS that it was once thought to be, as neurochemical studies on post-mortem material now reveal the degeneration to be selective for certain neuronal populations in the subcortical and cortical areas; other cell populations seem to be unaffected. Senile plaques and neurofibrillary tangles are the characteristic histological feature, found throughout the cerebral cortex and especially in certain regions of the limbic system (the amygdala and hippocampus), perhaps accounting for the memory loss so typical of the early phase of the disease. There is reduction of acetylcholine, noradrenaline, 5-HT and somatostatin in the subcortical areas in Alzheimer's disease. Superimposed upon the mental retardation of Down's syndrome, in all who are over 40 years of age, is dementia—with a pathology identical to that seen in patients with Alzheimer's disease.

As with the other illnesses presenting predominantly or exclusively with mental symptoms that are dealt with in this section, there is evidence of involvement of many of the neurotransmitter systems, though whether as cause or effect (or both), remains unclear.

NEUROENDOCRINOLOGICAL ASPECTS OF PSYCHIATRIC DISORDERS

Puerperal Psychosis[9]

In the first 4 weeks post partum there is a 20 times higher incidence of psychotic illness than in the 2 years before; there is, at this time, a rapid fall in circulating oestradiol and progesterone, both of which (unlike many other hormones) have direct access to the brain structures. Monoaminergic and dopaminergic neurotransmitter systems are modulated by oestrogens; in consequence, it has been suggested that puerperal psychosis is precipitated by the rapid withdrawal of oestrogens at this time.

Depression[10]

In depression there is 'overdrive' of the hypothalamic–pituitary–adrenal axis with early 'escape' from the serum cortisol suppression normally produced by a single dose of dexamethasone in the dexamethasone suppression test; in addition, there is blunting of the serum thyroid-stimulating hormone (TSH) response to thyrotrophin-releasing hormone. The true positive rate for these two tests is 44% and at least 20–30%, respectively; if both tests are carried out on patients with endogenous depression then 67% are abnormal on one or both tests. There is also blunting of the serum growth-hormone response to stimulation by precursors of 5-HT (i.e. tryptophan and 5-hydroxytryptophan). The serum prolactin response mediated by 5-HT is also reduced in depression; this is not, however, on account of an abnormality of prolactin function as there is a normal prolactin secretory response to the dopamine antagonist, metoclopramide—hence, the decreased amounts are most likely to be accounted for by a functional deficit in 5-HT neurotransmission.

Dexamethasone suppression test for depression[11]

The normal response of serum cortisol suppression, following a standard dose of dexamethasone given orally, is absent in approximately 50% of patients suffering from affective disorders with a significant element of endogenous depression; this is due to failure of negative feedback to suppress limbic system activity. Before performing this test on either in-patients or outpatients, there should be no treatment with glucocorticoid drugs (including topical preparations) for several weeks; mineralocorticoids do not interfere with the test. Blood is collected for assay of serum cortisol at 0900 h and 1600 h on the first day.

On the same evening at 2300 h, dexamethasone (1.0 mg) is given orally. A further blood test is taken at 0900 h and 1600 h on the following day.

In a normal individual the base-line 0900 h serum cortisol value on the first day should be within the reference range (140–460 nmol/L). There is marked suppression of the 0900 h serum cortisol value on the second day (i.e. 10 h after the dexamethasone dose); this remains low at 1600 h (< 180 nmol/L) and persisting for a total period of 24 h.

A significant proportion (44%) of patients with depression (in whom there is loss of the normal diurnal variation in serum cortisol) show early 'escape' from the suppression of serum cortisol normally seen at 1600 h on the second day, as evidenced by a concentration of more than 180 nmol/L, or of greater than 50% of the value found at 1600 h on the first day. However, many patients with depression fail to show this early 'escape' by exhibiting a low serum cortisol concentration at this time, i.e. a false-negative result. A recent study of patients with endogenous depression revealed the sensitivity (true positive rate) in the dexamethasone suppression test to be 44%; the specificity (true negative rate) was over 90% (when compared with normal controls) and 77% (when compared with patients suffering from other psychiatric disorders).

There is continuing discussion and some difference of opinion about the value of the dexamethasone suppression test in depression, and some authorities advocate a prolonged suppression test, in which there is an increased significance of a positive result. Other hormone tests that often yield abnormal results in patients suffering from depression include the thyrotrophin-releasing hormone stimulation test and the clonidine stimulation test, neither of which is, however, very informative.

Mania and Hypomania

In acute mania, the highest serum concentrations of the stress hormones cortisol and prolactin are found in the most psychotic patients; in young males there is also elevation of serum luteinizing hormone.

Stress

Psychological stress is characterized mentally by changes in cognitive processes, affect and behaviour, but there is also the accompanying impact on physiological mechanisms. There will be variability of response between individuals and there may even be changes in the same person at different times. Also influential are genetic inheritance, the past experience of an individual and the current state of health.

The psychological response to a stressful situation is closely integrated with a change of motor activity, stimulation of the autonomic nervous system and an endocrine response.

The autonomic nervous system has sympathetic

and parasympathetic components. Stimulation of the sympathetic nervous system leads to many physiological changes including an increase in heart rate and myocardial contractility, vasodilatation in skeletal muscle and constriction of blood vessels in the skin and gastrointestinal tract—hence deviating blood supply to skeletal muscle, the heart and the brain (i.e. the organs required in the 'fight, flight and fright' response), at the same time as temporarily conserving the blood supply to organs of lesser need (e.g. the skin and gastrointestinal tract). Stimulation of the parasympathetic nervous system may not only cause emotional fainting (involving the vagus nerve), but also can provoke the onset of hyperventilation, which can itself contribute to states of panic.

The neuroendocrine response to stress involves not only changes in the hypothalamic–pituitary–adrenocortical axis (the most important being the increased secretion of adrenocorticotrophic hormone (ACTH), which secondarily determines the adrenocortical response) but also alteration in the sympathetic–adrenomedullary system (causing catecholamines to be released from the adrenal medulla).

Psychological stress also promotes secretion of other hormones (e.g. growth hormone, prolactin, insulin and testosterone). In addition, there is involvement of the opioid peptide system; opioid secretion may serve as a mechanism for preventing too much activation of the sympathetic nervous system at times of stress, thereby limiting catecholamine secretion.

PSYCHIATRIC DISORDERS AND CLINICAL CHEMISTRY

The information supplied in the previous sections of this chapter provides some understanding of the anatomical and physiological basis of the equilibrium between mind and its chemistry. Many more aspects other than neurotransmitters themselves could have been discussed, since neurotransmitters are themselves influenced by yet other chemical processes. Oestrogens, for instance, are known to modulate CNS monoaminergic and dopaminergic neurotransmitter systems, melatonin (physiologically involved in the light–dark cycle) is integrally involved in the generation of seasonal affective disorder (SAD), and increase of CNS serotoninergic activity is effective not only in suppressing dietary carbohydrate intake but also in producing a favourable clinical response in SAD.

Endocrine Disorders

It is well known that emotional changes occur at certain times of life with greater frequency. Many of these are related to functional changes in the endocrine system. Puberty, menstruation, pregnancy and the menopause are physiological stresses which might underlie such behavioural changes. There should be no surprise that endocrine disturbances of a pathological nature are also associated with mood changes (e.g. Addison's disease and depression; hypothyroidism and depression; thyrotoxicosis and hyperdynamism; exposure to anabolic steroid drugs and aggression). In this context it is important to note that thyroxine is so fundamental to the proper development of cerebral structure and function, that without it (i.e. cretinism) there can be no normal intellectual development. Clearly, there is a close relation between endocrinology and psychiatry, but reference must also be made to the endocrine consequences of some primary emotional disturbances (e.g. the missed menstrual period at a time of anxiety; the increased sympathetic activity with rise of the associated circulating hormones at times of anger and tension).

Hyperthyroidism[12,13]

The typical mood changes comprise irritability, nervousness and restlessness, together with increased dynamism and tremulousness. Emotional lability may occur and depression is sometimes a feature; apathetic thyrotoxicosis is a rare presentation. Thyrotoxic crisis (with its accompanying delirium), although very rare, constitutes a grave emergency; it can be precipitated by acute infection, surgery for thyrotoxicosis and may even follow soon after severe stress, injury or an emotional crisis. The difficulty is being certain that the initial emotional reaction did not occur on the basis of overactivity of the thyroid gland, already present but unrecognized. Affective and schizophrenic psychoses sometimes occur, with mania being more likely than depression.

The cause of the mood changes is probably increased circulating thyroxine (T_4); cerebral catecholamines are also intimately involved. The pronounced adrenergic manifestations of thyrotoxicosis include sweating, tremor and tachycardia; all these can be relieved by therapy with propranolol.

Maintenance of the Na^+/K^+-ATPase pump requires much of the total energy utilized by a cell, together with oxygen and thyroid hormone. Excessive amounts of the latter lead to increased oxidative phosphorylation, thereby leading to elevated oxygen consumption with associated enhanced ATP utilization. Thyroid hormone also produces a positive nitrogen balance, by increasing protein synthesis; it also enhances transcription of the growth hormone gene (leading to the production of more growth hormone) and is involved in developmental processes (e.g. intrauterine and neonatal thyroid development, in the absence of which cretinism results).

Hypothyroidism[12,13]

A prime reason for the diagnosis of this condition being so often missed in the early stages is its usual insidiously slow onset. There is both mental and physical slowing, with progressive difficulty in understanding, loss of initiative, onset of lethargy and development of apathy; initially, the patient may have insight to the changes taking place, at the time when forgetfulness and failure to recall events are just beginning. Depression, dementia and organic psychoses can all occur, these usually being of gradual onset. Intellectual impairment is reversible if the condition is not left untreated for too long; depression, too, is often relieved by thyroid replacement therapy. 'Myxoedema madness' could include dementia, depression or schizophrenia. Myxoedema coma is the end-stage of the condition if left untreated, although precipitating factors include infection, injury, exposure to cold and administration of CNS depressants. Hypothyroidism in children may present as poor school performance, and in the first weeks of life cretinism can be the basis of impaired mental development.

Deficiency of circulating thyroxine (T_4) and increased thyrotrophin (TSH) occur, together with decreased cerebral blood flow (caused by reduction in cardiac output), anaemia and relative cerebral hypoxia. Dilutional hyponatraemia with cerebral hydraemia may contribute to mental symptoms—and so, too, may carbon dioxide retention in myxoedema precoma/coma. In early life, thyroxine is necessary for brain development.

Cushing's Syndrome[12,13]

Psychiatric features are often found in Cushing's syndrome, depression being the most common. Other symptoms sometimes seen include fatigue, emotional lability, irritability, agitation, restlessness and anxiety. Less commonly present are the more severe disorders of confusion, paranoia, frank schizophrenic psychosis and stupor. It is relatively uncommon, however, for any of the severe psychiatric features to accompany adrenal adenoma or carcinoma; it is in Cushing's disease (excessive production of ACTH by the pituitary gland) that depression is so typical. Elevation of mood is often observed when steroids (in pharmacological doses) or ACTH therapy are given, some patients even becoming hypomanic when the dose is excessively high. The treatment of Cushing's syndrome usually leads to concomitant improvement of both biological and mental symptoms.

The aetiology of the mental symptoms may relate to changes in electrolyte and water distribution within the brain; there is, however, evidence in some patients of cerebral atrophy and ventricular enlargement. No doubt, an element of reactive depression is also involved as a result of embarrassment felt by the patients in view of their facial and other body changes. It is possible, too, that there is a close link, in some way, between the origin of both Cushing's disease and endogenous depression; indeed, not only is there in endogenous depression an 'overdrive' of the hypothalamic–pituitary–adrenocortical axis (thus suggesting a link with the limbic system), but also there is a high incidence of factors predisposing to depression in patients with Cushing's disease.

Addison's Disease[12,13]

There is nearly always some mental involvement at initial presentation, the most typical features being apathy, lethargy, negativism and poverty of thought. Sometimes there is up to 2 years of psychiatric illness (e.g. depression) preceding the diagnosis. There can also be lack of drive and initiative, perhaps with rapid changes of mood, irritability, anxiety, restlessness, drowsiness and insomnia. More severe features, although less often seen, are paranoia and delusions.

Prior to an Addisonian crisis there may be exacerbation of certain mental feelings—such as apprehension, increasing irritability and even panic attacks. As the condition unfolds there is the onset of shock, with accompanying clouding of consciousness, delirium and stupor; at this point the clinical signs of shock are very apparent (for further information, *see* Chapter 41).

There is increased secretion of corticotrophin-releasing factor and ACTH in this disorder, accompanying the glucocorticoid deficiency; these factors could be the basis for neurotransmitter imbalance which, in turn, might influence β-adrenergic receptors and serotoninergic pathways. Electrolyte disturbances, found in the later states of the disorder, may also contribute to the neuropsychiatric presentation.

Phaeochromocytoma

The biological presentation of a phaeochromocytoma, whether it be located within the adrenal medulla, ectopically situated in relation to the sympathetic ganglia, part of the multiple endocrine neoplasia (MEN) syndrome (MEN type II, Sipple's syndrome) or as a component of von Recklinghausen's neurofibromatosis, comprises hypertension, profuse sweating, palpitations, pallor or flushing, and sometimes nausea and/or vomiting and diabetes mellitus; the symptoms may be either episodic or permanent. There is usually some mental accompaniment, however, taking the form of anxiety, intense fear, apprehension or a feeling of impending doom (*angor animi*). Attacks can last for a few minutes or even a few hours; as the disease advances, however, they increase in frequency, duration and severity. After an attack the patient may suffer excitability or confusion and then feel exhausted for several hours or days. Not all attacks are severe, and some consist only of feelings of faintness and mild anxiety. The close relatives and even the patient may regard such symptoms as being neurotic. Phaeochromocytomas are generally slow-growing tumours and some may have remained undiagnosed for in excess of 10 years; if sited in the urinary bladder they may present with headache and the other symptoms already described, episodically—every time urine is voided.

These tumours synthesize, store and secrete catecholamines; these are not released, however, by way of neural stimulation as there is no innervation of these tumours. Both noradrenaline and adrenaline are secreted by most tumours; noradrenaline is the main secretion of those tumours of extra-adrenal origin, but occasionally adrenaline is the sole secretion (e.g. particularly in association with the MEN syndrome).

Hypopituitarism[12]

The majority of patients manifest at least some psychiatric component, with depression being particularly prominent. Often there is apathy, anergia, lethargy, drowsiness, and lack of initiative, with drift towards self-neglect, indifference, stupor and finally coma. In contrast to these features, irritability is sometimes seen, with episodes of delirium and, rarely, hallucinations. Memory impairment also occurs. Hypopituitarism is not often associated with a functional psychosis; on the other hand, acute organic reactions are not uncommonly seen in association with the metabolic disturbance. Coma is a rare complication of stressful biological events (e.g. infection, hypoglycaemia).

Deficiencies of ACTH (with its consequential reduction of adrenocortical activity), TSH (leading to hypothyroidism), and follicle-stimulating and luteinizing hormones (leading to sex hormone depletion) are the main hormonal abnormalities upon which other biochemical disturbances are founded; the psychiatric features are secondary to these.

Metabolic Encephalopathies[3,14]

Hypoxia[3]

Inattentiveness and defects of judgement characterize mild hypoxia; more severe depletion can cause coma in as little time as 10 s, although if oxygen is given within 4 min the process is completely reversible. Should the oxygen lack be for a longer period, then irreparable damage ensues, affecting particularly the globus pallidus, hippocampus and parts of the parieto-occipital cortex; persistent severe hypoxia leads to a decerebrate state, although if the patient recovers, confusion or dementia may remain.

Anoxic/ischaemic encephalopathy can be caused by local pathology (e.g. cerebral thrombosis, embolus or haemorrhage), or by lesions outside the CNS—such as those of cardiac origin (e.g. myocardial infarction, cardiac arrest, congestive cardiac failure), shock (e.g. haemorrhagic, infective, traumatic) and respiratory problems (e.g. suffocation, paralysis of respiratory muscles and carbon monoxide poisoning).

The oxygen content of room air is normally about 21%; if it falls there is compensatory increased cerebral blood flow. It can, however, fall to 10% before any noticeable behavioural effects are seen, but not until it falls below 7% is there an increase in glycolysis and a 300% increase in lactate formation. Energy production in the form of ATP is, however, maintained.

Mild hypoxia decreases the activity of aromatic amine hydroxylases, thereby causing interference with synthesis of dopamine, noradrenaline and 5-HT. Continued hypoxia leads to impaired energy production, secondarily affecting electrolyte transport and repolarization; finally, there is structural damage to the mitochondria.

Hypercapnia

If carbon dioxide retention is of acute onset, or if there is an acute exacerbation of chronic hypercapnia, then intense and persistent headache develops, accompanied by inattention and indifference to events in the environment. There is also weakness, irritability and lassitude, progressing to drowsiness, confusion, stupor and coma. Entry to a high or very high carbon dioxide-containing atmosphere can produce rapid coma and death.

When hypoxaemia and hypercapnia occur simultaneously the neurological effects of each may be indistinguishable. Chronic hypercapnia by itself may produce no symptoms provided the respiratory acidosis is fully compensated.

Hyperventilation Syndrome[15]

The most common presentation of this syndrome is among female patients who, though unaware of over-breathing, may admit to sighing or feeling apprehensive. In the acute disorder, light-headedness is typical and panic attacks occur either for no very obvious reason, or in some instances, may be provoked by identifiable circumstances. In the chronic disorder there are feelings of unreality, difficulties in concentrating, anxiety and attacks of panic; an interesting feature is that symptoms are sometimes more marked at rest than during moderate exercise.

In acute hyperventilation the arterial P_{CO_2} is reduced without any change in the plasma bicarbonate as there has been insufficient time for compensatory processes to take place. In chronic hyperventilation there is compensated respiratory alkalosis; both arterial P_{CO_2} and plasma bicarbonate are reduced, but blood pH is relatively normal. The low arterial P_{CO_2} may account for neuronal hyperexcitability and vasoconstriction, with consequent reduction in cerebral blood flow, possibly accounting for the fainting, giddiness and blurred vision so often observed. Adrenaline release may be the basis for some of the cardiovascular symptomatology in these patients.

Hypoglycaemia

The mood changes of neuroglycopenia comprise lethargy, lack of concentration, poor judgement, faintness and dizziness; the condition may proceed further to convulsions and coma. If, however, the blood glucose has fallen very rapidly the sympathetic nervous system may be stimulated, with resulting agitation, tremor, sweating, tachycardia, palpitations and pallor.

Hyperglycaemia

The acute metabolic complications of diabetes mellitus are diabetic ketoacidosis and hyperosmolar coma. In both of these there is hyperglycaemia; in the former, associated with type 1 diabetes mellitus (insulin-dependent diabetes mellitus), ketoacidosis is dominant—with the hyperglycaemia sometimes being of minimal degree; in the latter, associated with type

2 diabetes mellitus (non-insulin-dependent diabetes mellitus), there is no metabolic acidosis but the hyperglycaemia is gross.

Liver Failure

Hepatic encephalopathy is characterized by episodes ranging from mild mental dulling to increased or decreased psychomotor activity, confusion, drowsiness and coma.

Acute hepatic encephalopathy has many causes and can unfold over as little as a few days or as long as a few weeks. It may be the presenting feature of acute liver failure. Chronic hepatic insufficiency with portacaval shunting of blood, chronic alcoholic cirrhosis and chronic hepatitis can also cause hepatic encephalopathy, which is characterized neuropathologically by an increase in both the number and size of protoplasmic astrocytes in the cerebral cortex.

The biochemical basis of hepatic encephalopathy is uncertain. Cerebral oxidative metabolism is impaired, and both oxygen uptake and glucose utilization are reduced, but this may be consequential rather than causative.

Ammonia (NH_3), formed from the breakdown of amino acids or (together with other amines) derived from gastrointestinal urease-containing organisms, has been incriminated, especially in the presence of a portacaval shunt, but is not now thought to be the main causal mechanism.

Changes in the synthesis and metabolism of neurotransmitters, or false neurotransmitters (e.g. octopamine and phenylethanolamine) may play a part. A rise in the amount of the inhibitory neurotransmitter, GABA, has also been suggested as an explanation for the mental sequelae of hepatic disease.

Uraemia

Initially, the psychiatric manifestations of acute uraemic encephalopathy comprise apathy, fatigue, inattentiveness and irritability; later, there is confusion, hallucinations, stupor and coma. These features are sometimes episodic. In the 'disequilibrium syndrome', which sometimes complicates haemodialysis or peritoneal dialysis, the patient develops headaches, irritability, agitation, drowsiness and convulsions, commencing several hours after the onset of dialysis (occasionally up to 2 days after the procedure) and of several hours' duration. There is also a less common manifestation, 'dialysis encephalopathy', in which there is a change of personality and episodes of psychosis with intellectual decline; at first these episodes last for a few hours and occur soon after dialysis, but later, as they progress, they become more persistent and finally achieve permanency.

The rise in blood urea and creatinine are not the basis of the mental features, the exact cause of which is unknown. Glucose and oxygen consumption by the brain are decreased, and concentrations of ATP and phosphocreatine in the brain are increased, suggesting a defect in energy utilization.

In the disequilibrium syndrome there is a shift of water into the brain tissues. Dialysis encephalopathy is characterized by mild, diffuse microcavitation of the upper layers of the cerebral cortex; aluminium has been found in higher amounts in the cerebral grey matter of such patients when compared with those who were dialysed but who did not have encephalopathy. The aluminium is derived not only from dialysate fluid but also from orally administered aluminium-containing gels. It has been suggested, therefore, that aluminium intoxication is the basis of these disorders.

Ethyl Alcohol[16,17]

Alcohol ingestion produces mood changes and neuropsychiatric symptoms which vary according to the circumstances. Alcohol toxicity in the short term is associated, initially, with progression from inebriation to the slowing of thought processes, being unable to concentrate, and displaying an unreliable memory, loss of restraint, irregular behaviour, drowsiness—and finally coma; should 'pathological intoxication' occur, then irrational outbursts of anger (with the accompanying danger of physical violence) may be expressed. 'Alcoholic black-outs' may take the form of amnesia for significant events taking place during the bout of drinking, lasting from a few hours up to several days; subsequent exposure to alcohol may aid recall of those events. Hypoglycaemia, symptomatic or asymptomatic, sometimes occurs—commencing a few hours after the alcohol ingestion, lasting even for 36 h or so.

There may be long-term complications such as the neuropsychiatric accompaniments of cirrhosis of the liver or severe hepatitis. The nutritional consequences of alcohol ingestion comprise vitamin B_1 deficiency and the consequent Wernicke's encephalopathy and Korsakoff's psychosis. Alcohol may also induce falls and head injuries; it is always important to consider taking an X-ray of the skull or doing a computerized tomographic scan. The administration of certain drugs concomitantly with the alcohol (e.g. benzodiazepines, barbiturates) can produce profound clinical consequences. Withdrawal of alcohol leads to fits, hallucinations and delirium tremens. Chronic alcoholics can develop a variety of endocrine disorders including, very rarely, Cushing's syndrome, which quickly resolves on withdrawal from alcohol.

Neuropathological changes occurring in patients with a high alcohol intake include slight reduction in the weight of the brain with increased pericerebral space, the changes of Wernicke's encephalopathy, cerebral atrophy of the dorsolateral aspect of the frontal lobes in particular, and enlargement of the frontal horns of the lateral ventricles. Histologically, there is arachnoidal thickening and cell degeneration with partial destruction of the myelin sheath.

Approximately 70% or more of ingested alcohol, assuming that the serum alcohol concentration does not exceed 20 mmol/L (92 mg/100 mL), is metabolized in the liver via alcohol dehydrogenase to acetaldehyde, which is then converted by aldehyde dehydrogenase to acetate; both enzymes require NAD as cofactor, NADH being produced in the process. Hence, the ratio NADH:NAD rises—which, in turn, influences the rate of activity of other metabolic reactions; this ratio is responsible, therefore, for many of the metabolic derangements caused by high alcohol consumption. Should the alcohol in the blood rise above about 20 mmol/L, then the NADP-dependent microsomal ethanol oxidizing system assumes increasing importance, accounting for up to 10% or more of the amount metabolized. There is a third pathway, the catalase pathway, involved in alcohol metabolism when blood concentrations are high, but it is thought to be comparatively unimportant.

In general, alcohol metabolism proceeds at around 7 g/h in an adult but is in part dependent upon the blood alcohol concentration, though very little upon body size.

Alcohol acts initially on the reticular formation in the brainstem, thereby stimulating increased excitability of the cerebral cortex. Following on from this, however, comes the direct toxic inhibitory action of the compound on the cerebral cortex. Alcohol is, therefore, a CNS depressant which causes inhibition of neuronal activity. Even moderate exposure to alcohol influences neurotransmitter systems; in 'alcoholic dementia' and cerebral atrophy, post-mortem studies yield evidence for a reduction in cholinergic function, somewhat similar to the findings in Alzheimer's disease. Moreover, acetaldehyde formed during the metabolism of alcohol possesses toxic effects of its own; it is more toxic than alcohol and its effects are narcotic.

Electrolyte and Water Disorders[18]

Disorders of electrolyte and water balance, and the accompanying disturbances in osmolality, produce changes in brain volume and determine the mode of clinical expression, the most important of which are fits and coma.

Water Intoxication

This hypo-osmolar syndrome can be due to numerous causes: infusion postoperatively with low sodium-containing fluids, administration of analogues of antidiuretic hormone (ADH, vasopressin), compulsive water drinking and the syndrome of inappropriate antidiuresis. In the early stages of water intoxication the patient passes through a period of being less alert than usual, followed by lassitude, lethargy, apathy, restlessness, confusion, delirium, headache, stupor, convulsions and, eventually, coma. A slow fall in plasma osmolality permits accommodation to take place so that even very low plasma sodium concentrations may be tolerated with only minimal symptoms. Compulsive water drinking may be episodic, and itself has many causes. There is not only the conse-

quential mood change, but also the psychiatric origin of the disorder to consider; the individual may be neurotic (e.g. anxiety state), psychotic (e.g. delusions, schizophrenia) or have a personality disorder (e.g. depression, hypochondria). There may be variation in fluid intake over the course of the day, unlike diabetes insipidus. It must be distinguished from diabetes insipidus, in which the osmolality of the extracellular fluid is high. In compulsive water drinking the cell water content rises in the brain as elsewhere, leading to a rise in intracranial pressure with all the attendant problems.

Water Depletion

Water depletion (causing a hyperosmolar state) can be caused by reduction or cessation of water intake for any reason. Dehydration is less overt than in sodium depletion on account of the loss being from the whole of the body water rather than mainly from the extracellular compartment. As the water depletion progresses there is increasing lethargy, mental confusion, delirium, stupor and coma. The elderly, who have a lessened ability to accommodate to such changes, and some patients who lack the sensation of thirst, are particularly at risk.

A steady rise in plasma sodium, chloride, urea and other metabolite concentrations leads to hyperosmolality which, in turn, affects the CNS, producing disturbance of electrical transmission.

Hypernatraemia

Clinical expression of severe hypernatraemia takes the form of thirst, lethargy, weakness, disorientation, confusion and, eventually, coma; in cases of lesser severity, alteration in the level of consciousness may be the only sign.

Hypertonicity within the extracellular space causes loss of water from the neurons. Brain volume decreases and is responsible for the symptomatology, with the possibility of haemorrhages caused by shrinkage of cerebral tissue leading to mechanical tearing of cerebral blood vessels. Post-mortem studies reveal both brain and meningeal haemorrhages, and capillary thromboses.

Vitamin Disorders[19]

Both fat-soluble and water-soluble vitamins, either in excess or deficiency, are indirectly implicated (by way of secondary biochemical changes) in mood alterations or frank psychiatric disorders; there may also, of course, be other accompanying clinical features.

Vitamin B₁ (Thiamine) Deficiency

Wernicke's encephalopathy is a cerebral form of thiamine deficiency presenting either acutely or unfolding rapidly over several days. It is most commonly seen in chronic alcoholics. They may be deficient in thiamine for several reasons (e.g. nutritional insufficiency, impaired gastrointestinal absorption of the vitamin, inability of the liver to store and utilize the vitamin). Vitamin B_1 deficiency is also found in cases of starvation, malnutrition, administration of inadequate parenteral nutrition in gastrointestinal problems and persistent vomiting.

There may be prodromal symptoms in the form of mild delirium, agitation, inability to sleep and hallucinations. The patient may become apathetic, be inattentive, sleepy, confused and disorientated; occasionally there may be progression to stupor and coma. Amnesia for new information may sometimes be found. In response to treatment with thiamine, confusion may slowly improve over a few days or weeks, perhaps allowing any memory defect to come to light; the defect itself would take longer to improve, although some patients may be left with a residual memory defect, i.e. Korsakoff's amnesic syndrome (Korsakoff's psychosis).

Korsakoff's psychosis is characterized by defective ability to form new memories (anterograde amnesia), difficulty in recalling recent memories (retrograde amnesia), disorientation in both time and place, and confabulation. Although immediate memory recall is excellent, just a few minutes later those memories will not be recalled. Judgement, however, remains intact.

Thiamine pyrophosphate (TPP) acts as coenzyme for certain enzyme reactions in the metabolism of carbohydrate and amino acids, e.g. the decarboxylation of pyruvate to acetyl coenzyme A (CoA) via pyruvate dehydrogenase (providing the connection between the anaerobic glycolytic pathway and Kreb's tricarboxylic acid cycle), the transketolase reaction (in the hexose monophosphate shunt), the decarboxylation of α-ketoglutarate to succinate via α-ketoglutarate dehydrogenase (in Kreb's cycle) and branched-chain α-ketoacid dehydrogenase. Cells deficient in thiamin are unable to utilize glucose aerobically; the CNS in particular is in danger because of its absolute dependency on the delivery of glucose for energy needs. In addition to its role as coenzyme, thiamine and TPP may also function in maintaining neuronal membrane electrical activity.

Vitamin B_{12} (Cobalamin) Deficiency

Vitamin B_{12} deficiency giving rise to pernicious anaemia is a disease of insidious onset, with or without neuropsychiatric accompaniment which can precede the onset of anaemia. The mild depression and lassitude often present are not always recognized by the patient, but the marked feeling of well-being which develops within 24 h of the first therapeutic dose of intramuscular vitamin B_{12} brings with it realization that the patient had not felt as well as had been thought. There may also be progression to irritability, a tendency to paranoia and nocturnal confusion. The psychiatric presentation may indeed antedate other features of the illness by up to 2 years. Progressive dementia may occur, although it is unusual in the absence of neurological signs; affective disorders,

schizophrenia, disorientation and delirium have all been documented as consequences of vitamin B_{12} deficiency.

The cerebral pathology comprises progression from demyelination to axonal degeneration and neuronal death, by which stage the condition is no longer reversible with vitamin B_{12} therapy; there is very little gliosis or neuronal damage.

Vitamin B_{12} is a cofactor in two different enzyme systems. Methylcobalamin serves as coenzyme to N5-methyltetrahydrofolate homocysteine methyltransferase, which donates its methyl group to homocysteine during methionine synthesis, tetrahydrofolate being regenerated at the same time. Another coenzyme, 5'-deoxyadenosylcobalamin, is involved in the methylmalonyl–CoA mutase reaction in which succinyl CoA is generated. The activity of both enzymes is reduced when vitamin B_{12} is deficient. In consequence, there is lack of methionine formation (which not only serves as a substrate for protein synthesis, but also is a precursor for transmethylation reactions in, for example, neurotransmitter, phospholipid and protein metabolism) and failure to convert methylmalonate to succinyl CoA (with increased urinary excretion of methylmalonic acid).

Vitamin B_3 (Niacin, Nicotinic Acid) Deficiency[19]

Pellagra results from nutritional deficiency of vitamin B_3 or, rarely, the carcinoid syndrome, in which tryptophan is metabolized via the 5-HT pathway, and Hartnup disease, in which there is defective intestinal and renal transport for certain amino acids.

The classical features of pellagra are dermatitis, diarrhoea and dementia—with death as the ultimate consequence. Mental changes occur early. Initially there is simply insomnia and fatigue. Later, the patient becomes irritable and nervous and there is anxiety with depression. Mental processes slow down and memory impairment becomes evident; disorientation, confusion, confabulation, episodic violent outbursts, paranoia and delusions are late features. Therapy with vitamin B_3 induces improvement, within hours or days, of many of the psychiatric symptoms, but dementia, once it has developed, is not reversible.

Nicotinic acid derivatives are precursors of NAD and NADP, which are essential participants in many oxidation and reduction reactions, but this does not explain the specific neuropsychiatric symptoms associated with vitamin B_3 deficiency.

Vitamin B_6 (Pyridoxine) Responsiveness[19]

Oral contraceptives can cause depression in some women, a proportion of whom demonstrate disturbances in tryptophan metabolism which return to normal after pyridoxine therapy. There is, however, no evidence of vitamin B_6 deficiency in these women, in whom the therapeutic response is clearly a pharmacological response to the vitamin rather than correction of a nutritional deficiency.

It is thought that the mechanism of action is by

way of stimulating tryptophan pyrrolase, which is the rate-limiting enzyme in the kynurenine pathway.

Vitamin A Toxicity

Chronic vitamin A toxicity is associated with signs and symptoms of neural dysfunction, including irritability, fatigue, anorexia, drowsiness, difficulty in concentration and a rise of intracranial pressure. Even a single massive dose of vitamin A may cause drowsiness, irritability, somnolence and headache. In infants, vitamin A toxicity causes elevated intracranial pressure, associated with a bulging anterior fontanelle.

Some patients with hypervitaminosis A develop hypercalcaemia and a raised serum alkaline phosphatase that responds rapidly to treatment with hydrocortisone. However, withdrawal of the vitamin is normally all that is required for treatment of both the somatic and psychiatric manifestations of vitamin A intoxication.

Folic Acid Deficiency[20]

Deficiency of folate, accompanied by depression and dementia, is thought to occur in up to 30% of psychiatric inpatients and an even higher percentage of psychogeriatric patients. Folate deficiency such as can be induced by anticonvulsant therapy in children is associated with mood change, with neuropsychiatric symptoms and possibly a fall in IQ. Neurotic disturbance, depression, dementia and schizophrenic-like psychoses have also been observed.

It is probable that methylfolate exerts a modulatory role on neurotransmission and that this is in some way responsible for the symptoms observed.

Mineral Disorders

Mental changes may result from either deficiencies or excesses of various minerals.

Zinc Deficiency

Apart from the manifestations of skin disease that characterize zinc deficiency, mental apathy or depression is prominent. Zinc is an intrinsic part of many metalloenzymes; it is essential for protein, DNA and RNA synthesis. Dietary zinc deficiency, however, is very rare, as is the inborn error of metabolism associated with its malabsorption.

Hypercalcaemia[21]

Severe psychiatric changes usually occur only when the serum calcium is grossly raised. Nevertheless, depression may be the presenting symptom of hypercalcaemia, and also irritability and anxiety. Occasionally there may be paranoia, mania or hallucinations. Stupor and coma are the consequences of untreated progressive hypercalcaemia. There does seem to be some relation, in general, between serum calcium concentrations and symptoms; lack of initiative, drive and affective disorder occur at around 3.0–4.0 mmol/

L, delirium and organic encephalopathy at 4.0–4.75 mmol/L and stupor and coma at greater than 4.75 mmol/L. However, these values are somewhat variable, some patients having relatively few, if any, symptoms at a concentration at which others are frankly unwell. Calcium plays a part in neural transmission, nerve excitability and neurotransmitter secretion. Hyperpolarization occurs when extracellular calcium concentration rises.

Hypocalcaemia[21]

Hypocalcaemia is much less common than hypercalcaemia, and the symptoms associated with the increased neural excitability to which it gives rise, namely paraesthesiae of the extremities and circumoral areas, muscle cramps, laryngeal spasm and convulsions, are less likely to be attributed to mental disease. Nevertheless, symptoms of lassitude, tension, irritability, emotional lability, difficulty in concentration, depression, impaired intellect, and sometimes frank psychosis, can result from insidious hypocalcaemia such as may follow thyroidectomy and damage to the parathyroid glands.

Increased neural excitability is to be expected when there is lowering of the extracellular calcium concentration, accounting for parasthesia, muscle spasms and convulsions.

Magnesium Deficiency[21,22]

Magnesium is an essential component of many enzyme systems; it is vital not only for cell membrane permeability, neuromuscular excitability, and muscular contraction, but also for protein, nucleic acid and fat synthesis.

Magnesium deficiency is rare, and virtually never solely of dietary origin. It is associated with symptoms of lethargy, fatigue, decreased mentation and depression, which are, however, also features of magnesium intoxication.

Manganese Toxicity[16,22]

Manganese is a trace element that serves as an enzyme activator and is also a component of metalloenzymes. Miners who inhale manganese dust over many months or years may develop, in addition to extrapyramidal features, irritability, euphoria and emotional instability, followed by onset of lethargy, apathy and somnolence.

Lead Poisoning[16,22]

Inorganic lead salts can cause lead poisoning via ingestion or inhalation; pica (eating lead-containing paint chips) is often the basis in infants and children in particular and this, in turn, is often secondary to iron deficiency. A subclinical form of plumbism, with none of the general symptoms, can later present clinically with irreversible mental retardation when the growing brain is exposed to high amounts of lead; the consequences are failure of language development, disorders of cognitive function and abnormalities of behaviour. In children, mental changes occur if the condition is of sufficient severity, toxicity being indicated by irritability, lethargy, convulsions and coma; cerebral oedema is an important factor in development of the encephalopathy.

In adults, lead poisoning may cause memory loss and other signs of nervous dysfunction. It is, however, unusual for encephalopathy to develop at this time of life, except after exposure to tetraethyl lead, when convulsions and confusion may occur.

Lead poisons enzyme systems by binding to disulphide groups, and when present in high concentration may cause denaturation of intracellular proteins. Cell death with tissue inflammation follows. Blood lead concentrations are elevated.

Iron Deficiency[23]

Even mild iron deficiency can lead to subtle behavioural changes with diminution of work performance, listlessness, fatigue and pica; all are rapidly reversible by correction of the iron deficiency state. In children with iron deficiency there may be impairment of learning ability, which is often irreversible; the degree of reversibility depends on the severity of iron deficiency and the age of the child.

Depletion of iron-containing enzymes and cofactors in tissue metabolism may be important in the development of these symptoms. As a component of haemoglobin, iron has a vital role in the transport of oxygen in the blood. Iron is also a component of monoamine oxidase, an enzyme that plays a central role in the production of several neurotransmitters, namely dopamine, noradrenaline, adrenaline and 5-HT. There is evidence that iron is essential for normal development and functioning of dopaminergic neurons, and it may be that deficiency of iron in early life could cause permanent damage to this system; animal experiments have revealed that rats with low iron content had fewer D_2 receptors. Iron is distributed unevenly in the brain, but it does seem to be found in relation to those neurons producing the inhibitory neurotransmitter GABA. Low concentrations of iron are thought either to interfere with GABA degradation or to impair normal performance of dopaminergic neurons.

Mercury Poisoning[16,24]

Clinical mercury poisoning can be acute or chronic and is due to the inhalation of mercury vapour or to the ingestion of inorganic or organic 'salts' of mercury. The nature of the mercurial compound determines the symptom complex to which it gives rise. Acute metallic mercury toxicity causes increased excitability, whereas chronic mercury-vapour poisoning causes lassitude and anorexia initially; later there is mercurial erethism, characterized by timidity, emotional lability, excitability, loss of memory, insomnia, delirium, suicidal tendencies and psychosis. It was erethism that accounted for the problems encountered in the past by felt hat-makers who inhaled hot mercuric nitrate fumes—hence the phrase 'as mad as a hatter'. Low-grade chronic inorganic mercury poisoning is the basis of acrodynia (pink disease) in children, who typically developed irritability after exposure to mercury-containing teething powder, ointments and medicaments. Acute and chronic organic mercury toxicity cannot easily be distinguished; postnatally, apart from other CNS involvement, there is memory loss, erethism, stupor and coma.

Mercury has a particular affinity for thiol groups and consequently poisons enzymes that rely upon them.

Selenium Toxicity[25]

Excessive exposure to selenium fumes or overindulgence in selenium 'food supplements' can cause symptoms of apathy, lassitude, nervousness and depression, although these symptoms soon disappear on reduction of exposure to the toxin.

Selenium is an essential trace element involved in the function of glutathione peroxidase.

Thallium Poisoning[16]

Acute thallium poisoning produces delirium whilst subacute poisoning leads to confusion, hallucinations, sleep disorders, convulsions, psychosis and dementia. Both forms of poisoning are almost always deliberate. Chronic industrial thallium exposure may cause residual memory loss.

Thallium binds strongly to the sulphydryl groups that are often present in enzyme systems, thus interfering with their functions. Thallium also enters cells in exchange for potassium.

Vanadium Toxicity[22]

Industrial exposure to vanadium can cause lassitude and depression, which lessens when exposure is reduced. Vanadate (the pentavalent ion of vanadium) inhibits Na^+/K^+-ATPase which, in turn, inhibits the sodium pump.

Inherited Metabolic Disorders[26]

Acute Intermittent Porphyria (AIP)

AIP is a rare inborn error of metabolism of autosomal dominant inheritance which is dealt with in detail elsewhere (*see* Chapter 24). Psychiatric symptoms are sometimes dominant. Disorientation, confusion, delirium, coma and convulsions are the extreme manifestations, but restlessness, emotional lability, histrionic behaviour, severe depression and emotional instability may be observed. Psychiatric disorders resembling schizophrenia and paranoid reactions are well recognized. As regards the general personality it has been claimed that emotional instability and functional disturbances are typical. Probably less than 1:3 of all individuals showing the enzyme deficiency ever have symptoms of AIP, which are provoked by certain drugs (e.g. barbiturates, alcohol, anticonvulsants), hormones (e.g. oestrogens, oral contraceptives), other agents and circumstances (e.g. starvation, infections). Other mechanisms may also be involved in the genesis of the psychiatric state (e.g. development of the inappropriate antidiuresis syndrome; features of the latter disorder, superimposed upon the other metabolic disturbances, may create a complex situation.

Metachromatic Leucodystrophy
This disorder is of autosomal recessive inheritance and normally presents in childhood, but 1:4 cases present in adult life during the second to fifth decade. There is a male:female ratio of 2:1. Initially, there may be a falling off in intellectual performance at school or college, with forgetfulness and irrational behaviour; emotional difficulties, suspiciousness, delusions and general personality problems also emerge. In adults the initial presentation may be in the form of a psychosis and dementia. Over the years the psychiatric state gradually deteriorates, with dementia being the end-result.

This is a lysosomal storage disease caused by a deficiency of arylsulphatase-A (cerebroside sulphatase), leading to accumulation of cerebroside sulphates (galactosyl sulphatide) in the Schwann cells, the myelin sheath and in other parts of the body; as a result there is an increase in urinary sulphatide and presence of metachromatic material in the urine. Neuropathologically, there is demyelination.

Adrenoleucodystrophy (X-linked Schilder's Disease)
This is one of a group of disorders known as leucodystrophies which include metachromatic leucodystrophy, globoid cell leucodystrophy, Pelizaeus–Merzbacher disease and Canavan's disease, as well as adrenoleucodystrophy itself. This slowly progressive disorder presents with Addison's disease and/or cerebral involvement in which there is intellectual deterioration leading to dementia. Although adrenal corticoid therapy improves the Addison's disease, it does not influence the cerebral component of the illness which is progressive. The disease is associated with greatly increased excretion of urinary C_{22}–C_{26} fatty acids.

Adult GM$_2$-gangliosidosis
The clinical presentation is predominantly neurological, although sometimes behavioural change, intellectual decline and a slowly developing dementia are found.

This condition is caused by accumulation of GM_2-ganglioside in the engorged lysosomes of the neurons in both the central and autonomic nervous system and is only one of several types of GM_2-gangliosidoses including Tay–Sachs disease, Sandhoff's disease, and juvenile GM_2-gangliosidosis. GM_2-gangliosidosis is an autosomal recessive disorder due to defi-

ciency of hexosaminidase A, the enzyme which catalyses conversion of GM_2-ganglioside to GM_3-ganglioside. Usually presenting as Tay–Sachs disease at around 6 months of age, it is occasionally observed in young adults.

There are a number of lipid storage diseases of autosomal recessive inheritance which present in adolescence or early adult life; these neurolipidoses include sphingomyelin lipidosis (Niemann–Pick disease), glucosyl ceramide lipidosis (Gaucher's disease), and the various gangliosidoses. Further details can be found in the specialist literature devoted to them.

PSYCHIATRIC SIDE-EFFECTS OF DRUG THERAPY

Psychiatric changes attributable solely (or in part) to commencement, continuation or cessation of drug therapy range from mere changes of mood to much more florid clinical presentations. The interactions of a drug, not only with the personality but also with physiological status and metabolic inheritance (i.e. pharmacogenetic aspects) of the individual, are fundamental to the actual clinical expression of toxicity; the dosage, too, is a vital consideration. The elderly often have cerebral atherosclerosis and may be more sensitive to the effects of drugs; moreover, alcohol and other drugs may produce an additive effect—or just complicate the presentation. With a psychiatric illness in particular it is often very difficult to be certain that the patient's symptoms are related to the drug therapy—as opposed to being due to an exacerbation or phase of the original clinical problem; this applies whether it is the presence of the drug or its withdrawal that is being incriminated.

The psychiatric manifestations of adverse responses both to psychotropic and non-psychotropic drugs and also to drugs of abuse include schizophrenic-like reactions, paranoia, depression, hypomania, hallucinations, delirium, confusion, sleep disturbance and drowsiness. Symptoms of lesser severity are, however, very common and may collectively be incapacitating. In addition to these definitive reactions there are those even less well-defined complaints where the patient claims that 'the tablets made me feel awful'.

MUNCHAUSEN'S SYNDROME AND OTHER FACTITIOUS ILLNESSES[27]

Factitious disorders comprise deliberate production of physical and/or psychological symptoms, but without either an obvious external incentive or identifiable reward; there just seems to be, psychologically, a requirement to perpetuate the scenario of 'sickness'. Munchausen's syndrome is an extreme form of the disorder, with the seeking of attention for some reason (e.g. the patient may need love, care, attention, or sympathy, hence choosing to 'create illness' in order to achieve this end). Such individuals are not aware of their motivation, but fully realize that they are faking a clinical presentation. In the 'Munchausen's syndrome by proxy', it is usually a parent (often the mother or sometimes a carer) who seeks medical help, falsely representing the child's symptoms, sometimes even making false physical signs and interfering, too, with biological specimens to be sent for laboratory analysis (e.g. they might add glucose or other substances to the urine sample).

Laboratory Investigations[28]

The diagnosis of Munchausen's syndrome may be made in the chemical pathology department of the hospital, or on account of a test result that then permits the clinician to confirm a previous suspicion. Diuretic compounds may be being taken in order to cause loss of weight, purgatives to produce diarrhoea and/or loss of weight, anticoagulants to precipitate haematuria and bruising, chlorpropamide to produce hypoglycaemia, insulin to cause fits, or sleeping tablets to create drowsiness; the appropriate biochemical assays will assist in their detection. On the other hand, a patient may contaminate a biological specimen such as urine with blood, lactose, glucose, sucrose, organisms (from a faecal source) or egg albumin and proudly present it to the laboratory for analysis. Renal stones, supposedly passed by the patient but in reality picked up from the path on the way to the hospital, and which consequently do what no stone of biological origin ever does, namely damage the pestle and mortar used for crushing the stone before analysis, can be another mode of presentation of Munchausen's syndrome. In this context perhaps the 'rattle test' should be added to the routine list of investigations of renal stones; this cheap test consists of simply rattling the pot in which the stone has been sent to the laboratory—the sharp sound of granite or flint on the sides of the jar is unmistakable and cannot be confused with the sound of any stone of biological origin. Faecal fat analysis, too, may provide the final clue to the diagnosis; on alkaline hydrolysis a glorious regal red colour indicates consumption of the laxative phenolphthalein—the cause of the diarrhoea that precipitated the request for the analysis in the first place!

'Munchausen's syndrome by proxy' is where the parent of a child causes either diagnostic confusion or actual harm by giving it something and then taking it to hospital for investigation. A typical feature is that the parent is 'always' present, hardly ever leaving the child—giving an impression of utter devotion. There may be only a subtle difference between creating such a situation for the purpose of attention seeking and using almost the same scenario for malicious intent.

Munchausen's syndrome may not be the final diagnosis; the sequence of events may proceed to suicide (e.g. the patient who initially presents with hypogly-caemia following non-prescribed dosage with chlorpropamide and who is later found dead from taking another agent or by some other means), or the patient who, having taken anticoagulants to achieve attention for some reason, is found dead in a car full of exhaust fumes with a suicide note expressing great concern about cancer, but for which no evidence had ever been found during life—or, indeed, at postmortem examination. In a similar way, 'Munchausen's syndrome by proxy' can end in murder. However, many patients with Munchausen's syndrome continue to present with monotonous regularity at different clinics, in different hospitals in the country, and over a period of many years.

Investigation of both Munchausen's syndrome and 'Munchausen by proxy' is extremely difficult and depends upon the diligence of both laboratory and clinical staff, and awareness that the conditions exist.

LABORATORY INVESTIGATIONS OF PSYCHIATRIC DISORDERS[28]

All the varied laboratory investigations appropriate in any clinical situation may be relevant to the diagnosis and follow-up of a psychiatric illness, especially if the mood change forms only part of the clinical presentation as a whole. Nevertheless, a great deal of clinical information, whether confirmatory, non-confirmatory or exclusory, of a particular diagnostic

TABLE 8.1
LABORATORY INVESTIGATIONS OF PSYCHIATRIC DISORDERS

Investigation	Routine Procedures	Other Procedures	Drugs
URINE	Glucose Protein Cells Organisms	Electrolytes Osmolality Volume Porphyrins Porphobilinogen Vanillylmandelic acid (VMA)	Amphetamines Morphine Methadone Cannabis Cocaine Benzodiazepines Barbiturates Codeine Dihydrocodeine Heroin
BLOOD	Electrolytes and urea Osmolality Glucose Liver function tests Calcium γ-glutamyl transferase Prothrombin time	Vitamin B_{12} Folic acid Ferritin Alcohol Cortisol Thyroxine/TSH Insulin and C peptide Magnesium Lead Adrenaline Noradrenaline Dexamethasone suppresion test	Lithium carbonate
FAECES	Occult blood	Phenolphthalein Porphyrins	

possibility, can be attained by performing a relatively small range of basic tests (see Table 8.1).

CONCLUSIONS

The foregoing account of the biochemical and mental aspects of psychiatric disorders has covered some of the more florid conditions (e.g. schizophrenia, depression, mania/hypomania, anxiety and Alzheimer's disease), in addition to the mood changes and psychiatric consequences of biochemical derangements, pharmacological agents and toxicological factors.

It should be reiterated that the disorders discussed in this chapter have been, essentially, biochemically induced or based. The mental accompaniments of physical lesions (e.g. the depression associated with space-occupying lesions of the brain) and of those disorders of microbiological origin (e.g. the fatigue that may precede or accompany viral hepatitis and which may, in subclinical cases, be the only symptom; the dementia of human immunodeficiency virus infection) have been specifically excluded; nevertheless, all of them need to be considered during differential diagnosis.

REFERENCES

1. Thudichum J.L.W. (1884). Preface. In *A Treatise on the Chemical Constitution of the Brain*, London: Baillière, Tindall and Cox, pp. vii–xiii.
2. Young J.Z. (1979). Learning as a process of selection and amplification. *J. Roy. Soc. Med.*, **72**, 801.
3. Iversen L.L. (1979). The chemistry of the brain. *Sci. Am.*, **241**, 118.
4. Bloom F.E. (1985). Neurohumoral transmission and the central nervous system. In *The Pharmacological Basis of Therapeutics* (Gilman A.G., Goodman L.S., Rall T.W., Murad F. eds.) New York: MacMillan, pp. 236–259.
5. Perry E.K. (1991). Neurotransmitters and diseases of the brain. *Br. J. Hosp. Med.*, **45**, 73.
6. Laurence D.R., Bennett P.N. (1987). Central nervous system III: Drugs and mental disorder: psychotropic and psychoactive drugs. In *Clinical Pharmacology*, Edinburgh: Churchill Livingstone, pp. 343–369.
7. Thompson C. (1991). Mood disorders. *Med. Int.*, **94**, 3904.
8. Gelder M. (1991). Diagnosis and management of anxiety and phobic disorders. *Med. Int.*, **94**: 3913.
9. Kendell R.E., Chalmers J.C., Platz C. (1987). Epidemiology of puerperal psychosis. *Br. J. Psychiatry*, **150**, 662.
10. Cowen P.J., Anderson I.M., Gartside S.E. (1990). Endocrinological responses to 5-HT. *Ann. N.Y. Acad. Sci.*, **600**, 250.
11. Lascelles P.T., Donaldson D. (1989). Dexamethasone suppression test (DST)—single low dose for depression.

In *Diagnostic Function Tests in Chemical Pathology*, Dordrecht: Kluwer, pp. 43–44.
12. Lishman W.A. (1987). Endocrine diseases and metabolic disorders. In *Organic Psychiatry, the Psychological Consequences of Cerebral Disorder*, Oxford, Blackwell Scientific, pp. 428–485.
13. Fava G.A., Sonino N., Morphy M.A. (1987). Major depression associated with endocrine disease. *Psychiatr. Dev.* **4**, 321.
14. Bachelard H.S. (1990). The molecular basis of coma and stroke. In *The Metabolic and Molecular Basis of Acquired Disease* (Cohen R.D., Lewis B., Alberti K.G.M.M., Denman A.M. eds.) London: Baillière Tindall, pp. 1354–1380.
15. Patten J. (1977). Attacks of altered consciousness. In *Neurological Differential Diagnosis: An Illustrated Approach*, London: Harold Starke, pp. 231–237.
16. Lishman W.A. (1987). Toxic disorders. In *Organic Psychiatry, the Psychological Consequences of Cerebral Disorder*, Oxford: Blackwell Scientific, pp. 508–544.
17. Marks V. (1983). Clinical pathology of alcohol. *J. Clin. Pathol.*, **36**: 365.
18. Lambie A.T. (1987). Disturbances in water and electrolyte balance and in hydrogen ion concentration. In *Davidson's Principles and Practice of Medicine*, Edinburgh: Churchill Livingstone, pp. 84–99.
19. Lishman W.A. (1987). Vitamin deficiencies. In *Organic Psychiatry, the Psychological Consequences of Cerebral Disorder*, Oxford: Blackwell Scientific, pp. 486–507.
20. Trimble M.R., Corbett J.A., Donaldson D. (1980). Folic acid and mental symptoms in children with epilepsy. *J. Neurol. Neurosurgery Psychiatry*, **43**, 1030.
21. Alberti K.G.M.M. (1978). Metabolic comas and confusions. *Med. Int.*, **10**, 507.
22. Linter C.M. (1985). Neuropsychiatric aspects of trace elements. *Br. J. Hosp. Med.*, **34**, 361.
23. Schafer A.I., Bunn H.F. (1987). Anaemias of iron deficiency and iron overload. In *Harrisons' Principles of Internal Medicine* (Braunwald E., Isselbacher K.J., Petersdorf R.G., Wilson J.D., Martin J.B., Fauci A.S. eds.) New York: McGraw-Hill, pp. 1493–1498.
24. Graef J.W., Lovejoy F.H. (1987). Heavy metal poisoning. In *Harrisons' Principles of Internal Medicine* (Braunwald E., Isselbacher K.J., Petersdorf R.G., Wilson J.D., Martin J.B., Fauci A.S. eds.) New York: McGraw-Hill, pp. 850–855.
25. Falchuk K.H. (1987). Disturbances in trace element metabolism. In *Harrisons' Principles of Internal Medicine* (Braunwald E., Isselbacher K.J., Petersdorf R.G., Wilson J.D., Martin J.B., Fauci A.S. eds.) New York: McGraw-Hill, pp. 418–421.
26. Stern J. (1983). Hereditary and acquired mental deficiency. In *Biochemistry in Clinical Practice* (Williams D.L., Marks V. eds.) London: Heinemann Medical, pp. 489–523.
27. Sakula A. (1978), Munchausen: fact and fiction. *J. R. Coll. Physicians*, **12**, 286.
28. Donaldson D. (1981) Laboratory investigations in psychiatric disorders. *Faculty News* (North and West London Faculty of the Royal College of General Practitioners), **1**, 4.

9. The Clinical Biochemistry of Neoplasia

C.R. Tillyer

Introduction
The metabolic effects of malignancy
  Carbohydrate metabolism
  Fat metabolism
  Protein metabolism
  Energy metabolism
  Mineral metabolism
  Endocrine system
  Renal system
  The biochemical consequences of neoplasia
    on other systems
Tumour products as markers of malignancy
  Oncofetal proteins
  Non-oncofetal proteins
  Cancer antigens

INTRODUCTION

The biochemical effects of cancer are simply divided into direct and indirect effects.

Direct effects are caused by the infiltration into normal tissue by, and expansion of, primary and secondary tumours. This may result in the obstruction of the venous, lymphatic or arterial supply of that tissue, causing oedema, infarction, retention of secretions or excretions, which may also lead to secondary infection or an inflammatory response. Obstruction of the ducts draining an organ, such as the bile duct in the liver or the ureters from the kidneys, has profound metabolic consequences. The continued expansion of the tumour eventually leads to the replacement of the normal tissue and gradual loss of its normal function, which can have drastic secondary metabolic effects, particularly when an endocrine tissue or the bone marrow is affected. The cells of most tissues and organs, however, can tolerate a substantial amount of tumour infiltration before function is lost. The first manifestations of tumours and their deposits usually occur clinically as a simple swelling, as a result of interruption of the arterial supplies with loss of function or necrosis, infection and haemorrhage, or obstruction of secretory or excretory ducts with retention of products. Direct effects account for by far the majority of the metabolic effects of cancer, if only because the outcome of most cancers is, unfortunately, metastatic spread. These effects are directly related to the bulk of the tumour or the degree to which it has metastasized and it is interesting to note that tumours rarely reach a size greater than 5% of total body weight.

Indirect effects, those that are associated not with direct tumour invasion of normal tissue but with the production of hormones, peptides, or other biologically active factors acting at a site remote from the tumour, are much less common. They are commonly referred to as 'paraneoplastic' effects or syndromes and are estimated to occur with a frequency of 7–15% in cancer patients.[1] This is probably an underestimate, however, as the nature of the factor causing the effect is commonly unknown. For instance, there is some evidence that the cachexia and anaemia of cancer may be caused by such factors. Those syndromes due to the secretion of known hormones by tumours are further classified depending on whether the hormone is secreted by tumours arising in a tissue or site that normally produces that hormone (a *eutopic* hormone), or in a tissue or site not normally associated with the production of that hormone (an *ectopic* hormone). Another term used to describe a tumour product is *oncodevelopmental*, which refers to the production by a tumour of the product of a gene that is normally completely shut off in adult life.[2] *Oncofetal* and *carcinoplacental* are more specific terms relating to the same process. It should be noted that oncodevelopmental genes are commonly activated transiently by a proliferative stimulus to a normal tissue, as in regeneration or inflammation; it is only in tumours that the proliferative stimulus is irreversible.

This division of effect is not to be considered absolute, however, as some of the more common metabolic syndromes associated with cancer have causes that may be due to direct effects, and dependent on tumour bulk and 'aggressiveness', or due to the secretion of known and unknown tumour products acting at a local or systemic level. A good example is the hypercalcaemia of malignancy, which can be associated with extensive tumour bulk and bony metastases eroding normal bone tissue, but which can also be associated with a small, non-metastatic tumour secreting a parathyroid hormone-like, humoral factor.

Finally, it should be noted that many of the metabolic complications encountered in cancer patients in hospital are caused by the highly intensive and toxic treatments used, in particular chemotherapy, and I have included these where they are important or well known. The combined effect of a malignant tumour and the secondary effects of highly cytotoxic chemotherapy often result in a complex metabolic picture which it is difficult to explain by one simple mechanism.

THE METABOLIC EFFECTS OF MALIGNANCY

Carbohydrate Metabolism

Hyperglycaemia

Glucose intolerance in association with malignancy

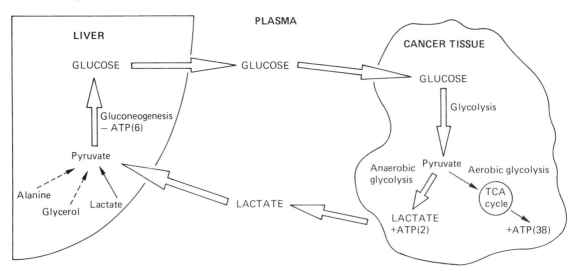

Figure 9.1 The Cori cycle: lactate and glucose cycling between neoplastic tissue and the liver results in a net loss of four molecules of ATP per molecule of glucose cycled and is therefore an energy-consuming process.

was first described in 1885.[3] Endocrine tumours secreting ectopic or eutopic hormones normally associated with blood glucose elevation (cortisol by pituitary adenomas and adrenocortical carcinoma; growth hormone by pituitary adenomas and lung carcinoma; glucagon by pancreatic tumours; catecholamines by phaeochromocytoma and neuroblastoma) may be expected to manifest themselves with hyperglycaemia, but these are rare. The presence of glucose intolerance, defined by the oral glucose tolerance test, has a prevalence of 36.7% in patients with all malignant tumours as compared to 9.3% in benign tumours.[4] The mechanism for this effect is not absolutely clear. There is an increased rate of endogenous glucose production and turnover in cancer that is apparently influenced by tumour stage, type and is associated with cachexia. There are four possible mechanisms involved.

1. *The Warburg effect and the Cori cycle.* Otto Warburg in 1930 noted an excess lactate production by tumour cells due to anaerobic glycolysis in spite of an apparently adequate oxygen availability.[5] Excess lactate production by tumour is taken up by the liver and used to produce glucose, which is then passed back into the circulation and may be reused for glycolysis—the *Cori cycle*[6] (Fig. 9.1). This is an energy expending or 'futile' cycle and its flux is increased in both disseminated and localized tumours.[7,8]

2. *Insulin resistance.* Marks and Bishop in 1956[9] noted that the fall in glucose in response to intravenous insulin was significantly smaller in patients with carcinoma, leukaemia and lymphoma. These findings have been confirmed and there is no apparent defect in insulin receptors, but it is not clear whether this a specific

effect of cancer rather than the effect of associated weight loss or sepsis.

3. *Impaired insulin secretion.* There is a decreased insulin response to glucagon and the oral glucose tolerance test in cancer but again this is only seen inassociation with weight loss; malnutrition *per se* is also associated with insulin resistance.

4. *Increased gluconeogenesis.* The gluconeogenic hormones, insulin, cortisol and growth hormone show consistent increases in cancer patients but there is evidence that gluconeogenesis in cancer is substrate-led, presumably from lactate (due to the Warburg effect) and alanine rather than glycerol.[10–12]

On balance the excessive Cori cycle activity combined with a defect in insulin response or action would seem to be the most likely explanation for glucose intolerance in cancer. The contribution of factors such as weight loss, sepsis and bedrest associated with cancer is difficult to assess but when present such factors probably contribute significantly.

Glucose intolerance secondary to destruction of β-cells in the pancreas by primary or secondary tumours occurs, but this also appears to be unusual in spite of a well-recognized association between carcinoma of the pancreas and glucose intolerance or diabetes (an incidence of 81% in one series).[13]

Treatment of malignant disease by high doses of steroids and oestrogens, asparaginase and cyclophosphamide, and pancreatic resection can also induce glucose intolerance and diabetes.

Hypoglycaemia
Tumour-associated hypoglycaemia is also a long-recognized syndrome. The incidence is much less

than hyperglycaemia and the cause in the majority of cases is also not entirely clear. Insulin hypersecretion either eutopically by an insulinoma or ectopically by a pancreatic carcinoma or carcinoid tumour is an uncommon cause. Most cases are associated with low concentrations of insulin, the most common tumour types being fibrosarcomas (26%), hepatomas (16%), carcinomas (19%), mesotheliomas (10%), lymphomas (6%), haemangiopericytomas (4%), leiomyosarcomas (3%) and others forming a large, highly heterogeneous group (19%).[14] The association with haemangiopericytomas is particularly high.

Two different types of patients with hypoglycaemia were delineated in hepatoma:[15] *type A*, the majority, with mild hypoglycaemia and easily treated with glucose supplements, who were in the terminal stages of the cancer and cachectic: and *type B*, who had severe hypoglycaemia which presented earlier in the disease, which was difficult to control and who did not have cachexia. Type A tumours were rapidly growing and poorly differentiated and type B tumours slow growing and well differentiated. The latter group is more suggestive of secretion of a specific, insulin-like, hypoglycaemic factor by the tumour, and there are a number of possible mechanisms at work in these tumours:[16]

1. *Inappropriate glucose utilization.* Many of these tumours are very large, particularly hepatomas and the fibrosarcomas, which are generally retroperitoneal, intra-abdominal or in the pleural cavity, and can reach 2–4 kg (3–6% of body weight). Glucose consumption by such a large tumour could be high but rarely high enough to exceed the liver output of glucose. Some hepatomas require 0.5–2 kg of glucose per day to maintain normoglycaemia but the glucose uptake caused by these tumours can be peripheral, not directly by the tumour, owing to a paraneoplastic effect.

2. *Hepatic destruction by metastases.* This is rather more unlikely than (1); hypoglycaemia is rare in tumours, even when there are extensive metastases. Extensive surgical hepatic resection for non-malignant conditions does not result in hypoglycaemia and the degree of liver destruction required by a tumour would probably never be achieved before the patient's demise from other causes.

3. *Decreased hepatic glucose production.* There is often a decreased hepatic output of glucose in the presence of hypoglycaemia in these tumours, which can be increased with the administration of exogenous glucagon. Also, the blood lactate can be elevated, suggesting an inadequate gluconeogenic response, and deficient glucagon release has been demonstrated in some cases. This all points to the secretion by the majority of tumours of a factor that interferes with normal hepatic glucose production.

The balance of evidence would suggest that tumour-associated hypoglycaemia not due to excessive insulin secretion is mediated, in many cases, by an as yet uncharacterized factor or factors released by the tumour. A possible candidate is non-suppressible insulin-like activity (NSILA) in blood. NSILA refers to the bioassayable, insulin-like activity that remains after insulin has been removed from plasma by anti-insulin antibodies. It consists of a number of peptides, two of which have been well characterized and sequenced: insulin-like growth factors (IGF) I and II. Their molecular masses are about 7500 Da and they show a great degree of homology with proinsulin. They have potent growth-stimulating activity and an insulin-like effect on glucose oxidation but with only a fraction of its activity. However, specific radioimmunoassays for these peptides have failed to demonstrate any consistent elevations above normal of either IGF-I or IGF-II in tumour-associated hypoglycaemia; in fact they are both usually at low or normal concentration. Raised amounts of IGF-II and its mRNA have been demonstrated in specific tumours but, after resection, IGF-II concentrations in serum have not changed even though the hypoglycaemia has resolved.

Hypoglycaemia should be sought in any cancer patient with confusion, aggressive or unusual behaviour, fits, lapses of consciousness or unexplained coma (which are commonly due to cerebral metastases), bearing in mind its particular associations with certain uncommon tumours. In a cancer patient, fasting hypoglycaemia in association with normal concentrations of plasma insulin, C-peptide and cortisol is usually sufficient to establish a diagnosis.[4,16] Finally, it should be noted that hypoglycaemia may be due to a secondary effect of a primary or secondary tumour directly obliterating normal endocrine tissue and resulting in a hormone-deficiency syndrome (e.g. hypopituitarism, adrenocortical failure) and that resection of a phaeochromocytoma can result in a severe 'rebound' hypoglycaemia.

Lactic Acidosis

This condition, defined as the development of a metabolic acidosis in association with a raised blood lactate, is an uncommon association with cancer. The most common form is type A, associated with circulatory collapse, owing to immunosuppression, infection, septicaemia and shock. In hospital this is most commonly caused by the immunosuppressive effects of radiotherapy or chemotherapy, but it can occur purely in association with an untreated malignancy. Type B lactic acidosis, in the absence of shock, occurs much less commonly but is associated with acute myeloid leukaemia, lymphoma, and Hodgkin's disease, and also occasionally with lung, breast and colonic carcinoma, and osteosarcoma. This type is often more stable and chronic but may be progressive. Diagnosis requires the demonstration of low blood pH and/or respiratory compensation (tachypnoea and a normal, slightly lowered or slightly elevated pH) and elevated blood lactate (>2 mmol/L (>0.22 mg/dL)).

The mechanisms responsible for lactic acidosis in cancer patients do not appear to be different from those in any other disorders, but are particularly associated with large tumours and a degree of liver impairment.

Fat Metabolism

Cancer appears to have little direct effect on fat metabolism. There is an increased rate of fat mobilization as determined by rates of release of free fatty acids and glycerol into plasma but this is seen only in patients with weight loss.[17] Fat oxidation is increased in cancer patients, but is usually associated with, and may be secondary to, weight-loss or cancer cachexia.

Plasma Lipids

Hypertriglyceridaemia and low concentrations of high-density lipoprotein–cholesterol have been described in association with breast, lung, and gastric cancer in women when compared with appropriate age- and sex-matched controls, but resection of the tumours appeared to have no effect on the blood lipid concentrations.[18]

Cancer treatment can have quite marked effects on lipid metabolism. Tamoxifen, an oestrogen antagonist used for the treatment of breast cancer, can lower blood cholesterol, apolipoprotein-B and low-density lipoprotein–cholesterol, particularly in post-menopausal women. This effect is probably due to an oestrogen agonist effect on liver protein synthesis.[19] Cyclosporin, an immunosuppressive compound used in bone-marrow transplantation, can also cause marked hypertriglyceridaemia.[20]

Protein Metabolism

There is very little evidence that cancer *per se* has any effect on protein metabolism. Although a net increase in protein turnover may be demonstrated in some cancer patients when compared with suitably matched controls with equivalent weight loss, and although there may be a net increase in protein catabolism, these are not universal features in cancer but more related to cancer cachexia.

Plasma Proteins

Hypoalbuminaemia can be a very prominent feature of most cancers; the albumin is decreased more in malignancy than in non-malignant conditions[21] and apparently precedes the clinical manifestations of cancer by some years. The reasons for this are poorly understood. In the past, a low albumin has been attributed to malnutrition in cancer, but poor nutrition does not generally have any great effect on albumin concentrations. Experimentally, albumin degradation rates are apparently normal, fractional synthetic rates are increased and transcapillary escape rates are also increased, which would argue for a capillary leak of albumin as being the main factor causing hypoalbuminaemia in cancer, as in the acute-phase response to sepsis and trauma.

Total protein concentrations in plasma may be elevated in malignancy, owing to immune stimulation with or without superadded sepsis, or to secretion of monoclonal protein by the tumour (as in myeloma and related malignancies). More often, total protein is decreased in association with hypogammaglobulinaemia due to extensive obliteration of bone marrow by tumour or intensive chemotherapy. Serum electrophoresis will often show a typical acute-phase response, which may be related to sepsis but may also be mediated by cytokines secreted by a tumour, although there is very little evidence for this. Sometimes an oligoclonal pattern, which is often associated with severe infection, generally viral and hepatitic, is seen during or after intensive chemotherapy; a similar picture may be seen with no obvious evidence of infection, although usually in advanced malignancy. Bone marrow recovery after high-dose chemotherapy and immunosuppressive therapy in transplantation is also associated with an oligoclonal response.

Surprisingly few of the routinely assayed, specific plasma proteins, other than those associated with the acute-phase response, myeloma and B-cell malignancies, are affected by malignancy in any significant way, and these have only been reported as being elevated in a few specific malignancies where their value as tumour markers has been assessed.

Energy Metabolism

Cachexia

Weight loss is commonly a presenting feature of cancer and a significant sign that malignant disease is present. Where weight loss is severe and the patient has anorexia, lethargy, muscle wasting, loss of body fat, hypoproteinaemia, anaemia and oedema the syndrome is called *cachexia*. The principal changes in body composition in cancer cachexia are a 70% or more loss of body·fat and skeletal muscle.[22] The degree of weight loss found at presentation of the cancer varies quite considerably; for example, patients with breast cancer and sarcoma have a low incidence (30–40%) and those with pancreatic and gastric cancer a high incidence (80–90%), such differences not being entirely due to the fact that the more occult tumours present at a later stage. The speed at which cachexia develops also seems to vary depending on the tumour type, carcinomas of the lung, oesophagus and stomach being particularly prone to rapid wasting. Weight loss is simply due to a failure of energy input to match energy output and there are several possible factors responsible for this in cancer.[22,23]

1. Reduced Energy Input

This could be due to:

(a) *Mechanical obstruction.* Obstruction may be due to primary tumours of the gastrointestinal tract (oesophageal, gastric, pancreatic and colonic carcinomas) or secondary tumours invading the gut, preventing or delaying the absorption of food. This is easily identifiable and certainly not the cause in the vast majority of cancers. Rapid intestinal transit with diarrhoea is a possible mechanism, as in the carcinoid syndrome, but this is more often associated with surgical treatment of gastrointestinal malignancy and has to be particularly severe to cause cachexia.

(b) *Reduced food intake.* This may be due to anorexia, nausea and vomiting. This is very common and anorexia can be a complaint of as many as 40% of patients in an oncology clinic and 70% of cancer patients with weight loss. Although an almost universal feature of cytotoxic chemotherapy it is also a feature of many untreated cancers, for ill-understood reasons. Altered taste sensation, depression and anxiety can all affect intake but anorexia can occur for no obvious reason and it may be a paraneoplastic effect in many patients.

(c) *Inadequate absorption or utilization of carbohydrate, fat and protein by cells.* There is no real evidence for any gross defect in the utilization of basic fuels. In spite of the prevalence of glucose intolerance, frank diabetes with weight loss is unusual in cancer, and some associations of mild hyperlipidaemia with certain cancers do not imply any gross defect in fat utilization in the vast majority of cancers (see above). There may, however, be a defect in protein anabolism, as it is known to be difficult to replace lean body mass using parenteral nutrition in cancer patients, despite provision of adequate calories.

2. Increased energy output.

Increased energy expenditure is also undoubtedly a feature of many tumours, but the difference is not so obvious when the sufferers are matched with patients having similar weight loss due to benign disease. There is certainly a heterogeneity of metabolic response; some tumours (sarcomas, leukaemias and carcinoma of the bronchus) produce a hypermetabolic response, others a hypometabolic response (pancreatic, hepatobiliary tumours) and some have no effect on metabolic rate. Possible mechanisms are:

(a) increased demand by the tumour (large tumours);

(b) increased utilization of energy-wasting metabolic cycles such as the Cori cycle and protein turnover;

(c) toxic effects on cells which, in combination with inadequate replenishment or conservation of protein, cause nitrogen loss.

It is still not clear which of these mechanisms is responsible, either alone or in combination with any other factors, for significant weight loss in most cancers.

The metabolic response to cancer in the presence of weight loss very closely resembles the metabolic response to sepsis and trauma and it is possible that similar underlying mechanisms may be involved, mediated by the same classes of cytokines implicated in the acute-phase response and inflammation. The fact that there is experimental evidence for a number of energy-wasting metabolic changes remote from the site of a tumour, such as the increase in whole-body protein turnover, and that these can occur in patients with apparently small tumours, provides circumstantial evidence for a humoral mediator for cachexia in at least some cases. Attention has been directed mainly to factors that may cause accelerated protein turnover or nitrogen loss, or which activate fat stores.

Cachectin or tumour necrosis factor is a 17 000 Da polypeptide, secreted by macrophages, that apparently causes endotoxic shock and, from consideration of animal experiments, has been postulated as a mediator of cachexia in cancer and sepsis.[25] Its effect when infused into human subjects is to cause nitrogen loss, but this is rather surprisingly thought to be due to the anorexia it causes rather than any effect on metabolism.[26] There is also some evidence for 'lipolytic' factors such as toxohormone in some tumours, but no clear evidence or theory that relates these to any mechanism of weight loss in cancer.

Mineral Metabolism

Hypercalcaemia

Hypercalcaemia is a common complication of malignancy, with as many as 20% of patients experiencing it at some stage in the course of their disease. As a cause of hypercalcaemia, malignancy accounts for the majority of cases in most hospital series[27,28] but slightly less in population surveys where hyperparathyroidism predominates (primary hyperparathyroidism due to the eutopic or ectopic production of parathyroid hormone (PTH) by tumours of the parathyroid glands is dealt with below). The most commonly associated tumours are breast and bronchial tumours (Table 9.1), which are also the most common neoplasms found in the general population; these tumours are also usually metastatic. However, some types of tumour are associated with hypercalcaemia far more commonly than might be expected from their population prevalence and frequency of metastatic spread. Myeloma is an uncommon malignancy but has the highest prevalence of hypercalcaemia (33%), five times that of the next most prevalent,

TABLE 9.1

MALIGNANCIES ASSOCIATED WITH HYPERCALCAEMIA (DATA FROM TWO MAJOR SURVEYS)

Tumour site	Total cases (%)	
	Mundy et al. (1985)[29]	Fisken et al. (1980)[28]
Lung	35	25
Breast	25	20
Myeloma	7	6
Lymphoma	6	5
Head and neck	6	7
Renal	3	3
Prostate	3	1
Unknown	7	5
Others	8	28*

* This group included 7% ureters, bladder and urethra; 6% female genital tract; 6% oesophagus as well as large bowel, thyroid, liver and biliary, melanoma, testis, osteosarcoma and pancreatic tumours.

oesophageal cancer (6.5%). Myeloma is always associated with extensive metastatic spread, but cancers such as oat-cell carcinoma of the bronchus also commonly metastasize to bone and rarely cause hypercalcaemia. The tumour types causing hypercalcaemia can be divided into three clinical categories:[29]

1. *Solid tumours with metastases* (70% cases). This group includes carcinoma of the breast, kidney, ovary, thyroid and adrenal. They usually present with hypercalcaemia at a late stage with widespread bony deposits.

2. *Solid tumours without metastases* (10% cases) (humoral hypercalcaemia of malignancy). This group includes squamous-cell carcinomas of the lung, oesophagus, head and neck, skin; carcinomas of the pancreas, liver, colon, ovary, bladder and prostate, renal-cell carcinoma and melanoma. These tumours present with hypercalcaemia at an early stage and bony deposits, as determined by radiology or bone scan, are absent.

3. *Haematological malignancies* (20% cases). This group is dominated by myeloma but also includes adult T-cell leukaemia/lymphoma and rarely Hodgkin's lymphoma, non-Hodgkin's lymphoma and chronic myeloid leukaemia. Myeloma frequently presents with hypercalcaemia and widespread bony deposits whereas the others are more heterogeneous in presentation.

Mechanisms of Hypercalcaemia in Malignancy. Plasma calcium concentrations are regulated in the short-term in normal people by PTH, which is released by the parathyroids in response to a fall in calcium in the extracellular fluid. The action of PTH is to promote osteoclastic resorption of calcium, renal resorption of calcium and loss of phosphate, and to stimulate the synthesis of 1,25 dihydroxy vitamin D (1,25(OH)$_2$D), which in turn, and more slowly, promotes calcium absorption from the gut. Hypercalcaemia of malignancy can be explained by the shifting balance between these normal homeostatic processes of bone resorption, renal clearance and intestinal absorption of calcium. There seem to be clear differences in their relative contributions, leading to the recognition of three groups of tumours listed above and further described below.

Increased bone resorption seems to be the primary process causing hypercalcaemia in malignancy and is probably the *sine qua non* for all but a few, very rare cases. However, excess calcium is adequately cleared by the kidneys if normal regulating mechanisms operate, up to a maximum of about 15 mmol/day (600 mg/day). A certain degree of impairment of renal clearance of calcium must therefore be present before hypercalcaemia is manifest unless the renal calcium load is extremely high. Intestinal absorption of calcium is generally decreased in malignancy hypercalcaemia secondary to suppression of PTH, although this may be an important factor in some of the rarer haematological malignancies where 1,25(OH)$_2$D may be synthesized.

In group 1—*solid tumours with metastases*—there is extensive bone resorption probably mediated by (i) a direct effect of the tumour on bone demineralization or (ii) activation of osteoclasts directly by the tumour or cells activated in response to the tumour. There is now growing evidence that a number of cytokines (interleukin-1$\alpha\beta$, tumour necrosis factor-α (cachectin), tumour necrosis factor-β (lymphotoxin) or growth factors (transforming growth factor-α) with potent hypercalcaemic actions secreted by the tumours or by cells activated by the tumours are responsible for this, acting in a paracrine or autocrine fashion.[30,31] All of these factors stimulate osteoclastic bone resorption *in vitro* and growth of osteoclasts or their precursors *in vitro*, as well as causing hypercalcaemia when injected or infused into mice, but none, as yet, has been shown to be elevated in the serum of any patients with malignancy and they seem unlikely to produce any distant (endocrine) effects. Prostaglandins of the E series have long been implicated in this group; they do stimulate bone resorption *in vitro* and have been found to be elevated in some tumours. Indomethacin, a prostaglandin inhibitor, has rarely been reported to be effective in cases of hypercalcaemia, but the effects of some of the cytokines may be mediated by prostaglandins. Renal impairment of calcium clearance must also play a part in precipitating hypercalcaemia, as the patients often have advanced disease and infection, haemorrhage, vomiting and dehydration, which will all tend to reduce glomerular filtration rate (GFR) and calcium excretion.

In group 2—*solid tumours without metastases*—there are no disseminated deposits to account for the significant degree of local bone resorption, and the

TABLE 9.2

THE BIOCHEMICAL FEATURES OF HYPERCALCAEMIA OF MALIGNANCY AND PRIMARY
HYPERPARATHYROIDISM (1° HPT)

	Group 1	Group 2	Group 3		
		HHM	Myeloma	Lymphoma	1°HPT
Serum					
Calcium	↑	↑	↑	↑	↑
Phosphate	N or ↑	↓	N or ↑	N or ↑	↓↓
Chloride	N	N	N		↑
ALP	↑↑	N or ↑	N	N or ↑	N or ↑
PTH	↓	↓	↓	↓	↑
1,25(OH)$_2$D	N or ↓	N or ↓	↓	↑	↑/↑↑
Urine					
Cyclic AMP	↓	↑	↓	↓	↑

Abbreviations: ALP, alkaline phosphatase; 1,25(OH)$_2$D, 1,25 dihydroxy vitamin D; HHM, humoral hypercalcaemia of malignancy; N, normal; PTH, parathyroid hormone.

secretion by the tumour of a humoral PTH-like factor has been suggested to account for hypercalcaemia. The biochemical features of these tumours (Table 9.2) provide strong circumtantial evidence for a substance with effects similar to PTH on calcium resorption from bone and renal clearance. This was originally thought to be ectopic PTH but as more reliable immunoassays for biologically active PTH have been introduced, it has become obvious that PTH is not raised but rather is low in almost all cases of malignant hypercalcaemia. The cardinal biochemical feature of humoral hypercalcaemia of malignancy (HHM) is an increase of nephrogenic cAMP in the urine, which can be produced by the action of PTH on the renal tubule. It has long been known that there is a factor in the tumour and serum of patients with HHM that stimulates renal tubule adenyl cyclase and increases glucose-6-phosphate dehydrogenase activity but which is inhibited by synthetic inhibitors of PTH. This factor has been purified by a number of groups from squamous and breast carcinomas, and from cell cultures of human squamous and renal carcinoma lines, and has been found to consist of two peptides of 6000–9000 Da and 16 000–18 000 Da.[32,33] Eight of the first 13 amino-acids of the N-terminal fragments of the peptides were found to be identical to the N-terminal fragment of PTH, hence its name—*parathyroid hormone-related protein* (PTHRP). Its mRNA has been cloned as cDNA, and mapped to the short arm of chromosome 12 (the *PTH* gene maps to chromosome 11), and its sequence determined. It appears to consist of 177 amino acids, of which 141 appear in the mature peptide. The rest of the molecule shows little homology with PTH. Peptides, synthesized from the deduced sequence, have identical effects to PTH on kidney and bone, stimulating osteoclastic bone resorption *in vitro* and *in vivo*. It is produced by normal keratinocytes, lactating mammary glands, the placenta, parathyroid

glands and the central nervous system. Immunoradiometric and radioimmunoassays to the biologically active N-terminal end (1–74) of the molecule show that PTHRP is elevated above normal in 83% of cases of HHM and in no cases of local osteolytic hypercalcaemia (these were three cases of myeloma, four of breast carcinoma and one lung tumour—groups 1 and 3), hyperparathyroidism, or non-malignant hypercalcaemia. Some non-hypercalcaemic patients (2 out of 23) and one patient with chronic renal failure had elevations of PTHRP above normal. Concentrations were particularly high in breast milk. The C-terminal assay (109–138) showed elevations in all patients with chronic renal failure and more patients with local osteolytic hypercalcaemia.[34] Its role as the mediator of HHM seems well established. More extensive surveys of PTHRP are required to evaluate fully its role in groups 1 and 3.

Hypercalcaemia in group 3—*the haematological malignancies*—is dominated by myeloma, which accounts for most cases. The mechanism in myeloma appears to be similar to that in group 1, in that the hypercalcaemia is usually associated with widespread metastases, and myeloma is particularly likely to present at a metastatic stage. A locally secreted factor, termed osteoclast activating factor, was thought to be responsible, but this term is now regarded as including a variety of putative compounds or cytokines as described above. As in group 1, bone resorption is not the only operative factor; hypercalcaemia in myeloma is rarely manifest unless there is a significant degree of renal impairment, implying that the excess plasma calcium is adequately excreted by the kidney until GFR is reduced. Renal disease is also a very common complication of myeloma, owing to the direct toxic effects of monoclonal immunoglobulins and light-chain deposition in the kidney. Hypercalcaemia in Hodgkin's disease and non-Hodgkin's lymphoma is unusual, even though bone involvement is not uncommon; the incidence ranges from as low as 0.5% and 3%, respectively, in small series to as high as 5.4 and 13% in large series of patients. In contrast, adult T-cell leukaemia-lymphoma, which is associated with the human T-cell lymphotrophic retrovirus type 1, and cutaneous T-cell lymphoma have very high frequencies of hypercalcaemia (24–100%). Although most cases with hypercalcaemia have extensive bone involvement, there is now strong circumstantial evidence that in those cases without significant metastatic disease, hypercalcaemia is also an indirect effect mediated by a humoral factor, in this case 1,25-dihydroxycholecalciferol (1,25(OH)$_2$D). Breslau et al.[35] reported elevated concentrations of 1,25(OH)$_2$D in three patients with non-Hodgkin's lymphoma, and there have been further reports of elevated 1,25(OH)$_2$D in this and Hodgkin's disease. The patients tend to have significant degrees of renal impairment, no or very little evidence of bone disease on bone scan or marrow biopsy, low PTH concentrations (or lower than expected for the degree of renal impairment), and, where measured, normal or low nephrogenic cAMP, low renal tubular maximum reabsorptive rates for phosphorus (Tm$_P$/GFR), high fasting calcium excretion, and high mean fractional ^{47}Ca absorption. Activity of 'osteoclast activating factor' was also absent when tested on cell cultures in one patient and urinary excretion of prostaglandin E has been usually low normal. Glucocorticoids, chemotherapy and even surgical removal of primary tumour have all resulted in restoration of serum calcium and 1,25(OH)$_2$D to normal. One patient showed an elevation of calcium and 1,25(OH)$_2$D in response to ultraviolet irradiation, the response disappearing after chemotherapy and clinical remission of the tumour.[36] The similarity of the humoral effect to the hypercalcaemia of sarcoidosis suggests that the mechanism may be excess production of 1,25(OH)$_2$D by 1-α hydroxylase present in the tumour, causing increased intestinal absorption and increased bone resorption of calcium. As with myeloma it is clear that these cases usually have renal impairment along with the hypercalcaemia.

Effects of Therapy. Tamoxifen and oestrogens used in the treatment of breast cancer in some patients cause an acute hypercalcaemia on initiation of therapy. This coincides with an acute exacerbation of tumour symptoms and signs. The mechanism is not entirely clear but appears to be related to a transient stimulation of tumour deposits acting locally in bone to cause hypercalcaemia.

Hypocalcaemia
This is not seen in association with cancer except where it is due to treatment, usually an effect of therapy due to:

(a) cytotoxic chemotherapy causing hypoparathyroidism;

(b) cis-platinum;

(c) L-asparaginase;

(d) secondary to hyperphosphataemia in the tumour lysis syndrome

The Tumour Lysis Syndrome. This syndrome occurs after the treatment of certain particularly sensitive or large tumours, usually lymphoblastic malignancies such as Burkitt's lymphoma, lymphoblastic lymphoma and acute lymphoblastic leukaemia.[37] It is thought to be caused by the rapid and massive release of phosphate, potassium, uric acid and other intracellular substances into the circulation by the lysing tumour cells. It occurs within the first 5 days of therapy and patients show weakness, cardiac arrhythmias and sometimes acute renal failure, presumably due to hyperkalaemia and hyperuricaemia precipitating an acute uric-acid nephropathy. There is a marked hyperphosphataemia which secondarily causes a hypocalcaemia and which can lead to tetany especially if bicarbonate has been given to prevent precipitation of uric acid in the kidney. Acute renal failure will also exacerbate the hyperphosphataemia and hyperkalaemia. It is now usually avoided in these tumours by giving allopurinol 24 h before therapy.

Phosphate
Hyperphosphataemia is usually due to renal failure associated with cytotoxic therapy or the direct effects of advanced cancer, or, more rarely, to the tumour lysis syndrome.

Hypophosphataemia is a feature of the rare and apparently paraneoplastic syndrome of tumour-associated osteomalacia.[38] It is associated predominantly with mesenchymal tumours (haemangioma, haemangiopericytoma, bone tumours) and presents clinically as a hypophosphataemic osteomalacia with generalized bone pain and weakness, a low serum and high urinary phosphate with a reduced tubular resorption of phosphate, a normal serum calcium, PTH and 24,25-dihydroxy vitamin D$_3$, low concentrations of 1,25(OH$_2$)D, a raised serum alkaline phosphatase, and a normal creatinine clearance and urinary calcium. It resembles inherited hypophosphataemic rickets most closely, and is usually best treated by removal of the tumour.

Magnesium
Neoplasia has no direct or indirect effect on magnesium metabolism. However, hypomagnesaemia is associated with the therapeutic use of cisplatin or aminoglycoside, which both cause a renal tubular loss of magnesium.

Endocrine System
Hormonal Excess Syndromes
The endocrine system has major effects on metabolism and many of the indirect or paraneoplastic effects of neoplasia on metabolism are due to hyper-

TABLE 9.3
MULTIPLE ENDOCRINE NEOPLASIA (MULTIPLE ENDOCRINE ADENOMATOSIS)

Type I (MEA I)	Type IIA (MEA II)	Type IIA (MEA III)
Tumours		
Parathyroid adenoma/ hyperplasia	Bilateral MTC* (relatively benign)	Bilateral MTC (relatively aggressive)
Pancreatic-islet adenomas (β or non-β cells)	Phaeochromocytoma (bilateral or extra-adrenal)	
Pituitary adenomas (functioning or non-functioning)	Parathyroid hyperplasia	
Adrenocortical adenomas		
Thyroid adenomas		
Lipomas		
Carcinoid (foregut)		
Clinical Features		
	Autosomal dominant inheritance	Mucosal neuromas Marfanoid body habitus Optic nerve abnormal

* MTC, medullary thyroid carcinoma.

secretion of hormones by ectopic or eutopic tumours; in this sense many of the hormonal excess syndromes can be described as paraneoplastic. Ectopic hormone secretion is probably more common than eutopic hormone secretion because endocrine tumours, particularly malignant ones, are quite rare and tumours of the lung, which are commonly responsible for ectopic secretion (in particular small-cell carcinoma of the lung) are much more common. Even though the incidence of hormone excess syndromes in these tumours is quite low, excess hormones are often detected in the serum, with an incidence estimated to approach 50% for lung cancer, which indicates that the hormone can be present pre- or subclinically in many cases. Some of the reasons for this may be:

1. The hormones assayed are not always the active ones, having been released in a different form (as larger precursor molecules, partially degraded or with different carbohydrate content).
2. The modified hormones have a shorter active half-life.
3. The clinical syndromes take a long time to develop when compared to the time for the tumour to manifest.

The APUD Cell System and Ectopic Hormone Synthesis. Cells that secrete large amounts of polypeptide and peptide hormones and biologically active amines share common cytochemical and ultrastructural characteristic, which has led to the concept that they have a common embryological origin from the neutral crest and form part of a 'diffuse' endocrine system. The cells are called APUD cells, an acronym from *a*mine *p*recursor *u*ptake and *d*ecarboxyla-

tion.[39] Only some of these cells are now thought to be of neural crest origin (thyroid C-cells, chromaffin cells of the adrenal medulla and sympathetic ganglia) and others not (anterior pituitary, pancreatic islet, gastrointestinal tract). The concept is of use in classifying and accounting for the origin of the syndromes of multiple endocrine neoplasia (MEN) (or multiple endocrine adenomatosis (MEA), where there is a hereditary disposition to the development of multiple tumours in endocrine organs and tissue apparently derived from these cells (Table 9.3).[40] However, some of the tumours in these syndromes (parathyroid, thyroid and adrenocortical adenomas) are not APUD cells. APUD cells are thought to be widely distributed in organs derived from the embryonic gut and it is interesting that the majority of tumours that synthesize ectopic hormones show great similarity to APUD cells or cells of neural crest origin and arise in either the embryonic midgut (e.g. carcinoid tumours of the appendix, ileum and jejunum) or foregut (e.g. small-cell carcinomas or carcinoid of bronchus, pancreatic tumours).

The hormonal excess syndromes associated with malignancy are summarized in Tables 9.3, 9.4 and 9.5. The reader is referred to Bone[40] for details of the laboratory diagnosis of the MEN syndromes, to individual chapters on each hormone in this volume for the diagnosis of eutopic hormone-secreting tumours, and to the general references given at the end of this chapter for further details. Only the three most common ectopic hormone syndromes, the ectopic adrenocorticotrophic hormone (ACTH) syndrome, the syndrome of inappropriate antidiuresis (SIAD) and the carcinoid syndrome, will be considered in detail here.

TABLE 9.4

EUTOPIC HORMONE SECRETION BY TUMOURS

Hormone	Tumour	Presentation
Pituitary Tumours		
Growth hormone	Chromophobe adenoma	Acromegaly
Prolactin	Prolactinoma	Galactorrhoea
		Amenorrhoea
		Infertility
Adrenocorticotrophic hormone	Basophilic adenoma	Cushing's syndrome
		MEA I*
Human chorionic gonadotrophin	Choriocarcinoma, hydatidiform mole	Pregnancy
Thyroid Tumours		
Calcitonin	Medullary carcinoma of the thyroid (C cells)	Lump in neck
		Diarrhoea
		MEA II, III
Thyroglobulin (precursor of T_4, T_3)	Papillary and follicular carcinoma	Lump in neck
		MEA I
Pancreatic Tumours		
Insulin (β-cell)	Insulinoma (10% malignant)	Psychiatric, hypoglycaemia
Gastrin	Gastrinoma (60% malignant)	peptic ulcer, diarrhoea
Vasoactive instestinal peptide (VIP)	VIPoma	Watery diarrhoea, hypokalaemia achlorhydria (WDHA syndrome)
Glucagon (α-cell)	Glucagonoma	Weight loss
		Impaired glucose tolerance
		Migratory necrolytic erythema
Somatostatin (δ-cell)	Somastatinoma	Gallstones
		Diabetes mellitus
		Steatorrhoea
Pancreatic polypeptide (PP-cells)	PPoma	Abdominal mass
		Obstruction
Adrenal Medulla/Sympathetic Nervous System Tumours		
Noradrenaline, adrenaline	Phaeochromocytoma (10% malignant)	Sweating, anxiety, palpitations
		Hypertension
		MEA III
		Neurofibromatosis
Noradrenaline, adrenaline, dopamine	Neuroblastoma, ganglioneuroma, ganglioneuroblastoma	Abdominal swelling
Adrenal Cortical Tumours		
Cortisol	Adrenal cortical adenoma or carcinoma (50%)	Cushing's syndrome
Oestrogens		Precocious puberty
Androgens		MEA I
		Virilization, feminization
Aldosterone	Adrenal cortical adenoma (carcinoma, very rare)	Hypertension
		Hypokalaemia
Others		
Parathyroid hormone	Parathyroid adenoma or carcinoma (11%)	Hypercalcaemia
		MEA II
Oestrogens	Ovarian germ-cell	Precocious puberty
		Virilization
Androgens	Testicular germ-cell	Precocious puberty
		Feminization

* MEA, multiple endocrine adenomatosis.

The Ectopic ACTH Syndrome. The first ectopic hormone syndrome described was a case of Cushing's syndrome associated with an oat-cell carcinoma of the lung in 1928[41] and it is now known that the syndrome is associated with many other tumours, usually those of presumptive neuroectodermal or APUD origin.

Tumours Associated with Ectopic ACTH. In 50% of cases these are small-cell (oat-cell) carcinomas of the lung. Carcinoid tumours (bronchial, thymic, and rarely of other sites), pancreatic islet-cell adenocarcinomas, medullary carcinoma of the thyroid, phaeochromocytoma and rarely others account for the rest.

TABLE 9.5
ECTOPIC HORMONE SECRETION BY TUMOURS

Hormone	Tumour	Presentation
Tumours Derived from Neuroectoderm or APUD Cells		
ACTH,LPH,MSH, POMC	SCLC etc. (*see text*)	Muscle weakness, weight loss, oedema, hypertension, hypokalaemia
CRF	SCLC Carcinoid Medullary thyroid carcinoma Pancreatic islet-cell Nephroblastoma Colonic carcinoma	Cushing's syndrome
ADH	SCLC	SIAD
Neurophysin	SCLC	Acromegaly
GH/GHRF	Carcinoid	
Somatostatin	SCLC Medullary thyroid carcinoma	Asymptomatic
Calcitonin	SCLC Carcinoid Breast carcinoma	Asymptomatic
Gastrin	SCLC Ovarian	Peptic ulcer
VIP	SCLC	Watery diarrhoea
Insulin	Carcinoid Pancreatic carcinoma	Asymptomatic
Glucagon	SCLC Carcinoid	Asymptomatic
Non-neuroectodermal or Non-APUD Cell Origin		
PTH	Hepatoma Renal carcinoma Bronchial carcinoma	Hypercalcaemia
GH	Bronchial carcinoma Gastric carcinoma	Osteoarthropathy
Prolactin	Bronchial carcinoma Renal carcinoma	Galactorrhoea Amenorrhoea Infertility
hCG	Bronchial carcinoma Hepatoma Testicular	Gynaecomastia
Erythropoietin	Renal cell, liver and uterine carcinoma	Erythrocytosis

Abbreviations: ACTH, adrenocorticotrophic hormone; ADH, antidiuretic hormone; CRF, corticotrophin-releasing factor; GH, growth hormone; GHRF, GH releasing factor; hCG, human chorionic gonadotrophin; LPH, lipotrophic pituitary hormone; MSH, melanocyte-stimulating hormone; POMC, pro-opiomelanocortin; PTH, parathyroid hormone; SCLC, small-cell lung carcinoma; SIAD, syndrome of inappropriate antidiuresis; VIP, vasoactive intestinal peptide.

It was not until 1962 that the hormonal activity responsible for it, ACTH, was described.[42] Yalow and Berson[43] first recognized that the ACTH secreted ectopically was of much larger molecular mass (22 kDa) than that secreted from pituitary-dependent tumours and with only 4% of the biological activity. It is now known that this form is the ACTH prohormone ('big' ACTH or pro-opiocortin), which gives rise to the physiologically active molecule after tryptic cleavage, and the generation of ACTH and its related peptides from the pro-opiomelanocortin gene is now well established (Fig. 9.2). It is also apparent that many more tumours secrete the precursors (20–30%) than manifest the syndrome. However, concentrations of these precursors or measured ACTH activity do not in general correlate well with clinical stage, course or prognosis, and their value as markers is limited. The same is apparently true of peptides such NPOC (*N*-pro-opiomelanocortin), which are also secreted by these tumours.

Clinical Features. The release of 'big' ACTH rather than ACTH 1–39 probably accounts for the unusual features of the ectopic ACTH syndrome compared to

TABLE 9.6

COMPARISON OF ECTOPIC ACTH SYNDROME WITH CUSHING'S SYNDROME

	Ectopic ACTH	*Cushing's syndrome*
History	Short (days to weeks)	Long (1–12 months)
Presenting features	Muscle weakness, weight loss, oedema, hypertension	Centripetal obesity, cutaneous striae, buffalo hump, moon face
	Male	Female
Hypokalaemic Metabolic alkalosis	+ +	+
ACTH	> 300 ng/L	< 300 ng/L
Abnormal glucose-tolerance test	+ +	+
Cortisol		
0900 h	400– > 10 000 nmol/L (14– > 362 μg/dL)	450–4000 nmol/L (16–145 μg/dL)
Midnight	300– > 10 000 nmol/L (11– > 362 μg/dL)	300–4000 nmol/L (11–145 μg/dL)
Urinary free cortisol	Very high (more than 10–20 × ULN*)	High (less than 10–20 × ULN)

* ULN, upper limit of normal range.

classical Cushing's syndrome, but there is very little hard experimental evidence for this. The main differences between the two syndromes are shown in Table 9.6.

Although small-cell carcinoma of lung accounts for about 50% of reported cases of the ectopic ACTH syndrome, only 2.8–7.2% of cases have the clinical features. Those cases due to bronchial and thymic carcinoids, pancreatic tumours, phaeochromocytoma and the rarer tumours, in contrast, often present in the same way as classical Cushing's syndrome, with a long (1–12 month) history, and with neuropsychiatric symptoms, the cushingoid habitus, hypertension, pigmentation, hypokalaemia, as well as less of a male predominance.

Diagnosis of Ectopic ACTH. There is no absolute way of making a biochemical differentiation between ectopic and eutopic ACTH production. The investigation of patients presenting as suspected Cushing's has been well reviewed elsewhere.[44] The ectopic syndrome in small-cell carcinoma of lung is often based on the association of clinical and biochemical features described above with a history or evidence of a lung malignancy on radiographs, computerized tomographic scan or biopsy. The treatment of, and prognosis in, small-cell carcinoma with ectopic ACTH is poor and identifying the origin of the immunoreactive ACTH less important, but surgical resection and cure are possible with some of the less common tumours, and as these present more commonly mimicking Cushing's, differentiation between ectopic and eutopic sources can be of some use and importance. Treatment is then directed to removal of the tumour, where possible (e.g. bronchial carcinoid, phaeochromocytoma) and correction of the metabolic abnormalities.[45,46]

Syndrome of Inappropriate Antidiuresis (SIAD). This syndrome was first described in 1957 by Schwarz et al.[47] in a bronchogenic carcinoma as hyponatraemia, urinary salt wasting and impaired urinary dilution.

Clinical Features. Bartter and Schwarz[48] defined the principal features of the syndrome as:

1. Hyponatraemia and inappropriately low plasma osmolality.
2. Urine osmolality greater than plasma osmolality.
3. Excessive renal excretion of sodium.
4. Absence of hypotension, hypovolaemia and oedema-forming states (heart failure, cirrhosis, nephrotic syndrome).
5. Normal renal and adrenal function.

If patients are secreting inappropriate amounts of antidiuretic hormone (ADH; vasopressin) and they continue to drink, then they develop a hypotonic hyponatraemia with water intoxication and central nervous effects. This presents clinically as lethargy, confusion or psychosis leading to fits, coma and death. Plasma osmolality is always low (< 280 mosmol/kg) and the plasma sodium is always low and often below 130 mmol/L (about 50% of cases are between 130 and 120 mmol/L); concentrations below 120 mmol/L require immediate intervention.

Tumours Associated with SIAD. These are: small-cell (oat-cell) carcinoma of the lung (approximately 80% of cases), carcinoma of pancreas, bladder, ureter, prostate and duodenum, thymoma, mesothelioma, lymphoma, Hodgkin's disease, leukaemia, Ewing's sarcoma and carcinoid.

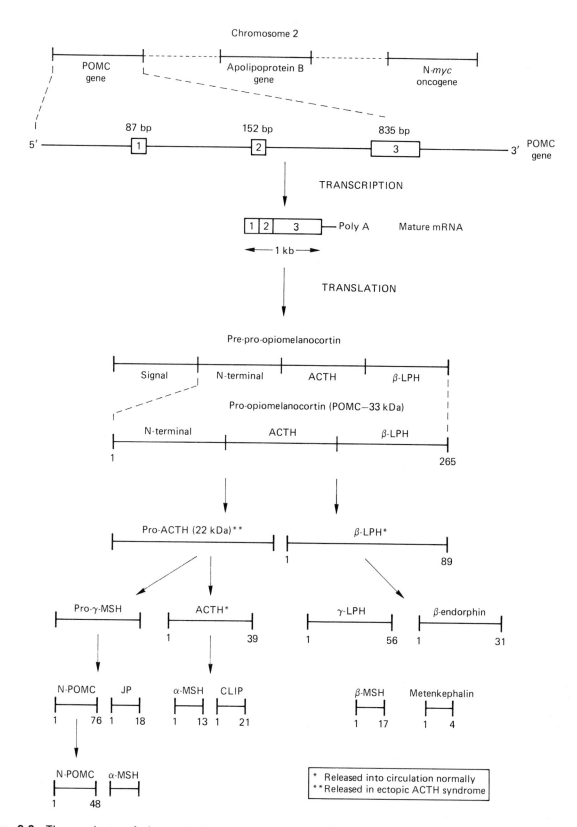

Figure 9.2 The products of the pro-opiomelanocortin (POMC) gene on chromosome 2 and the resulting polypeptides and peptides in serum. *Abbreviations:* bp, base pair; kb, kilobase; ACTH, adrenocorticotrophic hormone; LPH, lipotrophic hormone; MSH, melanocyte-stimulating hormone; JP, joining peptide; CLIP, corticotrophin-like, intermediate-lobe peptide. Numbers of amino-acids are shown under each peptide.

Mechanism of Inappropriate ADH Secretion in Malignancy. As in the ectopic ACTH syndrome, small-cell carcinoma of lung is the tumour found with the highest frequency in this syndrome, with 9% of cases showing the clinical syndrome and direct assay of ADH revealing a far higher incidence of excess hormone in the blood (32–44%). If the response to water-loading tests is examined, abnormal responses are found in 41–69% of small-cell carcinomas and only half have raised ADH with hypotonic plasma. If patients with malignant and non-malignant disease and an apparently typical clinical syndrome are studied, plasma concentrations of arginine vasopressin are not elevated in 80% of cases and the ADH response to hypertonic saline infusion and water loading shows four patterns:[49,50]

1. *Erratic release of ADH* (37% patients). ADH concentrations show wide fluctuations and bear no relation to plasma osmolality. This might be a more appropriate mechanism for random release from a tumour but the pattern is seen in malignant and non-malignant conditions.

2. *Reset osmostat* (33%). Osmotically sensitive ADH release occurs but the regression of ADH on osmolality is shifted to the left (i.e. plasma ADH is completely suppressed at a lower osmolality—270 mosmol/kg). This is also seen in malignant and non-malignant disease.

3. *ADH leak* (16%). An inability to suppress ADH release completely in spite of a normal ADH/osmolality response in the normal range. This is not often seen in malignant disease.

4. *Normal* (14%). These patients have an entirely normal ADH response to changes in osmolality, namely a normal ADH/osmolality ratio and an ability to suppress ADH secretion completely.

Although (1) above may be the most appropriate mechanism for SIAD in malignancy where there is ectopic secretion of ADH by the tumour, there are a number of other causes of SIAD in malignancy:

1. *Eutopic ADH secretion from the neurohypophysis.* Schwartz et al.[47] originally thought that the origin of ADH in their two patients with lung cancer was the pituitary, rather than a tumour product. Many non-malignant conditions that are also associated with SIAD *per se* occur as complications of malignancy, namely meningitis, pneumonia, and space-occupying lesions of the brain (primary or secondary tumours, abscesses).

2. *Effects of chemotherapy.* Some cytotoxic drugs can cause SIAD (vincristine, vinblastine and high-dose cyclophosphamide) and vomiting is a potent stimulus to ADH release: prolonged nausea and vomiting due to chemotherapy, radiotherapy or directly by the tumour could lead to SIAD.

Finally, it should be noted that it is quite difficult to be absolutely sure that the criteria are fulfilled; for example detecting significant degrees of hyper- and hypovolaemia is not always easy clinically, and some cases of hyponatraemia due to 'SIAD' may be misdiagnosed; also, ADH assays are routinely difficult to obtain and confirmation of the appropriateness of ADH concentrations after water loading are rarely obtained in practice. In advanced malignancy, renal and adrenal function may also be impaired and oedema-forming states may be present, due to ascites or lymphatic obstruction, which will make SIAD due to a specific effect of the tumour more difficult to diagnose.

Diagnosis and Treatment of SIAD. The diagnosis still rests primarily on strict adherence to the clinical criteria of Barrter and Schwarz.[48] Measurement of ADH is not routinely used and, owing to the large number of non-tumour specific causes of inappropriate ADH secretion, it is unlikely to be of much use for tumour diagnosis or monitoring. ADH, like ACTH, is synthesized as a larger precursor, neurophysin I, but there is little evidence for it as a major circulating form in malignancy, although a radioimmunoassay for ADH-associated neurophysins has been shown to reflect the clinical course.

Treatment is that of the underlying carcinoma, which is usually small-cell carcinoma of lung and, unfortunately, has a poor prognosis. To alleviate symptoms and prevent the cerebral effects of water intoxication, water restriction is the usual procedure followed by appropriate chemo- or radiotherapy for the tumour where possible. Demeclocycline, an ADH-blocking antibiotic, or frusemide diuresis plus sodium supplements can also be used unless hyponatraemia is severe (< 120 mmol/L) and there is a danger of fitting or coma; hypertonic saline is used in this situation to achieve negative water balance.

Carcinoid Tumours and the Carcinoid Syndrome. 'Carcinoid' was a term coined by Obendorfer in 1907 to describe a tumour of the small intestine that was apparently less aggressive than carcinoma. It was later established that the tumours were composed of argentaffin cells and therefore presumed to be derived from Kulschitsky cells and much later (1953) they were shown to contain 5-hydroxytryptamine (5-HT; serotonin).

They were classified according to the embryonic origin of the site of the carcinoid and biochemical differences in the secreted product (Table 9.7). It was then discovered that they also produced polypeptides such as kallikrein and polypeptide hormones, and Pearse[39] included them as part of the APUD series of tumours (carcinoid apudomas) on the basis of immunocytochemical staining (e.g. strongly positive α-glycerophosphate dehydrogenase, non-specific esterase), classifying many histological carcinoids as insulinomas, vipomas, gastrinomas and other depend-

TABLE 9.7

CLASSIFICATION OF CARCINOID TUMOURS BY EMBRYONIC
ORIGIN AND BIOCHEMICAL PRODUCTS

Origin	Product
Midgut	
Lower duodenum, ileum, jejunum, appendix, caecum	Histologically 'typical' Usually secrete only 5-HT
Foregut	
Bronchus, stomach, biliary tract, pancreatic ducts	Histologically 'atypical' Often secrete only 5-HTP
Hindgut	Biochemically inactive
Rectum	

Abbreviations: 5-HT, 5-hydroxytryptamine; 5-HTP, 5-hydroxytryptophan.

ing on the particular hormones they secreted. In fact, less than half of the tumours Pearse studied had cytochemically detectable 5-HT.

The Carcinoid Syndrome. The carcinoid syndrome is the group of signs and symptoms associated with carcinoid tumours. The syndrome generally occurs in relation to carcinoids that have metastasized to the liver or lung (and are therefore malignant) and the most common site for a primary tumour is the terminal ileum. Carcinoids of the appendix or rectum are rarely malignant and almost never cause the syndrome. Its features are:

1. *Flushing.* This occurs in the face, neck and sun-exposed areas and is frequently accompanied by facial and periorbital oedema, tachycardia and hypotension. The nature of the flushing varies with the site of the primary tumour but that associated with the commonest ileal tumour is episodic, red and cyanotic, and lasts about 30 min. The flushing can be precipitated by various stimuli such as food, alcohol, and pain.

2. *Diarrhoea.* With abdominal pain, tenesmus and even obstruction.

3. *Right heart failure.* This is due to endocardial fibrosis causing stenosis of pulmonary and tricuspid valves. The fibrosis is generalized and can affect the great vessels, the peritoneum (causing retroperitoneal fibrosis and ureteric obstruction), and the pleurae.

4. *Bronchospasm.* This is initially episodic, but can develop into permanent wheezing dyspnoea.

Pathophysiology. The syndrome becomes apparent generally only after the tumour metastasizes because monoamine oxidase in the liver rapidly clears any 5-HT secreted by a tumour draining into the portal circulation, as most intestinal carcinoids do. Bronchial carcinoids release 5-HT directly into the general circulation and more frequently present with the syn-

drome before they metastasize. The diarrhoea and fibrosis are thought to be a direct effect of large quantities of 5-HT in the circulation. Methysergide, a 5-HT antagonist, can cause a very similar pattern of fibrosis, presumably due to partial agonist effects. It is generally the right side of the heart that is affected because the lung also contains large quantities of monoamine oxidase. The cause of the flushing is less clear. It is apparently not 5-HT; α-adrenergic catecholamines are potent stimulators of the flush and it is controlled by antiadrenergic drugs. Prostaglandins and other vasoactive peptides such as bradykinin mediate this effect. The unusual flush seen in gastric carcinoids, with raised wheal-like lesions, may be related to the secretion of histamine by this type.

Patients can also suffer from:

(a) weight loss secondary to malabsorption caused by the diarrhoea and a direct tumour effect (tumour cachexia);

(b) pellagra (nicotinamide deficiency), which is thought to be due to a combination of poor nutrition and diversion of dietary tryptophan to 5-HT production by the tumour and away from the kyneurenine–nicotinic acid pathway (Fig. 9.3);

(c) episodes of hypotension, thought to be due to 5-HT.

Some patients, particularly those with bronchial carcinoids, show the features of ectopic hormone syndromes due to PTH, gonadotrophins, ACTH, insulin and other secreted hormones.

Treatment is by surgical removal for localized tumours. Metastatic tumours are treated surgically to decrease their bulk and the symptoms of carcinoid syndrome alleviated. Flushing is relieved using α-adrenergic receptor-blocking drugs (phentolamine), phenothiazines, which block the action of bradykinin, or sometimes indomethacin, which blocks the synthesis of prostaglandins. Diarrhoea is relieved with 5-HT antagonists (methysergide, cyproheptadine) or with diphenoxylate hydrochloride. Occasionally parachlorophenylalanine, an inhibitor of 5-hydroxytryptophan decarboxylase and tryptophan 5-hydroxylase, is used. Chemotherapy is only used in advanced cases and can precipitate a 'crisis' of severe asthma, diarrhoea and flushing due to rapid tumour destruction.

Biochemical Detection. The main breakdown products of 5-HT in the urine are depicted in Fig. 9.3. Some indole acetic acid and 5-hydroxyindole acetic acid (5-HIAA) is produced by the action of microorganisms in the intestine, particularly if there is a delay or defect in tryptophan absorption. The major urinary metabolite is 5-HIAA and the detection of this in the urine by a colorimetric method using nitrosonaphthol or by high-performance liquid chromatography (HPLC) is still the best way of detecting and monitoring these tumours. Some gastric carci-

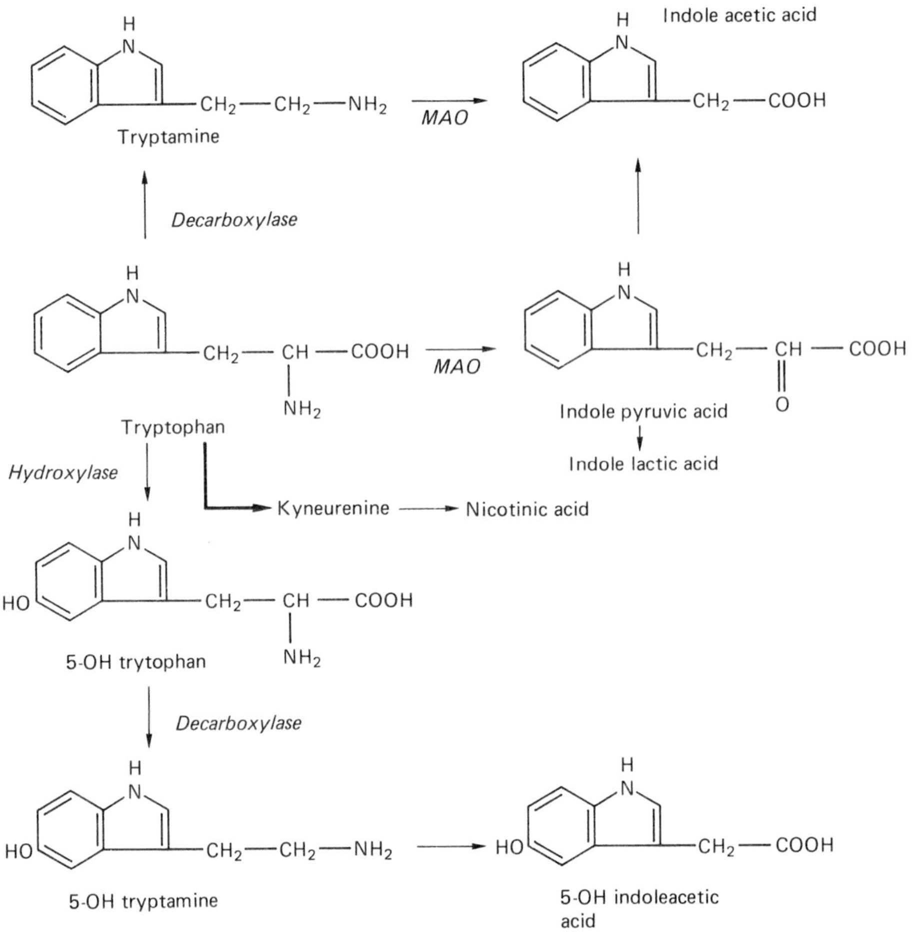

Figure 9.3 The main pathways of tryptophan metabolism in the normal individual: most is normally consumed by the kyneurenine–nicotinic acid pathway; diversion to 5-OH tryptamine synthesis in carcinoid can result in pellagra due to nicotinamide deficiency.

noids secrete 5-hydroxytryptophan, owing to a lack of the 5-HT decarboxylase, and this metabolite appears in the urine; 5-HIAA and 5-HT are still produced in these tumours, due to metabolism of the 5-hydroxytryptophan by the kidney. HPLC can detect the 5-hydroxytryptophan in these tumours.

The assays are subject to positive interference by a wide range of 5-HT-containing foods (bananas, pineapples, walnuts, red plums, avocados, tomatoes), glyceryl guaiacolate in cough preparations (in the colorimetric assay) and reserpine (a physiological effect); and negative interference by phenothiazines.

Hormone-Deficiency Syndromes
Primary and secondary tumours can directly affect endocrine tissue through their expansion, obliteration of the blood supply and destruction of normal tissue resulting in endocrine hypofunction. Endocrine hypofunction is quite rare, although the presence of extensive metastases in endocrine organs is quite commonly seen at autopsy. Unless the blood supply to an endocrine organ is particularly susceptible to obliteration, as in the pituitary, most endocrine organs

can apparently function adequately with a large part of their tissue replaced by tumour deposits. Endocrine hypofunction syndromes due to the direct effects of tumours are summarized in Table 9.8.

Renal System
Malignancy has a number of effects on the kidney and ureters, which manifest in a number of ways but usually result in renal failure. Direct infiltration of renal tissue causing renal failure is, in fact, unusual, even though the kidneys receive about 20% of the cardiac output and may therefore be expected to be a common site for metastatic tumours. Non-Hodgkin's lymphoma is found to infiltrate the kidneys in about 30% of cases, but only half of these show any evidence of renal impairment, which is not necessarily due to the infiltration *per se*. However, direct obstruction of the ureters leading to secondary renal failure is a much more common complication. Other effects are indirect and most commonly associated with myeloma; the secretion of monoclonal proteins, light chains and amyloid deposition and could therefore

TABLE 9.8

HORMONE-DEFICIENCY SYNDROMES CAUSED BY TUMOURS

Hormone	Tumour	Presentation
Pituitary Hormones		
ACTH, GH FSH, LH, TSH and ADH	1. Hypothalamic tumours: Primary—craniopharyngioma (benign), commonest Gliomas, germinomas (malignant) Secondary—metastases from breast and lung carcinomas (uncommon) 2. Pituitary tumours: Primary—adenomas (benign), uncommon Carcinoma (malignant), very rare Secondary—metastases from breast and lung, most common cause	Hypopituitarism of varying degrees and diabetes insipidus
Adrenal Cortisol	Secondary—metastases from lung, breast, kidney, pancreas, stomach and melanoma Rare, even though adrenal metastases from lung tumours are common (28–42% incidence)	Adrenal failure

Abbreviations: ACTH, adrenocorticotrophic hormone; ADH, antidiuretic hormone; FSH, follicle-stimulating hormone; GH, growth hormone; LH, luteinizing hormone; TSH, thyroid-stimulating hormone.

be regarded as paraneoplastic effects of this malignancy. There is also evidence that the immunological response to some tumours leads to indirect renal damage as immune complex disease.

Obstructive Uropathy

Certain primary pelvic tumours that arise close to the bladder—such as carcinomas of the colon, cervix, uterus, ovaries, bladder, urinary tract and prostate—and primary and secondary retroperitoneal tumours that adjoin the ureters—such as lymphoma, carcinoid and sarcomas—are often associated with ureteric obstruction and renal failure. Patients may present with acute renal failure with anuria or with chronic renal failure with nocturia, thirst and polyuria, or, if obstruction is incomplete, intermittent polyuria and oliguria. Anaemia in these patients can be particularly severe, owing to the combination of malignancy and renal failure. Distal tubular dysfunction is a feature of this uropathy, either during or following relief of the obstruction, with:

(a) salt wasting;[51]

(b) the two varieties of hyperkalaemic distal renal tubular acidosis (type IV—hyporeninaemic hypoaldosteronism—and that due to an intrinsic tubular defect) which cause a hyperchloraemic metabolic acidosis;[52]

(c) a diminished urinary concentrating ability.

Uric Acid Nephropathy

This occurs typically with the tumour lysis syndrome but it can occur in patients who have lymphoproliferative disorders before therapy.[53] It is generally an acute uric-acid nephropathy, due to a combination of high serum concentrations of uric acid (> 1 mmol/

L (20 mg/dL)), low tubular pH and high tubular sodium causing precipitation of uric acid in the distal tubules and collecting ducts, and acute intrarenal obstruction and oliguric renal failure. Treatment and prevention of this complication with allopurinol, a xanthine oxidase inhibitor, has also led to the development of a *xanthine* nephropathy due to accumulation of uric acid precursors.

Myeloma

This malignancy is the one most commonly associated with renal disease, due in particular to the nephrotoxic effects of the monoclonal light chains secreted in gross excess by the neoplastic plasma cells. Their deposition, or deposition of their complexes with other proteins, within glomerular vessels, glomeruli, tubular cells and lumina, leads to proliferative glomerulonephritis, membranous nephropathy, amyloid formation, and obstructive nephropathy. These effects are exacerbated by hypercalcaemia and infection, which are both common in myeloma. About 50% of patients have renal impairment at some stage; 50–70% have evidence of renal disease at autopsy, and renal failure is the second most common cause of death (infection being the first).

The renal syndromes associated with myeloma are:[54,55]

1. *Chronic renal failure* (18–60% of patients). This is associated in 80–90% of cases with Bence–Jones proteinuria, in 40–60% with hypercalcaemia, in 10% with amyloid, and also hyperuricaemia and pyelonephritis. Direct plasma-cell infiltration is, as in other malignancies, an uncommon cause.

2. *Acute renal failure* (7–10% of cases). This is associated with hypercalcaemia, dehydration,

infection, hyperviscosity syndrome (rare in myeloma), the use of nephrotoxic antibiotics and of intravenous pyelography, all of which add to the nephrotoxic effects of the light chains.

3. *Proteinuria and the nephrotic syndrome.* Over 90% of patients have some degree of proteinuria, of which 75% have Bence–Jones proteinuria and 25% predominantly albuminuria. The latter have predominantly glomerular disease, which includes those with amyloidosis due to deposition of AL amyloid fibrils (which are derived from light chains). Some of these develop nephrotic syndrome with marked albuminuria and high molecular-weight protein loss, although this is a relatively uncommon syndrome.

4. *Proximal tubular defects.* Fanconi syndrome can occur rarely, with glycosuria, aminoaciduria, phosphaturia and proximal (type II) renal tubular acidosis. Myeloma is probably the major cause of this type of renal tubular acidosis in adults. It is associated with the presence of light-chain crystals in the cytoplasm of the tubular cells. Low molecular-weight proteinuria also occurs as a result of proximal tubular damage with increased excretion of retinol-binding protein, β_2-microglobulin, N-acetyl β-glucosaminidase, and other low molecular-weight proteins and tubular enzymes.

5. *Distal tubular defects.* Renal tubular acidosis types I and IV, nephrogenic diabetes insipidus and salt-wasting occur uncommonly in myeloma, but it is difficult to exclude the effects of hypercalcaemia and general renal failure in many of these patients.

Nephrotic Syndrome

Apart from myeloma there are a number of associations between benign and malignant tumours and various renal nephropathies, usually a membranous nephropathy with the development of proteinuria, the nephrotic syndrome, and the finding of immune complexes in the glomerular basement membrane.[55] They are usually quite rare, but can have a relatively high incidence in some tumours (e.g. 2.3% in carcinoma of the bronchus). In some cases, tumour-specific antigens have been found in the deposits; in others the nephropathy may disappear and relapse along with removal and relapse of the tumour, suggesting a tumour-specific antigen as the cause. Specific tumours have the following associations:

1. Carcinoma of the bronchus, colon and stomach and some benign tumours (e.g. the carotid-body tumour): membranous nephropathy and rarely minimal-change nephropathy. Renal-cell carcinoma (hypernephroma) and carcinomas of the lung, gut, urogenital tract, and melanoma are associated with reactive systemic amyloidosis,

due to the deposition of AA amyloid fibrils, which is also a cause of proteinuria and the nephrotic syndrome.

2. Lymphomas: Hodgkin's disease is associated with amyloid deposition in the kidney and also a minimal-change nephropathy. Amyloid in this disease is now quite rare, owing to better treatment. The amyloid fibrils are AA, not the AL type associated with monoclonal proteins. Minimal-change nephropathy is not associated with immune-complex deposition, but it may also disappear and relapse with treatment and relapse of the malignancy. Patients with type II cryoglobulinaemia may have a proliferative glomerulonephritis with purpura, arthralgia, hypertension, proteinuria, and renal failure. This type is associated with a low serum C3.

Cancer Treatment

Most cytotoxic drugs used in cancer treatment have nephrotoxic effects with secondary metabolic effects; they have been summarized by Boulton-Jones.[55]

The Biochemical Consequences of Neoplasia on Other Systems

Tumours and their secretions have effects on all other body systems and it is not possible to cover all the conceivable biochemical consequences, many of which are described in the chapters on individual systems. The effects are mostly mediated by the general mechanisms and toxic effects of particular tumour products described and illustrated above, and mention should be made of the following systems.

Cardiovascular System

Indirect effects of tumours, such as amyloid deposition secondary to myeloma, excess growth hormone from a pituitary adenoma, excess catecholamine secretion by a phaeochromocytoma, excess 5-HT secretion by a carcinoid tumour and excess PTH secretion by a parathyroid adenoma, can all cause hypertension and progressive heart failure, which may lead to a myocardial infarction and a rise in cardiac enzymes in plasma, but little else of biochemical interest.

Gastrointestinal System

1. *Obstructive jaundice* with raised bilirubin, and raised liver enzyme activities is caused by the *direct* effect of primary or secondary tumour deposits, usually from gastrointestinal, breast or lung malignancies, blocking the bile ducts inside or outside the liver.

2. *Ascites*: this is from a combination of *direct* effects (lymphatic obstruction by tumour—usually carcinoma of the colon, stomach, pancreas or ovary—and raised portal venous pressure due to extensive liver tumour deposits) and low

albumin probably owing to an *indirect* tumour effect causing an increased transcapillary escape rate. It is associated with low plasma albumin and sodium, with marked secondary hyperaldosteronism producing hypokalaemia.

Haematopoietic System

1. *Anaemia*: iron deficiency anaemia (usually as a result of haemorrhage), folate and vitamin B_{12} deficiency (in advanced malignancy), leucoerythroblastic anaemia (due to tumour encroaching on bone marrow) and, rarely, haemolytic anaemias occur in malignancy. The characteristic anaemia of malignancy is the anaemia of chronic disease—with low haemoglobin, serum iron and iron-binding capacity, a normochromic normocytic blood film, an increase in stainable iron in the marrow, and increased erythrocyte sedimentation rate. There is a defect in the utilization of iron in this condition and it may reflect an inflammatory reaction to the presence of tumour.

2. *Porphyria*: cutaneous porphyria has been described in association primarily with primary hepatic carcinoma, but also with liver secondaries and benign hepatomas. It presents as porphyria cutanea tarda with photosensitivity, skin lesions, hair growth and increased pigmentation, and the tumours have been shown to secrete large amounts of urinary coprophyrin, uroporphyrin and faecal porphyrins. Cirrhosis has been found in association with some of these tumours, but the origin of the porphyrins appears to be the malignant tissue itself.

TUMOUR PRODUCTS AS MARKERS OF MALIGNANCY

The products of tumours may serve to signal the presence of that tumour and be of use in its detection and treatment. In the context of clinical biochemistry, it is only those products that are capable of detection in the body fluids by biochemical means that are of interest but the detection of tumour products in tissue sections by biochemical means in histopathology overlaps quite considerably with this area.

The potential clinical requirements for such a tumour marker are as follows; it should ideally:

(a) assist in the detection and diagnosis of primary cancer and facilitate screening of selected groups;
(b) assist in the early detection of recurrence;
(c) assist in predicting the response to therapy and the assessment of prognosis; thus patients may be grouped so that different and perhaps more successful modes of therapy may be used in appropriate groups;

(d) help in the assessment of the response to therapy, that is, help determine if the tumour has been completely or partially eliminated;
(e) help in the localization of metastases, for example to detect central nervous metastases by concentrations of the marker, in cerebrospinal fluid.

The ideal biochemical criteria that a potential tumour marker must fulfil can be considered to be as follows:

1. The marker should be highly specific for the tumour of interest—it should not be elevated above normal in any individuals when the tumour is absent.
2. The marker should be highly sensitive for the tumour of interest—it should always be elevated above normal when the tumour is present in an individual.
3. It should bear a high degree of correlation with the tumour burden.
4. It should be measurable with an analytical imprecision sufficiently low to fulfil criteria (1–3) and within currently acceptable analytical goals.
5. It should possess a sufficiently low intraindividual imprecision to fulfil criteria (1–3).
6. It should possess a sufficiently low interindividual imprecision to fulfil criteria (1–3) on a population basis. A marker with a high interindividual imprecision and a low intraindividual imprecision can still be useful once base-line levels are established.
7. It should be a robust marker—easily and inexpensively measured.

Almost every substance detected in the body fluids has been assessed at one time or another as a tumour marker. In practice, however, very few potential markers satisfy any of the biochemical criteria sufficiently well and do not fulfil any of the clinical requirements to be used on a routine basis. Only three markers, alpha-fetoprotein in the management of hepatoma, the β subunit of chorionic gonadotrophin in the management of molar pregnancy, and the monoclonal immunoglobulins secreted in myeloma approach the ideal and occupy a key role in the clinical management of patients. Some markers, however, meet one or a few of these criteria sufficiently to give them a useful role *in certain well-defined clinical situations*, such that they have found a place in current clinical practice, and these are described below. The reader is referred to the general references for a more complete account of the vast literature on tumour markers and to specific references for those described.

Oncofetal Proteins

Alpha-fetoprotein [56–58]
Alpha-fetoprotein (AFP) was discovered in 1963 by Abelev as a protein normally present in the blood of

newborn or pregnant mice which was also present in mice with transplanted hepatocellular carcinomas. A similar protein was found in serum from human subjects with hepatocellular carcinoma. It was later characterized and found to be very similar to albumin in its amino acid content, molecular mass (70 000 Da in man), isoelectric point (4.8–5.2) and carbohydrate content (4%). It displays some heterogeneity in its carbohydrate content, depending on its tissue of origin.

AFP originates in the embryonic yolk sac, which is derived from the endodermal germ layer of the blastocyst, and which produces AFP within 3 days of conception. The liver, which is also derived from the yolk sac, becomes the major source of AFP as soon as it is recognizable until birth, when albumin synthesis starts and AFP declines. Other fetal organs derived from the yolk sac produce only traces of AFP.

Causes of Elevated Serum AFP. The normal concentration of AFP in serum is less than 5 μg/L (equivalent to 5 ku/L of World Health Organization standard), with a range of less than 2 to less than 10 μg/L depending on the sensitivity of assay used. The plasma half-life is 4–7 days. Serum AFP is elevated in the following conditions (the approximate frequency of this elevation is shown in parentheses).

1. *Neoplastic disease*:
   (a) germ-cell tumours of yolk-sac origin, namely the endodermal-sinus tumour (or pure yolk-sac tumour or orchioblastoma) and embryonal carcinomas (including teratocarcinomas) (40–90%);
   (b) hepatomas and hepatoblastomas (65–90%);
   (c) gastrointestinal carcinomas in organs closely related to the yolk-sac in development viz. biliary tract, stomach, pancreas, colon (7–23%);
   (d) lung and breast tumours (uncommon);
   (e) sarcomas and other non-germinal carcinomas (rarely).

2. *Non-neoplastic diseases*: hepatitis, regenerating liver (after resection), toxin-stimulated liver (e.g. CCl$_4$ poisoning), cirrhosis, tyrosinosis, ataxia telangiectasia, hepatitis surface-antigen carriers, abnormal development of the fetus in pregnancy (multiple pregnancy, neural tube defects, congenital nephrosis, oesophageal atresia).

3. *Normal subjects*: familial raised AFP.

Most of the non-neoplastic elevations are due to liver disease, but the elevations are rarely more than 400 μg/L, except in the case of the inborn error tyrosinosis where they can be very high.

Clinical Use.
1. *Screening and diagnosis.* Although concentration of AFP is elevated in a variety of non-malignant liver diseases, an elevation of more than 400 μg/L in a child or non-pregnant adult has a very high degree of specificity (60–99%) for hepatocellular cancer and yolk-sac tumours. Where cancer of the liver is endemic (China, Alaskan Eskimos), AFP has been used successfully to screen populations for hepatoma, with some evidence of improved survival due to the early detection of small tumours.

2. *Prognosis.* Teratoma patients with AFP of more than 500 μg/L are less likely to have the tumour eradicated by those therapeutic regimens that are successful in patients with a lower AFP.

3. *Monitoring.* The apparent half-life of AFP in blood can give an estimate of the effectiveness of tumour 'kill' by therapy. If AFP concentrations do not decline with the expected normal half-life or a further rise is shown, these are indications of incomplete tumour 'kill' or regrowth of tumour and second-line therapy may be adopted. This has been shown to be of value in hepatoma after hepatectomy and in yolk-sac tumours after first-line treatment. AFP is very sensitive for detection of recurrent tumour, but it should be noted that markers may be lost in recurrence, particularly in germ-cell tumours.

Human Chorionic Gonadotrophin [57–59]
Aschheim and Zondek in 1927 discovered a gonadotrophin in the urine of pregnant women which stimulated the ovaries of rats, mice and rabbits; over the next 4 years it was discovered that this gonadotrophin was also excreted in the urine of individuals with gestational and non-gestational neoplasms. The normal source of human chorionic gonadotrophin (hCG) is the syncytiotrophoblast in pregnancy, appearing in maternal serum at 6–9 days after conception, rising exponentially, peaking at about 8–12 weeks after the last menstrual period, decreasing to a nadir at 17–22 weeks, and remaining constant in the last part of pregnancy. Its early rise and extremely high sensitivity for the trophoblast make it the most reliable marker of pregnancy, and agglutination or colorimetric immunoassays for hCG or β-hCG form the basis of most modern pregnancy tests.

Structure. hCG is a glycoprotein consisting of two subunits: the α-subunit (92 amino acids, 28% carbohydrate, 14 500 Da), which is nearly identical to the α-subunits of thyroid-stimulating hormone (TSH), follicle-stimulating hormone (FSH) and luteinizing hormone (LH) from the anterior pituitary, and the β-subunit (145 amino acids, 28–36% carbohydrate, 22 200 Da), which shows some homology to the β-subunits of those hormones but much less so than the α-subunits. Both subunits are necessary for full biological activity and immunoassays using antiserum raised against the β-subunit distinguish hCG from TSH, FSH and particularly LH, which has 80% of the first 115 amino acids of the molecule at identical positions to the β-subunit of hCG. More recent assays are directed to the 30 carboxyterminal amino acids of β-hCG, which are not present in LH. hCG has intrinsic TSH, FSH and LH activity, owing to its homology, and its biological action is to stimulate the granulosa, luteal and interstitial cells of the ovary and the interstitial cells of the testes.

Causes of Elevated Serum β-hCG. Normal concentrations of β-hCG in the serum of males and non-pregnant females range from 5 to 10 iu/L (1–2 μg/L) depending on the assay, and its serum half-life is 24 h. The degree of cross-reactivity of the assay with physiological levels of LH is of importance for its use as a marker for tumours and pregnancy, particularly in relation to the menstrual cycle. It is elevated in the following conditions (at approximate frequencies shown in parentheses).

1. *Neoplastic disease*:
   (a) gestational trophoblastic disease—hydatidiform mole, invasive mole, choriocarcinoma (100%);
   (b) germ-cell tumours of the testis—seminomas (13%), non-seminomas (54%) (includes embryonal carcinomas (51%)), teratocarcinomas (35%), choriocarcinomas (100%));
   (c) non-trophoblastic tumours (11%)—islet cell (45%), ovarian (epithelial) (39%), carcinoid (29%), non-ovarian gynaecological (27%), breast (26%), gastrointestinal (21%), ear, nose, throat (21%) and many others at lower frequencies. Concentrations in non-trophoblastic tumours are generally quite low (5–25 iu/L).

2. *Non-neoplastic diseases*—benign diseases of lung, breast, gastrointestinal tract, and female genital organs (3%).

3. *Normal subjects* (1%).

Clinical Use. Assay of hCG is most useful in the following tumours.

Gestational Trophoblastic Tumours. β-hCG is used primarily for the detection and monitoring of choriocarcinoma, in which role it approaches the ideal as a tumour marker:

1. *Screening and diagnosis*: elevated serum β-hCG is a highly sensitive marker for trophoblastic tissue but it will not distinguish between a normal pregnancy and gestational trophoblastic tumours (hydatidiform mole, invasive mole and choriocarcinoma). Gestational trophoblastic tumours affect 1 in 1400 normal pregnancies in the UK and are usually detected by clinical history, examination and ultrasound. A clue to their presence is particularly high β-hCG concentrations in blood (> 200 000 iu/L) or urine (> 30 000 iu/24 h), or the failure of hCG to decline after the 8–12 week peak of a normal pregnancy. The real value of the marker becomes apparent in the detection of the 5–10% of patients who progress to an invasive mole or choriocarcinoma after evacuation of a hydatidiform mole, and its measurement forms the basis of a (British) national screening programme.

2. *Prognosis*: the level of hCG is an important prognostic factor in gestational trophoblastic tumours and is used to stratify patients into different groups for more effective forms of therapy. Serum β-hCG of more than 40 000 iu/L is a poor prognostic sign and these high-risk patients receive combination chemotherapy, which results in higher remission rates than are achieved using the single-agent chemotherapy or surgery more appropriate for the low-risk group.

3. *Monitoring*: concentrations of urinary hCG or serum β-hCG are very sensitive to changes in the status of gestational trophoblastic tumours, there being a high correlation between tumour burden as measured by radiology or radionucleotide assessment of the size of metastases and hCG in serum or urine. The rate of fall of β-hCG may be used to judge the effectiveness of therapy, a rate greater than the expected half-life or a rise indicating residual tumour, regrowth of tumour or the development of drug resistance, so allowing further therapy, which, when successful, results in a fall in hCG to undetectable concentrations. Recurrences of trophoblastic tumours are always detected by elevations in urinary hCG concentrations, there being apparently no false negatives. All elevations are worthy of further investigation.

   β-hCG can also be used to localize tumour deposits: cerebral metastases may be detected by measuring the serum:cerebrospinal fluid ratio, which is less than 45 in the presence of metastases. The serum concentration of β-hCG usually greatly exceeds that in the cerebrospinal fluid.

Germ-cell Tumours of the Testis. Measurement of serum β-hCG has a useful role in the diagnosis and monitoring of testicular tumours, where it is thought to reflect the activity of tumour cells of trophoblastic origin (in contrast to AFP, which is a marker of tumour cells of yolk-sac origin). Urinary hCG is too insensitive as a marker for these tumours. Serial measurements of β-hCG and AFP are used to monitor the effectiveness of therapy, but the correlation with tumour burden is not as high as with gestational trophoblastic tumours, and testicular tumours can frequently lose their markers as the tumour relapses or progresses. Also, the response of these markers when secreted by the same tumour can be completely different, probably reflecting their different cellular origin. The use of different markers in germ-cell tumours and other tumours of the testis is summarized in Fig. 9.4.

Non-trophoblastic Tumours. The secretion of β-hCG

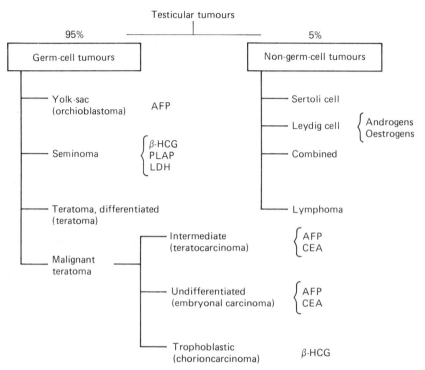

Figure 9.4 The major tumour markers secreted by different testicular tumours; secretion of AFP is usually taken as evidence of yolk-sac elements and β-hCG as evidence of trophoblastic elements in most germ-cell tumours. *Abbreviations:* AFP, Alpha-fetoprotein; β-hCG, β-human chorionic gonadotrophin; PLAP, placental alkaline phosphatase; LDH, lactate dehydrogenase.

by these tumours may be regarded as ectopic but the wide range of tumours which do so and the low concentrations of marker generally present have not led to the adoption of β-hCG as a marker for non-trophoblastic tumours.

Hormones as Tumour Markers. hCG is almost the ideal tumour marker, and happens to be a hormone. The hormones secreted by endocrine tumours might be expected to act as rather good tumour markers, as they tend to be quite specific products of endocrine tissues, have very marked clinical and metabolic effects when produced in excess, and sensitive and specific assays exist for their detection. For most eutopic and benign tumours they act as very good markers, facilitating diagnosis, relating to tumour burden, and assisting in the diagnosis of recurrence. They are rather less good for malignant and ectopic hormone-secreting tumours, due primarily to the infrequency of association with these tumours but also to the different forms of these hormones secreted by such tumours, a problem that can also affect eutopic hormonal tumours. Larger hormonal precursors are commonly secreted in malignancy (e.g. big ACTH, pro-insulin) and may not react in conventional assays, may be secreted more intermittently and may be degraded more rapidly, which could all result in a failure to detect them. Hormonal and other markers

that are of use in endocrine malignancies have been well reviewed by De Lellis.[60]

Carcinoembryonic Antigen[61–63]
Carcinoembryonic antigen (CEA) was discovered in 1965 as an antigen from perchloric acid extracts of human colonic tumours and has been demonstrated, using an antibody prepared in rabbits, in extracts of all tumours from endodermally derived, digestive-system epithelium and in embryonic gut, pancreas and liver cells in the first two trimesters of gestation. With more sensitive immunological techniques it has been shown to be present at low concentrations in the adult gastrointestinal tract and a wide variety of prenatal and adult tissues. CEA appears to be normally secreted into the lumen of the gut but in cancer into the blood and lymphatics, resulting in an increased serum concentration.

Structure. CEA is a glycoprotein of about 180 000 Da with β-mobility on electrophoresis at pH 8.2–8.6. It has a carbohydrate content of about 50%, which shows considerable variation in different tumours and probably accounts for its extensive charge heterogeneity. CEA consists of a single polypeptide chain with six disulphide bridges and the major amino acids are aspartate, asparagine, glutamate and glutamine. Most of the major antigenic determinants are on the protein part of the molecule and the main epitopes are *not* blood-group antigens. There are other normal antigens that cross-react with radioimmunoassays and the CEA family consists of up to 36 glycoproteins. The other principal member of the family is non-specific cross-reacting antigen (NCA), which is of lower molecular mass (60 000 Da) and lower carbohydrate composition (30%) but similar amino-acid composition. These cross-reacting antigens do not generally interfere with competitive radioimmunoassays and more specific polyclonal or monoclonal antiserum preparations are now used to prevent interference with the CEA assay. There are about 10 genes for CEA forming two clusters on chromosome 19 and it is now thought that *CEA* and *NCA* genes form part of the immunoglobulin gene 'superfamily'.

Causes of Elevated Serum CEA. The normal concentration of CEA is 2.5–10 μg/L, depending on the assay used. The serum half-life is unknown but its disappearance by 2 weeks after apparently curative surgery suggests a fairly rapid catabolism. It is elevated in the following conditions (at the approximate frequencies shown in parentheses):

1. *Neoplastic disease*:
(a) carcinoma of colon and rectum (65–90%), carcinoma of stomach (50–70%), carcinoma of pancreas (80–90%), hepatoma (50–60%), carcinoma of lung, breast, gynaecological cancers (30–50%);
(b) lung (non-small-cell carcinoma; about 60%), (small-cell carcinoma; about 30%).

2. *Non-neoplastic disease*:
(a) gastrointestinal—ulcerative colitis, Crohn's disease, polyps, gastroduodenal ulcers, chronic pancreatitis, cirrhosis, acute hepatitis, cholestasis (0–60%);
(b) pulmonary emphysema (50–60%);
(c) benign gynaecological diseases (0–5%)
(d) also trauma, infarction, renal impairment, collagen diseases.

3. *Normal subjects*:
(a) smokers (10–20%);
(b) blood donors (0–4%).

Although the elevation of CEA is often low in non-cancerous diseases (< 10 μg/L), and the highest concentrations are associated with tumours, high concentrations are found in many non-gastrointestinal malignancies.

Clinical Use

1. *Diagnosis.* It is now obvious that CEA has a low specificity for gastrointestinal malignancy, in contrast to optimistic indications from the early studies, and it has very little, if any, diagnostic role. It is only suggestive of colorectal cancer if present at more than 20 μg/L, and can

be suggestive of carcinoma developing in a colonic polyp if greater than 5 times the upper limit of normal, but the clinical possibilities in these circumstances are fairly limited and the diagnosis already partially made.

2. *Monitoring.* CEA has found a role after surgery and radiotherapy for colorectal cancer and for some other CEA-positive cancers. A high concentration postsurgically or only a partial decrease is strong evidence for residual tumour or metastases; if treatment is successful, concentrations generally fall to normal by 1 month. CEA can predict recurrence 4–6 months before clinical detection for colorectal carcinoma but surgically resectable tumours are not often found and rises in CEA do not seem to be reliable enough to base second-look surgery on.

3. *Prognosis.* A raised preoperative CEA is a poor prognostic sign in colonic carcinoma, and the survival of patients is worse if the CEA does not fall to normal after surgery, but these associations do not seem to be high enough to base any treatment strategies on.

Placental Alkaline Phosphatase[64,65]
The placental isoenzyme of alkaline phosphatase (PLAP) is a membrane-bound glycoprotein produced at a gene locus separate from the intestinal and liver/bone isoenzymes. It is highly polymorphic and there are three alleles at the locus giving rise to six common phenotypic variants on electrophoresis, owing to its dimeric structure. With conventional electrophoretic and enzyme heat-inhibition techniques, it is usually only detected in the serum of pregnant females, being produced by the syncytiotrophoblast of the placenta from the 12th week of pregnancy, and disappearing after delivery. In 1968, Fishman discovered the presence of a placental-like isoenzyme in serum from a patient with carcinoma of the bronchus—the Regan isoenzyme. Since then the presence of several other tumour-associated alkaline phosphatase isoenzymes has been noted, similar to the term placental (the Nagao variant), the first-trimester placental (the non-Regan variant) or the fetal intestinal isoenzymes (the Kasahara variant); these are assumed to be expressions of oncofetal or oncodevelopmental proteins by the cancer. PLAP is found with a low frequency (9.5%) in the serum of a variety of cancer patients. With the development of very sensitive radio- and enzyme immunoassays for PLAP these results have been confirmed and the isoenzyme has been found in various tumours, trophoblastic and non-trophoblastic in origin, particularly seminoma (43% at diagnosis and 75–90% with metastatic disease) and ovarian cancer (30–40%, mainly associated with serous cystadenocarcinomas), endometrial (20%), breast (6%) and lung (2%) carcinoma. It can be detected in the blood of normal subjects not only in pregnancy but also in smokers, where significant

elevations are found. Despite this, PLAP may have a useful role in the diagnosis and monitoring of therapy in seminoma because it is frequently elevated in this tumour but not in the other germ-cell tumours, and because its concentration does appear to reflect tumour response.

Non-oncofetal Proteins

Prostate-specific Antigen[66-68]

Prostate-specific antigen (PSA) was discovered and purified in 1979 using an antibody prepared by injecting crude extracts of human prostate into rabbits and simultaneously as a specific protein on acrylamide gel electrophoresis in seminal plasma. It is a 34-kDa glycoprotein, consisting of a single polypeptide chain of 240 amino acids and 7% carbohydrate. It is functionally and antigenically distinct from prostatic acid phosphatase, and is a serine protease. It is quite specific to prostatic tissue and is found in the normal prostatic epithelial lining cells of the acini and ducts.

Causes of an Elevated Serum PSA. The normal concentration of PSA in serum in the most widely used assay is 0–4 μg/L. The decay of PSA in serum after surgery shows a biphasic, logarithmic curve; the initial phase from 0 to 6 h has a half-life of 12.6 $\pm$ 19.7 h and the second phase from 12 h has a half-life of 2.2 $\pm$ 0.8 days, the latter being the main determinant of PSA elimination. Elevations of PSA above the upper limit of normal are seen in the following conditions (at the approximate frequencies shown in parentheses):

1. *Neoplasia*:
   (a) carcinoma of the prostate (80%);
   (b) non-prostatic malignancy (3%)—gastrointestinal, lung (5%), renal (4%), genitourinary (2%), breast (1%).

2. *Non-neoplastic disease*: benign prostatic hypertrophy (20%), genitourinary disease (7%) (including orchitis, prostatitis, urethritis, renal disease), gastrointestinal, cardiovascular, liver, pulmonary, infections, endocrine, immunological disease (2%).
   Acute retention of urine, which is a frequent complication of benign prostatic hypertrophy, also causes an elevation of PSA.

3. *Normal subjects*: female (0%), male (1%), male < 40 years (0%), male $\geqslant$ 40 years (3%).

4. *Surgical procedures*: prostatic massage increases serum PSA by 1.5–2 times at 60 min after massage and needle-core perineal biopsy and transurethral resection of the prostate elevate it 57 times; these effects are transient.

The absolute concentration of serum PSA increases and elevated concentrations of PSA occur with increasing frequency through the clinical stages of pros-

tatic cancer; the logarithm of the serum PSA is very significantly related to the logarithm of the intraprostatic tumour volume as determined by tumour sectioning.

Clinical role. Assay for PSA has some role in diagnosis and monitoring of prostatic cancer.

1. *Diagnosis*. In spite of having a very high degree of specificity for prostatic disease as compared to non-prostatic disease, estimation of PSA is not sufficiently sensitive or specific for prostatic cancer to justify its use in population screening. When used to screen for prostatic cancer at all ages the sensitivity of PSA ranges from 68 to 90% and specificity from 79 to 91%; in the context of a prevalence of 35/100 000 for prostatic cancer in the white male population, the accuracy of detection of prostatic neoplasia by PSA would be far too low to justify screening and unlikely to be better than clinical examination, even in selected age groups. Clinically, however, discrimination between benign prostatic hyperplasia and carcinoma in an elderly man presenting with symptoms of outflow obstruction is the usual diagnostic problem in which a tumour marker is expected to help. Even here, PSA does not sufficiently distinguish between the two at the upper limit of normal (4 μg/L) and 20% or more patients with benign enlargement will have concentrations of PSA that exceed this. For this reason a cut-off of 10 μg/L is used in practice; even at this level, 5–10% of prostatic carcinomas will be missed. However, a PSA of more than 10 μg/L in a patient without urinary retention carries a high probability of prostatic cancer and this could be used to prioritize patients for surgery.

2. *Monitoring.* PSA has an undoubted role in monitoring the success of therapy and recurrence of tumour. A failure of PSA to fall to normal or undetectable concentrations after surgery is associated with an increased risk of tumour recurrence, and elevations of PSA are seen some 6–95 months before clinical recurrence. PSA behaves in a similar way after hormone therapy, with remissions being more prolonged if PSA declines to low, normal or undetectable concentrations, but it is thought that PSA concentrations may be unreliable with this mode of therapy as the expression of PSA appears to require testosterone or dihydrotestosterone, and it is possible that anti-androgen therapy may decrease the expression of PSA in recurrent tumour.

PSA and Prostatic Acid Phosphatase as Markers for Prostatic Cancer. An elevation of acid phosphatases in the serum of patients with metastatic carcinoma of the prostate was first demonstrated in 1938 by Gutman and Gutman. The prostatic isoenzyme (prostatic acid phosphatase; PAP) responsible for this is a glycoprotein of 100 kDa produced by prostatic epithelial cells and secreted into prostatic fluid to a concentration of up to 500–1000 u/L, compared with its usual serum concentration of less than 2–4 u/L. There are a number of ways of measuring its enzymatic activity in serum, using different substrates that are variably specific for the prostatic isoenzyme, or using a specific inhibitor of the prostatic enzyme, commonly L-tartrate. Immunoassays specific for the prostatic isoenzyme have been developed since 1975, in the hope that they would be more sensitive and specific for prostatic cancer. In general, assays for PAP are more specific but less sensitive than those for PSA for the detection of prostatic cancer, and PAP enzyme assays (PAP-EA) are marginally less sensitive and less specific than PAP immunoassays (PAP-IA). Sensitivity and specificity are very dependent on the cut-off value used for classification, however, and the accuracy of classification of a test into diagnostic groupings is better assessed by a receiver (or relative) operator characteristic curve; using this, PSA is better than PAP-IA and PAP-IA better than PAP-EA for its accuracy of diagnostic classification.[68] Clinically there may be some degree of independence between the enzyme and the antigen such as to merit the assay of both, particularly for patients on antiandrogen therapy.

Lactate Dehydrogenase

Lactate dehydrogenase has long been known as a non-specific indicator of malignancy, being raised in 65% of patients with liver metastases and 20–60% of those without. In spite of its non-specificity it has recently found a clinical role in the assessment of prognosis in non-Hodgkin's lymphoma, and to detect recurrence and response to therapy in melanoma and seminoma.[65,69]

Neuron-specific Enolase[65,70]

Neuron-specific enolase (NSE) was found during the study of proteins localized in neural tissue and isolated as a soluble acidic protein from brain called 14-3-2. It later became known as neuron-specific protein, then neuron-specific enolase when its enzymic activity was discovered. A further, different enolase activity was then discovered in glial cells and called non-neural enolase (NNE). The differences between these enzymes were resolved as a difference in subunit composition; it is now known that three different gene loci produce three different subunits α, β, γ, and that each isoenzyme consists of two subunits which are $\gamma\gamma$ in NSE and $\alpha\alpha$ in NNE. Other isoenzymes are found in liver ($\alpha\alpha$), heart ($\alpha\beta$) and muscle ($\beta\beta$), but the γ gene is only expressed in neurons. There appears to be a switch from NNE to NSE in the developing brain, and NSE concentrations rise only after birth. NSE is found in all classes of nerve cells, in APUD cells and in other tissues depending on the amount of neural or APUD tissue they contain. Interest has centred around its use as a possible marker in APUD tumours—pancreatic islet-cell tumours, carcinoids, neuroblastoma and small-cell lung carcinoma. It has not proved sensitive or specific enough in any of these tumours to be of clinical use for diagnosis or monitoring, but very high concentrations are associated with a poor prognosis in neuroblastoma, which may be of clinical value in patient stratification for therapy.

Cancer Antigens

Many tumour markers are specifically developed for a particular tumour by raising polyclonal or monoclonal antibodies in hybridomas to extracts of excised tumours or cell lines derived from those tumours. The major antigenic-determinant fractions in these preparations are often membrane glycoproteins or mucins; as the antibodies produced are screened for specificity by their reaction to formalin-fixed sections of the tumour of interest and normal tissue, many of them are directed to the carbohydrate portions of these molecules because these tend to retain their configuration after fixing.

Carbohydrate Antigens

CA 125. This is an antigen in an ovarian carcinoma cell line identified by a monoclonal antibody (OC 125). The antigen is a high molecular-weight glycoprotein but the detailed structure of the epitope is still unknown. The antigen is detectable by immunocytochemical means in the epithelium of the fallopian tubes, endometrium, cervix, mesothelial cells (pleura, pericardium, peritoneum), Müllerian epithelium, fetal serosa and amniotic fluid but *not* in normal or fetal ovarian tissue.

The normal mean serum concentration of CA 125 is 8.7–11.2 u/mL with a standard deviation (SD) of 8.9–5.4 and the upper limit of normal is conventionally taken as 35 u/mL, as only 0–1.8% of normals exceed this value. Females have values 1–3 u/mL higher on average. It is elevated in 60–85% of ovarian carcinomas, the serous type usually having greater concentrations (2000–4000 u/mL) than the mucinous type (100–200 u/mL), but is also elevated in other gynaecological malignances (carcinoma of the fallopian tubes, cervix and endometrium) and in non-gynaecological malignancies (pancreatic, biliary tract, lung and breast carcinoma, mesotheliomas and Krukenberg tumours), although the concentrations are not generally as high as in ovarian carcinoma. Unfortunately, CA 125 is also elevated in a wide variety of non-malignant diseases or conditions both gynaecological (pregnancy, menstruation, endometriosis, pelvic inflammatory disease, uterine fibroids) and non-gynaecological (cirrhosis, ascites, hepatitis, pancreatitis, peritonitis, autoimmune disorders, endocrine disorders), although the elevations are usually not much greater than 65 u/mL. This seriously undermines the usefulness of CA 125 alone as a screening test or as a diagnostic aid for gynaecological disorders or malignancy when it is only slightly elevated but does not exclude its use in combination with other screening procedures. However, in a patient with ovarian carcinoma, CA 125 is related to tumour size, stage of disease and type of tumour, and it probably has a role in the monitoring of this malignancy. Concentrations correlate with clinical course in 92–94% of cases on chemotherapy; it has a sensitivity of 97% in follow-up and a lead time of 1–17 months in recurrence. It is superior to CA 19–9 and CEA in these respects, and these latter markers do not add any further useful information.

CA 19–9. CA 19–9 was an antigen detected in the cell membrane of a human colon carcinoma growing in culture by a monoclonal antibody raised to extracts of that tumour. Its antigenic determinant has now been shown to be the sialylated form of the Lewis oligosaccharide, a blood group antigen (sialylated lacto-*N*-fucopentanose II). It is found in a wide variety of normal tissues (pancreas, liver, gallbladder, lung) and body fluids (pancreatic and gastric juice, milk, saliva, cervical mucus).

The mean serum concentration ($\pm$ SD) is 8.4 ± 7.4 u/mL and a cut-off of 37 u/mL is taken as the upper limit of normal, with only 0.4% of normal subjects showing higher concentrations. It is elevated mainly in gastrointestinal malignancy; in one series it was elevated in pancreatic (76%), biliary tract (73%), gastric (42%) and liver (22%) carcinoma, but it was also raised in benign conditions of those organs in 16%, 36%, 0%, and 15% of cases. These results have been confirmed in subsquent studies. It is also elevated in colorectal carcinoma, carcinoma of the cervix, ovary, breast, thyroid and kidney, and in some germinomas. Its role as a marker is dubious at present, being no more effective than AFP as a marker in hepatoma and adding little extra. It is perhaps slightly more specific than CEA for pancreatic carcinoma but no more sensitive diagnostically. In colorectal cancer it is no more sensitive but more specific than CEA diagnostically and adds little in combination with CEA, and is no better than CEA for monitoring treatment. Its role in gastric cancer is as yet unclear. Furthermore, CA 19–9 is not synthesized in patients who are Lewis a$^-$ b$^-$, which is about 5% of the population.

Other Carbohydrate Antigens. Most of the other carbohydrate antigens have not been studied as well as CA 125 or CA 19–9 or are insufficiently investigated to have any clear role as yet as tumour markers.[63,71]

REFERENCES

1. Leonard R.C.F. (1988) Metabolic complications of malignant disease. In *Medical Complications of Malignant Disease*, vol. 2 of *Baillière's Clinical Oncology* (Kaye S.B., Rankin E.M. eds.) London: Baillière Tindall, pp. 261–282.
2. Ibsen K.H., Fishman W.H. (1979). Developmental gene expression in cancer. *Biochim. Biophys. Acta*, **560**, 243.
3. Freund E. (1885). Zur Diagnos des Carcinoms. *Wien. Med. Bull.*, **8**, 268.
4. Clark A.J.L. (1984) Glucose homeostasis. In *Endocrine Problems in Cancer: Molecular Basis and Clinical Management* (Jung R.T., Sikora K. eds.) London; Heinemann, pp. 71–87.
5. Warburg O. (1930). *The Metabolism of Tumours*, London: Constable.
6. Cori C.F. (1931). Mammalian carbohydrate metabolism. *Physiol. Rev.*, **11**, 143.
7. Eden E. et al. (1984). Glucose flux in relation to energy expenditure in malnourished patients with and without cancer during periods of fasting and feeding. *Cancer Res.*, **44**, 1717.
8. Burt M.E., Aoki T.T., Gorschboth C.M., Brennan M.F. (1983). Peripheral tissue metabolism in cancer-bearing man. *Ann. Surg.*, **198**, 685.
9. Marks P.M., Bishop J.S. (1956). The glucose metabolism of patients with malignant disease and normal subjects as studied by means of an intravenous glucose tolerance test. *J. Clin. Invest.*, **35**, 254.
10. Waterhouse C. (1974). Lactate metabolism in patients with cancer. *Cancer*, **33**, 66.
11. Waterhouse C., Jeanpetre N., Keilson J. (1979). Gluconeogenesis from alanine in patients with progressive malignant disease. *Cancer Res.*, **39**, 1969.
12. Lundholm K. et al. (1982). Glucose turnover, gluconeogenesis from glycerol and estimation of net glucose cycling in cancer patients. *Cancer*, **50**, 1142.
13. Schwartz S.S. et al. (1978). A prospective study of glucose tolerance, insulin, C-peptide and glucagon responses in patients with pancreatic carcinoma. *Dig. Dis.*, **23**, 1107.
14. Doege K.W. (1930). Fibrosarcoma of the mediastinum. *Ann. Surg.*, **92**, 955.
15. McFadzean A.J.S., Yeung R.T.T. (1969). Further observations on hypoglycaemia in hepatocellular carcinoma. *Am. J. Med.*, **46**, 220.
16. Marks V. (1981). Extra-pancreatic neoplasms. In *Hypoglycaemia*, 2nd edn (Marks V., Rose F.C. eds.) Oxford: Blackwell Scientific, pp. 246–266.
17. Shaw J.H.F., Wolfe R.R. (1987). Fatty acids and glycerol kinetics in septic patients with gastrointestinal cancer; the response to glucose infusion and parenteral feeding. *Ann. Surg.*, **12**, 286.
18. Dilman V.M. et al. (1981). Peculiarities of hyperlipidaemia in tumour patients. *Br. J. Cancer*, **43**, 637.
19. Powles T.J. et al. (1990). Prevention of breast cancer with Tamoxifen—an update on the Royal Marsden Hospital pilot programme. *Eur. J. Cancer*, **26**, 680.
20. Carreras E. et al. (1989). Hypertriglyceridaemia in bone marrow transplant recipients: another side-effect of cyclosporine A. *Bone Marrow Transplant.*, **4**, 385.
21. Fleck A. Personal communication.
22. Fearon K.C.H. (1988) Nutritional and gastrointestinal complications of malignant disease. In *Medical Complications of Malignant Disease*, vol. 2 of *Baillière's Clinical Oncology* (Kaye S.B., Rankin E.M. eds.) London: Baillière Tindall, pp. 375–395.
23. Douglas R.F., Shaw J.H.F. (1990). Metabolic effects of cancer. *Br. J. Surg.*, **77**, 246.
24. Douglas R.F., Shaw J.H.F. (1989). Metabolic effects of sepsis and trauma. *Br. J. Surg.*, **76**, 115.
25. Beutler B., Cerami A. (1987). Cachectin: more than a tumour necrosis factor. *N. Engl. J. Med.*, **316**, 379.
26. Michie H.R. et al. (1989). Chronic TNF infusion causes anorexia but not accelerated nitrogen loss. *Ann. Surg.*, **209**, 19.

27. Heath H.W., III, Hodgson S.F., Kennedy M.A. (1980). Primary hyperparathyroidism: incidence, morbidity and potential economic impact on the community. *N. Engl. J. Med.* **302**, 189.

28. Fisken R.A., Heath D.A., Bold A.M. (1980). Hypercalcaemia—a hospital survey. *Q. J. Med.*, **44**, 405.

29. Mundy G.R., Martin T.J. (1982). The hypercalcaemia of malignancy: pathogenesis and management. *Metabolism*, **31**, 1247.

30. Mundy G.R., Ibbotson K.J., D'Souza S.M. (1985). Tumour products and the hypercalcaemia of malignancy. *J. Clin. Invest.* **76**, 391.

31. Gutierrez G.T. et al. (1990). Mechanisms of hypercalcaemia of malignancy. In *Endocrine Aspects of Malignancy*, vol. 4 of *Baillière's Clinical Oncology* (Shalet S.M. ed.) London: Baillière Tindall, pp. 119–138.

32. Broadus A.E., Mangin M., Insogna K.L. (1988). Humoral hypercalcaemia of cancer. Identification of a novel parathyroid hormone-like peptide. *N. Engl. J. Med.*, **319**, 556.

33. Martin T.J., Suva L.J. (1989). Parathyroid hormone-related protein in hypercalcaemia of malignancy. *Clin. Endocrinol.*, **31**, 631.

34. Burtis W.J. et al. (1990). Immunochemical characterization of circulating parathyroid hormone-related protein in patients with humoral hypercalcaemia of cancer. *N. Engl. J. Med.*, **322**, 1106.

35. Breslau N.A. et al. (1984). Hypercalcaemia associated with increased calcitriol levels in three patients with lymphoma. *Ann. Intern. Med.*, **100**, 1.

36. Davies M. et al. (1985). Abnormal vitamin D metabolism in Hodgkin's lymphoma. *Lancet*, **i**, 186.

37. Cohen L.F. et al. (1980). Acute tumour lysis syndrome: a review of 37 patients with Burkitt's lymphoma. *Am. J. Med.*, **64**, 486.

38. Davie M.W.J. (1984). Disorders of mineral metabolism. In *Endocrine Problems in Cancer: Molecular Basis and Clinical Management* (Jung R.T., Sikora K. eds.) London: Heinemann, pp. 103–5.

39. Pearse A.G.E. (1968). Common cytochemical and ultrastructural characteristics of cells producing the polypeptide hormones (the APUD) series and their relevance to thyroid and ultimobranchial C cells and calcitonin. *Proc. R. Soc. (B)*, **170**, 71.

40. Bone H.G., III. (1990). Diagnosis of the multiglandular endocrine neoplasias. *Clin. Chem.* **36**, 711.

41. Brown W.H. (1928). A case of pluriglandular syndrome: diabetes of bearded women. *Lancet*, **ii**, 1022.

42. Meador C.K. et al. (1962). Cause of Cushing's syndrome in patients with tumours arising from non-endocrine tissue. *J. Clin. Endocrinol. Metab.*, **22**, 693.

43. Yalow R.S., Berson R.A. (1971). Size heterogeneity of immunoreactive human ACTH in plasma and in extracts of pituitary gland and ACTH-producing thymoma. *Biochem. Biophys. Res. Commun.*, **44**, 439.

44. Howlett T.A., Rees L.H. (1985). Is it possible to diagnose pituitary-dependent Cushing's disease? *Ann. Clin. Biochem.*, **22**, 550.

45. White M.C. (1984). The ectopic ACTH syndrome. In *Endocrine Problems in Cancer: Molecular Basis and Clinical Management* (Jung R.T., Sikora K. eds.) London: Heinemann, pp. 188–215.

46. White A., Clark A.J.L., Stewart M.F. (1990). The synthesis of ACTH and related peptides by tumours. In *Endocrine Aspects of Malignancy*, Vol. 4 of *Baillière's Clinical Oncology* (Shalet S.M. ed.) London: Baillière Tindall, pp. 1–27.

47. Schwartz W.B., Bennett W., Curelop S., Bartter F.C. (1957). A syndrome of renal sodium loss and hyponatraemia resulting from inappropriate secretion of antidiuretic hormone. *Am. J. Med.*, **23**, 529.

48. Bartter F.C., Schwartz W.B. (1967). The syndrome of inappropriate secretion of antidiuretic hormone. *Am. J. Med.*, **42**, 790.

49. Zerbe R.L., Stropes L., Robertson G.L. (1980). Vasopressin function in the syndrome of inappropriate antidiuresis. *Annu. Rev. Med.*, **31**, 315.

50. Robertson G.L., Aycicena P., Zerbe R.L. (1982). Neurogenic disorders of osmoregulation. *Am. J. Med.*, **72**, 339.

51. Witte M.H., Short F.A., Hollander W., Jr. (1964). Massive polyuria and natriuresis following relief of urinary tract obstruction. *Am. J. Med.*, **37**, 320.

52. Battle D.C., Arruda J.A.L., Kurtzman N.A. (1981). Hyperkalaemic distal renal tubular acidosis associated with obstructive uropathy. *N. Engl. J. Med.*, **304**, 373.

53. Lynch R.E., Kjellstrand C.M., Coccia P.F. (1977). Renal and metabolic complications of childhood non-Hodgkin's lymphoma. *Semin. Oncol.*, **4**, 325.

54. Coward R.A. (1986). Renal complications. In *Multiple Myeloma and Other Paraproteinaemias* (Delamore I.W. ed.) Edinburgh: Churchill Livingstone, pp. 239–306.

55. Boulton-Jones J.M. (1988). Renal complications of malignant disease. In *Medical Complications of Malignant Disease*, vol. 2 of *Baillière's Clinical Oncology* (Kaye S.B., Rankin E.M. eds.) London: Baillière Tindall, pp. 347–373.

56. Sell S. (1980). Alphafoetoprotein. In *Cancer Markers: Diagnostic and Developmental Significance* (Sell S. ed.) Clifton NJ: Humana, pp. 249–293.

57. Lange P.H. (1983). Markers for germ cell tumours of the testis. In *Oncodevelopmental Markers: Biologic, Diagnostic and Monitoring Aspects* (Fishman W.H. ed.) London: Academic, pp. 241–258.

58. Rustin G.S. (1987). *Circulating Tumour Markers in the Management of Human Cancer* (Daar A.S. ed.) Oxford: Blackwell Scientific, pp. 204–227.

59. Braunstein G.D. (1983). hCG expression in trophoblastic and non-trophoblastic tumours. In *Oncodevelopmental Markers: Biologic, Diagnostic and Monitoring Aspects* (Fishman W.H. ed.) London: Academic, pp. 351–372.

60. De Lellis R.A. (1990). Tumour markers in endocrine malignancies. *Clin. Lab. Med.*, **10**, 39.

61. Burtin P., Escribano M.J. (1983). The carcinoembryonic antigen and its cross reacting antigens. In *Oncodevelopmental Markers: Biologic, Diagnostic and Monitoring Aspects* (Fishman W.H. ed.) London: Academic, pp. 315–334.

62. Zamcheck N. (1983). In *Oncodevelopmental Markers: Biologic, Diagnostic and Monitoring Aspects* (Fishman W.H. ed.) London: Academic, pp. 335–350.

63. Sell S. (1990). Cancer markers of the 1990s. Comparison of the new generation of markers defined by monoclonal antibodies and oncogene probes to prototypic markers. *Clin. Lab. Med.*, **10**, 1.

64. Horwich A., Tucker D.F., Peckham M.J. (1985). Placental alkaline phosphatase as a tumour marker in seminoma using the H17E2 monoclonal assay. *Br. J. Cancer*, **51**, 625.

65. Schwartz M.K. (1989). Enzymes in cancer. *Clin. Lab. Med.*, **9**, 757.
66. Stamey T.A. et al. (1987). Prostate specific antigen as a serum marker for adenocarcinoma of the prostate. *N. Engl. J. Med.*, **317**, 909.
67. Lange P.H. et al. (1989). The value of serum prostate specific antigen determinations before and after radical prostatectomy. *J. Urol.*, **141**, 873.
68. van Dieijien-Visser M.P. et al. (1988). A comparative study on the diagnostic value of prostatic acid phosphatase (PAP) and prostate specific antigen (PSA) in patients with carcinoma of the prostate gland. *Clin. Chim. Acta*, **174**, 131.
69. Goldberg D.M., Brown D. (1987). Biochemical tests in the diagnosis, classification and management of patients with malignant lymphoma and leukaemia. *Clin. Chim. Acta*, **169**, 1.
70. Cooper E.H. et al. (1987). Serum neuron-specific enolase in children's cancer. *Br. J. Cancer*, **56**, 65.
71. Duffy M.J. (1989). New cancer markers. *Ann. Clin. Biochem.*, **26**, 379.

GENERAL TEXTS AND REVIEWS

Cancer

Souhami R., Tobias J. (1986). *Cancer and Its Management*, Oxford: Blackwell Scientific.

Metabolic Effects of Neoplasia

Jung R.T., Sikora K. eds. (1984). *Endocrine Problems in Cancer: Molecular Basis and Clinical Management*, London: Heinemann.
Kaye S.B., Rankin E.M. eds. (1988). *Medical Complications of Malignant Disease. Baillière's Clinical Oncology*, vol. 2, London: Baillière Tindall.
Shalet S.M. ed. (1990). *Endocrine Aspects of Malignancy, Baillière's Clinical Oncology*, vol. 4, London: Baillière Tindall.

Tumour Markers

Daar A.S. ed. (1987). *Tumour Markers in Clinical Practice: Concepts and Applications*, Oxford, Blackwell Scientific.
Fishman W.H. ed. (1983). *Oncodevelopmental Markers: Biologic, Diagnostic and Monitoring Aspects*, London: Academic.
Ghosh B.C., Ghosh L. eds. (1987). *Tumour Markers and Tumour-associated Antigens*, New York: McGraw-Hill.
Sell S. ed. (1980). *Cancer Markers: Diagnostic and Developmental Significance*, Clifton NJ: Humana.

10. Clinical Biochemistry in Intensive and Postoperative Care

A. C. Ames

Introduction
The inflammatory response: clinical consequences
The effects of hypoxia on cell metabolism
Phasing of the general metabolic response to injury
Endocrine changes after trauma
Carbohydrate metabolism
Fat metabolism
Protein metabolism
Changes in plasma proteins after injury
    Acute–phase proteins
    Albumin
Water, sodium and potassium metabolism
Magnesium, calcium, phosphate and zinc metabolism
Acid–base disturbance
    Lactic acidosis
Acute renal failure

INTRODUCTION

Shock, trauma, burns, surgery, infection and postoperative complications activate physiological defence reactions. If, however, the degree of stress involved is overwhelming and these reactions are inadequate, the protective responses are replaced by damaging pathological events that involve other tissues and organs, and the patient becomes critically ill. Single or multiple organ failure is a possible consequence and the association with complex metabolic disturbances carries a poor prognosis and increased mortality.

Shock can be conveniently divided into three main types, namely hypovolaemic, cardiogenic and septic. The initial physiological responses serve to maintain homeostasis, but if these fail, progressive deterioration of tissue perfusion, cellular hypoxia and the accumulation of toxic metabolites lead to profound haemodynamic and metabolic disturbances. The situation is complicated by the liberation of vasoactive substances that increase capillary permeability and the leakage of fluid into the interstitial space, which exacerbate hypovolaemia. The development of disseminated intravascular coagulation (DIC) causes further regional ischaemia and tissue hypoxia, while splanchnic ischaemia may facilitate the dissemination of micro-organisms from the gut, leading to endotoxaemia or septicaemia. At this stage, the clinical distinction between the various types of shock becomes blurred and features of all three, hypovolaemia, myocardial failure and septicaemia, may occur in the same individual.

THE INFLAMMATORY RESPONSE: CLINICAL CONSEQUENCES

The acute inflammatory response to tissue injury and infection lacks specificity and there are extensive interactions between each of the component subsystems. These include common activating enzymes, modulators and inhibitors and overlapping effects on the cellular elements of inflammation, any resulting imbalance being potentially detrimental to the individual. While the activation of lymphocytes and macrophages is intricate, the activation of the subcellular components of acute inflammation is induced by collagen, bacteria, viruses, fungi and damaged cells. Although cell-mediated immune effectors require attachment to the target before exerting their toxic effects, cytotoxic effectors of the response are released into the extracellular fluid phase and, being able to diffuse widely, there is the risk of destruction of otherwise healthy tissues. When the local inflammatory response is not contained, it can have far-reaching effects in distant sites, being responsible for non-infectious complications like the adult respiratory distress syndrome (ARDS), suppression of the immune system and acute renal failure. Much of the current pharmacological management of critically ill patients is based on the prevention of inflammation-related disease.

The non-cellular mediators of inflammation depend on surface or contact activation by protein surfaces such as basement membrane collagen and vascular endothelium.[1] Contact activation of plasma is caused by surface binding of a molecular complex of four plasma proteins, Hageman factor, high molecular-weight kininogen, prekallikrein and factor XI. Activated Hageman factor (AHF) stimulates the *coagulation cascade*, which, although necessary for local haemostasis, may progress to DIC. The excessive consumption of coagulation factors and platelets in this process can lead to either a generalized haemorrhagic state or end-organ failure following occlusion of the microcirculation by thrombus. The kidney is most susceptible to ischaemic damage, but the brain, heart and adrenals can also be seriously affected.

Kallikrein, a weak activator of plasminogen, is also released from its precursor by AHF and *fibrinolysis* is initiated. It also triggers the release of several different kinins, the most notable being bradykinin. Kinins cause profound vasodilation and hypotension, increased capillary permeability with oedema, and myocardial depression. When the principal source of kinins is the intestinal tract, they are particularly important in the mediation of endotoxic shock. The lung can also play a significant role in shock, as it is not only a source of kinin production but also responsible for its inactivation.

The complement system is the direct link between the humoral and cellular host defence mechanism. The *complement cascade* is activated by either antigen–antibody complexes via the classical pathway or through the alternative pathway by damaged tissues, bacteria, toxins and AHF to produce C3a, C4a and C5a.[2] These are potent anaphylotoxins, causing venous constriction, increased capillary permeability and histamine release. Release of lysosomal enzymes, cytolysis, proteolysis, opsonization and neutrophil aggregation are also stimulated, processes that are vital to the success of the inflammatory and immune response. Uncontrolled activation produces major damage, but a series of inhibitors exists to prevent such an event. However, massive complement activation in prolonged endotoxaemia contributes significantly to the development of shock by mechanisms not completely understood, as both C3a and C5a are capable of producing hypotension. The same products increase neutrophil aggregation, which, by embolization, can cause microvascular plugging in the lungs. Activated neutrophils produce large amounts of toxic oxygen radicals,[3] which, by damaging vascular endothelium, promote the exudation of protein-rich fluid from lung capillaries and pulmonary oedema. These events are features of ARDS, a dangerous complication of endotoxic shock, and of acute pancreatitis, where complement activation is mediated by the direct action of proteases such as trypsin. Complement activation can also enhance the coagulation cascade in endotoxaemia leading to DIC.

Phospholipids released from damaged cell membranes, platelets and white cells by phospholipase A_2 are a source of arachidonic acid from which leucotrienes and prostanoids (eicosanoids) are synthesized in the *arachidonic acid cascade* system. Leucotrienes cause vasoconstriction, bronchoconstriction and increased capillary permeability. The prostanoids consist of two groups of prostaglandins with opposing actions. Thromboxane A_2 and prostaglandin F_1 are vasoconstrictors, while prostaglandins I_2, E_1 and E_2 are vasodilators. Platelet aggregation is activated by thromboxane A_2 and prostaglandin E_2, but is inhibited by prostaglandins I_2 and E_1. The vasomotor properties of this group of substances and their influence on platelet aggregation are of considerable importance in the pathogenesis of shock and in the development of pulmonary hypertension in endotoxaemia.

THE EFFECTS OF HYPOXIA ON CELL METABOLISM

The ability of cells to resist the effects of hypoxia generally depends upon their blood supply and the concentration of cellular glycogen. In the central nervous system, the length of time cells can withstand hypoxia is measured in seconds, while the liver may function anaerobically for several hours. Although the myoglobin in skeletal muscle helps to overcome the immediate effects of hypoxia, longer resistance depends on anaerobic glycolysis. Although whole-body oxygen consumption (V_{O_2}) may be sub-basal during shock, vital organs are protected by vascular shunting at the expense of those resistant to hypoxia, such as skin, fat and skeletal muscle. These tissues have low resting oxygen requirements and more robust mitochondria, while muscle can produce adenosine triphosphate (ATP) anaerobically.

As the oxygen supply diminishes, aerobic metabolism of glucose and ultimately pyruvate by the Krebs cycle and electron transport system decreases. Anaerobic glycolysis becomes established to meet the energy requirements but lactate, the end-product, accumulates in the cells causing intracellular acidosis. As the normal glycolytic pathway is blocked, glucose diffuses from the cells.

The change from aerobic to anaerobic glycolysis reduces the generation of ATP within the mitochondria from 30 mol to 2 mol of ATP per mole of glucose which, in turn, reduces the transmembrance potential of muscle cells by 30%. As the ionic gradients cannot be maintained across the cells, disturbances of ionic balance occur. Movements of Ca^{2+} and Na^+ across the cells, and the maintenance of the normal Ca^{2+}–Na^+ ionic gradient are effected by specific ion pumps that are ATP dependent. Failure of ATP production reduces the active extrusion of Ca^{2+}; this accumulates in the cells causing mitochondrial damage, further inhibition of ATP release and activation of phospholipases, which cause cell membrane degradation.[4] In the myocardium, persistently raised intracellular calcium will result in failure of muscular relaxation and arrest in systole. The disorganization of ATP synthesis leads to an increase in intracellular phosphates and a loss of nucleosides by diffusion.

The Na^+–K^+ pump is similarly affected and, as membrane potentials fall, sodium and water are able to enter the cell and potassium diffuses out. This influx of sodium may be partly responsible for the 'sick cell syndrome', which is associated with cellular oedema and hyponatraemia. It has been calculated that in severe and prolonged shock, nearly 2 L or 10% of the extracellular fluid (ECF) water moves into the cells.

Plasma concentrations of cyclic AMP (adenosine 3′,5′-phosphate) fall, and may be responsible for modifying the effects of insulin, glucagon, catecholamines and possibly corticosteroids on cell receptors. Autolysis by leaking lysosomes and oxidation of phospholipids in the cell membrane by free radicals damage their receptor systems. Exceptionally high concentrations of insulin may be necessary to stimulate glucose uptake if the insulin receptors are

TABLE 10.1

PHYSIOLOGICAL, ENDOCRINE AND METABOLIC RESPONSES IN RELATION TO THE
EBB AND FLOW PHASES AFTER INJURY OR MAJOR SURGERY

	Shock or ebb phase	Flow phase	
		Early catabolic	Anabolic
Metabolic rate	↓	↑	↑ or N
Body temperature	↓	↑	N
Cardiac output	↓	↑	N
U. catecholamines	↑	↑	N
U. 17-oxogenic steroids	↑	↑	N
P. insulin	↓	↑	↑ or N
P. glucagon	↑	↑	N
P. growth hormone	↑	↑	↑ or N
B. glucose	↑	↑	↑ or N
P. free fatty acids	↑	↑	↓
Nitrogen balance	Negative	Negative	Positive

B, blood; P, plasma; U, urine.

affected, and this combination of events may partly explain the phenomenon of 'insulin resistance' and the impaired uptake of glucose in severe shock.

If cellular metabolism continues to deteriorate, progressive morphological changes involving the cytoplasm and mitochondria occur, with autodigestion and cell necrosis caused by leaking lysosomes. These changes may be prevented if normal tissue perfusion and oxygenation can be restored.

PHASING OF THE GENERAL METABOLIC RESPONSE TO INJURY

The response is conveniently subdivided into an early 'ebb' phase lasting 24–48 h, which corresponds to the initial period of shock, and a longer 'flow' or recovery phase lasting several days or weeks. The flow phase can be further subdivided into a catabolic period lasting 3–7 days, which eventually progresses into another variable period of progressive and active anabolism (Table 10.1).

The ebb phase is one of depressed metabolic activity, oxygen consumption, body temperature and cardiac output. In severe trauma, if these effects persist, there is continuing deterioration culminating in terminal necrobiosis.

In the flow phase, metabolic activity slowly increases but during the catabolic period, protein and fat reserves are mobilized to provide energy, resulting in loss of body weight and a negative nitrogen balance. During the subsequent anabolic period, nutritional reserves are restored, nitrogen balance becomes positive and wound healing is accelerated. The homeostatic, metabolic and nutritional changes are largely influenced by the immediate and sustained hyperactivity of numerous endocrine systems in a complex but coordinated response essential for the survival of the individual.

ENDOCRINE CHANGES AFTER TRAUMA

Many stimuli such as hypotension, hypovolaemia, acidosis, hypoxia and hypercapnia are responsible for increasing the plasma concentration of *catecholamines*, noradrenaline being secreted by the sympathetic nervous system, with mainly adrenaline from the adrenal medulla. In haemorrhagic shock, plasma adrenaline rises rapidly to a concentration 50 times normal, while noradrenaline increases more slowly up to 10 times the upper limit of the normal range. Apart from their action on the cardiovascular system, catecholamines have a marked effect on carbohydrate metabolism (Fig. 10.1), stimulating glycogenolysis and glucagon production while suppressing insulin secretion, and on lipid metabolism by stimulating lipolysis.[5] Adrenaline has greater metabolic activity than noradrenaline.

All stressful situations stimulate the release of *adrenocorticotrophic hormone* (ACTH) from the anterior pituitary and *cortisol* from the adrenal cortex, plasma cortisol being transiently raised for 24–48 h with variable increases in urinary free cortisol. Cortisol facilitates the release of catecholamines and their vascular effects, and the retention of sodium and excretion of potassium by the kidney. It has an important influence on carbohydrate metabolism by inhibiting insulin secretion, in addition to its immunosuppressive and anti-inflammatory functions. Critically ill patients with inappropriately low plasma cortisol concentrations respond poorly to resuscitative measures and have a high mortality unless corticosteroid therapy is given, but even this measure does not always alter the poor prognosis.

Trauma and sepsis stimulate *glucagon* secretion and plasma concentrations remain elevated for several days, the pancreatic islets responding to sympathetic nervous stimulation, cortisol, growth hor-

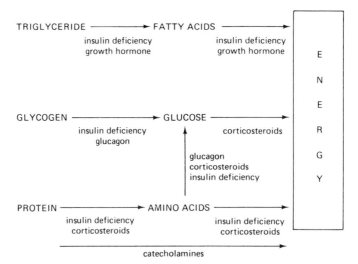

Figure 10.1 The mobilization of energy reserves by catecholamines indicating the relationship with other hormones that augment catabolism.

mone, hypoglycaemia and hyperaminoacidaemia. Its glycogenolytic and gluconeogenic effects are diametrically opposed to that of insulin, but by interaction they balance increases in the production and utilization of glucose. Glucagon also stimulates lipolysis and enhances renal blood flow and cardiac output.

Plasma *growth hormone* remains elevated for a few days, rapidly returning to normal. It plays a minor role in carbohydrate and fat metabolism, potentiating the lipolytic effect of catecholamines and exerting anabolic effects during recovery in the presence of insulin.

Insulin release is inhibited initially, but in the flow phase, plasma concentrations rise. However, the combined actions of catecholamines, cortisol and glucagon oppose the cellular uptake of glucose by insulin, ensuring high concentrations of plasma glucose are maintained through the ebb and early flow phases.

Hypotension, hypovolaemia, hyperosmolality, hypoxia and pain stimulate the release of arginine *vasopressin* (AVP, earlier known as antidiuretic hormone, ADH) from the posterior pituitary. Vasoconstriction and water retention produced by VP act synergistically with other compensatory mechanisms to restore ECF volume and blood pressure. Highest plasma concentrations of VP are seen in haemorrhagic shock and burns, but occasionally inappropriately high concentrations of VP are secreted, even in the presence of low plasma osmolality, with the development of severe hyponatraemia. This syndrome can occur with head injuries and pulmonary infections, representing possible malfunction of hypothalamic osmoreceptors or large-vessel baroceptors, respectively. Conversely, trauma to the base of the brain may impair VP release, resulting in diabetes insipidus with hypernatraemia and polyuria.

When hypotension, hypovolaemia or renal vaso-constriction reduce renal blood flow the *renin–angiotensin–aldosterone* pathway is activated. Renin is released from the juxtaglomerular apparatus in the kidney and cleaves the α-globulin precursor angiotensinogen to form angiotensin I, which is further modified by angiotensin-converting enzyme to angiotensin II. In addition to being a powerful vasoconstrictor, it stimulates the release of aldosterone from the adrenal cortex. Promotion of salt and water retention by the kidney is at the expense of potassium loss, but assists in the restoration of the ECF (Fig. 10.2). As a further example of the complex interrelations between the compensatory mechanisms, angiotensin II is a stimulus for ADH and ACTH release.

If fluid overload with hypervolaemia occurs, *atrial natriuretic peptide* (ANP) is released from the atria of the heart and plasma concentrations of guanosine $3',5'$-cyclic monophosphate increase. ANP is a potent natriuretic, counteracting the effects of aldosterone and cortisol.

In the critically ill patient, little useful information in relation to clinical management is obtained by measuring the hormones involved in these complex compensatory processes.

Severe illness, burns, starvation, infection, renal failure and liver disease are sometimes accompanied by unexpected abnormalities in *thyroid function* tests, even though the patient is clinically euthyroid. These are referred to as the 'sick euthyroid syndrome', which involves two distinct abnormalities. The first presents with low serum free tri-iodothyronine (T_3) due to decreased extrathyroidal conversion of thyroxine (T_4) to T_3. Free T_4 may be normal or high. This is observed more frequently in the elderly and may be due to the increased concentrations of cortisol, which inhibit enzymic conversion. During recovery, the concentration of T_3 reverts to normal. The second is

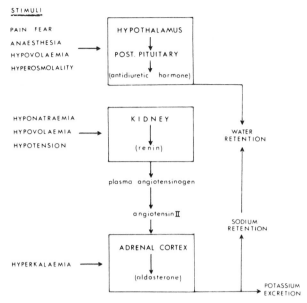

Figure 10.2   The stimuli and endocrine responses associated with salt and water conservation after trauma.

associated with low serum free T_4 and low free T_3. This form is seen in more severe illness with an increased mortality and is due to general depression of the hypothalamic–pituitary–thyroid axis. It is distinguished from primary hypothyroidism by the presence of normal serum thyroid-stimulating hormone.

The situation can be complicated by the choice of method for serum T_4 assay. With some assays, if the serum albumin is low, as it often is in acute illness, an artefactual underestimation of free T_4 is obtained. With newer assays unaffected by albumin, the converse may occur, namely raised serum free T_4. This is yet another form of 'sick euthyroid syndrome', which has to be distinguished from hyperthyroidism. To avoid unnecessary confusion, thyroid function tests should only be made if overt clinical signs of thyroid disease are present.

CARBOHYDRATE METABOLISM

In the early post-traumatic phase, blood glucose concentrations rise to 8 mmol/L or above in response to the stimulation of hepatic glycogenolysis by catecholamines, aided by increased secretion of glucagon and corticosteroids. The initial suppression of insulin secretion by increased α-adrenergic activity assists the development of hyperglycaemia (*see* Fig. 10.1). Hepatic reserves of glycogen are sufficient to supply about 3.36 MJ (800 kcals) and become rapidly depleted within 12 h. At this stage, hepatic gluconeogenesis becomes responsible for maintaining a high circulating glucose. This involves the metabolism of lactate, pyruvate, glycerol, alanine and other glucogenic amino acids through the stimulus of corticosteroids and glucagon.

During the catabolic period of the flow phase, hyperglycaemia can persist in the presence of hyperinsulinaemia. This results from uninhibited and sustained gluconeogenic activity, which becomes an important pathway for the clearance of the increasing concentration of substrates, notably lactate and amino acids, that cannot be used for protein synthesis. This is associated with glucose intolerance, which used to be called 'traumatic diabetes', with reduced utilization and oxidation of glucose. In hypoxic shock it has been shown experimentally that damage to insulin receptors is partly responsible, but after trauma this insensitivity or resistance to the action of insulin appears to be caused by the glucocorticoid response and the peripheral actions of adrenaline in limiting glucose utilization.[6] If the injury is not too severe and as the levels of counterregulatory hormones decline, hyperglycaemia can be expected to disappear by the seventh day. Occasionally insulin resistance persists for longer and in these instances, increased protein catabolism is responsible.

Hypoglycaemia may be observed in the terminal stages of endotoxaemic shock with poor cardiac output and hypotension. Although it has been suggested that endotoxins have insulin-like effects, the hypoglycaemia is usually due to depletion of hepatic glycogen and impaired gluconeogenesis. Paradoxically, there is increased utilization of the small amount of glucose made available, but this contributes to the terminal decline, with increased production of lactate and progressive acidosis.

FAT METABOLISM

As catecholamine concentrations rise and that of insulin falls, lipolysis of adipose-tissue triglyceride by lipases with the release of glycerol and free fatty acids (FFA) occurs (*see* Fig.10.1). Transport of FFA in plasma is dependent on binding to albumin, but as the perfusion of adipose tissue is reduced after injury or haemorrhagic shock, release of FFA into the general circulation may be impaired. FFA undergo β-oxidation in nearly all tissues, but as this increases there are two important consequences. Firstly, the uptake and oxidation of glucose by muscle are suppressed. Secondly, the overproduction of acetylcoenzyme A (CoA) exceeds the capacity for its oxidation via the Krebs cycle, which results in the condensation of acetyl CoA units in the liver with the production of acetoacetate and 3-hydroxybutyrate (ketogenesis). Carnitine acyl transferase plays a significant role in fatty acid oxidation and ketogenesis, but if carnitine synthesis by the liver is inadequate, the energy potential of these sources may not be realized. Most extrahepatic tissues can oxidize ketone bodies, and the heart and brain can obtain a significant proportion of their energy requirements by the process of ketoadaptation. After injury a modest ketonaemia occurs, but concentrations rarely exceed 1 mmol/L. Ketonuria invariably occurs during starvation. With septicaemia and endotoxaemia, the release and oxidation of FFA and ketogenesis can be depressed. Several factors including hyperinsulinaemia, which inhibits lipolysis, high lactate concentrations, which encourage re-esterification of FFA within the adipocyte, and hypoalbuminaemia may be contributory.

PROTEIN METABOLISM

Protein reserves have been estimated as being able to provide 104 MJ (24 000 kcals) of energy in an average man, either by direct oxidation of amino acids or by oxidation of glucose produced from amino acids by gluconeogenesis. The stimulus to proteolysis comes from the increased liberation of catecholamines, glucagon and corticosteroids with reduced secretion of insulin (*see* Fig. 10.1). The response also appears to be assisted by increased concentrations of 'proteolysis-inducing factor', which is a circulating cleavage product of interleukin-1. During recovery amino acids are required for protein synthesis and wound healing, with increased insulin secretion providing the necessary anabolic stimulus.

Following trauma and sepsis the principal source of amino acids is muscle, their plasma concentrations rising to three or four times that found in the postabsorptive state. When starvation coexists, amino acids are also mobilized from protein in the liver, kidney, pancreas and intestine. Loss of protein from the intestine leads to mucosal atrophy, which not only impairs its secretory and absorptive properties but also removes the mucosal antibacterial barrier, making it easier for bacteria to enter the portal system and leading to septicaemia, endotoxaemia and multisystem organ failure.

Proteolysis in muscle mobilizes leucine, isoleucine and valine (branched-chain amino acids), asparagine, aspartate and glutamate, which, before they can be oxidized, must be deaminated. This is achieved by transamination with pyruvate to produce alanine and with α-ketoglutarate to form glutamine. Alanine and glutamine, together with 3-carbon intermediates including lactate, pyruvate and other amino acids, are then transported to the liver to undergo gluconeogenesis (Fig. 10.3) in a process termed the 'alanine shuttle'.

As the rate of hepatic conversion of amino acids to glucose and urea increases, the net result is a negative nitrogen balance, which rises to between 20 and 40 g nitrogen per day. Urea can form 85% of the very high urinary non-protein nitrogen excretion, the remainder being amino acids, ammonia, creatine and creatinine. The normal urine creatine : creatinine ratio, which is less than 0.1, increases dramatically after trauma, indicative of increased muscle catabolism. As 1 g of nitrogen is equivalent to 6.25 g of protein or 25 g of muscle, this can involve the loss of up to 1 kg of muscle each day, especially in hypercatabolic states involving burns and multiple injuries.

CHANGES IN PLASMA PROTEINS AFTER INJURY

Acute-phase Proteins

After trauma and infection, serum electrophoresis shows increases in α_1- and α_2-globulins, which include several distinct proteins forming part of the 'acute-phase response', notably C-reactive protein (CRP), α_1-acid glycoprotein (orosomucoid), haptoglobin, α_1-antitrypsin, α_2-macroglobulin, caeruloplasmin and fibrinogen. The functions of acute-phase proteins are exceptionally varied, modifying the cellular and humoral inflammatory response in diverse ways. Taking CRP as an example, it is synthesized in the liver and after an initial delay of 6 h the plasma concentration can rise from 10 mg/L to 300 mg/L within 48 h. With resolution of the injury or inflammation, its decrease is equally dramatic. It can activate complement, enhance phagocytosis, inhibit platelet aggregation, and act as a regulator of cellular and humoral immunity.

Albumin

Several plasma proteins including prealbumin, transferrin and retinol-binding protein decrease after trauma, but the fall in albumin concentration is clinically the most important, values decreasing by 30% between the third and sixth days. This is only partly explained by a slight increase in catabolism and depression of hepatic synthesis of albumin. The most important cause is the shift of albumin from the intravascular to the extravascular space, owing to the increased premeability of the microvasculature, by processes previously discussed. Considerable 'leak-

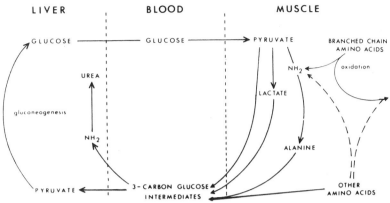

Figure 10.3 Hepatic gluconeogenesis from 3-carbon glucose intermediates derived from muscle (alanine shuttle).

TABLE 10.2

NORMAL DAILY VOLUME AND AVERAGE IONIC COMPOSITION IN MILLIMOLES PER LITRE OF GASTROINTESTINAL SECRETIONS

	Na^+	K^+	Cl^-	HCO_3^-	Mg^{++}	Ca^{++}	H^+	Volume (mL)
Gastric	60	10	120	10	0.5	2	70	500–2500
Biliary	145	5	100	40	0.7	2.5		700
Pancreatic	140	5	65	110	0.1	1.5		800
Ileal	130	11	110	30	0.5	2.0		3000
Diarrhoea	75	40	60	50	Variable	Variable		

age' occurs in septic shock and multiple injuries, which by increasing the oncotic pressure in the extravascular space result in oedema. One of the potentially most dangerous sequelae in a critically ill patient is the development of pulmonary oedema. In shock, visceral or splanchnic pooling of blood may also contribute to the loss of albumin from plasma. It should be remembered that recumbency itself promotes a 15% decrease in plasma albumin following the redistribution of water, which returns to the vascular compartment as the hydrostatic pressure in the legs falls.

WATER, SODIUM AND POTASSIUM METABOLISM

As a comprehensive account will be found in Chapter 4, only brief reference will be made here to those fluid and electrolyte disorders that can complicate postoperative or post-traumatic recovery.

Within hours the increased secretion of AVP overrides the normal osmoreceptor regulation and free water is reabsorbed by the kidney. The stimulus of hypovolaemia following haemorrhage or gastrointestinal fluid losses also overrides any osmolar effects to produce water retention. The excessive water retention in these circumstances is included in the syndrome of inappropriate antidiuresis (SIAD). This syndrome is encountered occasionally in postoperative patients with complications such as pneumonia, peritonitis, septicaemia, and during artificial ventilation and also following cerebral damage. The injudicious infusion of excessive volumes of hypotonic solutions in these conditions can be dangerous, leading to pulmonary and cerebral oedema with hyponatraemia and plasma hypo-osmolality. Neurological symptoms are associated with plasma sodium concentration less than 120 mmol/L.[7] Combined water and sodium retention must be anticipated in congestive cardiac failure and hepatic cirrhosis with portal hypertension due to increased ADH and aldosterone secretion. The development of hypo- or hypernatraemia depends on the relative amounts of salt and water retained.

In acute oliguric or chronic renal failure, water overload may be iatrogenic if the volume of fluid given exceeds the ability to excrete the excess water, the plasma sodium concentration being dependent on the relative amounts of salt and water given.

Water and sodium depletion are a consequence of inadequate intravenous replacement therapy when there are large fluid losses from gastroduodenal aspiration, fistulae, ileostomy or fluid sequestration in paralytic ileus (Table 10.2). As the plasma volume falls, compensatory water and salt retention occur, but although the total body sodium becomes progressively and dangerously depleted, with virtual absence of sodium from the urine, the plasma sodium concentration may be normal.

When water losses are relatively greater than sodium after profuse sweating or gastric aspiration and water depletion exceeds 3 L, hypernatraemia occurs, plasma sodium concentrations greater than 150 mmol/L being virtually diagnostic unless hypertonic saline has been infused. Urine output falls below 500 mL/day, becoming hyperosmolar with a high urea concentration. In the postoperative state, the increased solute load from tissue catabolism and the potential impairment of renal function make a minimal urine output of more than 500 mL/day necessary to maintain plasma osmolality between 280 and 295 mosmol/kg.

Other causes of water depletion with accompanying hypernatraemia are diabetes insipidus after head injury, 'encephalogenic hypernatraemia' in brian injury due to resetting of the hypothalamic osmoregulatory receptors, and osmotic diuresis in diabetes mellitus or after high-nitrogen parenteral feeding. Hypernatraemia may also result from the infusion of 8.4% sodium bicarbonate in the treatment of metabolic acidosis or cardiac arrest, and from treatment with large doses of corticosteroids. Plasma sodium concentrations above 155 mmol/L in adults may produce neurological symptoms; concentrations above 170 mmol/L are dangerous.

Hyponatraemia occurs when excessive hypotonic solutions are infused in the immediate postoperative period, in the SIAD, with inadequate replacement of gastrointestinal losses of sodium, and in the 'sick cell' syndrome when cell membrane damage allows an intracellular shift of sodium; also in patients with malignancy, liver disease, chronic infection or malnutrition who are subjected to surgery. This may be due to haemodilution or hypoalbuminaemia.

Caution should be exercised if hyponatraemia is diagnosed in a patient receiving intravenous nutrition containing lipid, if the plasma sodium is measured by flame photometry. Hyperlipidaemia may, by diluting plasma water, result in apparent or pseudohyponatraemia, unless sodium is measured with an ion-selective electrode that will give a concentration corresponding to its osmotic activity.

For several days after trauma, there is increased urinary excretion of potassium of about 120–140 mmol/day, partly due to the effect of aldosterone on the kidney but also due to clearance of the additional potassium load derived from hypercatabolism of muscle, necrotic tissue or reabsorption of blood from the intestine and haematoma. For every gram of nitrogen released from cells, 2.7 mmol of potassium enters the ECF. Unless renal function and water intake are adequate, hyperkalaemia may occur.

If potassium is continually lost from the gastrointestinal tract or during diuretic or corticosteroid therapy, without adquate replacement severe body depletion and hypokalaemia will develop. Hypokalaemia is often a feature of metabolic or respiratory alkalosis, or of glucose and insulin infusion, which enhance intracellular movements of potassium. Plasma concentrations below 2 mmol/L cause muscle weakness, confusion and potentially dangerous electrocardiographic abnormalities.

MAGNESIUM, CALCIUM, PHOSPHATE AND ZINC METABOLISM

After uncomplicated surgery there is increased uri-nary excretion of magnesium derived from hepatic and muscle catabolism, which rises to a maximum by the third day and slowly declines. This will be exacerbated by any sustained losses of magnesium in gastrointestinal secretions through suction, fistulae or ileostomy, but, as the concentrations are less than 1 mmol/L, a significant negative balance requires large losses of these fluids. The use of diuretics, aminoglycoside antibiotics, carbenicillin and amphotericin will induce additional renal losses and unless magnesium replacement is adequate, hypomagnesaemia will occur.[8] Concentrations below 0.5 mmol/L are usually asymptomatic but below this muscular weakness, tetany, arrhythmias, neurological and psychiatric disturbances may appear.

Hypocalcaemia is almost invariably associated with hypomagnesaemia as low concentraions of magnesium suppress parathyroid function. As their clinical symptoms are similar, it is difficult to distinguish between them. Hypoalbuminaemia is frequently associated with low serum calcium and it is therefore essential to correct for variations in albumin by adding 0.025 mmol/L to the measured serum calcium for every gram per litre the serum albumin is below 40 g/L. If the corrected serum calcium is low, the most common causes are renal failure, acute pancreatitis and rhabdomyolysis. When massive transfusion of blood containing citrate as an anticoagulant is given, a reduction in ionized calcium and hypocalcaemia may develop rapidly. Low ionized calcium in respiratory alkalosis due to hyperventilation or following treatment of metabolic acidosis with bicarbonate may precipitate symptoms, although the total serum calcium may remain normal.

Hypercatabolic states, extensive tissue trauma and rhabdomyolysis liberate large amounts of phosphate; if renal function is impaired, plasma concentrations rise. Otherwise, phosphaturia occurs with a transient fall in serum phosphate for a few days, which may be compounded by an intracellular shift of phosphate from the ECF, especially if large amounts of glucose are being infused as a calorie source. During recovery, as nitrogen balance becomes positive, increased amounts of phosphate are incorporated into the cells, which may give rise to hypophosphataemia. Concentrations below 0.4 mmol/L are likely to cause neuromuscular irritability, confusion and hyperventilation. Equally important, but clinically inapparent, is the fall of red-cell ATP to 15% of normal with depletion of 2,3-diphosphoglycerate. This allows a 'shift to the left' of the oxygen dissociation curve, which increases the affinity of the red cell for oxygen while diminishing the amount of oxygen available to the tissues, an undesirable event in hypoxic states.

Zinc metabolism is altered in response to injury and infection, muscle catabolism releasing zinc bound to metalloproteins, which is then excreted in the urine as zinc–amino acid complexes. Excretion parallels the increase in urinary nitrogen and creatinine becoming maximal after 8–10 days, coincident with

TABLE 10.3
METABOLIC DISTURBANCES AND PREDISPOSING CAUSES OF ACID–BASE IMBALANCE AFTER SHOCK,
TRAUMA AND SURGERY

	Metabolic disturbance	Predisposing cause
Metabolic acidosis	Ketonaemia	Starvation
		Hypercatabolic states
		Diabetes mellitus
	Hyperlactataemia (type A)	Shock
		Congestive cardiac failure
		Open heart surgery
		Hypothermia
	Hyperlactataemia (type B)	Intravenous fructose, sorbitol, ethanol
	H^+ ion retention	Acute and chronic renal failure
	Loss of base	Biliary, pancreatic fistulae
		Ileostomy (recent)
	Infusion of acid	Amino acid solutions
	Hyperchloraemia	Ureterosigmoidostomy
Metabolic alkalosis	Loss of acid	Vomiting, gastric aspiration
	Infusion of base	Sodium bicarbonate
		Blood and plasma transfusion (citrate)
	Potassium depletion	Gastrointestinal fluid losses
		Diuretic phase of acute renal failure
		Diuretics, corticosteroids
Respiratory acidosis	Retention of CO_2	Bronchial obstruction, pneumothorax
		Pulmonary oedema, collapse, consolidation
		Thoracotomy, chest wall injury
		Medullary depressant drugs, muscle relaxants
		Inadequate ventilation
Respiratory alkalosis	Excessive loss of CO_2	Pain, septicaemia
		Head injury, brain damage
		Overventilation

high uptake of zinc at the wound site.[9] Zinc deficiency impairs wound healing and it is therefore essential to replace postoperative losses. As zinc is excreted in bile and pancreatic secretion, considerable losses of these fluids through aspiration or fistulae will further deplete zinc reserves.

When there is prolonged gastrointestinal failure, deficiencies of a wide range of essential biological (trace) elements including copper, iron, zinc, chromium, manganese, cobalt and iodine can arise unless maintenance requirements are satisfied by parenteral nutrition.

ACID–BASE DISTURBANCE

Any acid–base disturbance in the post-traumatic or postoperative period is most likely to be due to a mixed metabolic or respiratory acidosis or alkalosis, rather than a single disorder.[10] It may be caused by a combination of any of the precipitating factors listed in Table 10.3. Compensatory mechanisms may achieve complete or partial correction depending on the magnitude of the initial imbalance, but these may be compromised if renal or pulmonary function is impaired or if postoperative metabolic complications are not recognized and treated.

Correct interpretation of acid—base laboratory results cannot be done without taking into consideration the overall clinical status, including any treatment the patient may be receiving.

Lactic Acidosis

Lactate homeostasis and the maintenance of a normal serum lactate between 0.4 and 1.3 mmol/L depends on a balance being achieved between lactate production and removal. This is disturbed in the presence of clinically evident shock, hypoxia and poor tissue perfusion, which generates large amounts of pyruvate and lactate by anaerobic glycolysis. Removal of increased amounts of lactate in the liver by gluconeogenesis will be impaired by hepatocellular disease, but occult regional underperfusion before overt shock is recognized is probably contributory, causing actual generation of lactate. Imbalance results in hyperlactataemia and lactic acidosis, which can be defined as clinical acidosis in an ill patient with blood lactate concentration persistently above 5 mmol/L and with arterial pH at less than 7.25. Lactic acidosis in hypoxic states is classified as type A, which distinguishes it from type B that occurs in a variety of conditions where there is adequate tissue perfusion and oxygena-

TABLE 10.4

INVESTIGATIONS TO DISTINGUISH PRERENAL FROM
ESTABLISHED INTRINSIC ACUTE RENAL FAILURE (ARF)

	Prerenal ARF	Established intrinsic ARF
Urine osmolality (mosmol/kg)	> 400	< 400
Osmolality ratio (urine:plasma)	> 1.5:1	< 1.5:1 often 1.1:1
Urea ratio (urine:plasma)	> 10:1	< 10:1 often 4:1
Urine sodium (mmol/L)	< 20	> 30
Effect of intravenous mannitol or diuretic	Diuresis	No diuresis

tion. Included in type B is lactic acidosis associated with diabetes mellitus, acute liver failure, chronic liver disease, renal failure and septicaemia. Alcohol and methanol intoxication, ethylene glycol and paracetamol poisoning, large fructose and sorbitol infusions for nutritional purposes can all be associated with lactic acidosis, which is a very serious complication however caused. There is a progressive rise in mortality as the arterial lactate increases, with a 90% mortality when it exceeds 9 mmol/L. The prognosis is especially poor when lactic acidosis develops in bacteraemic shock. When there is an unexplained metabolic acidosis with an 'anion gap' greater than 10 mmol/L, plasma lactate measurement should be obligatory.

ACUTE RENAL FAILURE

Acute renal failure (ARF) after trauma or surgery requires prompt diagnosis and careful management. Oliguria is a common but not invariable presenting feature, as about 20% of cases have normal or increased urinary output. Table 10.4 indicates the simple laboratory investigations that are useful in differentiating prerenal and established ARF, but they are not unfailingly discriminatory in every instance. In prerenal ARF there is active conservation of water and salt involving ADH and aldosterone to maintain the ECF volume. Consequently, the urine has a high osmolality and urea concentration, but a low sodium. In established oliguric ARF, the urine:

plasma urea and osmolality ratios are low, with a high sodium concentration. Intravenous diuretic or mannitol therapy promotes a spontaneous diuresis in prerenal ARF, which can usually be reversed by vigorous fluid replacement.

Other associated features of ARF are increases in plasma creatinine and urea, hyperkalaemia, metabolic acidosis, hypocalcaemia and salt and water overload if replacement of either was excessive before diagnosis. Nitrogen retention is not as dangerous as hyperkalaemia, and concentrations of potassium above 6–6.5 mmol/L need urgent treatment to prevent cardiac arrhythmias and arrest. The large amount of potassium liberated by muscle crush injury and rhabdomyolysis and uncompensated metabolic acidosis will exacerbate the situation. Myoglobinuria should be anticipated in the muscle conditions.

REFERENCES

1. Solomkin J.S., Simmons R.L. (1983). Cellular and subcellular mediators of acute inflammation. *Surg. Clin. North Am.*, **63**, 225.
2. McPhaden A.R., Whaley K. (1985). The complement system in sepsis and trauma. *Br. Med. Bull.*, **41**, 281.
3. Dormandy T.L. (1989). Free-radical pathology and medicine—a review. *J.R. Coll. Phys. Lond.*, **23**, 221.
4. Heath D.F. (1985). Subcellular aspects of the response to trauma. *Br. Med. Bull.*, **41**, 240.
5. Hawker F. (1988). Endocrine changes in the critically ill. *Br. J. Hosp. Med.*, **39**, 278.
6. Frayn K.N. (1985). Substrate turnover after injury. *Br. Med. Bull.*, **41**, 232.
7. Jamieson M.J. (1985). Clinical algorithms: hyponatraemia. *Br. Med. J.*, **290**, 1723.
8. Brenton D.P., Gordon T.E. (1984). Fluid and electrolyte disorders: magnesium. *Br. J. Hosp. Med.*, **32**, 60.
9. Hallbrook T., Hedelin H. (1977). Zinc metabolism and surgical trauma. *Br. J. Surg.*, **64**, 27.
10. Bihari D.J. (1986). Disturbed homeostasis: metabolic acidosis. *Br. J. Hosp. Med.*, **35**, 89.

FURTHER READING

Bihari D., Semple S.J.G. eds. (1987). *Critical Care*, vol. 2 of *Medicine International*, Oxford: Medical Education (International), p. 38.
Tinker J., Rapin M. eds. (1983). *Care of the Critically Ill Patient*, 1st edn, Berlin: Springer Verlag.
Barton R.N. (1985). Trauma and its metabolic problems. *Br. Med. Bull.*, **41**, 201.

11. Clinical Biochemistry and Transplantation Surgery

G.A. Maguire and A.K. Trull

Introduction
General factors
    Assessment of potential donors
    Immunosuppression and cyclosporin
Kidney transplantation
    Selection of patients
    Pre- and perioperative monitoring
    Postoperative monitoring
    Immunosuppression
Heart transplantation
    Selection of patients and preoperative
        assessment
    Perioperative monitoring
    Postoperative monitoring
Heart and lung transplantation
    Preoperative assessment
    Peri- and postoperative monitoring
    Immunosuppression in heart and heart-lung
        transplant recipients
Liver transplantation
    Patient selection and preoperative
        assessment
    Perioperative monitoring
    Postoperative monitoring
    Immunosuppression
Pancreatic transplantation
    Selection and assessment of patients
    Perioperative monitoring
    Postoperative monitoring
Multiple organ transplants
Biochemical detection of rejection
Future perspectives

INTRODUCTION

The first successful human organ transplant operation was performed by Joseph E. Murray at the Peter Bent Brigham Hospital, Boston, Massachusetts in 1954. He transplanted a kidney from one of a pair of identical twins to the other. Thus began the modern era of organ transplantation. For this work, Joseph E. Murray was awarded the 1990 Nobel prize for medicine jointly with E. Donnall Thomas, the pioneer of clinical bone marrow transplantation.

Today the success rate of organ transplantation is impressive (Table 11.1, Fig. 11.1) and organ transplantation is widely recognized as being a viable treatment option for organ failure involving kidney, heart, lung or liver. Pancreatic transplantation is an established procedure, but not as widely adopted. Intestinal and skin transplantation have yet to become established. Corneal transplantation has been established for many years and bone transplantation has recently entered orthopaedic practice. Bone marrow transplantation is increasingly being successfully used in lymphoproliferative and other disorders. Only the transplantation of solid organs with a significant impact on clinical biochemistry will be considered here.

The term 'transplantation' is used here to mean the transplantation of an organ from one individual to another. The transplanted organ in these cases is an allograft. Homografts are grafts where the tissue comes from the recipient individuals themselves, for example coronary artery bypass grafts or skin grafts. These will also not be considered further.

Clinical biochemistry is used to a greater or lesser extent in the assessment of potential donors, the selection and assessment of patients for transplantation, and in perioperative and postoperative monitoring. Transplantation surgery requires some special biochemical support but many of these demands are not unique to this situation. Some of the postoperative requirements for intensive care of cardiac and liver transplant recipients will be similar to those of other patients, particularly in the (nowadays rare) case when multiorgan failure occurs (*see* Chapter 10).

TABLE 11.1
SURVIVAL OF TRANSPLANT RECIPIENTS

Organ	Year of transplant	No. of transplants	1-year patient survival (%)	4-year patient survival (%)	5-year patient survival (%)
Kidney	1985	942	90		78
	1988	1147	94		
Heart	1985	119	65	60	
	1988	274	74		
Heart-lung	1985	35	54	40	
	1988	83	60		
Liver	1985	56	43	34	
	1988	195	50		

Data taken with permission from the UK Transplant Registry Annual Report 1990.

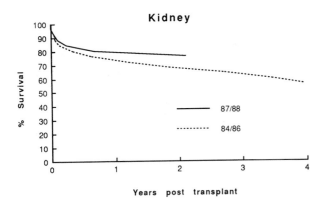

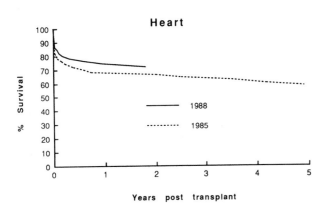

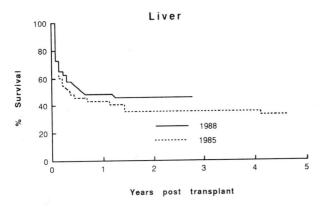

Fig. 11.1 Survival of grafted organs: the results are taken with permission from the 1990 annual report of the UK transplant service.

The monitoring of organ function of renal and hepatic transplant recipients will be similar to that of those with reversible failure of these organs (*see* Chapters 19 and 22). A major role of clinical biochemistry in these patients is in the monitoring of immunosuppressive therapy, which will be considered here in detail.

GENERAL FACTORS

Assessment of Potential Donors

Organs for transplantation may be harvested from living, related donors or from donors who are certified as brain dead and are being maintained on a respirator. Kidneys are the only organ universally accepted as being ethical for living relatives to donate. After unilateral nephrectomy the remaining kidney undergoes hypertrophy to compensate. Although the loss of renal reserve might be expected to make the donor more susceptible to renal disease, there has been no increase in clinically significant renal disease in donors followed for 10–20 years. Partial donation of liver and pancreas from living relatives is possible but involves risk to the donor. Partial pancreas donors have gone on to develop impaired glucose tolerance[1] and complications (including death) from partial liver donation have led to only a limited adoption of this procedure.

The causes of brain death are usually cerebral trauma as a result of a road-traffic accident, subarachnoid haemorrhage, primary brain tumour, or cardiac or respiratory arrest. Biochemical tests are vital if a diagnosis of brain death is being considered. They are necessary to exclude other causes of deep coma such as drugs or metabolic factors. Thus measurement of drug concentration will be required in a comatose patient previously treated with phenobarbitone or phenytoin. Measurement of glucose and electrolytes will be required to exclude metabolic causes such as hypoglycaemia.

It is also necessary to establish that the organ(s) being donated are healthy. Thus renal, liver and lung function should be assessed when harvesting of these organs is contemplated. Monitoring and correction of electrolyte abnormalities are important before harvesting to prevent possible deterioration of the donor organ(s). These tests will usually be made at the hospital where the potential donor is situated; consequently any laboratory may be requested to do these tests and not just laboratories at hospitals where transplant operations are performed.

Immunosuppression and Cyclosporin

The ideal immunosuppressive drug would selectively inhibit allograft rejection while leaving the rest of the immune system intact. Predictably the ideal drug does not exist. The first drugs to be used clinically were azathioprine (a derivative of 6-mercaptopurine) and adrenal corticosteroids. Although these non-specifically inhibit cellular and humoral immunity, they can be and were used successfully in renal transplantation. By the late 1970s, renal transplantation had become an accepted treatment for patients in end-stage renal failure. However considerable doubt remained about the future of other organ transplants. Fortunately, in 1978 the more selective immunosuppressive agent, cyclosporin, was introduced into clinical practice[2] and the survival rates now achieved (*see* Fig. 11.1) are in no small measure the result of the use of this drug. The frequency and severity of rejection crises are generally reported to be less in patients treated with cyclosporin than in those treated with the earlier drug regimens. Use of cyclosporin also allows lower doses of steroids to be used. This 'steroid sparing' is particularly advantageous in childhood recipients of transplants, in whom normal growth can be achieved, and in diabetic recipients, in whom steroids can aggravate the glucose intolerance.

Cyclosporin is a metabolite isolated from *Tolypocladium inflatum* Gams. It is a neutral, lipophilic cyclic undecapeptide with a molecular weight of 1202.6. It has a selective mode of action, inhibiting the early events in T-helper lymphocyte activation, so preventing lymphokine-driven differentiation and proliferation of effector T- and B-cells.[3]

One major disappointment that emerged from the clinical use of cyclosporin was that in man, in contrast to many of the animal species studied, therapeutic doses caused a number of adverse side-effects. The major side-effect is renal impairment; others are hepatic dysfunction, hypertension, neurotoxicity, lymphoma, abnormal glucose homeostasis, hypertrichosis and gingival hypertrophy. Some degree of renal impairment is seen in virtually all patients receiving cyclosporin, and it is this attendant nephrotoxicity that limits its clinical application.

Unlike the earlier-used immunosuppressants, the efficacy and degree of toxicity of the drug are highly variable between individuals. Pharmacokinetic studies have revealed that this is at least partly due to substantial intra- as well as interindividual variability in absorption, distribution and clearance of cyclosporin.[4,5] The variation is so great that standard dosing protocols based on median population values are not appropriate for the majority of patients and most centres have adopted the strategy of monitoring blood concentrations of cyclosporin with appropriate dosage adjustment to compensate for interindividual variability.

Several factors can complicate the interpretation of cyclosporin assays. Cyclosporin is metabolized to a number of compounds that may have immunosuppressive and/or toxic activity and that may be detected by some immunoassays for cyclosporin. Furthermore, the distribution of the drug between plasma and red cells changes with time and temperature. This has led to widespread debate as to which choice of assay (specific for the parent drug or cross-reacting with metabolites) and which choice of sample (whole blood or plasma) provides the better guide to efficacy and toxicity in monitoring cyclosporin. The consensus is that the drug should be measured when it is at its lowest concentration in blood (i.e. the 'trough'), that assays should be specific for the parent drug, and that whole blood should be used for its measurement.[6,7,8] Specific and reliable

whole-blood assays for cyclosporin are now widely available.

Cyclosporin is usually given orally but absorption is slow, incomplete and erratic. The bioavailability of cyclosporin is usually only 30%[9] and may be considerably lower in patients with external biliary drainage, cholestasis, gastrointestinal disease and reduced pancreatic exocrine section. In patients with external biliary diversion, intravenous cyclosporin infusion is currently the only means of achieving therapeutic blood concentrations. A new microemulsion oral formulation of cyclosporin, which may be less dependent upon bile salts for its absorption, is now under evaluation. Preliminary results in a liver transplant recipient with cholestasis and impaired absorption of the conventional oral cyclosporin formulation indicate that absorption of the microemulsion formulation is substantially greater.[10]

Poor and highly variable absorption of oral cyclosporin is a particular problem in the first weeks after transplantation. During this period, the recommended frequency of monitoring trough cyclosporin blood concentrations is every 2 days. Daily monitoring may be warranted in some patients, particularly children, or during coadministration of drugs known to interfere with the pharmacokinetics of cyclosporin. High dosage requirements can present physical problems of administration, especially in children, and also have important financial implications because the drug is expensive.

At 37°C most cyclosporin in the plasma is bound to high-, low- or very low-density lipoproteins (34%, 34% and 10% respectively) and to chylomicrons.[11] Since lipoproteins serve as a reservoir for cyclosporin, probably directly transferring the drug into plasma membranes, lipid binding may buffer its effects. The neurotoxicity of cyclosporin has been found to be enhanced if serum cholesterol concentrations are below 3.1 mmol/L.[12]

Cyclosporin elimination occurs predominantly by metabolism in the liver, the rate of metabolism being limited by the fraction of the drug that is unbound and the capacity of the metabolizing enzymes within the liver and to a lesser extent by the rate of delivery of cyclosporin to it, which is itself determined by the hepatic blood flow. About 6% of a given dose appears in urine. Therefore renal failure does not significantly alter cyclosporin clearance. As most of the circulating cyclosporin is lipoprotein bound, haemodialysis also has no appreciable effect on clearance.

Many drugs are known to interfere with the metabolism of cyclosporin. Of particular importance are drugs such as phenytoin and rifampicin that induce the activity of those hepatic cytochrome P450 enzymes responsible for cyclosporin metabolism, so reducing its blood concentration and potentially precipitating rejection. This enzyme induction may take several days to affect concentrations demonstrably. In contrast, drugs that are believed to compete with cyclosporin for the hepatic enzyme pool, such as

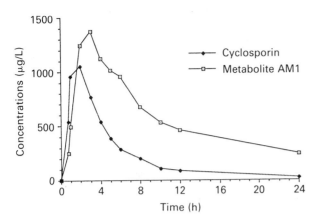

Fig. 11.2 Mean cyclosporin and primary metabolite (AM1) concentrations measured by high-pressure liquid chromatography in 10 healthy volunteers following a single oral dose (5 mg/kg) of cyclosporin.

erythromycin and ketoconazole, can cause an increase in cyclosporin concentrations far more quickly. Sometimes it is not possible to avoid the use of such interacting drugs and close monitoring of cyclosporin is extremely important under such circumstances.

The total number of possible cyclosporin metabolites is now known to exceed 30, although fewer than six appear to be present in the blood in significant amounts. The drug is converted into more polar metabolites that retain the cyclic structure.[13] Primary metabolite concentrations are usually greater than parent cyclosporin concentrations in trough whole-blood samples (Fig. 11.2) and some tissue samples.[14,15] Metabolites are eliminated mainly (90%) by secretion into bile, and thus cholestasis causes an increase in metabolite concentrations in blood.

To what extent the metabolites of cyclosporin have immunosuppressive activity is critical to our application of therapeutic drug monitoring in the optimization of cyclosporin dosage. Immunosuppressive activity—albeit less than that observed for parent cyclosporin—has been found *in vitro* for metabolites AM1, AM9 and AM4N.[16–18] Currently cyclosporin metabolites are not routinely measured. Whether there might be a case for so doing in certain circumstances requires further study.

Provision of a Cyclosporin Assay Service
As discussed above, cyclosporin should be measured in whole-blood samples by means of a method that is specific for the parent drug. Various methods are available, including high-pressure liquid chromatography, fluorescence polarization immunoassay and radioimmunoassay. Each has its own advantages and disadvantages with regard to speed, convenience and cost. The level of service provision will vary between transplant centres and will depend on the types of transplant(s) being carried out. Given the requirements for monitoring discussed below, the service

needs to be available at least three times per week and preferably every day from Monday to Friday. It is not usual to require the measurement of cyclosporin concentrations at weekends, although samples may be taken for retrospective assessment of any changes, especially in the early postoperative period. This may assist with the targeting of the therapeutic range when dosage is increasing daily. Occasionally, an urgent request for blood cyclosporin measurement is warranted at weekends, particularly if an important drug interaction is likely to reduce blood concentrations precipitously over this period. A member of staff should be available 'on call' to cover such eventualities.

Transplant patients often live well away from the transplant centre but are followed-up there. To avoid the need to travel to the transplant centre for blood monitoring, samples are often taken locally. To ensure that the same assay procedure, sample matrix and sample collection protocols are used during follow-up, it has been the practice for samples to be posted to the laboratory at the transplant centre. This is now probably no longer strictly necessary as the use of similar protocols is now widespread. However, the consequences of inappropriate dosage adjustment in the event that the wrong method of measurement is used are potentially so dangerous that it may still be wise to continue this practice. Samples may be sent by a next-day delivery postal service without freezing by the patient's own practitioner or local hospital, the EDTA anticoagulant also serving as an effective bacteriostatic agent in the short term.

Newer Immunosuppressive Agents
Given the nephrotoxic and other side-effects of cyclosporin, it is not surprising that other selective immunosuppressive agents have been sought. Only one, FK506, has so far been widely used in humans and is currently undergoing extensive clinical trials. Preliminary results from clinical trials of its use in liver transplantation suggest that it is not free from side-effects, including nephrotoxicity, and that monitoring of its blood concentration will be necessary to avoid these. As was the case with the early experience in the use of cyclosporin, the choice of sample matrix and collection time as well as the ideal assay method remain to be determined.

KIDNEY TRANSPLANTATION

Transplantation is arguably the treatment of choice for end-stage renal failure which is inevitably the end-point of the chronic renal failure that can result from a variety of renal diseases. Some, such as acute glomerulonephritis, rarely progress to chronic failure; others, such as adult polycystic disease, invariably do. However, acute glomerulonephritis is much more common than polycystic disease and therefore causes more patients to develop end-stage failure (Table 11.2). Renal transplantation is done heterotopically;

TABLE 11.2
CAUSES OF END-STAGE RENAL FAILURE (PERCENTAGES)

Glomerulonephritis	21
Pyelonephritis	16
Polycystic disease	10
Renal vascular disease	12
Diabetes mellitus type 1	9
Diabetes mellitus type 2	3
Others	29

that is, the transplanted kidney is placed at a site (the right iliac fossa) different from its natural position.

Selection of Patients

Chronic renal failure is progressive and irreversible. As the disease progresses, the number of functioning nephrons diminishes. This is manifested by steadily falling creatinine clearance. By definition, end-stage failure is reached when the creatinine clearance is less than 5 mL/min. At this stage, renal replacement therapy is required, of which there are two forms, renal transplantation and dialysis. These two are not mutually exclusive: it is usual for a patient to undergo a period of dialysis while waiting for a suitable donor and patients may return to dialysis if the transplant is not successful.

Once the diagnosis of end-stage renal failure has been made, the decision on whom and when the transplant should be performed is taken not on biochemical grounds but on the availability of a suitably matched donor organ, presence of a disease not well managed on dialysis (such as, some would argue, diabetes), age and patient's preference. Although the quality of life after a renal transplant is generally considered to be better than that on dialysis, not all suitable patients actually desire a transplant.

Pre- and Perioperative Monitoring

Before transplantation the patient will usually be receiving maintenance haemodialysis or continuous ambulatory peritoneal dialysis. It is important to check electrolytes, particularly potassium, before operation because of the danger of cardiac arrhythmias arising from hyperkalaemia. If the potassium concentration is greater than 5.5 mmol/L, then it will need to be brought down by dialysis. In any case, dialysis will be required if it has not been done in the previous 24 h. If the patient is diabetic, good glycaemic control will have to be established. Thus urgent preoperative assays of glucose and electrolytes will be required.

Changes in electrolytes can occur intraoperatively and potassium monitoring where possible has been recommended by some. In practice, intraoperative monitoring is rarely required. However, there will always be occasions when urgent potassium measurement is required.

Postoperative Monitoring

The aim of postoperative monitoring is to detect failure of the donated organ as well as secondary complications of the operation itself or the subsequent therapy. Organ failure may be the result of a poor donor kidney, technical problems of the operation (e.g. leakage, ureteric obstruction or thrombosis) or rejection. Biochemical tests will detect organ failure but cannot distinguish the cause. Primary organ non-function is rare but electrolyte abnormalities can sometimes develop very quickly (e.g. with acute tubular necrosis of the transplanted kidney, which occurs in 60% of donor kidneys subjected to more than 24 hours', ischaemia). Therefore immediate postoperative measurement of electrolytes may be required, particularly if a diuresis has not been established (urine flow less than 30 mL/h). Hyperkalaemia may be monitored continuously but crudely from an electrocardiogram. A potassium concentration greater than 7.0 mmol/L will lead to detectable electrocardiographic changes. Control of postoperative fluid balance consists basically of replacing known and estimated fluid and electrolyte losses. Fluid losses are sometimes enormous. One transplant recipient at our hospital produced up to 16 L of urine per day. The monitoring of postoperative fluid balance for the duration of the hospital stay consists of daily measurement of serum electrolytes and regular (thrice weekly has proved sufficient) measurement of the 24-h urinary excretion of sodium, potassium and protein, with calculation of the creatinine clearance.

At one time, patients were kept in hospital for a month; nowadays the stay is normally for about 10 days. The incidence of acute rejection is greatest between the second and fourth postoperative weeks and therefore rejection may occur after the patient has left hospital. There are no specific biochemical tests for transplant rejection. However, deteriorating renal function as evidenced by rising serum urea and creatinine and falling creatinine clearance is an indication for renal biopsy from which the histological diagnosis of rejection is made. A deterioration in renal function is less likely to be due to rejection if urinary protein excretion is normal.

Ideally, daily electrolyte measurements should be made in order to detect rejection as soon as possible so that necessary treatment can be started without delay. This may not be easy to arrange if the patient has left hospital. A practical compromise is the twice-weekly measurement of serum and urine electrolytes, creatinine clearance and protein excretion for the first month. As the likelihood of acute rejection recedes, electrolyte monitoring can be relaxed, as indicated in Table 11.3.

Late complications after transplantation are (in order of prevalence) hypertension, infection, malignancy, anaemia, chronic hepatitis, diabetes, peptic ulcer, myocardial infarction and tertiary hyperparathyroidism. Biochemical tests to detect or help in the differential diagnosis of some of these are

TABLE 11.3
SUGGESTED POST RENAL-TRANSPLANT ELECTROLYTE MONITORING

Period post operation	Serum electrolytes	Urine electrolytes
Days 0–10 (inpatient)	Daily	Thrice weekly
Days 10–30	Ideally daily; minimum twice weekly	Twice weekly
Weeks 4–8	Weekly	Weekly
Months 3–5	Every 6 weeks	Every 6 weeks
Months 5–24	Every 3 months	Every 3 months
Thereafter	Twice yearly	Twice yearly

available. Cyclosporin nephrotoxicity is discussed below.

Hypertension occurs in about 50% of transplant recipients. The mechanisms are various and incompletely understood. Most patients will be controlled by drugs but surgical intervention is necessary in a few. Measurement of plasma renin activity in samples collected after selective venous catheterization may be helpful. Higher concentrations in veins draining the native kidney compared with the transplanted kidney indicate that the diseased native kidney is the cause of the hypertension, although similar concentrations from both kidneys do not rule it out. When transplant arterial stenosis can be ruled out, removal of the native kidney in hypertension that is refractory to medical treatment will usually control the hypertension. If renal arterial stenosis of the transplanted kidney is suspected, the plasma renin activity may be high but the diagnosis is usually made by arteriography.

Immunosuppressive therapy would be expected to render the transplant recipient more prone to infection and 20–30% of recipients experience a clinically important infection.[19] The natural history of infection with hepatitis B is different in these immunocompromised patients. The majority who are infected go on to develop chronic active hepatitis and half of these may die of liver disease.[20] Conventional liver function tests measured biannually are used to help to detect and monitor this complication.

Tertiary hyperparathyroidism, although less common in transplant recipients than in those on dialysis, is a well-recognized complication. The autonomous production of parathyroid hormone leads to hypercalcaemia and thus monitoring of calcium concentrations is required. Treatment by parathyroidectomy requires careful postoperative monitoring of calcium, as profound hypocalcaemia can develop.

The incidence of steroid-induced diabetes (as well as of steroid-induced cataracts) is declining as steroid doses have declined. Reduction of the steroid dose will correct the diabetes. Measurement of blood glucose at annual review will detect this potential complication.

Immunosuppression

The nephrotoxicity of cyclosporin was recognized soon after its introduction into clinical practice[21] and it was recommended that its administration should be delayed until diuresis had been established. The relatively high (compared with current practice) doses given to kidney transplant recipients, superimposed on the unavoidable ischaemic damage to a cadaveric donor kidney, were found to predispose to the development of interstitial fibrosis in the late phase.[22] The increased susceptibility of the transplanted kidney to cyclosporin nephrotoxicity is responsible for the almost classical clinical dilemma over cyclosporin management in the early postoperative period. That is, the nephrotoxicity of the drug is greatest at a time when there is the highest risk of acute rejection requiring especially effective immunosuppression. New therapeutic strategies had to be devised either to reduce the dosages of cyclosporin required for effective immunosuppression or to reduce its nephrotoxic side-effects. The former strategy has been the most widely applied over the last decade, reduced doses of cyclosporin being given with various combinations of supplementary immunosuppressive agents.

Most kidney transplant centres use one of a variety of cyclosporin-based, combination immunosuppressive regimens. 'Triple therapy' (cyclosporin, azathioprine and prednisolone) is regarded as particularly beneficial in patients with impaired renal function as a result of prolonged 'cold ischaemia' time and in those with cyclosporin-induced nephrotoxicity.[23] Patients who cannot tolerate the full dose of azathioprine or steroids may also benefit from a reduction in the required doses of these less selective immunosuppressive agents.

Immunosuppressive Combination Therapy as Induction Treatment

In general, very low oral doses of cyclosporin are given in the immediate postoperative period and the dose is slowly increased until satisfactory blood concentrations are attained over about a 7-day period. In patients with delayed graft function, any increase in dose is usually delayed until the serum creatinine has fallen to a reasonable level (e.g. 200 μmol/L).

During the first week, antithymocyte globulin is commonly used to provide effective immunosuppression while blood concentrations of cyclosporin remain subtherapeutic. This protocol, when used in combination with steroids and azathioprine, is often referred to as quadruple therapy. Double (cyclosporin and steroids), triple and quadruple induction treatment protocols have been devised.[24] Most are designed to introduce cyclosporin slowly and judiciously, particularly in patients with delayed kidney function, while providing effective immunosuppressive cover with alternative agents.

Despite the reduction in the effective dosage requirement for cyclosporin made possible by triple or quadruple regimens, significant nephrotoxicity is still seen with doses as low as 1.5–2.0 mg/kg. Regular monitoring of blood cyclosporin concentrations and renal function is particularly advocated in the early postoperative period, which is characterized by unstable graft function, extreme interindividual variability in response to cyclosporin therapy and heightened risk of both acute rejection and nephrotoxicity. Shaw et al.[8] reviewed the therapeutic ranges for solid-organ transplantation from several centres in Canada and the United States where whole-blood and selective cyclosporin assays are used. Most kidney transplant centres have target ranges between 50 and 200 μg/L higher in the first 3 months than in subsequent months.

Ideally, cyclosporin should be monitored at least every other day in the first few weeks following transplantation and, indeed, close monitoring should be continued for 3 months to compensate for documented changes in the pharmacokinetics of the drug during this period. In kidney recipients the absolute bioavailability may range from less than 5% to 68%, with a mean of 27%,[25] indicating the necessity for individual dosage adjustment based on blood concentration measurements. A three- to fivefold increase in bioavailability over time has been noted.[26] Clearly, without regular and careful adjustment of dosage in the early postoperative period, increased bioavailability would lead to increased blood cyclosporin concentrations and nephrotoxic damage to the allograft.

Immunosuppressive Combination Therapy as Maintenance Treatment

Although early graft loss is not always attributable to rejection, it is well recognized that the risk of acute rejection is highest during the first 3 months after kidney transplantation. The mechanism(s) underlying this apparently steady decrease in alloreactivity (i.e. immunoreactivity of the allograft) with time is not clearly understood but most management protocols have been designed to take into account the need for greater immunosuppression during the immediate postoperative period.

The major impact of cyclosporin on renal allograft survival is within the first 3 postoperative months.[27]

It is therefore prudent to maintain careful monitoring of cyclosporin concentrations throughout this period. Lindholm and coworkers[28] concluded that, overall, the selective monoclonal antibody-based radioimmunoassay (Sandoz) of the whole-blood matrix provided the best means of distinction between patients who respond well and poorly to cyclosporin treatment – in terms of rejection, nephrotoxicity and infection. Shaw and coworkers[29] selected 200 μg/L as the optimum cyclosporin concentration, minimizing the incidence of both rejection and nephrotoxicity. Routine cyclosporin monitoring is particularly valuable in kidney transplant recipients, as a rising serum creatinine can be the result of either rejection or nephrotoxicity, a high blood cyclosporin concentration more often being associated with cyclosporin nephrotoxicity than allograft rejection.

The time of blood sampling in relation to the time of dose is crucial to the interpretation of cyclosporin concentration. The trough level (i.e. the concentration immediately before the next dose) is invariably used but sampling at other times has been considered. Preliminary data from Johnston[30] suggest that a single value, taken at 5 (t_5) or 6 (t_6) hours after cyclosporin administration, but not the trough (t_0), correlate with the average drug concentration during the dosing interval. Cantarovich[31] has also shown that plasma cyclosporin concentrations measured by polyclonal (non-selective) radioimmunoassay 6 h after oral administration (t_6) correlate with clinical events better than t_0. The t_6 concentration also coincides with the median peak steady-state concentration in clinically stable renal transplant recipients on chronic oral dosing (Fig. 11.3). It could be, for instance, that, as for gentamicin, t_0 gives a guide to efficacy and t_6 gives a guide to toxicity. Prospective clinical studies are required to assess whether, in practice, measurement of drug concentrations at times other than t_0 are useful.

Immunosuppression in Patients with Chronic Renal Dysfunction

One of the main problems with cyclosporin therapy in kidney transplant recipients is related to chronic renal dysfunction due to chronic rejection, chronic nephrotoxicity, or both. In cases of predominantly chronic nephrotoxicity, a modified triple-drug therapy—consisting of low or even ultra-low cyclosporin doses combined with azathioprine and prednisolone—may be tried. If this is unsuccessful, conversion to azathioprine/prednisolone seems to be the last resort to overcome this problem. However, the potential risk of conversion-induced rejection has to be kept in mind.

In cases of predominantly chronic rejection, again a modified triple-drug protocol should be considered. This consists of an increased cyclosporin dose adjusted to target concentrations at the upper limit of the therapeutic range, in combination with azathioprine and prednisolone, which should also be given

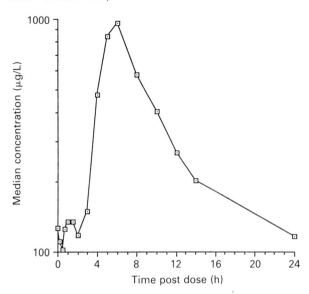

Fig. 11.3 Median steady-state cyclosporin concentrations (Cyclo-trak SP; Incstar Corp.) measured in whole blood from 15 clinically stable kidney transplant recipients on chronic oral dosing. All patients were receiving cyclosporin doses to achieve trough blood concentrations within the range of 80–150 μg/L.

at transiently increased doses. It must be stressed, however, that the prognosis for chronically rejected organs is usually very poor, regardless of what rescue efforts have been made.

Cyclosporin Monotherapy

In some kidney transplant centres in the UK, cyclosporin monotherapy is still the treatment of choice. For monotherapy to succeed, it may be particularly important to achieve adequate blood concentrations of cyclosporin as quickly as possible.[32] Salaman[33] commences treatment with oral cyclosporin at a dose of 15 mg/kg, reducing this dose once satisfactory whole blood concentrations have been attained. Rejection episodes are relatively common, but usually respond rapidly to a short course of high-dose methylprednisolone.

Cyclosporin monotherapy can, of course, also be instituted by discontinuation of all other immunosuppressive agents apart from cyclosporin. Conversion to cyclosporin monotherapy is compatible with the concept of a reducing risk of rejection with time after transplantation. Steroid withdrawal should reduce the risk of potentially serious side-effects without precipitating rejection but, in practice, rejection episodes have been observed,[34,35] although they have usually responded to treatment. Cyclosporin monotherapy is not generally considered appropriate for other organ transplants because of the more serious consequences of organ failure. It is conceivable, however, that patients with established grafts might be converted to monotherapy so that they can benefit

from the very low infection rate associated with this type of treatment.

HEART TRANSPLANTATION

Although the first successful heart transplant operation in man was performed in 1968, it was done with more enthusiasm than experience and was followed by a series of disastrous operations worldwide in which 80% of 150 recipients died soon after surgery. It was not until the introduction of immunosuppression with cyclosporin in the late 1970s and early 1980s and the work of Norman Shumway in Stanford, that the impressive results shown in Fig. 11.1 above were obtained.

Selection of Patients and Preoperative Assessment

Clinical biochemistry does not feature heavily in the selection of patients for heart transplantation as biochemical changes are not used to assess the severity of the diseases for which transplantation is indicated, the vast majority of which are for either cardiomyopathy or ischaemic heart disease. However, it is important to investigate the possible presence of coexistent disease that may be an absolute or relative contraindication to transplantation. The contraindications have changed as experience has grown. Thus, although hepatic disease should be excluded, renal disease and diabetes are not now considered absolute contraindications. For instance, retransplantation of the heart may be accompanied by renal transplantation where the nephrotoxicity is the result of immunosuppression.

Perioperative Monitoring

During the transplant operation the functions of the patient's heart and lungs are transferred to a heart-lung machine. During this 'bypass' procedure, monitoring of its effectiveness is achieved by measuring blood gases. During bypass the patient's plasma potassium usually starts to fall and potassium infusions may be required, the aim being to maintain the plasma potassium above 4.0 mmol/L. Acidosis or acidaemia can also occur. Thus, immediately before and every 30 min during the bypass, monitoring of blood gases and electrolytes is necessary. Care must be taken in the interpretation of the blood gas results, as pH and P_{O_2} are temperature dependent and the patient is cooled to 30°C during bypass. As the results are required quickly and relatively frequently, analysis close to the theatre is preferable. The less acceptable alternative is to have a courier to transport specimens to the laboratory. Analysers that will measure blood gases (pH, P_{O_2}, P_{CO_2}) and electrolytes (Na$^+$, K$^+$, Ca^{2+}) on a single arterial specimen are available. They may be used successfully by non-laboratory personnel and may be sited within the theatre suite to allow instantaneous monitoring of these vari-

TABLE 11.4

SUGGESTED BIOCHEMICAL MONITORING PROTOCOL FOR HEART AND HEART-LUNG
TRANSPLANT RECIPIENTS

	Biochemical investigations
Immediate preoperative	U + E, LFT, glucose, uric acid, TIBC
Days 1–3 postoperative	Daily U + E, LFT, glucose, LFT, gases, calcium and phosphate, serum and urine osmolality
Days 4–10 postoperative	Daily U + E, LFT, cyclosporin; thrice weekly 24-h urine
Days 10–intermediate discharge (i.e. ~14–28 days)	Thrice weekly, U + E, LFT, cyclosporin, 24-h urine
Intermediate discharge – full discharge (i.e. ~21–35 days)	Thrice weekly U + E, LFT; weekly glucose
At 6 weeks	U + E, LFT, uric acid, glucose, cyclosporin
At 2 months	As above
At 3 months	As above
At 4 months	As above
Every 3 months thereafter	As above
Every 6 months thereafter	As above plus fasting glucose and lipids

Protocol taken with permission from the Guidelines for the Management of Transplant
Patients, Papworth Hospital, Cambridge.
Abbreviations: LFT, liver function tests; TIBC, total iron-binding capacity; U + E, urea and
electrolytes.

ables. The potential problems of the use of analysers
not in the laboratory are outside the scope of this
chapter.

Postoperative Monitoring

There are no biochemical means of monitoring cardiac function but possible damage to other organs
either from the operation itself or from the medication must be looked for. Thus daily measurement of
electrolytes will be required to monitor the intravenous drip regimens and to detect possible renal
damage occurring as a result of the operation or as
a consequence of immunosuppression (*see below*).
A suggested monitoring protocol as used in Papworth Hospital, Cambridge (UK) is given in Table
11.4.

Early graft failure (at less than 9 days) is usually
due to acute rejection but the most common cause of
late failure (at more than 1 year) is coronary occlusive
disease. This is thought to be due to multiple minor
rejection episodes. However, hyperlipidaemia is associated with cyclosporin therapy and therefore occurs
commonly after heart transplantation. The contribution of abnormal lipid concentrations to the coronary
arterial disease is not known but such abnormalities
are taken sufficiently seriously in some centres to
prompt intervention. Thus monitoring of lipid concentrations is part of the long term follow-up of these
patients (Table 11.4).

Immunosuppression of heart transplant recipients is
considered later.

HEART AND LUNG TRANSPLANTATION

Heart and lungs are usually transplanted together as
a set and this is currently the most common procedure. However, transplantation of lungs alone is
now becoming an accepted procedure for limited
applications such as for pulmonary emphysema. If
the recipient of a heart-lung has good preoperative
cardiac function, then the recipient's heart can in
turn be used to transplant into a patient requiring
heart transplant alone—the 'domino' procedure. Potential donors of heart and lung require careful evaluation of their suitability. This includes standard pulmonary function tests and blood gas measurement. A
P_{O_2} of greater than 15 kPa should be achieved with
an inspired O_2 concentration of 30%.

Preoperative Assessment

As discussed above for heart transplantation, clinical
biochemistry is used to detect coexistent disease. For
heart-lung transplantation, clinical biochemistry can
help to assess the severity of the disease. Thus cystic
fibrotic patients with elevated P_{CO_2} (> 6.5 kPa) have a
greater mortality while awaiting transplantation than
those with a normal P_{CO_2}. However, as with other
transplant groups, the choice of recipient is dependent on compatible blood group, cytomegalovirus
serology and physical size, the last being particularly
important. In effect the 'donor selects the recipient'.
However, where there is more than one potential
recipient, the severity of the disease will influence the
choice.

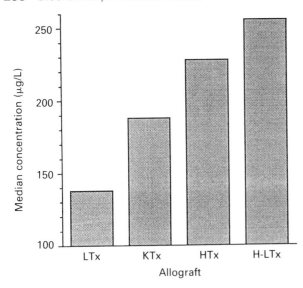

Fig. 11.4 Median whole-blood cyclosporin concentrations measured in the first 3 postoperative months in 30 liver (LTx), 30 kidney (KTx), 24 heart (HTx) and 8 heart-lung transplant (H-LTx) recipients.

Peri- and Postoperative Monitoring

This is similar to that described above for heart transplantation.

Immunosuppression in Heart and Heart-lung Transplant Recipients

In general, the management of immunosuppression in heart and heart-lung transplant recipients is similar to that of kidney recipients. However, the use of steroids is controversial. Some centres do not use long-term steroids for maintenance immunosuppression so as to avoid many of the potentially serious attendant side-effects of chronic steroid treatment. In other centres, steroids and azathioprine are given intraoperatively to heart transplant recipients. Steroids retard healing of the tracheal and bronchial anastomoses in heart-lung recipients and their administration should be delayed until 2 weeks after transplantation. However, it is sometimes started earlier to treat acute rejection. In recent years at Papworth Hospital the concern over the effects of steroids on healing have been allayed by improvements in surgical technique and organ preservation. The introduction of cyclosporin did, however, permit an overall reduction in the use of steroids. Indeed, this steroid-sparing effect during the early postoperative period was largely responsible for initiation of the first heart-lung programme in Stanford in the spring of 1981.

Heart and heart-lung transplant recipients at Papworth do not usually receive cyclosporin (2–5 mg/kg) until the first day after transplantation. Pre- and intraoperative administration of cyclosporin to heart recipients was found to be associated with severe nephrotoxicity in patients whose renal function had often already been compromised by preoperative cardiac failure. In the first few postoperative days, cyclosporin doses are gradually increased to achieve therapeutic steady-state blood concentrations within a week. During this time, or until the patient is clinically stable, daily measurements of the blood concentration may be warranted to compensate carefully for interindividual variability in pharmacokinetics. Cyclosporin is given more cautiously or even delayed in patients with very poor postoperative renal function until the urine output increases and the serum creatinine concentration falls to an acceptable level as a result of improved cardiac output and renal perfusion.

The requirements for a particularly high level of immunosuppression in the early postoperative period, when the risk of rejection is greatest, are accentuated further in heart and heart-lung transplant recipients. Although there has been no carefully controlled comparison of rejection rates in recipients of different solid organs on identical immunosuppressive regimens, it has been suggested that heart transplant recipients do need relatively more prophylactic immunosuppression than kidney transplant recipients.[36] Almost all heart-lung transplant recipients at Papworth develop some acute rejection within the first 2 weeks after transplantation. Whether or not the thoracic organs are genuinely capable of eliciting a greater acute allogeneic immune response than the kidney in the transplant recipient, the consequence of intractable acute rejection in heart or heart-lung recipients is usually death, whereas the kidney recipient can be supported by dialysis if retransplantation is not an immediate option. The major clinical priority in heart and heart-lung recipients is, therefore, the prevention of rejection and, under some circumstances, this may be at the expense of deteriorating renal function due to cyclosporin-induced nephrotoxicity.

The greater risk of under-administering cyclosporin in heart or heart-lung recipients may be responsible for a tendency to maintain these patients on higher blood cyclosporin concentrations than kidney transplant patients. In one study the median cyclosporin concentrations during the first 3 postoperative months in heart and heart-lung recipients were 50–120 μg/L higher than those measured in kidney and liver recipients (Fig. 11.4). Unfortunately, one penalty for the excellent survival rate in this series was a high incidence of acute cyclosporin-induced nephrotoxicity, although there appeared to be considerable heterogeneity in the susceptibility to this side-effect.[37] Indeed, it has been argued that effective cyclosporin immunosuppression is not achieved without some degree of overt nephrotoxicity.

It has been intuitively assumed that excessive cyclosporin immunosuppression could predispose the transplant recipient to opportunistic infection, although there has been little objective evidence for this. Cytomegalovirus (CMV) infection is the most important infection affecting heart transplant recipients and many transplant centres have embarked on a CMV antibody-matching policy, matching CMV antibody-negative donor organs with antibody-negative recipients. Patients are monitored serologically after transplantation for evidence of primary infection, reinfection or reactivation of latent virus. In a longitudinal study of 95 heart transplant recipients, blood cyclosporin concentrations greater than 550 μg/L in the first two postoperative months were found to increase the susceptibility to CMV infection (more than fourfold rise in CMV antibody titre) and symptomatic disease.[38]

During the first 3–6 months after transplantation, the aim is to achieve blood cyclosporin concentrations of 200–400 μg/L in heart transplant recipients and 350–550 μg/L in heart-lung transplant recipients. With the passage of time after operation and, in the absence of rejection, the target concentration of cyclosporin can usually be reduced quite safely to 100–200 μg/L. The most common indication for a reduction in dose is a slow but progressive fall in creatinine clearance. However, the degree to which a reduction is possible depends upon the perceived short-term and long-term risks of inadequate cyclosporin dosage, including death from acute rejection. It has even been suggested that under some circumstances it may be necessary to sacrifice renal function in order to maintain adequate immunosuppression.[39]

The pharmacokinetic approach may be of value in reducing the nephrotoxicity of cyclosporin while maintaining effective immunosuppression. Fashola and coworkers[40] have found that, in prospective heart transplant recipients, a peak whole-blood cyclosporin concentration exceeding 750 μg/L is more likely to be associated with a decline in renal function after transplantation than a peak below this value. It was suggested that modification of dosage (e.g. from twice to three times daily) to minimize such high peak cyclosporin concentrations might be of value in avoiding this adverse effect.

More serious than the acute nephrotoxicity described above, however, is the development of chronic, irreversible, cyclosporin-induced nephrotoxicity. This has been described as the most significant complication associated with long-term use of cyclosporin in heart transplant recipients at Papworth Hospital.[41]

The development of chronic cyclosporin-associated nephrotoxicity is probably a cumulative process; the result of repeated or persistent exposure to nephrotoxic concentrations of cyclosporin in combination with a multitude of other predisposing factors. These may include preoperative renal dysfunction, age, infections and the use of other, additively nephrotoxic antibiotics such as aminoglycosides and amphotericin B. As with other transplant groups, regular monitoring of cyclosporin in heart and heart-lung transplant

recipients beyond 3 months is essential. This should be accompanied by appropriate dosage adjustment and further measurements under the new steady-state conditions 2 or 3 days later. Careful, long-term management of cyclosporin should also reduce the risk of opportunistic infections and repeated rejection episodes.

Analogous to the relation between acute and chronic nephrotoxicity, recurrent episodes of acute rejection are believed to be responsible for the development of chronic rejection. Chronic rejection is the major cause of death of long-term survivors of heart-lung transplants but inadequate immunosuppression is unlikely to be the cause. In a multivariate logistic regression analysis of 31 heart-lung transplant recipients it was found that the relative risk of rejection decreased with increasing blood cyclosporin concentrations within the first three postoperative weeks.[42] After this time there was no relation between blood cyclosporin concentrations and the risk of rejection, probably because maintenance immunosuppression in these patients is too high to confer any further protective effect. High variability in blood cyclosporin concentrations was, however, associated with an increased risk of rejection after 3 months. Therefore, there may be no precedent for increasing maintenance immunosuppression in this group beyond what is probably already more than adequate, even in the face of recurrent rejection. Instead, efforts should be concentrated on maintaining stable blood cyclosporin concentrations and perhaps, with time, even reducing maintenance immunosuppression to lower the incidence of infection and chronic nephrotoxicity.

Another long-term penalty of the relatively high levels of immunosuppression maintained in the heart, and particularly heart-lung, transplant groups may be a higher incidence of lymphomas than in other transplant groups. In a study from Pittsburgh, lymphomas occurred in 1% of kidney transplant recipients but in 1.8% of cardiac transplant recipients and 4.6% of recipients of heart-lung allografts.[43]

Individualization of cyclosporin dosage with the aid of blood concentration measurements is particularly important in the cystic fibrotic subgroup of heart-lung transplant recipients. On average, these patients require twice the daily dose of cyclosporin given to age- and sex-matched non-cystic recipients (Fig. 11.5) in order to achieve the equivalent blood cyclosporin concentration (Fig. 11.6). Preliminary results of a more formal comparison of cyclosporin pharmacokinetics in patients with cystic fibrosis and Eisenmenger syndrome awaiting heart-lung transplantation showed that cyclosporin bioavailability was lower and both clearance and steady-state volume of distribution were higher in the cystic fibrotic group. Clearly, without careful cyclosporin monitoring and appropriate dosage adjustment, recipients with cystic fibrosis would tend to be under-immunosuppressed on the dosage regimens used for other heart-

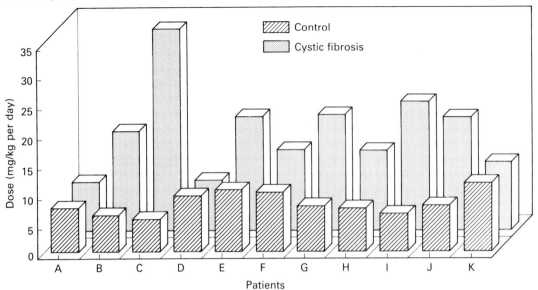

Fig. 11.5 Mean daily dosage of cyclosporin in cystic fibrosis and control patients.

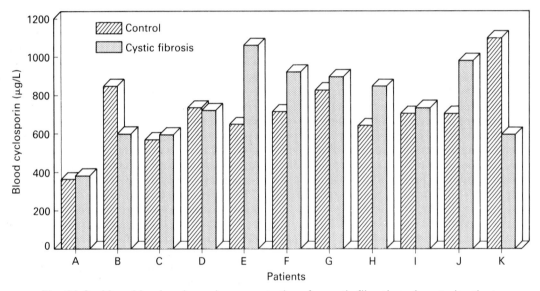

Fig. 11.6 Mean blood cyclosporin concentrations for cystic fibrosis and control patients.

lung transplant subgroups. The high dosage requirement in cystic fibrotic patients has prompted the use of dosing three or even four times a day—mainly to resolve the practical problem of physically taking such large oral doses of cyclosporin. As suggested earlier, this may have the additional benefit of reducing toxicity associated with high peak concentrations in patients on twice-a-day dosing, although this remains conjecture until carefully controlled comparisons are made between different dosing regimens.

LIVER TRANSPLANTATION

As with transplantation of other organs, the early history of liver transplantation was one of failure. In 1964, of the first six orthotopic liver transplant opera-tions performed by Professor Tom Starzl in Denver, Colorado, the longest survivor lived for only 23 days. No further operations were done for 3 years until 1967 when the programme was restarted in Denver and in Cambridge (UK) by Sir Roy Calne. Results have gradually improved and now it is considered to be a viable treatment option for a number of liver diseases (Table 11.5), although the overall results are less successful than those for kidney and heart transplants (*see* Table 11.1).

Of the transplantation operations performed, that of the liver perhaps poses the greatest challenge to the surgeon, anaesthetist, physician and biochemist. It is the most metabolically active organ—and manipulating, monitoring and artificially reproducing these metabolic functions all form a part of pre-,

TABLE 11.5
INDICATIONS FOR LIVER TRANSPLANTATION

Adult	*Childhood*
Primary biliary cirrhosis	Biliary atresia
Chronic active hepatitis	α_1-Antitrypsin deficiency
Primary hepatic malignancy	Metabolic, e.g. tyrosinosis
Acute liver failure, e.g. hepatitis A, B, drug reactions	
Metabolic, e.g. primary hyperoxaluria, Wilson's disease	

peri- and postoperative management. It poses special problems for the biochemistry laboratory, generating an enormous additional workload, particularly for urgent and semiurgent analyses, and sometimes for analytes that in most other circumstances would almost never be considered urgent.

Patient Selection and Preoperative Assessment

Biochemical investigation is required in the selection and assessment of suitable patients for transplantation and may contribute to the timing of the subsequent operation. The diseases listed in Table 11.5 as being indications for liver transplantation all give rise to abnormal results for liver function tests. However, the abnormalities are not characteristic for individual diseases and they cannot be used to distinguish between diseases that are suitable and those that are not suitable for transplantation. But, they can be used to monitor the progress of the disease, particularly those with fairly predictable courses such as primary biliary cirrhosis. The transplantation can then be done when progression to severe liver failure is imminent.

Preoperatively the most important biochemical tests are not liver function tests but, as with the other transplant groups, are those used to detect those secondary complications of the liver disease or other coexistent disease that may be a contraindication to transplantation. Thus blood gases should be measured. A low arterial P_{O_2} (<6.6 kPa) would be an indication of the presence of arteriovenous shunts or pulmonary fibrosis. These secondary complications of liver cirrhosis are absolute contraindications to transplantation because they are irreversible. Similarly, severe renal failure must be excluded. Patients may be malnourished and parenteral feeding may be necessary to bring them up to the required fitness before operation. It is widely believed that low albumin is a sign of malnutrition. This is not the case. However, very low albumin may be used as a contraindication to surgery, not because it indicates malnutrition but rather that the patient is ill.

Perioperative Monitoring

The operation has several distinct stages, each of which imposes different metabolic strains on the recipient with consequent biochemical changes. These changes are predictable and efforts are taken to forestall some of them. The operative stages are identified by the letters A–F.

Stage A is preoperative, when the patient is still on the ward; B is dissection of the diseased liver; C is the anhepatic phase, that is, when the recipient's liver has been removed; D is when the donor liver is perfused; E is when the gallbladder is anastomosed; and F is when the wound is finally closed.

During stage B and throughout the operation the patient is slightly overventilated to achieve a mild respiratory alkalosis. This helps to compensate for the metabolic acidosis occurring during the operation. Stages C and D are where the metabolic load is greatest. During the anhepatic phase (C), normal liver metabolism ceases. Before this, even with the most diseased liver, some metabolism (albeit at a reduced rate) of drugs, hydrogen ion, lactate, citrate, etc. can occur. The metabolism of citrate is particularly important as a large citrate load is given in transfused blood—3 g (approx. 100 mmol) per unit—and often around 15 units are transfused! This load could be metabolized by a normal liver but in its absence citrate complexes to calcium, leading to a low ionized calcium (Fig. 11.7). This lowering during the anhepatic phase is despite the infusion of 1% calcium chloride. The ionized calcium results illustrated in Fig. 11.7 were obtained after correction to a hydrogen ion concentration of 40 nmol/L. It is important to do this, as the value is used to estimate the amount of calcium to infuse and the hydrogen ion concentration is adjusted towards normal at the same time (either by infusion of bicarbonate or by metabolism once the donor liver is functioning). Eventual metabolism of the citrate by the donor liver leads to postoperative metabolic alkalosis.

During stage D the donor liver is introduced into the recipient's circulation. Although care is taken to flush out the liver before making the final connections and unclamping the inferior vena cava, there will be a bolus of acid and potassium released into the recipient's circulation at this stage. This is self-limit-

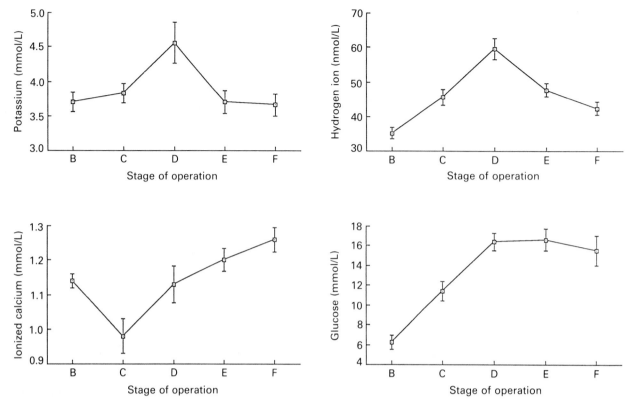

Fig. 11.7 Metabolic changes during liver transplantation. The results are the means ± SEM of 25 consecutive liver transplants performed at Addenbrooke's Hospital, Cambridge during May and June 1989. Reference ranges: ionized calcium, 1.18–1.30; potassium, 3.5–5.0; hydrogen ion, 35–45; glucose, 3.5–9.0.

ing but potentially lethal as the hyperkalaemia can lead to cardiac arrest. This is forestalled by correction of any disturbance of acid–base and ionized calcium before perfusion of the donor liver (Fig. 11.7).

During the course of the operation, despite the forced absence of hepatic gluconeogenesis and glycogenolysis, the glucose concentration increases. This is probably due to the stress of the operation with a small contribution from the dextrose contained in the transfused blood. In any case, no attempts are made to correct this.

From the foregoing it will be obvious that monitoring of blood gases, potassium and ionized calcium are mandatory during the operation. Monitoring of glucose is not essential because, although it changes, no action is necessary. As discussed above for heart transplantation, instruments for measuring these analytes are available and are best located in the operating theatre suite.

Postoperative Monitoring

After transplantation it is necessary to monitor the patient both to assess the function of the transplanted liver and to detect the development of postoperative complications. A monitoring protocol is suggested in Table 11.6.

There are no specific biochemical tests for rejection but deteriorating liver function is an indication for urgent liver biopsy from which the histological diagnosis is made. Of the traditional liver function tests, those of hepatocellular damage are the most useful in monitoring. Thus daily (including weekend) measurement of transaminases is important. There are of course two potential enzymes, AST (aspartate transaminase) and ALT (alanine transaminase), that could be measured. ALT is the more sensitive enzyme in this situation but, unlike AST, modest elevations are common after transplantation.

Post-transplant bilirubin concentrations of $1000 \mu mol/L$ are common in these patients and this places a severe strain on the analytical accuracy of other biochemical tests. This is particularly the case with creatinine measurements. Significant interference in creatinine assay by the standard Jaffe method is evident in samples containing bilirubin concentrations greater than $180 \mu mol/L$.[44] With some methods, creatinine measurement is impossible and ^{57}Cr EDTA clearance has to be done instead of creatinine clearance. Similarly, colorimetric magnesium may be impossible. Any laboratory supporting liver transplantation has to assess all its methods in relation to interference from high concentrations of bilirubin. Most literature and product information on bilirubin

TABLE 11.6

POSTOPERATIVE BIOCHEMICAL MONITORING OF LIVER TRANSPLANT RECIPIENTS

Period post operation	Biochemical investigations
0–6 days (ITU stay)	Daily: U + E, LFT, 24-h excretion of Na, K, urea and creatinine As required: serum and urine osmolality, blood gases
6–28 days (inpatient stay)	Daily: U + E, LFT Thrice weekly: 24-h excretion of Na, K, urea and creatinine Weekly: magnesium, zinc, lipids
2, 4, 8 weeks post discharge and every 8 weeks thereafter	U + E, LFT and cyclosporin A

Abbreviations: ITU, intensive therapy unit; remainder as in Table 11.4.

interference is usually only available up to bilirubin concentrations of 340 μmol/L.

Immunosuppression

The management of immunosuppression in liver transplant recipients is particularly complex. This is perhaps not surprising, considering the predominantly hepatic metabolism of cyclosporin. It is now well established that hepatic dysfunction not only alters the elimination of cyclosporin but also impairs its absorption. The impairment of cyclosporin pharmacokinetics varies with the degree and cause of hepatic dysfunction and, therefore, individualization of cyclosporin dosage based upon regular blood concentration measurements is crucial in patients with hepatic insufficiency.[45] In the early postoperative period, external biliary diversion causing fat malabsorption leads to extremely poor absorption of orally administered cyclosporin, necessitating the use of the intravenous formulation.

The management of cyclosporin therapy in liver transplant recipients, as with other transplant groups, differs considerably between centres. Indeed, even within a single unit, the protocol is constantly being modified and fine tuned as experience with immunosuppression is gained. There are differences in the management of cyclosporin treatment for adult and childhood subgroups. According to current practice at Addenbrooke's, Cambridge (UK) in adults cyclosporin therapy is begun within 12 h of transplantation provided that urine output is satisfactory (>60 mL/h). If urine output is poor (<40 mL/h), treatment is delayed until adequate renal function is achieved. Initially the drug is infused continuously, permitting early discontinuation of dosage should urine output fall significantly due to cyclosporin nephrotoxicity. Withdrawal of treatment might also be prompted at this time by a rise in serum potassium or urea. Creatinine tends to be an insensitive indica-

tor of renal failure in the early postoperative period, particularly in the cachectic patient with low muscle mass or in the presence of high bilirubin, which, as mentioned above, can interfere with creatinine measurement. If urine output is good in the face of an abnormal or rising urea, cyclosporin may also be discontinued on the suspicion of polyuric renal failure. If the concentration of urea is normal or near normal and urine output is good, then the patient is converted to 2-h infusions of cyclosporin within a day or so of starting treatment. The target cyclosporin concentration range at this stage is 100–150 μg/L in patients with poor renal function and 100–200 μg/L in patients with good function. An inspection of the external bile drainage T-tube is made by cholangiogram at about 10 days after transplantation. If there is good bile flow the tube is clamped off so that normal bile drainage into the gastrointestinal tract can occur. After clamping an improvement in oral cyclosporin absorption can be anticipated. The intravenous dose is, therefore, halved and the equivalent dose of the oral formulation given. After 24–48 h the intravenous dose is stopped and the full oral dose given at about two or three times the original intravenous dose. The therapeutic range for maintenance cyclosporin immunosuppression in adult liver transplant recipients remains at 100–200 μg/L.

The target therapeutic concentration range for cyclosporin in the childhood group has been increased from 100–200 μg/L to 150–250 μg/L in recent years, this increase being associated with a decrease in the incidence of acute and chronic rejection. In order to avoid toxic side-effects, this level of immunosuppression is attained gradually during intravenous cyclosporin administration. Currently, this slow attainment of optimum cyclosporin concentrations is compensated for by the use of quadruple immunosuppressive therapy for a full 10 days after transplantation. Cyclosporin is introduced on the second day after transplantation with a 6-h intravenous infusion (a dose of 1 mg/kg given twice a day). This slow rate of infusion compared to that in adults is thought to minimize the risk of side-effects due to acutely high blood concentrations. Therapy is delayed if the patient is oliguric (< 1 mL/kg an hour), the urea is high or rising (e.g. > 20 mmol/L) or the creatinine exceeds 100 μmol/L (note age-dependent normal range). Some children are given an internal stent for internal bile drainage and these patients may start immediately on the full oral cyclosporin dose (usually 4 mg/kg, twice a day) after the first week. In children with external bile drainage, the T-tube is clamped on day 14; for half the time at first (6 h clamped and 6 h unclamped) and then continuously when bile flow to the gut has satisfactorily resumed. Being fat soluble, the absorption of cyclosporin is dependent on the presence of bile salts and blood cyclosporin concentrations may increase after clamping of the external bile drainage t-tube.[46] Absorption of oral cyclosporin may, however, remain impaired until good bile flow into the gut is achieved and attaining therapeutic blood cyclosporin concentrations can require very high doses at this time. This difficulty is accentuated in children where both poor absorption and high clearance may act in concert to increase dosage requirements. There was once a slow transition between intravenous and oral cyclosporin dosage. However, dosage adjustment of the different formulations to maintain therapeutic blood concentrations of cyclosporin during this transition proved difficult to manage accurately, even with daily monitoring, and now there is an instant switch to the oral drug at a dose of 4 mg/kg (twice a day), equivalent to about four times the former intravenous dose. In some cases it may be necessary to give oral cyclosporin doses of up to 250 mg three times a day. This is equivalent to 100 mg/kg a day in an 8-kg child—over 10 times the average dosage requirement of adult kidney transplant recipients. Dosage requirements may change rapidly with time after transplantation and sometimes for no obvious reason, although large changes are usually associated with gastrointestinal disturbances such as diarrhoea. This again illustrates the importance of regular, individualized monitoring and dosage adjustment for cyclosporin.

Blood cyclosporin concentrations are monitored daily in the first 2 weeks and then at least every other day up to the end of the first month. As outpatients the children are monitored weekly for the first 2 months, every 2 weeks between the second and fourth month, and monthly between the fourth and sixth months. After the first 3 postoperative months, assuming that the patient has successfully stabilized, the target cyclosporin therapeutic range is reduced to 100–150 μg/L for maintenance immunosuppression. The frequency of monitoring is further decreased to once every 2 months between the sixth and twelfth month, every 3 months during the second year, and then every 4 months as indicated. As with other

transplant groups it is evident that patients require less and less cyclosporin with time after transplantation.

Chronic rejection remains the most serious late complication of liver transplantation. Despite the difficulties encountered in managing cyclosporin immunosuppression after liver transplantation, this drug has largely been responsible for the steady improvements in 1-year survival over the last decade to more than 90% in some centres. In the childhood group at Addenbrooke's Hospital, 1-year actuarial survival in the first 100 children was 71% but since August 1988 this has increased to 86%.[47] As with other transplant groups, this increased survival has brought with it increasing concern about the attendant short- and long-term adverse effects of cyclosporin therapy. However, most of the cyclosporin-associated side-effects after liver transplantation are self-limiting or easily treated.[48] Refractory hypertension and progressive nephrotoxicity—serious concerns in kidney and heart transplant recipients treated with cyclosporin—are not major problems after liver transplantation when cyclosporin concentrations are monitored frequently and maintenance immunosuppression minimized.

Serious neurological complications in the postoperative period have been documented in about one-third of liver transplant recipients. Cyclosporin has been implicated in the development of such complications, especially fits,[49] although a number of other predisposing or synergistic factors also appear to be involved and it is by no means certain that cyclosporin is the culprit. Indeed, cyclosporin does not appear readily to cross the blood–brain barrier and less than 1% of the blood concentration is found in the central nervous system.

PANCREATIC TRANSPLANTATION

Currently, pancreatic transplantation is a viable treatment option for only a very few diabetics. Most are very successfully treated by insulin or oral hypoglycaemic agents. While the idea of replacing lifelong insulin injections by a single operation is superficially attractive, the present reality is quite different. Even if the operation was 100% successful and excellent glycaemic control was achieved, the risks from the immunosuppressive therapy are, for most patients, worse than the risk from their diabetes. Overall graft survival is 50% at 2 years.

Unlike for other organs that may be transplanted, there is a variety of operative techniques for pancreatic transplantation. Both partial and complete organs can be transplanted, either paratopically or heterotopically. There are also three ways of dealing with the unwanted donor pancreas *exocrine* function: duct occlusion, enteric drainage or bladder drainage. The two most popular techniques are partial transplantation with enteric drainage (where donation from a living, related donor is involved) and transplantation of a complete cadaveric organ with bladder drainage. The latter technique has the advantage of providing a means of monitoring organ function.

Selection and Assessment of Patients

The criteria for selecting patients for pancreas and kidney transplantation include those used in selecting patients for kidney transplant alone (*see above*). Currently, in the UK, pancreatic transplantation is reserved for poorly controlled (i.e. 'brittle') type 1 diabetics with renal failure and retinopathy who require a kidney transplant. Elsewhere transplantations have been done on poorly controlled, non-uraemic diabetics when the risks from the diabetes have been considered to outweigh the risks from immunosuppression. Interestingly, graft survival was poorer in this category of transplant.[50]

Thus the degree of glycaemic control as evidenced by measurements of blood glucose and haemoglobin A_{1C} will be an additional feature in the selection.

Perioperative Monitoring

Kidney-pancreas transplants require the same perioperative monitoring as kidney transplants.

Postoperative Monitoring

The usual biochemical test for pancreatic damage, serum amylase, has not proved to be useful in assessing the integrity of a transplanted pancreas. If normoglycaemia is achieved as a result of the transplant, then organ failure will be manifested by a deterioration in glucose control. However, when bladder drainage is used, organ failure can be detected some 2–3 days in advance of this by measurement of urinary amylase. In a healthy transplanted pancreas, endocrine and exocrine systems will both continue to function. The exocrine secretions will drain into the bladder and high urinary amylase concentrations will result. If pancreatic function deteriorates, then the exocrine secretions will slow down and the urinary amylase concentration will decrease.

MULTIPLE ORGAN TRANSPLANTS

In some diseases, transplantation of more than one organ is required. In primary oxaluria, kidney and liver are transplanted together. A new kidney is required for the renal failure resulting from stone formation. The new liver supplies the missing enzyme and normalizes oxalate excretion, and thereby prevents damage to the new kidney. Dual heart and liver transplants have been done for homozygous familial hypercholesterolaemia and dual heart and kidney transplants when a heart transplant recipient has developed renal failure as a result of the nephrotoxicity of cyclosporin A. The biochemical monitoring

requirements of these patients are the sum of those for each of the organs involved.

BIOCHEMICAL DETECTION OF REJECTION

A transplant recipient is at risk from a technical failure of the operation, primary organ non-function, rejection or infection. The first two are early complications and do not constitute a great diagnostic problem. The last two are difficult to diagnose and distinguish but it is crucial to do so because the treatments are so different. A simple biochemical marker to diagnose these conditions would be extremely useful and such markers have been sought. A whole host of cytokines or soluble cytokine receptors has been investigated but their specificity has not been established and so far none has entered routine clinical practice.

FUTURE PERSPECTIVES

From the foregoing it will be obvious that transplantation surgery makes great demands upon clinical biochemistry. The particular demands, as presented above, will be different depending on the organ transplanted. They will also be different depending on the particular clinical practice observed. Clinical practice changes with technological advances and there are several avenues of research currently being explored that may have a great impact on transplantation. Methods are being investigated of inducing 'tolerance' to the transplanted organ. This would render immunosuppressive therapy unnecessary. The possibility of using organs from different species ('xenografts') for transplantation is being investigated. This would make organs available to all who needed them. Artificial organs are being developed. If these proved practical, they would combine the advantages of non-immunogenicity with potentially unlimited availability. These advances might, perhaps, change, but would not abolish, the demands on clinical biochemists.

REFERENCES

1. Kendall D.M., Sutherland E.R., Najaran M.D., Goetz F.C., Robertson R.P. (1990). Effects of hemipancreatectomy on insulin secretion and glucose tolerance in healthy humans. *N. Engl. J. Med.*, **32**, 898.
2. Calne R.Y. et al. (1978). Cyclosporin A in patients receiving renal allografts from cadaver donors. *Lancet*, **ii**, 1323.
3. Thomson A.W., Duncan J.I. The influence of cyclosporin A on T cell activation, cytokine gene expression and cell-mediated immunity. In *Cyclosporin: Mode of Action and Clinical Application* (Thomson A.W. ed.)
4. Kahan B.D. et al. (1982). Immunopharmacologic monitoring of cyclosporin A treated recipients of cadaver kidney allografts. *Transplantation*, **34**, 36.
5. Kahan B.D. (1989). Cyclosporin. *N. Engl. J. Med.*, **321**, 1725.
6. Shaw L.M. (1987). Critical issues in cyclosporine moni-

toring: report of the task force on cyclosporine monitoring. *Clin. Chem.*, **33**, 1269.

7. Kahan B.D., Shaw L.M., Holt D., Grevel J., Johnston A. (1990). Concensus Document: Hawk's Cay Meeting on Therapeutic Drug Monitoring of Cyclosporine. *Clin. Chem.*, **36**, 1510.

8. Shaw L.M. et al. (1990). Canadian Concensus Meeting on Cyclosporine Monitoring: Report of the Concensus Panel. *Clin. Chem.*, **36**, 1841.

9. Ptachcinski R.J., Venkataramanan R., Burckart G.J. (1986). Clinical pharmacokinetics of cyclosporin. *Clin. Pharmacokinet.*, **11**, 107.

10. Trull A.K., Tan K.K.C., Uttridge J., Bauer T., Alexander G.J.M., Jamieson N. (1993). Cyclosporin absorption from microemulsion formulation in liver transplant recipient. *Lancet*, **341**, 433.

11. Gurecki J., Warty V., Sanghvi A. (1985). *Transplantation Proc.*, **17**, 1997.

12. de Groen P.C., Aksamit A.J., Rakela J., Forbes G.S., Krom R.A.F. (1987). Central nervous system toxicity after liver transplantation: the role of cyclosporine and cholesterol. *N. Engl. J. Med.*, **317**, 861.

13. Bertault-Peres P., Bonfils C., Fabre G., Just S., Cano J.P., Maurel P. (1987). Metabolism of cyclosporine A. II. Implication of the macrolide antibiotic inducible cytochrome P-450 3c from rat liver microsomes. *Drug Metab. Dispos.*, **15**, 391.

14. Lensmeyer C., Wiebe D., Carlson I. (1987). Identification and analysis of nine metabolites of cyclosporine in whole blood by liquid chromatography. 2: Comparison of patients' results. *Clin. Chem.*, **33**, 1851.

15. Lensmeyer C., Wiebe D., Carlson I. (1988). Deposition of nine metabolites of cyclosporine in human tissue, bile, urine, and whole blood. *Transplantation Proc.*, **20**, 614.

16. Zeevi A. et al. (1988). Sensitivity of activated human lymphocytes to cyclosporine and its metabolites. *Hum. Immunol.*, **21**, 143.

17. Rosano T., Freed B., Cerill J. (1986). Immunosuppressive metabolites of cyclosporine in the blood of renal allograft recipients. *Transplantation*, **42**, 262.

18. Copeland K.R., Yatscoff R.W., McKenna R.M. (1990). Immunosuppressive activity of cyclosporine metabolites compared and characterized by mass spectroscopy and nuclear magnetic resonance. *Clin. Chem.*, **36**, 225.

19. Rubin R.H., Wolfson J.S., Cosimi A.B., Tolkoff-Rubin N.E. (1981). Infection in renal transplant recipients. *Am. J. Med.*, **70**, 405.

20. Parfrey P.S. et al. (1985). The impact of renal transplantation on the course of hepatitis B liver disease. *Transplantation*, **239**, 610.

21. Calne R. et al. (1981). Cyclosporin A in clinical renal allografting. *Transplantation Proc.*, **13**, 34921.

22. Thiel G. (1986). The use of cyclosporin blood level measurements in renal transplantation. In *Cyclosporin Issues of Today* (*Proceedings of the Wishaw Workshop*), Oxford: Medical Education, pp. 12–19.

23. Slapak M. (1987). Triple and quadruple immunosuppressive therapy in organ transplantation. *Lancet*, **ii**, 958.

24. Land W. (1987). Immunosuppressive combination therapy. In *Optimal Use of Sandimmun in Organ Transplantation*, (W. Land ed.) Berlin: Springer-Verlag, pp. 8–10.

25. Ptachcinski R.J. et al. (1985). Cyclosporin pharmacokinetics in renal transplant recipients. *Clin. Pharmacol. Ther.*, **38**, 296.

26. Kahan B.D., Ried M., Neuburger J. (1983). Pharmacokinetics of cyclosporine in human renal transplantation. *Transplantation Proc.*, **1**, 446.

27. Bradley B.A., Wilks W.R., Gore S.M. (1988) Cyclosporine: its use in the UK and its time of impact on graft survival. In *Cyclosporin Five Years On* (*Proceedings of the Wishaw Workshop*) Abingdon: Medicine Group, pp.16–22.

28. Linholm A., Dahlqvist R., Groth G.G., Sjoqvist F. (1990). A prospective study of cyclosporin concentration in relation to its therapeutic effect and toxicity after renal transplantation. *Br. J. Clin. Pharmacol.*, **30**, 443.

29. Shaw L.M. et al. (1990). Adjustment of cyclosporin dosage in renal transplant patients based on concentration measured specifically in whole blood: clinical outcome results and diagnostic utility. *Transplantation Proc.*, **22**, 1267.

30. Johnston A. et al. (1990) A limited sampling strategy for the measurement of cyclosporin AUC. *Transplantation Proc.*, **22**, 1345.

31. Cantarovich F., Bizollon C.H., Cantarovich D., Lefrancois N., Dubernard J.M., Traeger J. (1988). Cyclosporin plasma levels six hours after oral administration. *Transplantation*, **45**, 389.

32. O'Donovan R., Compton F., Verbi V., Bewick M., Parsons V. (1985) Higher cyclosporin levels in the first three days post-transplantation are associated with fewer rejection episodes, lower serum creatinines and significantly improved graft survival at 12 months. *Kidney Int.*, **28**, 398.

33. Salaman J.R. (1991). Cyclosporin monotherapy—who needs it? *Clin. Exp. Perspect. Sandimmun Ther.*, **1**, 1.

34. Brown M.W., Forwell M.A. (1985). Rejection reaction after stopping prednisolone in kidney transplant recipients taking cyclosporin. *N. Engl. J. Med.*, **314**, 183.

35. Reisman L., Lieberman K.V., Burrows L., Schanzer H. (1990) Follow-up of cyclosporin treated renal allograft recipients after cessation of prednisone. *Transplantation*, **49**, 76.

36. Wallwork J. (1986). *Cyclosporin: Issues of Today*, Oxford: Medical Education, pp.39–44.

37. Trull A.K. Cross-correlation between cyclosporin concentration and biochemical measures of kidney and liver function in heart and heart-lung transplant recipients. *Clin. Chem.*, **36**, 1474.

38. Best N., Trull A.K., Tan K.K.C., Spiegelhalter D.J., Wreghitt T.G., Wallwork J. (1994). Cyclosporin-based immunosuppression and cytomegalovirus infection following heart transplantation in man. (in press).

39. Scott J.P., Wallwork, J. (1992) Practical problems in immunosuppression: Heart and heart-lung transplantation. *Prescribers' J.*, **32**: 63–69.

40. Holt, D. (1990). Blood cyclosporin absorption profiles and renal function in heart transplant recipients. (Abstract.)

41. Hakim M., Siegelhalter D., English T.A.H., Caine N., Wallwork J. (1988). Cardiac transplantation with cyclosporin and steroids: medium and long-term results. *Transplantation Proc.* **20** (suppl. 3), 327.

42. Best N.G. et al. (1992) Blood cyclosporine concentrations and the short term risk of lung rejection following heart lung transplantation. *Br. J. Clin. Pharmacol.*, **34**, 513.

43. Nalesnik M.A., Makowka L., Starzl T.E. (1988). The diagnosis and treatment of post-transplant lymphoproliferative disorders. *Curr. Probl. Surg.*, **25**, 365.

44. Hue D.P., Maguire G.A. (1990). Can creatinine be accurately measured in icteric samples? *Proceedings of the ACB National Meeting*, p.73.

45. Takaya S. et al. (1987). Effect of liver dysfunction on cyclosporin pharmacokinetics. *Transplantation Proc.*, **19**, 1246.

46. Venkataramanan R. et al. (1985). Biliary excretion of cyclosporin in liver transplant patients. *Transplantation Proc.*, **17**, 286.

47. Salt A. et al. (1992). Liver transplantation in 100 children: Cambridge and King's College Hospital series. *Br. Med. J.*, **304**, 416.

48. Grant D., Wall W., Duff J., Stiller C., Ghent C., Keown P. (1987). Adverse effects of cyclosporin therapy following liver transplantation. *Transplantation Proc.*, **19**, 3463.

49. Adams D.H. et al. (1987). Neurological complications following liver transplantation. *Lancet*, **i**, 949.

50. Sutherland D.E.R., Moudry-Munns K.C. (1989). Summary of clinical data on pancreas transplants. In *Organ Transplantation: Current Clinical and Immunological Concepts* (Brent L., Sells R.A. eds.) London: Baillière-Tindall, pp.219–228.

12. Nutrition of the Sick Patient

J.W.T. Dickerson and Jane B. Morgan

Introduction
The nutritional support team
Nutritional assessment
Appetite
Providing nutritional support
  Enteral nutrition
  Total parenteral nutrition
Patient monitoring
Examples of patients requiring nutritional
   support
  Elderly surgical patients
  Patients with burn injuries
  Patients with head injuries
  Patients with cancer
Conclusion

INTRODUCTION

It cannot be taken for granted that patients in hospital receive an adequate diet. The problems highlighted by Platt and his colleagues in their survey of 'Food in Hospitals'[1] still largely exist today. Malnutrition exists in some hospital patients, and may be created or exacerbated by their stay in hospital—'hospital-induced malnutrition'. The cause of malnutrition is simple—insufficient food to meet requirements. The factors responsible for a low food intake may differ in individual patients and it is only when these factors are identified that adequate nutrition can be provided in a manner suited to the patients' needs. Individuals in hospital for a short time are generally not at risk. Those receiving special diets for metabolic conditions, such as diabetes mellitus, are also usually well cared for. Those most at risk are the critically ill with diseases affecting the alimentary tract, patients with cancer and those who have suffered multiple injuries. A previously healthy young man involved in a road accident is equally at risk as a frail old lady with a broken femur.

Some patients are malnourished when they are admitted to hospital. This is particularly true of those with debilitating disease affecting the alimentary tract. Cancer patients may have had a progressive dysphagia and anorexia with consequent reduction in food intake and fall in body weight. It is recognized that some old people are susceptible to malnutrition, such as the recently bereaved (particularly widowers) and the socially isolated. Consumption of an adequate amount of food is no guarantee that they will not be suffering from vitamin deficiency caused by a diet lacking in variety, or low in vitamin content due to losses in preparation and cooking or, in the case of vitamin D, lack of exposure to sunlight. Deficiencies of thiamin, vitamin C and folic acid are common in elderly persons admitted to hospital, including in those admitted with femoral fractures (Table 12.1). These nutritional deficiencies are likely to persist unless specific supplements are given because the nutrient content of hospital diets is probably adequate for maintenance only.

Food should be suitable for and acceptable to patients. Uneaten food, however excellent, is of no nutritional value. Anorexia, taste aberrations and physical handicap lead to low food consumption. Poor food preparation and presentation lead to poor food acceptability. Subjecting a patient to phlebotomy or carrying out other investigations at meal times is not conducive to maintaining food intake.

The nutrition of patients often presents a challenge and clinical biochemists can make important contributions to patient assessment and monitoring. In this chapter we outline methods of patient investigation, the means of supplying food to sick patients, and give some examples of the problems associated with four vulnerable groups.

THE NUTRITIONAL SUPPORT TEAM

The feeding of all patients in hospital involves several persons. Even if patients do not have a nutritional problem, supplying them with appetizing, nutritionally adequate meals involves catering officers and cooks in food preparation, porters in distribution from the kitchen and ward orderlies in delivery on the wards. When patients have particular feeding problems or are critically ill, the number of persons involved increases. It is to meet the needs of such patients that nutritional support teams have been formed in many large or specialist hospitals. Although the contribution of such teams to the nutrition of patients has tended to focus on the provision of total parenteral nutrition (TPN), the team can make a real contribution to the care of patients requiring special enteral diets, whether these are taken orally or given by a fine-bore tube.

It is now generally accepted that the involvement of a support team or a specially trained nutrition nurse reduces the rate and risk of complications, and results in more regular monitoring and in the administration of the prescribed amounts of nutrients. The composition of a formal team depends on the team's activities and responsibilities. These may vary from providing a purely consultative service to the acceptance of full responsibility for the nutritional management of referred patients. It may be formalized, with regular meetings and patient reviews, or meet on an *ad hoc* basis when problems arise. The minimum of persons involved in such a team would be a physician, pharmacist, dietitian, clinical biochemist and nurse. Assessment of the patient and estimation of requirements would involve the physician and dietitian with

TABLE 12.1
VITAMIN STATUS OF ELDERLY WOMEN WITH FRACTURES ON ADMISSION TO HOSPITAL

	Normal range	Mean range	% below lower level of normal
Vitamin C (Plasma concentration; mg/100 ml)	0.5–1.5	0.34 (0.03–1.27)	82
Vitamin B₁ (Red cell transketolase; thiamin pyrophosphate %)	< 15%	23.0 (0.0–62.5)	70
Vitamin A (Plasma retinol; μg/100 ml)	50–150	28.6 (13.9–50.1)	97
Retinol-binding protein (Plasma concentration; mg/100 ml)	3–4	3.5 (1.2–6.5)	51

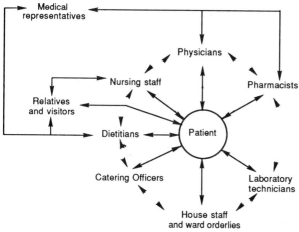

Fig. 12.1 Schematic outline of the relation between members of the nutritional support team.[2]

support. Modification of oral feeds could be done by the dietitian in collaboration with a catering manager. Enteral or parenteral feeds would be prescribed by the physician in collaboration with the dietitian and pharmacist. Administration of these feeds would be controlled by the nurse. The nurse, in collaboration with the physician and biochemist, would be responsible for monitoring the patient. Monitoring is a vital part of the management of patients receiving TPN, who can develop severe metabolic disturbances.

For the satisfactory nutritional care of most critically ill patients it is realistic to consider that rather more persons actually contribute to the work of the team (Fig. 12.1).[2] Involvement of relatives and visitors can be important whilst patients are in hospital, but is certainly important when previously nutritionally compromised patients are discharged. Much of the value of attempts to maintain or restore the nutritional status of critically ill patients can be lost if support is not continued when patients leave hospital. For those patients in whom enteral feeding is to continue at home, the general practitioner and community nurse must be considered members of the team and given the information necessary for continu-

ing this aspect of the care. For some patients who have been critically ill, nutritional support may be at least as important to survival as drug prescriptions.

NUTRITIONAL ASSESSMENT

Accurate assessment of the patient is a prerequisite to the provision of all forms of care and treatment. Nutritional assessment aims to:

(i) define nutritional status at a particular time and elicit a history of recent nutrient intake;
(ii) detect evidence of nutritional deficiencies and identify individuals needing support;
(iii) assess the amounts of energy and nutrients to be given;
(iv) monitor the patients' responses.[3]

Much has been written about the methods available to achieve these aims. The outline given here concentrates on those of practical value in the nutrition of sick patients and those in which the clinical biochemist may be involved. Whatever methods are used, it is important that values are recorded sequentially in the patient's notes to facilitate evaluation.

Deterioration of nutritional status may occur before admission to hospital. Indeed, weight loss may be the first sign in some patients that they are ill. Other patients become malnourished whilst in hospital for a variety of reasons that cause them to consume too little food to meet their requirements. It is useful to be able to distinguish on admission those patients whose nutritional status is already compromised and those who are likely to become malnourished. Non-invasive methods are preferable. Pertinent aspects of the patient's history can be incorporated into a nutritional risk questionnaire, which can be used to obtain a nutritional risk quotient (NRQ).

Body weight is a simple measurement. Weight on admission to hospital can be compared with the patient's own 'healthy' weight or with population standards for age in the two sexes. Comparison with the patient's own healthy weight is preferable. Although it is usual to assess the significance of weight

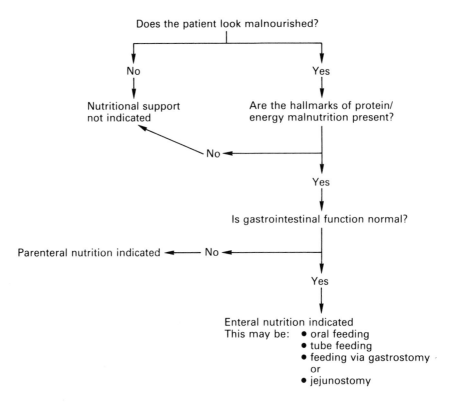

Fig. 12.2 Patient selection for total parenteral nutrition.[12]

loss in relation to the period of time over which the loss has occurred, a weight loss of 10% or more over any time period is significant. Losses in excess of 30% body weight increase postoperative morbidity and mortality regardless of initial body weight.

Measurements of skinfold thickness can be used to assess body fat content and standards are available for triceps skinfold thickness and males with values of 7.5 mm and females with values of 9.9 mm are severely depleted. Mid-arm muscle circumference (MAMC) can be used as a measure of muscle mass. Values of 15.2 cm for men and 13.9 cm for women indicate that the patient is severely depleted. MAMC is of limited value in the elderly and it has been suggested that abdominal girth may be the most valuable variable to measure in this group. Measurement of grip strength (dynametry) may provide another useful, non-invasive method of assessing muscle reserves. Control values quoted are 48.8 ± 7.0 kg for males and 34.4 ± 4.7 kg for females. Values below 85% of this have been taken as indicating 'appreciable' protein depletion.

Of the biochemical indices that may be used (see below), serum albumin has probably been used most, but is the least satisfactory because it is essential to exclude reasons other than malnutrition for a low value. Moreover, albumin has a long half-life (19 days) and is therefore a poor indicator of acute change in nutritional status. Thyroxine-binding prealbumin (half-life 2 days) and retinol-binding protein (half-life 12 h) are much more useful as indicators of nutritional status. Assessments of immunocompetence, including the lymphocyte count, have been used but are now seldom used as a routine.

Methods for the assessment of vitamin and trace element status are described elsewhere. Use of the above methods of assessment provides a quantitative expression of a patient's nutritional status.[4] For some patients the use of such techniques is quite unnecessary in order to determine the need for nutritional support (Fig. 12.2). It is necessary only to examine the patient. However, quantitative assessments provide a baseline against which to compare future measurements to assess deterioration or improvement. The clinician should also take into account the patient's diagnosis and programme of treatment in order to assess risk of malnutrition and hence the need for continuing observation. If possible, patients needing nutritional support should be fed enterally. It is usually sufficient to follow general guidelines in the assessment of requirements for this type of feeding (see below) and only rarely is it necessary to attempt to obtain a more precise estimate. However, this is not the case for the more critically ill patients who receive TPN, and generally speaking the more sick the patient the greater the care necessary in the assessment of requirements (see below).

Whether the patient is being fed enterally or parenterally, certain treatments may modify requirements for vitamins and minerals. Drug therapy may alter the type and amount of food eaten, change the absorption of nutrients and alter nutrient metabolism and excretion. Surgery increases requirements for vitamins C and K.

APPETITE

Appetite is described in the *Concise Oxford Dictionary* as 'desire to satisfy natural necessities, especially hunger'. In health, appetite is part of the complex physiological control of energy balance.[5] However, there are a number of conditions where appetite is suppressed and individuals become anorexic. More uncommon is hyperphagia (overeating)—sometimes a symptom of depression, particularly in women.

Change of appetite can be related to drug therapy, anxiety, sepsis and fever, radiotherapy and as an effect of ageing. Subsequently there is a reduced intake of nutrients. If anorexia is suspected, dietary intake should be assessed. If there is doubt about the accuracy of the information an independent check is needed. The most practical of these is the 24-h urinary nitrogen output, which can be compared with the reported nitrogen (protein) intake.[6]

Appetite can be either increased or decreased by drug administration. Anticancer drugs such as cyclophosphamide, non-steroidal anti-inflammatory drugs such as indomethacin, biguanides, glucagon, morphine and the digitalis group all decrease appetite. Alcohol, insulin, thyroid hormone, steroids, some antihistamines, the sulphonylureas and psychotropic drugs increase appetite.

Patients in the immediately preoperative and postoperative states are also vulnerable to changes in appetite. The majority of surgical patients are anxious and unsure about surgical procedures. Some will have physical difficulty with eating, pain and nausea, all of which affect appetite. As a result there is a risk of preoperative malnutrition, particularly if poor appetite is associated with dysphagia, prolonged malabsorption, malignancy or inflammatory bowel disease. Nutritional support (provision of appetizing meals, supplements, nasoenteric tube feeding or TPN) in the perioperative phase should aim to enhance wound healing, reduce postoperative complications, reduce the period of convalescence and prevent further deterioration of the nutritional state.

After a general anaesthetic, gastric mobility and emptying are delayed. Anorexia is frequently seen on general surgical wards, and regular monitoring should be carried out to identify patients at risk. Nutritional support, as has been previously described, should be considered as a routine part of postoperative care.

Many sick patients are discharged from hospital before their natural appetite has returned. Nutritional advice should be given, and continue in the community and in general practitioner clinics if possible.

PROVIDING NUTRITIONAL SUPPORT

The consequences of malnutrition are well known— loss of body weight, impaired immunocompetence with increased susceptibility to infection, increased incidences of wound breakdown, oedema, apathy and increased mortality. Superimposed on the effects of low food intake, traumatized patients suffer concomitant metabolic changes—the metabolic response to injury. This involves complex neuroendocrine changes that result in the breakdown of protein, particularly muscle protein to provide amino acids for the synthesis of increased amounts of acute-phase reactant proteins, such as C-reactive protein, and non-essential amino acids for gluconeogenesis. Body fat is utilized as a source of energy and there is an increase in plasma free fatty acids and ketone bodies. Water and sodium are retained and the patient becomes oliguric and may be anuric. There is a rise in resting metabolic energy expenditure (RMEE) and an increase in urea excretion.

The magnitude of these changes is greater in well-muscled males than in females and in younger persons than older. The magnitude of the changes also increases with the severity of the injury and is greater in patients with burns than in other patients. The exception is patients with head injuries (see below), in whom the response may be similar to that in patients with burns.

The trigger mechanisms for the neuroendocrine changes involve cytokines, a range of polypeptides produced in response to inflammatory stimuli.[7]

The aim of nutritional support is to maintain or restore body composition and well-being and to facilitate convalescence. Food can be provided enterally, using the gastrointestinal tract, or parenterally as solutions or emulsions directly into the circulation.

Enteral Nutrition

Enteral diets are those which are taken by mouth or introduced by a tube into the gastrointestinal tract. Oral feeding is always the method of choice, being 'natural' and generating pleasurable sensations associated with the taste and texture of food. 'Likes and dislikes' can be catered for and this can have important psychological effects on the patient, increasing the sense of being 'cared for'. By comparison, tube feeds are somewhat impersonal but have the advantage of bypassing appetite and being nutritionally of more certain adequacy.

Oral Feeding

The success of hospital feeding may depend on the patient's response to psychological influences, the environment, lack of exercise, handicap (physical and mental), cultural background, and the acceptability, presentation, temperature and variety of meals.

A disturbed psychological state is common in those who are sick and is likely to be marked in the critically ill. Lack of progress or experience of pain may cause depression and indifference to food. A peaceful environment with a carer's encouragement may have an important effect on food consumption and well-being. Lack of exercise does not stimulate appetite. An adequate food intake may only be achieved by giving food 'little and often'. Acceptability is the key to successful catering. The presentation of food, its colour, variety and temperature are all important factors.

When the voluntary food intake falls below about 80% of the amounts of energy and protein recommended for healthy individuals of the same age and sex, the patient should be encouraged to take sip feeds. Prescribed amounts of feeds used as tube feeds should be consumed between meals. A variety of suitable feeds (see below) is available and it may be necessary to use a range of feeds in patients requiring long-term sip feeds because of tiredness of the taste, texture or mouth-feel of individual feeds. Accurate records of the types of feed offered and the volume consumed should be kept so that they can be used in monitoring the patient.

Tube feeds

The amounts of energy and nutrients to be given as a tube feed should be calculated in the same way as for TPN. Homogenized meals are unsuitable for tube feeds because of their variable nutrient content and the need for a wide-bore Ryle's tube for their administration. A range of commercially produced feeds is available.[8] The feed chosen for a particular patient may depend on the absorptive capacity of the gastrointestinal tract and it may be necessary to prescribe feeds that are lactose-free, low-fat/high medium-chain triglycerides, or low osmolarity.[4] Feeds with high N:calorie ratios are becoming available for patients whose requirements for protein are increased, e.g. those with burns. It has been found that for most patients, feeds supplying about 12 g N (75 g protein/day) and 1500–2000 kcal (6.3–8.4 MJ) are satisfactory, but there are those for whom more precise estimates need to be made. All commercial feeds contain electrolytes, vitamins, minerals and trace elements. Individual patients may need additional supplements of vitamins and trace elements. Most liquid diets contain 1.0 kcal (4.2 kJ) per ml of formulation. The osmolality is important and should be close to 285–300 mmol/L.

There are a number of simple, or weighted, fine-bore (1–2 mm) tubes available. The tubes contain a guide wire to assist their insertion and a radiograph is necessary to ensure correct positioning of the simple, fine-bore nasogastric tubes, but not normally for the insertion of the more expensive, weighted tubes. Simple tubes may also be inserted through a gastrostomy or jejunostomy. Patients may be fed continuously, with the rate controlled by a pump or simply by gravity. Patients who are tube fed at home usually rely on a gravity feed. Babies' tube feeding is

not now very common and is more difficult with a fine-bore tube. Nausea, abdominal distension and diarrhoea are the most common side-effects and can usually be controlled by reducing the flow of feed into the intestine. The feeds can be given by simple, or weighted fine-bore tubes inserted nasogastrically or through a gastrostomy or jejunostomy.

Total Parenteral Nutrition

TPN is the delivery of all nutritional components, in aseptic conditions, into the circulatory system. Parenteral nutrition should only be instituted when enteral feeding is impossible or when requirements are so great that insufficient food can be given enterally. The administration of TPN requires considerable expertise and a more complete commitment of back-up services (medical, nursing, pharmacy, laboratory, nutritional) than for enteral nutrition.

The incidence of clinical malnutrition in acute hospital admissions can be as high as 45–50%, although only 15% will require aggressive nutritional support—and of these about one-third will require parenteral nutrition.[9]

Indications for the Use of TPN

There are generally four clinical conditions where parenteral nutrition is necessary. First, when the gastrointestinal tract is inaccessible, e.g. oesophageal stricture; secondly, when complete rest of that tract is required (e.g. fistula); thirdly when the tract, although accessible, cannot be used for enteral feeding (e.g. postoperative cleanse); finally when, as noted above, requirements exceed enteral capacity (e.g. in patients with burns). In the present-day climate of improved parenteral feeding and the development of the 'big bag' system, which provides complete, mixed, nutritional support, partial parenteral nutrition should not be considered as a form of protein-sparing therapy.

The conditions described above are the common ones requiring TPN. There are, however, interesting case reports of individuals with these conditions who have become pregnant and have been maintained on TPN throughout the pregnancy.[10]

Route of Access and Administration

TPN solutions are hyperosmolar and therefore it is often necessary to infuse them through a central vein. Usually a catheter is inserted via the subclavian vein into the superior vena cava. There are circumstances, however, when a peripheral vein is used preferentially, as for instance in the neonate, and for short-term (up to 10 days) feeding in the adult. More detailed accounts of the establishment and maintenance of access can be found elsewhere.[11]

Problems with stability of the solutions used in the provision of TPN, including calcium precipitation in the presence of amino acid solutions, mean that solutions are now mixed shortly before delivery. Al-

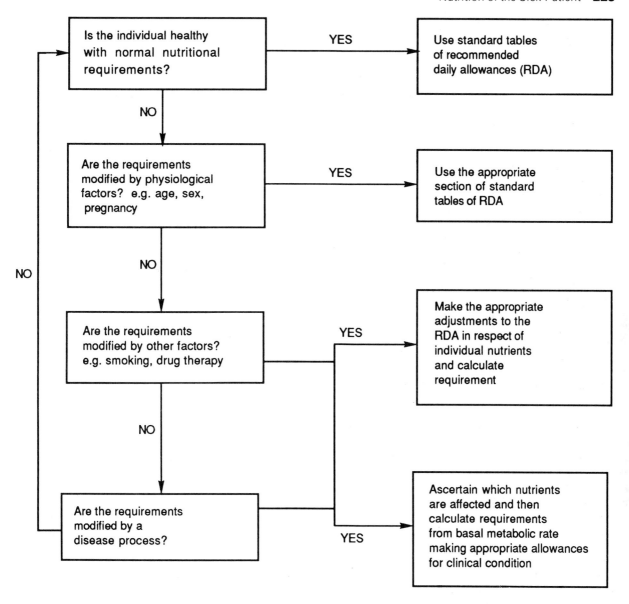

| Is the individual healthy with normal nutritional requirements? | → YES → | Use standard tables of recommended daily allowances (RDA) |

↓ NO

| Are the requirements modified by physiological factors? e.g. age, sex, pregnancy | → YES → | Use the appropriate section of standard tables of RDA |

↓ NO

| Are the requirements modified by other factors? e.g. smoking, drug therapy | → YES → | Make the appropriate adjustments to the RDA in respect of individual nutrients and calculate requirement |

↓ NO

| Are the requirements modified by a disease process? | → YES → | Ascertain which nutrients are affected and then calculate requirements from basal metabolic rate making appropriate allowances for clinical condition |

NO (loop back)

Fig. 12.3 Nutritional requirements.[12]

though this could be seen as tedious, and open the way to errors, it allows flexibility in the provision of nutrients, and each patient can have a tailor-made TPN regimen, which can be adapted as the individual's nutritional requirements change.

There are three basic methods of administration— the sequential single-bottle regimen, the multiple-bottle regimen, and the 'big bag' regimen. The introduction of the 'big bag' has revolutionized the administration of TPN. The clinician, with the guidance of his or her nutritional support team, provides information on the 24-h nutritional requirements of the patient, and this regimen (in a 2 or 3L bag) is produced (in the UK) by the Pharmacy Sterile Production Unit. This affords great advantages as it incorporates the scientific skills of a pharmacist who has knowledge of precipitation, stability and miscibility. The

'big bag' regimen also saves nursing time, reduces infection, improves metabolic tolerance, and optimizes the use of substrate over 24 h. There are problems, however, with this regimen, including cost and stability. For the long-term and home TPN patient, bags with a shelf life of 90 days can be purchased that require the addition of lipid and vitamins only.

Nutritional Requirements

The primary aim of parenteral feeding, particularly in a very sick individual, is to provide sufficient essential nutrients to promote and maintain good health. Essentially each patient should be considered as an individual in the estimation of his or her requirements (Fig. 12.3). There are five basic objectives that must be considered:

(i) achieving positive nitrogen balance, or, at the very least, nitrogen equilibrium;

(ii) minimization of weight loss—and there is general acceptance that no patient (if overweight) should be prescribed a weight-reducing regimen when seriously ill, because of the possibility of loss of lean body mass;

(iii) the provision of vitamins and minerals;

(iv) maintenance of fluid balance;

(v) prevention of overfeeding.

To achieve these objects, each patient should be assessed in terms of his or her nutritional requirement.

Energy Requirements

Energy requirements, conventionally, for the sick patient are based on his or her basal (or resting) metabolic rate (BMR), with additional modifications. Many units do not have the facility to measure the actual BMR of an individual using an indirect calorimeter, in which case BMR can be derived from standard tables as follows:[12]

1. BMR
2. Activity
   (a) ventilator   BMR − 15%
   (b) unconscious   BMR
   (c) bed-bound and awake BMR + 10%
   (d) sitting in a chair   BMR + 20%
   (e) walking round ward   BMR + 30%
3. Thermic effect of feeding BMR + 10%
4. Weight gain   300 kcal (1255 kJ)/day (approximately)
5. Pyrexia   1°C increase in body temperature results in 10–12% rise in BMR.

The main sources of energy in TPN are lipid and carbohydrate (see next section), with a guide to energy requirement of 30–35 kcal (125–145 kJ)/kg per day.

Protein Requirements

Protein requirements for patients on TPN are provided in the form of amino acid solutions and conventionally described in terms of grams of nitrogen. This, in our opinion, can lead to confusion, as in every other condition of nutritional assessment grams of protein are the terms adopted. Having said that, requirements are ideally assessed by the measurement of protein (nitrogen) intake and nitrogen output (including urinary, faecal and other minor/major losses). A typical N excretion formula is:

$$\text{Nitrogen excretion} = \frac{\text{mmol urinary urea over 24 h}}{30}$$

Thus, the amount of nitrogen required to maintain N balance can be assessed. Alternatively a value can be based on arbitrary energy : nitrogen ratios (Table 12.2). Nitrogen input should never be less than 0.16 g (1 g protein)/kg per day.[12]

The normal energy:nitrogen ratio is providing a regimen with a protein:energy ratio (PER) of 10%, whereas in the case of severe catabolism the PER is 40%. This is an extremely high PER (more than double the customary PER profile of individuals in the UK). The justification of providing such highly concentrated nitrogen regimens over any period of time should be questioned, as there may be a risk of metabolic complications. Advances in our knowledge of the nutritional requirements of infants with low birth weight have made possible the use of tailor-made TPN solutions for their nutrition; detailed information on parenteral nutrition in these infants can be found elsewhere.[13]

Table 12.3 provides a summary of energy and nitrogen requirements in different kinds of patients on TPN.

Vitamins and Minerals in TPN

Requirements of vitamins and minerals are generally in line with national guidelines[14] (Table 12.4). However, there are reports of deficiencies on long-term TPN for certain trace elements (zinc, copper, chromium and selenium) and vitamins (vitamins A and D, and biotin). Selenium deficiency has been reported recently in four children receiving TPN.[15] Biotin deficiency has also been reported in a group of infants.[16] TPN in infants with short-gut syndrome resulted in biotin deficiency and an abnormal fatty acid profile in serum phospholipids. Biotin therapy (100 μg/day) changed the profile, but not sufficiently to match control values. All patients responded positively to biotin. Obviously infants on TPN should receive biotin.

There exist no guidelines for the assessment of individual needs for the micronutrients generally. Today, vitamins and minerals are usually given according to the local clinical practice. Requirements for zinc, copper and manganese are well understood, and for feeding for under 6 weeks there is no need to give chromium or selenium. Mineral requirements are more complicated. In the neonate, requirements for calcium and other minerals may be compromised by metabolic diseases. Recently, guidelines on micronutrients for infants and children on TPN have been provided from the USA.[17]

There are a number of commercial preparations on the market that provide a full profile of vitamins, and there also exist commercial preparations of electrolyte and trace element sources.[12]

Preparations and Sources of TPN

(For a comprehensive review, see Thomas[12])

In the preparation of the energy source of TPN, glucose and lipid (as an emulsion) are favoured today. Glucose concentrations may range from 5 to 50%, and the solution may or may not contain amino

TABLE 12.2

COMMONLY USED ENERGY:NITROGEN (E:N) RATIOS (UNITS USED—KCAL/G) IN PARENTERAL NUTRITION

	Total ratio E:N		Non-nitrogen ratio E:N
Normal	250–350:1	(10% PER)	225–335:1
Convalescence	200:1		175:1
Mild catabolism	150:1		125:1
Moderate catabolism	125:1	(30% PER)	100:1
Severe catabolism	100:1	(40% PER)	75:1

PER, protein:energy ratio.

TABLE 12.3

APPROXIMATE REQUIREMENTS FOR ENERGY AND NITROGEN IN DIFFERENT PATIENTS ON A PARENTERAL FEEDING REGIMEN

	Normal	Catabolic	Non-catabolic
Energy requirements			
MJ/day	11–14	15–18	7–9
kcal/day	≈3000	≈4000	≈2000
*Optimal ratio**			
kJ/g	1365	630	1050
Non-protein energy/ nitrogen (kcal/g)	325	135	250
N requirement for equilibrium	8.5	25	7.5

* Non-protein energy ratio.
Normal men are used for comparison.[12]

TABLE 12.4

SUGGESTED MICRONUTRIENT REQUIREMENTS FOR ADULT MALE PROVIDED WITH PARENTERAL NUTRITION

	Values per day	
Nutrient	DRV[14]	Adult[12]
Ca (mmol)	17.5	7.7–14.0
Fe (μmol)	200.0	19.5–70.0
Zinc (μmol)	145.0	37.5–100.0
Selenium (μmol)	0.9	0.4
Thiamin (mg)	1.0	3.0
Nicotinic acid (mg)	17.0	40.0
Folic acid (μg)	200.0	500.0
Biotin (μg)	N/A	60–200.0
Vitamin C (mg)	40.0	100–500.0
Vitamin A (μg)	700.0	1000.0
Vitamin D (μg)	N/A	5.0

DRV, dietary reference value.

acids or electrolytes. A 5% glucose solution cannot be used for TPN; provision of 1000 kcal would require 5L! The only lipid emulsion available in the UK is Intralipid (KabiPharmacia (UK)) as 10% or 20% emulsions. Unless lipid is contraindicated, a rule of thumb is to limit glucose to between 30 and 70% of non-amino acid energy, the remainder being provided by lipid.

The choice of an amino acid source is dependent on several factors, not least cost. A practical consideration is related to the use of the 'big bag', particularly if lipid is to be used as well, and stability must also be taken into account. All nitrogen sources sold in the UK are crystalline amino acid solutions, with an essential to non-essential amino acid profile of 1:3.

Some Complications Associated with TPN

Much has been written about the potential complications of TPN, and comprehensive accounts can be found in a number of texts.[9,11,18] However, an interesting phenomenon is the changes that occur in gastrointestinal morphology during parenteral nutrition. If adequate nutrition is provided by the intravenous route, the intestine atrophies. This implies that the presence or absence of nutrients in the gut lumen, rather than the availability of nutrients to the body as a whole, affects gut structure and function. Lo and Walker[19] in a review highlighted this problem in patients with small-bowel resection. In such patients, the remaining segment can adapt by increasing in length and mucosal adaptive area. Adaptation may be mediated by the presence of luminal nutrients, e.g. glutamine, and also gastrin, cholecystokinin and glucagon. This response depends on the provision of enteral feeding. If TPN is prolonged, hypoplasia of the mucosa occurs. Thus, the reviewers concluded that in the management of short-bowel syndrome, enteral feeding should be added to TPN as soon as feasible.

TABLE 12.5
MONITORING PROGRESS DURING PROLONGED NUTRITIONAL
CARE IN HOSPITAL

Daily
Visual assessment
Body weight
Fluid intake/output

Twice a week
Urea and electrolytes
Urine for sugar (or blood glucose)

Once a week
Full blood count
Serum Ca, Mg, phosphate
Serum proteins

Once a month
Full baseline

Additional tests for those requiring long-term TPN
Tests of vitamin and trace element status

Other useful tests
Triceps skinfold thickness (TST)
Mid-arm muscle circumference (MAMC)
Retinol-binding protein (RBP)

TPN, total parenteral nutrition.
Modified from Neale.[4]

This phenomenon emphasizes the need for a gradual transition from TPN to enteral feeding when TPN is to be stopped. Abrupt removal of a central venous line is likely seriously to interrupt the patient's feeding.

PATIENT MONITORING

Monitoring is an essential part of the provision of nutritional support for the sick. The extent of the monitoring depends on the condition of the patient and the form of support provided. Broadly, there are three objectives:

- assessment of the nutritional status of the patient;
- detection of metabolic abnormalities;
- detection of excess or deficiency of nutrient elements supplied.

Monitoring should be systematic, with records kept in a form in which visual comparison of results can be made easily. Practically, it is desirable that a limited number of persons should be responsible for making measurements, taking the appropriate samples and recording the results.

Anthropometric measurements are the usual method of monitoring nutritional progress and it is essential that all measurements are made under standard conditions. If skinfold thickness and anthropometric measurements are made, the person making them should be carefully trained in order to obtain reliable and reproducible results.

Tests that may be used (together with their fre-

quency) for monitoring the progress of patients during prolonged nutritional care in hospital are shown in Table 12.5. Metabolic complications in patients receiving enteral support are largely due to the clinical condition. Hypophosphataemia is an important problem, owing to the increased requirement for phosphate caused by the metabolism of large amounts of carbohydrate.

The infusion of nutrient solutions directly into the circulation is a potentially dangerous procedure. Patients are often critically ill and their progress rather more uncertain. Furthermore, there is a reduced physiological control because the flow of nutrients into the circulation is not controlled by the intestine or by first pass through the liver. For these reasons there must be much more attention to the results of laboratory monitoring, with appropriate modification of the infused solution. Maintenance of fluid balance is the keystone of the management of the acutely sick patient. Particularly critical conditions requiring careful monitoring of fluid balance are those in which there is tissue breakdown (gross sepsis, malnutrition). Monitoring of body weight and serum osmolarity regularly are vital.[12,18]

EXAMPLES OF PATIENTS REQUIRING NUTRITIONAL SUPPORT

Elderly Surgical Patients

Many elderly patients admitted to hospital with acute illness develop serious complications, occupy hospital beds for long periods of time, and require intensive nursing and medical treatment. Amongst these are patients admitted for surgery for treatment of proximal femoral fracture. The incidence of this condition in elderly women in the UK has been said to have reached epidemic proportions. These patients have a high death rate and of those who survive, one-quarter never return to former mobility or independence. Many of these patients are malnourished on admission to hospital and more than half of them may suffer from subclinical vitamin deficiencies (see Table 12.1).

Measurements of the postoperative voluntary food intake of elderly patient with fractures showed a wide range of energy and nutrient intakes, with some consuming only about 250 kcal and 7 g of protein 14 days after surgery.[20] Using the gastrointestinal tract is usually not a problem in these patients. In any case, long-term TPN might be contraindicated, if only because of the number of patients that might be involved and the cost of the solutions.

There are three possible ways in which the food intake of this sort of patient might be increased. They might be encouraged to eat more food and thus their voluntary food intake increases. This is likely to be expensive on nursing time because the patient might need to be fed. An alternative would be to enlist the assistance of a relative. The voluntary food intake might also be increased by offering sip-feed supplements. Williams et al.[21] reported results of a controlled trial of these in elderly orthopaedic patients identified as being at high risk of malnutrition by means of a nutritional risk questionnaire. The compliance was relatively poor, with a significant number of patients consuming less than one can of supplement per day, and there was no change in clinical outcome after 3 weeks' supplementation.

Tube feeding is a more reliable and certain way of giving a dietary supplement. Bastow et al. studied 744 elderly patients with fractures, who were classified on admission as well nourished, thin or very thin.[22] Patients who were thin or very thin were randomly allocated into control and tube-fed. The tube-fed patients were given 1000 kcal and 28 g protein by nasogastric tube overnight. The very thin derived the greatest benefit, in terms of time taken to achieve independent mobility. As with the study by Williams, this study underlines the importance of assessment and the value of concentrating on those patients who have a nutritional problem.

Reference has been made above to the need for nutritional follow-up in patients whose nutrition has been at risk in hospital. Elderly patients with fractures who have been at high risk of malnutrition may lose weight on discharge if support is not continued.

Patients with Burn Injuries

Severe burn trauma is usually defined as a body surface area burn of more than 30% of total body surface area (TBSA). A major burn is defined as more than 10% of TBSA in the child and more than 15% of TBSA in an adult, or if there is an inhalation injury. The biphasic metabolic response to burn injury was first described by Cuthbertson[23] and is similar in its characteristics to that which follows other serious injuries. The ebb phase from the time of burning up to 36–48 h after coincides with the resuscitation period. Historically, no routine nutritional support was given during this period, because it was thought that the need to prevent hypovolaemia by giving plasma and other fluids should take precedence. However, the trend now is to provide early nutritional support (within the first 24 h); early enteral feeding may prevent paralytic ileus and functional gut atrophy, improve nitrogen balance and more rapidly normalize visceral proteins. The flow, or hypercatabolic phase, begins at about 48 h after the burn and the depth of the burn determines its duration. It is characterized by an increase in energy expenditure (up to 150% of predicted RMEE), effected by an increase in plasma catabolic hormones—catecholamines, glucocorticoids and glucagon. In addition there is accelerated protein and fat breakdown, negative nitrogen balance and altered carbohydrate metabolism. The maximum catabolic response usually occurs 10–15 days after the burn.

After this period, healing of partial-thickness burns, and early excisions and grafting of deep burns reduce the wound size and thus the exogenous demands for nutrients. The patient then enters the anabolic phase, which is associated with improved appetite. As with other injuries the aim of nutritional therapy is to restore muscle mass and strength, and return to normal function.

During the initial period of resuscitation the amount of fluid required can be predicted[24] from well-used formulae such as:

$$\text{Water loss (mL/h)} - (25 + \% \text{ burn}) \times \text{body surface area (m}^2).$$

Dextrose and colloids are used for resuscitation. Few data are available on target intakes for glucose and nitrogen during this period.

Sutherland has pioneered studies of nutritional requirements in burns and her (modified) formulae for adults and children with respect to protein and energy requirements are still widely used:

- **Adults** (modified from Sutherland[25])
  Energy = 20 kcal (84 kJ)/kg + 70 kcal (294 kJ)/% burn;
  Protein = 1g/kg + 2g/% burn.
  This would provide for a 65 kg male (30% burn): energy 3400 kcal (14.2 MJ); protein 155 g (PER = 17).

- **Children** (modified from Sutherland and Batchelor[26])
  Energy = 60 kcal (250 kJ)/kg + 35 kcal (146 kJ)/% burn;
  Protein = 3g/kg + 1g/% BSA burn

In the intervening two decades since Sutherland's studies, more information has come to light regarding protein and energy requirements, and some units are now using different formulae. Cunningham et al.[27] have argued the case for retaining the rule of thumb of $2 \times$ RMEE for energy requirements. Although data from his group indicate that metabolic energy expenditure declines by 15% per month (30–50% TBSA) and 6% per month (76–98% TBSA), he states that to reduce nutritional support on the basis of expenditure at rest must be tempered by compensation for increased energy needs due to increased activity with convalescence. This debate will obviously continue, as will similar debates concerning children. In practice it has been very difficult to meet the high nutritional requirements of the Sutherland formula across the age range, and in larger burns. Investigators working in paediatric burns units have suggested other formulae based on recently published data and personal experience.[28,29]

Requirements for vitamin C, thiamin, iron, and zinc are higher in patients with burns than in those without, and supplements may be required. In the case of vitamin C (dietary reference value, 40 mg[14]), requirement could be as high as 500–1000 mg because of its known role in collagen synthesis. Urinary zinc excretion may be greatly increased and serum zinc an unreliable indicator of zinc status.

Enteral feeding is always preferred to parenteral feeding in patients with extensive burns. Parenteral feeding is associated with a high incidence of septicaemia, even if the feeding line does not go through the burn area. The advantages of enteral over parenteral feeding are that it is cheaper, more physiological because the liver is not bypassed, and requires less biochemical monitoring. The feed should be given at up to 2L in the first 24 h and gradually increased in volume to target requirements. Enteral feed should continue until either all the burns have healed, with minimum weight loss, or the burns have healed and biochemical variables are within normal limits. Patients should be encouraged to eat and drink—they are invariably fed nasogastrically overnight as their oral intake improves during the day. The same nutritional principles apply to TPN as to enteral feeding. Fat-free regimens are not acceptable, as a patient with burns cannot oxidize glucose at as great a rate as healthy individuals, and fat (intralipid) is an important source of energy.

Patients with Head Injuries

The brain is unique in many ways. Though it contains considerable amounts of lipid, this is present as complex lipids in myelin and cell membranes. The amounts of glycogen and neutral fat in the brain are very small and hence the organ is dependent on a continuous supply of exogenous fuel. The major fuel is glucose, which in an adult is used at the rate of 0.3–1.00 mmol/kg per min, with more than 90% being metabolized by glycolysis. The brain of a newborn baby can readily use ketones, but in an adult the use of ketones is dependent on their circulating concentrations and their passage through the blood–brain barrier. Ketones act as brain fuel in conditions of starvation, and ketone production after injury, 'ketone adaptation', can be an important factor in survival.

Besides their role in protein synthesis, brain amino acids act as neurotransmitters and as precursors of neurotransmitters. Energy-dependent specific mechanisms control the passage of amino acids across the blood–brain barrier. Serotonin (5-hydroxytryptamine, 5-HT) in serotonergic neurons is synthesized from tryptophan. The passage of this amino acid into the brain is controlled by the ratio of its concentration to the sum of the concentrations of other large neutral amino acids and this sum is, in turn, controlled by insulin. Thus, 5-HT synthesis is affected by both dietary protein and carbohydrate. Other dietary precursors of neurotransmitters are phenylalanine and tyrosine (noradrenaline and dopamine, respectively) and lecithin and choline (acetylcholine).

Vitamins and minerals involved in brain metabolism include thiamin, nicotinic acid, pyridoxine, vitamin B_{12}, folic acid and vitamin C, magnesium, zinc and manganese.

When the brain is injured these processes may be interfered with to a degree that depends on the age of the patient, and the severity and location of the injury. The metabolic response to injury has been described above. Cytokines[7] play an important role in this response and lead to the production of fever and anorexia. Increased ventricular activity of the cytokine, interleukin 1 (IL-1) has been reported in head-injured patients,[30] and it has been suggested that small amounts of strategically located IL-1 in the brain of head-injured patients might also cause a profound systemic metabolic response in man.[31] These investigators showed that 25 patients had a profound acute-phase response for the period of study, 21 days. An earlier study had suggested that hypermetabolism might persist for up to 1 year after brain injury.

In the majority of head-injured patients, achieving a positive nitrogen balance may be difficult. In a study of steroid-treated comatose patients,[32] the RMEE varied from 70 to 190% of normal, according to age, sex and body surface. Patients who achieved nitrogen balance received 161–240% of RMEE with externally administered formulae. The metabolic response in these patients was similar to that of patients with 20–40% body surface burns. Failure to meet the hypermetabolic response is likely to precipitate malnutrition, with risks of infection and death. Wasting of body mass may occur even when food intake appears adequate. Furthermore, glucose, the brain's normal energy source, may not be the best fuel to provide energy during the immediate post-injury period.[33] Nutrition in the recovery and rehabilitation of the head-injured patient has been reviewed elsewhere.[34]

Patients with Cancer

Protein–energy malnutrition is common in patients with cancer and may precede the diagnosis and bear no relation to the size of the tumour. 'Cancer cachexia' is a syndrome of complex aetiology,[35] characterized by emaciation, debilitation and inanition associated with anorexia, early satiety, anaemia and marked asthenia. Establishing and maintaining adequate nutrition in the face of the interplay of biochemical, physiological and psychological consequences of cancer is often difficult.

Inadequate food intake may be caused by anatomical obstruction, anorexia and early satiety, taste aberration, food aversion or methods of treatment. Anorexia may vary from mild to severe and its severity may go unnoticed by the patient. Many factors, none of them mutually exclusive, may act synergistically to exacerbate the problem.[35] These factors include toxic substances or 'hormones' produced by the tumour, changes in the hypothalamic control of feeding behaviour, psychological and emotional responses to the

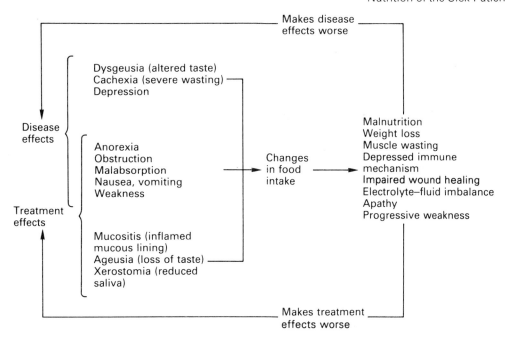

Fig. 12.4 Nutritional implications of cancer and cancer therapy.

disease and its treatment, metabolic abnormalities of uncertain origin and the effects of treatments.

Vitamin deficiencies are common and may be attributed to poor food intake, abnormal losses and possible drug-induced increases in requirements.

The treatment of neoplastic disease may cause many significant nutritional disabilities, which may be superimposed upon, and exacerbate, those caused by the disease (Fig. 12.4).

There is no justification for withholding food from cancer patients under the mistaken notion that it will accelerate tumour growth. However, nutrition is supportive and not therapeutic. It may well have an adjunctive role, increasing the effectiveness, or decreasing the side-effects, of specific antitumour regimens. Nutritional support of the right kind, be it enteral or parenteral, can have an important effect on the patient in restoring or maintaining some sense of well-being, physical or psychological. The role of nutritional support in maintaining or improving the quality of life in cancer patients merits further study. The need for support often continues long after the possibilities for active anticancer treatment have been exhausted, and its provision may affect the survival curve.[36]

Nutritional support for the cancer patient should follow the principles established for the management of any malnourished patient; it should be seen as part of the patient's therapeutic programme and suitably planned. Oral feeding may require modification of food items in order to increase nutrient density and tempt a poor appetite. Prepared enteral feeds may be incorporated to achieve these goals. True

enteral feeds may be given via the nasogastric, gastrostomy or jejunostomy route with a fine-bore tube. Cancer patients may need nutritional support before surgery or other anticancer treatment. Sometimes TPN is the method of choice, e.g. in patients with oesophageal cancer, but TPN for less than 5 days is probably quite ineffective (as well as expensive!). On discharge from hospital, many cancer patients benefit from nutritional advice contained in specially prepared, attractive booklets.

CONCLUSION

Optimal nutrition is important to the sick patient and should be viewed as part of total care and treatment. Its provision can be achieved if the correct guidelines are followed to assess the patient's nutritional status, appetite, and nutritional requirements. Patients should always be fed enterally if possible. If parenteral feeding is necessary, it should be instituted as soon as possible. The administration of parenteral nutrition requires considerable expertise and the complete commitment of, ideally, a nutritional support team. In large hospitals there are major advantages to the team approach, not only in the early instigation of appropriate feeding regimens and regular monitoring but also in the reduction of life-threatening complications. Each sick patient should be assessed as an individual.

REFERENCES

1. Platt B.S., Eddy T.P., Pellett P.L. (1963). *Food in Hospitals*, Oxford: Nuffield Provincial Hospital Trust.

2. Tredger J. (1982). Feeding the patient—a team effort. *Nursing*, **2**, 92.

3. Goodinson S.M., Dickerson J.W.T. (1988). Assessment of nutritional status. In *Nutrition in the Clinical Management of Disease*, 2nd edn (Dickerson J.W.T., Lee, H.A. eds.) London: Arnold, pp. 456–485.

4. Neale G. (1988). *Clinical Nutrition*, London: Heinemann Medical.

5. Passmore R., Eastwood M.A. (1986). *Davidson and Passmore Human Nutrition and Dietetics*, 8th edn, Edinburgh: Churchill Livingstone, pp. 88–89.

6. Bingham S., Cummings J.H.C. (1984). Urine 24 hour nitrogen excretion as an independent measure of the habitual dietary protein intake in individuals. *Proc. Nutr. Soc.*, **43**, 80A.

7. Grimble R.F. (1990). Nutrition and cytokine action. *Nutr. Res. Rev.*, **3**, 193.

8. Lee H.A. (1988a). Enteral feeding. In *Nutrition in the Clinical Management of Disease*, 2nd edn (Dickerson J.W.T., Lee H.A. eds.) London: Arnold, pp. 486–495.

9. Lee H.A. (1988b). Parenteral nutrition. In *Nutrition in the Clinical Management of Disease*, 2nd edn (Dickerson J.W.T., Lee H.A. eds.) London: Arnold, pp. 496–511.

10. Leading article (1988). Maintenance of pregnancy by total parenteral nutrition. *Nutr. Rev.*, **46**, 220.

11. Grant A., Todd E. (1987) *Enteral and Parenteral Nutrition*, 2nd edn, Oxford: Blackwell Scientific.

12. Thomas B. (1988). *Manual of Dietetic Practice*, Oxford: Blackwell Scientific.

13. Kovar I.Z., Morgan J.B. (1990). Parenteral nutrition in the preterm infant. *Clin. Nutr.*, **9**, 57.

14. Department of Health (1991). *Dietary Reference Values for Food Energy and Nutrients for the United Kingdom* (Report on Health and Social Subjects No. 41) London: HMSO.

15. Leading article (1989a). Newly recognised signs of selenium deficiency in humans. *Nutr. Rev.*, **47**, 117.

16. Leading article (1989b). Biotin deficiency due to total parenteral nutrition alters serum fatty acid composition. *Nutr. Rev.*, **47**, 121.

17. Green H.L., Hambidge K.M., Schanler R., Tsang R.C. (1988). Guidelines for the use of vitamins, trace elements, calcium, magnesium and phosphorous in infants and children receiving total parenteral nutrition. *Am. J. Clin. Nutr.*, **48**, 1324.

18. Phillips G.D., Odgers C.L. (1986). *Parenteral and Enteral Nutrition*, 3rd edn, Edinburgh: Churchill Livingstone.

19. Lo C.W., Walker W.A. (1989). Changes in the gastrointestinal tract during enteral or parenteral nutrition. *Nutr. Rev.*, **47**, 193.

20. Dickerson J.W.T., Fekkes J., Goodinson S.M., Older J. (1985). Postoperative food intake of elderly fracture patients. In *Nutrition, Immunity and Illness in the Elderly* (Chandra R.K. ed.) Oxford: Pergamon, pp. 247–252.

21. Williams C.M., Driver L.T., Older J., Dickerson J.W.T. (1989). A controlled trial of sip-feed supplements in elderly orthopaedic patients. *Eur. J. Clin. Nutr.*, **43**, 267.

22. Bastow M.D., Rawlings J., Allison S.P. (1983). Benefits of supplementary tube feeding after fractured neck of femur: a randomised controlled trial. *Br. Med. J.*, **287**, 1589.

23. Cuthbertson D.P. (1930). The disturbance of metabolism produced by bony and non-bony injury with notes on certain abnormal conditions of bone. *Biochem. J.*, **24**, 1244.

24. Wilmore D.W., McDougal M. (1977). Nutrition in burns. In *Nutritional Aspects in Care of the Critically Ill* (Richards J.R., Kinney J.M. eds.) Edinburgh: Churchill Livingstone.

25. Sutherland A.B. (1976). Nitrogen balance and nutritional requirements in the burn patient; a reappraisal. *Burns*, **2**, 238.

26. Sutherland A.B., Batchelor A.D.C. (1968). Nitrogen balance in burned children. *Ann. N.Y. Acad. Sci.*, **150**, 700.

27. Cunningham J.J., Hegarty T., Meara P.A., Burke J.F. (1989). Measured and predicted calorie requirement of adults during recovery from severe burn trauma. *Am. J. Clin. Nutr.*, **49**, 404.

28. Cunningham J.J., Lyden M.K., Russell W.E. (1990) Calorie and protein provision for recovery from severe burns in infants and young children. *Am. J. Clin. Nutr.*, **51**, 553.

29. Shalaby S., Morgan J.B., Tanner N.J.B., Marks V. (1990). Protein and energy requirements of children with burn trauma. *J. Enteral Parenter. Nutr.*, **9**, 52P.

30. McClain C.J., Cohen D., Ott L., Dinarello C.A., Young B. (1987) Ventricular fluid interleukin-1 activity in patients with head injury. *J. Lab. Clin. Med.*, **110**, 48.

31. Young B., Ott L., Beard D., Dempsey R.J., Tibbs P.A., McClain C.J. (1988). The acute phase response of the brain-injured patient. *J. Neurosurg.*, **69**, 375.

32. Clifton G.L., Robertson C.S., Grossman R.G., Hodge S., Foltzk F., Garza C. (1984). The metabolic response to severe head injury. *J. Neurosurg.*, **60**, 687.

33. Robertson C.S., Goodman J.C., Haragan R.K., Contant C.F., Grossman R.G. (1991). The effect of glucose administration on carbohydrate metabolism after head injury. *J. Neurosurg.*, **74**, 43.

34. Dickerson J.W.T. (1992). Recovery of function: nutritional factors. In *Recovery from Brain Damage—Reflections and Directions, Advances in Experimental Medicine and Biology*, Vol. 325 (Rose F.D., Johnson D.A. eds.) New York: Plenum Press, pp. 23–33.

35. Holmes S., Dickerson J.W.T. (1987a). Malignant disease: nutritional implications of disease and treatment. *Cancer Metastasis Rev.*, **6**, 357.

36. Dickerson J.W.T., Williams C.M. (1988). Nutrition and cancer. In *Nutrition in the Clinical Management of Disease*, 2nd edn (Dickerson J.W.T., Lee H.A. eds.) London: Arnold, pp. 350–373.

SECTION 3
CLINICAL BIOCHEMISTRY OF PREGNANCY AND CHILDHOOD

13. Prenatal Screening for Neural Tube Defects and Down's Syndrome
J. Wong

Introduction
Neural tube defects
  Prevalence
  Why screen?
  What tests?
  When and how to screen
  Raised maternal serum AFP
  Twin pregnancies
  Conclusion
Down's syndrome
  Screening
  Maternal biochemical markers
  Conclusion
Epilogue

INTRODUCTION

The criteria for a successful screening programme are well established. These include:

1. The disease is an important health issue for both individual and community.
2. The disease history is well documented.
3. A specific and sensitive screening test is available.
4. There are facilities and resources available for definitive diagnosis and treatment.
5. There is an agreed treatment policy.
6. The disease can be favourably treated on detection.
7. The screening programme is cost effective.

Alas, the prenatal screening programmes for neural tube defects (NTD) and Down's syndrome do not satisfy all the conditions. The screening procedures are controversial but have become well established. Screening for NTD came about in the middle of the 1970s, whilst detection of Down's syndrome utilizing maternal serum markers has only been practised since late 1980s. Arguments are especially rife in the screening of Down's syndrome.

NEURAL TUBE DEFECTS

NTD encompasses three conditions:

- anencephaly
- encephalocoele
- spina bifida.

Anencephaly and spina bifida make up 95% of the cases, with encephalocoele accounting for the final 5%. The neural tube is the embryonic precursor of the brain and spinal cord. It is the failure of surrounding and wrapping of the central nervous system by meninges and skin that causes an NTD. This sealing of the tube is complete by the 30th day of gestation.

Prevalence

The aetiology of NTD is still undetermined. Undoubtedly, hereditary and environmental factors are involved. The genetic component could be a mutant gene or chromosomal abnormality. It is more common in females, has greater propensity to recur in siblings, and is subject to ethnic variation. There are geographical pockets of high incidence, e.g. Northern Ireland, different rates of occurrence in social classes, and latterly some evidence for beneficial effects of nutritional supplements, which point to environmental factors. Overall the prevalence of the condition is falling, which cannot be fully explained by its detection and termination because of the screening programme.

The risk of NTD is very much increased where a positive maternal history exists. It is 10 times greater with one affected child, 20 times with two and 30 times with three. The probability is also increased for children of affected parents. Most NTD babies (90–95%), though, are born to families with no trait.

Figure 13.1 shows the rate of NTD live births in England and Wales. The decade has shown a steady decline. In the region where the author works the incidence of NTD is 2 per 1000 births. Of those that go to full term, approximately 40% are stillbirths, 20% die in the neonatal period, and 5–10% succumb between 4 weeks to a year.

Why Screen?

Anencephalic fetuses are not viable. Detecting the abnormality early in pregnancy with subsequent termination shortens the period of emotional suffering by the parents.

The natural history of spina bifida is quite variable. The clinical state does depend on the site of the lesion. A graver prognosis is found with a high lesion (in the spinal cord) than one that lies low. Spina bifida can cause paralysis and weakness of the lower limbs, both urinary and faecal incontinence, hydrocephalus and is sometimes associated with mental retardation. The financial consequences of dealing with it, such as hospital admissions for special care

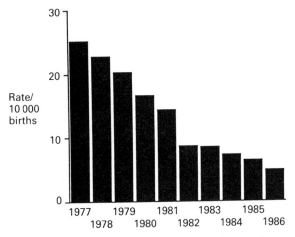

Fig. 13.1 Live births with neural tube defects (anencephaly and spina bifida: England and Wales (1977–1986).

facilities and surgical procedures, are very expensive. It is certainly economic to establish a screening programme. Anencephaly, being fatal at birth, does not consume such resources.

What Tests?

There are now three established ways of detecting NTD:

(i) maternal serum α-fetoprotein (MAFP) and amniotic fluid α-fetoprotein (AAFP);
(ii) amniotic fluid acetylcholinesterase (ACHE);
(iii) ultrasonography.

AFP and ACHE are biochemical markers. AFP is the mainstay of the programme. At present, though, as in the author's hospital, MAFP and ultrasound scanning are the best combination for detection.

AFP is a glycoprotein of approx. 64 000 Da. During serum electrophoresis it migrates in the α-1 fraction. Its function is undermined. In pregnancy, AFP is formed in the yolk sac, fetal liver and mucosa of stomach and small bowel. The yolk sac atrophies by the end of the first trimester. The major portion of AFP is then produced by the fetal liver.

ACHE is present in cerebrospinal fluid (CSF). In a fetus with a NTD a second ACHE isoenzyme is found in the amniotic fluid. The ACHE isoenzyme in CSF is usually detected by polyacrylamide slab-gel electrophoresis. The confirmation of this screening pointer can be substantiated by its sensitivity to an inhibitor. There are two chemical inhibitors available, BW284C51 and Lysivane, which specifically inhibits the NTD ACHE. When the ACHE isoenzymes are found the NTD fraction must always be confirmed with an inhibitor. The inhibitor deletes the specific ACHE band due to the lesion. This dual combination ensures that the correct conclusion is drawn on the presence of ACHE in amniotic fluid.

Ultrasound scanning is now available in most hospi-

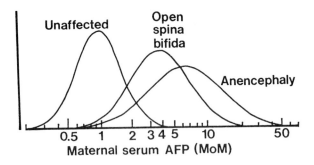

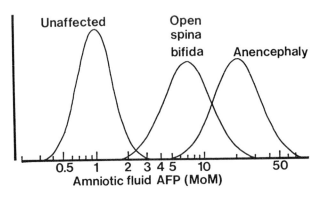

Fig. 13.2 Distribution of α-fetoprotein (AFP) in maternal serum and amniotic fluid in relation to neural tube defects (MoM, multiples of the median).

tals. The advent of high-resolution scanning has made it possible to have a detailed look at the central nervous system of the fetus. Ultrasonography has also been valuable in dating the gestational age of the fetus.

The basis of the screening programme is the determination of AFP in maternal serum. AFP concentration is 150 times greater in the fetus than in amniotic fluid, which in turn, is 350 times more than in maternal serum. AFP concentrations are in equilibrium between fetus, amniotic fluid and mother's serum. An escape of AFP from the fetus is reflected by a raised circulating concentration in maternal serum. This is the position with an open NTD, anencephaly and encephalocoele. Only an open NTD will cause an elevated MAFP. An open NTD is defined as a lesion not covered by skin or a thick opaque membrane. Essentially an open NTD has no barrier for the diffusion of AFP from fetus to amniotic fluid and the maternal circulation.

When and How to Screen

All studies have shown that the best detection rate is achieved by screening between 16 and 18 weeks of gestation. It is also at a stage in which organ details can be seen by ultrasound scanning. In the UK the new abortion law allows terminations only up to 24 weeks of gestation. Therefore it is appropriate that

TABLE 13.1

CAUSES OF A RAISED MATERNAL SERUM α-FETOPROTEIN

Incorrect gestational age

Multiple pregnancy

Fetal death, miscarriage, threatened abortion

Neural tube defects

Chromosomal disorders:
  Turner's syndrome
  Trisomies 13, 18

Renal disorders:
  Polycystic kidneys
  Renal agenesis
  Urethral obstruction
  Finnish-type nephrosis

Gastrointestinal disorders:
  Oesophageal atresia
  Duodenal atresia

Anterior abdominal-wall anomalies:
  Gastroschisis
  Omphalocoele

the screening procedure takes place between 16 and 18 weeks of pregnancy.

Figure 13.2 shows the AFP distribution profile between normal and fetuses with NTD. It is clear that in maternal serum there is an overlap between normal and abnormal fetuses. A better discrimination is obtained in AAFP, which thus has greater predictive value than MAFP. Using a cut-off point of 2.5 multiples of the median (MoM) for maternal serum it is possible to detect 88% of anencephalics and 79% of open spina bifida when the test is carried out between 16 and 18 weeks of gestation. For AAFP (using figures from the UK Collaborative AFP Study) a series of cut-offs was established: 2.5 MoM for 13–15 weeks, 3.0 MoM for 16–18 weeks, 3.5 MoM for 19–21 weeks, and 4.0 MoM for 22–24 weeks of gestation enables a detection rate of 98% for anencephaly and open NTDs.

The results are expressed in terms of MoMs rather than mass units for several reasons. Medians are easy to derive from small numbers and the estimations are reliable, simple to calculate and mathematically sound (as the derivation will not be skewed by the occasional rogue value). MAFP also rises during pregnancy and expressing the result as MoM is sensitive to this variation, i.e. it allows for a steady baseline in the face of rising concentrations of AFP in maternal serum. Finally, the expression has made it possible to compare measurements between different laboratories in the face of varying measurement techniques, AFP standards and units of quantitation.

Raised Maternal Serum AFP

There are various reasons for increased concentra-

tions of MAFP. These can be physiological or pathological. Table 13.1 lists the most common causes of a raised MAFP.

Although the differential diagnosis is wide, most cases are explained by incorrect gestational age, multiple pregnancy, NTDs and fetal death. The mother herself could also be responsible for excess MAFP. The most likely reason is maternal hepatitis.

AAFP will also be elevated in the anomalies of Table 13.1. ACHE is very helpful in confirming a diagnosis of NTD. These days, ultrasound scanning will and can confirm many of the malformations mentioned.

Twin Pregnancies

A multiple pregnancy is associated with raised MAFP. In the unaffected, normal twin pregnancy the MAFP is approximately twice the MoM expected for a singleton. There is a lack of data to be definite for decisions on 'cut-off' levels. It is very probable that only one twin is affected. It is now possible and feasible with the guidance of ultrasound scanning to perform selectively a single fetocide. Because of being uncertain about 'normal' concentrations for MAFP in regard of twins, most screening centres do not advise on the risk of NTD.

Conclusion

The procedure for NTD screening is now well established. The first line is determination of MAFP between 16 and 18 weeks of gestation. Should the MAFP be raised, amniocentesis is then done for measuring AAFP and/or establishing the presence of ACHE. With the recent advent of high-resolution ultrasound scanning there is less need for amniocentesis. The latest screening position is probably to determine MAFP and use ultrasonography. The scan offers synergy with MAFP as it helps date the gestation and will show a multiple pregnancy. High-resolution scans will detect most of the physical anomalies. This is true of NTD.

Amniocentesis is not without danger. It can result in fetal loss. Though the risk is small, in the region of 0.5–1.0%, it is avoidable. Amniocentesis is emotionally quite traumatic and also expensive of manpower and resources consumed.

It is the practice, in the author's centre, to screen for NTD by MAFP and ultrasound. We do not use amniocentesis for analysis of amniotic fluid. Since the introduction of high-resolution scanning, and disregarding examination of amniotic fluid, we have not missed a case of NTD.

DOWN'S SYNDROME

This syndrome is the most frequently occurring chromosomal abnormality and is responsible for about a third of the severe mental handicap population.

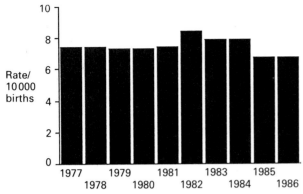

Fig. 13.3 Live births with Down's syndrome: England and Wales 1977–1986.

There are two chromosomal abnormalities in Down's syndrome. The first, trisomy 21 (non-dysjunctional, regular-type Down's), accounts for 95% of cases. In this the child has 47 chromosomes. The other 5% have 46 chromosomes (translocation-type Down's) where there is an exchange of genetic material in part of the autosomal short arms. Down's babies of the translocation, 46-chromosome type are usually born to the younger mother, with a very pronounced chance of inheritance.

Down's syndrome is characterized by physical characteristics of facial appearance, a single palmar crease and a wide spacing between the large and second toes. The condition is associated with infections, especially of the ears and lungs, congenital heart disease and high gastrointestinal abnormalities. The one common feature is that they are all mentally deficient. Successful treatment of the infections and neonatal surgery has meant an increased longevity, now averaging 60 years. They eventually develop pathological brain changes very similar to Alzheimer's disease.

Figure 13.3 shows the rate per 10 000 live births in England and Wales. The prevalence in pregnancy is higher than at birth. There is a high rate of fetal loss through miscarriages. Therapeutic termination of pregnancies has also kept the numbers lower.

Screening

Increasing maternal age correlates positively with the incidence of the trisomy 21 anomaly after 35 years of age. For example, the incidence at birth for a woman aged 35 is 1.2%, rising to 8.2% at 46 years of age. Up to 35 years the incidence does not vary much, except there is evidence that women under 20 years also have a higher incidence of Down's babies. Therefore the profile does seem to be a J-shaped curve. The relation between increasing maternal age and Down's syndrome is well documented and there are also data to show that increasing paternal age behaves similarly.

Mothers over 35 years have always been considered a high-risk group, along with those who have had babies born with Down's of the translocation type. As trisomy 21 is so prevalent, we have always concentrated on the group of older mothers. These women have generally been given the choice of an amniocentesis to determine fetal karyotype. Thus a limited screening programme is in existence. The take-up, though, has historically been running at about 50% of expected numbers. This group of mothers, who make up 7.5% of total pregnancies, is responsible for 30% of babies born with Down's syndrome. Therefore the large majority, i.e. mothers below 35 years, producing 70% of Down's children, are deprived of a detection scheme because facilities and resources are not available for amniocentesis and cytogenetic studies.

There are four possible ways of screening for Down's:

(i) amniocentesis with karyotyping of fetal cells;
(ii) chorionic villus sampling;
(iii) ultrasonography;
(iv) biochemical markers in maternal serum.

Amniocentesis can be done at any time in gestation between 10 weeks to term. It is usually carried out at about 16 weeks. The procedure allows the harvesting of fetal cells, found in the amniotic fluid, to be grown in cell culture medium. It is these cultivated fetal cells that are examined for their chromosomal content. The procedure has its risks, including the induction of miscarriage (0.5–1%), damage to the placenta and injury to the fetus. These risks are minimal when the procedure is carried out with real-time ultrasound. Other problems associated with amniocentesis are the failure of fetal cell growth (probably less than 1%), maternal cell contamination and mosaicism.

Chorionic villus sampling is the biopsy of the placenta to obtain trophoblast cells. These cells reflect the chromosomal constitution of the fetus. This technique can be used from about 8 weeks of gestation but is traditionally done between the 10th and 12th week. The cells harvested can be either examined directly or cultured. The risks associated with chorionic villus sampling are miscarriage (approximately 2%) and infection. This procedure needs clinical and laboratory expertise to obtain and analyse the tissue. It is more expensive as a technique than amniocentesis. It is, therefore, not · suitable for screening purposes.

Ultrasound scanning can recognize Down's fetuses. Features sought include brachycephaly, decreased femur length, and an increased nuchal thickening. These features are variable. Thus at present ultrasound scanning has no place in screening for Down's. The technique has a very low predictive value.

In 1984 the association between Down's syndrome and low concentrations of MAFP was first reported. Ironically the impetus to the seminal paper was a mother who gave birth to a trisomy 18 (Edward's syndrome) baby, whose persistent abnormality during pregnancy was an undetectable MAFP. Her

TABLE 13.2
CAUSES OF LOW MATERNAL SERUM α-FETOPROTEIN

Overestimated gestational age

Trisomy syndromes:
Trisomy 21 (Down's)
Trisomy 18 (Edward's)
Trisomy 13 (Patau's)

Heavier, bigger mothers

Insulin-dependent diabetic mothers
40% lower than expected for their gestational age

Spontaneous abortion

Choriocarcinoma

Hydatidiform mole

Not pregnant

TABLE 13.3
DETECTION RATES FOR DOWN'S SYNDROME

Factors considered	Detection rate (%)
Age alone (> 35 years only)	30
Age + MAFP	35
Age + MAFP + UE3	45
Age + MAFP + UE3 + HCG	60

HCG, human chorionic gonadotrophin; MAFP, maternal serum α-fetoprotein; UE3, unconjugated oestriol.

insistent questioning persuaded the obstetrician to review their cases of trisomy aneuploidy and MAFP. This was responsible for launching the idea of biochemical markers in maternal serum to screen for Down's syndrome.

Maternal Biochemical Markers

Recently the search has been on to find a reliable biochemical pointer of Down's syndrome. Amongst the candidates are:

(i) α-fetoprotein (AFP);
(ii) human chorionic gonadotrophin (HCG);
(iii) free HCG;
(iv) unconjugated oestriol (UE3);
(v) CA 125;
(vi) pregnancy-specific β_1-glycoprotein (SP-1);
(vii) urea-resistant neutrophil alkaline phosphatase activity.

At present, AFP, HCG and UE3 have a role in screening. The place of determining free HCG is still unresolved. The measurement of alkaline phosphatase activity in neutrophils after urea treatment is promising, the activity being greater in Down's than normal controls. The measurement technique, however, is laborious and until an automated or simpler

way is found for assessing activity it will have no place in a screening.

MAFP, as described above, is already a marker for NTD. It was thus attractive to use also for Down's. Concentrations of MAFP are at the extremes of the spectrum, being high in NTD and low in Down's. This can give rise to problems in that the assay range may sometimes not be wide enough to satisfy the dual screen. Low MAFP is not specific to Down's syndrome (Table 13.2).

Low MAFP is an independent risk factor for Down's, as is increasing maternal age. Thereby combining the two will positively affect the efficiency of a screening. Latterly, HCG and UE3 have also been shown to be independent variables in the predictive stakes. By combining all four factors—age, MAFP, HCG and UE3—it is possible to compute a likelihood ratio (risk probability) of a fetus being born with Down's syndrome. This factor can be further refined by considering the mother's weight and presence of maternal diabetes mellitus.

In the UK, the present position of offering amniocentesis to all mothers over 35 years will detect 30% of affected newborns. In reality, with the low acceptance rate for amniocentesis (50%), only 15% are found. Screening all mothers over 35 years will mean amniocentesis for 7.5% of pregnancies *in toto*. By considering the markers mentioned, and retaining a 5% absolute amniocentesis rate, the detection rates are shown in Table 13.3.

A personal-computer software package is now available for determining the probability ratio of Down's syndrome at birth from the values of MAFP, HCG, UE3 and maternal age. The calculation also considers the prevalence of Down's in the area of residence, mother's weight and presence of diabetes mellitus. It is then possible to express the computed result as screen negative or positive. To maintain a 5% amniocentesis rate in the UK, a risk ratio of 1:250 is required, ie. a risk of greater than 1:250 is considered a positive screen and less than 1:250 is negative. This 'cut-off' point can be changed to suit any screening programme but should reflect the balance between the predictive value and amniocentesis rate.

Now we have a means of screening, by maternal biochemical markers, to improve the detection of Down's. This is to cover the whole pregnant population. It must be remembered that the maternal serum tests are only acting as a gatekeeper to amniocentesis. The confirmation of Down's will still have to come from examining the fetal cells obtained.

The optimal time for biochemical maternal screening is 16–18 weeks' gestation. This coincides with the screen for NTD. Amniocentesis will then be indicated in the high-risk pregnancies. The karyotyping will take a further 1–2 weeks. Therefore, timing is crucial in the conduct of a Down's fetus screen.

Conclusion

It is feasible to screen for Down's syndrome. The most economic and fruitful method is by examining biochemical markers in maternal serum. By using and considering mother's age, MAFP, UE3 and HCG it is possible to detect 60% of Down's. This would consist of screening all pregnancies whilst maintaining an amniocentesis rate of 5%. Amniocentesis with cytogenetic typing will need to follow this 'pre-screen' by biochemical markers. There is presently no place for its detection either by chorionic villus sampling or ultrasonography.

EPILOGUE

It has been estimated that approximately 6000 babies per year (one in every 100 live births) are born with a serious impairment of a physical or chromosomal nature. This is in spite of nearly 2000 planned therapeutic terminations for reasons of anomalies. The benefits of screening are financial and other more esoteric reasons. The second benefit is rather difficult to quantify but includes a provision of information to the family, relief from uncertainty, expansion of personal choice, and support during a period of crisis.

All screening procedures have their risks and harmful effects. The ultimate risk is the loss of a normal baby. Other harmful effects include the worries during the period of confirmatory testing, distress from false positives, and an illusory reassurance from false negatives.

Undoubtedly we can now screen for NTD and Down's syndrome. This can be done simultaneously, by analysis of a maternal blood sample taken between 16 and 18 weeks of gestation for markers of the abnormalities. Further testing may need to be done if the initial screen is positive. In recent times, ultrasound scanning has been very beneficial with the screening programme. Screening for NTDs is certainly well accepted. It is now practical to screen for Down's syndrome but is still controversial.

Considering the major problem of the two conditions in our society, the good probability of detecting both Down's syndrome and NTD with the same sample of maternal blood should be made available to all families.

FURTHER READING

Lilford R. J. ed. (1990). *Prenatal Diagnosis and Prognosis*, London: Butterworth.

King's Fund Forum Consensus Statement (1987). *Screening for Fetal and Genetic Abnormalities*, London: King's Fund.

Wald N. J. ed. (1984). *Antenatal and Neonatal Screening*, Oxford University Press.

14. Prenatal Diagnosis of Inherited Metabolic Diseases

J. B. Holton and L. Tyfield

Introduction
Obtaining a sample for prenatal diagnosis
Problems and risks with the procedures
  Amniocentesis
  Chorionic villus biopsy
  Fetal blood and liver samples
Prenatal diagnosis by biochemical methods
  Enzyme assay using amniotic fluid cells
  Enzyme assay using chorionic villi
  Metabolite assay in amniotic fluid
    supernatant
Prenatal diagnosis using DNA analysis
How DNA analysis is used
  Gene tracking
  Identifying specific mutations
  Fetal sexing with the PCR
Prenatal diagnosis or gene therapy?

INTRODUCTION

In developed countries, where there has been a reduction in diseases due to infection and nutritional deficiencies, disorders that are wholly or partly genetically determined are acquiring greater significance in all branches of medicine. In aggregate, genetic diseases are common. About 2–3% of all couples are at high and recurrent risk of having a child with an inherited disorder and 1% of all live births are associated with single-gene disorders.[1] Most genetic diseases are not amenable to effective treatment and so, until gene replacement becomes a reality, the only approaches to the control of genetic diseases are prevention and avoidance. This is achieved by identifying couples and testing pregnancies at risk.

For many congenital disorders (neural tube defects and most chromosomal abnormalities, for example), preventive measures can be initiated only during the pregnancy itself. Because screening tests are available that are reliable, relatively non-invasive and pose no undue risk to the fetus, it should be possible to test all pregnancies in any population for several of these conditions. For the single-gene disorders, on the other hand, it is necessary to predetermine the pregnancies at risk. This is because there is a very large number of diseases (more than 4300 distinct genetic conditions have been recognized) and most of them occur at a very low frequency. Furthermore, the prenatal diagnostic tests are specific for each of them and the tests have to be made on a sample obtained by invasive techniques such as amniocentesis or chori-

onic villus biopsy, which carry a finite risk of fetal loss. It is certain that, in the absence of any preselection of pregnancies at high risk for a particular genetic disease, the risk of fetal loss associated with prenatal sampling far outweighs the risk of the fetus being affected with the disease.

Because of this relative infrequency of individual mutant genes, the identification of 'at risk' individuals or couples invariably relies on a previous family history, and for the rarer recessive disorders a couple usually first becomes aware of the disorder and their increased risk at the birth of an affected child. In these circumstances, prenatal diagnosis can be offered in subsequent pregnancies if the appropriate tests are available because, according to Mendelian inheritance, the couple would stand a 1 in 4 chance at each conception of having another affected child, a risk that is considerably higher than the risk of fetal loss associated with the prenatal sampling.

In contrast to this, in some populations or ethnic groups the frequency of a specific mutant gene is particularly high and so the background risk to couples of producing an affected child is considerably increased. In these situations, screening for carrier status using biochemical or molecular genetic techniques may be feasible, and with this knowledge there should be a better understanding of the reproductive options that are available. However, carrier detection programmes that aim to test individuals either premaritally or preconceptually have been disappointing and so carrier testing is usually undertaken on a pregnant woman at her first antenatal check-up.

In the face of an increased risk of having a child with a disease for which there is no known treatment, prenatal diagnosis offers a couple the assurance of having their own unaffected children by avoiding the birth of affected ones. It is essential, of course, to have a precise diagnosis of the condition for which the couple (or the woman in the case of an X-linked disorder) is at risk and some estimate of the extent of the risk of another child being affected. Some disorders are clinically difficult to distinguish and this can be a major pitfall for meaningful genetic counselling and prenatal diagnosis. Once the diagnosis is confirmed, prenatal diagnosis can change a probability statement about recurrence risk (1 in 4 for autosomal recessive conditions) to one of virtual certainty as to whether another child is affected or not.

One of the objectives of prenatal diagnosis as recommended by the Royal College of Physicians' working party on prenatal diagnosis[2] is to provide reassurance and reduce the level of anxiety associated with reproduction. This recommendation encompasses the decision of couples who would opt for prenatal diagnosis but for whom termination would not be considered an option. Knowing the outcome in an 'at risk' pregnancy may be psychologically beneficial in these circumstances, whether the indications are of a normal or an affected fetus. However, it is not universally agreed that the risks to the fetus and the financial cost of prenatal diagnosis can be justified for such purposes.

For a very few disorders, early prenatal treatment may prevent some adverse effects on the developing fetus. Prenatal diagnosis might be undertaken to ascertain the genotype of the fetus and so determine whether treatment should be considered or not. This approach has been used successfully by offering first-trimester dexamethasone treatment to prevent the development of ambiguous genitalia in female fetuses homozygous for 21-hydroxylase deficiency.[3] Prenatal treatment has also been used to protect a female fetus heterozygous for X-linked ornithine carbamoyl transferase deficiency from intrauterine hyperammonaemia by giving arginine supplementation and a diet low in protein to the mother.[4]

OBTAINING A SAMPLE FOR PRENATAL DIAGNOSIS

In order to carry out a prenatal diagnosis it is necessary to have either cells of fetal origin or a fluid in which abnormal metabolites that are produced by an affected fetus may be found. Nowadays there is a great deal of flexibility in the strategies that can be used for prenatal diagnosis and the approach taken is dependent on the variety of sampling methods available as much as on developments in laboratory techniques.

Amniocentesis, which was introduced about 30 years ago, was the first means of obtaining a sample for prenatal diagnosis. The procedure is usually done between 16 and 18 weeks' gestation and the amniotic fluid cells, which are derived from the external membranes of the fetus, are normally grown in culture medium. The cultured cells can be used for enzyme analysis or as a source of DNA. Sometimes, diagnosis can be made without culturing the cells, provided that abnormal metabolites can be detected directly in the amniotic fluid supernatant when an affected fetus is present.

For some inherited metabolic disorders, however, prenatal diagnosis cannot be undertaken using amniotic fluid because either the diagnostic enzyme is not expressed in amniotic fluid cells or abnormal metabolites do not accumulate, and so alternative techniques have to be found. These include molecular genetic methods or fetal blood and liver sampling. The last two procedures, which are difficult and more hazardous, are used less often now as more genes are being cloned and specific mutations characterized. Nevertheless, some situations remain in which enzyme analysis on fetal blood or on a liver biopsy is necessary.

The main disadvantage of second-trimester amniocentesis and fetal tissue sampling is that diagnoses are available and terminations done relatively late in the pregnancy. The development and routine availability of real-time ultrasound scanning has been a significant factor in making prenatal sampling precise and safe and has led to major developments in first-trimester prenatal diagnosis including chorionic villus biopsy[5] and early amniocentesis.[6]

First-trimester amniocentesis is the latest major development in prenatal diagnosis. Relatively small volumes of amniotic fluid (2–11 mL) can be obtained between 10 and 13 weeks' gestation and viable fetal cells grown successfully in cultured medium. Moreover, it has been demonstrated that, for some disorders, abnormal metabolites accumulate in the fluid early in pregnancy and appear to allow fast and accurate diagnoses to be made.[7] A chorionic villus biopsy is also generally taken between 10 and 12 weeks' gestation and can be used with or without culture for direct enzyme analysis or for DNA extraction.

Sometimes maternal blood and urine contain substances that clearly have been derived from an affected fetus and have crossed the placenta into the maternal circulation.[8] Although this phenomenon has been exploited to good effect in the preliminary screen for neural tube defects, it has not been used reliably for the diagnosis of inherited metabolic disease. The ability to detect male fetuses by the detection of Y chromosome-specific DNA sequences in a sample of maternal blood[9] will have wide application in the investigation of pregnancies at risk for X-linked conditions because a completely non-invasive technique can be used to determine the sex of the fetus. It seems unlikely, however, that this approach will be used for the diagnosis of autosomally inherited diseases in the near future.

PROBLEMS AND RISKS WITH THE PROCEDURES

Amniocentesis

The aim of amniocentesis is to obtain a 10–20 mL sample of clear liquor. It has always been preferable to obtain the sample by transabdominal rather than a transplacental route because of a reduced risk of infection, and in recent years this has become easier to achieve with advances in ultrasound imaging. The risks associated with amniocentesis vary from centre to centre, but a recent large randomized study of second-trimester amniocentesis[10] found a spontaneous abortion rate of 1.7% after the procedure compared with a rate of 0.7% in a control population, thereby increasing the relative risk by 2.3-fold. Transplacental amniocentesis was associated with an increased fetal loss of 2.6-fold and any discoloration of the fluids, not necessarily due to blood, signals an approximately 10-fold increased risk of fetal loss. The greater incidence of fetal limb deformation found in an earlier study[11] was not confirmed, but the increased risk of neonatal respiratory problems, regardless of gestational age at birth, was similar.

The main problem associated with amniotic fluid

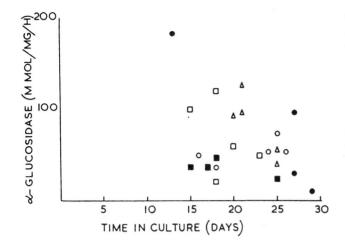

Fig. 14.1 Variations in the activity of α-glucosidase in primary amniotic-fluid cell cultures, expressed in terms of the amount of protein; results shown with the same symbol are from primary cultures grown from the same amniotic fluid (reproduced from Niermeijer et al.[13]).

sampling is the risk of contamination with maternal cells. This is one reason that amniotic fluid cells should not be used directly but should be cultured first because it is less likely that maternal cells will contaminate cells that have been harvested after several cycles of culture. The risks associated with early amniocentesis may be no different to those for second-trimester amniocentesis but further work is necessary to confirm this.

Chorionic Villus Biopsy

This procedure was first used for the diagnosis of an enzyme defect in 1982. It was at first done by passing a small endoscope through the cervix to enable direct visualization of the trophoblast before taking the biopsy. The techniques required a high degree of skill and complications were relatively high. Nowadays the biopsy is taken under ultrasound visualization either transcervically with the passage of a fine catheter into the trophoblastic tissue, or transabdominally with a fine needle attached to a syringe for aspirating trophoblastic tissue. The latter procedure is very similar to amniocentesis. The disadvantage of the transabdominal route is that a small tissue biopsy is obtained and multiple insertions may be necessary, particularly for enzyme assays, which frequently require as much as 30 mg of material.

The overall fetal loss following chorionic villus biopsy is about 3–5% compared to a rate of spontaneous loss of 2–3% at 9–12 weeks' gestation.[12] This is not significantly different from the risks of a second-trimester amniocentesis, although the transabdominal biopsy may be marginally safer than the transcervical. The availability of chorionic villus biopsy has been a major advance in the diagnosis of congenital abnormalities and genetic disease; how-

ever, its direct use in the assay of some enzyme activities has a number of limitations. These will be dealt with in a later section.

Fetal Blood and Liver Samples

Early methods of blood sampling were accompanied by high fetal loss, but since then considerable refinements have been made to the technique. The development of fibreoptic systems enables a small fetoscope to be introduced into the uterus transcervically under local anaesthetic and, more recently, percutaneous insertions have been made into the cord either by a transplacental or transamniotic route, a technique now known as cordocentesis. The most common puncture site into the cord is close to the placenta, and 2–5 mL of pure fetal blood can be obtained routinely. The risk of fetal loss is not excessive and is estimated to be 1–2% compared to a spontaneous loss of less than 1% at 18–20 weeks' gestation.

Fetal liver biopsies may be taken after 19 weeks' gestation by aspiration under fetoscopic or ultrasound guidance. Experience of the techniques is not widespread and, therefore, the precise risks of the procedure are difficult to assess. In skilled hands, there is no reason to believe that they should be any greater than those associated with cordocentesis.

PRENATAL DIAGNOSIS BY BIOCHEMICAL METHODS

Most prenatal diagnoses by biochemical methods use enzyme assays on cells derived from the amniotic fluid or chorionic villi. More rarely, erythrocytes or liver cells are used but techniques involving the latter two sources are being superseded in many cases by molecular genetic techniques. Very sensitive enzyme assay techniques are needed because the amount of biological material is small. This sensitivity is usually achieved by the use of fluorometric or radioisotopically labelled substrates and, of course, by careful optimization of the conditions of the enzyme assay.

Enzyme Assay Using Amniotic Fluid Cells

Enzyme analyses can be made directly on uncultured amniotic cells but for diagnostic purposes cultured cells should be used. This is because the amniotic cells that are collected by centrifugation may contain some contaminating maternal cells and those that are derived from the fetus are very heterogeneous in terms of their integrity and origin. These are all factors that will affect the concentration and activity of the enzymes being assayed.

A primary cell culture is obtained by incubating the amniotic fluid cells in medium containing essential nutrients and growth factors. The cells harvested from a confluent primary culture are also heterogeneous in their morphology and enzyme composition (Fig. 14.1), and so the harvested cells should be

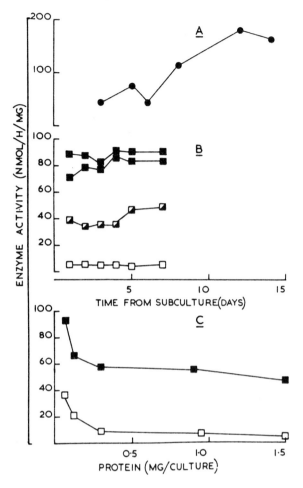

Fig. 14.2 Different patterns of change of enzyme activity with time in amniotic-fluid cell cultures after the first passage. Enzyme activity is expressed per mg of protein in all cases. (A) α-Glucosidase activity assayed from 3 to 15 days after subculture of the primary culture shown with the same symbol as in Fig. 14.1. (B) Galactose-1-phosphate uridyl transferase activity (gal-1-P converted/h) on days 1–7 after subculture of amniotic fluid cells: ■ normal homozygote cells; ◪ normal/galactosaemic heterozygote cells; □ galactosaemic homozygote cells. (C) Galactose-1-phosphate uridyl transferase activity (gal-1-P converted/h) after subculture with increasing cell growth measured as mg protein/culture; symbols as in (B) (reproduced from Fensom and Benson[14]).

subcultured one or more times in order to produce a homogeneous growth and a sufficient number of fibroblast-like cells (amniocytes) that can be used in the enzyme assay.

Even though subculturing produces a more homogeneous population of cells, the activities of different enzymes vary with the length of time of subculturing. Because of this, the optimum time for harvesting cells must be established to give consistent results for any single enzyme that is being studied (Fig. 14.2). However, despite every precaution being taken, the activity of a particular enzyme can be so variable that an erroneous result can still be reported if

enzyme activity is expressed relative to variables such as cell number or protein concentration. One way of avoiding this potential for diagnostic error is to express the activity of the diagnostic enzyme as a ratio with the activity of a control enzyme that (ideally) has the same subcellular location and is known to behave similarly in subculture. Control cell lines should always be assayed in parallel with the test, but cell lines do grow at different rates and sometimes it may be difficult to examine test and control cells under the same conditions.

The main drawback of using culture of amniotic fluid cells, particularly after a second-trimester amniocentesis, is the lapse of time before a result is available. If cell growth is very slow the time required to reach a diagnosis can delay the decision to terminate a pregnancy to unacceptable limits. Enzyme assay following first-trimester amniocentesis reduces this disadvantage considerably.

Enzyme Assay Using Chorionic Villi

Enzyme methods for amniocytes have been applied without modification to chorionic villus specimens either directly on the biopsy material or after cell culture. All the enzymes normally measured in amniocytes are expressed in chorionic villus, but the relative activities of different enzymes vary considerably between cells derived from the two sources.[15] Direct assay is especially useful because it reduces much of the delay that is associated with cell culture; however, if an enzyme has very low activity by direct assay, cultured cells have to be used. In addition, some enzymes not detected in amniocytes can be assayed in uncultured chorionic villus material and so first-trimester prenatal diagnosis can be offered for the disorders that arise from these enzyme defects. This approach has been used in prenatal diagnosis of non-ketotic hyperglycinaemia, in which the glycine cleavage enzyme is defective, and in enzyme defects that cause disorders of the urea cycle. Until recently, the only means of prenatal diagnosis for these disorders had been to use fetal liver.

One of the main problems associated with the direct use of chorionic villus material is contamination from maternal cells, which are mostly decidua. It is essential that the biopsy be carefully cleaned under a microscope by an experienced person to ensure that only chorionic villus is used. The dangers are exemplified by reference to direct karyotyping using chorionic villus where there is estimated to be a 1% risk of a false-positive prediction of a female fetus. With regard to particular inherited metabolic diseases, normal levels of α-iduronidase activity have been reported when a fetus was affected by Hurler's disease, and in another instance, the A isoenzyme of hexosaminidase was reported in chorionic villus material when a fetus was affected with Sandhoff disease. In both cases, the falsely normal results were presumed to have arisen because of the presence of maternal cells in the material that was assayed.

In assaying particular enzymes for diagnosing certain metabolic disorders, more specific problems can occur. In metachromatic leucodystrophy, for example, a diagnostic deficiency of arylsulphatase A can be masked by a high concentration in chorionic villus material of one of its isoenzymes, arylsulphatase C, and for reasons that are not apparent, unreliable results can be obtained when enzyme assays are made directly on chorionic villus material in the diagnosis of methylmalonic or propionic acidaemia.[16] Difficulties have also been encountered in diagnosing the lysosomal storage disorder, I-cell disease, on a chorionic villus biopsy. In this disorder, there is a defect in the post-translational attachment of a recognition marker to a broad spectrum of enzymes that targets them to the lysosomes. Patients with the defect have a reduced concentration of the enzymes in the lysosomes, but in the cell supernatant or body fluids enzyme concentrations are higher than normal. These altered enzyme concentrations are seen in the cellular fraction or the culture medium, respectively, when cultured amniocytes are used for prenatal diagnosis but attempts at using the same approach directly on chorionic villus material have been unsuccessful. However, a recent report has shown that the enzyme, N-acetylglucosamine-1-phosphotransferase, which is responsible for the attachment of the recognition marker, can be measured directly on a chorionic villus biopsy, and low activities of the enzyme may be indicative of the disease.[17]

Metabolite Assay in Amniotic Fluid Supernatant

From early in fetal life, small molecular-weight substances can equilibrate readily between mother, fetus and the amniotic sac, and from 12 weeks' gestation the fetus passes urine into the amniotic fluid in significant amounts. Thus, provided the biochemical effects of the gene defect are present in the fetus at the time of amniocentesis, prenatal diagnosis by metabolite assay in amniotic fluid supernatant should be possible. This approach has been used in the second-trimester diagnosis of some organic acidurias, disorders of galactose metabolism and congenital adrenal hyperplasia due to 21-hydroxylase deficiency, but in other disorders such as phenylketonuria the technique is not applicable. Although the principal advantage of the method is speed because a result can be obtained within a few hours, it has been the practice to confirm the result by enzyme analysis on amniocytes.

The key to reliability of the metabolite method lies in the assay techniques. It is essential that the analysis be highly sensitive and specific for any single disorder, and this condition is usually met by the use of gas chromatography/mass spectrometry with or without the use of isotope dilution.

It has become apparent that the technique can be used on amniotic fluid obtained in the first trimester. Surprisingly, for some disorders, the concentrations of metabolites appear to be as high, or even higher, in the first trimester than in the second.

PRENATAL DIAGNOSIS USING DNA ANALYSIS

DNA analysis in prenatal diagnosis has been invaluable for those disorders in which the molecular defect is not expressed in amniotic or chorionic villus cells. For some conditions it has superseded fetal blood sampling or fetal tissue biopsy as the means of prenatal diagnosis and so has reduced the risks of fetal loss whilst at the same time making an earlier diagnosis possible. More recently, the extreme versatility of the polymerase chain reaction (PCR) has expanded its applications[18] and fetal sexing by DNA analysis can now be done directly on preimplantation embryos[19] or on the maternal circulation, with no risk to the fetus.[9]

Chorionic villi are an excellent source of fetal genetic material. However, if a woman presents too late for chorionic villus sampling, DNA can also be obtained from cultured amniocytes, although the yield may be smaller and culturing the cells will obviously impose an additional delay of 2–3 weeks.

DNA analysis in prenatal diagnosis is undertaken in one of two ways. The first encompasses digestion of total genomic DNA, electrophoresis, transferring the DNA to a nylon or nitrocellulose membrane, and hybridizing the membrane with a labelled probe. A yield of about 1 μg DNA per mg wet weight of villus material is usually obtained. Five μg of undegraded genomic DNA is required for each digest and so, for an average-sized villus sample of about 35 mg, seven digests can be made. A minimum of 4 days is required before a result is available but 7–10 days is usually a more realistic time-scale.

The second approach involves DNA amplification of a fragment of a specific gene locus using the PCR. The technique uses a set of primer DNA sequences that flank a segment of the gene of interest, thermostable DNA polymerase enzyme, all four deoxynucleotides and a portion of the DNA under investigation. By subjecting the reaction mixture to several cycles of temperature alterations, which permit DNA denaturation, annealing and extension, the sequence of genomic DNA can be amplified several million-fold and the amplified product can be examined in a variety of different ways. One main advantage of DNA amplification in prenatal diagnosis is that a very small amount of target DNA is required and degraded DNA can also be used. A typical 100-μl reaction mix requires only 100 ng of genomic DNA, but even smaller amounts are used, particularly when analysing fetal DNA in the maternal circulation or in preimplantation embryos. Another advantage of the PCR technique in prenatal diagnosis lies in its speed. Most thermocyclers can go through 30 cycles of amplification within 4 h and, depending on the method of characterizing the amplified DNA, results can be available in as little as 24–48 h. Because of the extreme sensitivity of the technique, however, every precaution must be taken to prevent contamination of

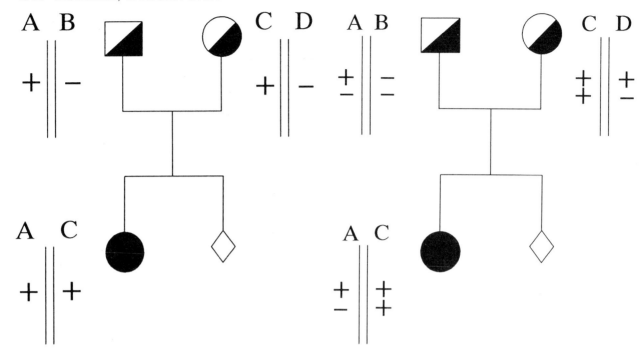

Fig. 14.3 Gene tracking illustrating a situation in which a family requesting prenatal diagnosis is fully informative with one probe/enzyme combination. Plus indicates the presence of the polymorphism; minus represents its absence. In this family, the mutation in both parents is found on the allele carrying the polymorphic marker. Circles are females, a square is male; the diamond is the fetus.

Fig. 14.4 A situation in which it is necessary to use two different restriction enzymes with one or two probes to make a family fully informative for prenatal diagnosis. With the first enzyme/probe combination it is not possible to differentiate between the maternal chromosomes; with the second, the father is uninformative. Combining the individual results into a haplotype makes the family fully informative and prenatal diagnosis could be offered. Symbols are the same as in Fig. 14.3.

the specimen or the reaction mix with exogenous DNA, which could result in a false-negative result.

HOW DNA ANALYSIS IS USED

Gene Tracking

Some genes that encode the enzymes involved in particular metabolic disorders have been cloned but for many disorders the specific mutations that can give rise to the disease state have not been identified. As a result, DNA analysis in prenatal diagnosis often involves linkage studies or gene tracking. Family studies must be done and in the case of autosomal recessive disorders, DNA from an affected child is always required. The aim in gene tracking is to differentiate between homologous chromosomes at the same gene locus in carrier parent(s) and then by reference to the affected child, to identify which chromosomes carry the mutant alleles. The genotype of the fetus is determined according to whether the DNA from the chorionic villus biopsy (or cultured cells) has one, neither or both alleles in common with the affected child.

In X-linked disorders, family studies are complicated by the fact that the carrier status of the mother of an affected son is not always certain because of germinal mosaicism and the high frequency of new mutations. Even if it is possible to establish which maternal X chromosome the affected son has inherited, in the absence of any previous family history non-affected male siblings should also be studied. If an affected and non-affected son have inherited the same allele from their mother, her risks of being a carrier of the mutation would be reduced to one of germinal mosaicism.

At the moment, it is usual to use restriction enzymes to highlight polymorphisms in gene tracking. Figure 14.3 shows a situation in which a family is fully informative using only one restriction enzyme. Provided there is not a recombination between the polymorphic marker and the site of the mutation, prenatal diagnosis can be offered on the basis of this result. Sometimes, however, only one or other parent is informative using a single enzyme but, when the individual results of two or more enzymes are combined into a haplotype, the family then becomes fully informative. The fetal DNA must then be digested using the various enzymes that make up the haplotype (Fig. 14.4). Inevitably, however, there are some families in which one or both parents are homozygous at all polymorphic sites and so it is not possible to establish which parental chromosomes carry the mutant gene. When this occurs, alternative techniques would have to be found. One of these includes the identification of repeat elements near to or within the gene sequence of interest. The Alu repeats[20] or CA_n dinucleotide repeats[21] are abundant repetitive DNA elements that are distributed essentially at random throughout the human genome. Both types exhibit length polymorphism according to the number of repeats within the sequence. These polymorphisms are analysed by amplifying a small segment of DNA that contains the repeat elements using the PCR, and then sizing the amplified fragments on polyacrylamide gels. They are usually multiallelic at any given locus and so are rich sources of highly informative genetic markers.

Sometimes when polymorphic markers are used for gene tracking, it becomes apparent that in one of the children a recombination has occurred between the site of the polymorphism and the site of the mutation. This usually happens when the marker is not within the gene sequence itself but is some distance away, in a region of DNA that is closely linked to the gene of interest. For the inherited metabolic disorders, the polymorphic markers are generally in the uncoded regions (introns) within the gene and because most of these genes do not span an enormous amount of DNA, intragenic recombinations are a rare occurrence. Nevertheless, on the few occasions that they are found, if it is not possible to establish which individual carries the recombination, other approaches would have to be used if a prenatal diagnosis was requested.

Identifying Specific Mutations

For clinical and diagnostic purposes of most inherited metabolic diseases, there is often no great advantage in knowing which mutations give rise to the clinical phenotype. However, for some families, identifying the specific mutation(s) that cause the disorder may be the only means by which a prenatal diagnosis can be offered. This would arise where an affected child is no longer alive, a parent is homozygous at all sites using polymorphic markers, or additionally, in X-linked disorders, the carrier status of the mother is uncertain.

Within any single genetic disorder the clinical phenotype can be caused by several different mutations at the same gene locus. This allelic heterogeneity is almost certainly the rule rather than the exception, although for a particular genetic disorder, one or two mutations may predominate in an individual population or race. In Tay–Sachs disease, for example, although 13 mutations have been described at the hexosaminidase-B gene locus on chromosome 15, in the Ashkenazi Jewish population a 4-bp insertion[22] and a splice mutation[23] are the most common, whereas in the French Canadian population, the most common mutation is a deletion in exon 1.[24]

For autosomal recessive disorders, affected individuals are often compound heterozygotes: that is, they carry a different mutation at the same gene locus on each homologous chromosome, one having been inherited from each parent. Because the identification of specific mutations usually involves DNA amplification it is very often necessary to amplify and characterize two separate parts of the gene. When this approach is used, prenatal diagnosis is undertaken by amplifying the relevant parts of the gene in the DNA extracted from the chorionic villus biopsy and determining whether it has one, both or neither of these mutations.

When the clinical phenotype of an X-linked disorder is caused by a deletion of part of the gene locus, the deletion can be identified in the DNA from the affected boy using either Southern blotting and hybridization with locus-specific probes[25] or DNA amplification.[26,27] However, it is often not possible to determine whether the mother of the affected boy also carries the deletion because the presence of a complete gene sequence on one of her X chromosomes will mask the absence of part of the gene on the other. In these situations, prenatal diagnosis must always incorporate fetal sexing and the genotype of a male fetus determined by establishing whether the DNA from the chorionic villus biopsy has the same pattern of deletions or not.

Fetal Sexing with PCR

The great potential of PCR is being realized in the application to fetal sexing either in maternal blood[9] or in preimplantation embryos.[19] The technique uses primer sequences that will amplify a Y chromosome-specific sequence if a male fetus/embryo is present. Extreme sensitivity in detection is achieved by using two rounds of amplification (generally with fewer cycles in the second round), the second round using a set of 'nested' primers, that is, sequences which are internal to those used in the first round. This results in a double amplification of the Y-specific sequence if it is present.

The ultrasensitivity of the approach, however, is also one of its major drawbacks because contamination of the PCR reaction by carry-over from previously amplified DNA, from cloned DNA which is in the laboratory or from fragments of genomic DNA from the skin surfaces of operators can lead to false-positive results. Because of this, a strict anticontamination protocol must be adhered to and this must include doing the procedures under class II containment.

The success of this technique has immediate implications for prenatal diagnosis of X-linked conditions. Fetal sexing using maternal blood eliminates the risks to the fetus associated with the more invasive techniques and, although male fetuses would have to be investigated further to determine the presence or absence of the abnormal gene, further genetic investigation of female fetuses can be deferred until after delivery. Sexing of preimplantation embryos enables the transfer only of female embryos to mothers who are known carriers of serious X-linked disorders. This avoids the decisions posed by prenatal diagnosis later in gestation of having to terminate a much wanted pregnancy. Although detection of a single-copy fetal DNA sequence has also been achieved,[28] further developments are necessary before the technique can be applied to the prenatal diagnosis of non-sex-linked conditions.

PRENATAL DIAGNOSIS OR GENE THERAPY?

It is worth considering, albeit briefly, whether by the end of the century prenatal diagnosis will become obsolete because it will be possible to 'treat' individuals born with a genetic disease by replacing the defective gene with a normal one whose expression in appropriate cells is well regulated. Currently, the technology is available for isolating genes and their important regulatory sequences and introducing them into foreign cells. Experiments using recombinant retroviruses have demonstrated that gene transfer can be achieved in intact mice and there are hints that a technique which involves site-directed recombination rather than one which involves random integration may be a more logical approach to the correction of genetic disease. However, despite continued encouraging successes there are still enormous technical difficulties to be overcome and so it seems likely that in the immediate future at least, prenatal diagnosis will still be an approach that is used in the prevention of inherited metabolic disorders. A more complete discussion of different approaches to gene therapy and the ethical issues that the technique raises is provided by Weatherall.[1]

REFERENCES

1. Weatherall D.J. (1991). *The New Genetics and Clinical Practice*, 3rd edn, Oxford University Press.
2. Royal College of Physicians (1989). Prenatal diagnosis and genetic disease. Community and service implications. *J. R. Coll. Physicians London*, **23**, 215.
3. Speiser, P.W. et al. (1990). First trimester prenatal treatment and molecular genetic diagnosis of congenital adrenal hyperplasia (21-hydroxylase deficiency). *J. Clin. Endocrinology Metab.* **70**, 838.
4. Pembrey M.E., Old J.M., Leonard J.V., Rodeck C.H., Warren R., Davies K.E. (1985). Prenatal diagnosis of ornithine carbamoyl transferase deficiency using a gene specific probe. *J. Med. Genetics*, **22**, 462.
5. Kazy Z., Rozovsky I.S., Balkarev F.A. (1982). Chorion biopsy in early pregnancy: a method for early prenatal diagnosis of inherited disorders. *Prenat. Diagn.*, **2**, 39.
6. Nevin J. et al. (1990). Early amniocentesis: experience of 222 consecutive patients, 1987–1988. *Prenat. Diagn.*, **10**, 79.
7. Chadefaux B. et al. (1989). Eleventh week amniocentesis for prenatal diagnosis of metabolic diseases. *Lancet*, **i**, 849.
8. Gompertz D. et al. (1974). Prenatal diagnosis of methylmalonic aciduria. *Pediatr.*, **54**, 511.
9. Lo Y-MD. et al. (1989). Prenatal sex determination by DNA amplification from maternal peripheral blood. *Lancet*, **ii**, 1363.
10. Tabor A. et al. (1986). Randomised controlled trial of genetic amniocentesis in 4606 low risk women. *Lancet*, **i**, 1287.
11. Medical Research Council Working Party on Amniocentesis: an assessment of the hazards of amniocentesis. (1979). *Br. J. Obstet. Gynaecol.*, **85** (suppl. 2), 1.
12. Anon (1989). Early prenatal diagnosis. *Br. Med. J.*, **299**, 1211.
13. Niermeijer M.J. et al. (1976). Prenatal detection of genetic disorders. *J. Med. Genet.*, **13**, 182.
14. Fensom A.H., Benson P.F. (1975). Assay of galactose-1-phosphate uridyl transferase in cultured amniotic cells for prenatal diagnosis of galactosaemia. *Clin. Chim. Acta*, **62**, 189.
15. Fowler B., Giles L., Cooper A., Sardharwalla I.B. (1989). Chorionic villus sampling: diagnostic uses and limitations of enzyme assays. *J. Inherited Metab. Dis.*, **12** (suppl. 1), 105.
16. Rolland M.O. et al. (1990). Early prenatal diagnosis of propionic acidaemia with simultaneous sampling of chorionic villus and amniotic fluid. *J. Inherited Metab. Dis.*, **13**, 345.
17. Ben-Yosef Y., Mitchel D.A., Nadler H.L. (1988). First trimester prenatal evaluation for I-cell disease by *N*-acetyl-glucosamine-1-phosphotransferase assay. *Clin. Genetics*, **33**, 38.
18. Eisenstein B.I. (1990). The polymerase chain reaction. A new method of using molecular genetics for medical diagnosis. *N. Engl. J. Med.*, **322**, 178.
19. Handyside A.H., Kontogianni E.H., Hardy K., Winston R.M.L. (1990). Pregnancies from biopsied human pre-implantation embryos sexed by Y-specific DNA amplification. *Nature*, **344**, 768.
20. Orita M., Sekiya T., Hayashi K. (1990). DNA sequence polymorphisms in Alu repeats. *Genomics*, **8**, 271.
21. Weber J.L., May P.E. (1989). Abundant class of human DNA polymorphisms which can be typed using the polymerase chain reaction. *Am. J. Hum. Genetics*, **44**, 388.
22. Myerowitz R., Costigan F.C. (1988). The major defect in Ashkenazi Jews with Tay–Sachs disease is an insertion in the gene for the alpha-chain of β-hexosaminidase. *J. Biol. Chem.*, **263**, 18587.
23. Arpaia E. et al. (1988). Identification of an altered splice site in Ashkenazi Tay–Sachs disease. *Nature*, **333**, 85.
24. Myerowitz R. (1987). A·deletion involving Alu sequences in the β-hexosaminidase alpha-chain gene of French-Canadians with Tay–Sachs disease. *J. Biol. Chem.*, **262**, 15396.
25. Rozen R. et al. (1985) Gene deletion and restriction fragment length polymorphisms at the human ornithine transcarbamylase locus. *Nature*, **313**, 815.
26. Grompe M., Caskey C., Fenwick R.G. (1991). Improved molecular diagnostics for ornithine transcarbamylase deficiency. *Am. J. Hum. Genetics*, **48**, 212.
27. Gibbs R.A. et al. (1990) Multiplex DNA deletion detection and exon sequencing of the hypoxanthine phosphoribosyltransferase gene in Lesch–Nyhan families. *Genomics*, 7, 235.
28. Lo Y-MD. et al. (1990). Detection of single-copy fetal DNA sequence from maternal blood. *Lancet*, **i**, 1463.

15. Neonatal Screening for Biochemical Disorders

J. B. Holton and L. Tyfield

Introduction
Reason for screening
  Benefit to the individual
  Benefit to the family
  Benefit to society
Practical aspects of screening
  Collecting the sample
  The test
  Action on screening results
  Cost
Notes on established and pilot neonatal
  screening programmes
  Phenylketonuria
  Congenital hypothyroidism
  Galactosaemia
  Maple-syrup urine disease
  Homocystinuria
  Cystic fibrosis
  Duchenne muscular dystrophy
  Congenital adrenal hyperplasia
  Biotinidase deficiency
  Glucose-6-phosphate dehydrogenase
    deficiency
  Hypercholesterolaemia type II

INTRODUCTION

Population screening programmes of various kinds have been in operation over many years. The earliest was introduced into the UK almost 50 years ago in order to reduce the morbidity and mortality that was associated with pulmonary tuberculosis, which was prevalent at the time. The disease was curable only when an early diagnosis was made and this was achieved by means of a mass chest X-ray programme. The programme was eventually abandoned because of its success in reducing the prevalence of the disease and also because modern methods of treatment made early diagnosis less essential.

This historical perspective illustrates well the main objectives of a population screening programme. Principally, the aim is to select from within a defined population (determined by geographical area, race and/or age) a relatively small number of individuals with a high risk of having (or developing) a particular disease from the majority whose risk is negligible.[1] These programmes should aim to screen for a specific disease because only then can the cost–benefit and ethical issues be properly assessed. Programmes in which broad biochemical profiles have been used to

screen with poorly defined diagnostic objectives have generally fallen into disrepute.

The disease itself must meet two requirements: first, that it be ubiquitously distributed throughout the population being tested and, therefore, everyone starts with an equal risk of having it; and secondly, that appropriate action can be taken once a diagnosis is confirmed. This is usually seen as the introduction of effective treatment. Also implicit in the concept of population screening is that a diagnosis is made presymptomatically.

Phenylketonuria screening, the first neonatal programme, fulfils completely this criterion, as does the programme for congenital hypothyroidism. However, justifications for many other screening programmes that have been introduced permanently or developmentally are more polemic. Whether the broader reasons for screening are accepted depends very much on whether one's approach is that of the 'snail' or the 'evangelist'.[2] Specific arguments are presented below in the sections on individual diseases.

Screening and treatment of affected individuals in the neonatal period has been part of the management of genetic diseases for about 30 years and no doubt will remain so for some time yet. However, in the long term it is likely that its role will be less prominent than it is now. For example, in some disorders for which early treatment was originally thought to be highly successful it is now known that the long-term outcome is not as good as was expected. Carrier detection and counselling for prenatal diagnoses, diagnosis in the preimplanted embryo and gene therapy[3] may be the options that are more acceptable in the future.

REASONS FOR SCREENING

It is generally understood in population screening that early, presymptomatic diagnosis is of direct benefit to the individual concerned. However, when justifying the introduction of screening programmes for various conditions, consideration must also be given to possible benefits to the rest of the family and to society in general.

Benefit to the Individual

For some disorders the full potential of treatment is realized only if it is started soon after birth and before any of the clinical consequences of the untreated disease are evident. Provided it is possible to identify affected neonates by biochemical methods, population screening in the neonatal period for these conditions is fully justified.

With other disorders, such as those that cause most of their damage in the developing fetus or those for which the treatment is only palliative, early diagnosis and treatment may not alter the clinical outcome. Nevertheless, biochemical screening for some of these disorders may be justified on the grounds

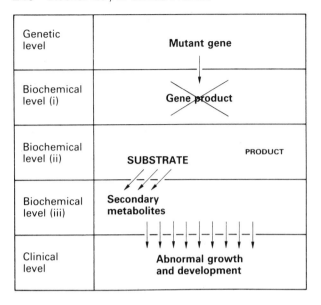

Genetic level	Mutant gene
Biochemical level (i)	Gene product
Biochemical level (ii)	SUBSTRATE PRODUCT
Biochemical level (iii)	Secondary metabolites
Clinical level	Abnormal growth and development

Fig. 15.1 The biochemical and clinical effects of some gene mutations and the various levels at which a diagnosis can be made. Diagnosis at the gene requires molecular genetic techniques. Laboratory screening usually is undertaken at one of the three biochemical levels: (i) by measuring enzyme activity or protein concentration in a readily accessible tissue; (ii) by assessing substrate accumulation or product depletion in body fluids; or (iii) by determining the presence of secondary metabolites that are not normally present in body fluids. Diagnosis at the clinical level is often least desirable because irreversible damage in physical or mental development may already have taken place.

that it eliminates the delays in making an accurate diagnosis when a sick infant presents repeatedly with non-specific symptoms or signs of developmental delay.

Some diseases present very acutely in the neonatal period and sometimes a diagnosis either comes too late to institute life-saving measures or is missed completely. Screening for these conditions may prevent morbidity and mortality but all aspects of the screening programme must be extremely efficient to produce a diagnosis in time to be effective.

Benefit to the Family

For X-linked and autosomal recessive disorders, parents usually become aware of the disease and their increased risk at the diagnosis of an affected child. The advantage to the family of early diagnosis through a neonatal screening programme is that appropriate genetic counselling can be given to the parents. With this, they learn of their risks of having other affected children and the reproductive options that might be available to them. In the absence of an early diagnosis, some families might already have other children, some of whom could also be affected. A less tangible but equally important benefit of early

diagnosis lies in reducing the anxiety and stress that a family experiences when there is a prolonged period of uncertainty about the diagnosis in their sick child.

Screening for autosomal dominant disorders such as familial hypercholesterolaemia could have ramifications for the rest of the family that might not be wholly beneficial. Early diagnosis through neonatal screening would result in early treatment in the index case, but this is also seen as a simple and effective means of tracing numerous cases in the extended family. Family members may become unwittingly involved and the knowledge of their increased risk of developing coronary heart disease might precipitate considerable family disharmony as well as appreciable mental and physical stress to the high-risk individuals.

Benefit to Society

There are inevitably financial advantages in diagnosing and treating from a very early age children who otherwise would suffer chronic or irreversible damage to their mental and physical development and thereby require prolonged hospitalization or long periods of institutional care. However, sometimes screening programmes are undertaken for research purposes, even when there might be no immediate benefit to the individual or to the family. For example, if it is necessary to investigate the early course of a disease in which diagnosis is usually delayed, and perhaps to carry out a trial of treatment, one way of achieving this is to recruit patients from a neonatal screening programme. Such an objective would be seen by most as perfectly ethical. However, it is incumbent upon the research workers to obtain the consent of parents, who are made fully aware of the true purpose of the screen.

Samples collected in a neonatal screening programme can also be part of an epidemiological study. This is currently being carried out in parts of the UK in order to assess the incidence and distribution of AIDS in the newborn population, so as to obtain some indication of the impact of this lethal disease on public health resources in the near future. Unlike the situation mentioned above, where family consent must be obtained, it is essential that this sort of study be performed totally anonymously.

PRACTICAL ASPECTS OF SCREENING

For many biochemical disorders, mutations at the level of the gene are manifest as gross disturbances of metabolism and development (Fig. 15.1). It is often least desirable to make a diagnosis at the clinical level, and so if a presymptomatic diagnosis is to be made, screening must be done at one of the biochemical levels or even at the level of the gene.

Collecting the Sample

Which sample to collect (cord blood, capillary blood or urine) and the optimum time to take it depend

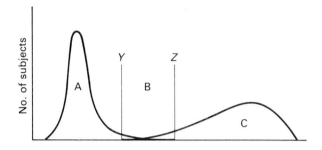

Fig. 15.2 The distribution of values of a screening test that is being used to differentiate populations with and without a disease. When two cut-off points are used values less than Y have a very high specificity for normality whereas values above Z have a very high specificity for the disease. Infants with results between Y and Z require repeat tests to differentiate them further (*see* Fig. 15.3).

very much on the condition being screened and the pattern of metabolic disturbance that accompanies it in the neonatal period. In those in which enzymes are normally expressed in red blood cells or in which biochemical expression of the disease is fully developed at birth, very early diagnosis using cord blood would be both possible and desirable, especially if early, acute clinical symptoms may be life threatening. With others, although the primary metabolic defect (for example, loss in enzyme activity) is present at birth, the enzyme may not normally be expressed in readily accessible cells. It may take several days or weeks for the secondary biochemical effects to accumulate in body fluids and a delay in screening would be necessary until an appropriate test could detect the disorder unequivocally in affected infants.

In the UK, where daily home visits from midwives are mandatory for the first week of an infant's life, capillary blood is collected by heel prick usually between 6 and 10 days of age. In other countries, such as in parts of the United States, difficulty in tracing an infant once it is discharged from hospital has made earlier screening more widespread. Ideally, one aims to screen, confirm a diagnosis and start therapy before an infant is 3 weeks old.

The Test

The particular test that is used in a population screening programme should meet a number of stringent criteria (Fig. 15.2). First, it should be highly sensitive so that it identifies all affected individuals. False negative results reduce the overall efficiency of a screening programme, but more importantly, they can have disastrous consequences for the undiagnosed patients and their families. Secondly, the test should be highly specific so that there are few false-positive results. The false-positive cases will be classified correctly upon further investigation, but a screening test with low specificity generates considerable extra work for the community health-care staff, and the laboratory, as well as causing appreciable parental anxiety.

Action on Screening Results

When screening programmes measure concentrations of metabolites in body fluids two cut-off levels are usually used (Fig. 15.2). A flow chart showing the subsequent course of action for results in each of the three zones is shown in Fig. 15.3.

Results below the lower cut-off (area A, Fig. 15.2) have a high specificity for the normal individual and no further action is taken except the reporting of a negative result. Results above the high cut-off (area C, Fig. 15.2) are highly indicative of the infant having the disorder and an immediate referral to a specialist for further investigation is essential. When results are between the two limits, in an 'intermediate' range (area B, Fig. 15.2), a second screening sample is required immediately from the infant. After the second screening test, some infants will be reclassified as normal because the finding will have fallen below the lower cut-off but in others the levels will still be raised and these infants should be referred without delay to a specialist for further clinical and biochemical investigation. Some infants will have results persistently in an 'intermediate' range, which will be caused by a variety of physiological, or genetic, factors. Decisions about management of these infants are often difficult and so regular clinical assessment and monitoring of the appropriate biochemical variables are imperative.

Cost

Before implementing a population screening programme for a specific disorder, consideration must be given to the financial implications for the health care services. The total cost of population screening, measured in terms of clinical and laboratory staff, laboratory equipment and reagents can be calculated easily and accurately, but the cost of making a single positive diagnosis is the important figure. This requires an exact knowledge of the incidence of the disorder in the population being tested and is of prime importance in determining whether a screening programme might be cost effective or not.

The economic advantages of early diagnosis, which can lead to successful treatment of patients and so prevent long-term institutional care, have already been mentioned, but the cost effectiveness of screening for disorders for which treatment is only palliative is more difficult to assess.

NOTES ON ESTABLISHED AND PILOT NEONATAL SCREENING PROGRAMMES

In developed countries, neonatal screening programmes for phenylketonuria and congenital hypothyroidism are well established and fulfil the main criteria for screening. Recommendations for screening other diseases have been made by some individuals,[4] but the case for these has not been universally accepted.

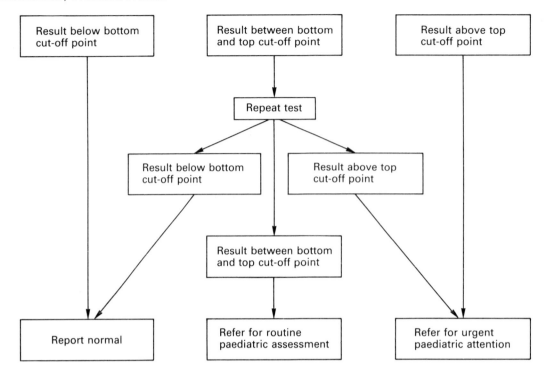

Fig. 15.3 Courses of action of screening test results when two cut-off points are used (*see* Fig. 15.2).

The following is a brief consideration of many of the disorders for which screening programmes have been set up on a permanent or research basis, with arguments for and against each of them.

Phenylketonuria

The basic defect in phenylketonuria (PKU) is a loss in the activity of the hepatic enzyme phenylalanine hydroxylase. In most countries that screen for PKU the incidence varies between 1 in 5–15 000, although in Japan, Sweden and Finland, where screening programmes also exist, the incidence is much lower (about 1 in 100 000 in Finland). Affected infants appear well and tend not to have any characteristic clinical symptoms in the first months of life, and so in the absence of screening in the neonatal period, a diagnosis is usually not made before the child is over 1 year old when irreversible damage to mental development will already have taken place. As a direct consequence of this delay in diagnosis, the majority of patients would tend to have an eventual intelligence quotient (IQ) of less than 50. Patients screened and treated from the neonatal period usually have an IQ within the normal range, but the overall clinical outcome is determined very much by the quality of dietary phenylalanine control up to teenage years,[5] which itself may be dependent upon the specific mutations that the affected individual carries at the gene locus.[6]

Screening is done by measuring the concentration of phenylalanine in blood collected on to filter paper or into capillary tubes. Most laboratories use methods that are specific for phenylalanine and the remainder use chromatographic techniques that may pick up other amino acid abnormalities as well. Current practice in the UK is to collect blood from neonates some time between 6 and 14 days of age, thereby ensuring the infant is well established on an adequate protein intake. However, it appears that this is not essential because in some parts of the United States, screening is done on the first or second day of life. In order to detect patients at these earlier ages, a lower cut-off value must be used.[7]

Patients with minor degrees of phenylalanine hydroxylase deficiency who have non-PKU hyperphenylalaninaemia are also detected in the screening programme and now it is becoming the practice to treat patients with all but the mildest forms of hyperphenylalaninaemia (less than about 400 μmol/L).

A very small number of patients with some degree of hyperphenylalaninaemia have a defect in the synthesis of tetrahydrobiopterin, the cofactor for phenylalanine hydroxylase.[8] Because the clinical management is quite different, it is essential to test all patients who are manifesting permanent hyperphenylalaninaemia for defects in cofactor synthesis.

Congenital Hypothyroidism

The prevalence of congenital hypothyroidism (CHT) is surprisingly uniform in most screened populations, being about 1 in 4000 live births. The aetiology of the disease is varied, and includes thyroid dysgenesis (aplasia, hypoplasia and ectopy), dyshormonegenesis, hypothalamic–pituitary deficiency and transient hypothyroidism, which is usually induced by iodine, maternal drug therapy for hyperthyroidism or the presence of maternal antibodies in the infant's blood. The proportions of these causes are about 75:10:5:10, respectively.

Newborn screening is well established in most economically affluent countries and is currently being introduced into some less well-developed countries in parts of Eastern Europe, South America, Asia and Africa. It is estimated that worldwide, 10 to 12 million babies are screened each year.[9] In the absence of a neonatal screening programme, CHT is a significant cause of mental retardation, but with early screening and treatment IQ is within the normal range in most cases, although neurological problems have been reported in some treated children. A small number of severely affected babies who show cretinous features at birth are believed to have sustained irreversible brain damage *in utero* and are subnormal on long-term follow-up.

In North America the most popular screening method is the measurement of serum thyroxine (T_4) in blood spots. The specificity of this as a primary screen is low, and 10–20% of the lowest results must be followed with a test for thyroid-stimulating hormone (TSH). Measuring capillary TSH concentration as a primary, or secondary, test is extremely sensitive and specific for primary hypothyroidism, but obviously misses cases of hypothyroidism due to TSH deficiency. In centres that use this approach, it is not regarded as a great disadvantage because the incidence of secondary hypothyroidism is very much lower. Blood spots are best obtained after the third day of life. In samples taken before this a higher false-positive rate is experienced because of the physiological surge in TSH production in the newborn.

The incidence of CHT in screened populations is usually about twice that reported before its introduction.[10] The discrepancy may be accounted for by patients who are clearly hypothyroid but in whom the diagnosis is long delayed or missed; patients who have biochemical hypothyroidism but show no clinical signs; patients with an adequately functioning ectopic thyroid that fails in later childhood; and those with a long-term transient abnormality. In order to avoid unnecessary lifelong treatment it is recommended that treatment be discontinued for a trial period between the first and second year of life.

Galactosaemia

Screening for galactosaemia is done in many countries, with widely varying incidences—from 1:26 000 in the Republic of Ireland to 1:667 000 in Japan. Cord blood or capillary blood collected on to filter paper can be used to assay galactose-1-phosphate uridyl transferase (Beutler method) or galactose-1-phosphate plus galactose by a microbiological technique (Paigen method). The latter is used more widely because it gives fewer false-positive results and will also detect the other disorders of galactose metabolism (galactokinase and uridine diphosphate-epimerase deficiencies).[11] Some galactosaemic patients may be detected by applying one of the above screening assays to samples that have shown a moderately raised phenylalanine on PKU screening. However, the sensitivity of the approach is not likely to be high and the result may be too late to prevent neonatal morbidity and mortality.

There is still some doubt over the validity of population screening for galactosaemia. The available evidence indicates that the long-term complications (mental retardation, speech disorder, growth retardation and ovarian dysfunction in females) are not alleviated by early diagnosis and treatment.[12] Neither is it certain that screening will significantly affect the neonatal mortality rate, which has been estimated as 20% of affected babies. A survey in the UK suggests, however, that clinical diagnosis is being made quite promptly now[13] and neonatal deaths are rare. In fact, they may occur as frequently in screened populations unless screening is undertaken very early and acted on very rapidly.

Maple-syrup Urine Disease

Maple-syrup urine disease (MSUD) has a wide range of clinical presentations. It can present acutely in the neonatal period or, in an intermittent form, throughout infancy and childhood. In an 'intermediate' variant and in a thiamine-responsive form, the disease course is typically more chronic with severe psychomotor delay. Most patients are at risk of a life-threatening episode brought about by a stress-induced, severe catabolic state.

Screening for MSUD is undertaken in some parts of the United States and Europe using a Guthrie-type bacterial inhibition assay for leucine.[14] The programmes will be too late to detect the neonatal, acutely presenting cases; however they should have a place in diagnosing other variant forms of the disorder. With early diagnosis, treatment and awareness, it may be possible to avoid the life-threatening events.

That MSUD screening is not done widely is largely due to the rarity of the condition. Although the incidence is as high as 1:760 in an inbred population of Mennonites, it is closer to 1:2 000 000 in most other populations studied in the United States and Europe.

Homocystinuria

Homocystinuria is a progressive disease causing a wide range of physical and mental handicap.[15] Treatment with a low methionine diet, or by administration of vitamin B_6 in the vitamin-responsive form, is most effective if begun early. Screening has been done using a bacterial inhibition assay for methionine; the amino acid chromatography method used to screen for PKU in some areas of the UK also identifies raised methionine concentrations. The evidence, however, is that the severe, non-vitamin responsive form may be detected but milder, vitamin B_6-responsive cases do not have a raised methionine in the neonatal period. Because of incomplete detection a specific screen for the condition is rarely undertaken.

Cystic Fibrosis

At present the treatment of cystic fibrosis is palliative and, although it has been possible to extend the life expectancy very considerably, there is no indication that screening and early treatment significantly affect clinical outcome.

Nevertheless, advocates of screening for cystic fibrosis point to a number of other advantages. First, an early, accurate diagnosis would reduce the numbers of irrelevant investigations and trial therapies that are undertaken in an ill child and would ensure that the correct treatment is given. Furthermore, it is well established that early-diagnosed patients require fewer hospital visits and stays during the first 2 years of life compared to an unscreened group. This should reduce the amount of physical and mental stress to the patient and to the family. Secondly, a screening programme can be cost effective. In Caucasians, this is the most common single-gene disorder, affecting one person in 2500. The cost of screening is less than the cost of increased medical care and laboratory testing, particularly of sweat electrolytes, that is required in affected, unscreened patients during the first 2 years of life. Finally, the identification of the molecular defects in cystic fibrosis has enabled effective prenatal diagnosis to be offered to most couples with an affected child. Early diagnosis would enable appropriate genetic counselling to be given to the parents so that they know not only their risks of having another affected child, but also the reproductive options that are available to them.

Screening is currently being done most commonly by blood-spot immunoreactive trypsin (IRT) assay. Patients who show a repeat blood test above the cut-off are investigated further, clinically and biochemically. Unfortunately the test has a high false-positive and false-negative rate. The latter, which may be around 14%,[16] seems to be partly the result of affected individuals having a raised IRT on the first screen but a normal result on the repeat specimen.[17]

An interesting alternative approach to screen for affected infants is to use a 2-tier system in which, first, all samples are screened by IRT and then the highest 1% of results is screened on the same blood collection for the two most common mutations by direct gene analysis.[18] It has the advantage of not requiring a second blood sample to complete the

screen and would be less costly than an approach that screens all samples using molecular genetic techniques. It remains to be seen what the sensitivity of the combined procedure will be.

Duchenne Muscular Dystrophy

This is the most common X-linked disorder, affecting about 1 in 3000 males. Clinical diagnosis of affected males is often not made for several years and at the moment no effective long-term treatment is available. Screening the neonatal male population can be undertaken by measuring creatine kinase (CK) on blood spots.[19] This detects males with a persistently raised CK that is confirmed of the MM isoenzyme. The unavoidable low false-positive rate is due to transient rises in CK in the neonatal period and to a permanent increase in the BB isoenzyme in some cases, the latter being of no known pathological significance.

Despite the ability to detect affected males in the neonatal period, population screening for this disorder is not widely practised. Opponents to screening question the charity of telling a family their infant son has an incurable disease. However, highly sensitive molecular genetic techniques now make it possible to detect the specific molecular lesion in most affected males, to identify carrier females in the family and to carry out definitive prenatal diagnosis.[20,21] As a result, the principal objective in early screening would be to investigate further the families of the affected boys, to offer appropriate genetic counselling, and to provide some reassurance to the parents and other female relatives of having unaffected male offspring in the future.

Congenital Adrenal Hyperplasia

Ninety per cent of cases of congenital adrenal hyperplasia are caused by 21-hydroxylase deficiency. It is possible to screen for this disorder using an immunoassay for 17-α-hydroxyprogesterone. The test will probably detect the early-presenting forms of the disorder and will help to prevent the morbidity and mortality that are associated with severe salt loss, incorrect gender assignment, and abnormal growth and development in the simple virilizing forms. There are two main problems with the assay: first, it will probably not identify the milder forms that present in later life, but that still may cause considerable morbidity; and secondly, there is a significant number of false-positive results in sick, particularly preterm, babies.

Paediatricians who oppose screening for this condition maintain that, with the exception of males with the simple virilizing form, early clinical diagnosis is both possible and desirable because a screening result may be available too late to save the life of infants with severe salt loss. World-wide experience shows a higher incidence with screening (1:14 000 as opposed to 1:32 000) and a more equal sex ratio in affected cases. This suggests that male cases are missed in non-screened populations.

Biotinidase Deficiency

A deficiency of biotinidase causes a depletion of biotin, the cofactor for a number of carboxylase enzymes. The clinical manifestations include skin rash, conjunctivitis, alopecia and progressive neurological damage. Administration of biotin causes an immediate improvement in the symptoms, apart from the neurological abnormalities, which remain permanent. It is probable that treatment begun in the neonatal period would prevent the neurological sequelae of the condition.

The blood-spot assay for biotinidase is stated to be simple, sensitive and specific. A survey of over 4 million screened births has given an incidence of 1 in 61 000.[23] However, further testing reveals that only slightly more than half of these have a complete enzyme deficiency and the remainder a partial deficiency (about 30% of normal), which is not associated with biotin depletion. The low cost of the test may make screening justifiable, even though the numbers who would require and benefit from treatment are very low.

Glucose-6-Phosphate Dehydrogenase Deficiency

This X-linked recessive trait occurs quite rarely in north European populations but has a high frequency in parts of the Mediterranean, the Middle East, the Indian subcontinent, South-East Asia and in the black population of the United States. Affected males generally enjoy normal health but they may suffer serious haemolytic episodes in the neonatal period and sporadically throughout life. The factor(s) that cause a crisis in the neonate are unknown, but severe jaundice with neurological problems and death may result. In the adult the drugs and dietary factors that cause a crisis are well established. Serious anaemia and death may occur.

Screening for the enzyme deficiency on blood spots is possible using a simple method with a sensitive, fluorometric end-point.[24] One problem is that an affected baby with a moderate haemolysis and reticulocytosis at the time of screening may give a false-negative result. It is unlikely that newborn screening will have any impact on the early presentation of the disease. However, it will enable appropriate counselling to be given to parents who could prevent the child's exposure to the environmental triggers.

It has been claimed that crises should always be handled medically whenever they occur and, therefore, screening programmes are not necessary.[3] This may be true in some countries with the resources for well-developed medical services, but in poorer countries in which the incidence of the condition is very high, screening might be justified. Unfortunately, such a screening programme and supportive counselling services may not receive the high financial priority that is required.

Hypercholesterolaemia Type II

Neonatal screening for hypercholesterolaemia type II (HCII), an autosomal dominant condition with a frequency of 1:500 in many populations, has been piloted using immunoassays for apolipoprotein B (apoB) on blood spots. It is not easy to define a satisfactory cut-off for the assay, as the distribution of values is skewed to the left, although the specificity for the disorder can be improved by taking birth weight, sex and age at screening into consideration. Measuring a broader apolipoprotein profile (A1 and (a) in addition to apo B) would most probably make the assay specificity more acceptable.[25]

The major question, however, is whether the neonatal period is the right time to screen for the condition. The extent of atherosclerosis in children with proven HCII who have died accidentally supports the proposition that treatment should start as early as possible. How practical and effective it is to begin treatment in infancy has to be discovered. Some see neonatal screening as a unique opportunity that can lead to the diagnosis in the extended family in an autosomal dominant condition. On the other hand, this is seen by others as a fundamental problem, pointing to both the ethical issues involved and the practical difficulty of providing adequate counselling to all those concerned.

REFERENCES

1. Sacket D.L. (1975), Laboratory screening: a critique. *Fed. Proc.*, **34**, 2157.
2. Sacket D.L., Holland W.W. (1975). Controversy in the detection of disease. *Lancet*, **ii**, 357.
3. Modell B. (1990). Biochemical neonatal screening: preconceptual and antenatal screening may be preferable in some cases. *Br. Med. J.*, **300**, 1667.
4. Bickel H. (1981). Neonatal mass screening for metabolic disorders. *Eur. J. Pediatr.*, **137**, 133.
5. Smith I., Beasley M.G., Eades A.E. (1991). Effect on intelligence of relaxing the low phenylalanine diet in phenylketonuria. *Arch. Dis. Child.*, **66**, 311.
6. Okano Y. et al. (1991). Molecular basis of phenotypic heterogeneity in phenylketonuria. *N. Engl. J. Med.*, **324**, 1232.
7. Doherty L.B., Rohr F.J., Levy H.L. (1991). Detection of phenylketonuria in the very early newborn blood specimen. *Pediatr.*, **87**, 240.
8. Scriver C.R., Kaufman S., Woo S.L.C. (1989). The hyperphenylalaninaemias. In *The Metabolic Basis of Inherited Disease* (Scriver C.R., Baudet A.L., Sly W.S., Valle D. eds.) New York: McGraw Hill, pp. 495–546.
9. Fisher D.A. (1991). Management of congenital hypothyroidism. *J. Clin. Endocrinology Metab.*, **72**, 523.
10. John R. (1987). Screening for congenital hypothyroidism. *Ann. Clin. Biochem.* **24**, 1.
11. Holton J.B. (1990). Galactose disorders: an overview. *J. Inherited Metab. Dis.*, **13**, 466.

12. Waggoner D.D., Buist N.R.M., Donnell G.N. (1990). Long-term prognosis in galactosaemia: results of a survey of 350 cases. *J. Inherited Metab. Dis.*, **13**, 802.

13. Green A., Holton J.B., Honeyman M., Leonard J.V. Galactosaemia: results of the British Paediatric Surveillance Unit Survey, 1988–90. *Arch. Dis. Child.*, **69**, 339.

14. Naylor E.W., Guthrie R. (1978). Newborn screening for maple syrup urine disease. *Pediatr.*, **61**, 262.

15. Mudd S.H. et al. (1985). The natural history of homocystinuria due to cystathionine 5-synthase deficiency. *Am. J. Hum. Genetics*, **35**, 1.

16. Chatfield S., et al. (1991). Neonatal screening for cystic fibrosis in Wales and the West Midlands: clinical assessment after five years of screening. *Arch. Dis. Child.*, **66**, 29.

17. Rack M.J., Mischler E.H., Farrell P.M., Wei L.J. (1990). Newborn screening for cystic fibrosis is complicated by an age-related decline in immunoreactive trypsinogen levels. *Pediatr.*, **85**, 1001.

18. Ranieri E. et al. (1991). Neonatal screening strategy for cystic fibrosis using immunoreactive trypsinogen and direct gene analysis. *Br. Med. J.*, **302**, 1237.

19. Plancher H. et al. (1987). Systematic neonatal screening for Duchenne muscular dystrophy: results of a ten year study in Lyon, France. In *Advances in Neonatal Screening* (Therrell B.L. ed.) Amsterdam: Excerpta Medica, pp. 371–374.

20. Darras B.T. et al. (1988). Intragenic deletions in 21 DMD/BMD families studied with the dystrophin cDNA: location of breakpoints on *Hind*III and *Bg*III exon-containing fragment maps, meiotic and mitotic origin of the mutations. *Am. J. Hum. Genetics*, **43**, 620.

21. Chamberlain J.S. et al. (1988). Deletion screening of the Duchenne muscular dystrophy locus via multiplex DNA amplification. *Nucl. Acids Res.*, **23**, 11141.

22. Pang S. et al. (1989). Worldwide newborn screening update for classical adrenal hyperplasia. In *Current Trends in Infant Screening* (Schmidt B.T., Diament A.J., Loghin-Gross, N.S. eds.) Amsterdam: Excerpta Medica, pp. 307–312.

23. Wolf B., Heard G.S. (1990). Biotinidase deficiency in newborns. *Pediatr.*, **85**, 512.

24. Shusheela K., Grimes A., Scopes J.W. (1985). Prevalence of glucose-6-phosphate dehydrogenase deficiency. *Arch. Dis. Child.*, **60**, 184.

25. Wang X.L., Wilcken D.E.L., Dudman N.P.B. (1990). Neonatal apo A-1, apo B and apo(a) levels in dried blood spots in an Australian population. *Pediatr. Res.*, **28**, 496.

16. Inherited and Acquired Mental Deficiency

J. Stern and A. H. Wilcox

Introduction
  Size of the problem
  Aetiology—pathogenetic factors
Detection of metabolic disorders causing mental handicap
  Laboratory investigations for mentally retarded patients
Encephalopathies of environmental origin
  Hypoxia–ischaemia, ventricular haemorrhage, hypoglycaemia
  Kernicterus and electrolyte disturbance
  Epilepsy
  Nutrition
  Vitamins, teratogens, drugs and poisons
Degenerative diseases of the nervous system with mental handicap—storage disorders
  Diagnosis
  Approaches to treatment
Aminoacidurias
  Phenylketonuria (PKU)
  Histidinaemia
  Non-ketotic hyperglycinaemia
  Homocystinuria
  Hyperammonaemias
  Other aminoacidurias
  Disorders of GABA metabolism
Organic acidurias
  Disorders of pyruvate and lactate metabolism
  Mitochondrial respiratory-chain disorders
  Other organic acidurias
Peroxisomal disorders affecting the brain
Other neurometabolic disorders
  Galactosaemia
  Endocrine disorders
  Hereditary disorders of trace-metal metabolism
  Disorders of purine and pyrimidine metabolism
Down's syndrome—chromosomal disorders
Ethical considerations—genetic counselling
  Problems and dilemmas
  Genetic counselling
  Other medico-ethical issues

INTRODUCTION

Many mentally retarded patients have evidence in their histories of biochemical disturbance before or after birth, but its contribution to the pathogenesis of the mental defect is often difficult to assess (Table 16.1). In some neurodegenerative disorders, deficiency of a single enzyme leads inexorably to progressive intellectual deterioration. Here the metabolic factor is decisive. In an infant with antenatal brain damage, consequent loss of intellectual potential is sometimes compounded by perinatal anoxia, hypoglycaemia and jaundice. Here biochemical abnormalities may play a significant part in determining intelligence. In phenylketonuria, there is a clear causal connection between the metabolic defect and the mental retardation. However, in several other aminoacidopathies, assumption of a causal relation between the biochemical abnormality and the mental defect has proved unfounded. Frequently, biochemical abnormality either has no bearing on an observed intellectual deficit or is only one of several pathogenic factors.

In all cases it is, therefore, important to ascertain

(1) if any observed biochemical abnormalities do in fact affect cognition,

(2) by what mechanism,

(3) to what extent.

Answers to these questions can only be given with confidence when reliable biochemical data are matched by sound clinical and psychological assessment.

Size of the Problem

Mental retardation (*synonyms*: mental deficiency, mental handicap, subnormality, learning disability) is a permanent impairment of the intellect sufficiently severe to prejudice normal existence in the community. Mental retardation is thus a social as well as a psychopathological concept; it is a function both of the inadequacy of the brain of an affected individual and of the complexity of the society in which he lives.[1,2]

The World Health Organization distinguishes:

- *Impairment*, loss or abnormality of psychological, physiological or anatomical structure or function
- *Disability*, any restriction on performance caused thereby
- *Handicap*, the disadvantage for a given individual resulting from an impairment or disability.

Contemporary methods of assessing intelligence are based on verbal and non-verbal responses to standardized tasks. The results are expressed as intelligence quotients (IQ), which essentially compare the performance of an individual to that of the population of which s/he is a member. Commonly used intelligence scales such as the Stanford–Binet or Wechsler are so constructed that the distribution of IQs roughly conforms to the pattern of distribution commonly found for continuously variable biological measures such as height. For a mean population IQ of 100 with a standard deviation (SD) of 15, half the population will have an IQ in the range 90–109 and a

TABLE 16.1

EXAMPLES OF METABOLIC DISORDERS DETECTED IN MENTALLY RETARDED PATIENTS

Aminoacidurias	Phenylketonuria, homocystinuria, non-ketotic hyperglycinaemia, urea-cycle disorders
Organic acidurias	Methylmalonic acidurias, propionic acidaemia, multiple carboxylase deficiencies, acyl-CoA dehydrogenase deficiencies
Other inborn errors	Galactosaemia, Lesch–Nyhan disease, Wilson's disease, Menkes' disease
Hormonal disorders	Congenital hypothyroidism
Lysosomal disorders	Mucopolysaccharidoses, mucolipidoses, sphingolipidoses, leucodystrophies
Mitochondrial disorders	Cytochrome oxidase deficiency
Peroxisomal disorders	X-linked adrenoleucodystrophy, acyl-CoA oxidase deficiency
Environmental causes	Hypoxia–ischaemia, bilirubin encephalopathy, electrolyte imbalance, drugs, mineral or organic poisons, burns, encephalopathy, malnutrition

quarter will have an IQ of less than 90. Individuals with an IQ of 70–50, more than 2 SD below the mean, are classed as mildly retarded, but most do not need medical care or special educational provisions. They make up approximately 1.8% of the population. If mental retardation is defined as an IQ more than 2 SD below the mean for the population, the proportion of individuals classified as retarded will be somewhat higher because the mean IQ for the population using standard tests is currently greater than 100. Approximately 0.4% of the population are severely retarded, with an IQ below 50. This group invariably requires special educational provision and often medical care in hospital or in the community.[1,2]

The above figures refer to prevalence—the number of patients living at any time as a fraction of the general population. The prevalence of many disorders associated with severe mental retardation is considerably lower than their incidence at birth because of the high mortality amongst the severely subnormal.

Aetiology—Pathogenetic Factors

Genetic or environmental factors will impair intelligence if they act at the molecular level to produce structural or metabolic defects in the brain that preclude normal function. Genetic disorders such as tuberous sclerosis or untreated homocystinuria, some chromosomal disorders such as the fragile X syn-

drome, and conditions of environmental aetiology such as rubella embryopathy or lead poisoning may present a whole range of mental defect from virtual normality to the grossest handicap. The view that intelligence and mild mental retardation are largely determined by polygenes is no longer favoured.[3]

At autopsy it is found that biochemical disturbances sufficiently severe to result in permanent intellectual deficits are almost invariably associated with identifiable structural changes in the nervous system. The distribution of these changes is often topographically uneven, and most observed neuropathological changes are non-specific; the repertoire of structural changes in the nervous system is rather limited in relation to the great variability of adverse metabolic factors to which it may be exposed. Genetic and environmental factors may act via *common pathological pathways*. For example, a high concentration of unconjugated bilirubin may occur in premature infants in whom glucuronyl transferase production is immature. High concentrations may also occur in blood-group incompatibilities when so much bilirubin is formed from haemoglobin that the conjugating enzyme is overwhelmed, or in the Crigler–Najjar syndrome in which there is hereditary deficiency of the enzyme. Brain damage with kernicterus may be seen in all three conditions.

Severe mental handicap may result from the effect of a single gene or a well-defined environmental hazard such as meningitis or head injury (Table 16.2). More often, the aetiology of the mental defect is multifactorial, as a result of the interaction of several genetic and environmental factors, and such interactions are, indeed, the basis of biological variation. Rather than argue the relative importance of heredity and environment we should aim to identify pathogenetic factors, be they genetic or environmental, and to counteract their harmful effects. In a significant proportion of cases the cause of the mental defect cannot be reliably classified (Table 16.2).

The vulnerability of the brain at critical periods of its development has been stressed by Dobbing.[5] On this view, it is the severity and duration of growth-restricting factors and, crucially, the developmental stage of the brain and blood–brain barrier that determine the extent of the ultimate intellectual deficit, rather than the precise nature of the insult. Early in pregnancy, metabolic upsets or teratogens may produce malformations, and in mid-trimester neuronal multiplication is at risk. The period from the last trimester of pregnancy to 18 months or 2 years after birth has been called the 'brain growth spurt'. This is the period of glial multiplication, dendritic arborization and synaptogenesis, and of a high rate of myelination when the brain is particularly vulnerable to malnutrition, to endogenous and environmental poison, and to hormonal imbalance. Damage sustained by the brain during early development may only become apparent months or years later, as de-

TABLE 16.2
AETIOLOGICAL FACTORS IN MENTAL RETARDATION

	Severe mental retardation (n = 73)	Mild mental retardation (n = 91)	Comments
Prenatal			
Genetic:			
Chromosomal	21	4	Higher incidence in patients with mild retardation found in a later Swedish study[4]
Mutations	4	1	Contribution of inborn errors to prevalence of mental retardation is comparatively modest
Environmental:			
Alcohol		7	Fetal alcohol syndrome
Infections	5		TORCH (toxoplasma, rubella, cytomegalovirus and herpes) most pertinent
Other	1		Fetal exposure to drugs and poisons (see Table 16.12)
Unknown:			
Specific syndromes		2	Syndromes of unknown aetiology, many described in Jones[6]
Non-specific, multiple anomalies	9	7	Cerebral developmental abnormalities often found at autopsy
Perinatal			
Placental insufficiency, asphyxia, anoxia	9	15	With better antenatal care the incidence of perinatal brain damage is decreasing
Infections of the nervous system	2	1	Meningitis, encephalitis
Postnatal	8	2	Includes head injuries, battered baby syndrome, infections of the central nervous system
Psychosis	1	2	
Unidentified			
Epilepsy, cerebral palsy	8	5	The size of this group depends on intensity of biomedical 'work-up' and criteria for classification; in some series it has been as high as 40–50% of total
Without epilepsy or cerebral palsy	5	45	

Adapted from Swedish studies (Hagberg and Hagberg).[1,2]

mands on the nervous system increase and ability for abstract reasoning is tested. On the other hand, the effects of an early metabolic insult may be mitigated if the infant is subsequently reared in a favourable environment.

Of great importance in shaping the disease pattern of hereditary disorders is the phenomenon of *genetic heterogeneity*. More than one mutation may occur at the locus involved in an inborn error, or a mutation may affect the pathway from gene to gene product. Often this results in variable residual enzyme activity. In general, the higher the residual activity the milder the disorder, and the lower the risk to the nervous system. Mutations may affect the stability of an enzyme, its kinetics, or its cofactor requirements.

Sometimes enzyme activity is reduced to a small fraction of normal but this residual activity may be sufficient for normal development. However, those affected may exhibit enhanced *vulnerability* to environmental hazards such as infections, in whose presence the underlying defect is unmasked. Inborn errors such as medium-chain acylCoA dehydrogenase defi-

ciency or intermittent maple-syrup urine disease may present in this way, and constitute a difficult problem to clinician and laboratory staff, as prompt and specific treatment may prevent death or mental deterioration. Between attacks the disorder is not always detectable by routine examination of the body fluids, but will always be demonstrable by assay of the affected enzyme.

Determinants and mechanisms of pathogenesis in inborn errors are listed in Tables 16.3 and 16.4. Because of the multiplicity of factors involved it is seldom possible to identify a unique pathogenetic process. Such processes may differ in patients with the same disorder, and also in the same patient at different stages of development.

Excess or deficiency of endogenous or exogenous metabolites can overwhelm the adaptive capacity of the brain and result in mental retardation. In the past, biochemical causes of mental retardation had to be inferred from scanty data recorded at irregular intervals. Today, we have comprehensive biochemical profiles and frequent, sometimes continuous, monitoring of the metabolism of the patient. The new imaging

TABLE 16.3

DETERMINANTS OF THE VULNERABILITY OF THE BRAIN IN HEREDITARY DISORDERS

Nature of the defect	Disorder generally more serious if enzyme deficiency is on a major metabolic pathway, or if synthesis or metabolism of neurotransmitters or neuropeptides is affected
Genetic heterogeneity	Disorder generally more serious if deficient enzyme occurs in more than one organ or if more than one isoenzyme is affected; more benign if enzyme deficiency is only partial
Other genes	Effects of an inborn error may be alleviated by operation of alternative pathways
Environmental factors	Hypoxia and hypoglycaemia, infections, malnutrition or inappropriate diet, drugs, lack of stimulus in environment enhance vulnerability
Developmental stage of brain	Brain particularly vulnerable in early pregnancy and during the 'brain growth spurt' from last trimester of pregnancy to end of second year of life

TABLE 16.4

SOME PATHOGENETIC MECHANISMS THAT MAY AFFECT THE BRAIN

Function affected	*Examples*
Interference with neurotransmission	Hypoxia–ischaemia, hyperammonaemia, non-ketotic hyperglycinaemia, malignant phenylketonuria
Interruption of energy supply in cells	Hypoxia–ischaemia, hypoglycaemia, pyruvate dehydrogenase deficiency, some organic acidaemias
Interruption of metabolic pathways	Untreated phenylketonuria, maple-syrup urine disease, urea-cycle disorders
Failure to synthesize or degrade large molecules	Glycogen synthetase deficiency, most lysosomal disorders, some peroxisomal disorders
Failure to maintain blood–brain barrier	Hypoxia–ischaemia, many organic acidaemias, Reye's encephalopathy
Failure of integrity and function of membranes or intracellular organelles	Some mitochondrial encephalopathies, Schindler disease, Zellweger syndrome
Uptake, transport or renal conservation of essential metabolites	Some variants of methylmalonic acidaemia, Menkes' disease, Wilson's disease
Failure to detoxicate products of metabolism, or poisons	Bilirubin encephalopathy, galactosaemia, urea-cycle disorders, fetal alcohol syndrome

Several mechanisms may operate simultaneously and synergistically

techniques permit us to follow the evolution and sometimes the regression of lesions in the brain. All those dealing with the mentally retarded, in whatever capacity, should be alert to the possibility and signs of a metabolic disturbance in these patients and know where to turn for help with appropriate investigations.

DETECTION OF METABOLIC DISORDERS CAUSING MENTAL HANDICAP

Most countries have introduced mass screening for phenylketonuria and hypothyroidism. Antenatal detection of Down's syndrome and neural-tube defects is also widely available; screening for galactosaemia and sickle-cell disease is more controversial.

Most cases of neurometabolic disorders are diagnosed in children who have signs of nervous system involvement or delayed physical or mental development. It is not possible to carry out diagnostic tests for every possible disease on every patient. Preliminary tests will often suggest the need for further investigations or referral to a specialized centre. Some retarded children have definite somatic abnormalities. These may be obvious from birth and sometimes form a recognizable pattern of clinical signs as, for example, in the Zellweger or the de Lange syndromes ('Amsterdam dwarfs').[6,7]

Ocular findings and deafness are common in severely retarded children. Nystagmus, strabismus, optic atrophy and microphthalmia do not suggest specific biochemical investigations but metabolic dis-

TABLE 16.5
OCULAR FINDINGS IN SOME METABOLIC DISORDERS ASSOCIATED WITH MENTAL RETARDATION [9,10]

Ocular finding	Disorder	Comment
Cataracts	Galactosaemia	Cataracts also seen in galactokinase deficiency
	Lowe's syndrome	Other signs include glaucoma and buphthalmos
	Cerebrotendinous xanthomatosis	See also Table 16.13
	Pseudohypoparathyroidism	Not always associated with mental retardation
	Dystrophia myotonica	Variable phenotype; gene on chromosome 19; dominant
Corneal opacities	Many mucopolysacchari- doses and mucolipidoses	See Table 16.13
	Fabry's disease	Most patients not mentally retarded
	Wilson's disease	Kayser–Fleischer rings rarely seen before age 7 years
Retinal degeneration	Hyperornithinaemia	Ornithine transaminase deficiency; gyrate atrophy of choroid and retina
	Abetalipoproteinaemia	Preventable by vitamin E therapy
	Laurence–Moon–Biedl syndrome	Associated with abnormalities of sex hormones
	Peroxisomal disorders	Widespread ocular changes in Zellweger syndrome and related disorders; prominent in Refsum's disease
	Respiratory-chain disorders	Kearns–Sayre syndrome and related disorders
	Sjögren–Larsson syndrome	Fatty-alcohol oxidoreductase deficiency; ichthyosis, spasticity
	Some lipidoses	See Table 16.13
Cherry-red spot on macula	Some lipidoses and mucolipidoses	Useful particularly in GM_2 and GM_1 gangliosidoses and sialidoses
Dislocation of lens	Homocystinuria	See p. 274
	Sulphite oxidase deficiency	More severe course than homocystinuria, also occurs in molybdenum cofactor deficiency
Conjunctiva	Ataxia telangiectasia	Teleangiectasis of conjunctiva, immune deficiencies

TABLE 16.6
DEAFNESS IN SOME METABOLIC ENCEPHALOPATHIES [9,10]

Disorder	Comments
Mucopolysaccharidoses I, II and III	Neurosensory and conduction mechanisms may be involved
Mucolipidosis I (sialidosis and mucolipidosis II	Deafness is a comparatively frequent finding in these disorders
Mannosidosis	Deafness is a feature of both the α and β variants
Peroxisomal disorders	Prominent in Refsum's disease, also present in Zellweger syndrome and often in X-linked adrenoleucodystrophy
Respiratory-chain disorders	Sensorineural hearing loss found in some mitochondrial encephalomyopathies
Aspartoacylase deficiency	Hearing loss reported in some patients
Biotinidase deficiency	Hearing loss may not be preventable by vitamin therapy

orders may be associated with the signs listed in Table 16.5. A significant role for biochemical factors in the aetiology of most cases of deafness has not been established. Exceptions are encephalopathies such as Hunter's syndrome, and the Pendred syndrome in which deafness and thyroid dyshormonogenesis are often associated with mental retardation (Table 16.6). Disorders in which mental retardation is associated with abnormalities of skin or hair, or peculiar odours, are shown in Tables 16.7 and 16.8. Examples of neurological signs characteristically seen in neuropsychiatric disorders are shown in Table 16.9. Abnormal movements, dyskinesia and dystonia are frequently associated with neurometabolic disorders.

TABLE 16.7
ABNORMALITIES OF SKIN AND HAIR IN MENTALLY RETARDED PATIENTS[9,10]

Disorder	Abnormality	Comments
Menkes' (kinky hair) disease	Pili torti and trichorrhexis nodosa	Low serum copper and caeruloplasmin; death in early infancy; a few patients less severely affected but mentally retarded
Argininosuccinic aciduria	Brittle hair	Wide spectrum of severity; urinary amino-acid chromatogram diagnostic
Homocystinuria	Hair sparse and brittle, malar flush	Marfan-like appearance and ocular signs
Hartnup disease	Pellagra-like rash	Many patients not retarded; urinary amino-acid chromatogram shows transport defect of mono amino-acids; psychiatric symptoms intermittent
Multiple carboxylase deficiency	Extensive skin rash, alopecia	May be due to biotinidase deficiency or holocarboxylase synthetase deficiency; whole range of clinical manifestations; biotin supplements mandatory
Phenylketonuria	Dry skin, sometimes with eczema, dilution of hair colour	Symptoms improve on a low phenylalanine diet
Tyrosinaemia type II	Hyperkeratotic plaques on palms, soles and elbows	Mental retardation seen in Richner–Hanhart syndrome (cytoplasmic tyrosine transaminase deficiency)
Fabry's disease	Angiokeratoma	See also ocular signs, Table 16.5
Farber's disease	Subcutaneus nodules over joints	Lipogranulomatosis, ceramide lipidosis; variable course
Cerebrotendinous xanthomatosis	Xanthoma of Achilles tendon	Cholestanol storage in nervous system, plasma cholestanol concentration elevated, plasma cholesterol low
Ataxia telangiectasia	Telangiectasia	Telangiectasis of conjunctiva

TABLE 16.8
METABOLIC DISORDERS ASSOCIATED WITH PECULIAR ODOURS[9,10]

Disorder	Smell	Comments
Phenylketonuria	Musty (phenylacetic acid)	Noticeable only in some older, untreated patients
Maple-syrup urine disease	Burnt sugar (branched-chain ketoacid derivatives)	Many variants; in classical form a neonatal emergency
Isovaleric aciduria	Sweaty feet (isovaleric acid)	Smell diagnostically helpful in sick neonate
3-Methylcrotonyl glycinuria	Cat's urine (3-hydroxyisovaleric acid)	Clinical presentation variable
Multiple acyl-CoA dehydrogenase deficiency	Sweaty feet (organic acids)	Severe and mild variants
Oasthouse disease	Musty (2-hydroxybutyric acid)	Very rare; methionine malabsorption defect
Tyrosinaemia type I	Cabbage (methionine)	Only noticeable in a few severely affected cases with high blood methionine
Trimethylaminuria	Fishy (trimethylamine)	Not associated with mental retardation

TABLE 16.9
SOME NEUROLOGICAL SIGNS IN THE MENTALLY RETARDED[9,10]

Clinical sign	Comment
Hypotonia without significant weakness	
Non-specific mental retardation	Very common in unclassified mental retardation; often variable and tends to get less severe with age
Down's syndrome	Treatment with 5-hydroxytryptophan of no benefit; some trisomies show increased tone
Amino acidurias	Hypotonia is marked in hyperlysinaemia and non-ketotic hyperglycinaemia
Organic acidurias	Hypotonia is seen in a number of organic acidurias, see Table 16.18
Prader–Willi syndrome	Adiposity, hypogenitalism, endocrine abnormalities; deletions on chromosome 15
Zellweger syndrome	See text
Other metabolic disorders	Hypotonia is found in hypercalcaemia of infancy, and untreated hypothyroidism
Muscle weakness with incidental hypotonia	
Congenital myopathies	Mitochondrial encephalomyopathies; Pompe's disease
Congenital myotonic dystrophy	Mental retardation common but non-progressive; serum creatine kinase and cerebrospinal-fluid protein normal; electromyogram shows 'dive bomber' effect
Congenital muscular dystrophy	Often associated with mental retardation; serum creatine kinase raised in early stages
Duchenne muscular dystrophy	Non-progressive mental retardation found in some patients, notably in those with large chromosomal deletions; plasma creatine kinase very high in early stages of the disease
Peripheral neuropathies	Lower motor neurons affected in most lysosomal and peroxisomal disorders, abetalipoproteinaemia, familial dysautonomia, and the infectious polyneuropathies; protein concentrations in cerebrospinal fluid diagnostically useful
Ataxia	
Environmental aetiology	Subacute sclerosing panencephalitis, encephalomyelitis; anticonvulsants, phenothiazines, lead intoxication
Aminoacidopathies	Late-onset urea-cycle disorders, hyperornithinaemia with gyrate atrophy, Hartnup disease
Organic acidaemias	Intermittent maple-syrup urine disease (branched-chain ketoaciduria) glutaric acidaemia I, methylglutaconic aciduria, pyruvate dehydrogenase deficiency, mitochondrial encephalomyopathies
Other metabolic disorders	Ataxia telangiectasia, Lesch–Nyhan disease, Wilson's disease, abetalipoproteinaemia, cerebrotendinous xanthomatosis, Refsum's disease
Neurodegenerative disorders	Juvenile variants of some lipidoses, mucolipidoses and leucodystrophies
Dyskinetic–dystonic syndromes	Abnormal movements such as chorea and athetosis and defective control of tone, signs of extrapyramidal dysfunction
Aminoacidopathies	Tetrahydrobiopterin-deficient phenylketonuria; rare complication in Hartnup disease and homocystinuria
Organic acidurias	Glutaric aciduria I, branched-chain organic acidurias, propionic acidaemia, pyruvate dehydrogenase deficiency (rare complication)
Lysosomal disorders	Krabbe's disease, metachromatic leucodystrophy, Gaucher's disease (acute neuropathic variant); late, rare complication in the gangliosidoses
Miscellaneous metabolic disorders	Lesch–Nyhan disease, hypoparathyroidism and pseudohypoparathyroidism (rare complication), Wilson's disease, xeroderma pigmentosum (some cases), Huntington's chorea, Crigler–Najjar syndrome
Psychiatric presentation	Wilson's disease, late-onset metachromatic leucodystrophy, homocystinuria, Hartnup disease

Of special interest is the infant or child with hypotonia. Hypotonia and weakness may result from a disorder of the motor unit but may also be secondary to upper motor-neuron lesions.

Growth disorders are common in the mentally retarded. Primary growth deficiency may be caused by teratogens, by intrauterine infections, chromosomal aneuploidy, and by mutant genes that may affect both brain and skeleton as in the mucopolysaccharidoses. Secondary growth deficiency is also common in mentally retarded children but in contrast to primary growth deficiency can be reversed by appropriate management. Examples are malnutrition and psychosocial deprivation. Renal, cardiac and respiratory disease, and especially chronic infection, are common in the mentally handicapped and also retard growth.

Mild, stereotyped, self-injurious behaviour occurs in over 10% of mentally retarded patients, and results in irreversible brain injury in about 0.1 per thousand. Biochemical factors may be involved; the γ-aminobutyric acid (GABA) analogue baclofen can reduce this behaviour temporarily. Self-mutilation is a diagnostic sign in Lesch–Nyhan disease.

Behavioural problems are common in mentally retarded patients. Severe behavioural problems have been noted in two out of three patients with γ-glutamyl transferase deficiency, and overproduction of phenylethylamine has been reported in aggressive psychopaths. Autistic features are sometimes found in neurometabolic disorders, for example in untreated phenylketonuria, homocystinuria and some lipidoses. In general, biochemical approaches have not been fruitful in childhood autism.[8]

Chromosomal disorders, antenatal infections and drugs or poisons ingested in early pregnancy are well-known causes of congenital malformation. Most inborn errors, in contrast, exert their effects postnatally. Exceptions are some peroxisomal disorders, notably the Zellweger syndrome, and some organic acidurias in which the energy supply for cell division and growth of the embryo may be restricted. Examples are multiple acyl-CoA dehydrogenase deficiency and 3-hydroxyisobutyryl-CoA deacylase deficiency.

Maternal phenylketonuria is a neurometabolic disorder that carries a high risk of mental retardation in the mother. The very small and decreasing number of undiagnosed women in the community who are retarded but able to bear children does not justify mass screening of pregnant women. Tests for metabolic disorders should be considered in a woman of child-bearing age who is mentally retarded or has other neuropsychiatric symptoms, has a family history of metabolic disease, mental retardation or microcephaly, or has one or more children with microcephaly, growth retardation or congenital malformations. Hereditary metabolic disorders in the mother are rare as a cause of mental retardation in the offspring compared with the fragile X syndrome or environmental factors acting on the fetus via the mother.

Hereditary disease severe enough to produce a life-threatening crisis usually manifests itself in the first few days of life but may present at any age. Examples are organic acidaemias, urea-cycle disorders (pp. 275 and 299) and galactosaemia (p. 285). Symptoms are often accompanied by infection, and may include acidosis, dystonia, vomiting, lethargy, fits and coma. Most of these signs are non-specific, and more often result from severe infection or cerebral pathology. Timely and vigorous treatment is essential to prevent death or handicap. When a patient dies undiagnosed, body fluids and tissue should be preserved for metabolic studies, and the brain examined by a neuropathologist so that the parents can be offered genetic counselling. For many neurometabolic disorders antenatal detection is now possible, and heterozygotes may be identified. For discussion of these topics, see below.

Laboratory Investigations for Mentally Retarded Patients

Most mentally retarded patients now live in the community in the care of parents or social services. The pathology services can contribute to their care by regular monitoring of patients on long-term medication with anticonvulsants or psychoactive drugs, to provide early warning of hypocalcaemia or liver damage. Haematological and microbiological screens may also be required. Thyroid function is abnormal in a considerable proportion of mentally retarded adults, particularly in those with Down's syndrome. Monitoring thyroid status and renal function is essential in patients on lithium therapy. Abnormal levels of sex hormones are seen in conditions associated with hypogonadism such as Klinefelter's syndrome or the Prader–Willi syndrome.

Problems in the diagnosis of neurometabolic disorders may arise because of shortcomings of methodology or lack of experience in the interpretation of the biochemical findings in these conditions. Chromatography of amino acids, carbohydrates, phenolic acids, purines and pyrimidines on thin layers of cellulose or silica gel is within the scope of some laboratories. Blood and urine should be examined at the same time, as this will indicate if excess of a urinary metabolite is an overflow or nephrogenic phenomenon. Chromatography is often supplemented by urine spot tests. Guthrie bacterial inhibition assays are still widely used in mass screening for amino acid disorders and in monitoring the dietary treatment of phenylketonuria. Other techniques are offered by a small number of specialized laboratories. For quantitative amino acid analysis, ion-exchange chromatography, for long the reference method, is being displaced by high-performance liquid chromatography, offering increased sensitivity and specificity based on new derivatives and detectors. Gas chromatography is the method of choice for the investigation of organic acidurias. Fast-atom bombardment mass spectrometry and, more recently, tandem mass spectrometry permit the assay of metabolites present in concentration below 1 nmol/L.

For definitive diagnosis of a neurometabolic disorder, assay of the affected enzyme will usually be required. Often, it is also necessary to ascertain its organ specificity, cofactor requirements, kinetics and stability. The enzyme defect may only be unmasked after separation by electrophoresis, heat inactivation or pH inactivation of interfering isoenzymes. Full characterization of the enzyme is essential if antenatal diagnosis is to be attempted in a subsequent pregnancy. Immunoassay techniques, both isotopic and non-isotopic, have helped to clarify the nature of enzyme deficiencies in neurometabolic disorders, while in the past decade the techniques of molecular biology have made possible, in favourable circumstances, the identification of both homozygotes and heterozygotes, often with a very high level of confidence. Other tissues/samples sometimes required for diagnosis are cerebrospinal fluid, liver, muscle, intestine and peripheral nerve. Brain biopsy is rarely justified except in some leucodystrophies and cerebral degenerative disorders.

The causal relation between the disturbance of amino acid metabolism and the mental defect in phenylketonuria, homocystinuria and citrullinaemia is widely known. It is tempting to try to attribute aetiological significance to any abnormal amino acid pattern found in body fluids of a mentally retarded patient or infant with neurological symptoms. Amino acid abnormalities are, in fact, produced by a wide variety of hereditary and environmental factors, many of which have no neuropsychiatric significance. Artefacts may be produced by drugs. Urinary excretion of aromatic amino-acid derivatives is affected by the intestinal flora and is abnormal in protein malnutrition. The excretion of phenolic acids is markedly affected by diet. Urinary excretion of amino acids is enhanced in the first few weeks of life, particularly in infants with low birth weight. These infants may also show raised blood concentrations of tyrosine and methionine, particularly when their protein intake is high.

Disorders may be missed in preliminary tests when the concentration of abnormal metabolites is too low to be detected by routine screening tests, when the abnormality is not expressed in the body fluids normally examined, or when the metabolic pattern characteristic of the disorder only develops with time. Homocystinuria illustrates these difficulties. Screening aims to detect an elevated blood methionine or urinary homocystine by the nitroprusside test. Both methods miss a high proportion of cases. In most affected individuals, methionine is not sufficiently elevated to be detected by screening tests, while the concentration of homocystine in urine is often below the limit of detection by the nitroprusside test. Furthermore, sulphur-containing amino acids are unstable in alkaline urine, and their excretory pattern may be distorted by bacterial action. Homocystine in plasma may be lost during storage and processing. In the mucopolysaccharidoses, bacterial degradation may invalidate urinary screening tests. Glycosaminoglycan (mucopolysaccharide) excretion is strongly age dependent, and as the excretion products are partially degraded they may differ in their physicochemical properties from commercially available standards. Urine organic-acid profiles are particularly liable to artefacts, such as benzoic acidaemia caused by bacterial action. Sophisticated techniques, including computerized mass spectrometry, are necessary to interpret urine organic-acid excretion patterns.

Biochemical abnormalities detected in mentally retarded patients, particularly those in unsatisfactory living conditions, are more often caused by malnutrition, chronic infection or iatrogenic factors, than by neurometabolic disorders. Inappropriate responses to stress and poor homeostasis are frequent findings.

These abnormalities are often the consequences of the way mentally retarded patients live, and are found less frequently as the care of retarded patients improves. As in other branches of medicine, laboratory investigations should start from the clinical signs and history of the patient and proceed via initial tests to specialized studies.[9,10] Local resources will determine where the line between initial and specialized tests is drawn. In the United Kingdom, lists are published and regularly updated of centres offering specialized assays. A scheme for the investigation of mentally retarded patients is shown in Fig. 16.1; similar schemes will be found in a number of recent publications.[9–14]

ENCEPHALOPATHIES OF ENVIRONMENTAL ORIGIN

Hypoxia–ischaemia, Ventricular Haemorrhage, Hypoglycaemia

Hypoxic–ischaemic brain injury is an important cause of mental handicap originating in the perinatal period. The brain can be deprived of oxygen by a diminished oxygen concentration in the blood (*hypoxaemia*) or by reduced tissue perfusion (*ischaemia*). Both may occur as a result of *asphyxia*, impairment of the respiratory exchange of oxygen and carbon dioxide.[15,16] Hypoxaemia is associated with accelerated uptake of glucose by the brain, increased glycolysis and lactic acidosis, diminished production of high-energy phosphates, changes in membrane physiology and breakdown of the blood–brain barrier, brain oedema and ultimately widespread destruction of brain tissue. The excitatory neurotransmitter glutamate and reactive free radicals generated in the hypoxic–ischaemic process enhance cellular damage.[17,18] Neurotransmitter synthesis, notably that of acetylcholine, is so sensitive to hypoxia that brain function may be severely affected before major changes in energy metabolism have occurred. The biochemical effects of ischaemia on the nervous system are similar to those of anoxia. Commonly both occur together, before and during birth.

The brain has an absolute requirement for glucose, and *hypoglycaemia*[19] has long been recognized as a cause of mental retardation (Table 16.10). There is a margin of safety in the supply of glucose to the brain at normal blood concentrations but if its minimum requirements cannot be met, hypoglycaemic coma will ensue. During fasting, glucose is mobilized from liver glycogen, and glycerol and fatty acids from fat. Excess fatty acids are oxidized to ketone bodies, which, if availability of carbohydrate is reduced, constitute a major source of energy for the brain, particularly in infants. Glycerol can be transformed to glucose via the gluconeogenic pathway, as can alanine and other glucogenic amino acids of muscle. Deficiency of any enzyme of gluconeogenesis or fatty acid metabolism will thus predispose to hypoglycae-

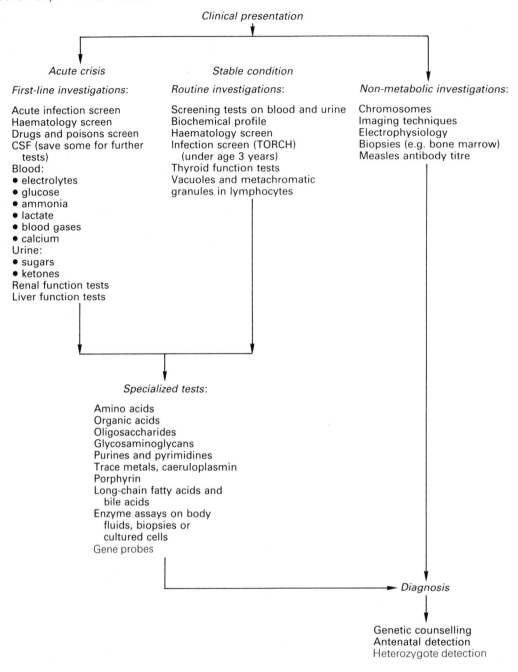

Fig. 16.1 Scheme for the investigation of mentally retarded patients.

mia. While an uncontrolled increase in the concentration of ketone bodies, lactic acid and many organic acids can be life threatening, the risk of brain damage is greater in hypoglycaemia without ketosis (as for example in hyperinsulinism due to nesidioblastosis) than in ketotic hypoglycaemia.

Neonatal hypoglycaemia (<2.0 mmol/L may be asymptomatic but may nevertheless prejudice intellectual development and must be promptly treated. Before feeding is established, the infant depends on endogenous glycogen and fat. Infants with low birth weight, particularly those who are small for gesta-

tional age, may have low glycogen and fat reserves. Also, production of ketone bodies is reduced because of the slow maturation of the enzyme systems involved. The demand for glucose is thereby increased at a time when the transport system carrying glucose into the brain is not fully developed.

In the newborn, particularly in the preterm infant, *ventricular haemorrhage* may result from trauma or circulatory disturbance, or as a consequence of perinatal or postnatal hypoxia, particularly in the respiratory distress syndrome. The association between low birth weight and mental handicap has long been

TABLE 16.10

Environmental
Asphyxia, anoxia, hypothermia, hyaline membrane disease
Shock, haemorrhage, intracranial injury
Septicaemia, meningitis, Reye's encephalopathy
Intrauterine malnutrition
Liver failure
Alcohol, salicylate, paracetamol ingestion

Endocrine
Hyperinsulinism (maternal diabetes, nesidioblastosis)
Deficiency of insulin antagonists (thyroid, adrenal,
    pituitary)
Beckwith–Wiedermann syndrome

Hereditary
Defects in gluconeogenesis
Defects in glycogenolysis, glycogen synthetase deficiency
Galactosaemia, fructose intolerance
Some organic acidaemias
Defects in oxidation of fat or in ketone-body formation

known. Infants of low birth weight due to intrauterine growth retardation are more likely to develop hypoglycaemia, while respiratory distress syndrome and intraventricular haemorrhage are more common in preterm babies. The risk of intellectual deficit is greater for small-for-dates infants than for preterm infants. The former include infants with severe intrauterine malnutrition, chromosomal disorders and congenital malformations of the brain; the low birth weight and perinatal problems may then be the consequence of pre-existing damage rather than its cause, but will pose an additional threat to the infant's intellectual progress.

Clinically, newborn infants are assessed by the Apgar scoring system of heart rate, respiration, muscle tone, reflexes and colour. Fetal hypoxia may be detected by observation of the fetal heart rate and during labour by analysis of blood gases. The risk of mental handicap and neurological sequelae is high if a full-term infant has a low Apgar score or neonatal convulsions coupled with severe intrapartum difficulties (e.g. placenta praevia, cord around the neck, intrapartum haemorrhage), or postnatal difficulties (e.g. respiratory distress, repeated periods of apnoea, abnormal electrocardiogram). For the past 40 years, paediatricians have striven to prevent mental handicap in low birth-weight infants. Prevention of perinatal trauma and asphyxia, and normalization of physiological variables that affect cerebral blood flow (P_{O_2}, P_{CO_2}, blood pressure, haematocrit), help to reduce the incidence of ventricular haemorrhage. Hypothermia and infection must be avoided and adequate nutrition provided by the appropriate route. Oxygen administration has to be carefully monitored as its excess is one of the factors that can disturb the delicate retinal circulation of the infant and produce retinal damage.

Modern techniques for the study of cerebral lesions include computerized tomographic scans, ultrasound, nuclear resonance imaging, positron emission tomography, single-photon emission computerized tomography and cerebral blood-flow studies by xenon clearance or transcutaneous Doppler ultrasound. These techniques have provided the means to observe the brain and its metabolic activity, localize lesions and monitor their evolution. There have been concomitant advances in neurological assessment and electrophysiological investigation, notably auditory brainstem-evoked potentials and visual-evoked responses. A sound basis therefore exists for prospective studies. Nevertheless, any prognosis based on perinatal observations is still subject to considerable uncertainty. A nationwide, high-technology service for intensive neonatal care will reduce infant mortality and the prevalence of mental handicap, but ultimately, medical care, no matter how excellent, will not compensate for poor antenatal care, inadequate maternal nutrition, low income, bad housing and lack of education, all prime determinants of low birth weight. The quality of the environment in which an infant grows up after an insult to the brain may also profoundly affect the outcome. Permanent handicap often results from the cumulative effect of several adverse factors, each of which acting on its own might have been withstood.[20,21]

Kernicterus and Electrolyte Disturbance[15,16]

Severe jaundice of the newborn may damage widely scattered areas of the brain, particularly the basal ganglia, brainstem, cerebellum and spinal cord. The early lesions are bright yellow, hence the term kernicterus (*kern* is the German for nucleus, meaning the subcortical formations of grey matter). Classical kernicterus is characterized by athetosis, deafness and mental retardation. Unconjugated bilirubin in plasma is free or bound to albumin, and it is the small, free fraction that is largely responsible for kernicterus. In the full-term infant with haemolytic disease, kernicterus is more likely to occur when the concentration of unconjugated bilirubin exceeds 340 μmol/L. In sick, premature infants, albumin binding may be severely depressed; furthermore, breakdown of the blood–brain barrier may allow the flow of albumin-bound bilirubin into the brain. The risk of kernicterus is increased by factors such as anoxia, acidosis and drugs, notably sulphonamides and sodium fucidate, which reduce the binding of bilirubin to albumin. Nevertheless, even in small high-risk infants (birthweight < 1250 g), bilirubin concentrations of < 170 μmol/L are not thought to cause long-term neurological impairment. It follows that therapy (phototherapy or exchange transfusion) will be decided upon in the light of the overall risk situation. Attempts to relate poor intellectual development to bilirubin concentrations, and to define 'safe' concentrations, have proved unsuccessful.

The pathogenesis of the brain damage is poorly understood. *In vitro*, bilirubin inhibits many enzymes of respiration, glycolysis, lipid and protein metabolism, but this may not be relevant to *in vivo* events. Rhesus (Rh) haemolytic disease in the newborn has been largely eliminated by administration of anti-D γ-globulin after the birth of Rh-positive infants to Rh-negative mothers. Bilirubin encephalopathy continues to occur in prematurity, respiratory distress and severe infections; the pattern of lesions in the brain of these infants may be unlike that seen in classical kernicterus.

Improvements in infant feeding and in the management of fluid balance in sick infants have reduced the role of *hypernatraemia* in the causation of mental handicap. Hyperosmolar dehydration in association with hypernatraemia can lead to intravascular stasis, infarction of brain tissue and haemorrhage. If rehydration is too rapid, oedema may result, followed by convulsions some hours after the start of therapy. Brain capillary failure has an important role in the pathogenesis of brain oedema and haemorrhage.

Neonatal hypocalcaemia occurs either at the age of 1 week as a result of excessive phosphate intake in milk, or more seriously, during the first 2 days of life, particularly in low birth-weight infants. While the outlook for infants with convulsions due to neonatal hypocalcaemia (serum concentrations < 1.75 mmol/L) is better than that for infants with hypoglycaemic fits, some are left with handicap.

Epilepsy[20]

In the mentally retarded, fits themselves or their consequences, such as cerebral hypoxia–ischaemia, asphyxia or vascular disturbances and associated biochemical changes, may be the primary cause of brain injury. Sometimes a vicious circle occurs, the lesions caused by fits producing further fits. Alternatively, seizures and retardation may both be the result of an underlying metabolic disorder such as a storage disease, or they may be iatrogenic, caused, for example, by withdrawal of an anticonvulsant or administration of drugs that interfere with the metabolism of anticonvulsants. Cognitive retardation may also be the consequence of injudicious anticonvulsant therapy rather than seizures. There is a well-recognized link between folate deficiency, intellectual deterioration and psychiatric disorder in patients on long-term anticonvulsants. Investigations appropriate in these cases are listed in Table 16.11. Excitatory amino acids and ingress of calcium ions into neurons play an important part in the genesis of the paroxysmal depolarization shifts that underlie seizures at the cellular level.[22] Within the cell, accumulation of calcium ions during prolonged fits results in mitochondrial failure and activation of hydrolytic enzymes that injure the cell and produce the appearance of ischaemic cell damage. Excess of intracellular cations also leads to activation of protein kinase C and gives rise to an environment that promotes

virus replication and thus susceptibility to viral encephalitis.

About one-third of the severely retarded have fits, compared with 0.5–1.0% of the general population. These patients benefit from careful attention to nutritional status to prevent vitamin D and folate deficiencies, and monitoring of anticonvulsant levels; as eliciting neurological signs of intoxication are often difficult to detect in these patients.

Nutrition[23]

The adult brain can withstand extreme and prolonged starvation without inevitable effects on intelligence. Malnutrition is most dangerous during the brain growth spurt from the start of the third trimester of antenatal life to the second birthday. In humans, the greater part of this spurt takes place after birth. Intrauterine malnutrition is therefore correctable to some extent in the postnatal period, unless the damage is compounded by postnatal malnutrition, or if biological deficits are reinforced by a poor environment and lack of stimulation. Vitamin supplementation of the diet of pregnant women in poor populations has been recommended but results are difficult to interpret.

Postnatally, primary nutritional deficiencies as a source of mental retardation are probably very rare in Britain, except as a form of child abuse. In the Third World they still constitute an important, preventable cause of educational underachievement, mental handicap and death in childhood. Neurological abnormalities such as mental changes, hyporeflexia and reduced nerve-conduction velocities are sometimes seen in protein–calorie malnutrition. While usually insidious in onset, kwashiorkor may present with acute encephalopathy. Tremors and other neurological signs may persist for some time after dietary correction. Many children so affected remain mentally retarded. Generally, the younger the child during the acute phase, the greater the risk of mental handicap. Malnutrition may also be the result of brain damage. For example, children with cerebral palsy may be incapable of coping with a normal diet. Improvement in nutritional status results when the consistency of the diet is adjusted to their ability to chew and swallow.

A major difficulty has been to isolate the effects of malnutrition as a specific cause of mental handicap from other adverse environmental factors.[24,25] In a group of deprived Jamaican children, dietary supplementation had a positive effect on cognitive development observable from the ages of 12 to 36 months. It is not known if these effects persist when supplementation ceases.[26] Early diet in pre-term babies affects their developmental status at 18 months.[27] In animals, malnutrition results in reduced brain size, in itself not of great significance. However, certain formations, for example the cerebellum, are selectively affected. Biochemical analyses have shown a reduc-

TABLE 16.11

INVESTIGATION OF MENTALLY RETARDED PATIENTS WITH CONVULSIONS OR SUSPECTED DEGENERATIVE DISEASE OF THE NERVOUS SYSTEM

Test	Comments
Urea, creatinine, electrolytes	Should include anion gap; sometimes abnormal due to vomiting, failure to drink or polydipsia
Blood gases	pH, P_{CO_2}, HCO_3; patients with organic acidurias are not always acidotic
Urine screen	Smell, ketones, glucose, reducing substances, blood, protein
Blood calcium, phosphate, alkaline phosphatase, magnesium	Onset of hypocalcaemia may be insidious in pseudohypoparathyroidism, mild rickets common particularly in patients on anticonvulsants; magnesium assays have low priority after 3 months of age
Liver function tests	Commonly abnormal in Wilson's disease before appearance of neurological signs, often abnormal due to long-term effects of drugs or infections
Blood copper and caeruloplasmin	Caeruloplasmin is not invariably low in Wilson's disease; copper assay useful in diagnosis of Menkes' disease
Blood lead	Regression and convulsions only rarely attributable to lead intoxication; concentration of lead commonly raised in retarded patients with pica, but not the cause of their mental retardation
Blood glucose (fasting)	Often as low as 2.2 mmol/L, even in older patients, but not identifiable as the cause of fits or mental retardation
Blood lactate and pyruvate	Preferably measured 1 h after a meal; good screen for disorders of carbohydrate metabolism and mitochondrial defects, but low specificity
Blood ammonia	Elevated concentrations may be found in late-presenting variants of urea-cycle disorders, in female carriers of ornithine carbamyl transferase deficiency and in some patients with Rett's syndrome (see Table 16.15)
Blood and urine amino acids and organic acids	Important to examine blood and urine amino acids to identify the often transient, non-specific aminoacidurias, said to be common in the mentally retarded; intermittent organic acidurias may be difficult to diagnose when asymptomatic
Very long-chain fatty acids and bile acid intermediates	For detection of peroxisomal disorders, usually assayed in reference laboratories
Urine uric acid:creatinine ratio	Screen for Lesch–Nyhan disease, patients with self-mutilation; preferred to plasma urate assay
Urinary oligosaccharides, glycosaminoglycans, intracellular metachromasia	Screen for some lysosomal disorders; may help in selecting enzyme assays or blood cells or fibroblasts
Blood film and bone marrow	Abnormal inclusions and vacuoles in blood and bone marrow cells useful in detecting some lysosomal disorders; may suggest need for electron microscopy
Enzyme assays	For definitive diagnosis of inborn errors, usually assayed in reference laboratories
Infection screen	Includes haematological and microbiological tests and tests for TORCH (toxoplasma, rubella, cytomegalovirus and herpes) under age 3 years, measles antibody titre for diagnosis of subacute sclerosing panencephalitis (SSPE)
Electroencephalogram (EEG)	Diagnostic in SSPE, some late-onset lipidoses, non-ketotic hyperglycinaemia; note that up to 10% of normal children have abnormal EEGs
Electrophysiology	Nerve conduction useful when peripheral neuropathies present. Visual-, auditory- and somatosensory-evoked potentials test integrity of respective pathways; electroretinography used in disorders with retinal degeneration
Imaging	Computerized tomographic scans; ultrasound imaging (while fontanelles open) and nuclear magnetic resonance imaging to follow brain development and evolution of lesion; positron emission tomography and single-photon emission computerized tomography for studying brain function *in vivo*

tion in myelin lipids, brain proteins and glycos-aminoglycans. The reduction in cell number as reflected by DNA analysis is not striking, but synaptic ultrastructure is affected, as are many enzymes, including some involved in neurotransmitter synthesis.

Vitamins, Teratogens, Drugs and Poisons[15,16,20]

Vitamins are involved in enzyme systems as coenzymes and a deficiency may therefore result in disturbance of nerve function. Beriberi caused by thiamine deficiency may present in infants as an acute encephalopathy; pellagra, nicotinic acid deficiency, may result in dementia; pyridoxine deficiency in convulsions. Hypocalcaemic convulsions may complicate vitamin D deficiency; folate deficiency may lead to brain

TABLE 16.12

SUBSTANCES THAT MAY CAUSE OR POTENTIATE CONGENITAL BRAIN ABNORMALITIES

Substance	Comments
Hydantoin	Craniofacial and distal limb anomalies, growth retardation and mental deficits
Trimethadione	Craniofacial, cardiac and genitourinary anomalies, microcephaly, growth retardation, delayed mental development
Valproate	Craniofacial abnormalities, increased risk of neural-tube defects, developmental delay
Barbiturates	In experimental animals, cell proliferation affected; no conclusive human data
Primidone	Craniofacial abnormalities, psychomotor retardation
Narcotic analgesics	In experimental animals, cell proliferation and neurotransmitter synthesis affected; no conclusive human data
Heroin	Low birth weight, small head size, developmental delay, decreased sensitivity of opiate receptors of locus coeruleus, possibility of mental retardation
Benzodiazepines	Intrauterine growth retardation, dysmorphic features, psychomotor retardation
Alcohol	Characteristic facies, microcephaly, growth retardation, mental handicap
Tobacco	Reduced birth weight; reading, mathematics and general ability retarded by 3 months at age 7 years
Caffeine	Fetus not at risk unless extremely large quantities ingested daily
Isoretinoin	Characteristic facies, cardiac defects, extensive central nervous system involvement
Vitamin A	Restricted intake advised during pregnancy
Aminopterin	Dysmorphic features of head and face, mental retardation seen when used unsuccessfully in early pregnancy to procure abortions
Coumarin derivatives	Nasal hypoplasia, epiphyseal changes, central nervous system abnormalities, fetal bleeding, mental retardation
Mercury	Psychomotor retardation and cerebellar ataxia described in children exposed *in utero*; methylmercury particularly toxic
Lead	Some evidence but inconclusive proof that small amounts of lead delivered transplacentally affect the intelligence of the offspring
Carbon monoxide	Mental retardation and congenital cerebral defects in offspring described after carbon monoxide poisoning during pregnancy

damage and vitamin B_{12} deficiency to subacute degeneration of the chord. Vitamin E deficiency can produce neuroaxonal dystrophy and is responsible for the neurological lesions of abetalipoproteinaemia.

Postnatally, in advanced countries, inadequate intake is probably rare as a cause of overt vitamin deficiency except in alcoholic, psychiatric and psychogeriatric patients. Patients on anticonvulsants may require vitamin D or folate supplements. Vitamin intake may be suboptimal in some groups of children but the case for supplementation as a means of increasing intelligence remains unproven.[27,28]

A few individuals have a constant specific requirement for a particular vitamin and may need up to several hundred times the recommended intake; they exhibit *vitamin dependency*. This is found in a small minority of patients with inborn errors. Untreated it often carries a high risk of death or mental retardation. Examples are variants of homocystinuria, some organic acidurias, and pyridoxine-dependent seizures in neonates. These vitamin-dependent individuals form only a minute section of the population; there is therefore no justification for massive and indiscriminate vitamin supplements beyond the recommended norms. An adequate vitamin intake during pregnancy is a significant factor in reducing the incidence of neural-tube defects in susceptible individuals, especially in areas of high prevalence.[29] Folate supplements are now recommended during the first trimester of pregnancy. It has also been suggested that folinic acid supplements may reduce the fragility of the X chromosome in the fragile X syndrome *in vivo* as well as *in vitro*. Tetrahydrobiopterin metabolism is disturbed in a number of neuropsychiatric disorders. Hydroxycobalamin and folinic acid are involved in the *in vitro* synthesis of this cofactor.

Drugs and poisons can interfere with prenatal development by disturbing embryogenesis or by acting on individual fetal organs, resulting in deformities. A single teratogen can be responsible for a wide range of defects; identical malformations may result from diverse pathogenetic processes.[6,7] Conclusive proof of teratogenicity is often difficult and requires laborious investigations. The timing of the insult may determine the form of the malformation as much as the agent responsible. Table 16.12 lists some substances which may have adverse effects on the developing nervous system. Anticonvulsants may increase the incidence of malformation in the offspring of pregnant epileptic women and some effects on the intelligence of these offspring may have occurred, but fits themselves are probably more dangerous to the fetus than the anticonvulsants. Antimitotic drugs may be teratogenic. On the other hand, a small number of women who have had renal transplants and who received steroids, azathioprine and folic acid antagonists throughout their pregnancy did not appear to have an increased incidence of malformed babies.

The possibility that *maternal alcoholism* might harm the fetus was considered by a Select Committee of the House of Commons in 1834 but it is only recently that the role of alcohol as a teratogen has been firmly established. The pathogenetic process is not well understood but acetaldehyde, zinc deficiency and tryptophan pyrrolase deficiency have been implicated. Alcohol abuse in pregnancy is nearly always associated with other factors that have adverse effects on the fetus. The mothers are often heavy smokers and some are on psychotropic or addictive drugs. Current opinion is that mental handicap in the offspring of a healthy, well-nourished, non-smoker who consumed one or two units (10–20 mL alcohol) per day during pregnancy is unlikely to be caused by the alcohol. The previous recommendation of total abstinence during pregnancy has now been modified to allow a maximum of two units per week.

Some drugs taken in pregnancy do not cause recognizable malformations but affect intelligence or behaviour.[16] In particular, drugs that alter the balance of neurotransmitter activity can produce long-lasting functional disturbances in the developing brain. Examples of drugs influencing central neurotransmitter activity are the phenothiazines and adrenergic agonists and antagonists. Experimental work suggests that these drugs affect cell proliferation in the developing brain when given to pregnant animals.

It is difficult to decide to what extent pollutants, food additives and allergens adversely affect intellectual development.[20] Up to 20% of the population are atopic; allergic disorders are therefore extremely common. Very rarely, severe food allergy plays a part in the aetiology of a neuropsychiatric disorder, such as migraine or a behaviour disorder. A few individuals may show adverse behavioural or cognitive reactions to artificial food colouring. Occasionally, parents wrongly believe that their child's handicap is caused by food allergies; parental obsession with allergen avoidance may result in bizarre lifestyles and dangerous attempts to treat with oligoantigenic diets.

In 1979, comparison of the intelligence of children in the USA with high and low lead exposure as reflected by the lead content of dentine revealed a significant difference of 5 IQ points. These findings were not universally accepted. More recent studies in the UK were specifically designed to eliminate methodological differences and to account for confounding variables.[20] Only small effects attributable to lead were found; sometimes they became insignificant when account was taken of other variables. Lead may account for about 2% of the variation in intelligence, a minor contribution compared with genetic and other environmental factors. In a recent study in a predominantly middle-class area, no relation could be found with either IQ or teachers' behaviour ratings. These ambiguities cannot be blamed on shortcomings of analytical techniques. Modern mass spectrometric analyses not only yield profiles of a number of trace metals but the relative abundance of isotopes may provide clues to whether, for example, the lead in blood originates predominantly from petrol or drinking water. It is the complexity of interacting biological and social factors that is at the root of the problem. Some metals protect against the harmful effects of others, some potentiate the risk. Thus zinc will protect against the toxic effects of cadmium, selenium against those of arsenic and cadmium, while cadmium and lead reinforce each other's toxicity. Excess of iron decreases the toxicity of lead, while lead poisoning is aggravated by diets low in calcium and iron. Secondary deficiencies may be caused by a toxic metal when the supply of an interacting essential element is barely adequate. Therefore, even if an attempt is made to allow for social factors, studies in behavioural toxicology in which a single biochemical variable is measured are unlikely to yield conclusive results.

DEGENERATIVE DISEASES OF THE NERVOUS SYSTEM WITH MENTAL HANDICAP—STORAGE DISORDERS[9,14,30–32]

Some degenerative disorders of the nervous system are genetic and therefore presumably have a biochemical basis. Often it is difficult to decide whether or not a condition is progressive. Clinical signs will narrow the diagnostic options but in some cases longitudinal observation, supplemented by psychological assessment and electroencephalographic and imaging studies, is necessary to demonstrate slowing in acquisition of skills, then regressing. Pathological processes may be active before birth, resulting in perinatal complications. It must be remembered that the contribution of hereditary metabolic disease to neuropsychiatric symptomatology is relatively small compared to antenatal or perinatal injury. Loss of previously acquired milestones is seen in encephalopathies of diverse origin; examples of disorders of the nervous system associated with intellectual deterioration are:

- Tumours
- Infections (subacute sclerosing panencephalitis)
- Autoimmune and post-infectious disorders
- Chronic poisoning (lead, organic mercury)
- Degenerative inherited disorders
- Neurocutaneous disorders (tuberous sclerosis, Sturge–Weber disease)
- Spinal and spinocerebellar degenerations
- Storage disorders (sphingolipidoses, mucopolysaccharidoses)
- Leucodystrophies (Krabbe's disease, metachromatic leucodystrophy, adrenoleucodystrophy)
- Canavan's spongiform encephalopathy
- Neuroaxonal dystrophy (Schindler disease)
- Huntington's chorea
- Wilson's disease
- Childhood autism (some cases).

In suspected degenerative disorders every attempt is made to arrive at a diagnosis, even if this will not help the patient, so that the parents can, if possible, be informed of the chance of a subsequent child being affected. The incidence of rare recessive disorders is increased in consanguineous marriages and some rare genes have a much increased frequency in certain ethnic groups. In Tay–Sachs disease the mutant gene frequency is a hundred times higher in Jews of Eastern European origin than in other populations. Aspartylglucosaminuria and Salla disease occur almost exclusively in Finns. Awareness of the more random distribution of rare genes may help in diagnosis.

Traditionally, storage disorders have been classified by the composition of the substance stored. In the sphingolipidoses the stored substance is a sphingolipid consisting of ceramide, an ester of the amino alcohol sphingosine, linked to phosphorylcholine to form sphingomyelin, or to hexose and neuraminic acid residues to form gangliosides. The main lipids of myelin are the phospholipids, sphingomyelin, cerebrosides (ceramide with one hexose residue) and cholesterol; nerve cells and their processes contain less phospholipid and more ganglioside. Sphingomyelin is also a constituent of subcellular organelles and the plasma membrane. The acid glycosaminoglycans (mucopolysaccharides), the substances stored in the mucopolysaccharidoses, are macromolecules consisting of repeating units of sulphated hexosamine and hexuronic acid. They are found in various tissues; for example, the cornea, blood vessels and the ground substance of cartilage. Some disorders combining the clinical and biochemical features of the sphingolipidoses and mucopolysaccharidoses have been termed mucolipidoses. Our understanding of these disorders has its root in the delineation of distinct syndromes from careful clinical and morbid anatomical observations at the turn of the century. This was followed by isolation and analysis of the stored substances and finally by identification of the enzymes involved and revelation of their lysosomal origin. Hers first postulated that the storage disorders were the results of lysosomal enzyme deficiencies.

Lysosomes possess a range of specific hydrolytic enzymes for the degradation of sphingolipids and glycosaminoglycans. Loss of activity at any of the catabolic steps is followed by intralysosomal accumulation of the molecules, which cannot be broken down. There is hypertrophy of the lysosomes, and sometimes overspill into the cytoplasm. The rate of accumulation of stored material depends on the turnover of the substance that cannot be degraded in the course of cellular activity. The stored material will be heterogeneous if the bond resistant to hydrolysis occurs in more than one type of molecule. In the brain, storage leads to mechanical distortion of cells, interferes with their metabolic activity, and ends with their destruction.

There is great variability in age of onset and progression of these disorders, determined in large measure by genetic heterogeneity. In lysosomal disorders, mutations have been found to involve transcription of the gene, processing of messenger RNA, transfer of the gene product from its site of synthesis to the lysosomes, and the formation of activator or stabilizer proteins. The enzyme deficiency may be virtually complete in some cases; in others, some activity may be preserved. In general, low activity is associated with early onset and rapid deterioration. Some enzymes occur as isoenzymes that differ in activity and organ specificity and utilize different substrates. They may be under independent genetic control, when distinct clinical entities are associated with mutations affecting each isoenzyme. If one mutation affects several isoenzymes the resultant disorder combines the clinical and pathological features of the individual deficiencies. An example is provided by arylsulphatase A deficiency (metachromatic leucodystrophy), with no features of gargoylism, and arylsulphatase B deficiency (Maroteaux–Lamy disease), a mucopolysaccharidosis with mainly somatic manifestations. Mucosulphatitosis (multiple sulphatase deficiency), in which both enzymes are affected, combines features of both a leucodystrophy and gargoylism.

Diagnosis[9]

Although individually rare, the overall incidence of lysosomal storage disorders is about 1 in 2000 births in European populations. The clinical presentation is variable and does not always conform to classical textbook descriptions. Gangliosides play a part in the binding and release of neurotransmitters, and in the transport of signals into the cell. Excess accumulation is likely to prejudice synaptic neurotransmission. Disturbance of ganglioside metabolism is often associated with nerve-cell destruction expressed by psychomotor retardation, fits, a cherry-red spot on the macula, and later spasticity and paralysis. Disorders of the metabolism of sulphatide or cerebroside, which are important constituents of myelin, affect the peripheral as well as the central nervous system, giving rise to signs of peripheral neuropathy, spasticity and ataxia. Seizures may occur, but usually in the later stages. In the mucopolysaccharidoses, storage in the skeletal system gradually results in a characteristic appearance and bony changes. When a stored substance has a high turnover in liver or spleen, visceromegaly ensues.

In the mucopolysaccharidoses and some mucolipidoses the skeletal abnormalities, termed *dysostosis multiplex*, produce characteristic radiological changes. Histochemical studies and electron microscopy are helpful when the biochemical defect is ill defined or unknown, as in some late-presenting variants of amaurotic family idiocy, the cerebroretinal degenerations.[32] Skin biopsies that contain axons and Schwann cells can be used, obviating the need for brain biopsies. Electroretinograms and visual-evoked potentials are helpful in suspected neurolipidoses. Metachromatic inclusions and vacuoles in lymphocytes and abnormal cells in bone marrow occur in a number of lysosomal disorders. The approach to the diagnosis of these disorders must be multidisciplinary (*see* Fig. 16.1 and Table 16.11).

Most clinical laboratories offer screening tests for the detection of excess urinary glycosaminoglycans in mucopolysaccharidoses and oligosaccharides in some mucolipidoses. In many cases, characteristic patterns are seen on thin-layer chromatography or thin-layer electrophoresis. High-performance liquid chromatography of glycolipids in urinary deposits or plasma can identify, for example, cases of Fabry's, Gaucher's and Farber's disease. In all lysosomal disorders, identification, characterization and assay of the deficient enzyme are essential for a definitive diagnosis, and if possible, heterozygote detection. Artificial substrates can be used in many of the assays. Enzymes are usually assayed in leucocytes or fibroblasts; occasionally in plasma or urine.

Fibroblasts growing in culture incorporate ^{35}S-sulphate into acid glycosaminoglycans; accumulation is greatly enhanced in fibroblasts from patients with mucopolysaccharidoses. This excessive accumulation, due to inability to degrade the glycosaminoglycan, can be prevented by supplying secretions from any genotypically different fibroblasts. Genotypes can therefore be identified by cross-correction experiments, even if the precise defect is unknown. The 'correction factors' in the secretions are the lysosomal enzymes deficient in the patients.

The techniques of molecular biology have now helped to clarify, in some disorders, the mechanisms by which enzyme deficiencies arise and to explain anomalies in their expression. For example, very low activity of arylsulphatase A can occur in clinically normal individuals, posing serious problems in genetic counselling and antenatal diagnosis of metachromatic leucodystrophy; more so as the frequency of the 'pseudodeficiency allele' has been estimated to be as high as 7–15%. The gene for arylsulphatase has now been cloned and two mutations carried by the pseudodeficiency gene identified. Based on these findings a rapid assay has been developed for the detection of the pseudodeficiency allele, using the polymerase chain reaction and oligonucleotide-specific hybridization.[33] Selected neurodegenerative disorders are listed in Table 16.13.

Approaches to Treatment[30,31,33]

The pathophysiological and biochemical mechanisms by which the lysosomal enzymes are synthesized, transferred from ribosome to lysosome and further modified to yield active enzyme are in most cases well understood. It has proved very difficult to reverse the inexorable course of these disorders. Cells can take up enzymes by endocytosis into pinocytotic vesicles, which fuse with lysosomes. An exogenous enzyme can thus take part in the degradation of a stored substance. Lysosomal enzyme deficiencies have, therefore, been prime candidates for enzyme replacement therapy. In practice, results with infusion of enzymes have been disappointing, even when the enzymes were modified by linking them to recognition markers, which target them to the receptors on the storage cells, given in carrier erythrocytes, or entrapped in phospholipid bilayers (liposomes). An exception is the case of mannose terminated glucocerebrosidase in non-neuropathic Gaucher's disease.

A more promising approach has been to provide a continuous source of enzyme by tissue or organ graft. Early optimism about fibroblast transplants has not proved justified. Bone marrow transplants have a place in those disorders in which storage is primarily extracerebral, and have the advantage that there is extensive experience of this technique gained from treating patients with leukaemia and immunodeficiencies. Additional problems arise when storage occurs primarily in the brain. In animal experiments, bone marrow precursors can populate the brain with the cells of the macrophage line to become a local source of enzyme. In man, the situation is complex. For example, it is not clear in patients with metachromatic leucodystrophy who have undergone bone marrow transplantation whether the disease process has been stopped or whether deterioration has just been delayed. Similar reservations are pertinent for other neurolipidoses.[33]

In the future it may be possible to treat some storage disorders by somatic gene therapy.[33] Cultured cells may be transformed with recombinant genes using retroviral vectors, *viral-mediated gene transfer*. These vectors carry chimeric genes but have been rendered devoid of genes coding for viral functions. The expression of the gene requires a promoter to direct transcription of the integrated DNA into RNA and the signals for translation of the RNA into protein. The target tissue for therapy must be selected so that the gene product is viable in its new environment and capable of altering the biochemical phenotype of the patient. Most research in somatic gene therapy has been concentrated on introducing genes into the bone marrow. In several species it has been possible to reconstitute bone marrow with transformed cells. Many animal studies have also demonstrated function of hepatocyte transplants in liver for weeks or months. One problem is that few of the transplanted cells become vascularized and remain viable. In man, transplanting portions of liver currently appears to be a more promising treatment. Because the blood–brain barrier prevents infection with most viruses, the central nervous system is a difficult target for somatic gene therapy. The herpes simplex virus is being assessed as a possible carrier of genes in neurological tissue, as it can insert genes directly into neurons. There is evidence that in some lysosomal disorders, for example Tay–Sachs disease, the pathogenetic progress is active *in utero*. For treatment to be effective, stored ganglioside must be degraded, and no irreversible changes must have

TABLE 16.13
SELECTED NEURODEGENERATIVE DISORDERS

Disorder	Comment
Mucopolysaccharidoses (McKusick)	
Hurler (MPS IH)	α-L-Iduronidase deficiency: corneal clouding, visceromegaly, coarse facies, heart disease, disostosis multiplex; severe mental retardation
Scheie (MPS IS)	Corneal clouding, stiff joints, normal or near-normal intelligence; genetic compound MPS IH/S of intermediate phenotype between MPS IH and MPS IS occurs
Hunter (MPS II)	L-Iduronate sulphatase deficiency: clear cornea, deafness, otherwise like MPS IH; a mild, more slowly progressive variant occurs with normal intelligence; dermatan sulphate and heparan sulphate are the glycosaminoglycans affected
Sanfilippo A (MPS IIIA)	α-N-acetylglucosaminidase deficiency: somatic features mild initially, may be more pronounced in later stages of disease; severe mental retardation
Sanfilippo B (MPS IIIB)	α-N-acetylglucosaminidase deficiency: clinically indistinguishable from MPS IIIA
Sanfilippo C (MPS IIIC)	Acetyl CoA: α-glucosaminide acetyltransferase deficiency: clinically indistinguishable from MPS IIIA
Sanfilippo D (MPS IIID)	N-acetylglucosamine-6-sulphatase deficiency: clinically indistinguishable from MPS IIIA; heparan sulphate is the glycosaminoglycan affected in MPS IIIA, IIIB, IIIC and IIID
Morquio A (MPS IVA)	N-acetylgalactosamine-6-sulphatase deficiency: wide spectrum of clinical manifestations including corneal clouding, skeletal abnormalities, sometimes mild mental retardation
Morquio B (MPS IVB)	Keratan sulphate β-galactosidase deficiency: clinically indistinguishable from MPS IVA; keratan sulphate is the glycosaminoglycan affected in MPS IVA and IVB
Maroteaux–Lamy (MPS VI)	Corneal clouding, dysostosis multiplex, appearance resembles MPS I, but not mentally retarded; dermatan sulphate is the glycosaminoglycan affected in MPS VI
Sly (MPS VII)	β-Glucuronidase deficiency: wide spectrum of severity—visceromegaly, dysostosis multiplex, skeletal abnormalities, mental retardation; mild variants with normal intelligence have been described; dermatan sulphate, heparan sulphate, chondroitin-4-sulphate and -6-sulphate are the glycosaminoglycans affected
Neurolipidoses	
Pompe's disease	Acid α-1,4-glucosidase deficiency: cardiomegaly, hypotonia, large tongue, nervous system involvement; adult forms occur in which brain is not involved
Wolman's disease	Acid lipase deficiency: visceromegaly, adrenal calcification, steatorrhoea, mental deterioration; cholesteryl-ester storage disease is a less severe variant
Farber's disease	Acid ceramidase deficiency: hoarse cry, joint deformities, skin nodules; life expectation and severity of mental retardation are variable
Fabry's disease	α-Galactosidase deficiency: skin, eyes, and kidneys primarily affected; peripheral neuropathy; most patients mentally normal; X-linked
Gaucher's disease	Glucocerebrosidase deficiency: hepatosplenomegaly, early- and late-onset variants; many genotypes, some neuronopathic; Gaucher cells in bone marrow
Niemann–Pick disease (sphingomyelin–cholesterol storage disease)	Sphingomyelinase deficiency: acute, subacute and chronic forms; cherry-red spot on macula, hepatosplenomegaly; nervous system involvement and severe mental retardation present in acute form, less prominent in subacute and chronic forms; foam cells in bone marrow; normal enzyme activity in some patients
GM₂ gangliosidoses:	
Tay–Sachs (B variant)	Defect in α-subunit of hexosaminidase A: fits, hyperacusis, paralysis, dementia, cherry-red spot on macula; early- and later-onset variants, some with minimal signs and residual enzyme activity
Sandhoff (O variant)	Defective α- and β-subunits of the hexosaminidases; clinically similar to B variant
Tay–Sachs (AB variant)	GM₂ activator protein deficiency, clinically similar to B variant
Mucolipidoses with oligosacchariduria	
GM₁, gangliosidosis (Landing)	β-Galactosidase deficiency: infantile form resembles Hurler syndrome; juvenile and adult forms occur with slower mental and neurological deterioration
α-Mannosidosis	α-Mannosidase deficiency: severe infantile and juvenile–adult variants; resembles mucopolysaccharidoses; hearing loss, cataracts and corneal opacities
β-Mannosidosis	β-Mannosidase deficiency: hypotonia, angiokeratoma, hearing loss
Fucosidosis type I	α-Fucosidase deficiency: resembles Hurler syndrome; raised sweat sodium concentrations, rapid deterioration
Fucosidosis type II	α-Fucosidase deficiency: milder course than type I; skin lesions as in Fabry's disease
Aspartylglucosaminuria	Aspartyl glucosaminidase deficiency: Hurler-like appearance, coarse facies, clumsiness, hypotonia, mental retardation

TABLE 16.13 (*contd*)

Disorder	Comment
Schindler disease	α-*N*-acetylgalactosaminidase deficiency: mental and neurological deterioration, fits, glycopeptiduria, neuroaxonal dystrophy
I-cell disease (mucolipidosis II)	*N*-acetylglucosaminylphosphotransferase deficiency: abnormal lysosomal enzyme transport, resembles Hurler syndrome; rapid course, characteristic inclusion cells; milder variant occurs (pseudo-Hurler polydystrophy, mucolipidosis III)
Salla disease	Lysosomal transport of sialic acid defective: coarse facies, dystonia, ataxia; a rapidly progressive and more severe variant, infantile sialic acid storage disease, occurs
Sialidosis (mucolipidosis I)	α-Neuraminidase deficiency: cherry-red spot, myoclonus; ataxia, normosomatic and more severe dysmorphic variants occur
Galactosialidosis	Combined α-neuraminidase and β-galactosidase protective protein deficiency; cherry-red spots, corneal clouding, ataxia, myoclonus, dysmorphism
Sialolipidosis	Ganglioside sialidase deficiency (mucolipidosis IV); corneal clouding, retinal degeneration, mental and growth retardation
Leucodystrophies	
Krabbe's disease	Galactosylceramidase deficiency; progressive paralysis, fits, dementia; characteristic globoid cells in white matter
Metachromatic leucodystrophy	Arylsulphatase A deficiency: weakness, ataxia, spastic tetraparesis; late infantile, juvenile and adult forms; may be caused by deficiency of activator protein
Multiple sulphatase deficiency	Loss of activity of arylsulphatase A, B, and C: features of mucopolysaccharidoses and metachromatic leucodystrophy; ichthyosis, hearing loss, severe course
Adrenoleucodystrophies	Peroxisomal disorders: neonatal autosomal recessive and X-linked genotypes
Canavan disease	Aspartoacylase deficiency: hypotonia, megalencephaly, spongiform encephalopathy
Cerebrotendinous xanthomatosis	Deficiency of mitochondrial sterol 26-hydroxylase: tendon xanthomas, dementia, tremor, ataxia, cataracts, storage in brain of cholestanol and cholesterol

occurred in the brain before treatment is started. Other forms of treatment have a place in neurodegenerative disorders. Plasmapheresis has been used in Fabry's disease and, together with dietary treatment, in some peroxisomal disorders. Neurological deterioration in abetalipoproteinaemia (*see* Tables 16.5 and 16.9) can be prevented by vitamin E therapy.

In the foreseeable future the emphasis will rightly be on early diagnosis, genetic counselling and prevention. For example, in Tay–Sachs disease, heterozygotes may be detected by assay in serum of the affected enzyme, hexosaminidase A. Screening by antenatal diagnosis for at risk pregnancies is offered to high-risk populations in some countries.

AMINOACIDURIAS[14,31,34,35]

Many inherited disorders of amino acid metabolism have been described, and in some mental retardation is a constant or frequent finding. The pathogenesis of the mental defect has proved elusive, despite accumulation of a formidable body of biochemical and clinical data.

Phenylketonuria (PKU)[31,36,37]

The discovery in 1934 that mental retardation could be the result of a well-defined biochemical abnormality and the demonstration 20 years later that mental handicap could be prevented by timely treatment constitute a landmark in the history of mental deficiency. The disorder is transmitted as an autosomal recessive trait; heterozygotes are free from symptoms. In European populations the incidence varies from 1 in 5000 to 1 in 20 000 births.

The enzymatic block in PKU is in the hydroxylation of the essential amino acid phenylalanine to form tyrosine, catalysed by an enzyme complex consisting of the liver enzyme phenylalanine hydroxylase, a cofactor, tetrahydrobiopterin, and dihydropteridine reductase. The reductase is required to maintain adequate amounts of cofactor. Hydroxylation of phenalanine serves as a safety valve that prevents accumulation of the amino acid when intake exceeds requirements. As a result of the block in PKU, phenylalanine accumulates in body fluids and is diverted into pathways that in unaffected individuals are of only minor importance. Phenylpyruvic acid and other aromatic metabolites are excreted in urine. In non-phenylketonuric babies, particularly if premature or sick, blood phenylalanine concentrations may rise temporarily to two or three times the mean adult amount. By contrast, in PKU the concentration climbs steadily to settle at more than 10 times the adult level. *Classical PKU* is defined biochemically by a blood phenylalanine of 1200 μmol/L or higher on a free diet, with a low or normal concentration of tyrosine and the presence in the urine of characteristic phenolic acids. Most patients with classical PKU have less than 1% of normal activity of phenylalanine hydroxylase but variants with some residual enzyme activity, up to 5% of normal, and a blood phen-

TABLE 16.14
SOME ENZYME DEFICIENCIES OF PHENYLALANINE HYDROXYLATION

Enzyme affected	Comments
Phenylalanine hydroxylase	Genetically heterogeneous: over 100 genotypes identified; many patients have partial deficiency, many are compound heterozygotes; enzyme must be assayed in liver
Dihydropteridine reductase	Enzyme widely distributed in tissues; can be assayed on blood spots
GTP cyclohydrolase I	Can be differentiated from other cofactor deficiencies by analysis of urine pterins
Pyruvate tetrahydrobiopterin synthase	Genetically heterogeneous: severe and partial forms occur; enzyme can be assayed in erythrocytes

alanine usually below 1000 μmol/L are not uncommon, about one case being found for every three to four cases of classical PKU. These are termed *non-PKU hyperphenylalaninaemia*. *Transient hyperphenylalaninaemia*, attributed to slow maturation of the enzyme system, also occurs.

Patients with deficiency of phenylalanine hydroxylase respond to a diet low in phenylalanine. As phenylalanine is an essential amino acid, sufficient must be provided for growth and synthesis of essential derivatives, while avoiding dangerously high blood levels. A strict diet of a mixture of amino acids as a protein substitute is prescribed in classical PKU; less stringent regimens are acceptable in less severe hyperphenylalaninaemias. Most paediatricians will not treat infants with blood concentrations below 600 μmol/L on a free diet. Concentrations in the range 250–400 μmol/L are sometimes referred to as *benign hyperphenylalaninaemia*. These infants may, however, show dramatic increases in blood phenylalanine levels during a febrile illness or when their protein intake is increased on weaning. In treatment, a blood concentration of 120–360 μmol/L is optimal but rarely achieved consistently. Overtreatment can lead to deficiency states, which are particularly dangerous during the brain growth spurt, and must be avoided. To be effective, treatment of classical PKU should be started in the first 3 weeks of life. Most countries, therefore, operate neonatal mass screening schemes (*see* Chapter 15).

In up to 2% of phenylketonurics the mutation affects dihydropteridine reductase or cofactor synthesis (cofactor-deficient PKU) (Table 16.14). The reductase and cofactor are also essential for hydroxylation of tyrosine and tryptophan. In classical PKU due to phenylalanine hydroxylase deficiency, symptoms other than mental retardation (dilution of hair colour, skin problems, epilepsy) are usually not striking, and life expectancy is good. Patients with mutations involving the reductase or cofactor are generally much more severely affected. They do not respond to a low phenylalanine diet and exhibit progressive neurological deterioration, fits, dystonia and dysphagia. The neurological signs have been attributed to failure to form DOPA (dihydroxyphenylalanine) and 5-hydroxytryptophan, the precursors of the neurotransmitters dopamine, adrenaline, noradrenaline and serotonin (5-hydroxytryptamine). These amines are, in fact, reduced in the body fluids. Most of these patients have been treated by phenylalanine restriction, cofactor and neurotransmitter precursor (DOPA and 5-hydroxytryptophan) supplements, the monoamine oxidase inhibitor carbidopa, and, in the case of dihydropteridine reductase deficiency, folinic acid. Response to treatment has been variable. Genetic heterogeneity and the occurrence of partial and transient deficiencies further complicate interpretation of the results of treatment. In most countries, screening laboratories routinely offer tests to exclude cofactor deficiency for all newly diagnosed cases of hyperphenylalaninaemia.

Neonatal screening followed by dietary treatment has dramatically reduced the number of phenylketonurics who are retarded.[38,39] Unsolved problems include the nature of the pathogenetic process, the role of factors, other than dietary control, which may affect the outcome, the risk of relaxing the diet in the older child when brain development is assumed to be complete, and the management of mothers with hyperphenylalaninaemia. In spite of a large number of publications on the biochemistry of PKU, surprisingly little is known definitively about the pathogenetic process. Concentrations of phenylalanine persistently greater than 1200 μmol/L in early infancy almost invariably lead to moderate to severe retardation; no harmful effect of concentrations of 60–250 μmol/L has been demonstrated. Beyond that little is known for certain. Myelination is disturbed in untreated PKU. In high concentration, phenylalanine interferes at some stages of protein synthesis and inhibits the entry of other essential amino acids into the brain. Some metabolites present in abnormally high concentration have been shown *in vitro* to inhibit some enzymes of glycolysis and pyruvate metabolism, and in particular neurotransmitter synthesis. In cofactor-deficient PKU, neurotransmitter synthesis is more directly affected. Tyrosine, the metabolite subsequent to the block, is for phenylketonurics an essential amino acid. While there is no evidence of significant tyrosine deficiency in treated PKU, it has been suggested that tyrosine supplements may improve performance in neuropsychological tests by favouring the synthesis of neurotransmitters.

Very little is known about the effects on patients

with intermediate concentrations of phenylalanine in blood (400–1000 μmol/L), particularly as these infants were deliberately excluded from some of the most extensive clinical trials. There is good evidence that, in classical PKU, high blood concentrations of phenylalanine are harmful in older patients, although less so than during the brain growth spurt. Treatment is, therefore, recommended beyond age 8 years and into adult life, although some relaxation of the diet has usually to be tolerated.

The phenylketonuric fetus of a heterozygote mother is not exposed to elevated concentrations of phenylalanine during gestation and the phenylketonuric infant is essentially normal at birth. In the reverse situation, the heterozygous fetus of an untreated phenylketonuric mother is at risk from the high maternal phenylalanine. During the first trimester, phenylalanine is teratogenic, and cardiac and skeletal malformations are seen in some affected infants. All exhibit intrauterine growth retardation, microcephaly and mental retardation with a characteristic facies. To minimize risks to the fetus it is now recommended practice to monitor and control the concentrations of phenylalanine and tyrosine starting before conception and continuing throughout pregnancy, aiming at a blood phenylalanine below 400 μmol/L. Fetal phenylalanine concentrations are considerably higher than those in the maternal circulation. This increases the risk of failure of dietary control. Paternal PKU is not associated with abnormalities in the offspring.[40]

The success of treatment and the progress of patients have been assessed by monitoring changes in blood phenylalanine and relating them to IQ, taking into account pretreatment blood concentrations, and any delay before treatment. The results of dietary challenges and enzyme activities in liver biopsies are also considered where available. Increasingly, noninvasive, physiological and neuropsychological investigations and magnetic resonance imaging provide information about structural changes. The interpretation of this gamut of information is difficult. The benefits of the dietary treatment are beyond dispute. It is also established that the nearer to normal the mean blood phenylalanine over the first 4 years of life, the better is the outcome. The extent to which factors other than dietary control affect outcome is uncertain. Problems of language development and behaviour are common. Able, caring parents who provide a stimulating environment are also likely to succeed with dietary treatment. Failure to maintain progress when the diet is relaxed may be attributed to the increased phenylalanine intake but may also reflect damage to the brain sustained much earlier. It may be difficult to decide whether any deficits are the consequence of mild or moderate elevation of blood phenylalanine over long periods, or of gross elevations over short periods, which may occur during infections or other acute illness.

It has now been established by the techniques of molecular biology that human phenylalanine hydroxylase is encoded by a single gene on chromosome 12. The normal gene and several mutant genes have been cloned and sequenced.[37] PKU is genetically and phenotypically heterogeneous, caused by mRNA splicing and mutations and deletions that inactivate the gene product by a variety of mechanisms and to a varying extent. For example, the Arg-Glu mutation at codon 261 results in a mild variant with little or no mental retardation, but a blood phenylalanine concentration high enough to cause the maternal PKU syndrome. The correlation between enzyme activity and phenylalanine tolerance is not close at low levels of enzyme activity. This introduces uncertainty into the interpretation of results for cohorts of patients; these include unknown proportions of less severe variants, whose blood phenylalanine is easier to control and who are better able to tolerate dietary indiscretions. The less severe manifestation of the disorder in some populations might be explained by a higher prevalence of less severe mutations reinforced in some cases by traditional infant diets of low protein content.

Adult patients with phenylketonuria who wish to have children, their prospective partners, and the parents of an affected child may require genotyping or prenatal diagnosis. Relatively simple techniques have been evolved using appropriate oligonucleotide probes, the polymerase chain reaction and dot-blot hybridization, which allow identification of both homozygotes and heterozygotes in 90% of cases. A substantial proportion of parents of phenylketonurics reject prenatal diagnosis and are willing to accept another phenylketonuric child. This is attributed to efficiency of treatment but may also reflect a wish on the parts of the parents not to make a decision that could be interpreted as a rejection of their affected child.

Histidinaemia[31]

In this aminoaciduria there is a block in the first step in the catabolism of histidine, its transformation to urocanic acid. As a consequence, histidine accumulates in body fluids and there is excessive excretion of imidazole pyruvic acid and other imidazoles. The metabolic phenotype has many analogies with PKU and the first few cases described had neuropsychiatric deficits including delayed language development. The biochemical abnormality was therefore assumed to be responsible for the clinical findings, and mass screening of neonates and treatment with a diet low in histidine was started in some centres. However, both prospective and retrospective studies have led to the conclusion that the overwhelming majority of histidinaemic infants do not require treatment. Nevertheless, histidinaemia may carry with it enhanced vulnerability of the nervous system, such as a lowered seizure threshold, and treatment has to be considered in histidinaemic infants with neurological symptoms. Children born to histidinaemic mothers do not show any of the signs seen in maternal phenylketonuria and are not retarded. Blood histidine concentrations in histidinaemia tend to be considerably lower on a molar basis than blood phenylalanine levels in PKU, due perhaps to the lower histidine content of our diet and the higher renal clearance of histidine relative to phenylalanine. This may at least in part explain the benign nature of this disorder.

Non-ketotic Hyperglycinaemia[14,31,45]

In man, hyperglycinaemia occurs with ketosis in some organic acidaemias. This form of hyperglycinaemia is referred to as *ketotic hyperglycinaemia*. Hyperglycinaemia without ketosis, *non-ketotic hyperglycinaemia*, is associated with deficiency of the glycine cleavage system, a multi-enzyme complex in mitochondria consisting of four protein subunits and requiring NAD, pyridoxal phosphate, lipoic acid and tetrahydrofolate as cofactors. Mutations affecting three of these subunits have been identified. The enzyme system is present in liver and brain, and it is the almost complete lack of activity of the brain enzyme that results in extreme myotonia, myoclonic fits, apnoeic episodes and a characteristic electroencephalogram with paroxysmal bursts on an almost flat record. Symptoms usually start within hours or days of birth and more than half the infants die in the first 30 days. Survivors are nearly always severely retarded. Some patients with a somewhat less acute course may present at a later age, and very rarely as adults with slowly progressive motor-neuron disease. A significant biochemical finding is a marked increase in the cerebrospinal fluid : plasma glycine ratio.

The role of glycine as an inhibitory neurotransmitter in the brainstem and spinal cord is well established. In mammals, both the influx of glycine into the brain and its neurotoxicity are strongly age dependent, being much greater in the newborn. The higher influx is required for the highly active protein synthesis characteristic of the developing brain. The glycine cleavage system presumably acts as a safety valve to prevent undue accumulation of glycine, particularly where it might interfere with neurotransmission. Toxic amounts will build up if the delicate balance is upset between dietary intake and synthesis, the active transport systems for influx and efflux of the amino acid, and the cleavage system.

Glycine binds to a strychnine-sensitive receptor and causes increased chloride conductance and hyperpolarization. Recent evidence suggests that glycine is also an allosteric modulator at the N-methyl-D-aspartate (NMDA) receptor where it potentiates activity of excitatory amino acid neurotransmitters such as glutamate. It may also enhance NMDA-mediated neurotoxicity.

Attempts to treat have included removal of glycine by exchange transfusions, haemodialysis or high-dose benzoate, supply of cofactors for the glycine cleavage system, and use of glycine antagonists such as strychnine and benzodiazepines. Combination of these strategies has in some cases relieved symptoms and delayed progress of the disease but without lasting benefits. This is not surprising as it appears that the pathogenic processes start before birth. Reliable prenatal diagnosis is not yet available, nor are there reliable estimates of the incidence of the disorder, as an unknown proportion of patients die undiagnosed.

Homocystinuria[14,31]

Excess of homocystine in urine is found in several inborn errors of metabolism. Of these, deficiency of cystathionine β-synthase is the most important. This enzyme catalyses the formation of cystathionine from homocysteine in the trans-sulphuration pathway from methionine to cystine. Clinical signs are absent in the newborn or young infant. They develop with age and include long, thin limbs and other skeletal abnormalities reminiscent of Marfan's syndrome, sparse and brittle hair, a malar flush and, most characteristic, dislocation of the lenses, which usually presents by the age of 3 years. Excess of methionine and homocystine (formed by the condensation of two molecules of homocysteine) is found in the blood, and there is increased excretion of homocystine, methionine and other sulphur amino acids, notably the cysteine–homocysteine disulphide. Most patients are diagnosed clinically. The concentrations of methionine and homocystine are not sufficiently elevated in blood to permit reliable detection by routine screening of the newborn.

Less than half the patients with homocystinuria are severely retarded. Abnormal electroencephalograms, epilepsy or psychiatric disorders are found in many patients with homocystinuria, including those of normal or high intelligence. The pathogenesis of the mental defect is uncertain.

Homocystine interferes with the formation of the normal cross-links of collagen, resulting in damage to the intima of arteries, platelet adhesion to the damaged surface and thromboembolic episodes. At autopsy, multiple infarcted areas have been found in the brains of some patients; these may account for some of the intellectual deficits and gradual intellectual deterioration seen in this disorder. A causal relation between the inborn error and psychiatric illness has not been established. Homocysteic acid is present in excess in body fluids. It is an excitatory amino acid and therefore a potent agonist of the NMDA receptor and may be responsible for some of the neurological complications of homocystinuria. Recently developed competitive NMDA antagonists and non-competitive channel blockers may assume a role in treatment.

The disorder is genetically heterogeneous. This is shown by *in vitro* studies on the enzyme in fibroblasts, and a variable response of patients to treatment with pyridoxine: nearly half of them respond to pharmacological doses (100–500 mg/day) of the vitamin both biochemically and clinically. Pyridoxal phosphate is the cofactor of cystathionine synthase. The mechanism whereby cofactor supplementation restores or preserves enzyme activity is not clear.

A diet low in methionine and supplemented with cystine, and in some cases also with folate or betaine, corrects the biochemical abnormalities in all variants of the disorder and is the only effective treatment for pyridoxine-unresponsive patients. Normal or near-normal somatic and intellectual development has been reported for early-treated patients. The effects of treatment on the long-term sequelae—thromboembolism, dislocation of the lenses and osteoporosis—remain to be evaluated.

The remethylation pathway from homocystine to methionine is as important as the trans-sulphuration pathway. Inborn errors are known that affect two of the enzymes involved: N^5-methyltetrahydrofolate homocysteine methyltransferase and $N^{5,10}$-methylenetetrahydrofolate reductase. In these disorders, increased excretion of homocystine is accompanied by a normal or decreased blood methionine.

Transferase deficiency has been described in several patients, with a broad spectrum of clinical manifestations. The deficiency may be caused by a defect in the apoenzyme, by a defect in methylcobalamin synthesis leading to homocystinuria and hypomethioninaemia, or by a combined defect of methylcobalamin and adenosylcobalamin synthesis, which presents as homocystinuria, methylmalonic aciduria and hypomethioninaemia. Lesions of the central nervous system resemble those seen in severe vitamin B_{12} deficiency. Early, aggressive treatment with hydroxycobalamin is essential to prevent mental retardation; the long-term outlook for these patients is uncertain.

Reductase deficiency is also associated with a wide range of adverse consequences, especially mental retardation. The nervous system is at risk from both homocystinuria and folate deficiency. Treatment with folate derivatives, methionine, betaine, pyridoxine and cobalamin, singly or in combination, must start early. Results have been variable, influenced by the genetic heterogeneity of the disorder.

Hyperammonaemias[11,14,31,36]

Ammonia is a major product of nitrogen catabolism. It is formed endogenously by deamination of amino acids and the breakdown of purines and pyrimidines, or it may be absorbed from the alimentary tract, where it is produced by bacterial action. Ammonia is constantly produced in the brain, and in increased amounts during convulsions. High concentrations are extremely toxic to the nervous system. Detoxication occurs mainly in the liver by transformation to urea by the urea-cycle enzymes (Table 16.15). The cycle is not effective in the brain, owing to the virtual absence of the mitochondrial enzymes carbamyl phosphate synthase and ornithine carbamyl transferase. Ammonia can also be metabolized by the formation of glutamine from glutamate and glutamate from oxoglutarate. These mechanisms operate in the brain but large increases in brain glutamine may, by their osmotic effects, exacerbate brain oedema, while glutamate formation from oxoglutarate tends to deprive the citric acid cycle of one of its constituents. Most of the ammonia formed in brain must be transported to the liver for conversion into urea.

The mechanisms whereby ammonia exerts its toxic action on the brain are still conjectural.[41] Functional disturbances are observed well before measurable effects on the energy metabolism of the brain; reduction in high-energy phosphate compounds is pronounced in the late stages of severe poisoning associated with coma. Ammonia has an excitant effect exerted by interference with pre- and postsynaptic inhibition, and a repressant effect associated with reduced concentrations of the excitatory neurotransmitters glutamate and aspartate. Interpretation of neurological signs is rendered more difficult by the possibility of selective depletion of energy stores in vulnerable regions of the brain and compartmentalization of ammonia within the cell. Overall levels of brain ammonia and oxygen consumption are poor guides to an understanding of pathogenesis. The most severe damage is associated with brain oedema, due to failure of the mitochondria-rich endothelial cells of the brain capillaries to maintain the integrity of the blood–brain barrier, and astrocytic swelling exacerbated by raised intracellular concentrations of glutamine, and myelin oedema.[42,43]

Hyperammonaemia may occur as a primary event due to an inborn error of one of the urea-cycle enzymes, as a secondary phenomenon in liver disease, or in any disorder that prejudices the metabolic integrity of the mitochondrion in which some of the reactions of the urea cycle take place (Table 16.15). Complete blocks of the urea cycle are probably incompatible with life. Severely affected patients present in the neonatal period with lethargy, fits, vomiting, coma and death. Patients with less severe disease and some residual enzyme activity develop symptoms in infancy or childhood. Persistent vomiting, failure to thrive and mental retardation are common signs. Symptoms may be triggered by infection and exacerbated by high protein intake. Even mildly affected patients may have episodes of acute illness with ataxia, alterations in consciousness and other neurological signs. Some patients have died during such acute episodes, owing to the development of brain oedema. Hyperammonaemia should be excluded in any mentally retarded child who develops an encephalitis-like illness.

Among environmental causes of hyperammonaemia is *Reye's encephalopathy*.[32,43] In this syndrome, transaminases are usually greatly elevated and hypoglycaemia is a characteristic finding. Plasma lactate, free fatty acids, triglycerides and alanine are often raised, and prothrombin time prolonged, in the absence of jaundice. The syndrome usually follows a viral infection, but a similar clinical pattern is seen in

TABLE 16.15
THE HYPERAMMONAEMIAS

Cause	Comments
Primary deficiencies of urea-cycle enzymes	
N-acetyl glutamate synthetase	Mitochondrial enzyme: neonatal onset; extremely rare
Carbamyl phosphate synthetase	Mitochondrial enzyme: requires N-acetyl glutamate as activator
Ornithine carbamyl transferase	X-linked: partial deficiencies occur; heterozygotes detectable in informative families by RFLP[a]; or by assay of urine orotic acid after allopurinol load
Argininosuccinate synthetase	Citrullinaemia; cytosolic enzyme; mild and atypical cases occur
Argininosuccinate lyase	Argininosuccinic aciduria: cytosolic enzyme; variable presentation; detectable by amino acid chromatography; often by characteristic microscopic appearance of hair
Arginase	Vomiting, fits, spastic tetraplegia, mental retardation, argininaemia, dibasic amino aciduria, orotic aciduria, milder cases occur
Other hereditary disorders	
Hyperornithinaemia, hyperammonaemia, homocitrullinuria	HHH syndrome: diminished ornithine transport into mitochondrion; lethargy, vomiting, dyskinesia; improvement on low protein intake; variable intellectual development
Lysinuric protein intolerance	Renal and intestinal defect of cationic amino-acid transport: vomiting, diarrhoea, failure to thrive; variable mental development: dibasic amino aciduria; hyperammonaemia after protein ingestion
Some organic acidaemias	Hyperammonaemia notable particularly in propionic, methylmalonic and isovaleric acidaemias; metabolic acidosis
Secondary hyperammonaemias	
Reye's syndrome	See text: may be caused or simulated by numerous viruses, aflatoxins; hypoglycin, pesticides, sodium valproate; aspirin; urea-cycle enzyme deficiencies and many organic acidurias
Hypoxia–ischaemia	Plasma ammonia elevated in asphyxiated neonates
Shock	Elevated concentrations found in shock but may be absent in haemorrhagic shock encephalopathy
Intravenous feeding	Risk of hyperammonaemia higher in low birth-weight infants; may in part be due to insufficiency of arginine
Diffuse liver failure	Raised concentrations found in acute fulminating and advanced chronic liver disease
Sodium valproate therapy	Elevation of plasma ammonia variable
Transient hyperammonaemia of the newborn	Cause unknown: may be life-threatening and require prompt treatment; may be caused by poor perfusion of liver
Urinary tract infection	Urea-splitting organisms liberate large amounts of ammonia, which may be absorbed from urinary tract
Non-specific causes	Fits, severe infections and any systemic illness in young babies may be accompanied by mild to moderate elevation of the plasma ammonia

[a] RFLP, restriction fragment length polymorphism.

some organic acidurias, as a rare complication of treatment with some drugs (e.g. valproate), and after ingestion of some toxins. Signs include vomiting, stupor, hyperventilation and, in severe cases, coma, opisthotonus and cerebral oedema. With the best treatment survival is about 90% but some survivors are left with neurological and mental handicap. A high blood ammonia carries a poor prognosis. Salicylate appears to increase the risk of developing the disorder; withholding the drug from infants and children has been accompanied by a reduced incidence.

Clinically, it is difficult to distinguish hyperammonaemia in young infants from conditions such as intracranial haemorrhage or septicaemia, which may also present with vomiting, lethargy and coma. To complicate matters, hyperammonaemia due to an enzyme deficiency is often associated with intracranial haemorrhage. Nor is the interpretation of biochemical investigations straightforward, as the correlation between the plasma ammonia and neurological signs is poor.[11,44] In young infants, concentrations below 100 μmol/L are difficult to interpret; at 100–200 μmol/L vomiting and ataxia usually occur; at higher concentrations there is a risk of stupor and coma. Abnormal amino-acid patterns help in the diagnosis of deficiencies of the cytosolic enzymes argininosuccinic acid synthase, argininosuccinase and arginase. Carbamyl phosphate accumulates in all urea-cycle disorders, except in deficiencies of syncarbamyl phosphate synthase or acetyl glutamate synthase, and leads to excessive urinary excretion of pyrimidines, which are diagnostically useful, as are the urinary ammonia: urea and ammonia:creatinine ratios. For the definitive diagnosis of deficiency of the mitochondrial enzymes in particular, enzyme assays on a liver biopsy are required. Interpretation may be difficult as urea-cycle enzymes show adaptive changes to protein intake. The mitochondrial enzymes are labile, making their assay difficult. They are also low in conditions of mitochondrial injury caused by environmental as well as inherited factors, for example in Reye's syndrome.

Secondary hyperammonaemia is treated by dealing, where possible, with the underlying cause, correcting metabolic derangements and, in Reye's syndrome in particular, controlling intracranial pressure. Low-protein diets are effective in some mildly affected patients with urea-cycle disorders but are often inadequate in promoting normal growth. Supplements of essential amino acids or their keto-analogues, and of arginine, are beneficial; in these patients, arginine is an essential amino acid and in citrullinuria and argininosuccinic aciduria it facilitates removal of ammonia via ornithine, by excretion as citrulline and argininosuccinate, respectively. The most effective therapeutic agents are phenylacetic acid and benzoic acid, which promote the excretion of nitrogenous compounds. Treatment of comatose hyperammonaemic patients with benzoic acid has led to clinical improvement and a return of the plasma ammonia to normal, in some cases. Haemodialysis is a treatment of last resort in patients with grossly elevated concentrations of ammonia. The long-term outlook for patients who present neonatally is poor; in the less severely affected, the chances of preventing mental retardation by timely and vigorous treatment of hyperammonaemic episodes are better.

All urea-cycle disorders are inherited as autosomal recessive traits, except ornithine carbamyl transferase, which is X-linked. Female carriers can be detected by a protein-load test, or preferably by the safer and more sensitive allopurinol-load test. Symptoms in female carriers vary widely as a result, presumably, of the extent to which normal or deficient chromosomes are inactivated (Lyon hypothesis). Even mildly affected carriers may show a slight reduction in intelligence. Prenatal diagnosis of urea-cycle disorders by recombinant DNA technology is increasingly available.

Other Aminoacidurias

Selected aminoacidurias and their relation to mental handicap are listed in Table 16.16. A detailed treatment of these and other aminoacidurias will be found in several recent publications. Of special interest here are disorders in which nervous function appears directly affected. The most likely site of the defect in *β-alaninaemia* is the enzyme β-alanine-α-oxoglutarate transaminase. In this very rare disorder, excess GABA as well as β-alanine are found in brain and body fluids; both are inhibitory neurotransmitters at a number of synapses. Symptoms in a thoroughly studied case included somnolence, hypotonia, diminished reflexes, fits and early death, a pattern not unlike that in neonatal non-ketonic hyperglycinaemia. In both disorders, failure to deal with accumulation of neurotransmitters results in rapid neurological deterioration.

Glutathione (L-glutamyl-L-cysteinylglycine) is present in virtually all mammalian tissues and takes part in a variety of metabolic processes. It is synthesized and degraded via five enzymatic reactions forming the *γ-glutamyl cycle*. Mental retardation has been a feature of the majority of patients with severe *glutathione synthase* deficiency. These patients present with life-threatening acidosis due to accumulation of the acid 5-oxoproline, and low tissue concentrations of glutathione. Failure to control the acidosis results in progressive neurological deterioration and mental retardation. Even early and sustained correction cannot safeguard normal intellectual development. All patients show decreased glutathione concentrations that may prejudice cellular protection mechanisms in which glutathione is involved; most also show an increased rate of haemolysis.

Mental retardation has also been a feature of three patients so far described with *γ-glutamyl transferase* deficiency (glutathioninuria). The enzyme catalyses the initial step in glutathione degradation—the transfer of the γ-glutamyl moiety from glutathione to an amino acid or other acceptor. The γ-glutamyl amino acids are transported more readily into cells than other amino acids, but no generalized defect of amino acid transport has been observed in kidney or fibroblasts from patients. However, it has been suggested that γ-glutamyl transferase could have a more restricted but essential function in the nervous system, for example in the transport of biologically active peptides.

Disease-related changes in neuropeptides have been postulated in *carnosinaemia*, in which elevated concentrations of carnosine (β-alanyl histidine) are formed in the body fluids; and in *homocarnosinosis*, in which elevated concentrations of homocarnosine (γ-aminobutyryl histidine) are found in cerebrospinal fluid. It is now considered that both disorders are due to carnosinase deficiency. There is no proof that the mental retardation and other neurological symptoms found in the majority of patients are causally related to the enzyme deficiency. In the brain, peptides may function as neurotransmitters and modulators of synaptic processes; investigation of their role in neurological disease is attracting increasing attention.

Disorders of GABA Metabolism[45]

Most disorders of amino acids and organic acids have been discovered by investigation of blood and urine. Abnormalities confined to cerebrospinal fluid

TABLE 16.16

SELECTED AMINOACIDURIAS IN RELATION TO MENTAL HANDICAP

Disorder	Comment
Untreated disorder generally associated with mental handicap	See text
Phenylketonuria, homocystinuria, non-ketotic hyperglycinaemia, β-alaninaemia, urea-cycle disorders	
Hyperornithinaemia (HHH)	Ornithine transport into mitochondria deficient: associated with hyperammonaemia and homocitrullinuria; clinically resembles urea-cycle defects
Hypervalinaemia	Defective transamination of valine: extremely rare
Hyperleucine–isoleucinaemia	Defective transmination of leucine and isoleucine: extremely rare
Tyrosinaemia type II	Defect in cytoplasmic tyrosine amino transferase: oculocutaneous involvement
Pipecolic acidaemia	L-Pipecolic acid oxidase deficiency: part of generalized peroxisomal deficiency of Zellweger syndrome
Sulphite oxidase deficiency	Dislocation of lenses, fits, dystonia and dyskinesia; sulphite and S-sulphocysteine detected in urine
Methylene tetrahydrofolate reductase deficiency	Homocystinuria, fits, folate and neurotransmitter defects, low methionine concentrations
Methyl tetrahydrofolate homocysteine methyltransferase deficiency	Homocystinuria, megaloblastic anaemia, low methionine concentrations, defect in methylcobalamin synthesis; responds to B_{12} therapy
γ-Glutamyl transferase deficiency	Glutathioninuria, behaviour disorders: very rare
Glutathione synthase deficiency	Massive oxoprolinuria, hypoglutathioninaemia, haemolytic disorders
Lowe's syndrome	Generalized renal aminoaciduria, cataracts, buphthalmos, rickets, dwarfism
No causal relation to mental defect established but disorder may enhance vulnerability of nervous system	
Histidinaemia	See text
Sarcosinaemia	Sarcosine oxidase deficiency
Cystathioninuria	Cystathioninase deficiency: also caused by some tumours, liver disease, B_6 and B_{12} deficiency
Hyperprolinaemia type I	Proline oxidase deficiency
Hyperprolinaemia type II	Δ-Pyrroline-5-carboxylic acid dehydrogenase deficiency
Hydroxyprolinaemia	Hydroxyproline oxidase deficiency
Hyperlysinaemia-saccharopinuria	Defects in bifunctional 2-aminoadipic semialdehyde synthase: often asymptomatic
2-Aminoadipic aciduria	2-Ketoadipic acid dehydrogenase deficiency: no consistent clinical pattern
Carnosinaemia, homocarnosinosis	Carnosinase deficiency: benign disorder sometimes secondary to urea-cycle defect, liver disease or muscular dystrophy
Glutamate formimino transferase deficiency	Marked excretion of formiminoglutamic acid; clinical presentation variable; ascertainment bias
γ-Glutamylcysteine synthase deficiency	Low blood glutathione, aminoaciduria, spinocerebellar degeneration, extremely rare
Hartnup disease	Transport defect of monoamino monocarboxylic amino acids: symptoms of pellagra occasionally seen
Lysinuric protein intolerance	Transport defect of dibasic amino acids: postprandial hyperammonaemia, muscle hypotrophy, osteoporosis; low protein diet and citrulline supplements helpful

are less accessible to study yet are likely to be more directly related to dysfunction of the nervous system, particularly when neurotransmitters or their derivatives are involved. GABA is a major inhibitory neurotransmitter present in high concentration in the brain. It is mainly formed from glutamate (an excitatory neurotransmitter) by glutamate decarboxylase, and metabolized by GABA transaminase to succinic semialdehyde, then by semialdehyde dehydrogenase to succinic acid, which is oxidized in the citric acid cycle. In cerebrospinal fluid, GABA occurs both free and in the form of peptides, notably homocarnosine.

Pyridoxine-dependent convulsions are believed to be a consequence of a deficiency of GABA due to a defect at the pyridoxal phosphate binding site of glutamate decarboxylase. Convulsions may start before or soon after birth and are refractory to anticonvulsants. The defect is specific; other enzymes requiring pyridoxal phosphate are not affected. There is an immediate and sustained response to pharmacological doses of pyridoxine. Some patients present at a somewhat later age and with prolonged seizure-free intervals. A trial of pyridoxine is therefore recommended for all seizure disorders with onset before 18 months of age. Low concentrations of GABA and homocarnosine have been reported in a variety of neurological disorders, unresponsive to pyridoxine and not in all cases associated with convulsions. In some of these, symptomatic improvement was achieved by treatment with the anticonvulsant γ-vinyl GABA, an irreversible inhibitor of GABA transaminase.

Succinic semialdehyde dehydrogenase deficiency has been documented in over 15 cases. Clinical features include ataxia, hypotonia, varying degrees of mental retardation, and sometimes choreoathetosis and convulsions. The salient feature of the disorder is the presence in body fluids of 4-hydroxybutyric acid formed by the reduction of succinic semialdehyde; 4-hydroxybutyric acid has anaesthetic properties. An attempt to reduce its accumulation by γ-vinyl GABA resulted in sustained improvement in one case.

GABA transaminase deficiency is an extremely rare condition with severe psychomotor retardation, hypotonia, convulsions and hypersecretion of growth hormone resulting in abnormally accelerated linear growth. GABA concentrations in cerebrospinal fluid are grossly elevated and there are also increases in the levels of homocarnosine, other GABA peptides and β-alanine. Attempts at treatment with pyridoxine and picrotoxin, a non-competitive GABA antagonist, were unsuccessful. *β-Alaninaemia*, also extremely rare, is presumed to be caused by a genetically distinct transaminase with different substrate preference. The concentration of GABA in CSF is elevated but less so than β-alanine. Symptoms include fits unresponsive to pyridoxine or anticonvulsants.

ORGANIC ACIDURIAS[31,46-48]

Disorders of Pyruvate and Lactate Metabolism

Pyruvate occupies a key position in the metabolism of all animal cells. Even moderate impairment of its metabolism may result in profound biochemical abnormalities, neurological symptoms, mental retardation or death. The major pathways of pyruvate utilization are:

1 transamination to alanine;
2 reduction to lactate;
3 carboxylation to oxaloacetate;
4 oxidative decarboxylation via pyruvate dehydrogenase, the citric acid cycle and the respiratory chain.

The transamination is reversible and alanine and lactate may become a source of glucose. Pyruvate carboxylase is the first step in the gluconeogenic pathway; its product oxaloacetate is a neurotransmitter and a precursor of aspartate, which primes the citric acid cycle.

Pyruvate dehydrogenase is a multi-enzyme system made up of three catalytic complexes: E_1 (pyruvate decarboxylase), E_2 (dihydrolipoyltransacylase) and E_3 (lipoamide dehydrogenase) requiring thiamine, lipoic acid and riboflavin for activity. Pyruvate dehydrogenase is activated by pyruvate dehydrogenase phosphatase and deactivated when phosphorylated by pyruvate dehydrogenase kinase. There is relatively little excess of this enzyme system, particularly in the brain, and a small reduction in activity may lead to impaired production of acetyl CoA, enhanced glycolysis, accumulation of lactic and pyruvic acid, and eventually, lack of ATP. Impairment of pyruvate oxidation can compromise brain function by affecting the synthesis of acetylcholine and other neurotransmitters long before there is a drop in high-energy compounds. Formations of high metabolic activity, notably the basal ganglia and brainstem, are particularly vulnerable. Some cases have shown cerebral atrophy and generalized neuronal loss. In others, necrotic areas have been prominent in the brainstem and basal ganglia, lesions typical of *Leigh's encephalopathy*, subacute necrotizing encephalomyelopathy. These lesions also occur in conditions such as pyruvate carboxylase deficiency and cytochrome oxidase deficiency.

Over 60 cases with hereditary deficiency of pyruvate dehydrogenase have been described. The most common and best studied mutation is deficiency of complex $E_{1\alpha}$. All affected patients have been mentally retarded but age of onset and severity have varied very widely. Some patients succumb by the age of 6 months; in some, brain lesions and facial dysmorphisms suggest that the pathogenetic process was active before birth; in others hypotonia, fits and ataxia are seen; in milder cases symptoms are limited to poor coordination and ataxia. The severity of symptoms correlates well with the severity of the lactic acidosis but not with the residual enzyme activity; patients with 40–50% activity may be symptomatic. Elevation of lactate and pyruvate concentrations in blood may be only intermittent, even in symptomatic patients, but pyruvate is always high 1 h after a standard glucose load. Urine lactate may be markedly elevated, particularly during acute episodes.

In a few cases, mutations have affected the activating phosphatase or complex E_3. As complex E_3 also forms part of α-oxoglutarate and branched-chain α-oxoacid dehydrogenase, elevation of pyruvate and concentrations of lactate are accompanied by elevation of α-oxoglutarate and branched-chain amino acids in the body fluids of these patients, as well as some of the organic acids also seen in maple-syrup urine disease.

Deficiency of pyruvate dehydrogenase may be acquired, for example, because of thiamine deficiency or heavy metal poisoning, or due to the action of any toxin or metabolite that causes mitochondrial damage and a general decrease of mitochondrial enzyme activity.

Pyruvate dehydrogenase deficiency has been

treated by a high-fat, low-carbohydrate diet, to provide an alternative oxidative substrate for brain mitochondria; this may slow down but does not prevent or reverse neurological deterioration. Cholinergic agonists such as physostigmine have been used in an attempt to counteract inhibition of acetylcholine synthesis. Thiamin and lipoic acid, cofactors, and dichloracetate, an inhibitor of the deactivating enzyme pyruvate dehydrogenase kinase, have also been used, none with sustained benefit. One patient had a dramatic and sustained response to thiamin, and appears to have a true thiamin dependency.

Pyruvate carboxylase, a biotin-containing protein, occupies a key position in the control of gluconeogenesis in liver and kidney, and in the maintenance of constituents of the citric acid cycle in brain. Pyruvate carboxylase deficiency presents in two ways: a severe form with complete absence of the enzyme, neonatal presentation and early death, and a somewhat milder form with some residual enzyme activity, later presentation and long survival. Symptoms include fits, hypotonia, psychomotor retardation and occasionally hypoglycaemia. In the severe form, depletion of oxaloacetate is accompanied by depletion of aspartate. This affects the urea cycle, leading to citrullinaemia and hyperammonaemia, and the aspartate shuttle, resulting in intramitochondrial acidosis and a raised lactate:pyruvate ratio.

In both forms of the disorder, damage to the nervous system is severe and widespread. In particular, it appears that the *de novo* synthesis of the neurotransmitters glutamic acid and GABA is prejudiced, as well as replenishment of citric acid intermediates in neurons.

Mitochondrial Respiratory-Chain Disorders[31,49,50]

The primary function of the mitochondrion is to produce ATP by oxidative phosphorylation. Defects may occur in substrate transport or utilization, in the citric acid cycle, or in the reactions of the respiratory chain. The respiratory chain transfers electrons from reduced pyridine and flavin nucleotides to oxygen. It consists of five complexes made up of 67 protein subunits. The majority of these are encoded by nuclear DNA. However, 1% of total cellular DNA is contained within the mitochondrion in the form of a circular molecule of 16 569 bp (mtDNA), which encodes for 13 of the subunits. It has been shown that mitochondrial DNA is transmitted exclusively via the ovum, with no contribution from sperm.

The mitochondrial disorders are a clinically heterogeneous group of diseases characterized by abnormal mitochondrial proliferation in skeletal muscle and other affected cells. There is evidence that in some cases the defect may not be inherited, but can be caused by microangiopathy, viruses, poisons such as the 1-methyl-4-phenylpyridium ion, or autoimmune mechanisms. In many but not all patients, muscle biopsies stained with Gomori trichrome show 'red ragged fibres'. Mitochondrial dysfunction is accompanied by lactic acidosis, raised lactate:pyruvate ratios and acetoacetate:β-hydroxybutyrate ratios. No single clinical phenotype appears to be exclusive to any defect in the respiratory chain. Phenotypic expression is determined by the distribution and severity of the metabolic block in different organs. Differential tissue expression could be the result of tissue-specific isoenzymes or organ-specific regulation of enzyme activity.

Recently, three syndromes associated with cognitive deficits have attracted much attention. They are the *Kearns–Sayre* (KS) syndrome of progressive external ophthalmoplegia, pigmentary retinopathy, ataxia, deafness and high protein concentrations in cerebrospinal fluid; MERRFA (myoclonus epilepsy, red ragged fibres and ataxia); and MELAS (mitochondrial encephalomyopathy, lactic acidosis and stroke-like episodes).

In the majority of cases these syndromes are associated with mutations or deletions of mitochondrial DNA. Tests making possible the detection of these disorders in blood samples have recently been developed and will improve the diagnosis of these often ill-defined syndromes.

Disorders of lactate and pyruvate metabolism are summarized in Table 16.17.

Other Organic Acidurias

Organic acidurias are characterized by the excessive excretion in urine of aromatic or aliphatic carboxylic acids. These disorders are sometimes associated with overt metabolic acidosis and abnormalities of amino acid or carbohydrate metabolism. Organic acidurias are often hereditary and frequently present as life-threatening emergencies soon after birth. Less frequently they present later in the first year of life, with failure to thrive, vomiting, hypotonia and delayed milestones. Some patients develop normally until an infection, drug, starvation or dietary change precipitate metabolic crisis with involvement of the central nervous system. Clinical signs may include any of the following: fits, dystonia, ataxia and athetosis, neutropenia and thrombocytopenia, neurological deterioration and the characteristic symptoms of Reye's encephalopathy (p.301). Impairment of the mitochondrial function of the endothelial cells of brain capillaries may result from the combined effects of toxic metabolites, aciduria and infection, resulting in failure of the blood–brain barrier, brain oedema and irreversible brain damage. Congenital malformations may occur when there is interference with the energy supply to the developing embryo.

Organic acidurias do not lend themselves readily to screening by paper or thin-layer chromatography; gas chromatography with mass spectrometry or more sophisticated techniques such as fast-atom bombard-

TABLE 16.17
AETIOLOGY OF LACTIC ACIDOSIS

Cause	Comments
Environmental	
Microangiopathy, shock, cardiopulmonary disease	Poor delivery of oxygen to tissues
Uraemia, liver disease	Impaired metabolism and clearance
Acute infections, septicaemia	Assay of cerebrospinal fluid lactate has been used to diagnose meningitis
Diabetic ketoacidosis	
Inhibition of enzymes by drugs or poisons	Phenformin, cyanide, acetaldehyde, 1-methyl-4-phenylpyridium ion
Hereditary	
Disorders of pyruvate and lactate metabolism:	
Disorders of pyruvate dehydrogenase complex	Increased pyruvate; normal lactate : pyruvate ratio
Pyruvate carboxylase deficiency	Two variants: complete deficiency associated with hyperammonaemia and raised lactate : pyruvate ratio
2-Oxoglutarate dehydrogenase deficiency	Neurological deterioration, increased plasma 2-oxoglutarate; very rare
Fumarase deficiency	Developmental delay, excess succinate, fumarase and 2-oxoglutarate in urine; variable severity
Respiratory-chain disorders	Variable clinical presentation and prognosis; nervous system involvement and mental retardation common; mitochondrial DNA involved in some cases of KS, MERFFA and MELAS (see text)
Disorders of gluconeogenesis	See Table 16.10
Organic acidurias	'Secondary lactic acidosis' seen in propionic acidaemia, methylmalonic acidaemia and fatty-acid oxidation defects due to interference with CoA metabolism which affects pyruvate dehydrogenase

ment–mass spectrometry with stable isotope-dilution analysis are available. Proton nuclear magnetic resonance spectroscopy has also proved a powerful though technically complex method for the diagnosis and investigation of patients with organic acidurias. Because they are rare and carry a high mortality, organic acidurias do not contribute substantially to the prevalence of severe mental handicap. When the urine organic acids of 2000 severely retarded patients were examined, nearly all the observed abnormalities were attributable to drugs, diet or environmental factors.[51] An organic aciduria should nevertheless be considered in the differential diagnosis when the physician is confronted by a severe illness in a mentally retarded child that is of sudden onset and accompanied by biochemical findings such as refractory metabolic acidosis, hypoglycaemia with or without ketonuria, lactic acidosis, hyperammonaemia, and neurological signs. In most cases, meningitis, septicaemia or a cerebral catastrophe will provide an explanation for the symptoms. A screen for acute metabolic disorders will help to decide if advice from a specialized centre should be sought.

Selected organic acidurias are listed in Table 16.18. Few generalizations can be made about pathogenesis in these disorders but impairment of mitochondrial function plays an important part. Acyl-CoA derivatives competitively inhibit reactions involving acetyl CoA, a metabolite with a pivotal role in several metabolic pathways. For example, propionyl CoA can disrupt the citric acid cycle, particularly citrate synthesis and pyruvate oxidation, resulting in loss of energy and failure to thrive. Propionyl CoA also inhibits pyruvate carboxylase, for which acetyl CoA is a critical positive effector. The malate shuttle, essential for making oxaloacetate available for gluconeogenesis, is also inhibited. Gluconeogenesis is therefore seriously impaired and patients are prone to hypoglycaemia and lactic acidosis. Propionyl CoA also inhibits N-acetyl glutamate synthesis and carbamyl phosphate synthetase, reducing the effectiveness of the urea cycle (resulting in hyperammonaemia) and of the glycine cleavage system (resulting in hyperglycinaemia). Decreased production of acetyl CoA in carnitine deficiency or acyl-CoA dehydrogenase deficiency results in reduced pyruvate carboxylase activity, reduced gluconeogenesis and reduced ketone-body formation. The risk of hypoglycaemic brain damage is enhanced when ketone bodies are unavailable as an alternative fuel as in the Tildon–Cornblath syndrome or in β-hydroxy-β-methylglutaric acidaemia, or when ketogenesis is impaired because of a defect in mitochondrial β-oxidation of fatty acids.

Three distinct mitochondrial enzymes catalyse the dehydrogenation of long-, medium- and short-chain fatty acids. Of these, the long-chain dehydrogenase deficiency tends to be most severe, while that of the medium-chain dehydrogenase is most common. Classically, L-carnitine transports fatty acyl CoA as acylcarnitine into the mitochondrial matrix, to be reconverted to acyl CoA for β-oxidation. It also has a role

TABLE 16.18
SELECTED ORGANIC ACIDURIAS

Disorder	Comment
Involving gluconeogenesis and pyruvate metabolism	
Von Gierke's disease	Deficiency of glucose-6-phosphatase (GSD IA), glucose-6-phosphate translocase (GSD IB) or phosphotransferase (GSD IC): hypoglycaemia, lactic acidosis, hyperuricaemia, hepatomegaly, mental retardation preventable by control of hypoglycaemia
Fructose-1,6-bisphosphatase deficiency	Hypoglycaemia, lactic acidosis, ketosis after fasting; metabolic crises—preventable by dietary management
Pyruvate carboxylase deficiency	See text
Pyruvate dehydrogenase-complex disorders	See text
Phosphoenol pyruvate carboxykinase deficiency	Two isoenzyme forms: hypoglycaemia, hypotonia, hepatomegaly, mental retardation; extremely rare
Involving amino acid derivatives	
Maple-syrup urine disease (branched-chain amino acids)	Deficiency of branched-chain ketoacid dehydrogenase complex: acute neonatal, intermediate, intermittent and thiamine-responsive variants; treatment of severe variants mostly disappointing
Isovaleric acidaemia (leucine)	Isovaleryl-CoA dehydrogenase deficiency: acute neonatal and chronic intermittent presentation; characteristic odour; some patients mentally retarded; treatment by protein restriction, glycine and carnitine has greatly improved prognosis
3-Methylcrotonyl-CoA carboxylase deficiency (leucine)	Hypoglycaemia, acidosis, hypotonia; variable neurological presentation; treated by restriction of protein intake
3-Methylglutaconic aciduria (leucine)	Variable neurological presentation, acidosis not prominent; 3-methylglutaconyl-CoA hydratase involved but enzyme studies equivocal in most cases
3-Hydroxy-3-methylglutaryl-CoA lyase deficiency (leucine)	Severe acidosis, vomiting, hypotonia; resemble Reye's syndrome; lactic acidosis, deficient ketone-body production
Mevalonic aciduria (leucine)	Mevalonate kinase deficiency: variable neurological deficits; deficiency of vitamins A, D and E; very rare
2-Methylacetoacetyl-CoA thiolase deficiency (isoleucine)	Isoenzyme affected is mitochondrial and of high substrate specificity: episodes of acidosis, ketosis, vomiting and diarrhoea; treated by protein restriction; most patients of normal intelligence
Acetoacetyl-CoA thiolase deficiency (isoleucine)	Mitochondrial and cytosolic isoenzymes: variable neurological and biochemical presentation; very rare
3-Hydroxyisobutyryl-CoA deacylase deficiency (valine)	Multiple congenital malformations, possibly caused by accumulation in tissues of methacrylyl CoA, a teratogen in rats; exceedingly rare
Propionic acidaemia (valine, isoleucine)	Usually acute neonatal onset: caused by mutations in either of two carboxylase subunits; ketoacidosis, hyperammonaemia, hyperglycinaemia ('ketotic hyperglycinaemia'); prognosis generally poor
Methylmalonic acidaemias (valine, isoleucine)	Caused by two mutations involving methylmalonyl-CoA mutase, two involving synthesis of adenosylcobalamin and three involving adenosyl and methylcobalamin synthesis: findings include failure to thrive, lethargy and hypotonia; ketoacidosis, hyperammonaemia and hyperglycinaemia; severity of disorder variable; nearly half the patients are mentally retarded, some with defects in cofactor synthesis responsive to cobalamin supplements
2-Ketoadipic aciduria (lysine)	2-Ketoadipic acid dehydrogenase deficiency: clinical presentation variable; no causal relation to mental retardation established
Glutaric aciduria type I (lysine, tryptophan)	Glutaryl-CoA dehydrogenase deficiency: dystonia and athetosis; neurological deterioration; glutaric acid excretion may be intermittent (p. 279)
4-Hydroxybutyric aciduria (glutaric acid)	Succinic semialdehyde dehydrogenase deficiency: hypotonia, ataxia, variable degrees of mental retardation (see text)
2-Oxoprolinuria (glutathione)	Glutathione synthetase deficiency (see p. 277)
Miscellaneous	
Acyl-CoA dehydrogenase deficiencies	Very long, long, medium- and short-chain variants, variable severity of presentation: may resemble Reye's syndrome; episodes of hypoketotic hypoglycaemia, vomiting, coma may occur; mental retardation preventable in many cases by vigorous treatment of crises and avoidance of fasting

TABLE 16.18 (*contd*)

Disorder	Comment
Multiple acyl-CoA dehydrogenase deficiency	'Glutaric aciduria type II': due to defects in either electron transfer protein (ETP) or ETP–ubiquinone oxidoreductase (ETP–QO); presentation may be neonatal, severe with congenital malformations or milder with later onset; liver, kidney, brain and muscle affected; acidosis, hypoglycaemia, hypotonia, characteristic odour and increased urinary organic acids; very poor prognosis: some mild cases respond to riboflavin
Long-chain 3-hydroxyacyl-CoA dehydrogenase deficiency	Presentation often resembles Reye's syndrome; involvement of liver, heart and brain; high mortality but milder cases occur; hydroxydicarboxylic aciduria not diagnostic
Multiple carboxylase deficiency: Holocarboxylase synthetase deficiency	Early onset, hypotonia, fits, breathing and feeding problems, skin rashes, acidosis, hyperammonaemia, characteristic organic aciduria; neurological damage in many cases preventable by biotin supplements
Biotinidase deficiency	Fits, hypotonia, dyskinesia, deafness, optic atrophy, skin rash, mental retardation preventable by treatment with biotin; neonatal screening in operation in some countries
D-Glyceric acidaemia	D-Glyceric acid dehydrogenase deficiency: variable presentation includes mental retardation, acidosis, fits, hypotonia; may be associated with hyperglycinaemia
Systemic carnitine deficiency	Presentation may resemble Reye's syndrome; encephalopathic episodes, hypotonia, hypoglycaemia, dicarboxylic aciduria; in most cases secondary to fatty oxidation defects or excessive urinary losses
Tildon–Cornblath syndrome	Succinyl-CoA : 3-ketoacid-CoA transferase deficiency: intermittent severe ketoacidosis and hypoglycaemia; mental retardation preventable by prompt treatment
L-2 hydroxyglutaric aciduria	Progressive ataxia, mental retardation, leucoencephalopathy; L-2 hydroxyglutarate raised in CSF, plasma and urine; defect unknown

in detoxifying accumulating acyl groups. A metabolic block at any point in the pathway of β-oxidation results in excess excretion of dicarboxylic acids formed by ω-oxidation of the fatty acid above the block and of hydroxy acids by ω-1 oxidation. The metabolic pattern is complicated by peroxisomal oxidation of the initial products of ω- and ω-1 oxidation and glycine conjugates. In addition, there is an increased urinary excretion of acyl carnitines and a raised acyl carnitine:free carnitine ratio. The acyl carnitine profile provides valuable clues to the nature of the metabolic block in organic acidurias.

In all *acyl-CoA dehydrogenase deficiencies* the inability to oxidize fats effectively produces a tendency to fasting hypoglycaemia with inappropriately low ketonuria. Lethargy and vomiting, progressing in severe cases to coma, is a frequent presentation, which resembles Reye's syndrome. Some patients become ill and lose consciousness while normoglycaemic. It is significant that acyl compounds with more than three carbons have encephalopathic properties, and that octanoate, which is produced in patients with medium-chain acyl-CoA dehydrogenase deficiency, has been shown to damage brain mitochondria with impairment of energy metabolism and progression to cerebral oedema. Mortality has been high, particularly in undiagnosed patients, and some survivors have been left with mental retardation. Yet many patients are asymptomatic for long periods and attacks may be prevented by ensuring a regular caloric intake with a diet moderately high in carbohydrate and by guarding against fasting stress as in infections. L-Carnitine supplements are probably useful in preventing deterioration during infections. Investigation of asymptomatic siblings is mandatory.

Advances in the treatment of other organic acidurias have not been insignificant. For example, in isovaleric acidaemia a low protein diet has been combined with supplements of glycine to form isovaleryl glycine from toxic isovaleryl CoA. Carnitine supplements provide a further route for disposal as isovaleryl carnitine. Some patients with carboxylase deficiency improve when given biotin; they are 'cofactor responsive'. Patients with multiple carboxylase deficiency respond well; however, two patients with biotinidase deficiency were left with a hearing loss and optic atrophy. Four of six genotypes of methylmalonic acidaemia have a defect in cobalamin metabolism or transport and may respond to B_{12} therapy. Treatment with riboflavin, carnitine and a diet low in protein and fat has had some success in treating milder cases of multiple acyl-CoA dehydrogenase deficiency.

A diet low in branched-chain amino acids is life saving in branched-chain ketoaciduria. Cofactor unresponsive propionic and methylmalonic acidaemia have been treated by protein restriction, exchange transfusion, peritoneal dialysis and forced diuresis. Administration of large doses of carnitine has been instrumental in reversing episodes of decompensation

TABLE 16.19

CLASSIFICATION OF PEROXISOMAL DISORDERS

Nature of disorder	Comment
Impaired biogenesis of peroxisomes	All disorders in this group have multiple enzyme deficiencies
Zellweger's syndrome	Cerebrohepatorenal syndrome: characteristic appearance, rapid deterioration, recessive
Neonatal adrenoleucodystrophy	Recessive, slightly less severe than Zellweger's syndrome
Infantile Refsum disease	Least severe of this group; moderately dysmorphic, most patients survive infancy
Rhizomelic chondrodysplasia punctata	Severe shortening of proximal parts of limbs; incomplete impairment of peroxisomal biogenesis; some peroxisomal functions normal
Single peroxisomal enzyme defects	
X-linked adrenoleucodystrophy	Caused by defective activation of very long-chain fatty acids; lignoceryl-CoA synthase deficiency
3-Oxoacyl-CoA thiolase deficiency	Pseudo-Zellweger syndrome: phenotype resembles disorders with impaired biogenesis
Acyl-CoA oxidase deficiency	Pseudo-neonatal adrenoleucodystrophy, hypotonia, fits, mental retardation
Bifunctional enzyme deficiency	Defect confined to fatty acid oxidation
Refsum disease	Defect in phytanic acid oxidation: retinitis pigmentosa, ataxia, deafness, peripheral neuropathy
Hyperoxaluria I, acatalasaemia	Not associated with neurological signs or mental retardation

in methylmalonic aciduria. In general, the outcome for these, the most common organic acidurias, remains disappointing. The mortality is high and many of the survivors are mentally handicapped.

PEROXISOMAL DISORDERS AFFECTING THE BRAIN[31,45,52]

Peroxisomes are subcellular organelles, surrounded by a single membrane, which occur in all cells other than mature erythrocytes. They oxidize fatty acids, including the very long-chain fatty acids that are poorly handled by mitochondria, and have a key role in the synthesis of bile acids and plasmalogens (ether-linked glycerolipids). Plasmalogens are abundant in brain, especially in myelin. It is therefore not surprising that peroxisomal defects have been implicated in a number of disorders involving the nervous system. Peroxisomal function may be impaired if the organelles fail to be formed or maintained, or if there is hereditary deficiency of one or more peroxisomal enzymes. In the former, import of enzymes synthesized in the cytoplasm is defective; in single-enzyme defects the peroxisome structure is intact and the consequences will, as in other inborn errors, depend on the role of the enzyme affected (Table 16.19).

In the normal human brain between 7 and 10 weeks of gestational age, young neurons migrate to the cortical plate. Waves of later migration must pass through layers already formed. Neurons that do not migrate normally are at risk of stunting or early death. Defects in fatty acid oxidation in mitochondria and peroxisomes appear to interfere with neuronal migration. Absence of peroxisomes results in the striking and characteristic disorders of neuronal migration in Zellweger's syndrome; migrational defects and heterotopias are more variable in other peroxisomal disorders with impaired fatty-acid oxidation. Sudanophilic leucodystrophy is another pathological neurological disability, which is often most striking in neonatal adrenoleucodystrophy.

Disorders of peroxisome biogenesis or isolated defects of peroxisomal fatty-acid oxidation should be suspected in children who are dysmorphic and hypotonic and have neonatal seizures and psychomotor retardation. Other clues are retinal degeneration, impaired hearing, hepatomegaly with abnormal liver-function tests, renal cysts and chondrodysplasia punctata. All patients are mentally retarded but none of the other signs is obligatory; if two or more are present a peroxisomal disorder should be considered in the differential diagnosis. X-linked adrenoleucodystrophy, the most common peroxisomal disorder, may present with behavioural problems and learning difficulties at school; sometimes adrenal insufficiency is the first symptom. Biochemical investigation of the peroxisomal disorders is outlined in Table 16.20.

Prenatal diagnosis of peroxisomal disorders is well established using either chorionic villus samples or amniocytes. Heterozygotes for X-lined adrenoleucodystrophy can be detected by plasma C26:C22 fatty-acid ratios in most cases, or in informative families, by a tightly linked DNA probe. Dietary restriction of phytanic acid is beneficial in Refsum's disease; treatment of X-linked adrenoleucodystrophy by normalization of plasma very long-chain fatty acids, or bone marrow transplantation, is still experimental.

TABLE 16.20
PEROXISOMAL DISORDERS: BIOCHEMICAL FINDINGS

Plasma very long-chain fatty acids	Elevated in all disorders of peroxisome biogenesis and fatty acid oxidation, normal in adult Refsum disease and rhizomelic chondrodysplasia punctata; usually expressed as C26:C22 ratio
Plasmalogen concentrations in red cells or synthesis in fibroblasts	Abnormal in disorders of biogenesis and, characteristically, in rhizomelic chondrodysplasia punctata
Bile acids	Elevated levels of bile acid intermediates demonstrable in disorders of peroxisome biogenesis
Phytanic acid	Characteristic of adult Refsum disease also found in disorders of peroxisome biogenesis
Pipecolic acid	Nearly all patients with disorders of peroxisome biogenesis have elevated levels

OTHER NEUROMETABOLIC DISORDERS

Galactosaemia[31,33]

Most affected infants have life-threatening symptoms by the end of the first week of life. They include failure to thrive, vomiting, jaundice, liver disease progressing to cirrhosis, and aminoaciduria. Cataracts usually develop over a period of weeks, but some infants show signs of cataracts and cirrhosis at birth and these lesions are then not fully reversible. Mortality is high, even in rapidly diagnosed cases, as the metabolic defect is often aggravated by infection, notably *Escherichia coli* septicaemia. The disorder may be milder; some patients present at a later age with cataracts and mental retardation, while a few stay virtually symptom free and intellectually normal. The gene coding for galactose-1-phosphate uridyl transferase, the enzyme affected in galactosaemia, exhibits extensive polymorphism. Genetic heterogeneity accounts for the wide range of severity observed in the disorder.

The metabolic block in galactosaemia results in the accumulation of galactose and at least two potentially toxic derivatives, galactose-1-phosphate and galactitol. Many cases of galactosaemia have been detected when the finding of a non-glucose-reducing substance in the urine of a sick neonate was followed up. The disorder can also be readily detected in blood collected on filter paper by a variety of methods including fluorimetric assay of galactose-1-phosphate uridyl transferase, or detection of excess galactose and galactose-1-phosphate by enzymatic assay or thin-layer chromatography of eluates. Protocols suitable for mass screening of neonates have been validated but not widely adopted. Quantitative assay of galactose-1-phosphate uridyl transferase and studies of its stability, electrophoretic mobility and kinetic properties are required to distinguish variants of the enzyme. Some, like the Duarte variant, are benign and do not require treatment.

Treatment with a diet free from galactose is life saving and usually results in the reversal of acute symptoms, but it is very difficult to maintain a diet that contains no lactose, galactose or galactosides. Once mixed feeding is introduced, above abnormal concentrations of galactose-1-phosphate and galactitol persist. Uridine diphosphate galactose, an intermediary of galactose metabolism and an essential galactosyl donor in the synthesis of oligosaccharides, glycoproteins and glycolipids, is low in treated patients; uridine or inositol supplements have therefore been recommended to restore its concentration to normal. It has also been proposed, on the basis of animal experiments, that progesterone or folate supplements might enhance any residual enzyme activity to about 10% of normal, and thereby improve the outcome.

Unfortunately, even patients who are treated appropriately from soon after birth tend to have visiospatial difficulties and intellectual deficits of up to 20 IQ points compared to their unaffected siblings, and sometimes tremor and ataxia. Emotional and behavioural problems are common even in patients of normal intelligence. Retrospective analysis of the long-term results of treating several hundred patients in many countries showed that neither delay in diagnosis nor poor dietary compliance were related to the generally disappointing outcome.

Cataract formation in galactosaemia has been explained by accumulation of galactitol in the lens, which is associated with osmotic swelling. Cataract is the only consistently present clinical sign in *galactokinase deficiency*, and galactitol accumulation is the major metabolic abnormality in this disorder, which is not associated with mental retardation. The pathogenesis of the mental retardation in galactosaemia has not been satisfactorily explained. Pathogenetic processes have been shown to operate before birth. Any damage to the nervous system is likely to be made worse during the perinatal period, when liver and kidney function are impaired, and there is risk of cerebral oedema. The low availability of uridine diphosphate galactose may impair galactosylation. A reduction in cerebrosides and protein-bound hexosamine in the white matter has been reported in cases coming to autopsy. In galactosaemia there is also an increased incidence of dysfunction of the ovary, an organ with a high content of complexed galactose. Pending validation of new approaches to treatment, at-risk families are increasingly opting for prenatal diagnosis.

Endocrine Disorders

In the mentally retarded, endocrine disorders are more often the consequence of impairment of the nervous system than its cause. Exceptions are *congenital hypothyroidism* and *hypoparathyroidism*. Cretinism was once regarded as the main cause of backwardness. In French and German the words 'cretin' and idiot were used synonymously. Congenital hypothyroidism may be caused by maldevelopment or maldescent of the thyroid, inborn errors of metabolism of thyroid hormones, iodine deficiency, pituitary or hypothalamic disorders, and ingestion of goitrogens. In severe cases, symptoms include feeding difficulties, constipation, lethargy and prolonged jaundice; later, short stature and a characteristic facies. Affected neonates may, however, show few if any signs, and the diagnosis is frequently not clinically apparent.

Endemic cretinism has largely disappeared in developed countries. It is thought to be mainly due to severe maternal iodine deficiency at an early stage of fetal development but other factors are probably involved. Goitrous cretinism with mental retardation has been described in offspring of mothers who had excessive intake of iodine during pregnancy and in offspring of thyrotoxic mothers overtreated with antithyroid drugs. Mental retardation has also occurred in patients with several rare inborn errors of hormonogenesis, including iodide peroxidase defects, dehalogenase defects, and defects in thyroglobulin synthesis or disposal. Most frequent is non-goitrous cretinism associated with an absent, hypoplastic or aberrant gland. The overall incidence of congenital hypothyroidism is 1 in 3000 to 1 in 4000 births, making it the most common endocrine disorder in infants and an important, preventable cause of mental retardation.

Work on rats has established that thyroid deficiency *in utero* or early postnatal life leads to a reduction in brain growth and defective myelination. Cell acquisition, dendritic arborization, synaptic organization and the development of neurotransmitter systems are adversely affected, resulting in distortion of the 'chemical wiring' of the brain. In man, hypothyroidism is uncommon amongst the severely retarded. In a retrospective study a mean IQ of 80 was found for 141 hypothyroid children; 25 out of 90 children had an IQ below 75 on the WISC-R test.[53] Delay in diagnosis was associated with reduced intellectual performance, but other factors are also involved.[21] Thus, IQ was strongly correlated with parental social class, and there is some evidence that inadequate replacement therapy (TSH not normalized) results in suboptimal intellectual development. During preg-

nancy, maternal hormones cannot compensate for fetal thyroid deficiency. This results in morbidity in many aspects of cerebral function. Fortunately, the adverse effects of prenatal hypothyroidism are largely reversible in early-treated cases, and even late-treated cases may show significant improvement. Neonatal screening for congenital hypothyroidism has been introduced in most developed countries and has dramatically reduced the contribution by this disorder to the prevalence of mental handicap.

Mental retardation is not uncommon in *pseudo-hypoparathyrodism type Ia*[31] due to deficiency of the guanine nucleotide-binding protein that couples the hormone receptor to stimulation of adenylate cyclase. It is tempting to attribute the mental handicap to hypocalcaemia, a salient feature of the syndrome. However, in some late-onset cases, mental retardation and epilepsy precede the hypocalcaemia. In others, hypocalcaemia and the morphological features of the syndrome, such as short stature, round face, short neck and brachydactyly, may be present without mental retardation. It is thus not clear if the mental retardation is a consequence of the biochemical defect or of an associated heritable disorder.

The association of hypercalcaemia with mental handicap, a characteristic facies and supravalvular aortic stenosis or peripheral pulmonary aortic stenosis has been known for over 30 years. To distinguish the disorder from the hypercalcaemia due to excessive vitamin D intake, the condition is sometimes referred to as Williams' syndrome.[20] Correction of the hypercalcaemia by a diet low in calcium and vitamin D is not followed by improved intellectual progress. Mean IQs fall within the range 55–66. In Britain the incidence of the disorder is about 1 in 50 000 births. Its aetiology is obscure; it probably involves hemizygosity at the elastin locus of chromosome 7.

Hereditary Disorders of Trace-metal Metabolism

Wilson's disease[31] (hepatolenticular degeneration) is a rare autosomal recessive disorder in which copper accumulates in liver, brain, kidney, heart and cornea; in the cornea it produces the characteristic Kayser–Fleischer rings. Patients may present with hepatic disease, haemolytic anaemia, psychiatric symptoms or commonly with neurological signs largely attributable to dysfunction of basal ganglia. Biochemically, the concentration of caeruloplasmin, the major copper-transporting protein, is nearly always reduced, as is that of the total serum copper, while non-caeruloplasmin copper, which is much more loosely bound to protein, is raised. Biliary excretion of copper and its incorporation into caeruloplasmin are reduced, while urinary excretion is raised.

Early diagnosis is important, as effective treatment with copper-chelating agents is available. There are few diagnostic problems once symptoms have become established but early, presymptomatic diagnosis poses problems. Unexplained failure at school, such as poor concentration or deterioration in handwriting, may be an early sign in neurological cases. Differentiation of presymptomatic cases from heterozygotes may be equivocal as up to a quarter of these also have low concentrations of caeruloplasmin and copper, and are about a hundred times more common in the general population than homozygotes. A penicillamine challenge test is helpful in confirming the diagnosis. A liver biopsy or study of incorporation of radiolabelled copper into caeruloplasmin may be necessary for a firm diagnosis. The gene for Wilson's disease has been mapped to chromosome 13, and the underlying protein defect may soon be identified, paving the way to new approaches to precise diagnosis and treatment.

Menkes' syndrome, an X-linked disorder, is also caused by a defect in copper transport. Clinical signs include abnormal hair and facies, rapid neurological deterioration, changes in bone and blood vessels, hypopigmentation and hypothermia. The minority of patients who survive the first year of life are profoundly retarded. Serum copper and caeruloplasmin are low. Liver copper is reduced, as is that in most tissue except kidney and intestinal mucosa. Both absorption from the gastrointestinal tract and intracellular transport of copper are impaired, leading to failure of assembly of copper-containing enzymes. The clinical manifestations may largely be explained by failure of the copper-containing enzymes lysyl oxidase, dopamine β-hydroxylase, tyrosinase and superoxide dismatase. There is evidence that the pathogenetic process is already active *in utero*. Treatment with copper salts can normalize the serum copper but does not halt the neurological degeneration. Prenatal diagnosis is available and it has been suggested that affected fetuses might be treated *in utero* or after premature delivery. Milder variants have been described, including the *occipital horn syndrome* (previously known as X-linked Ehlers–Danlos syndrome or X-linked cutis laxa) with skin and joint laxity, diagnostic radiological changes and intelligence in the low normal to mildly retarded range.

More than a dozen patients have been described with a combined deficiency of the enzymes xanthine oxidase, sulphite oxidase and aldehyde dehydrogenase. All three enzymes share a pterin-derived cofactor. *Molybdenum cofactor deficiency*[14,31] is responsible for lack of activity of these enzymes in the presence of normal plasma concentration of molybdenum. Patients are severely mentally retarded, with dystonia, myoclonus, fits, xanthine stones and dislocated lenses. They excrete excess sulphite, thiosulphate, *S*-sulphocystein, xanthine and hypoxanthine, and very little urate and sulphate. At autopsy, the brain shows neuronal loss, demyelination, gliosis and status spongiosus, the lesions resembling those seen in isolated sulphite oxidase deficiency. Prenatal diagnosis is possible; treatment by restricting intake of sulphur amino acids and supplementation with sulphate and molybdate have not been successful.

Disorders of Purine and Pyrimidine Metabolism[14,31]

The *Lesch–Nyhan syndrome* is characterized by compulsive self-mutilation, choreoathetosis, spasticity, gout and severe mental retardation. The enzyme affected in this X-linked recessive disorder is hypoxanthine–guanine phosphoribosyl transferase (HGPRT). This enzyme plays a vital part in the feedback control of intracellular purine concentrations by purine salvage. Its deficiency results in overproduction and increased urinary excretion of purines (notably uric acid), urolithiasis and ultimately renal failure. Stone formation can be prevented by treatment with allopurinol. Unsolved problems are the pathogenesis and alleviation of the neurological symptoms. Of all tissues, the brain has the highest concentration of HGPRT, particularly in the basal ganglia. It has been suggested that this region of the brain has a limited capacity for *de novo* synthesis of purines and that failure of the salvage pathway results in depletion of some nucleotides, notably guanosine triphosphate, at periods of high demand such as the brain growth spurt, when nigrostriatal dopaminergic terminal arborization occurs. Synthesis of dopamine and serotonin may also be vulnerable, as formation of the precursors DOPA and 5-hydroxytryptophan requires a purine-derived cofactor.

The disorder is genetically heterogeneous and the severity of the symptoms correlates with the extent of the enzyme defect. Patients with a few per cent of normal enzyme activity develop gout at a comparatively early age but are otherwise unaffected. Lower enzyme activities have been found in patients with choreoathetosis and spasticity but without self-mutilation and with near-normal intelligence, while enzyme deficiency is nearly complete in the full-blown syndrome. Assay of the enzyme in filter-paper blood spots, fibroblasts and amniotic cells is offered by specialized centres, which also provide services for carrier detection and antenatal diagnosis. A useful, but not infallible, screening test is measurement of the uric acid:creatinine ratio in urine. The blood uric acid is usually elevated.

The hyperuricaemia of the disorder can be effectively controlled and urolithiasis prevented by treatment with the xanthine oxidase inhibitor allopurinol. Attempts to treat the neuropsychiatric dysfunction have so far been unsuccessful. Supplements of nucleotides have been ineffective, as have attempts to boost the adrenergic and serotonergic neurotransmitter system, by the precursors DOPA and 5-hydroxytryptophan, supplemented by the decarboxylase inhibitor carbidopa. Diazepam and other psychoactive drugs are at best palliative. Lesch–Nyhan syndrome is an attractive candidate for gene transplant therapy. The possibility has been mooted of inserting cloned normal cDNA into bone-marrow stem cells cultured from patients and reinserting the corrected cells into the marrow, in the hope that in due course the normal cells will replace the deficient cells. Even if successful, this might not be sufficient, as it may also be necessary to replace the gene in the brain. Introduction of the gene into mouse embryos has been shown to give rise to enzyme activity in the brain, but this approach is not acceptable in humans. Preimplantation diagnosis is an alternative approach.

Purines and pyrimidines play an important part in the immune system. Severe immunodeficiency is seen in *purine nucleoside phosphorylase deficiency* and, in about half those affected, may be associated with tremor, ataxia or quadriplegia and developmental delay, the neurological signs preceding in some cases the manifestations of the defects in cell-mediated immunity. In contrast to the Lesch–Nyhan syndrome, blood and urine concentrations of uric acid are low, those of inosine and guanosine and their deoxy counterparts increased.

Adenylosuccinase deficiency is a rare disorder presenting with severe mental retardation, and sometimes autistic features and fits. The enzyme involved catalyses the conversion of succinyl-amino-imidazole carboxamide ribotide to amino-imidazole-carboxamide ribotide, and of adenylosuccinate to adenosine monophosphate. The pathogenetic process is not understood. The body fluids contain excess of the dephosphorylated substrates of the enzyme succinyladenosine and succinyl-amino-imidazole carboxamide ribotide. The disorder may be detected by screening urine with the Bratton–Marshall test or by thin-layer chromatography using a stain for imidazoles.

Orotic aciduria is a disorder of pyrimidine metabolism in which the enzyme uridine-5-monophosphate synthase, a bifunctional protein in the *de novo* synthetic pathway, is deficient. Patients are usually referred because of a refractory megaloblastic anaemia, and slow mental and physical development. Immune defences may be impaired, as in patients with disorders of purine metabolism. There is also a high incidence of cardiac and other malformations. On standing, urine samples produce a flocculent precipitate of colourless, fine, needle-shaped crystals of orotic acid. The interruption of pyrimidine nucleotide synthesis creates a requirement in patients for pyrimidines, which can be met by supplements of uridine. The prognosis for treated patients is mostly good.

Ataxia telangiectasia combines cerebellar ataxia, choreoathetosis, mental retardation and telangiectases (dilatation of the capillaries in the conjunctiva, skin and other organs). Both hormonal and cellular immunity are impaired and there is a high incidence of malignancies attributed to spontaneous chromosomal abnormalities arising from defective DNA repair. The concentration of α-fetoprotein is persistently raised; this is attributed to a defect in tissue differentiation.

In patients with *xeroderma pigmentosum*, pigmented skin lesions are produced by ultraviolet light, and there is a high incidence of malignancies. The underlying defect is deficiency of an endonuclease involved in excision repair of DNA damage by ultraviolet rays or other radiation. Abnormalities of the central nervous system occur in 20–30% of patients.

The basic defect in *Fanconi's anaemia* appears to be an abnormality in repair of DNA cross-links. Pancytopenia, growth retardation, unusual pigmentation and a high frequency of congenital malformations are common findings. Mental retardation occurs in about 20% of patients. In *Cockayne's syndrome* of dwarfism, premature ageing, mental retardation, ataxia, retinal pigmentary degeneration and deposition of calcium in many tissues, repair of ultraviolet damage is normal but DNA replication and RNA synthesis fail to recover from inhibition by ultraviolet damage.

DOWN'S SYNDROME—CHROMOSOMAL DISORDERS[1,2,31]

Following the discovery of the chromosomal basis of Down's syndrome (trisomy 21), interest has focused on the effect of the extra chromosome on metabolism. Early work produced evidence of minor abnormalities in the concentrations of body-fluid constituents and of defective homeostasis, rather than of specific changes attributable to the aneuploidy. Several studies demonstrated impaired cellular and humoral immune capacity, but the deficiencies are only partial, vary from patient to patient, and their underlying cause remains unknown.

Adults and older children with Down's syndrome have an increased incidence of autoimmune disease affecting the thyroid, pancreas, adrenals and gastric mucosa. Congenital hypothyroidism is much more common than in the general population, and a markedly increased incidence of hypoparathyroidism is also found in adult patients. The incidence of goitre, thyroid autoantibodies and hyperthyroidism is also increased. Regular monitoring of thyroid function is therefore advisable. There is also evidence in the syndrome of defective end-organ response to ACTH, FSH and LH. Statistically significant deficiencies in trace metals and vitamins have been found, but are of doubtful clinical significance. Dietary supplementation with vitamins has been disappointing, but controlled, long-term studies in children have not yet been reported.

The crucial question of how the presence of the additional chromosome affects the brain remains largely unanswered. It has been known for over 40 years that patients with Down's syndrome show signs of premature ageing, with neuropathological findings of neurofibrillary tangles and amyloid-containing senile plaques, as also seen in Alzheimer's disease. In a minority of patients with familial Alzheimer's disease a point mutation in the amyloid precursor-protein gene has been located to chromosome 21. A mutation on chromosome 14, the apolipoprotein E genotype and environmental factors may also affect the age of onset of the disorder.

Three genes intervening in *de novo* purine synthesis have been mapped to chromosone 21, and it has been postulated that *de novo* purine synthesis is involved in the pathogenesis of the disorder.[55] Another gene located on chromosome 21 is that for superoxide dismutase (*SOD-I*), whose concentration is elevated by about 50% in Down's syndrome in blood cells, fibroblasts and also in fetal brain. It has been suggested that this leads to perturbation of the metabolism of oxygen derivatives, rendering the brain vulnerable to oxidative damage. Lipoperoxidation of polyunsaturated fatty acids is increased in preparations of Down's syndrome brain, and the polyunsaturated fatty acid composition of brain phospholipids is abnormal. This may affect the structure and function of cellular membranes. Products of lipoperoxidation may also affect neurotransmitter function, notably the cholinergic system, via their action on the regulators guanilate cyclase and guanosine monophosphate. As pyruvate dehydrogenase, with its close links to acetylcholine synthesis is also reduced in cells from patients with Down's syndrome, the vulnerability of this system appears enhanced. No specific treatment for Down's syndrome is currently envisaged, but biochemists are making an important contribution to the prevention of the disorder by antenatal screening.

Another chromosomal disorder that has recently attracted the attention of biochemists is the fragile X syndrome.[55] The clinical features (moderate mental retardation, long face with large everted ears, and macro-orchidism) were described nearly 50 years ago, and the chromosomal nature of the disorder was recognized in 1969. It affects more than 1 in 2000 of the population and accounts for at least one-third of X-linked mental retardation. Expression in culture is dependent on a medium deficient in folate and thymidine, and is enhanced by the folate antagonist methotrexate. The gene involved, FMR-1, contains a repeat trinucleotide sequence of variable size. Beyond a certain size the sequence becomes unstable, the resulting fragility leading to the clinical signs. Similar mechanisms are also found in myotonic dystrophy and Huntington's chorea. Folic acid has been used in treatment, as have central nervous stimulants and neuroleptics, so far with no tangible success. Prenatal diagnosis is possible by cytogenetic analysis or preferably by DNA analysis. Advanced cytogenetic banding techniques have demonstrated that some mental retardation–malformation disorders such as the Prader–Willi syndrome are caused by chromosomal microdeletions or microduplications.[1,2,31] The same cytogenic abnormality may give rise to distinct clinical entities depending whether it is of maternal or paternal origin. When microcytogenetic abnormalities obliterate genes, the condition combines the features of an inborn error and a chromosomal disorder. In some cases these deletions can be used to locate in the genome genes whose function is unknown ('reverse genetics').

ETHICAL CONSIDERATIONS—GENETIC COUNSELLING[56,57]

Problems and Dilemmas

Recent advances in diagnosis, treatment and prevention of both genetically and environmentally determined disorders associated with mental retardation have given rise to many ethical problems. However, some apparent ethical dilemmas are based on a misunderstanding of the epidemiology of rare recessive disorders. For example, concern has been expressed about the increased genetic burden created when treated patients marry and pass on the harmful gene. In fact, calculations based on gene frequencies show clearly that the effect on future generations will be small and that equilibrium will not be reached for very many generations.

Estimates of cost-effectiveness of treatment and prevention should not be accepted unreservedly. Not all values can be expressed in monetary terms. Prevention of mental handicap is worthwhile on ethical grounds, even if costly. However, resources are finite and there is a real dilemma in prioritizing the rival claims for the prevention of mental handicap and other equally worthy causes. Value judgements, subjective feelings, aspirations and prejudices of the lay public, caring professions and legislators determine how this dilemma is faced.

Genetic Counselling

Counselling the parents of a mentally retarded child requires considerable expertise and judgement. Of primary concern to the parents are the limits set by the handicap to their child's intellectual development, the possibilities of treatment, and the risk of recurrence in a subsequent child.

There is little doubt that even in cases with a well-defined biochemical aetiology and mode of inheritance, genetic counselling should initially be the responsibility of the consultant in charge of the case, although s/he may call in specialist advice in complicated cases. The consultant's first task will often be to try to allay the parents' feeling of guilt and self-reproach, which are common in their circumstances; then to explain the nature of the disorder, its prognosis, the scope for treatment and the risk of recurrence.

In dominantly and recessively inherited disorders the recurrence risk is clear. However, in X-linked disorders, and especially in dominantly inherited diseases, the mutation rate is significant. For example, in tuberous sclerosis, a dominantly transmitted disorder associated with epilepsy and characteristic skin lesions, most patients carry new mutations, neither parent is affected, and there is a negligible recurrence risk. For patients with mental retardation of unknown aetiology it is possible to give the parents an empirical estimate of recurrence of about 3%. The parents may be so confused, upset or angry that they cannot understand or accept what they are told and several counselling sessions may be necessary. Some parents later claim that they were 'kept in the dark', even though the records clearly show that this was not so. Others see a succession of specialists in the hope that an unacceptable diagnosis may be overturned.

The handicapped child and his or her parents may have frequent contact with the laboratory, both for diagnostic tests and for the monitoring of treatment. Collecting specimens from mentally retarded children can be both time consuming and exhausting for staff and parents, who are often acutely embarrassed. A caring and supportive attitude by laboratory staff can have a beneficial effect, but they should not discuss diagnosis, prognosis, recurrence risks or management—except when a patient is formally referred for this purpose. Even if what they say is fully in line with the views of the consultant in charge of the case, they may be misunderstood or their views quoted out of context, and therapeutic relationships may be undermined. For a more detailed discussion of genetic counselling the reader is referred to Harper.[56]

Other Medico-ethical Issues

When severely retarded patients are involved in complex investigations, clinical trials or research, it must be borne in mind that they are unable to give informed consent, and that parental consent by itself is not necessarily sufficient. It is therefore essential to submit full details of any project to the ethical committee of the patient's hospital and to apply for clinical trials' certificates to the Department of Health (in the UK) where appropriate.

Some new developments, such as improved methods of behaviour therapy or rehabilitation, may alleviate the condition of existing mentally handicapped patients but will not help establish the cause or facilitate prevention of the handicap. Long-term research on aetiology and metabolic disease may benefit future generations but seldom the patients taking part in the research project. A balance has to be struck between these types of research.

Laboratory investigations may set a limit to the expectation of life or intellectual potential of a fetus or child and thus critically affect decisions about termination of pregnancy, sterilization or recommendation for institutional care. The clinical biochemist cannot, therefore, be indifferent to the complex ethical issues involved. Except on religious grounds, the case for aborting a fetus with a fatal, untreatable, storage disorder is unanswerable. However, in some disorders those affected may be physically well and, in a caring environment, enjoy a happy if limited existence. The mother clearly has rights in arriving at a decision but so have the fetus, unaffected siblings whose prospects may be adversely affected by a handi-

capped child in the family, and society. These issues have been inconclusively debated by physicians, philosophers, lawyers and theologians. All one can say is that flexibility of mind and a sense of humility are desirable qualities in those giving advice. Rigid rules governing antenatal detection, termination of pregnancy and sterilization are liable to cause unnecessary hardship and distress in some cases. The best safeguard for patients and the public is the provision of adequate resources by the community, and access to professional workers with competence, compassion and common sense.

REFERENCES

1. Dobbing J. (ed.) (1984). *Scientific Studies in Mental Retardation*, London: Macmillan.
2. Clarke A.M., Clarke A.D.B., Berg J.M. (eds.) (1985). *Mental Deficiency: The Changing Outlook*, 4th edn, London: Methuen.
3. Akesson H.O. (1986). The biological origin of mild mental retardation; a critical review. *Acta Psychiatr. Scand.*, **74**, 3–7.
4. Gostason R., Wahlstrom J., Johannison T., Holmquist D. (1991). Chromosomal aberrations in the mildly mentally retarded. *J. Ment. Defic. Res.*, **35**, 240–246.
5. Dobbing J. (1981). The later development of the brain and its vulnerability. In *Scientific Foundations of Paediatrics*, 2nd edn, (Davis, J.A., Dobbing J., eds.) London: Heinemann, pp. 744–759.
6. Jones K.L. (1988). *Smith's Recognizable Patterns of Human Malformation*. 4th edn, Philadelphia: W.B. Saunders.
7. Winter R.M., Baraitser M. (ed.) (1991). *Multiple Congenital Anomalies*, London: Chapman and Hall Medical.
8. Gillberg C. (1992). Autism and autistic-like conditions: subclasses among disorders of empathy. *J. Child Psychol. Psychiat.*, **33**, 813–842.
9. Adams R.D., Lyon G. (1982). *Neurology of Hereditary Metabolic Disease of Children*, London: McGraw-Hill.
10. Cohn R.M., Roth K.S. (1983). *Metabolic Disease: A Guide to Early Recognition*, Philadelphia: W.B. Saunders.
11. Clayton B.E., Round J.M. (eds.) (1984). *Chemical Pathology and the Sick Child*, Oxford: Blackwell Scientific.
12. Harkness R.A., Pollitt R.J., Addison G.M. (eds.) (1989). Perspectives: Prenatal and Perinatal Diagnosis. *J. Inher. Metab. Dis.*, **12** (Suppl. 1), 1–246.
13. Green A. (1989). Guide to the diagnosis of inborn errors of metabolism in district general hospitals, ACP Broadsheet 120. *J. Clin. Pathol.*, **42**, 84–91.
14. Fernandes J., Saudubray J.M., Tada K. (eds.) (1990). *Inborn Metabolic Diseases; Diagnosis and Treatment*, Berlin: Springer.
15. Volpe J.A. (1987). *Neurology of the Newborn*, 2nd edn, Philadelphia: W.B. Saunders.
16. Levene M.I., Bennett M.J., Punt J. (eds.) (1988). *Fetal and Neonatal Neurology and Neurosurgery*, Edinburgh: Churchill Livingstone.
17. Rothman S.M., Olney J.W. (1986). Glutamate and the pathophysiology of hypoxic ischaemic brain damage. *Ann. Neurol.*, **19**, 105–111.

18. Schindley J.W. (1990). Free radicals in CNS system ischaemia. *Stroke*, **25**, 7–12.
19. Aynsley-Green A. (1992). Hypoglycaemia. In Davis J.T. (ed.) *Recent Advances in Paediatrics No. 10*, Edinburgh: Churchill Livingston.
20. Taylor E. (1991). Developmental neuropsychiatry. *J. Child Psychol. Psychiatry*, **32**, 3–47.
21. Rutter M., Casaer P. (eds.) (1991). *Biological Risk Factors for Psychosocial Disorders*, Cambridge: Cambridge University Press.
22. Olney J.W. (1989). Excitatory amino acids and neuropsychiatric disorders. *Biol. Psychiatry*, **26**, 505–525.
23. Dobbing J.H. (ed.) (1987). *Early Nutrition and Later Achievement*, London: Academic Press.
24. Susser M. (1989). The challenge of causality: human nutrition, brain development and mental performance. *Bull. N Y Acad. Med.*, **65**, 1032–1049.
25. Simeon D.T., Grantham-McGregor S.M. (1990). Nutritional deficiencies and children's behaviour and mental development. *Nutr. Res. Rev.*, **3**, 1–24.
26. Grantham-McGregor S.M., Powell C.A., Walker S.P., Himes J.H. (1991). Nutritional supplementation, psychosocial stimulation, and mental development of stunted children: the Jamaican study. *Lancet*, **338**, 1–5.
27. Lucas A., Morley R., Cole J.J., Gore S.M., Boon A.J., Powell R. (1990). Early diet in preterm babies and developmental status at 18 months. *Lancet*, **335**, 1477–1481.
28. Editorial (1991). Brains and vitamins. *Lancet*, **337**, 587–588.
29. MRC Vitamin Study Research Group (1991). Prevention of neural tube defects: results of the Medical Research Council Vitamin Study. *Lancet*, **338**, 131–137; 153–154.
30. Neufeld E.F. (1991). Lysosomal storage diseases. *Annu. Rev. Biochem.*, **60**, 257–280.
31. Scriver C.R., Beaudet A.L., Sly W.S. Valle D. (eds.) (1989). *The Metabolic Basis of Inherited Disease*, 6th edn, New York: McGraw-Hill.
32. Filipe M.I., Lake B.D. (eds.) (1990). *Histochemistry in Pathology*, 2nd edn, Edinburgh: Churchill Livingstone.
33. Endres W. (ed.) (1990). Carbohydrate and Glycoprotein Metabolism; Maternal phenylketonuria. *J. Inher. Metab. Dis.*, **13**, 313–672.
34. Bremer H.J., Duran M., Kamerling J.P., Przyrembel H., Wadman S.K. (1981). *Disturbances of Amino Acid Metabolism: Clinical Chemistry and Diagnosis*, Murwick: Urban and Schwarzenberg.
35. Edwards M.A., Grant S., Green A. (1988). A practical approach to the investigation of amino acid disorders. *Ann. Clin. Biochem.*, **25**, 129–141.
36. Lloyd J.K., Scriver G.R. (eds.) (1985). *Genetic and Metabolic Disease in Pediatrics*, London: Butterworth.
37. Woo S.L.C. (1989). Molecular basis and population genetics of phenylketonuria. *Biochemistry*, **28**, 1–7.
38. Smith I., Beasley M.G., Ades A.E. (1990). Intelligence and quality of dietary treatment in phenylketonuria. *Arch. Dis. Child.*, **65**, 472–478.
39. Smith I., Beasley M.G., Ades A.E. (1991). Effect on intelligence of relaxing the low phenylalamine diet in phenylketonuria. *Arch. Dis. Child.*, **66**, 311–316.
40. Fisch R.O., Matalon R., Weisberg S., Michals K. (1991). Children of fathers with phenylketonuria: an international survey. *J. Pediatr.*, **118**, 739–741.
41. Blei A.T. (1991). Cerebral edema and intracranial hypertension in acute liver failure: distinct aspects of the same problem. *Hepatology*, **13**, 376–379.
42. Klatzo I. (1987). Pathophysiological aspects of brain oedema. *Acta Neuropathol.*, **72**, 236–239.
43. Harkness R.A., Pollitt R.J., Addison G.M., Besley G.T.N., Green A. (eds.) (1991). The Liver and Inherited Metabolic Disorders. *J. Inher. Metab. Dis.*, **14**, 405–652.
44. Green A. (1988). When and how should we measure plasma ammonia? *Ann. Clin. Biochem.*, **25**, 199–209.
45. Jaeken J. (ed.) (1993). Inherited Metabolic Disorders and the Brain. *J. Inher. Metab. Dis.*, **16**, 614–811.
46. Harkness R.A., Pollitt R.J., Addison G.M. (eds.) (1987). Inborn errors of cellular organelles. *J. Inher. Metab. Dis.*, **10** (Suppl. 1), 1–200.
47. Tanaka K., Coates P.M. (1990). *Fatty Acid Oxidation: Clinical, Biochemical and Molecular Aspects*, New York: Alan Liss.
48. Bennett M.J. (1990). The laboratory diagnosis of inborn errors of mitochondrial fatty acid oxidation. *Ann. Clin. Biochem.*, **27**, 519–531.
49. Clark J.B. (ed.) (1990). Biogenesis and Assembly of the Mitochondrial Respiratory Chain. *Biochem. Soc. Trans.*, **18**, 503–528.
50. Brenton D.P. (ed.) (1992). Mitochondrial DNA and Associated Disorders; The X Chromosome. *J. Inher. Metab. Dis.*, **15**, 437–688.
51. Watts R.W.E., Baraitser M., Chalmers R.A., Purkiss P. (1980). Organic acidurias and aminoacidurias in the aetiology of long-term mental handicap. *J. Ment. Defic. Res.*, **24**, 257–270.
52. Moser H.W. (1989). Peroxisomal diseases. *Adv. Paediatr.*, **36**, 1–38.
53. Hulse (1984). Outcome for congenital hypothyroidism. *Arch. Dis. Child.*, **59**, 23–30.
54. Lejeune J. (1990). Pathogenesis of mental retardation in trisomy 21. *Am. J. Med. Genet.*, **37**, 20–30.
55. Hagerman R.J. (1992). Fragile X syndrome: advances and controversy. *J. Child Psychol. Psychiat.*, **33**, 1127–1139.
56. Harper P.S. (1988). *Practical Genetic Counselling*, 3rd edn, Bristol: Wright.
57. Brenton D.P., Seakins J.W. (eds.) (1988). The ethics of antenatal diagnosis and the termination of pregnancy. *J. Inher. Metab. Dis*, **11** (Suppl. 1), 110–129.

17. Neonatal and Paediatric biochemistry

V. Walker

Introduction
Reference ranges
  Origins and reliability
  Ranges for plasma constituents
  Ranges for urine
  Ranges for other body fluids
Renal function
  Development
  Assessment of glomerular function
  Renal tubular function
Plasma lipids in childhood
  Hyperlipidaemia
  Hypolipidaemia
Hypoglycaemia
  Inadequate glycogenolysis or
    gluconeogenesis
  Hyperinsulinism: nesidioblastosis ('leucine-
    sensitive hypoglycaemia')
  Investigation of childhood hypoglycaemia
Hyperammonaemia
  Clinical features
  Causes
  Inherited urea-cycle defects
  Reye's syndrome
  Other conditions presenting with a Reye's
    syndrome-like illness
  Other causes of hyperammonaemia
Children with short stature
  Causes
*The acutely sick child with a possible inborn
  error of metabolism*
Biochemistry for sick and preterm neonates
Respiratory distress
  Surfactant and the respiratory distress
    syndrome (RDS)
  The respiratory distress syndrome
Fluid balance disturbances
Jaundice
  1. Unconjugated hyperbilirubinaemia
  2. Conjugated hyperbilirubinaemia and
    neonatal liver disease
  3. The bronze baby syndrome
Glucose homeostasis
  Hypoglycaemia
  Hyperglycaemia
Disorders of minerals
  Calcium
  Hypomagnesaemia
  Metabolic bone disease of prematurity
*Biochemical disturbances associated with
  parenteral nutrition*
Provision of a paediatric biochemistry service

INTRODUCTION

Compared with adults, children as they grow are normally intensely anabolic; they become catabolic rapidly during intercurrent illness; they have an immature endocrine system as they lack gonadal steroids; their immune system is immature; in early infancy, some of the body organs are also still developing, notably the kidneys, liver and lungs. For these reasons, the biochemistry of children in health differs in many respects from that of adults, and the metabolic response to illness is often more acute and intense. In addition, a different spectrum of diseases occurs in childhood: infections predominate, often associated with metabolic or nutritional imbalance; congenital and inherited disorders are most often manifest in early life, and the types of cancers encountered are different. Degenerative disorders, such as atherosclerosis, are rare. Paediatric medicine, therefore, makes special demands of a hospital biochemistry service. In addition, the small size of many of the patients and their reluctance to cooperate tax the resourcefulness of the service to provide meaningful data on meagre biological samples.

After considering reference ranges, this chapter will focus on some biochemical disorders of particular importance in children. The unique problems of sick and preterm, newborn infants are considered in depth. Childhood hypocalcaemia is not considered separately, as its major causes are covered elsewhere: rickets, hypoparathyroidism (Chapter 30); chronic renal failure (Chapter 19).

REFERENCE RANGES

Origins and Reliability

Useful sources of paediatric ranges are Clayton et al.,[1] Meites[2] and Clayton and Round,[3] and ranges are included in most paediatric textbooks. However, there is often poor agreement between published reference values, and comprehensive data are still not available for many investigations. This is due largely to three problems, as follows.

1. The ethical difficulties of collecting samples from normal children when the analyses will not be a direct benefit to them. A practical expedient has often been to derive ranges from samples collected from hospitalized children at the time of other, necessary, clinical tests. These children may be stressed by intercurrent illness or homesickness, they are relatively inactive, and their diet is changed with admission.

2. The need for standardized conditions for sample collection has often been ignored.[4] Some important factors are time of day, a constant relation to food if affected by it, posture (samples from those under 1 year of age are generally collected when supine, and in older children, when sitting), drug therapy, physi-

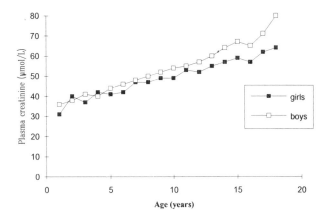

Fig. 17.1 Mean plasma creatinine concentrations in childhood and adolescence. Data from Schwartz G.J., Haycock G.B., Spitzer A. (1976), *J. Paediatrics*, **88**, 828 (with permission)

cal activity and stage of sexual development. Plasma lactate and ammonia concentrations are increased in struggling babies and during convulsions, and that of bicarbonate may decrease. Creatine kinase may be raised in adolescents undertaking strenuous sports activities. Diet is also important. Many published ranges for early infancy were derived when babies were fed high protein milks. Since 1974, lower-protein milk formulae have been used in the UK for term babies, and some of the earlier reference values are no longer appropriate.

3. The poor quality of biological samples from sick children used to derive ranges. This applies particularly to capillary blood samples from babies: haemolysis variably increases the plasma potassium, magnesium and lactate dehydrogenase and decreases the sodium and chloride; contamination with interstitial and cellular tissue fluids tends to decrease the protein, total calcium and potassium. Samples collected from an infusion site may also be contaminated. Twenty-four hour urine samples are often incomplete. Random urine samples may be faecally contaminated—especially if collected into cotton-wool balls, a common practice on neonatal wards.

Ranges for Plasma Constituents

Children
Outside the neonatal period, ranges for many analytes are the same as in adults. These include sodium, potassium, chloride, osmolality, total and ionized calcium, albumin, glucose, bilirubin, alanine and aspartate aminotransferases, creatine kinase, ammonia, lactate and most hormones. There are important differences, however.

The concentration of plasma *creatinine* is very low in young children and increases with age (Fig. 17.1).

Bicarbonate is lower (18–22 mmol/L) in the first months of life, reflecting renal immaturity (p. 295).

Phosphate changes during childhood: values are high neonatally, due to the combined effects of a high dietary phosphate, low glomerular filtration and increased secretion of growth hormone, which promotes renal tubular reabsorption of phosphate. Throughout childhood, values remain above the adult range and may increase a little during the adolescent growth spurt, probably reflecting increased growth hormone secretion. Finally, concentrations fall into the adult range in later puberty, an effect of steroid sex hormones.

Urate concentrations are below 0.40 mmol/L during childhood in both sexes, and increase in boys, but not girls at puberty.

Immunoglobulins change with age: IgG falls after birth to a nadir at between 2–3 months, and then increases steadily to reach the adult range at around 3 years of age. Low total protein concentrations in the first 3 months reflect the early decline. IgA is very low in the first 6 weeks and then increases slowly into the adult range by around 12 years. IgM is also decreased in early infancy, but achieves adult levels by 1 year.

Plasma *lipids* are discussed on p. 296.

Basal levels of *gonadotrophins* and *steroid sex hormones* are low until puberty.

Renin activity and *aldosterone* concentration, in contrast, are raised in early childhood.

Alkaline phosphatase (ALP) is increased above adult levels throughout childhood, due to release of bone isoenzyme by osteoblasts during growth. Laboratory ranges differ because analytical variables influence enzyme activity. Values increase rapidly from around the upper normal for adults at birth, to a peak at 1–6 months of age, averaging 3 times the adult upper limit. They then decline a little and during childhood do not exceed 2.5 times the adult limit. An increase occurs with the adolescent growth spurt, peaking at 10–12 years and 13–14 years in girls and boys, respectively. The growth rate is faster in boys, and their ALP is higher, possibly to three-and-a-half or four times the adult limit. In general, ALP activity exceeding five times normal adult values, at any age, may be pathological and should be investigated. Transient hyperphosphatasia[5] is observed sometimes in children under 5 years of age (median 14 months) without liver or bone disease. Some have been healthy, others had a variety of disorders, often recovering from a viral infection of the alimentary tract. ALP is 5- to 30-fold (or more) higher than the upper adult normal, and may remain elevated for several weeks. Two abnormal enzymes have been demonstrated. One may be an excessively sialylated liver isoenzyme and the other of bone origin. Impaired clearance of ALP from the circulation is a proposed explanation for the phenomenon.

Neonates
Published ranges vary considerably, particularly for preterm babies, probably because they have often been derived from poor samples from sick babies.

TABLE 17.1

GLOMERULAR FILTRATION RATE FROM INULIN CLEARANCE

Age	Glomerular filtration rate (ml/min per 1.73 m²)	
	Mean	Range (mean ± 2SD)
1–5.9 months	77	41–103
6–11.9 months	103	49–157
12–19 months	127	63–191
2–12 years	127	89–165
Adult male	131	88–174
Adult female	117	87–147

Data from Barratt (1982) (with permission).[7]

Although many published upper limits for plasma potassium, for example, are 6.5 mmol/L or higher, it seems likely that the physiological ranges should be lower, similar to those in older infants. Lower reference limits reported for albumin and total calcium are also probably not the physiological norm. True differences between neonates and older babies are: higher *phosphate*; higher total and free *thyroxine*, free *tri-iodothyronine* and *thyroid-stimulating hormone* (*TSH*) in the first week, due to a postnatal surge in TSH secretion; raised *17α-hydroxyprogesterone* (preterm babies); a low serum *copper* and *caeruloplasmin*, which increase slowly to the adult range by around 6 months of age; and differences in the activities of some enzymes: *amylase*, which is very low in the first month of life, only increasing to adult levels by 9 to 12 months; *creatine kinase*, which rises in the first 24 h of life and falls to normal by the second week; *aspartate aminotransferase* (AST) and *lactate dehydrogenase* (LDH), which may both be elevated to twice the normal adult upper limit in the first 72 h of life. In our experience, AST activity then falls into the adult range, but others report more persistent elevations of AST and LDH.

Pharmacokinetics in neonates differ markedly from older subjects,[6] yet there are few therapeutic drug ranges for newborns.

Ranges for Urine

Timed urine collections are universally unpopular. Samples are often lost and incomplete bladder emptying causes inaccuracy. The creatinine excretion is a measure of the completeness of a 24-h collection, and should fall within the range:[7]

0.132 + 0.004 × age(yr) ± 0.026(SD) mmol/kg body weight per 24 h.

Many tests are made on single-voided samples and are often related to urinary creatinine. Whilst generally useful, use of creatinine ratios may be misleading in malnourished children with poor muscle bulk, and also in the first weeks of life, when renal function is changing. An important practical consideration is that the volume of urine excreted by small children is low, and urine collection bottles should contain an appropriately reduced volume of preservative.

Ranges for Other Body Fluids

Adult ranges are applicable to cerebrospinal fluid (CSF) glucose and total proteins from 4 weeks of age for term babies. Until then, CSF protein ranges to 2–2.5 times the upper adult normal. Values are higher in preterm infants and often difficult to interpret. Sweat sodium is high (75–80 mmol/L) in the first 72 h of life, but then falls to low values maintained during childhood (mean 22–27 mmol/L). Values increase gradually from adolescence to the adult mean of 55 mmol/L.[1]

RENAL FUNCTION

Development[7]

By 36 weeks of gestation, the fetus has the full adult complement of nephrons, but these are small. At term birth, the mean glomerular diameter is approximately half that of adults, and the mean proximal tubular length around 10% of adult length. The loops of Henle descend less deeply into the renal medulla. Renal plasma flow is low compared with adults, but there are problems in its estimation because para-aminohippuric acid (PAH) is incompletely extracted neonatally. The mean glomerular filtration rate (GFR) of term babies in the first 24 h of life from inulin clearance was 3 ml/min or 20 ml/min per 1.73 m² (related to notional adult surface area) and by creatinine clearance, 1.40 ml/kg per min. It increases in the first few days, probably because of haemodynamic changes in the kidneys. Related to adult surface area, GFR increases to adult values by two years of age (Table 17.1). However, surface area is an unsatisfactory reference before 6 months. The GFR of preterm babies is lower at birth and rises only slowly to 34–36 weeks of gestational age, at which it increases steeply.[8]

Assessment of Glomerular Function

Plasma Urea

This is an unsatisfactory marker of GFR in childhood. Urea is a waste product of dietary and endogenous proteins. Dietary protein intake varies widely. Production from endogenous protein is low during rapid growth and high during catabolic, intercurrent illnesses. Plasma urea concentrations are also influenced by the state of hydration. In dehydration (common in sick children), solute and water flow through the distal tubule of the kidney is low and there is increased back-diffusion of urea from the tubule into the blood. Finally, plasma urea is insensitive because it does not rise until GFR has fallen to

40–50% of normal and then rises steeply with further small decrements of function.

Plasma Creatinine

This is a preferred index, but is still not ideal. Its main advantage is that it does not depend on protein intake, being a waste-product of creatine in skeletal muscle. In a steady-state, about 2% of muscle creatine is converted to creatinine daily. Production is therefore related to muscle mass and body weight, and increases with age. Plasma creatinine, similarly, increases with age (see Fig 17.1). It is important to be aware that reference values are much lower in early life, otherwise significant renal impairment may be missed.

Plasma creatinine is overestimated by analytical methods using the Jaffe alkaline picrate method (by around 13 μmol/L with modern analysers) because of interference from non-creatinine chromogens, e.g. methylguanidine. This causes a significant error at the low plasma creatinine concentrations found in young children.

Interference from acetoacetate causes spuriously high results in ketotic children. Nevertheless, serial plasma measurements are invaluable for monitoring changes in GFR. At birth, plasma creatinine reflects the maternal concentration because of equilibration across the placenta. Amounts fall during the first 2 weeks in term babies, and more slowly in preterm infants. Because there is a linear relation between GFR: surface area and height: plasma creatinine, GFR may be predicted for children over 6 months of age using the formula:[3]

GFR (ml/min per 1.73 m² surface area)

$$= \frac{40 \times \text{height (cm)}}{\text{plasma creatinine } (\mu\text{mol/L})}.$$

Clearance Studies[7]

Inulin clearance remains the definitive method for estimating GFR, but is unsuitable for clinical use. Creatinine clearance tests are unsatisfactory in young children because of incomplete bladder emptying and poor cooperation, leading to urinary losses, and because of the analytical error in measuring plasma creatinine (see Chapter 19 for further discussion of creatinine clearance tests). They are generally avoided, but may be necessary when children are oedematous or severely malnourished, with poor muscle bulk.

With methods measuring clearance of radiolabelled compounds there is no need for timed urine collections. The principle of single-injection techniques is that if a substance injected intravenously mixes rapidly within its volume of distribution and is only cleared by glomerular filtration, GFR can be estimated by the rate of fall of plasma concentration. Commonly, blood is taken 2 and 4 h after injection of a radiolabelled compound, [51Cr] edetic acid ([51Cr] EDTA) or [99mTc] diethylenetriaminepentace-tic acid ([99mTc] DTPA). The principle of constant-infusion techniques is that when a substance infused intravenously is cleared only by glomerular filtration then, at equilibrium, the rate of infusion equals the rate of excretion. GFR can be calculated from the plasma concentration and infusion rate.

Renal Tubular Function

Problems related to renal immaturity

Anatomically, glomerular development precedes that of the renal tubules and this may result in 'glomerulo-tubular imbalance' in early infancy. In addition, there is functional heterogeneity of the nephrons, as some are at a more advanced stage of development than others. Renal tubular immaturity is only clinically significant in the first months of life. Urinary concentrating ability is reduced because the loops of Henle are short and the renal medullary concentration gradient is low, as babies fed with breast milk or standard milk formulae produce relatively small amounts of urea. In response to exogenous arginine vasopressin or water depletion, the maximum urinary concentration is 600–700 mosmol/kg, compared with more than 1200 mosmol/kg water in children and adults. Sick infants may fail to conserve water despite dehydration.

The capacity for hydrogen ion excretion is diminished, owing to a lower renal bicarbonate threshold, low rates of phosphate excretion, low sodium concentrations available for H$^+$ exchange in the distal tubules and, probably, decreased tubular ammonia production. Healthy infants excrete H$^+$ ions at a rate close to the maximum, producing an acid urine. Plasma bicarbonate (18–22 mmol/L) is lower than in children. Metabolic acidosis develops rapidly if H$^+$ excretion is stressed, for example by high protein intakes.

Normal babies have an amino aciduria in the first weeks of life because of their lower tubular reabsorption of many amino acids than adults (values for adults exceed 98%). Increased excretion is commonly observed for glycine, serine, threonine, proline, histidine and, neonatally, cystine and lysine. Losses are accentuated during intravenous administration of amino acid solutions.

Pathological Disorders

Abnormalities of renal tubular function may be investigated using similar procedures to those in adults.[1,7] A concentrating defect is excluded if the urinary osmolality of a child deprived of fluid overnight exceeds 900 mosmol/kg water. If formal water-deprivation tests are carried out, body weight must be monitored, and the test terminated if loss exceeds 2–3%. The urinary concentrating response 3–6 h after intramuscular injection of D-deamino (8-D-arginine) vasopressin (DDAVP) (0.04 μg/kg body weight) distinguishes between lack of arginine vasopressin and resistance to it. Renal acidification is normal if the pH of an overnight urine sample is 5.3 or less, with normal or only slightly reduced plasma bicarbonate. Otherwise, an ammonium chloride load (4 g/m² body weight) may be given as an acid stress.

PLASMA LIPIDS IN CHILDHOOD

Hyperlipidaemia

Lipids are most often measured in children at risk of familial hypercholesterolaemia (Chapter 35) because a parent, grandparent, or first-degree relative has hypercholesterolaemia or premature coronary heart disease. On the basis of current evidence, it is reasonable to postulate that atherogenesis commences in childhood and is accelerated by hyperlipidaemia.[9] Therefore, there is a case for attempting to lower the plasma cholesterol of affected children. Mass screening of children for hypercholesterolaemia remains very controversial. As in adults, there are problems in defining reference ranges because the 'desirable' upper limits for plasma lipids are difficult to assess and likely to be significantly lower than the population mean.

In fetal life, plasma total cholesterol is low, as there is no dietary source and maternal lipoproteins do not cross the placenta. At birth (umbilical cord blood), mean values as indicated in many studies are:

- total cholesterol 1.8 mmol/L
- low-density lipoprotein (LDL) cholesterol 0.8 mmol/L
- high-density lipoprotein (HDL) cholesterol 0.9 mmol/L
- triglycerides 0.53 mmol/L.

[*Conversion factors*: cholesterol mmol/L ÷ 0.0259 = mg/dL; triglycerides mmol/L ÷ 0.0113 = mg/dL.]

Around half the cholesterol is carried on HDL. During the first weeks of life, total and LDL cholesterol concentrations increase rapidly. By 12 months of age, mean plasma concentrations approach those found throughout childhood. HDL cholesterol is similar in boys and girls until adolescence. Values in girls then remain steady, but fall in boys, so that the LDL:HDL cholesterol ratio is increased. Table 17.2 presents data from the Lipid Research Clinic Programme,[10] which included a large cross-sectional study of children in North America.

'Tracking' describes the tendency for serial measurements in an individual to follow a population percentile over a period of years. LDL cholesterol tracks well from early childhood (from 4 years of age, and possibly earlier). This means that high values in childhood are predictive of high values in adult life. Total cholesterol tracks significantly, but less well. Familial aggregation also occurs, with strong correlation between total, LDL and HDL cholesterol of parents and their children. This reflects genetic, cultural, socioeconomic and dietary factors. Obesity is associated with higher total and LDL cholesterol, and lower HDL concentrations. In infancy, the type of milk fed influences plasma lipids.[9]

Guidelines differ about when and how to test for hyperlipidaemia in children, and how to interpret the results. Cord blood may be tested at birth of a baby with a hypercholesterolaemic parent. Measurements of total cholesterol are not helpful (because of the high HDL contribution) but LDL cholesterol has more predictive power and apo-B measurements may prove superior. Dietary influences make measured lipid concentrations in the early months unhelpful, and testing after birth should be postponed until 1 year of age. There is, in any case, reluctance to introduce dietary modifications before 2 years of age (USA) and 5 years of age (UK), because of the risks of an unbalanced diet during rapid early growth. In families with hypertriglyceridaemia, fasting triglycerides may be measured at 1 year and, if normal, repeated once or twice during childhood, although an increased concentration is most likely to occur in adolescence.

Inherited primary hyperlipidaemias that manifest themselves in childhood are the familial hypercholesterolaemias and hypertriglyceridaemia due to hyperchylomicronaemia (*see* Chapter 36). Among causes of secondary hyperlipidaemia are diabetes mellitus, congenital biliary atresia, the nephrotic syndrome, chronic renal failure, hypopituitarism and anorexia nervosa.

Hypolipidaemia

Inherited hypolipidaemia[11] is extremely rare. The main disorders are as follows.

Abetalipoproteinaemia

This is an autosomal recessive condition due to a defect either in the post-translational modification of apo-B-100 or in its incorporation into lipoproteins. This results in the absence of lipoproteins containing apo-B from the plasma—chylomicrons, very low-density lipoprotein (VLDL) and LDL. Transport of both dietary and endogenous triglycerides is defective. The plasma triglyceride concentrations are extremely low and cholesterol is less than half normal, often only 0.5–1.2 mmol/L. HDL contains excessive amounts of free cholesterol and sphingomyelin, which it normally takes up from the tissues and transfers (the cholesterol now having been esterified) to apo-B-containing lipoproteins. The small-intestinal mucosal cells become distended with fat that they cannot export. This leads to severe fat malabsorption from early life, with failure to thrive and deficiencies of the fat-soluble vitamins A, E and K. As LDL normally transports vitamin E in the blood, the delivery of this vitamin to the tissues is also compromised. Vitamin E is an essential component of the tissue defences against oxygen-free radicals. Visual failure and progressive, ultimately fatal, neurological deterioration

TABLE 17.2
FASTING PLASMA LIPIDS

| | Plasma lipid (mmol/L) | | | | | | | |
| | 0–4 years | | 5–9 years | | 10–14 years | | 15–19 years | |
	Mean	Range	Mean	Range	Mean	Range	Mean	Range
Boys								
Total cholesterol	4.01	2.95–5.26	4.14	3.13–5.26	4.09	3.08–5.23	3.89	2.93–5.10
LDL cholesterol			2.41	1.62–3.34	2.51	1.66–3.42	2.43	1.61–3.37
HDL cholesterol			1.45	0.98–1.92	1.42	0.96–1.92	1.19	0.78–1.63
Triglycerides	0.63	0.33–1.12	0.63	0.34–1.14	0.75	0.36–1.41	0.88	0.42–1.67
Girls								
Total cholesterol	4.04	2.90–5.18	4.25	3.26–5.31	4.14	3.21–5.21	4.07	3.11–5.18
LDL cholesterol			2.59	1.76–3.63	2.49	1.76–3.52	2.46	1.55–3.50
HDL cholesterol			1.37	0.93–1.89	1.35	0.96–1.81	1.35	0.91–1.89
Triglycerides	0.72	0.38–1.27	0.68	0.36–1.19	0.85	0.42–1.48	0.81	0.44–1.40

5th–95th percentiles. Compiled with permission from the Prevalence Study of The Lipid Research Clinics Population Studies (North America), data collected 1972–76.
Values[10] shown for white boys and for white girls not taking sex hormones. Cholesterol mmol/L % 0.0259 = mg/dL; triglycerides mmol/L ÷ 0.0113 = mg/dL.

in this condition are attributed to free-radical damage. The red blood cells have a characteristic 'spiky' appearance (acanthocytosis) because the sphingomyelin:lecithin ratio is increased in their membranes, reflecting the abnormal plasma lipid environment.

Most patients die as young adults if untreated. Normal development is possible if treatment is started early, with a low fat diet, massive doses of vitamin E, and supplements of vitamins A and K.

Tangier Disease
This is an autosomal recessive disorder in which plasma concentrations of HDL cholesterol, apo-A-I and apo-A-II are very low, because of excessive catabolism of HDL. The synthesis and structure of apo-A-I and apo-A-II are normal. Concentrations of total and LDL cholesterol are also reduced, but those of triglycerides may be slightly raised, reflecting an abnormal VLDL composition.

Pathologically, macrophages laden with cholesteryl esters occur in many tissues, particularly the reticuloendothelial system. These scavenger cells normally take up cholesterol and cholesteryl ester from dead cells and lipoprotein remnants. However, it seems that HDL, also taken into the macrophages, carries cholesterol ester out of the cells and into the plasma so that it does not accumulate. There is evidence that this intracellular processing is defective in Tangier disease, and that HDL is 'trapped' within the cells and degraded.

Clinically, enlarged, yellow-orange tonsils are the most striking feature. There may also be hepatosplenomegaly and corneal clouding. Surprisingly, atherosclerosis is not increased under 40 years of age, but is manifest later. There is no treatment.

Familial Deficiency of Lecithin–Cholesterol Acyltransferase (LCAT)
This is another autosomal recessive condition in which the plasma concentration of HDL is low. However, in this disorder, the concentrations of total cholesterol and triglyceride are increased. VLDL, IDL (intermediate-density lipoprotein) and LDL particles are abnormal because they accumulate free cholesterol. There is a genetic defect in production of LCAT, the enzyme normally responsible for esterifying free cholesterol on the surface of HDL (see Chapter 37).

Clinical sequelae include:

- corneal opacities
- proteinuria and renal impairment, possibly progressing to uraemia
- haemolysis because of acanthocytosis of the red cells (target cells), whose membrane lipids are abnormal
- premature atherosclerosis.

HYPOGLYCAEMIA

In early life, the brain is large in comparison with body size and has a higher glucose consumption per kg of body weight than adults. This is met by a higher glucose production rate: 4–6 mg/kg per min in the newborn, falling gradually to the adult level of 2 mg/kg per min by around 6 years of age.[12] The brain is particularly vulnerable to hypoglycaemia. Convulsions occur readily and permanent brain damage results from recurrent or prolonged hypoglycaemia. Chapter 6 describes the physiological mechanisms that maintain a normal blood glucose. In children, the most common causes of hypoglycaemia are

TABLE 17.3

CAUSES OF HYPOGLYCAEMIA IN CHILDREN

Defective hepatic glycogenolysis and/or gluconeogenesis
Idiopathic ketotic hypoglycaemia
Severe liver damage:
  acute liver failure
  Reye's syndrome
Poisoning with alcohol, methanol, salicylates
Hormone deficiencies:
  glucocorticoids
  growth hormone
Inherited defects:
  fat oxidation defects
  glycogen storage diseases
  gluconeogenic defects
  organic acid disorders
  tyrosinaemia

Hyperinsulinism
Nesidioblastosis
(Isolated adrenal adenoma—very rare)
Administration of insulin or hypoglycaemic drugs

See Table 17.8 for neonates.

inadequacies of glucose production from glycogen stores and via gluconeogenesis when fasting (Table 17.3). Compared with adults, hyperinsulinism is rare, except among insulin-treated diabetics.

When healthy young children are fasted, the modest liver glycogen stores are exhausted within a few hours. As the plasma glucose begins to fall, growth hormone, cortisol and glucagon secretion increase, and insulin secretion is suppressed. Increased growth hormone, in conjunction with cortisol, stimulates lipolysis in the fat depots, and there is a large flux of free fatty acids to the liver. Here, β-oxidation and ketogenesis, driven by glucagon, produce acetyl CoA, NADH + H$^+$, ATP and the ketones, acetoacetate and 3-hydroxybutyrate.

Enhanced fatty acid oxidation is intimately linked to gluconeogenesis, the synthetic pathway by which 3-carbon (3-C) molecules are converted to glucose:

1. Increases in NADH + H$^+$:NAD, ATP:ADP and acetyl CoA:CoA ratios inhibit pyruvate dehydrogenase, thereby decreasing the flux of pyruvate into the tricarboxylic acid cycle, making it available for gluconeogenesis;
2. Acetyl CoA is a cofactor for pyruvate carboxylase, the first enzyme in the gluconeogenic pathway;
3. ATP and NADH + H$^+$ provide energy and reducing equivalents for glucose synthesis.
4. In addition, glycerol, released from triglyceride hydrolysis, provides 3-C substrate for gluconeogenesis.

The water-soluble ketones thus produced leave the liver and are used by the brain as an alternative fuel to glucose, so reducing the requirement for glucose.

Defective Hepatic Glycogenolysis and Gluconeogenesis

Idiopathic ketotic hypoglycaemia is the most common cause of hypoglycaemia after the newborn period. Typically, it affects active underweight children aged 2–6 years, who have missed breakfast. They may become stuporose or have fits. They smell ketotic, have ketonuria, and are often acidotic (plasma bicarbonate around 15 mmol/L). Plasma free fatty acids and ketones are high; lactate, pyruvate and alanine are low; and insulin is appropriately suppressed. Similar falls in glucose, and increases in free fatty acids and ketones have been observed in normal, fasted, young children, so it seems likely that ketotic hypoglycaemia is merely an exaggeration of the normal fasting response.

There is no evidence for an endocrine insufficiency or a gluconeogenic defect. The probable explanation is depletion of 3-C substrate molecules for gluconeogenesis.[13] Some of the glucose that leaves the liver is oxidized completely by the tissues (especially brain) to carbon dioxide, and carbon is thus lost from the body. A considerable proportion, however, is oxidized incompletely to 3-C intermediates by glycolysis, particularly in muscle. These return to the liver as pyruvate, lactate and alanine and, with energy provided by fat metabolism, are resynthesized to glucose (Cori cycle; Fig. 17.2). Recycled carbohydrate metabolites and not amino acid skeletons are the main gluconeogenic substrates. When glycogen reserves are poor, as in underweight children, less glucose is released from the liver during fasting and the return of 3-C intermediates for resynthesis to glucose will be very reduced.

Inherited defects of mitochondrial β-oxidation of fatty acids have been recognized since 1976. Defects of all the catalytic enzymes have been reported.[14]

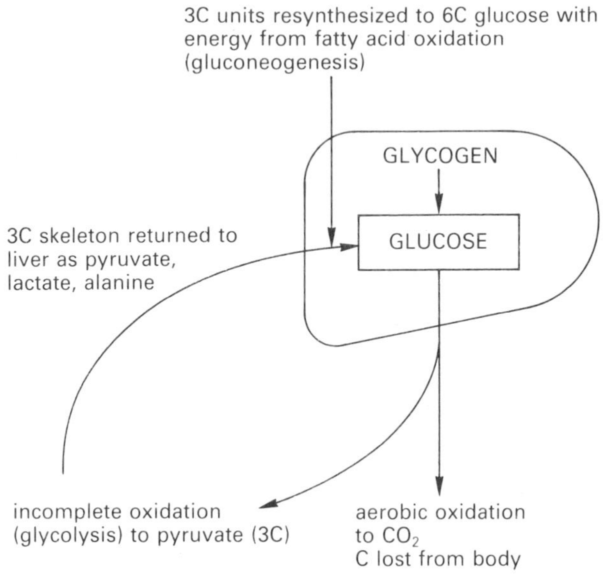

Fig. 17.2 The Cori cycle.

The most common disorder is medium-chain acyl-CoA dehydrogenase deficiency, with an incidence of at least 1 in 10 000 live births. Children with most of these defects are well when having regular meals with carbohydrate to provide energy. However, when calorie depleted, generally during an intercurrent infection, they develop an acute, life-threatening illness often clinically indistinguishable from Reye's syndrome (p. 301).

A minority of affected babies have had a cot death. The problem is that, when fasted, they use up their liver glycogen reserves quickly and then, like normal children, are dependent on fat oxidation to provide energy. Fatty acids are mobilized normally from the fat depots but are only partially degraded in the liver. An acute shortage of the normal products of fat catabolism develops. Decreased gluconeogenesis is a consequence and hypoglycaemia is common.

The liver enlarges rapidly because of fat accumulation, and liver function is disturbed. In addition, there is an acute cerebral disturbance with brain swelling, attributable to the combined deficiencies of ketones and glucose as energy sources, plus the toxic effects of circulating medium chain fatty acids. Plasma free fatty acids are appropriately raised for a fasting child, but plasma and urinary ketones are abnormally low. There is an organic aciduria with excretion of a wide range of medium-chain monocarboxylic and dicarboxylic acids.

Treatment is by glucose infusion, which promptly 'switches off' fat catabolism and leads to a rapid normalization of the biochemistry, with disappearance of the diagnostic urinary metabolites.

Inherited Disorders of Carbohydrate Metabolism. The glycogen storage disorders and hereditary fructose intolerance are discussed in Chapter 39. Defects of gluconeogenesis usually present in early infancy. The problem here is that the Cori cycle is defective: 3-C intermediates returning to the liver cannot be resynthesized to glucose. Fasting hypoglycaemia is associated with increased blood lactate, pyruvate and alanine and often a metabolic (lactic) acidosis.

Hyperinsulinism: Nesidioblastosis ('Leucine-sensitive Hypoglycaemia')[12]

Hyperinsulinism may have devastating effects on brain function in early childhood, explained by the simultaneous lack of the energy sources—glucose and the ketone bodies. In the majority of cases, it results from a developmental abnormality of the pancreatic islets, *nesidioblastosis*, in which the islet cells are increased in number and anatomically disorganized.

Presentation is during the first year of life. Insulin is raised inappropriately (generally above 10 mU/L) at the time of hypoglycaemia and C-peptide and proinsulin are raised. Plasma free fatty acids and 3-hydroxybutyric acid are low. The normal release of insulin in reponse to leucine (abundant in the milk protein, casein) is exaggerated, and most children formerly categorized as having 'leucine-sensitive hypoglycaemia' probably had this disorder.

Treatment with a combination of diazoxide and thiazide to inhibit insulin secretion may be effective, but surgical removal of 95% of the pancreas may be necessary. Islet-cell adenomas are extremely rare in childhood.

Investigation of Childhood Hypoglycaemia

Careful selection and planning of investigations is essential to avoid unnecessary risk. A thorough history and examination will narrow the diagnostic possibilities. The most useful samples are collected during hypoglycaemia: if possible, blood should be taken for glucose, insulin, cortisol, growth hormone, acid–base status, and lactate if indicated, and for later measurement of 3-hydroxybutyrate, free fatty acids and C-peptide if necessary. Urine should be tested for ketones and frozen, in case organic acid analysis is required.

It may be necessary to attempt to induce hypoglycaemia by fasting. The duration of the fast must be selected individually, guided by the history. For small babies, up to 8 h, and for older infants and young children up to 16 h is generally safe, with samples collected at 4, 6, and 8 h and 12, 14, and 16 h, respectively, for glucose, free fatty acids and 3-hydroxybutyrate, and at the end of the fast extra blood for hormone measurements and urine for organic acids. Older children may tolerate longer. Fasting should be done during the daytime, blood glucose monitored with stick tests, and an intravenous line should be sited to provide access in case of emergency.

The glucose response to glucagon stimulation in fasting and fed states is a helpful investigation for glycogen storage disorders.[1]

Provocative tests for hyperinsulinism using tolbutamide or leucine loading are hazardous and contraindicated. Glucose tolerance tests seldom have a place in the investigation of childhood hypoglycaemia.

HYPERAMMONAEMIA

There is a small number of serious disorders of childhood in which the plasma ammonia concentration is grossly elevated and contributes to an acute, and often life-threatening, illness. Except for the urea-cycle defect, ornithine transcarbamylase (OTC) deficiency, these very seldom present for the first time in adult life. Measurement of plasma ammonia is essential for diagnosis and management, and a hospital laboratory which serves a paediatric population must be able to offer this analysis at any time of day. When plasma ammonia is raised, other, specialist, laboratory investigations are required and appropriate samples must be collected at the time of the acute illness.

Ammonia is produced constantly by bacterial

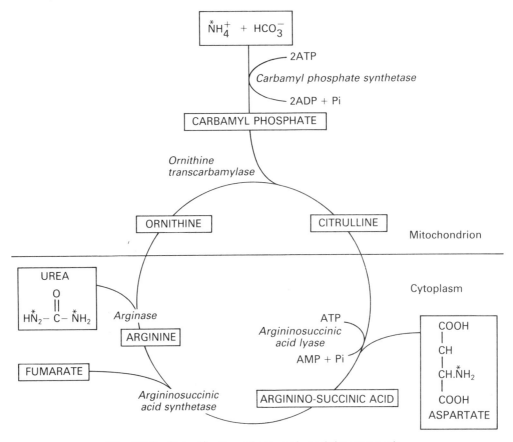

Fig. 17.3 Detoxification of ammonia and the urea cycle.

degradation of amino acids in the gut lumen. Production increases if there is haemorrhage into the gut, because of the high protein content of blood. Ammonia is absorbed into the portal circulation and detoxified in the liver by conversion to urea (Fig. 17.3). Plasma concentrations are normally maintained below 40 μmol/L.

The other important source is nitrogen from amino acids catabolized in the body. These may be dietary or from endogenous proteins. The pathways of production of ammonia from amino nitrogen are uncertain.[11] It was believed that most was channelled through glutamic acid, which was then deaminated by mitochondrial glutamate dehydrogenase. However, this has been challenged recently, and deamidation of glutamine in the gut mucosa and kidneys is proposed as a more important route.

Clinical Features

Severe hyperammonaemia in the newborn causes a gross neurological disturbance ('encephalopathy'). This commences with poor feeding and irritability but rapidly progresses, with development of fits, abnormal movements and muscle tone, coma and death. Ammonia stimulates respiration and may cause respiratory alkalosis. However, these features are not specific and may also occur, for example, following birth

asphyxia, brain haemorrhage and with a variety of inborn errors.

In later infancy and childhood, there is a range of severity from mild episodes with lethargy, confusion, unsteady gait, slurred speech and vomiting, to intractable fitting, coma and death. Again, these features overlap with those of other childhood encephalopathies. Recurrent or chronic elevation of ammonia may cause permanent brain damage.

Causes

Plasma ammonia analysis is generally requested when there is an unexplained encephalopathy suggestive of an inherited urea-cycle disorder or Reye's syndrome. Other, more common disturbances, however, may account for a raised value (Table 17.4). The quality of the plasma sample analysed cannot be overemphasized. The analysis aims to measure very low concentrations of ammonia in the presence of much greater amounts of protein and amino acids, all with the potential to liberate ammonia after sample collection, especially glutamine, which converts to glutamic acid. Haemolysed and clotted samples are unsuitable, and samples must be separated within 20 min of collection. Post-mortem samples are not acceptable. This analysis should be done at once. Samples may be stored at $-70°C$ but not at lower temperatures.

TABLE 17.4B
CAUSES OF HYPERAMMONAEMIA

Inherited defects of the urea cycle
Other inherited disorders:
    transport defects of urea-cycle intermediates
    organic acid disorders
Reye's syndrome
Liver failure

Others
Neonates:
    sick babies—non-specific increase
    birth asphyxia
    severe transient hyperammonaemia
Older infants and children:
    circulatory failure—'near miss' cot death
    salicylate poisoning

Ammonia is increased in blood from a struggling or fitting child because of release from muscles.

Inherited Urea-cycle Defects[15]

Defects of all steps of the cycle occur. Except for arginase deficiency, hyperammonaemia is the most common presentation. The clinical severity depends on the nature and completeness of the enzyme deficiency. In around one-third of cases, the liver is enlarged and plasma transaminases are raised. The most severe disorders present acutely in the first week of life, when plasma ammonia generally exceeds 300 μmol/L and plasma urea may be low. Less severe defects may not present until later childhood. This is particularly the case for girls who are carriers of the X-linked condition, ornithine transcarbamylase deficiency, which may even manifest for the first time in adult life. A few individuals with a mild, previously unsuspected, urea-cycle defect have become acutely ill with hyperammonaemia when treated with sodium valproate for epilepsy. This drug inhibits carbamyl phosphate synthetase. Even normal subjects may have a transient small increase in plasma ammonia (to around 60–70 μmol/L) when starting treatment. When there is, in addition, an inherited defect of urea production, the further 'brake' on the urea cycle by sodium valproate precipitates acute hyperammonaemia.

When a urea-cycle disorder is suspected, blood and urine must be collected for amino acid analysis and urine frozen at $-20°$C for measurement of orotic acid. Alanine and glutamine are increased non-specifically and are a useful clue. Increased citrulline, argininosuccinic acid and reduced or increased arginine help to localize the site of the defect. Orotic acid excretion is increased when carbamyl phosphate accumulates, as this is diverted to pyrimidine synthesis. Enzyme studies using skin fibroblasts, or, for some defects, liver biopsy material, confirm the diagnosis and DNA studies are useful in some kindreds. It is crucial that appropriate samples are collected from terminally ill children with these disorders, if the parents are to benefit from prenatal diagnosis of subsequent pregnancies (*see* Chapter 13). Siblings should be investigated.

Reye's Syndrome

This is a rare, serious, disorder of young children (UK: mean age 14 months). Typically, a previously healthy child has a common viral infection, apparently taking a normal course. Three to five days from its onset, however, there is profuse, effortless vomiting and lethargy, progressing to delirium and coma, sometimes with fits. There is a high mortality (UK, 1983–4: up to 50%) and survivors may have brain damage.

In the acute illness, the liver is enlarged and laden with fat. The liver mitochondria are abnormal in shape, swollen and have disrupted cristae. Low activities of mitochondrial enzymes are demonstrable: carbamyl phosphate synthetase and ornithine transcarbamylase (urea cycle), pyruvate carboxylase (gluconeogenesis) and tricarboxylic acid-cycle enzymes.[16] The brain is swollen and there may be pathological changes in the heart, skeletal muscles and kidney. The evidence points to an acute mitochondrial insult, affecting several body organs. Plasma transaminases are raised (3–30 times normal), bilirubin seldom exceeds 17 μmol/L, there may be hypoglycaemia, and ammonia is transiently (24–48 h) raised to 2–20 times normal. The urinary organic acid profile shows evidence of impaired mitochondrial oxidation of fatty acids. However, the liver disturbance is evanescent, and within 3 or 4 days the histology returns to normal.

The *aetiology* is unknown but is probably multifactorial, resulting from an abnormal reaction to a viral infection in a genetically susceptible host, perhaps modified by an exogenous toxin. Among those implicated are aflatoxins, insecticides, margosa oil and aspirin, frequently given to feverish children. Aspirin acts on mitochondria *in vitro* and epidemiological evidence from both the USA and UK, although inconclusive, supported a possible association with Reye's syndrome.[17] The incidence has decreased dramatically since 1984 (USA) and 1986 (UK), following recommendations not to give aspirin to febrile children under 12 years. With this decline, children *now* presenting with features of Reye's syndrome are likely to have an inherited defect and *must* be investigated (*see below*).

Other Conditions Presenting with a Reye's Syndrome-like Illness

Salicylate poisoning and, in rare instances, sodium valproate treatment have caused illnesses resembling Reye's syndrome. Urea-cycle defects may be a source of confusion clinically, although the pathology is distinct. Inherited fatty-acid oxidation defects (p. 298) may present as a 'typical' Reye's syndrome, and the

TABLE 17.5
CAUSES OF SHORT STATURE

Genetic
Racial
Familial
Chromosomal abnormalities:
　Turner's syndrome
　trisomies
Genetic defects:
　bone dysplasias
　metabolic disorders

Extrinsic
Intrauterine growth retardation
Nutritional:
　marasmus, kwashiorkor
　less severe malnutrition
　rickets
　malabsorption—gluten-sensitive enteropathy
Chronic disease:
　chronic renal failure
　asthma
　congenital heart disease
　mental retardation

Endocrine
Delayed puberty
Hypothyroidism
Excessive corticosteroids:
　iatrogenic
　Cushing's syndrome
Androgen excess:
　congenital adrenal hyperplasia
Growth hormone deficiency:
　Reversible:
　　emotional deprivation
　Permanent:
　　gene deletion
　　disturbed hypothalamic control
　　hypothalamic damage
Growth hormone insensitivity:
　Laron dwarfism

---

liver is enlarged and fatty. Other inherited organic-acid disorders may be confused. It is essential that blood and urine are collected *on admission* to investigate for a possible inherited disorder. The diagnostic abnormalities disappear very quickly with glucose therapy.

Other Causes of Hyperammonaemia

Sick newborn infants may have non-specific increase in plasma ammonia up to around 150 μmol/L, which need not be investigated. High values (even to 300 μmol/L) occur in the first 24 h following birth asphyxia, due to severe liver hypoxia, and similar increases are seen in older shocked babies, often following a 'near-miss' cot death. Liver hypoxia might also contribute to gross, transient, ammonia elevations in the first 48 h of life reported as a rare event in preterm infants with respiratory distress.

CHILDREN WITH SHORT STATURE

Growth rate and height are continuous variables. Generally, children are considered short if their height falls below the third centile (approximately 2 SD below the mean) on a growth chart—that is, less than that of 97% of children of the same sex, age, race, and sexual maturity. Growth rate (height velocity) is a better indicator of poor growth, with rates less than the twenty-fifth centile being subnormal, and below the third centile indicating severe growth impairment. It is estimated that as many as 2 or 3 in every 1000 children have short stature that is due to a treatable cause. Early identification and treatment are essential to achieve the maximal growth potential.

Causes

There are many causes (Table 17.5).[18]

The most extreme *racial variation* is seen in the African pygmies, who may have a defect of IGF-1 receptors. *Familial* short stature is common, and measurement of parental height is an essential investigation of a short child.

Turner's syndrome should be considered in all short girls. Typically the karyotype is 45XO but mosaicism and abnormalities of the X chromosome (e.g. ring chromosomes) also occur. These girls have a reduced 24-h growth hormone secretion and their height velocity increases with growth hormone injections.

Many *inherited disorders of bone* cause short stature, with skeletal disproportion if the trunk and limb bones are affected differently.

Children with other *inherited metabolic defects* are often small. This may be because of metabolic disturbances, for example acidosis in organic acid disorders and hypoglycaemia in glycogen storage disease, or because of a direct effect on bone turnover, as in pseudohypoparathyroidism and the mucopolysaccharidoses.

Severe fetal *malnutrition*, because of placental insufficiency, causes intrauterine growth retardation and, when this commences before 34 weeks of gestation, it may have a permanent effect on growth potential. Malnutrition in childhood is a common cause of poor growth worldwide. Despite raised basal plasma growth-hormone levels, IGF-1 production is low. Other hormonal changes (reduced tri-iodothyronine and thyroid-stimulating hormone, and insulin—depending on carbohydrate intake) may also contribute.

Endocrine Causes

By far the most common is *delayed puberty*, especially in boys. Growth rate normally slows during childhood (to around 5 cm/year) until puberty, when it accelerates dramatically (mean peak 10.5 cm/year and 9.0 cm/year in boys and girls, respectively), largely because of growth of the trunk. If appropriate, growth rate and sexual maturation may be accelerated by treatment with chorionic gonadotrophin (boys) or sex steroids, which increase the pulsatility of growth hormone release. Growth hormone may be added if secretion is still suboptimal.

Hypothyroidism in its less severe form, from developmental or biochemical disorders, may present with short stature during childhood, without intellectual deficits.

Corticosteroid excess most often occurs in children with a chronic disorder requiring steroid therapy—both factors contribute to poor growth.

Glucocorticoids decrease growth hormone secretion, protein anabolism, production of IGF-1, and possibly the end-organ response to it.

Increased *androgens* (e.g. in congenital adrenal hyperplasia) accelerate both growth rate and skeletal maturation. At first, children grow quickly, but the bone epiphyses fuse early, growth stops and the final height is small.

Growth Hormone Deficiency[19]

It is now clear that the variation of growth rate of children depends on how much growth hormone they secrete which, in turn, depends upon the number and amplitude of growth hormone pulses released into the blood over 24 h. There is a continuous spectrum of growth hormone secretion and, as with growth, there is not a clear separation between normal and abnormal. It is important to identify children with a persisting deficiency of growth hormone because they respond well to growth hormone therapy, if started early. Before 1985, growth hormone was in very short supply and had to be rationed to children with severe deficiencies. With the availability of synthetic growth hormone, produced by recombinant DNA technology, there is an unlimited supply, so that many more short children could be treated. Cost (several thousand pounds per year) is now the main restricting factor.

Reversible growth hormone deficiency occurs in emotionally deprived children who are rejected or unloved by their parents and lack social stimulation. At home, growth rate is very slow. When admitted to hospital, they respond to the attention on the ward, growth rate accelerates strikingly, only to fall again on return home. Poor growth is associated with decreased pulses of growth hormone secretion and the growth hormone response to insulin may be reduced at the time of admission. Both become normal in the ward setting.

Children with severe, *permanent*, growth hormone deficiency are typically very small, rather plump and have a round, immature face. Complete deficiency results from a rare inherited defect with a gene deletion. In the vast majority of cases, the deficiency seems to be due to disordered secretion of growth hormone-releasing hormone by the hypothalamus, which leads to abnormally small and disorganized pulses of growth hormone secretion by the pituitary gland. Gonadotrophins may also be deficient. The integrated, 24-h, growth hormone secretion is low. In a minority of children, large, but haphazard, pulses of secretion have been observed (neurosecretory dysfunction). A developmental cystic abnormality (craniopharyngioma) encroaching on the hypothalamus may cause deficiencies of growth hormone and other pituitary hormones. The very rare Laron dwarfs have high circulating concentrations of growth hormone but, because of an inherited defect of growth hormone receptors, do not synthesize IGF-1.

Diagnosis.[9] The initial assessment of a short child includes careful documentation of sitting and standing height and weight, and exclusion of causes such as chromosomal or inherited defects, chronic diseases, delayed puberty and hypothyroidism. Height is measured again, for example in 4 months, and the growth rate is assessed. If less than the third centile, growth hormone deficiency is investigated. If between the third and twenty-fifth centiles, growth rate may be followed for 1 year before investigating.

Because plasma growth hormone is normally very low, random measurements are useless and stimulation is required to show deficiency. A *physiological* stimulus may be used as first line: measurement of the plasma growth hormone rises following a standardized exercise test, or 1 and 1.5 h after sleep, when a normal surge of the hormone occurs. A value exceeding 15 mU/L (some prefer 20 mU/L) is normal.

Several *pharmacological* stimulatory tests are available:[3] insulin-induced hypoglycaemia, arginine infusion, a glucose-rebound rise test, and L-dopa, clonidine and glucagon tests. It is not known which is closest to physiological stimulation. Generally, results are clear-cut for severe deficiencies (growth hormone response less than 7 mU/L), but may be unhelpful in less severe cases. Children with a neurosecretory disorder may have a normal response.

In difficult cases, specialist growth units may investigate the 24-h growth hormone profile, by taking serial, 20-min, blood samples. More often now, a therapeutic trial of growth hormone is used. Measurement of overnight or 24-h urinary growth hormone excretion, or plasma IGF-1, is often unhelpful in less severe deficiencies, although values are clearly low in severe cases.

THE ACUTELY SICK CHILD WITH A POSSIBLE INBORN ERROR OF METABOLISM

Inborn errors of metabolism are rare causes of acute childhood illness, but they occur. The most severe defects often present neonatally.[20] It is important to act quickly. Untreated, inborn errors may damage the brain very rapidly—sometimes in as little as 1 or 2 days.

The aims of clinical management are to remove potentially toxic compounds from the body, to eliminate the substrate(s) for their production (for example, protein-containing foods), and to provide adequate calories as carbohydrate in order to suppress endogenous protein catabolism and provide fuel for brain metabolism. In addition, large doses of vitamin cofactors of defective enzymes may be given, in an attempt to increase enzyme activity.

Certain inborn errors of metabolism are so damaging that death is inevitable. It is then extremely important to establish a diagnosis in an affected child, so that the parents may be given accurate genetic counselling for subsequent pregnancies, and offered prenatal diagnosis for those conditions for which tests are available (see Chapter 13).

When such emergencies arise, the laboratory must take a leading role in coordinating investigations.[21] There is an enormous number of different defects, and their presentations overlap so much that it is hardly ever possible to make a precise diagnosis on clinical grounds alone. Senior staff must have a clear idea of the limits of the diagnostic services that they can provide for these conditions, and when and where to seek help.

Important clues often emerge from careful interpretation of routinely available tests. These should include plasma electrolytes, calcium, glucose, liver enzymes and bilirubin, arterial blood gases and acid–base status (with cognizance of the state of oxygenation and perfusion), and urine testing for smell, pH, ketones, glucose, reducing substances, and phenylketones (Ames Phenistix; ferric chloride test).

Haematological studies should include full blood count, including platelets, and clotting studies if liver damage is suspected. Blood and urine should be collected for amino acid analysis and urine frozen immediately, without preservative, in case organic acid analysis is required. Analysis of plasma ammonia is necessary if a urea-cycle defect is suspected.

Estimation of blood pyruvate, lactate, uric acid, 3-hydroxybutyrate, free fatty acids and carnitine may be indicated in some cases and samples may be taken and stored against this possibility. Spare cerobrospinal fluid from microbiological studies should be frozen.

All samples should be collected as soon as possible after the onset of illness, as the diagnostic biochemical disturbances in some disorders resolve very rapidly after instituting treatment. If transfusion is required, blood should be collected first, and plasma and washed red cells frozen. It is important to seek help from a more experienced laboratory early if there are analytical or interpretative problems.

In cases where there has been no time to make a diagnosis and death is imminent, appropriate samples must be taken before, or immediately after, death and stored for later analysis. These should include urine, plasma, whole blood for DNA studies (possible on frozen blood or, in some centres, transformed lymphocytes) and a skin biopsy for fibroblast culture. A percutaneous liver biopsy may be indicated if a defect of a liver enzyme is suspected,

which is not expressed in fibroblasts, and, rarely, a muscle biopsy. (See UK Directory[22] for practical details.)

BIOCHEMISTRY FOR SICK AND PRETERM NEONATES

The vast majority of babies are born at term, are of normal birth weight, and have no need for any biochemical investigations neonatally other than screening tests for phenylketonuria and congenital hypothyroidism. However, not all are as fortunate. Some babies become distressed during delivery, because of problems in labour, and are born in poor condition. In the worst cases, they suffer birth asphyxia—the heart beat and respirations cease, and central nervous system activity is severely depressed. Such babies require immediate, vigorous, resuscitation and even then may die neonatally or suffer long-term brain damage. Other babies have severe respiratory problems, are born with a congenital infection, or have a serious haemolytic disorder. A very small minority have an inborn error of metabolism that causes acute illness in the first days of life. All of these very sick newborns may have gross biochemical disturbances. They need intensive care, which must include close biochemical monitoring.

Another large group requiring intensive care is of those with low birth weight, that is, less than 2500 g. These account for around 7% of births in the UK. One-third are small because of intrauterine growth retardation, and two-thirds because of prematurity (birth before 37 weeks of gestation). Around 1% of infants weigh less than 1500 g and are defined as very low birth weight (VLBW); the majority of these are premature. With improvements in obstetric and neonatal care, survival rates are now around 50% for babies weighing between 750 and 1000 g and 90% or better for those between 1000 and 1500 g. However, around 10% of survivors weighing less than 1500 g have one or more persisting handicaps.

Most of the problems of preterm babies arise because of their immaturity. Maturation occurs rapidly, but until this happens these babies have to be supported with obsessional attention to detail.[23]

RESPIRATORY DISTRESS

Respiratory distress is the most common, serious problem of sick newborns. There are several different causes. However, in infants born before 35 weeks of gestation, by far the most common is the respiratory distress syndrome, also known as hyaline membrane disease, which is due to a deficiency of surfactant. The incidence is inversely related to gestational age (35–50% of babies born at 27–31 weeks of gestation are affected) and is increased in babies of diabetic mothers with poor diabetic control in pregnancy. Around 3 per 1000 live-born infants die from the syndrome.

Surfactant and the Respiratory Distress Syndrome (RDS)[24]

Surfactant is a complex mixture of lipids and proteins, synthesized by type II cells of the alveoli of the lungs from about 34 weeks of gestation. It is secreted into the thin layer of liquid that coats the alveoli, to form a covering surface monolayer. *In utero*, it diffuses from the lungs into the amniotic fluid.

Phospholipids are the major components, and contribute the important physical properties. In mature babies, phosphatidylcholine (lecithin) accounts for 80.9% of phospholipids, phosphatidylethanolamine 11.7%, phosphatidylglycerol 3.7%, and sphingomyelin 2.0%. Fifty per cent of the phosphatidylcholine contains two palmitic acid residues as the esterified fatty acid, and a further 10% has palmitic acid and one other saturated fatty acid. This high content of saturated long-chain fatty acids confers important structural properties to the surfactant.

About 10% of the total lipids are *neutral lipids*: free fatty acids, triglycerides and cholesterol. Three low molecular-weight *apoproteins* have also been identified.

Immature babies with RDS produce insufficient surfactant, and its composition is abnormal, with lower proportions of phosphatidylcholine and phosphatidylglycerol and increases in sphingomyelin, phosphatidylethanolamine and phosphatidylinositol. In addition, more of the fatty acids in phosphatidylcholine are unsaturated. Formerly, the amniotic fluid lecithin:sphingomyelin ratio, or, in some laboratories, palmitic acid, was used to assess fetal maturity and potential viability in complicated pregnancies where early delivery was contemplated. The need for this has now largely disappeared with the advent of ultrasound scanning for accurate assessment of gestational age.

The Respiratory Distress Syndrome

In utero, the alveoli of the term fetus are filled with aqueous fluid containing surfactant. Secretion increases sharply at birth, when the babies gasp and air enters the lungs. The surfactant spreads evenly over the alveolar surfaces and the phospholipid molecules align themselves at the air–water interface so that the fatty acids are in air and the head groups in water. This detergent action lowers the surface tension of the alveoli, which therefore distend easily and uniformly throughout the lungs during inspiration. It also prevents the alveoli collapsing during expiration.

When surfactant is deficient and abnormal, the surface tension is high, particularly in the smallest alveoli, and they cannot be inflated. There is uneven expansion and many alveoli collapse. The lining cells are damaged by high shearing forces during laboured respiration, and a proteinaceous fluid exudes into them, forming a 'hyaline' membrane, and decreases gaseous exchange further.

Within 3 h of birth, the babies are extremely distressed and struggling to breathe. They become hypoxic and cyanosed, and also have raised P_{CO_2} with mixed respiratory and metabolic (lactic) acidosis. In response to hypoxia and acidosis, the pulmonary arteries constrict and blood may be shunted away from the lungs, so that the blood–gas exchange becomes even worse. Bleeding into the brain (intraventricular haemorrhage) is a relatively common complication. The condition deteriorates over the first few hours of life, but improves after a few days, as surfactant production increases.

Ventilation of Babies with RDS

The aim is to support the infant until surfactant production is adequate, by maintaining oxygenation, which may necessitate intermittent positive-pressure ventilation with high concentrations of inhaled oxygen. It is crucial that the arterial oxygen tension (P_{O_2}) is maintained within tight limits (7–11 kPa). If the P_{O_2} is too low, the risk of permanent brain damage is increased. If P_{O_2} is too high, even for only a few hours, the retina may be damaged irreversibly, causing *retinopathy of prematurity* (retrolental fibroplasia) with blindness. In addition, high concentrations of inspired oxygen (more than 80%) may be one factor causing long-term lung damage (*bronchopulmonary dysplasia*).

It is possible that toxic superoxide O_2^- and hydroxyl $OH\cdot$ radicals are generated as hypoxanthine (increased in body tissues and fluids during hypoxia) is oxidized by xanthine oxidase when oxygen is supplied.[25] Protection against these damaging oxygen species may be suboptimal in very immature newborns because of deficiencies of the enzymes catalase, superoxide dismutase and glutathione peroxidase. Careful control of the P_{CO_2} (at 5–7 kPa) is also important: low tensions constrict the cerebral arteries and reduce blood flow through the brain; high ones cause arterial dilatation and may precipitate brain haemorrhage. Metabolic acidosis must be corrected.

Artificial surfactant is now available for replacement therapy. Given into the pharynx at birth and into the trachea during the first 24 h of life, it decreases the severity and mortality of RDS.

Blood Gas Monitoring

Frequent monitoring is essential. Small changes in ventilator settings may produce large fluctuations in blood gases of these babies, whose physiological state is unstable and whose disease processes are evolving. *In vivo* and *in vitro* monitoring are used in parallel.

During the first days of life, umbilical arterial P_{O_2} may be monitored continuously by insertion of a fine catheter with a polarographic, oxygen-sensitive electrode implanted into the tip. Blood is removed via the catheter at intervals, for full blood-gas analysis, to check calibration and assess acid–base status. These catheters are disposable but expensive. More often, blood is sampled repeatedly via indwelling arterial lines and analysed *in vitro*. Although blood gases are frequently still analysed in arterialized capillary blood collected by skin puncture, the measurements predict arterial Po_2, Pco_2 and pH poorly, particularly for babies with poor peripheral circulation.

Transcutaneous oxygen (Po_2(tc)) electrodes are used widely.[26] A small, polarographic, oxygen electrode, heated to 43°C, is applied to the skin. Oxygen diffuses from the capillaries through the skin (thin and poorly keratinized in premature babies) and then through the gas-permeable membrane of the electrode. It is necessary to check the calibration against *in vitro* arterial blood-gas measurements. Tight linear correlation of Po_2 (tc) and arterial Po_2 has been observed over the range 6–14 kPa, but Po_2 (tc) underestimates Po_2 at high oxygen concentrations.

Transcutaneous Pco_2 (tc) electrodes measure Pco_2 of arterialized capillary blood with a glass pH electrode, separated from the warmed skin by a hydrophobic membrane permeable to CO_2 but not H^+; CO_2 diffuses from the blood and into the electrode buffer, causing a pH change. A correction factor is used since Pco_2 (tc) measurements are approximately 27% higher than Pco_2: the skin produces CO_2 and local heating increases CO_2 release from the tissues. At higher values, Pco_2 is overestimated. Drift is also a problem. Transcutaneous monitoring is not reliable in shocked babies.

Pulse oximetry[27] provides information about the oxygen saturation of haemoglobin (Hb), which is related to Po_2 by the sigmoid Hb/oxygen dissociation curve. This, in turn, is influenced by arterial blood pH and the proportion of circulating fetal to adult Hb. The aim is to keep saturation within the range 90–95%. Oximetry is not a reliable means of monitoring for hyperoxaemia, as even large increases of Po_2 at high values induce insignificant increases in Hb saturation. It is very sensitive to small changes in Po_2 at low values, however. The method utilizes the differences in absorbance by oxyHb and Hb of light at the red end of the spectrum.

FLUID BALANCE DISTURBANCES[23]

Between 24 weeks and term, fetal body water decreases from 85% to 75% of body weight, and extracellular fluid volume (ECFV) from 60% to 45% (values at 1 year are around 60% and 27%, respectively). The newborn baby therefore has a relatively expanded ECFV. Fractional sodium excretion is high *in utero*—5% at 32 to 36 weeks, and 3.5% at term. At birth, the urinary flow rate decreases and urine osmolality increases, reflecting a transient increase in arginine vasopressin (AVP; antidiuretic hormone) secretion. Sodium is retained, fractional sodium excretion decreasing to 0.3%, probably because of high concentrations of renin and aldosterone.

In the first 4 h of life, plasma volume falls, as a result of a fluid shift from the vascular to extravascular compartments. Normally, over the next few days, there is a diuresis and natriuresis, which reduces the ECFV to around 40% of body weight by 7 days. Fluid loss is proportionately greater in preterm infants. Further reduction of ECFV occurs during the first 12 months of life.

Problems of fluid and electrolyte balance are frequently encountered in preterm and sick newborns, reflecting limited renal homeostatic function, relatively large, insensible water losses, losses from the gastrointestinal tract, and errors in fluid replacement therapy.

Renal compensation is limited by low glomerular filtration and tubular immaturity (p. 295). The response to sodium and water loading is blunted, partly because of decreased filtration but probably also because the outer cortical nephrons, normally concerned with sodium disposal, are immature. In the face of sodium depletion, normal newborn infants can retain sodium avidly: although proximal reabsorption of filtered sodium is proportionately less than in adults, this is compensated for by distal tubular reabsorption. However, some very immature babies have a diminished capacity for sodium retention and become hyponatraemic on low sodium intakes.

Salt wasting also occurs following renal tubular damage in birth asphyxia and if there is mineralocorticoid deficiency in congenital adrenal hyperplasia (*see* Chapter 41). The normal heavy dependence on aldosterone for sodium conservation neonatally may account for the gross salt wasting that occurs in newborn babies with this disorder.

Water depletion with hypernatraemia is a constant threat, particularly for preterm babies. Their insensible water losses from the skin are high compared with adults, as a result of increased skin permeability, increased skin blood flow, lack of subcutaneous fat, increased surface area:mass ratio and phototherapy (sweating is negligible before 35 weeks of gestation). Losses from the lungs may be increased if the breathing rate is rapid. Moreover, because of their decreased ability to concentrate urine (p. 295), newborns may lose water from the kidneys in the face of dehydration. Water retention with dilutional hyponatraemia also occurs frequently. Inappropriate AVP secretion is one cause, seen with brain damage, lung disease and during intermittent positive-pressure ventilation. Diagnostic criteria at this age are simultaneous plasma osmolality below 270 and urinary osmolality above 150 mosmol/kg water, in the absence of hypovolaemia or adrenal and renal insufficiency. Management is by fluid restriction—demeclocycline is not used neonatally. Indomethacin, used to treat patent ductus arteriosus, also causes water retention, perhaps through an interference with the tubular action of AVP. A third cause is administration of excessive amounts of aqueous, sodium-free fluids intravenously.

Fluid balance disturbances contribute to cardiovascular instability. Fluid overload may precipitate cer-

TABLE 17.6
PATHOLOGICAL CAUSES OF UNCONJUGATED
HYPERBILIRUBINAEMIA: NEONATES

Increased bilirubin load
Haemolytic disorders:
  Destructive red-cell antibodies:
    Rhesus incompatibility
    ABO incompatibility
    maternal autoimmune disease
  Structural red-cell defects:
    hereditary spherocytosis
    hereditary elliptocytosis
  Red-cell enzyme defects:
    glucose-6-phosphate dehydrogenase deficiency
    pyruvate kinase deficiency
Extensive bruising
Polycythaemia
Infections with intravascular coagulation and haemolysis

Decreased conjugation
Crigler–Najjar syndrome
Transient familial neonatal hyperbilirubinaemia
Dehydration
Pyloric stenosis
Congenital hypothyroidism
Breast-milk jaundice

Increased intestinal reabsorption
Intestinal obstruction

ebral bleeding and exacerbate brain oedema in asphyxiated babies. Meticulous clinical and biochemical monitoring is essential. In general, the aim is to keep plasma sodium between 135 and 145 mmol/L, and urinary osmolality between 150 and 400 mosmol/kg water.

JAUNDICE

1. Unconjugated Hyperbilirubinaemia

(a) Physiological Jaundice[23]
Some degree of jaundice due to unconjugated hyperbilirubinaemia is common in babies who are otherwise well. *In utero*, unconjugated bilirubin is cleared by the placenta, and umbilical cord blood bilirubin is normally less than 35 μmol/L. Bilirubin increases sharply from birth. In full-term babies, there is a peak of up to 180 μmol/L on days 2–4, then a rapid fall, generally to less than 34 μmol/L by 7 days of age. In preterm babies, peak values are higher (up to 270 μmol/L) and occur on days 5–7, with values then falling gradually, generally to below 34 μmol/L by 14 days.

The normal excretion of biliburin is discussed in Chapter 22. Physiological jaundice of the newborn is probably multifactorial, reflecting increased production of bilirubin compared with older children and adults, slower excretion and increased reabsorption from the small intestine. Carbon monoxide excretion in expired air is two- to threefold higher than in

adults. This is evidence of a higher rate of haem oxidation, probably accounted for by the shortened mean life-span of red blood cells neonatally (45–70 days compared with 120 days in adults), and by the relatively larger red-cell mass.

Factors contributing to impaired excretion of bilirubin are:

- deficiency of ligandin
- deficiencies of the enzymes uridine diphosphoglucose dehydrogenase and uridine diphosphoglucuronyl transferase, needed for bilirubin conjugation with glucuronic acid.

Disturbance of intrahepatic blood flow with poor perfusion of the hepatocytes is a further, theoretical, mechanism. Within the intestine, β-glucuronidases in the intestinal mucosa cleave conjugated bilirubin but the neonate initially lacks the appropriate intestinal bacteria to degrade bilirubin to urobilinogen. There is enhanced reabsorption of unconjugated bilirubin, particularly if gut motility is slower because oral feeds are withheld.

(b) Pathological Increases in Unconjugated Bilirubin
The common occurrence of 'physiological' jaundice indicates that even in healthy babies the bilirubin excretory pathway is overwhelmed in the first days of life. When a concurrent pathological process stresses the pathway further, the amount of unconjugated bilirubin in the plasma rises rapidly (Table 17.6).

The most dramatic increases occur in *haemolytic disorders* due to *blood-group incompatibilities*, sometimes referred to as 'haemolytic disease of the newborn'. The basic problem is that the baby inherits a red cell antigen from the father which the mother lacks. If fetal red cells get into her circulation, for example because of an antepartum haemorrhage or traumatic amniocentesis, the mother makes antibodies. These cross the placenta and destroy the red cells of her baby. Fetal red cells may also enter the maternal circulation during delivery. The antibodies produced then may damage the fetus of a succeeding pregnancy.

With severe red cell destruction *in utero* the baby becomes anaemic and develops heart failure with oedema ('hydrops fetalis'). Evidence of severe haemolysis at birth is a cord blood haemoglobin below 100 g/L, bilirubin above 70 μmol/L, and a progressive increase in bilirubin of more than 8 μmol/h. Rhesus (Rh) incompatibility was the most common cause of haemolytic disease, but the incidence has fallen dramatically with prophylactic administration of Rh antibody to Rh-negative mothers.

Neonatally, destruction of red cells because of inherited structural abnormalities (spherocytosis; elliptocytosis) may exacerbate jaundice. The X-linked enzyme defect glucose-6-phosphate dehydrogenase deficiency affects millions of individuals worldwide and may cause pathological jaundice neonatally if there is a coincident oxidant stress—for example, sepsis, or an oxidant drug administered to the baby or its mother. As circulating reticulocytes of an affected baby may produce normal blood-enzyme activities *in vitro*, the mother should also be investigated in suspected cases. The haemoglobinopathy, homozygous sickle-cell disease, only rarely presents with anaemia and jaundice neonatally. β-Thalassaemia generally presents after 3 months of age. Crigler–Najjar syndrome and Gilbert's syndrome are discussed in Chapter 22. It is uncertain whether Gilbert's syndrome contributes to neonatal jaundice.

Breast-milk jaundice is a frequent cause of concern. Around 2.5% of breast-fed infants have prolonged jaundice, with bilirubin concentrations of 255–360 μmol/L or higher, in the second or third weeks of life. They are generally well. Without intervention, bilirubin may remain elevated for several weeks, only declining to normal by 12–16 weeks. If breast milk is discontinued, plasma bilirubin falls to normal within 7 days and jaundice often does not recur when breast-feeding is resumed. Seventy-five per cent of siblings in these families are affected. The disturbance is not harmful, and mothers can be reassured, provided a pathological cause (particularly hypothyroidism) has been excluded. The cause is still debated. One proposed candidate is the steroid 3-α, 20β-pregnanediol found in the milk of some mothers. It has been shown that this inhibits glucuronide conjugation by guinea pig, although not human, liver *in vitro*. Increased free fatty acids in breast milk, perhaps reflecting increased mammary gland lipase activity, may inhibit conjugation. Alternatively, some abnormality of the breast milk may cause enhanced bilirubin reabsorption from the gut.

(c) Risks of Unconjugated Hyperbilirubinaemia

Unconjugated bilirubin in the circulation is normally bound tightly to albumin at a high-affinity binding site, which is probably shared by other endogenous anions and drugs. When plasma bilirubin concentrations become very high and the binding approaches saturation, free, unconjugated, bilirubin is able to cross the blood–brain barrier, because it is lipid soluble, and is deposited in the cells of certain deep-seated nuclei that have a very high metabolic activity. This causes a severe neurological disturbance in the neonatal period, 'kernicterus', which may be fatal.

Children who survive may have movement disorders, high-tone deafness and mental retardation. The risk of kernicterus begins to increase when plasma concentrations of unconjugated bilirubin exceed 360 μmol/L in full-term infants, and 290 μmol/L in otherwise normal preterm babies (lower in sick babies who are acidotic or hypoxic). However, the occurrence is very unpredictable and well, preterm babies have tolerated concentrations up to 410 μmol/L without damage. A lower affinity of albumin for bilirubin in preterm infants may increase their risk, and this is exacerbated by administration of drugs such as sulphonamides that compete for albumin binding. Dis-

turbance of the blood–brain barrier may also be contributory. *In vitro*, free bilirubin binds readily to cell membranes, including mitochondria, causing ion 'leakage', uncoupling of oxidative phosphorylation, inhibition of electron transport, and of DNA and protein synthesis. It also inhibits phosphofructokinase and other glycolytic enzymes. However, high concentrations have often been used, and the *in vivo* toxic mechanisms are unknown.

(d) Prevention of Kernicterus

Kernicterus is not treatable, but it can be prevented. Jaundiced babies must be monitored closely to anticipate the possibility of a toxic concentration. The results should be plotted serially on ward charts on which appropriate 'action limits' are marked. In the majority of cases, phototherapy effectively reduces the plasma bilirubin to safe levels. Cold blue light of wavelength 400–500 nm is directed on to the unclothed baby and penetrates the skin to around 2 mm. Unconjugated bilirubin circulating in the superficial blood vessels is converted to water-soluble compounds. The main change is probably photo-isomerization to a geometric stereoisomer (4(Z)-, 15(E)-bilirubin, (Z)-lumirubin, or photobilirubin) in which polar groups of the molecule are exposed. In this form, bilirubin may be excreted in bile without conjugation. A small amount of bilirubin undergoes photo-oxidation to water-soluble pyrroles excreted in urine. When plasma bilirubin concentrations are increasing rapidly, an exchange transfusion may be necessary in order to replace the infant's blood with non-jaundiced blood and red cells. This is a much more hazardous procedure.

(e) Monitoring Neonatal Jaundice

A bilirubinometer in a side-room of the ward, for use by clinicians, is an invaluable aid, providing that lipaemic, turbid and severely haemolysed samples are not analysed, and that bilirubin concentrations exceeding 250 μmol/L are confirmed by the laboratory. The instruments are insensitive below 34 μmol/L and loss of linearity is reported above 340 μmol/L. Mild to moderate haemolysis is corrected for, and there is no interference from phototherapy products. Transcutaneous bilirubinometry measures the yellow skin reflectance from a xenon lamp applied to the skin. This is linearly related to bilirubin. Measurements cannot be made on skin exposed to phototherapy. The method is best used to screen out babies with bilirubin below 170 μmol/L who do not, therefore, require a blood test.

2. Conjugated Hyperbilirubinaemia and Neonatal Liver Disease[28]

Jaundice with conjugated bilirubinaemia is always pathological, and is associated with disease of the liver or biliary tract (Table 17.7). Differentiation of the many causes is generally impossible on clinical grounds: hepatomegaly, cholestasis, abnormal liver

TABLE 17.7
CAUSES OF CONJUGATED HYPERBILIRUBINAEMIA: NEONATES

Hepatocellular damage with cholestasis
  Infective:
    septicaemia
    viral
    toxoplasmosis
Inherited defects
  Metabolic:
    galactosaemia
    hereditary fructose intolerance
    tyrosinaemia
  α-1-Antitrypsin deficiency
  Cystic fibrosis
  Peroxisome defects
  Trihydroxycoprostanoic acidaemia
  Storage disorders, e.g. Gaucher's disease; Wolman's
    disease
  Dubin–Johnson syndrome

Parenteral nutrition

Idiopathic neonatal hepatitis

Disorders of the biliary tree
  Intrahepatic biliary hypoplasia:
    normal chromosomes
    trisomy 13 or 18
  Extrahepatic biliary atresia
  Choledochal cyst

function tests and blood clotting, and raised α-fetoprotein are common features. (*Note*: α-fetoprotein is normally high, anyway, in newborn infants.)

There are four metabolic causes that must always be excluded as follows.

1. *Galactosaemia*, due to deficiency of galactose-1-phosphate uridyl transferase, presents after 3 or 4 days of life with poor feeding, rapidly increasing jaundice, hepatomegaly, bleeding, a neurological disturbance, and often Gram-negative septicaemia. Urine will be positive for reducing substances (Benedict's test or Clinitest), but negative for glucose (glucose stick test), providing the baby has received milk in the preceding few hours. Tests may be negative if milk has been withdrawn and, for example, a glucose infusion started. If the result is positive, the urine sample should be analysed by sugar chromatography and the milk changed to a galactose-free formula pending the result. The diagnosis is confirmed by analysis of red blood-cell galactose-1-phosphate uridyl transferase. If the baby has had a blood transfusion, the test must be postponed for 6 weeks.

2. *Tyrosinaemia* is caused by an inherited deficiency of fumaroacetoacetate hydrolase, an enzyme of the tyrosine degradative pathway. There is acute liver and renal tubular damage. Biochemically, plasma concentrations of tyrosine and methionine are very high, there is a generalized aminoaciduria, excretion of large amounts of phenolic acid metabolites of tyrosine and excretion of a diagnostic metabolite *succinylacetone*, identified by urinary organic analysis with gas chromatography–mass spectrometry.

3. *Hereditary fructose intolerance*, due to deficiency of aldolase B (fructose-1, 6-bisphosphate aldolase), is unlikely to present neonatally in the UK, as newborn babies should not be exposed to fructose in sucrose or fruit juices). However, a careful dietary history is essential.

4. *Liver disease due to α₁-antitrypsin* deficiency is associated with the abnormal Pi ZZ, PI SZ and Pi nul Z phenotypes. Swedish studies found that 11% of affected infants had prolonged jaundice and 6% anicteric hepatitis. A further 35% had abnormal liver function tests in the first months of life. Some babies present with bleeding due to clotting factor deficiencies. Serum α₁-antitrypsin concentrations below 1.0 g/L (reference 1.5–4.0 g/L) suggest deficiency. Phenotyping should be carried out when values are low or low–normal.

Extrahepatic biliary atresia causes severe liver damage with cirrhosis, fatal in early childhood. Surgery is the only effective treatment and must be done before 6 weeks of age for good results. Unfortunately it is often extremely difficult to differentiate between this condition and idiopathic neonatal hepatitis. Biochemical tests are not diagnostic, and even specialist radiological techniques (e.g. ^{131}I rose bengal test) are frequently unhelpful.

3. The Bronze Baby Syndrome

This syndrome, harmless in its own right, can cause considerable alarm. It is rare and occurs in newborns when three factors coincide:

(i) a primary liver disorder with cholestasis;
(ii) an increase in plasma unconjugated bilirubin, which necessitates
(iii) phototherapy.

Within 24 h of starting phototherapy, the babies' skin becomes bronzed-grey in colour and the plasma and urine are brown. The discoloration resolves when phototherapy is stopped, but it may take several weeks. Plasma and urine have a large peak of absorption at around 415 nm and absorbance at 600–700 nm. Fluorescent bands observed at 585, 619 and 670 nm were attributed to porphyrins.

The explanation remains conjectural. One hypothesis is that cholestasis leads to accumulation of copper-porphyrins in the blood. These are converted to brown pigments by transfer of an electron between photoexcited bilirubin and the Cu^{++} ion during phototherapy.

GLUCOSE HOMEOSTASIS

Normally, the fetus receives a constant supply of glucose across the placenta, and gluconeogenesis and

TABLE 17.8
CAUSES OF NEONATAL HYPOGLYCAEMIA

Deficient reserves of glycogen
Preterm infants
Intrauterine growth retardation

Excessive demands
Birth asphyxia
Sepsis
Respiratory distress
Cyanotic heart disease
Low environmental temperature

Hormone deficiencies
Growth hormone
Corticosteroids

Defective hepatic glycogenolysis and/or gluconeogenesis
Liver failure
Inherited:
    glycogen storage diseases
    gluconeogenic defects
    fat oxidation defects
    galactosaemia
    fructose intolerance

Hyperinsulinism
Transient:
    infants of diabetic mothers
    erythroblastosis fetalis
    Beckwith–Wiedemann syndrome
Persistent:
    nesidioblastosis
    (isolated adenoma—very rare)

glycogenolysis are probably inactive *in utero*. With birth, the glucose supply is withdrawn. Maintenance of a normal blood glucose then depends upon a correct balance between glucose entry into the blood, from the gut and from liver glycogenolysis and gluconeogenesis, and its utilization by the tissues. Even in healthy babies delivered at term, it may be 48 h before feeding is sufficiently established to meet glucose requirements. However, hepatic glucose production is 'switched on' at birth because of changes in metabolite concentrations, an increase in glucagon secretion and low amounts of insulin. Fatty acid mobilization and catabolism are also very active in the first 3 days of life, driven by high concentrations of circulating growth hormone and glucagon. This promotes gluconeogenesis and provides ketones as an energy source thus conserving glucose. Blood glucose of healthy babies may fall in the first 4–6 h after birth to around 2.5 mmol/L, but the concentration increases as feeding becomes established.

Hypoglycaemia[12]

Although newborn babies often tolerate a very low blood glucose without becoming symptomatic, it is now generally accepted that the plasma concentration should be maintained above 2.5 mmol/L. Clinical features include jitteriness and convulsions, and coma with permanent brain damage if severe hypoglycaemia is prolonged or recurrent. The aetiology is often multifactorial (Table 17.8).

Hypoglycaemia occurs most often in preterm babies, or those who are small for gestational age because of growth retardation *in utero*. Blood glucose is often normal at delivery, but then falls precipitously during the first 24 h if adequate glucose is not provided by feeding or intravenously, generally at a rate of 6–8 mg/kg per min. Their central problem is that they are born with small glycogen reserves, which are rapidly exhausted. Their brains are large in relation to body size and have a heavy glucose demand. Respiratory distress, and maintenance of body temperature in a cool environment, may also drain resources. It is speculated, but unproven, that decreased availability of fatty acids may contribute. Delay in activation of the key gluconeogenic enzyme, phosphoenolpyruvate carboxykinase, has also been proposed.

Babies who become hypoxic during labour and are asphyxiated at birth often have unrecordably low blood glucose concentrations within minutes of delivery. This is particularly likely if birth weight is low. In hypoxic conditions, glucose is metabolized anaerobically by glycolysis, which is greatly increased because of changes in intracellular redox potential and ATP:ADP ratios. The energy yield is low: two molecules of ATP per molecule of glucose compared with 36 from aerobic oxidation. The glycogen reserves are rapidly consumed. In addition, fatty acid catabolism, ketogenesis and ketone utilization, all oxygen-dependent processes, are depressed.

Hypoglycaemia in babies with cyanotic heart disease is accounted for by increased demand for glucose for accelerated anaerobic glycolysis and a rapid respiratory rate, together with poor feeding. Growth hormone deficiency may cause severe neonatal hypoglycaemia, perhaps because lipolysis and, therefore, ketogenesis are decreased. The inherited disorders causing hypoglycaemia are discussed on pp. 298–9 and Chapter 39.

Hyperinsulinism may cause severe symptomatic hypoglycaemia. Clinical features suggesting this diagnosis are: large body size, absence of hepatomegaly (seen in many inherited defects) and, particularly, difficulties in maintaining the blood glucose even with high infusion rates of glucose—for example, more than 12–15 mg/kg per min. The diagnostic biochemical features are listed on p. 299. Transient hypoglycaemia due to hyperinsulinism occurs in infants of poorly controlled diabetic mothers, often from around 1 to 4 h of life. A normal plasma glucose is generally attained within a few days, although hypoglycaemia may be more prolonged. Hyperinsulinism occurs because chronic stimulation by hyperglycaemia *in utero* leads to hyperplasia of fetal islet tissue. Hyperplasia, similarly, accounts for hyperinsulinism in babies with severe Rh incompatibility (erythroblastosis fetalis), although the mechanism is unknown. Babies with Beckwith–Wiedemann syndrome are very large and some develop hypoglycaemia, probably because of an increase in normal pancreatic-islet tissue. Prolonged hyperinsulinism is most often due to the condition 'nesidioblastosis' (p. 299).

It is mandatory that the blood glucose of all sick babies be monitored frequently from birth, but particularly when there is a known risk of hypoglycaemia, until the concentrations have stabilized. Glucose reagent strips are invaluable, as long as ward staff are carefully instructed in their use and low values are confirmed by the laboratory.

Hyperglycaemia

Hyperglycaemia is a much less common problem and is usually iatrogenic—generally because of excessive administration of glucose intravenously or, rarely, following aminophylline administration to preterm babies to stimulate breathing. Transient diabetes mellitus may occur neonatally and cause alarmingly high blood glucose values, but only mild ketoacidosis. The main problems are from the hyperosmolar state. Insulin therapy is required in only very small doses, if at all. The cause of the disturbance is unknown. Delayed development of the β-cells of the pancreatic islets is one possibility. Permanent diabetes mellitus is extremely rare under 6 months.

DISORDERS OF MINERALS

Calcium[29]

From week 28 of gestation, fetal plasma calcium is normally elevated, calcitonin is raised and parathyroid hormone (PTH) is low. Calcitonin and PTH do not cross the placenta, some 25-hydroxycholecalciferol is transported across, and the permeability to 1,25-dihydroxycholecalciferol is questionable. With ligation of the cord, the maternal calcium supply is withdrawn. Plasma ionized and total calcium concentrations fall, reaching a nadir at around 18 h of life, but then increase again to achieve the adult normal range (total calcium above 2.2 mmol/L) by 2–3 days of age.

The early fall may be accounted for, in part, by the abrupt cessation of the maternal calcium supply. Another factor may be the normal postnatal surge in the secretion of calcitonin, which reaches peak plasma concentrations at 12–24 h and then decreases after 36 h. It is speculated that this might limit calcium mobilization from bone. Assays for intact PTH and its active fragment (1–34 residues) have shown a two- to fivefold increase in PTH secretion in the first 48 h, which is probably an appropriate response to the falling calcium. Some studies have found poor correlation between total and ionized plasma calcium neonatally, perhaps because of the influence of pH and plasma protein concentrations. These are most likely to be disturbed in sick babies. In the future, measurement of ionized calcium may be preferable for this age group.

Hypocalcaemia

This is often asymptomatic in the newborn until the plasma total calcium concentrations falls below 1.75 mmol/L (ionized, below 0.63 mmol/L). Clinical features include irritability, twitching and convulsions, and poor cardiac contractility with a risk of sudden cardiac death.

Transient Early Hypocalcaemia. This occurs within the first 48 h of life, is common, and usually resolves spontaneously by 4–5 days of age. It affects preterm infants, infants of diabetic mothers, and babies with severe birth asphyxia.

The aetiology is multifactorial. In premature babies, it may be an exaggeration of the normal postnatal disturbance of calcium turnover. A more marked increase in plasma calcitonin has been reported. Evidence for a suboptimal response to PTH secretion to hypocalcaemia is conflicting. Demonstration of a significant calcaemic response to exogenous PTH argues against end-organ resistance to the hormone in bones. The renal phosphaturic and cAMP responses to PTH, on the other hand, are diminished. Preterm babies can hydroxylate vitamin D at birth, and deficiency of 1,25-dihydroxycholecalciferol is not the cause. Transient hypoparathyroidism, hypomagnesaemia and increased skeletal demand for calcium may all contribute to the hypocalcaemia of large babies of poorly controlled diabetic mothers. Following birth asphyxia, both PTH deficiency and resistance to its action may be implicated, together with hyperphosphataemia due to acute tissue damage.

Late Neonatal Hypocalcaemia. This type, presenting between 4 and 28 days of age, is much less common. Causes include:

- extension of early hypocalcaemia in pre-term babies
- transient hypoparathyroidism
- congenital permanent hypoparathyroidism
- congenital rickets
- hypomagnesaemia

Transient hypoparathyroidism occurs usually in sick hypoxic, acidotic babies, often with congenital heart disease. It often persists for up to 2 and, rarely, to 6 months of age. Biochemical features are hyperphosphataemia, inappropriately low plasma PTH, often a low plasma magnesium, normal plasma calcitonin and normal or moderately increased 1, 25-dihydroxycholecalciferol.

Another group is of babies born to mothers with hyperparathyroidism, as prolonged hypercalcaemia *in in utero* suppresses the fetal parathyroid glands. Measurement of the mother's plasma calcium is important when investigating prolonged neonatal hypocalcaemia.

Persistent hypoparathyroidism may be inherited, most often as an X-linked recessive disorder. It may also result from an embryological defect of the third and fourth pharyngeal arches, when associated features may be absence of the thymus gland with immunodeficiency and cardiovascular defects (Di George syndrome). Hypocalcaemia from pseudo-hypoparathyroidism (Chapter 30) generally presents after 3 years of age. Autoimmune hypoparathyroidism probably does not occur in the newborn.

Congenital rickets is uncommon in the UK and is due to maternal vitamin D deficiency in pregnancy. The rare, inherited, vitamin D-dependent rickets presents later in infancy. Formerly, hypocalcaemia frequently resulted from feeding with cow's milk, which has a high phosphate:calcium ratio. This has disappeared with the use of baby milks with proportionately less phosphate.

Hypercalcaemia

This is generally defined as total plasma calcium concentration above 2.65 mmol/L. However, raised values from capillary blood samples must be confirmed on a free-flowing venous sample, because of haemoconcentration from squeezing.

Severe, persistent hypercalcaemia causes feeding problems, weight loss, and calcification of the kidneys with renal failure. The most common cause of hypercalcaemia is *phosphate depletion* of premature babies (p. 313). The hypercalcaemia is generally modest and asymptomatic.

Neonatal hyperparathyroidism is extremely rare. It may occur transiently in babies of mothers with hypoparathyroidism, if prolonged hypocalcaemia *in utero* has led to fetal parathyroid hyperplasia.

Severe primary hyperparathyroidism, with life-threatening hypercalcaemia and bone disease, has occurred in some kindreds with familial hypocalciuric hypercalcaemia. Hypophosphatasia is another inherited disorder that may present neonatally with bone disease and hypercalcaemia. There is a deficiency of the tissue-nonspecific (liver, bone, kidney) alkaline phosphatase isoenzyme. Urinary excretion of phosphoethanolamine supports the diagnosis, but is not specific for the condition.

'Idiopathic hypercalcaemia' may be associated with a characteristic elfin facial appearance, cardiovascular abnormalities and mental retardation in Williams' syndrome. Calcium loading tests indicate that intestinal calcium absorption may be increased or that calcium 'clearance' is slow, and abnormalities of vitamin D metabolism and calcitonin secretion are speculated. However, hypercalcaemia may not persist, and some children with the syndrome have never been known to be hypercalcaemic. Deletions of the elastin gene have been identified.

Hypomagnesaemia

The only symptoms and signs reliably asociated with hypomagnesaemia in infancy are:

- increased muscle tone
- jitteriness
- exaggerated tendon reflexes
- fits.

Hypocalcaemia is often present too and may dominate the clinical presentation. This may be difficult to correct until a normal plasma magnesium concentration is restored, as magnesium deficiency inhibits PTH secretion and blunts the end-organ responses to it. Although hypomagnesaemia is fairly common in the newborn, it is generally mild (plasma magnesium, 0.5–0.7 mmol/L), asymptomatic, transient, and corrects spontaneously. It occurs most often in preterm infants and babies of diabetic mothers, in the first 3 days of life. It may follow an exchange transfusion or intestinal resection, or occur with hypocalcaemia in babies of mothers with hyperparathyroidism.

An extremely rare cause is the inherited disorder, *primary hypomagnesaemia*,[30] in which there is a defect in carrier-mediated transport of magnesium from the small intestine. Affected babies are well initially, but develop symptoms of severe hypomagnesaemia and hypocalcaemia with intractable fits from 3 to 4 weeks of age. Plasma magnesium is extremely low (0.15–0.30 mmol/L), and plasma calcium (generally as low as 1.2–1.6 mmol/L) cannot be corrected until magnesium therapy is given. Affected babies can absorb magnesium from the gut if given in large doses, possibly by simple diffusion. Plasma magnesium should be measured in any infant with persistent hypocalcaemia, especially if this cannot be corrected by the usual treatment, and in a normocalcaemic infant with unexplained intractable fitting or neonatal tetany.

Metabolic Bone Disease of Prematurity[31]

This is a problem of babies of very low birth weight, generally born before 33 weeks of gestation. It is also called osteopenia or rickets of prematurity, and covers a wide spectrum of bone disturbances of increasing severity: biochemical evidence, only, of increased bone turnover; decreased bone mineral (osteopenia) detectable by photon absorptiometry (not widely available); radiographic evidence of osteopenia; radiographic changes of rickets, and, finally, clinical rickets, sometimes with bone fractures.

Diagnosis of early rickets is subjective, and the true incidence is unknown. Compared with normal-term babies at birth, most infants of very low birth weight have osteopenia, seen by absorptiometry, when they reach the equivalent of 40 weeks' gestational age. Neonatal growth rate may slow down, and there is preliminary evidence that the ultimate height of the individual may be decreased.

The aetiology is probably multifactorial, but the dominant factor in most cases is deficiency of minerals—phosphate and/or calcium. Vitamin D deficiency may be contributory if vitamin D supplements are not given, as preterm babies have a small bile-acid pool and absorb fat-soluble vitamins poorly. There is no evidence that preterm babies cannot hydroxylate vitamin D to 1,25-dihydroxycholecalciferol.

Two groups of preterm infants, especially, become mineral deficient. (1) Babies fed solely on breast milk, which has a low phosphate content, may become *phosphate depleted*. Because of their rapid growth, they have a large requirement for phosphate, both for tissue protoplasm and for bone. The plasma phosphate concentration falls below 1.00 mmol/L (normal fasting, 1.20–2.78 mmol/L), and this triggers a cascade of events. Renal production of 1,25-dihydroxycholecalciferol is increased, which stimulates both calcium and phosphate absorption from the gut and bone turnover. This, and perhaps a direct effect of low phosphate on osteoblasts, causes an increase in plasma alkaline phosphatase. Plasma calcium rises, sometimes to hypercalcaemic levels, and PTH secretion is therefore suppressed. Hypercalciuria and renal phosphate retention result. Normal biochemistry is restored rapidly with phosphate supplementation. Many units now routinely give supplements to preterm babies fed with breast milk to prevent bone disease.

(2) Babies fed intravenously may become *deficient* in both *calcium* and *phosphate*. This occurs because the poor solubility of calcium and phosphorus limits the amounts that can be added to infusion fluids. The plasma calcium and phosphorus are often low and PTH is raised (secondary hyperparathyroidism). Bone turnover is accelerated and plasma alkaline phosphatase is raised.

Measurement of plasma alkaline phosphatase, for example at weekly intervals, is widely used as a preliminary screen to identify babies at risk. However, concentrations are higher in preterm than term babies and are further increased, physiologically, during rapid growth. There is no sharp cut-off between normal and abnormal. Commonly, a value exceeding five times the laboratory's upper limit of normal for adults is used as an arbitrary point at which to instigate radiological investigations for bone disease.

BIOCHEMICAL DISTURBANCES ASSOCIATED WITH PARENTERAL NUTRITION

Very sick infants—particularly those with severe respiratory or gastrointestinal problems—have to be fed intravenously.[23] In the majority of cases this is a short-term measure and is well tolerated. However, metabolic disturbances may be a problem. These are due, in part, to the small circulatory volume and to immaturity of the kidneys and liver, but also to our own ignorance of the optimal nutritional requirements. Moreover, the physiological state of the infants is so unstable that their requirements will fluctuate rapidly as their clinical state changes. Growth rate often slows, reflecting an inadequate calorie supply together with a catabolic illness.

Common metabolic disturbances include fluid and electrolyte imbalance, hyperglycaemia, sometimes with hyperosmolarity, glycosuria and dehydration, symptomatic hypoglycaemia if a dextrose infusion is terminated abruptly (because of transient hyperinsulinism), hypophosphataemia, hypoalbuminaemia and metabolic bone disease. If clearance of infused lipid is compromised, concentrations of plasma triglycerides and free fatty acids are raised and there is an increased risk of kernicterus in jaundiced babies, because free fatty acids may displace bilirubin from albumin. Carnitine, an essential requirement for fatty acid oxidation, is low in the blood and tissues of preterm infants receiving carnitine-free parenteral feeds. It is controversial, however, whether carnitine supplementation improves fat utilization.

The early amino-acid preparations used were protein hydrolysates. They sometimes produced disturbances in the plasma amino-acid profile, and caused hyperammonaemia. With modern crystalline L-amino acid mixtures, significant hyperammonaemia is rare and amino acid imbalance is generally not a problem. However, there is still uncertainty about the optimal mixture of amino acids. Because of enzyme deficiencies in the sulphur amino-acid pathway associated with immaturity, cysteine is probably an essential amino acid for preterm babies and taurine may be; methionine, on the other hand, accumulates if provided in excess. Very high plasma concentrations of phenylalanine have been observed in a minority of sick babies receiving an amino acid preparation of high phenylalanine content, reflecting deficiencies of the first two enzymes of tyrosine degradation—tyrosine aminotransferase and 4-hydroxyphenylpyruvate dioxygenase. There has been concern about possible brain toxicity from sustained, high concentrations of phenylalanine.

Symptomatic deficiencies of the trace elements zinc and copper may, rarely, complicate prolonged intravenous feeding. This has become less common with inclusion of trace-element mixtures in the feeding regimens. However, the optimal composition of these supplements is unknown. Selenium concentrations may fall in preterm babies, but apparently without adverse effects.

Cholestatic jaundice may occur, generally after 2–8 weeks of intravenous feeding, its incidence varying inversely with gestational age. It is usually transient and resolves within a few weeks of discontinuing parenteral nutrition. In a minority of cases, severe liver damage has resulted, culminating in liver failure. These babies have been very sick and many factors may have contributed: hypoxia, sepsis, toxins leached from central venous catheters, amino acid imbalance, excessive glucose intake, lack of intestinal stimulation of bile secretion (no oral intake), and inhibition of bile acid secretion by amino acids.

PROVISION OF A PAEDIATRIC BIOCHEMISTRY SERVICE

The condition of sick neonates can change rapidly and close biochemical monitoring is essential. Older babies and children may become acutely ill over a short time. Because of the immediacy of the clinical problems, a significant proportion of paediatric analyses are required out of hours. Some tests, notably plasma ammonia, lactate and magnesium, seldom required urgently in adult medicine, must be available on a 24-h basis. It is invaluable for neonatal and intensive care units to have side-room instrumentation, particularly a self-calibrating blood-gas analyser, microhaematocrit centrifuge and a bilirubinometer. Staff of the clinical chemistry laboratory must be closely involved in the choice and maintenance of instruments, and in training ward staff in their use, stressing particularly the importance of monitoring quality control and precautions to minimize the risks of infection.[32]

The total blood volume in infancy is only 80 ml/kg and small babies are difficult to bleed and often have a high haematocrit. Samples may be needed from sick, very low birth-weight babies several times per day. Although modern analysers typically use 5–10 μL of plasma per test, 25–60 μL is more often needed because of instrument dead-space. Investigations must be planned carefully. Plasma is preferred to serum when possible, as the yield after centrifugation is greater. Use of small collecting tubes of narrow diameter with an appropriate amount of anticoagulant, increases the recovery of plasma and reduces the surface area, and, therefore, losses by evaporation. With a microcentrifuge, separation is possible within 2 min.

Venepuncture of small babies is necessary when relatively large volumes of blood are needed or a baby is shocked and poorly perfused. Otherwise, arterialized capillary blood samples are generally preferred. These are best collected by phlebotomists trained in heel-prick techniques, for example nurses based in the laboratory. A single skin puncture yields an average of about 450 μL of blood, which may take 10 min or longer to collect. Artefacts from haemolysis occur with excessive squeezing (p. 293). Less than 5% of capillary samples collected in the first 2 weeks of life should be visibly haemolysed.[33] Sweat tests should also be undertaken by a small number of trained pathology-based staff who do them often enough to maintain their skills.

The key to providing a good paediatric biochemistry service is close coordination of all those concerned in planning, executing and interpreting the investigations, both on the wards and in the laboratory.

REFERENCES

1. Clayton B.E., Jenkins P., Round J.M. (1980). *Paediatric Chemical Pathology*, Oxford: Blackwell Scientific.
2. Meites S. (ed.) (1988). *Pediatric Clinical Chemistry*, 3rd edn, Washington DC: American Association for Clinical Chemistry.
3. Clayton B.E., Round J.M. (eds.) (1984). *Chemical Pathology and the Sick Child*, Oxford: Blackwell Scientific.
4. Lindblad B. et al. (1990). Recommendation for collection of venous blood from children, with special reference to production reference values. *Scand. J. Clin. Lab. Invest.*, **50**, 99.
5. Stein P., Rosalki S.B., Ying Foo A., Hjelm M. (1987). Transient hyperphosphatasemia of infancy and early childhood: clinical and biochemical features of 21 cases and literature review. *Clin. Chem.*, **33**, 313.
6. Rylance G.W. (1986). Neonatal pharmacology. In *Textbook of Neonatology* (Roberton N.R.C., ed.) Edinburgh: Churchill Livingstone, pp. 223–238.
7. Barratt T.M. (1982). Renal function. In *Paediatric Urology*, 2nd edn, (Williams D.I., Johnston J.H., eds.) London: Butterworth Scientific, pp. 1–9.
8. Arant S. (1984). Estimating glomerular filtration rate in infants. *J. Pediatr.*, **104**, 890.
9. Kwiterovich P.O. (1986). Biochemical, clinical, epidemiologic, genetic, and pathologic data in the pediatric age group relevant to the cholesterol hypothesis. *Pediatrics*, **78**, 349.
10. U.S. Department of Health and Human Services, National Institutes of Health (1980). *Lipid Research Clinics Population Studies Data Book*, Vol. I, *The Prevalence Study*, Washington DC: Government Printing Office.
11. Scriver C.R., Beaudet A.L., Sly W.S., Valle D. (eds.) (1989). *The Metabolic Basis of Inherited Disease*, 6th edn, New York: McGraw-Hill.
12. Aynsley-Green A., Soltész G. (1986). Metabolic and endocrine disorders. In *Textbook of Neonatalogy* (Roberton N.R.C., ed.) Edinburgh: Churchill Livingstone, pp. 605–621.
13. Senior B., Wolfsdorf J.I. (1979). Hypoglycemia in children. *Pediatr. Clin. North Am.*, **26**, 171.
14. Vianey-Liaud C., Divry P., Gregersen N., Mathieu M. (1987). The inborn errors of mitochondrial fatty acid oxidation. *J. Inherited Metab. Disease*, **10** (Suppl. 1), 159.
15. Brusilow S.W. (1985). Inborn errors of urea synthesis. In *Genetic and Metabolic Disease in Paediatrics* (Lloyd J.K., Scriver C.R., eds.) London: Butterworths, pp. 140–165.
16. Heubi J.E., Partin J.C., Partin J.S., Schubert W.K. (1987). Reye's syndrome: current concepts. *Hepatology*, **7**, 155.
17. Hall S.M. (1986). Reye's syndrome and aspirin: a review. *J. R. Soc. Med.*, **79**, 596.
18. Parkin J.M. (1989). The short child. In *Clinical Paediatric Endocrinology*, 2nd edn, (Brook C.G.D., ed.) Oxford: Blackwell Scientific Publications, pp. 96–117.
19. Brook C.G.D., Hindmarsh P.C. (1991). Tests for growth hormone secretion. *Arch. Dis. Child.*, **66**, 85.
20. Saudubray J.-M. et al. (1989). Clinical approach to inherited metabolic diseases in the neonatal period: a 20 year survey. *J. Inherited. Metab. Disease.*, **12** (Suppl. 1), 25.

21. Holton J.B. (1982). Diagnosis of inherited metabolic diseases in severely ill children. *Ann. Clin. Biochem.*, **19**, 389.
22. Holton J.B. (compiler) (1988). *U.K. Directory of Laboratories Diagnosing Inborn Errors of Metabolism*, 3rd edn.
23. Roberton N.R.C. (ed.) (1986). *Textbook of Neonatology*, Edinburgh: Churchill Livingstone.
24. Morley C.J. (1986). The respiratory distress syndrome. In *Textbook of Neonatology* (Roberton N.R.C., ed.) Edinburgh: Churchill Livingstone, pp.274–311.
25. Saugstad O.D. (1990). Oxygen toxicity in the neonatal period. *Acta Paediatr. Scand.*, **79**, 881.
26. Wimberley P.D. *et al.* (1990). Guidelines for transcutaneous P_{O_2} and P_{CO_2} measurement. *J. Int. Fed. Clin. Chem.*, **2**, 128.
27. Dear P.R.F. (1987). Monitoring oxygen in the newborn: saturation or partial pressure? *Arch. Dis. Child.*, **62**, 879.
28. Mowat A.P. (1987). *Liver Disorders in Childhood*, 2nd edn, London: Butterworths.
29. Salle B.L., Delvin E., Glorieux F., David L. (1990). Human neonatal hypocalcaemia. *Biol. Neonate*, **58** (Suppl. 1), 22.
30. Lombeck I. (1990). Genetic defects of the metabolism of magnesium, zinc, manganese, molybdenum and selenium. In *Inborn Metabolic Diseases* (Fernandes J., Saudubray J-M., Tada K., eds.) Berlin: Springer-Verlag, pp. 493–505.
31. Bishop N. (1989). Bone disease in preterm infants. *Arch. Dis. Child.*, **64**, 1403.
32. Marks V., Alberti K.G.M.M. (1985). *Clinical Biochemistry Nearer the Patient*. Edinburgh: Churchill Livingstone.
33. Meites S., Glassco K.M. (1985). Studies on the quality of specimens obtained by skin-puncture of children. 2. An analysis of blood-collecting practices in a pediatric hospital. *Clin. Chem.*, **31**, 1669.

18. The Chemical Analysis of Urine

G.S. Challand and J.L. Jones

Introduction
The type of urine sample
  Early morning sample
  Random sample
  Timed collections
Measurements derived from urine analyses
Biochemical screening using reagent pads
*Simple urine tests to screen for an inherited
    metabolic disease*
Protein analysis in urine
  Proteinuria
  Microalbuminuria in diabetes mellitus
  Measurement of individual urinary proteins
Urine electrolytes, urea and osmolality
Hormones and their metabolites in urine
Urinary drug screening
Other urine tests

FALSTAFF: *Sirrah, you giant, what says the doctor to my water?*

PAGE: *He said, sir, that the water itself was a good healthy water, but for the party that owned it, he might have more diseases than he knew of.*

William Shakespeare
King Henry IV, Part 1

INTRODUCTION

Prior to the development of the hypodermic syringe, urine was the most accessible bodily fluid and its physical examination and analysis has formed part of the physician's weaponry for many hundreds of years.[1] Even now, more urine samples are examined than blood samples.

Changes in the physical properties of urine, particularly the volume passed, the colour, smell and perhaps taste, were linked with disease processes several thousand years ago. In retrospect it is sometimes possible to link these to pathological abnormalities described today. The abnormal volume and sweet character of urine in diabetes mellitus were known in ancient Egypt, India, and China. In the fourth century BC, Hippocrates of Cos stated that a foaming urine (presumably linked to a high protein content) indicated kidney disease. Other early descriptions linked to high protein concentration were those of Theophilus, who precipitated a material by heating

urine; and Paracelsus, who used vinegar to accomplish the same feat.

Excessive claims were frequently made for the diagnostic information that could be obtained by examining a urine sample (often without seeing the patient) and in the early seventeenth century James Hart commented; 'Hence it comes to pass that any old trot cobbler or costard-monger will seem to pronounce some Delphian oracle by urine.' Thomas Brian[2] commented more caustically: 'She is indeed the dumb messenger betweene the Doctour and his patient: who (instead of passing the relation of his disease in writing or by some discreet messenger) pisseth his mind in his water, and expecteth an answer; but if I should write an answer in a letter written in the same language, I doubt if he would scarce read it.'

Most common constituents of urine were established in the eighteenth and nineteenth centuries. Bright demonstrated in 1827 the connection between dropsy, organic disease of the kidney, and proteinuria. The sugar in diabetic urine was found to be glucose by Peligot in 1838; and the first tumour marker—Bence-Jones' eponymous protein—was described in 1848.

By the early twentieth century the examinations of urine for protein and sugar were commonplace. But although blood analyses have now supplanted many of the older urine tests in a clinical biochemistry laboratory, the analysis of urine still offers some advantages:

- Urine is a more convenient sample for most patients than a blood sample, particularly for screening purposes.
- Urine is a concentrate for many substances of low molecular weight, so that their detection is easier than in blood.
- Urine is usually relatively free of interfering substances such as lipids and proteins, so that complex 'clean up' procedures are unnecessary before analysis.
- Timed collections of urine can be used to estimate production or excretion rates; and some hormone analyses in urine can be used as a convenient estimate of non-protein-bound hormone concentrations in plasma.
- Some patients present to their doctor solely because of unusual physical characteristics of their urine: abnormal volume, colour, or smell.

The chemical analysis of urine is likely to retain a place in laboratories and clinics for many more years.

THE TYPE OF URINE SAMPLE

Three types of urine sample are traditionally used for analysis and occasionally for calculation of derived variables.

Early Morning Sample

An early morning urine sample is usually the most concentrated of the day. Its use was therefore recommended when chemical methods of analysis lacked sensitivity and when an abnormal constituent present in low concentration was to be detected, the classical example being the early diagnosis of pregnancy. For many analytes, more sensitive methods of analysis have been introduced, so that now early morning samples offer little advantage.

Random Sample

A random urine sample obtained at the time of a clinic visit is convenient for patient and doctor, minimizes errors in the identification of sample, and helps to ensure that the sample is attributed to the correct patient (particularly important when analyses for drugs of abuse or misuse are requested). Such random samples, usually analysed by 'dipstick' techniques (urinalysis) are extensively used for screening purposes. Random urine samples are also common in paediatric practice when phlebotomy is difficult and timed urine collections are impracticable.

Timed Collections

These fall into two groups:

(i) a urine sample taken at a defined time (for example, as part of a glucose tolerance test);
(ii) a sample taken over a defined time interval, usually 24 h, although shorter times are used.

Other than in carefully controlled conditions, it is difficult to collect an accurate urine volume over a defined time period. Even in carefully controlled studies involving well-motivated volunteers, up to a fifth of all supposed 24-h collections have been deemed 'incomplete'; and every laboratory has received timed urine collections accompanied by the cryptic comment '200 cc missing'. The reasons for unsatisfactory collections are many. Common errors include both collecting too much urine (including the urine sample at the start of the time period rather than discarding it); and collecting too little (through forgetfulness, accidental spillage, or incomplete bladder emptying, particularly in the elderly).

The errors involved in measuring the volume of a timed collection should be small; but it is commonplace for volumes to be recorded to the nearest 50 mL, thus introducing an error of $\pm 2\%$; or to weigh the urine sample instead of measuring its volume, which produces similar errors through variations in urine specific gravity.

The advantages of collecting a urine sample of 24-h duration are that the output of many urine constituents can be measured over a period that minimizes both diurnal variation and that associated with dietary intake; and there are rather well-defined reference ranges for such output. The practical difficulties in collecting an accurate volume outweigh these advantages in a substantial minority of patients.

MEASUREMENTS DERIVED FROM URINE ANALYSES

These fall into two main groups. First, results from random samples are extrapolated to daily output on the basis of a concentration ratio with an analyte such as creatinine. Second, results from blood and from a timed urine collection can be combined to give a clearance.

All derived measurements are limited in usefulness by the propagation of errors. For any ratio or product of two numbers, the final CV is equal to the square root of the sum of the squared individual CVs. Small errors in each component of an equation accumulate to give a large error in the product of an equation.

Individual variability is a further problem with derived measurement. In extrapolating from an analyte:creatinine ratio to a calculated 24-h output, two assumptions are involved. The first is that the pattern of excretion of the analyte through the day exactly mimics that of creatinine (i.e. is independent of urine flow rate and not subject to physiological variation). This is unlikely to be true for the majority of analytes; and in practice, large discrepancies have been found.[3] The second assumption is that daily creatinine excretion is constant. It is often taken to be 1 g/24 h in adults. As creatinine excretion is dependent on muscle mass, considerable individual variation from this figure can be found (*see* Chapter 19). Where serial investigations are made on a single individual to monitor progress, this assumption is of little consequence; but where a single value is compared with a published reference range from other individuals, subsequent interpretation can be difficult.

In practice, the increasing accuracy and availability of measurements in plasma that has developed over the last 30 years has rendered many of the older urine tests and derived indices redundant. Plasma creatinine analyses have now replaced measurements of creatinine clearance in the majority of patients with renal impairment; and measurements of blood glycosylated haemoglobin and serum fructosamine have replaced the old 24-h urinary glucose measurements in the assessment of diabetic control. Much urine testing can now safely be dispensed with.

BIOCHEMICAL SCREENING USING REAGENT PADS

Biochemical screening of random urine samples using reagent pads ('dipsticks') is extensively used in clinics, wards, and by patients themselves. A review of the principles and practice has recently been produced by the Ames Division of Miles Ltd.[4] As with much of screening, the analytes measured are dictated more by the tests available in a pad format than by the clinical utility of such testing. Furthermore, quality assessments of these tests when they are used by inexperienced or untrained operators have shown alarmingly high proportions of incorrect results,[5] caused by many factors from inadequate technique and incorrect training to deteriorated or outdated reagent pads. As with all chemical analyses, training and good laboratory practice are essential if results of adequate quality are to be produced.

There are two main areas of proven clinical utility. If *protein* is detected, there is a strong suspicion of renal disease. The reagent-pad method is based upon dye binding, and is mainly sensitive to albumin. The sensitivity limit of around 200 mg/L albumin is rather above the upper reference limit for healthy adults; but is sufficient to detect orthostatic proteinuria and exercise- and pregnancy-related proteinuria as well as that associated with renal damage. A positive finding is not entirely specific for renal disease, and false positives can be obtained, for example in alkaline urine. In addition the test is insensitive to materials such as Bence-Jones protein. None the less it is still of value in screening, a positive result suggesting the need for further investigation. Urine protein detection has also proved of use in self-monitoring, either for patients with the nephrotic syndrome or for those prescribed potentially nephrotoxic drugs such as *cis*-platinum or penicillamine.

If *glucose* is detected in a random urine, there is a high probability of the patient having diabetes mellitus, particularly if ketones are also present; as with protein, the test is sufficiently sensitive to detect pregnancy-related glycosuria. It is also specific for glucose and is insensitive to other sugars in urine. Urine testing for glucose and ketones has been used for many years for self-monitoring by diabetics; this use is declining because of the increasing availability of inexpensive meters used in conjunction with reagent pads, which are capable of producing quite accurate blood glucose results.

Many different reagent pads have been developed, which are available either singly or in a strip combination. Multiple strips often include, in addition to protein and glucose, ketones, pH and 'specific gravity', blood, urobilinogen and bilirubin, and nitrite. Although many of these are of value in assessing or monitoring individual patients or selected groups, they are not of proven value in a screening programme for a relatively unselected population.

A further widely used application of reagent pads with urine samples is the early detection of *pregnancy*. Sophisticated chemistry using enzyme-linked antibodies specific for human chorionic gonadotropin has enabled the development of a range of pregnancy-testing kits. These are reasonably suitable for home monitoring or for use by small laboratories; and because of the great improvement in sensitivity are gradually supplanting the older agglutination tests despite being more expensive.

SIMPLE URINE TESTS TO SCREEN FOR AN INHERITED METABOLIC DISEASE

When an inherited metabolic disease is suspected, examination of urine, together with clinical information and blood tests, can lead to a preliminary diagnosis. It is usually necessary to confirm this using more expensive and time-consuming tests, best done at specialist centres. The use of urine tests in a local laboratory can often speed up the diagnostic process; and usually identifies normal samples, thus minimizing the work to be sent away.

Symptoms that give rise to a high degree of suspicion in a young child include:

- failure to thrive without apparent cause;
- unexplained mental retardation;
- episodic lethargy or vomiting;
- unexplained metabolic acidosis;
- sudden, catastrophic illness.

Both blood and urine samples should be available for investigation. Detailed clinical information should accompany the request to ensure that appropriate analyses are carried out. This should include:

- any relevant family history;
- any symptoms related to food intake;
- any association with infection, fasting, or surgery;
- the feeding regimen and drug therapy in the few days preceding sample collection.

It is for example pointless looking for galactose in the urine of a baby with suspected galactosaemia if galactose was withdrawn from the diet some days previously.

Urine samples for testing should be fresh, and early morning specimens are often preferable except when screening for mucopolysaccharidoses. Preservatives are best avoided because these can interfere with organic acid and glycosaminoglycan determinations. Some disorders can be picked up by very simple observations: the darkening of urine in cases of alkaptonuria is well known; as are the smells characteristic of disorders such as maple-syrup urine disease and isovalericacidaemia.

Multiple reagent-pad strips can often give useful information. Both pH and a nitrite test are of value in checking for bacterial contamination, which can give rise to false-positive or false-negative tests on further examination. Glucose can be found in the urine following renal tubular damage caused by inherited diseases such as tyrosinaemia and cystinosis. The presence of reducing substances in urine can be detected using Clinitest tablets (Ames Division of Miles Laboratories). This derivation of Benedict's test gives a positive result with most sugars (but not sucrose). Sugar chromatography[6] should be used on any urine that gives a positive result, but is negative on testing for glucose: galactosaemia, hereditary fructose intolerance, intestinal lactase deficiency, and the benign condition pentosuria can all be identified.

The excretion of galactose can be variable in galactos-aemia; and the measurement of galactose-1-phosphate uridyl transferase activity in blood may be required to confirm a diagnosis.[7]

The cyanide–nitroprusside test can be used for the detection of increased excretion of cysteine, cystine and homocystine. This test is positive in cystinuria and homocystinuria. Although a modification to the test allows differentiation between the two conditions,[8] it is preferable to subject the urine sample to chromatography, which not only enables the differentiation of the two amino acids but also allows identification of the other amino acids elevated in cases of cystinuria—ornithine, arginine and lysine.

Many amino acid abnormalities can be demonstrated using thin-layer amino acid chromatography, including those in which a single amino acid is excreted in excessive amounts, such as glycinuria and phenylketonuria; those in which a specific group of amino acids is produced, such as cystinuria or maple-syrup urine disease; and those in which a generalized increase in excretion of all amino acids occurs, such as congenital Fanconi syndrome. The patterns produced by thin-layer chromatography can be difficult to interpret; but provided a large enough number of samples is analysed to amass the necessary experience, and care is taken in interpretation, the method and equipment are simple enough for use in most laboratories.[9]

Amino acid excretion varies with both age and diet, and in particular the urine of neonates shows elevated excretion when compared with that of an older child. Some premature babies show patterns characteristic of amino acid abnormalities that are caused by immaturities in enzyme development rather than by inherited deficiencies. Some drugs, particularly antibiotics, may produce abnormal spots or bands. Any positive result obtained with thin-layer chromatography should be confirmed by more precise quantitation, high-performance liquid chromatographic techniques now probably being more popular than amino acid analysis on a specific analyser.

The mucopolysaccharidoses are a group of diseases characterized by storage of excessive amounts of glycosaminoglycans in organs, caused by inherited deficiencies in lysosomal enzymes. Glycosaminoglycans excreted in urine can be identified turbidimetrically in a screening test by their reaction with cetylpyridinium chloride. Preferable screening tests for these conditions are semiquantitative, and it is usually necessary to relate the result to urine creatinine, as the amount excreted varies with urine concentration and shows a marked age dependence.[10] Not all mucopolysaccharidoses are associated with an elevated glycosaminoglycan excretion; and as with amino aciduria, all positive findings should be confirmed by independent techniques, such as thin-layer chromatography or electrophoresis of glycosaminoglycans followed by enzyme studies.

PROTEIN ANALYSIS IN URINE

Even though the permeability limit for glomerular filtration of proteins is usually taken to be approximately 40 000 kDa, most plasma proteins can be detected in urine, albeit by sensitive immunoassay techniques. In addition, the proteins found in normal urine include some produced by the urinary tract itself (such as Tamm–Horsfall glycoprotein[11]) as well as proteins derived from plasma. The predominant proteins of urine in the normal individual are albumin and mucoproteins secreted by the renal tubule. A discussion of benign proteinuria appears in the next chapter.

Proteinuria

Excess protein in urine has traditionally been detected and quantitated by either dye-binding techniques (particularly sensitive to albumin) or by precipitation reagents such as sulphosalicylic acid. Quantitative results by the two methods are not necessarily comparable. In addition, the problems of quantitation are compounded by difficulties in standardization. For proteinuria *per se*, human serum should be used as standard with value assigned by the biuret reaction; but many laboratories still use animal serum or purified albumin preparations with values assigned by dye-binding techniques. A further difficulty is imposed by a lack of sensitivity of traditional assay methods: usually around 200 mg/L, despite frequently quoted upper reference limits for normal excretion of 100–150 mg/L.

Despite these problems, assessment of proteinuria has proved of considerable value in the diagnosis and subsequent assessment of subclinical renal disease. The proteinuria can be classified as either a loss of plasma proteins not normally present in the glomerular filtrate (glomerular proteinuria); or caused by a saturation or failure of the tubular reabsorption mechanisms (tubular proteinuria).

Glomerular proteinuria may be selective, consisting mainly of albumin; or unselective. It may result from an increase in glomerular pressure and flow rate; but is more often associated with an alteration in the permeability of the glomerular membrane to proteins, probably through changes in what is essentially an electrostatic barrier to protein loss.[12]

Tubular proteinuria is less common, and occurs when tubular damage prevents the reabsorption of filtered proteins. This may also be associated with other tubular reabsorption deficiencies (e.g. Fanconi syndrome). Alternatively, tubular proteinuria may occur when an increase in the production rate and filtration of a low molecular-size protein occurs, leading to a saturation of the normal tubular reabsorption mechanisms (e.g. Bence–Jones proteinuria).

Tubular proteinuria does not usually lead to protein losses of more than 2 g/24 h. Glomerular proteinuria can give a considerably greater output, which can lead to a low plasma albumin concentration and oedema (now known as the nephrotic syndrome).

Microalbuminuria in Diabetes Mellitus

Kidney disease is the major cause of morbidity and mortality, particularly in young insulin-dependent diabetics, and an early feature of this is an increased urinary excretion of albumin, possibly caused through depletion of the glycosaminoglycan content of the glomerular membrane reducing the electrostatic charge barrier to protein permeability.

Because physiological factors can increase urinary albumin excretion, microalbuminuria has been defined as a urinary albumin excretion rate of between 20 and 200 μg/min in an overnight or 24-h urine sample on at least two of three occasions within a period of 6 months.[13] This is approximately equal to an excretion of 30–300 mg/24 h. Samples should not be collected after undue exertion or after an acute fluid load.

Because microalbuminuria has been shown to be a strong risk factor for overt nephropathy in diabetics, and because therapeutic measures reduce the concentration of microalbuminuria, there has been a rapidly increasing demand for this analysis, even though its clinical utility in terms of improved morbidity or mortality is as yet unproven. An overview of microalbuminuria and diabetes mellitus, and recommendations as to the measurement of albumin in urine, have recently been published.[14] In essence, methods of assay should be immunological, and calibrants should be either human albumin or human serum, either of which should be checked for calibration against an independent secondary calibrator. Once microalbuminuria has been detected, there is a commitment to the subsequent monitoring of patients at periods of between 6 months and 2 years.[14]

Measurement of Individual Urinary Proteins

In some circumstances the quantitation of individual proteins in urine is of value.

Bence–Jones protein (free monoclonal light chains or light-chain fragments) is found in the urine of many patients with malignancy of B lymphocytes: it only accumulates in plasma if there is glomerular damage. It can be detected either immunologically or electrophoretically. Electrophoresis of urine, although only giving semiquantitative results, can provide some information on the severity of the glomerular lesion in the nephrotic syndrome, depending on the relative amounts of low and high molecular-size proteins. A more accurate measure is given by a differential protein clearance: usually the ratio in urine of IgG to transferrin or albumin. A low ratio implies lack of sensitivity and a poorer prognosis.

A red-coloured urine sometimes leads to requests for the assessment of *haemoglobin* in urine (usually indicative of haemolysis) or *myoglobin* (indicative of severe muscle damage). Both of these proteins, and their oxidation products, can be detected spectroscopically. As with proteinuria, haemoglobinuria can be induced by undue exertion (March haemoglobinuria), and it is occasionally detected in screening programmes using reagent pads.

Urine *enzyme activities* are now uncommon requests. Amylase estimation in a random urinary sample is of no value in assisting the diagnosis of acute pancreatitis. Of more theoretical value is the ratio of amylase clearance to creatinine clearance, using a random urine sample together with a blood sample. A ratio of less than 0.3 is considered normal, but considerable errors are inherent in the calculation, and renal disease can give confusing results.

URINARY ELECTROLYTES, UREA AND OSMOLALITY

The normal person achieves metabolic balance of water and sodium by ingesting excesses and excreting surpluses. The physiological mechanisms are the osmolal – arginine vasopressin (AVP; formerly antidiuretic hormone) system for control of water balance; and the renin–angiotensin–aldosterone system for control of sodium balance. The renal tubules operate by interchanging sodium and potassium, and physiological mechanisms and treatment designed to alter sodium excretion also affect potassium.

Requests for urinary electrolytes, urea and osmolality tend to be made more by rote than by thought: they are worthwhile in few cases of abnormal water or electrolyte imbalance. Requests for specific gravity measurement are now seldom encountered. In laboratories they have been replaced by measurements of osmolality; and although reagent strips have a pad supposedly measuring specific gravity, this is insensitive to non-ionized substances such as urea and glucose and would be more properly termed a measure of ionic activity.

Requests for urea and electrolyte analysis in 24-h urine collections are frequently made to give a guide to quantitative replacement. In the case of sodium and potassium this is not only unnecessary but may be dangerous, as urinary sodium excretion is related to renal blood flow rather than to body sodium content; and as exchange across cell walls and loss of potassium from damaged cells cannot be measured. Effective replacement must be based on plasma rather than urinary concentrations.[15] Urea analysis in 24-h urine collections is occasionally made to assess nitrogen balance in patients receiving total parenteral nutrition, the more accurate micro-Kjeldahl nitrogen analysis having disappeared from the repertoire of most laboratories.

The analysis of random samples of urine is occasionally helpful, usually in situations either of abnormal urine output or of abnormal plasma electrolyte concentration. However, the measurement of urinary electrolytes without some knowledge of dietary intake is of limited value.

If urine volume is high, the usual problem is whether the patient has an osmotic diuresis due to glycosuria (in which case a glucose estimation provides a diagnosis), or lacks AVP or is a compulsive water drinker (in both of which cases urine osmolality will be low), or has renal tubular damage (usually confirmable by the demonstration of proteinuria). The methods of distinguishing between these causes are detailed in Chapter 5.

Plasma concentrations of urea depend largely on glomerular function; urinary concentrations depend mainly on tubular function. A low urinary urea inappropriate to the state of hydration suggests tubular damage.

If urinary volume is low, the problem is to distinguish between damaged kidneys and normal kidneys responding well to AVP. A urine volume of less than 0.25 mL/min (350 mL/24 h) combined with a urine osmolality of less than 400 mosmol/kg indicates damaged kidneys. A urine osmolality of greater than 600 mosmol/kg suggests normal renal function. The finding of a high urine osmolality with a low plasma sodium concentration is found in the syndrome of inappropriate antidiuresis, which may follow injury or surgery.

Measurement of urinary sodium is occasionally helpful in deciding whether a sodium deficiency is due to insufficient intake (in which case urinary sodium concentration is low) or to too high an excretion. Potassium is conserved by the kidney less well than sodium; and it is debatable whether a urine potassium analysis is ever of any value. However, following prolonged hypokalaemia a urine potassium concentration of less than 20 mmol/L suggests that any cause of loss is not related to the kidney. In patients with elevated plasma sodium or potassium concentrations, analysis of urine electrolytes is valueless.

Requests for electrolytes other than sodium and potassium in 24-h urine samples are occasionally made, particularly in patients with renal calculi. Analyses such as urine calcium are likely to be of value only if the dietary intake is known: dietary intake of calcium in particular is markedly affected by the hardness of the local water.

The use of measurement of urinary creatinine as part of the creatinine clearance test is fully discussed in the next chapter.

HORMONES AND THEIR METABOLITES IN URINE

Assays in serum of total hormones, hormone-binding proteins and 'free' hormones have replaced most of the old urine hormone assays. Saliva has proved useful in the measurement of steroid hormones; and improvements in ultrasonics have made the old feto-placental function tests such as pregnancy oestriol redundant. In urine, there are only a few useful analyses remaining.

Urinary *hydroxymethoxymandelic acid* (HMMA) is still widely used in screening patients with idiopathic hypertension for phaeochromocytoma. Because of episodic excretion, it is traditional (but of doubtful mathematical validity) to collect three successive 24-h samples. The old colorimetric Pisano method was non-specific, and has been replaced by chromatographic techniques, either semiquantitative thin-layer or quantitative high-performance liquid chromatography. These methods often lack the sensitivity required for the detection of neuroblastoma in infants; and even in adults blood analyses for individual catecholamines and metabolites are usually requested when urinary HMMA concentration is high or when there is strong clinical suspicion of phaeochromocytoma, particularly if hypertension is paroxysmal.

Urinary *5-hydroxyindole acetic acid* (5-HIAA) is still the preferred method for screening patients with clinical features of the carcinoid syndrome. As with HMMA, excretion of 5-HIAA can be episodic, and it is conventional wisdom to use three successive random samples, or a single 24-h sample, in order to support a diagnosis. It is usually of more value to collect a urine sample during an acute clinical exacerbation.

The only urinary *steroid* analysis that has retained usage is the measurement of 24-h urinary 'free' cortisol. Usually measured by radioimmunoassay, this reflects overall daily secretion and is not subject to the diurnal variation of plasma cortisol; in cases of Cushing's syndrome, results are more markedly elevated than plasma cortisol. However, stress (including physical illness) can elevate urinary cortisol; it is unlikely that the test will remain indefinitely in the usual analytical repertoire as plasma steroid and ACTH assays improve.

The measurement of 24-h urinary 17-oxogenic steroids is still occasionally required in order to assess the response of a patient to the metyrapone test. This test, used in the investigation of possible disorders of the hypothalamic–pituitary feedback control of adrenocortical activity, is discussed in Chapter 42.

URINARY DRUG SCREENING

Dukes commented in 1939 that 'the detection and quantitative estimation of drugs and poisons may require a high degree of technical skill and considerable apparatus'.

In the diagnostic laboratory, there are two main situations in which drug analyses are requested: to investigate a drowsy, confused, or comatose patient whose symptoms may be induced by drugs; and to screen asymptomatic patients in order to see whether they are taking drugs. The latter group includes both testing for the presence of drugs of abuse and misuse, and checking for compliance with medication. Both urine and blood samples are valuable (together with stomach contents or gastric washings in the first group); urine is particularly useful in screening for unsuspected drugs because of the relatively high concentrations present, and the occurrence of metabolites that often assist identification. However, interpretation of results in a random urine sample is difficult; and blood samples are always preferable when quantitation is needed in order to assess possible therapeutic effects.

In the majority of patients presenting with a drug overdose, screening is of little clinical use. Treatment does not usually depend on the nature of the drug ingested (the most common exception being paracetamol). But a high proportion of multiple overdosess are complicated by ethanol ingestion; it is often difficult even for an experienced clinician to pinpoint an exact combination of drugs; and the information given by the patient or his colleagues after an overdose is notoriously inadequate. It is therefore usually good practice to obtain a urine sample soon after admission to save for drug analysis if required: either because the patient's condition fails to respond to therapy or because he dies.

Most laboratories can readily measure serum salicylate and paracetamol, and an approximate quantitation of ethanol can be obtained in emergency by measuring plasma osmolality. Even when these drugs are found, the possibility of other drugs being present is not excluded: combinations of paracetamol with other drugs, particularly dextropropoxyphene, are common.

A few simple spot tests on urine samples may prove useful information on drug groups ingested[16] and may detect drugs not easily detected by standard screening techniques (e.g. chloral hydrate). However, the majority of laboratories now use more sophisticated methods in routine practice. Most screening methods use initial extractions of urine at different pH values to separate acidic and basic drug groups. Subsequent thin-layer chromatography (now commercially available as Toxi-Lab, Mercia Diagnostics) has the disadvantage that to some extent chromatographic mobility is concentration dependent, but the advantage that multiple staining sequences can be followed to assist identification. Microcapillary gas chromatography is now becoming popular, many drugs and their metabolites being quite precisely identified by their retention times.[17] High-performance liquid chromatography tends to be used more for quantitation of a known drug than screening for an unknown drug, and mass spectrometry as an aid to drug identification is still expensive for most routine applications. No single method of screening is adequate for all drugs that may be ingested, and in cases of overdose appropriate clinical information on possible drug identity is essential: drugs such as lithium are not detectable by conventional screening methods.

In examining urine from subjects to check for the presence of illicit drugs, the problems are rather simpler. Broad-spectrum immunoassay techniques are useful to check for the presence of drug groups such as benzodiazepines, sympathomimetic amines or opiates. Any positive finding requires an alternative technique such as gas chromatography to give precise identification. In screening patients for compliance with methadone therapy, any technique must not only be able to identify methadone, but also metabolites of methadone (in order to identify samples 'spiked' with methadone); in addition the system must also be capable of identifying other opiates that may also have been ingested. It is important in this group of patients to check the integrity of the urine sample (guaranteed drug-free lyophilized urine is commercially available): sample temperature when produced, and osmolality may be helpful.

Laxatives are quite commonly misused: the simple test for phenophthalein is well known, and reasonably sensitive thin-layer chromatographic techniques are available for identification of anthroquinones and other laxatives. Either urine or faecal samples can be used.

Finally, there is periodic concern about environmental factors such as exposure to trace metals. Urine mercury and other trace metals are often monitored using 24-h urine samples. Because of problems with sample contamination and interpretation, particularly in screening, such analyses are best left to specialized centres using dedicated atomic-absorption techniques.

OTHER URINE TESTS

Many hundreds of spot tests for urine samples have been described over the last century: experimental details are often only described in older textbooks. Some spot tests have found an important place in the diagnostic laboratory; others are only occasionally of value.

A spot test for *porphobilinogen* can be of great value in the investigation of a patient with acute abdominal pain. Acute attacks of porphyria are always associated with an increased excretion of porphobilinogen: the urine sample may be initially normal in colour, but frequently darkens on standing. Other porphyrins may also be detected in urine; but adequate investigation of a case of porphyria also requires faecal and blood samples.

Colour changes in urine occasionally lead to requests for chemical analysis. Both increased *melanogen* in cases of melanoma and *homogentisic acid* in the rare inherited disease alkaptonuria can give rise to a urine sample that darkens on standing. The useful ferric chloride reagent can be used to identify and distinguish the two, although clinically such differentiation is usually unnecessary.

Pigments often give rise to coloured urine: vegetable dyes, colouring matter from food additives, etc. Simple tests for such ingested material include indicator properties (e.g. phenolphthalein) and characteristic fluorescence (e.g. eosin). After ingestion, a range of *sugars* can also appear in urine: these are occasionally of interest in investigating conditions such as hereditary fructose intolerance or essential pentosuria, and are best differentiated by thin-layer chromatography.

Tests for *urobilinogen* and *bilirubin* in urine are occasionally helpful in assisting the differential diagnosis of jaundice; but most other tests are seldom requested and rarely of clinical utility. Despite urine now having passed out of fashion as a worthwhile sample for analysis, the thoughtful analyst should remember a sixteenth century quotation: 'Amongst all signes of sickness and health whereby the skilful physician is led into the knowledge of the state of the body two are of most general and certain signification which are taken from the pulse and urine, without which all the knowledge of physicke besides is obscure, doubtful and uncertain.'[18]

REFERENCES

1. White W.I. (1991). A new look at the role of urinalysis in the history of diagnostic medicine. *Clin. Chem.*, **37**, 119.
2. Brian Thomas (1637). *The pisse-prophet or certain pisse-pot lectures*, London.
3. Shelley T.F. (1970). Estrogen creatinine ratios: clinical application and significance. *Obstet. Gynecol.*, **37**, 184.
4. Newall R.G., Howell R. eds. (1990). *Clinical Urinalysis: The Principles and Practice of Urine Testing in the Hospital and Community*, Stoke Poges, Bucks. Ames Division, Miles Ltd.
5. Challand G.S. (1987). Is ward biochemical testing cheap and easy? *Intensive Care World*, **4**, 9.
6. Smith I. and Seakins J.W.T. (1976). *Chromatogaphic and Electrophoretic Techniques*, 4th edn, vol 1, London: Heinemann Medical.
7. Holton J.B. (1982). Diagnosis of inherited metabolic diseases in severely ill children. *Ann. Clin. Biochem.*, **19**, 398.
8. Spaeth G.L., Barber G.W. (1967). Prevalence of homocystinuria among the mentally retarded: evaluation of a specific screening test. *Paediatr.*, **40**, 586.
9. Edwards M.A. et al. (1988). A practical approach to the investigation of amino acid disorders. *Ann. Clin. Biochem.*, **25**, 129.
10. Pennock C.A. (1980). Investigation of mucopolysaccharidoses. *Assoc. Clin. Pathol. Broadsheet*, **93**.
11. Tamm I., Horsfall F.L. (1952). A mucoprotein derived from human urine which reacts with influenza, mumps and Newcastle disease virus. *J. Exp. Med.*, **95**, 71.
12. Cameron J.S. (1984). Proteinuria and the nephrotic syndrome. In *The Oxford Book of Medicine*, Oxford University Press.
13. Mogensen C.E. et al. (1986). Microalbuminuria: an early marker of renal involvement in diabetes. *Uremia Invest.*, **9**, 85.
14. Rowe D.J.F. et al. (1990). Microalbuminuria in diabetes mellitus: review and recommendations for the measurement of albumin in urine. *Ann. Clin. Biochem.*, **27**, 297.
15. Zilva J.F. et al. (1988). *Clinical Chemistry in Diagnosis and Treatment*, 5th edn, London: Lloyd-Luke Medical.
16. Meade B.W. et al. (1972). Simple tests to detect poisons. *Ann. Clin. Biochem.*, **9**, 35.
17. Caldwell R., Challenger H. (1988). A capillary column gas-chromatographic method for the identification of drugs of abuse in urine samples. *Ann. Clin. Biochem.*, **26**, 430.
18. Fletcher J. (1541). *The Differences, Causes and Judgements of Urine*. London.

FURTHER READING

Curry A.L. (1988). *Poison Detection in Human Organs*, 4th ed, Springfield, IL: Charles C. Thomas.
Dukes C.E. (1939). *Urine: Examination and Clinical Interpretation*, Oxford University Press.
Harrison G.A. (1957). *Chemical Methods in Clinical Medicine*, London: Churchill Livingstone.
Hawk P.B. et al. (1952). *Practical Physiological Chemistry*, 12th edn, London: Churchill.
Hill A. et al. (1976). Difficulties and pitfalls in the interpretation of screening tests for the detection of inborn errors of metabolism. *Clin. Chim. Acta*, **72**, 1.
Thomas G.H. and Howell R.R. (1973). *Selected Screening Tests for Genetic Metabolic Diseases*, Chicago: Year Book Medical.

19. Tests of Kidney Function

R.B. Payne

Introduction
Glomerular function
    Glomerular filtration rate (GFR)
    Assessment of GFR
    Monitoring changes in GFR
    Glomerular ultrafiltration
Tubular function
    Tubular maximum
    Assessment of glycosuria
    Assessment of tubular phosphate handling
    Assessment of urine acidification
    Assessment of water reabsorption
    Tubular function in acute renal failure
Endocrine function
    Renin
    Erythropoietin
    1,25-dihydroxycholecalciferol
Renal function after transplantation

INTRODUCTION

The constancy of the chemical composition of the internal environment is largely determined by renal function. The extracellular fluid that bathes the cells is in equilibrium with plasma and the total plasma volume passes through the kidneys every 6 min. One-fifth of this plasma flow is ultrafiltered through the 1 000 000 glomeruli in each kidney. Of the 100 mL/min of almost protein-free filtrate that is formed, all but about 1 mL/min is reabsorbed. Thus, every 30 min the total plasma volume is filtered through glomeruli and reabsorbed through tubules that are able to alter its chemical composition in response to changes in the internal environment.[1]

With increasing age, even in the absence of overt disease, nephrons die and are replaced by fibrous tissue. By the age of 70 years only 60% may survive. Each surviving nephron has an increased blood supply and an increased glomerular filtration rate (GFR), but tubular function appears to be normal. Because of their reduced number and the increased filtered load, the tubules work closer to their full capacity and the rate of correction of a disturbance is slower. As a consequence the elderly show a greater change in the internal environment following a disturbance of body composition induced, for example, by an intravenous infusion or by an acidosis. Dietary protein increases GFR. It has been suggested that glomerular damage follows a sustained increase in glomerular filtration caused by the high protein content of the modern diet and that this is responsible both for these age-related changes and for the progressive nature of renal disease.[2] This view remains controversial.

When the number of functioning nephrons is substantially reduced by renal disease, the urinary excretion of normal quantities of waste products such as urea and creatinine is achieved at considerably elevated plasma concentrations (Fig. 19.1) and the urinary excretion of a normal acid load is achieved with a reduced tubular synthesis (and therefore filtered load) of bicarbonate. The total body water and plasma sodium concentration show a much wider variability than in health.

Tubular function is impaired in a number of clinical conditions in which there is little change in glomerular function. Depending on the site and nature of the lesion, there can be a combination of defects in the reabsorption of many substances or specific impairments, for example of acid–base or water balance.

As well as regulating the chemical composition of plasma and thus of the extracellular fluid, the kidneys also function as endocrine organs. Diseases that reduce glomerular perfusion alter the internal auto-regulatory endocrine system that, within limits, compensates for reduced blood flow, and also increase the secretion of renin into the circulation, so increasing the production of angiotensin and aldosterone. In chronic renal disease, the synthesis of the renal hormones erythropoietin and 1,25-dihydroxycholecalciferol may be impaired. Successful renal transplantation improves the quality of life of a patient in end-stage renal failure both by removing the necessity for regular dialysis and by relieving symptoms caused by deficiency of these hormones.

GLOMERULAR FUNCTION

Glomerular Filtration Rate

The principle underlying the measurement of GFR is to determine the rate of appearance in the urine of a substance that has a constant plasma concentration over the period of the test, that is freely filtered at the renal glomeruli and that is neither secreted nor reabsorbed by the tubules. The assumption is made that the concentration in the glomerular filtrate is the same as that in plasma, so it is important to use a marker substance that has no protein-binding. Ideally the plasma concentration should be measured in a plasma ultrafiltrate, or should be increased by a factor to account for the volume of plasma occupied by proteins and lipids that are not present in glomerular filtrate. (The aqueous phase occupies only 93% of normal plasma and less in hyperlipidaemic or hyperproteinaemic plasma.) Knowing the amount of the substance excreted in the urine in unit time and its concentration in the glomerular filtrate, the volume of glomerular filtrate formed in unit time is simply the former quantity divided by the latter. If the urine concentration is designated U, the urine formation

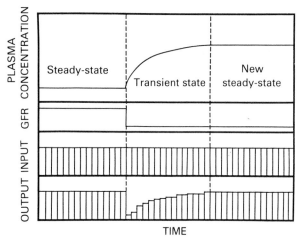

Fig. 19.1 Theoretical transient and steady-state changes in plasma concentration and urine output of a substance excreted by glomerular filtration following a reduction in glomerular filtration rate (GFR). The immediate fall in output causes a rising plasma concentration, which increases output until a new steady-state is reached with a constant raised plasma concentration and a normal output.

rate V, and the plasma concentration (in the same units) P, then:

GFR = urine excretion rate/plasma concentration
= UV/P.

This quantity is also sometimes called the clearance—an expression derived from the concept of the volume of plasma completely cleared of a substance in unit time. The final measurement is the sum of the filtration rates of all nephrons in both kidneys and may be misleading in, for example, unilateral renal disease. However, it is rarely necessary to use ureteric catheterization to measure individual kidney GFR because isotopic radiographic techniques are usually adequate.[3]

Assessment of GFR

Inulin Clearance
Inulin is a polysaccharide with a molecular weight of about 5000 that largely replaces starch in dahlia and Jerusalem artichoke tubers. It is the classical substance that fulfils the criteria for the measurement of GFR. However, because it is poorly soluble and its measurement is technically demanding, it is rarely used.

EDTA and DTPA Clearance
Other substances that fulfil the criteria are chromium-labelled ethylenediaminetetraacetic acid (^{51}Cr-EDTA) and technetium-labelled diethylenetri-aminepentaacetic acid (^{99}mTc-DTPA). The latter, a pure γ-emitter of moderate energy, is now the more widely used because it has a half-life of only 6 h, so reducing the radiation dose. Occasional commercial samples show some protein binding, so each batch

must be checked and plasma samples ultrafiltered if necessary. The standard method of infusing DTPA to achieve a constant plasma concentration has been replaced by bolus injection.[4] A plasma concentration curve is generated, allowing the filtered load during the urine collection period to be calculated. This method has been shown to correlate very closely with inulin clearance measured during continuous infusion to achieve a steady plasma concentration (Fig. 19.2a).[5] The DTPA method is most precise at GFR values close to normal. It becomes less precise at low GFR values, largely because of errors in calculating the plasma disappearance rate when the slope is very shallow. Direct measurement of GFR by this method is used in clinical practice to confirm normality in subjects with, for example, minor proteinuria or hae-maturia detected during employment or insurance examinations, and from time to time when plasma creatinine concentration is used to monitor renal function in patients.

A slightly less precise modification, which is of value in infants and children in whom urine collection is difficult, is to measure only plasma concentrations of DTPA over a period that is sufficiently long to ensure complete equilibration of body pools—this may be 6–8 h in children with renal failure. Under equilibrium conditions the disappearance rate from plasma must equal the excretion rate in urine. The method is unsuitable for patients with oedema, ascites or pleural effusions because equilibrium is not achieved, and it does not correlate as closely with inulin clearance as does the urinary clearance of DTPA.[5]

Endogenous Urea Clearance
Urea does not have a constant plasma concentration in subjects on a protein-containing diet. It is freely filtered at the renal glomerulus but it is reabsorbed with water in the renal tubule so that its clearance is related to the activity of arginine vasopressin (AVP; formerly known as antidiuretic hormone) and tubular function, decreasing as the rate of the urine formation falls. Endogenous urea clearance has been abandoned as a clinical measure of glomerular function.

Endogenous Creatinine Clearance
Because the renal clearance of creatinine does not depend on the rate of urine flow, it superseded urea clearance as a measure of glomerular function that did not require infusion of an exogenous substance. A urine collection period of 24 h has been used in clinical practice for many years to reduce some of the inaccuracies of shorter periods of collection. However, plasma creatinine concentration is not constant over 24 h if the diet contains meat. It has been shown to increase by up to 30% after an ordinary hospital meal and by up to 80% after a substantial goulash or stew. After 300 g of boiled beef, plasma creatinine was still raised 20 h later (Fig. 19.3).[6] During this elevation, urine excretion increases and so would

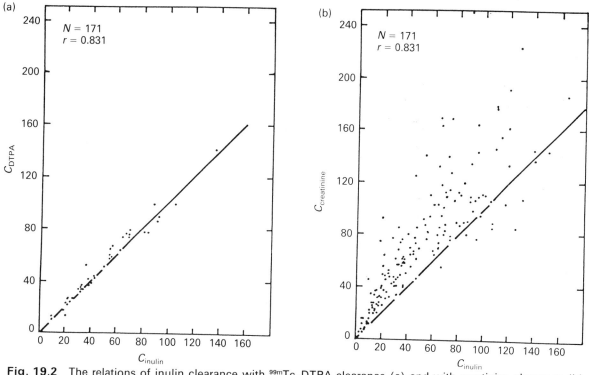

Fig. 19.2 The relations of inulin clearance with ^{99m}Tc-DTPA clearance (a) and with creatinine clearance (b) measured under experimental conditions in normals and subjects with chronic renal failure (reproduced from *Kidney International*[5] with permission).

spuriously elevate clearance if plasma creatinine were measured when its concentration was low. Even when outpatients receive expert instruction, the inaccuracies of urine collection combined with the effects of different diets lead to creatinine clearance values that can vary from day to day by more than 50% in either direction.

The evidence from research studies, conducted with carefully timed and repeated urine collections over short periods and with plasma creatinine measured by a specific method, is that creatinine clearance substantially and variably overestimates GFR by an average of more than 60% (*see* Fig. 19.2b).[5] Creatinine is actively secreted by renal tubules at all plasma concentrations and its secretion by surviving

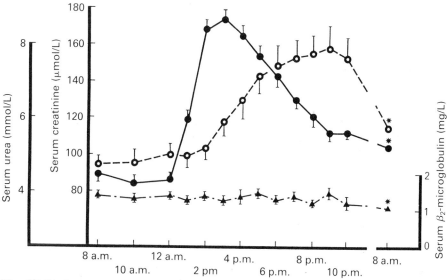

Fig. 19.3 Serum urea, creatinine and β_2-microglobulin concentrations over 24 h: a goulash containing 250–300 g of beef was eaten at 12 noon. ○, urea concentration; ●, creatinine concentration; ▲, β_2-microglobulin concentration (reproduced from the *Lancet*[6] with permission).

TABLE 19.1
SERUM CREATININE CONCENTRATIONS BETWEEN 8 AND 10 A.M.
IN 18 181 WORKING MEN RELATED TO AGE.[8]

| | | Serum creatinine concentration ($\mu mol/L$) | |
Age (years)	No. of subjects	Mean	95% limits
20–24	1989	87.5	63–112
25–29	2401	88.8	65–112
30–34	2354	88.0	64–112
35–39	2493	88.0	65–111
40–44	2506	87.5	63–112
45–49	2329	88.4	65–112
50–54	1707	89.2	65–113
55–59	1403	88.5	66–112
60–64	868	88.4	54–113
65–69	131	89.9	64–116

The serum creatinine concentrations of 17 456 working women averaged 9.6 $\mu mol/L$ less than that of men in each age group (reproduced with permission[9]).

nephrons increases as renal function is lost. As the plasma concentration rises there is also increasing extrarenal degradation of creatinine, largely in the gut. These changes vary from patient to patient, and it is apparent from Fig. 19.2(b) that GFR cannot be predicted from creatinine clearance with confidence in individual patients. Others have confirmed under similar experimental conditions that a normal creatinine clearance is not evidence of a normal GFR.[7]

Plasma Urea Concentration and GFR

Plasma urea concentration is determined by production rate and renal clearance. Production rate varies with the amount of protein eaten (*see* Fig.19.3) while renal clearance varies with both GFR and tubular water reabsorption. Vegans can be recognized by their remarkably low plasma urea concentrations. In clinical practice, plasma urea is used to assist in the assessment of the pathophysiology of acute renal failure rather than to predict GFR (see below).

Plasma Creatinine Concentration and GFR

The renal clearance of plasma creatinine is unaffected by tubular water handling, but its rate of entry to plasma depends both on release from muscle after non-enzymatic degradation of phosphocreatinine and on absorption of creatinine from ingested meat.

GFR falls progressively through adult life. Creatinine excretion rate also falls with increasing age, owing to a reduction in muscle mass and possibly to the ingestion of less meat. However, plasma creatinine concentration during adult life is largely independent of age (Table 19.1).[8] This close relation between GFR and muscle mass in the absence of overt disease has been confirmed by the demonstration that fasting plasma creatinine concentration is independent of lean body mass in health. As a consequence it is not possible to predict a patient's GFR

from a normal fasting plasma creatinine concentration. While a normal fasting plasma creatinine concentration, like a normal creatinine clearance, is not evidence of a normal GFR, it does indicate that the GFR is reasonably appropriate for the patient's age and muscle mass. It is therefore not surprising that, using measurements made under careful experimental conditions, calculation has shown that the reciprocal of plasma creatinine concentration is neither better nor worse than creatinine clearance at predicting measured GFR (Table 19.2).[9] It is simpler, cheaper, more convenient and more reproducible. Isotopic methods are necessary to establish the presence of minor reductions in GFR with confidence.

Plasma creatinine concentration falls substantially during the first year of life and then rises gradually through childhood and the teens to reach adult values in the early 20s (Fig. 19.4).[10] It falls again during pregnancy because there is a substantial increase in true GFR. A value in a specimen taken in the fasting state and on a meat-free diet that is normal by comparison with the appropriate reference range (for children, adult men or women, or pregnancy)[9,10] cannot exclude a minor degree of renal impairment. However, a raised fasting plasma creatinine concentration indicates a GFR that is lower than normal for age, sex and muscle mass if care has been taken to avoid interfering factors.

Plasma creatinine may be significantly raised by the inhibition of tubular secretion in patients taking salicylate, co-trimoxazole, trimethoprim or cimetidine (ranitidine appears not to have this effect). Its value may be spuriously elevated in patients with ketosis because acetoacetate interferes with the Jaffé reac-

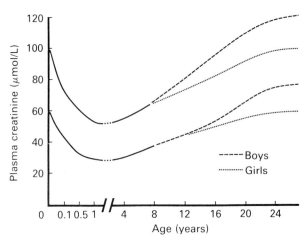

Fig. 19.4 Ninety-five per cent confidence limits of plasma creatinine concentration through infancy, childhood and adolescence, based on the data of T. M. Barratt and J. M. Round in *Paediatric Chemical Pathology: Clinical Tests and Reference Ranges* (1980) Oxford: Blackwell, pp. 60–61 (reproduced from the *Annals of Clinical Biochemistry*[9] with permission).

TABLE 19.2

CORRELATION COEFFICIENTS BETWEEN INULIN CLEARANCE AND MEASURES OF GLOMERULAR FUNCTION BASED
ON CREATININE IN FASTING SUBJECTS

Creatinine method	No. of subjects	Inulin clearance vs. creatinine clearance	Inulin clearance vs. reciprocal of plasma creatinine concentration
Manual picrate total chromogens	123	0.679	0.611
Manual picrate with Lloyd's reagent	116	0.616	0.648
Auto Analyser picrate	104	0.667	0.577

Re-analysis of data from normal men and men with renal disease.[7] The correlation coefficients do not differ significantly between columns (reproduced with permission[9]).

tion, even with reaction rate methods. The apparent values measured by the Jaffé reaction can also be raised by therapeutic concentrations of the cephalosporin antibiotics cefoxitin and cephalothin, while other cephalosporins, including cefotaxime, ceftazidime and ceftizoxime, are without effect. None interferes with enzymatic methods at therapeutic concentrations.

Plasma creatinine concentration can appear to be low in patients with marked jaundice because bilirubin causes a negative interference with some methods. Creatinine production rate is decreased in patients with marked muscle wasting, and this can lead to misleadingly low plasma concentrations.

The initial dose of some potentially toxic drugs that are eliminated largely by renal excretion must be reduced if GFR is significantly reduced. However, direct measurement of GFR is rarely used for this purpose and dosing regimens are based on the simple measurement of plasma creatinine.[11] The dose adjustment takes account of both the normal age-related fall in GFR that takes place with no change in the plasma creatinine concentration, and of an approximation of the fall in GFR due to renal disease reflected by an increase in plasma creatinine. These methods are adequate within the range of initial doses used in clinical practice.

Plasma β_2-microglobulin Concentration and GFR

Beta$_2$-microglobulin, a small protein with a molecular weight of only 11 800, is the short chain of the major histocompatibility antigen on the surface of the nucleated cells of the body. It is freely filtered at the renal glomerulus and normally reabsorbed by pinocytosis and catabolized in the proximal renal tubule. Its plasma concentration in health rises with age as GFR falls because its production rate, unlike that of creatinine, does not fall with decreasing muscle mass. Its production rate is, however, determined by the rate of body cell turnover, so in inflammatory and neoplastic diseases its plasma concentration rises in the absence of any change in GFR to the extent that it is used as a tumour marker in, for example, the lymphoproliferative disorders. Because of this difficulty, and because it is expensive to measure, it is little used for the assessment of renal disease. However, in the absence of inflammation or neoplasia its plasma concentration, unlike that of plasma creatinine, is directly related to GFR.

Monitoring Changes in GFR

Monitoring changes in GFR is not the same thing as monitoring the progression of renal disease; the loss of nephrons in chronic renal failure proceeds faster than the fall in GFR because the filtration rate of surviving nephrons increases. Frequent monitoring of GFR using EDTA or DTPA is impractical because of inconvenience and expense. Creatinine clearance is rarely used for monitoring progression because it has such a large variance in clinical practice. The use of plasma creatinine alone for assessment has been stimulated by the observation that in most patients the reciprocal of its concentration tends to decrease linearly with time. This allows the prediction of the time when 'action limits' may be reached—for example, the plan to construct an arteriovenous fistula when plasma creatinine concentration reaches, say, 600 μmol/L (6.8 mg/dL), allowing it to mature before the patient develops symptoms and needs to start on haemodialysis. An increase in slope suggests that a change in treatment or a clinical event has had an unfavourable effect on progression and vice versa (Fig. 19.5). However, the rate of fall of GFR measured using EDTA or DTPA cannot be predicted with accuracy from the reciprocal of plasma creatinine concentration.[12] It has been suggested that if clinicians supplement their routine plasma creatinine-based monitoring with the occasional determination of true GFR using DTPA, appropriate changes in therapy are more likely to be made.[5] Evaluation of new treatments designed to alter the rate of progression of chronic renal disease will certainly need to be monitored using isotopic methods.

Glomerular Ultrafiltration

Impaired function of the glomerulus as an ultrafilter results in glomerular proteinuria. There is normally about 50 mg/L of protein in glomerular filtrate.

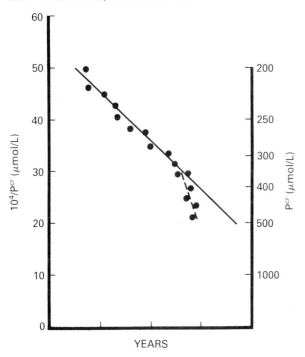

Fig. 19.5 An example of a nearly linear decrease of the reciprocal of plasma creatinine concentration P^{CR} with time during the progression of chronic renal failure, with an inflexion indicating an event causing more rapid progression.

Proteins of molecular weight less than 14 500 appear freely, while those of above 70 000 are virtually absent. (Free plasma haemoglobin, with a molecular weight of 68 000, is freely filtered and so appears to be an exception; it is a tetramer in equilibrium with small concentrations of dimer and monomer that pass through the glomerular membrane and reassemble on the other side.) Most filtered protein is taken into tubular cells by pinocytosis and catabolized; less than 2% of the filtered load appears in the urine. By far the most common cause of the incidental detection of proteinuria by dipstick during routine health screening is postural or orthostatic proteinuria. It is found in 12–40% of children aged 10–16 years and in about 5% of young adults.[13] The prevalence can be increased to 75% by placing youths in extreme lordosis; it is caused by pressure on the inferior vena cava increasing renal vein and thus glomerular filtration pressure. In postural proteinuria there is no increase in protein in the first urine collected after overnight bedrest. Benign proteinuria often follows exercise.

Rapid but transient impairment of the function of the glomerulus as an ultrafilter may be observed between 3 and 8 h after generalized trauma, burns or surgery, coincident with a reversible increase in generalized capillary permeability to proteins. A similar but more marked and longer-lasting generalized increase in capillary permeability, also leading to glomerular proteinuria, occurs after the onset of acute pancreatitis.

The microalbuminuria of early diabetes, a three- or fourfold increase above the reference range and below the sensitivity of most urine dipsticks, may revert to normal with insulin treatment and reappear with its withdrawal. The cause of diabetic renal disease is uncertain. It has been suggested that glomerular basement-membrane changes permit anionic molecules, particularly albumin, to reach the glomerular matrix where they cause mesangial proliferation. Microalbuminuria appears to precede the development of overt diabetic nephropathy. Present immunological methods for the quantitation of microalbuminuria are expensive. A sensitive urine dipstick has been developed commercially.

In the nephrotic syndrome a measure of the selectivity of the glomerular permeability to proteins is obtained by calculating the ratio of the renal clearances of proteins of different molecular size, for example IgG (150 000) and transferrin (90 000). If the urine concentration of IgG is U_g, that of transferrin is U_t, the plasma concentration of IgG is P_g and that of transferrin is P_t, then:

$$\text{IgG:transferrin clearance ratio} = \frac{U_g \times V}{P_g} \times \frac{P_t}{U_t \times V}.$$

Because the timed urine volumes V cancel out, the test can be done with an untimed urine specimen. Minimal histological change on renal biopsy with the likelihood of a favourable response to steroid therapy is associated with clearance ratios of 0.2 or less, but similar numbers of non-responders have such values. In contrast, a clearance ratio greater than 0.2 points to a high probability of failure to respond to steroids. This test has been largely superseded by renal biopsy.

TUBULAR FUNCTION

The renal tubules modify the composition of about 150 L of glomerular filtrate that are normally formed each day by removing water and other solutes and adding ammonia and hydrogen ion. In the steady state, the composition of the urine formed exactly balances the quantities absorbed from the gut and formed by metabolism. This remarkable feat is accomplished with the help of only four non-renal hormone feedback systems: AVP, aldosterone, atrial natriuretic peptide and parathyroid hormone (PTH). The remaining regulatory systems, including the regulation of acid excretion and bicarbonate synthesis, depend on intrarenal mechanisms.

A number of inborn errors primarily affect specific renal tubular transport mechanisms, for example:

- renal glycosuria,
- nephrogenic diabetes insipidus,
- cystinuria (affecting cystine and the dibasic amino acids),
- Hartnup disease (affecting neutral amino acids),
- iminoglycinuria (affecting glycine, proline and hydroxyproline),

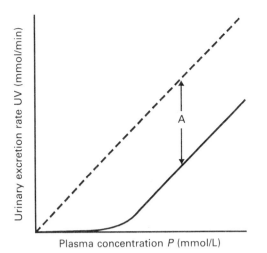

Fig. 19.6 The typical relation between the plasma concentration (P) and the urine excretion rate (UV) of a substance reabsorbed by the renal tubule. The slope of the line is the glomerular filtration rate (GFR) (UV/P). The tubular maximum reabsorptive capacity (Tm) is the distance on the y axis between the dotted line and the linear portion of the continuous line (A). Tm/GFR is the intercept of the linear part of the curve with the x axis.

- the proximal and distal forms of isolated renal tubular acidosis,
- the hypophosphataemias.

The *Fanconi syndrome* is a generalized disturbance of the proximal renal tubule affecting reabsorption of amino acids, glucose, phosphate, urate and low molecular-weight proteins.[14] Because proximal reabsorption of water, sodium, potassium, calcium and magnesium are also impaired, regulation by the distal tubule can become inadequate when stressed. The syndrome can be inherited or acquired. The inherited variety occurs alone or results from the accumulation of cystine in cystinosis, fructose in fructose intolerance, galactose in galactosaemia, tyrosine in tyrosinaemia or copper in Wilson's disease. The syndrome can also occur in vitamin D-dependent rickets and in glycogen storage disease type I. In Wilson's disease there may be an associated distal renal tubular acidosis (RTA). Severe phosphate depletion from any cause can also lead to the Fanconi syndrome and distal RTA. The Fanconi syndrome is sometimes seen in patients with Bence–Jones proteinuria. It results from damage to proximal tubular cells by enzymes released from lysozomes, which are vastly increased in number because of massive pinocytosis of immunoglobulin light chains.

Tubular Maximum

The typical relation between the plasma concentration (P) and the urine excretion rate (UV) of a substance reabsorbed by the renal tubule is illustrated in Fig. 19.6. At low plasma concentrations the filtered load is entirely reabsorbed. As the concentration increases there is a gradual curvilinear increase in urinary excretion rate and then a linear increase which parallels the relation that would hold if there were no tubular reabsorption or excretion (dotted line). The slope of the line is the GFR (UV/P). The curved portion or 'splay' is a consequence of the normal range of maximum reabsorptive capacities of individual nephrons; the relation becomes linear when each is working at its maximum. Thus, the tubular maximum reabsorptive capacity (Tm) is the distance on the y axis between the dotted line and the linear portion of the continuous line. This value, like GFR, is the sum of the capacities of all the nephrons in both kidneys.

Assessment of Glycosuria

It is not usual to measure the tubular maximum for glucose (Tm_G) in clinical practice, but rather to examine the relation between plasma glucose and the appearance of glucose in the urine in a less formal way. Normally there are only trace amounts of glucose in urine and significant amounts appear only when the plasma concentration exceeds about 10 mmol/L (180 mg/dL). This point is represented approximately by the intercept of the extension of the straight part of the line in Fig. 19.6 with the x axis and is sometimes called the 'threshold'. It is more correctly designated Tm_G/GFR (mmol/L of glomerular filtrate), because it can be derived from the distance between the lines, Tm_G, divided by the slope of the lines, UV/P or GFR.

Significant glycosuria, more than 5 mmol/L (90 mg/dL), can be detected by urine dipsticks. It is of renal origin if it occurs while the plasma glucose concentrations after a 75-g oral glucose load are within normal limits. Its most common cause is the substantial increase in GFR during pregnancy. The slope of the lines in Fig. 19.6 (GFR) becomes steeper and the plasma 'threshold' or Tm_G/GFR falls with no change in Tm_G. In non-pregnant adult patients, isolated renal glycosuria is more common than the Fanconi syndrome, and the acquired causes of the syndrome outlined above are usually clinically evident. However, if in children the urine shows both glycosuria and aminoaciduria, amino acid excretion should be measured and tests for cystinuria and other inborn errors carried out.

Assessment of Tubular Phosphate Handling

The shape of the curved portion or 'splay' for phosphate was found to be the same in all normal fasting individuals when variation due to GFR was removed. Because Tm_P/GFR completely described the variation between individuals it became possible to construct a nomogram to determine Tm_P/GFR from plasma phosphate and the ratio of UV to GFR.[15]

Kenny and Glen[16] were able to fit a rectangular hyperbola to the primary data for the splay, so that Tm_p/GFR can be derived mathematically without recourse to a nomogram. The tubular reabsorption of phosphate (TRP) as a decimal fraction is calculated from:

$$TRP = 1 - \frac{P_c \times U_p}{U_c \times P_p},$$

where P_c and U_c are the plasma and urine concentrations of creatinine and P_p and U_p the plasma and urine concentrations of phosphate measured in the same units in fasting specimens (after discarding the overnight urine). If TRP < 0.86, then:

$$Tm_P/GFR = TRP \times P_p.$$

If TRP > 0.86 then, using the algorithm of Kenny and Glen:

$$Tm_P/GFR = \frac{(0.30 \times TRP)}{(1 - (0.8 \times TRP))} \times P_p.$$

Adult 95% reference values are 0.80–1.35 mmol/L (2.5–4.2 mg/dL). Values during childhood are considerably higher, approximately 1.15–2.44 mmol/L (3.6–7.6 mg/dL) between 2 and 15 years. It should be noted that there are a number of approximations in the calculation of Tm_p/GFR, including the assumption that the plasma concentration of phosphate is equal to its concentration in the glomerular filtrate, and that creatinine clearance is a close approximation to GFR. However, these assumptions also apply to the reference data.

The tubular reabsorption of phosphate is reduced by PTH, so Tm_p/GFR was widely used at one time for the differential diagnosis of hypercalcaemia. However, it was inefficient because PTH-related peptide produced by some malignant tumours also decreases Tm_p/GFR. Thus, the test cannot be used to diagnose hyperparathyroidism but only to exclude it when high normal or raised values of Tm_p/GFR consistent with secondary hypoparathyroidism are found. Now that measurement of intact whole-molecule PTH is available, Tm_p/GFR is little used for this purpose, but remains useful in the hypophosphataemias,[17] in the Fanconi syndrome,[14] and in the detection of proximal tubular damage by toxins, drugs or metabolites.

Assessment of Urine Acidification

Urine is acidified at two sites in the renal tubule: proximally by exchange of hydrogen ion for sodium ion together with reabsorption of bicarbonate ion, and distally by a second sodium/hydrogen ion exchange mechanism. In the proximal tubule, 90–95% of the filtered load of bicarbonate disappears, partly entering the tubular cell along the electrochemical gradient created by the active reabsorption of sodium, and partly by reaction with excreted hydrogen ion to form carbon dioxide and water, intracellular synthesis of hydrogen ion from carbonic acid having formed an equivalent quantity of bicarbonate. The fine tuning of urinary acid secretion and tubular bicarbonate synthesis takes place in the distal tubule in response to the acid–base status of the blood. The distal sodium/hydrogen ion exchange behaves as though it were in competition with an associated sodium/potassium exchange mechanism for luminal sodium, both pumps being stimulated by aldosterone. Part of the excreted hydrogen ion reacts with the remaining 5–10% of filtered bicarbonate, part combines with ammonia derived from glutamine to form ammonium ions, part reacts with phosphate and other buffers in the luminal fluid, and a small fraction lowers fluid pH itself. Each day, normal kidneys reabsorb or resynthesize the total filtered load of bicarbonate, about 3600 mmol, and in addition excrete about 50–100 mmol of urinary acid as buffered hydrogen ion and ammonium ion, simultaneously replacing an equal quantity of bicarbonate that has been used up during normal metabolism.[18] The mechanisms for the acidification of urine are further discussed in Chapter 3.

Diseases that limit the rate of acidification of the urine thus result in a reduced rate of bicarbonate regeneration. As a consequence the plasma bicarbonate concentration falls. Less hydrogen ion secretion is required to reabsorb the reduced filtered load of bicarbonate, so in the steady state the normal metabolic acid load can be excreted. The key feature of renal tubular acidosis (RTA) is therefore a reduced plasma bicarbonate concentration with no increase in the anion–cation gap, so-called hyperchloraemic acidosis. The plasma potassium concentration may suggest the site of the lesion.

RTA affecting the proximal tubular excretion of hydrogen ion is usually a manifestation of the Fanconi syndrome, may sometimes be associated with vitamin D deficiency and may rarely occur as an isolated acidification defect. In these conditions the plasma potassium concentration is usually normal. In addition, in the Fanconi syndrome there is hypophosphataemia as well as glycosuria, aminoaciduria and phosphaturia, and in vitamin D deficiency there is often hypocalcaemia and hyperphosphatasaemia.

RTA affecting the sodium/hydrogen ion, but not the sodium/potassium exchange mechanism in the distal tubule is commonly associated with low plasma potassium concentration because a greater proportion of distal tubular sodium reabsorption takes place in exchange for potassium. This is predominantly a disorder of adult women, probably of an autoimmune nature, that may present suddenly with profound hypokalaemic muscle weakness, particularly in the post-partum period. It sometimes occurs in association with a systemic illness and less commonly in infancy or childhood as an autosomal-dominant inherited defect.

Aldosterone controls both distal exchange mechanisms. RTA with a raised plasma potassium concentration is usually the result of hypoaldosteronism either due to Addison's disease or, more commonly, to the syndrome of hyporeninaemic hypoaldosteronism (see below). Hyperkalaemic RTA may also result from failure to respond to aldosterone because of distal tubule damage in obstructive renal disease.

The acidosis of chronic renal failure is usually hyperchloraemic (and so falls within the definition of RTA) until the GFR falls to about 20 mL/min, when the increasing plasma concentrations of phosphate, urate and other substances increase the anion–cation gap. The acidosis can be hyperkalaemic but is usually normokalaemic because of increased potassium excretion both into urine from the renal collecting ducts and into the colon.

Urine Acidification Test

If the pH of the first fasting morning urine after discarding the overnight urine is less than 5.5, distal RTA is excluded and the urine acidification test of Wrong and Davies[19] is unnecessary. The test requires the oral administration of ammonium chloride in a dose of 100 mg/kg body weight. When it is given as enteric-coated capsules or tablets, absorption may be incomplete. The powder has a nauseating, bitter taste and is best administered, after collecting an initial venous blood sample, in iced solution along with food and plain water. Urine samples are collected about once an hour for the next 8 h, and then a second blood specimen is taken. The plasma bicarbonate concentration should have fallen by 3 mmol/L or more. If none of the urine specimens has a pH of 5.3 or less, the patient has distal renal tubular acidosis. Assuming that the indication for the test was a hyperchloraemic acidosis, if the patient achieves a urine pH of 5.3 or less a proximal tubular lesion is likely and the renal handling of glucose, phosphate and amino acids should be examined.

Ammonium chloride provides an acid load because hepatic metabolism of ammonium ions to urea consumes bicarbonate ions. In patients who cannot tolerate ammonium chloride and those with liver disease an alternative is to give calcium chloride orally.[20] Calcium combines with bicarbonate in the intestinal secretions to form insoluble calcium carbonate. Plasma bicarbonate falls because chloride rather than bicarbonate is reabsorbed from the gut.

Bicarbonaturia

Should the urine acidification test indicate a proximal tubular defect and the patient has none of the features of the Fanconi syndrome, the presence of an isolated proximal RTA can be proved by the oral or intravenous administration of sodium bicarbonate. The increased filtered load will result in the appearance of bicarbonate in the urine, which becomes alkaline at a time when the plasma bicarbonate concentration may not have reached even a low normal concentration.

Assessment of Water Reabsorption

With ageing and during the progression of chronic renal disease the ability of the tubules to remove water from the glomerular filtrate under maximum stimulation from AVP is reduced, so that the stress of fluid deprivation produces higher plasma osmolality and lower urine osmolality than in a healthy youth. If all fluid intake is avoided and only dry foods eaten for 18 h, young men can achieve urine osmolalities of at least 750 mosmol/kg and the elderly about 600 mosmol/kg. In advanced chronic renal disease the urine osmolality differs little from the plasma osmolality. The decreased concentrating ability seems to be due in part to the increased GFR of the surviving nephrons delivering to each of them an increased solute load that passes through the medullary countercurrent mechanism more rapidly. In experimental animals, excision of one kidney and half of the other is followed by failure of the surviving, presumably normal, nephrons to produce concentrated urine; and the production of diuresis by expansion of the extracellular fluid volume in intact animals results in the production of dilute urine even if the plasma AVP is maintained at very high concentrations by infusion. In renal disease it is also likely that the surviving nephrons in a disordered architecture are unable to maintain a normal medullary hypertonicity.

Nephrogenic diabetes insipidus is sometimes a familial disorder with variable expression but is much more commonly acquired.[21] Nephrogenic diabetes insipidus together with the Fanconi syndrome can follow heavy-metal poisoning. The broad spectrum antibiotic demeclocycline (dimethylchlortetracycline) causes diabetes insipidus by inhibiting the action of AVP on the renal tubules, and is sometimes used in the treatment of the syndrome of inappropriate antidiuresis. Lithium, even at therapeutic concentrations of less than 0.8 mmol/L, sometimes causes nephrogenic diabetes insipidus and this may be associated with a distal RTA. Hypokalaemia or hypercalcaemia from any cause can impair tubular function and cause polyuria, often as a presenting clinical symptom.

Diabetes mellitus, chronic renal failure, hypokalaemia, hypercalcaemia and lithium therapy must all be excluded before diabetes insipidus is considered, and failure to produce a normally concentrated urine after overnight fluid deprivation should be demonstrated before proceeding to a formal test of renal concentrating ability.

Tubular Function in Acute Renal Failure

Acute renal failure is a sudden reduction in GFR that is followed by increasing plasma concentrations of substances normally excreted in urine, such as urea and creatinine. It is usually, but not invariably, accompanied by a reduced urine output. Simple tests on plasma and, if some urine is being produced, on a random urine sample can help to distinguish between prerenal, glomerular, tubular and postrenal (obstructive) causes. The distinction is not always clear cut in practice. Prerenal, glomerular and postrenal causes can all lead to tubular necrosis if they are sufficiently severe and persist long enough because the blood supply to the tubules, which derives entirely from the glomeruli, is impaired.

It may well be obvious from the clinical situation that acute renal failure is primarily prerenal in origin, and the question may then be whether it has progressed to *acute tubular necrosis* (ATN). It is unusual for the reduced renal perfusion that occurs in oedematous conditions such as congestive cardiac failure, the nephrotic syndrome and chronic hepatic disease to progress from prerenal failure to ATN in the absence of another precipitating factor, but any cause of acute circulatory failure can do so. These causes include haemorrhage, acute pancreatitis, crush injuries, rhabdomyolysis, burns and severe diarrhoea and vomiting. ATN can also be caused by a wide variety of nephrotoxic drugs and chemicals.

Reduced renal perfusion increases the production rate of renin and thus of angiotensin and aldosterone, while hypovolaemia is a potent stimulus to AVP production. The basis of the biochemical assessment of tubular survival is to determine whether the tubules are able to respond to aldosterone and AVP by modifying the glomerular filtrate.

The tubular response to aldosterone in prerenal failure is shown by a reduction in the urine concentration of sodium to less than 20 mmol/L and often to less than 5 mmol/L, while in ATN and acute obstruction it is usually over 40 mmol/L. The response to AVP is shown in prerenal failure by a ratio of the concentration of creatinine in urine to that in plasma of usually well over 30; in ATN, whether oliguric or polyuric, and in acute obstruction, the ratio is less than 20. Because tubular function is usually well preserved in acute glomerulonephritis the values are similar to those seen in prerenal failure. However, the condition is readily distinguished by urine microscopy: a centrifuged deposit of urine shows large numbers of red cells together with red-cell and granular casts. Cells and large numbers of casts are also present in the urine deposit in ATN.

In prerenal failure the increase in plasma urea concentration is proportionally greater than that in plasma creatinine. Because urea is freely diffusible, it is reabsorbed with water when the tubules are able to respond to AVP. Plasma urea concentrations may reach 40–60 mmol/L (240–360 mg/dL), while plasma creatinine concentrations do not often exceed 250 μmol/L (2.8 mg/dL). A similar relation between plasma urea and creatinine concentrations is found in dehydration and early acute glomerulonephritis.

The increase in *plasma potassium* that is almost invariable in acute renal failure is partly due to impaired distal tubular secretion, partly due to a shift from cells caused by acidosis, and may be greatly contributed to by release of potassium from necrotic cells if the renal failure is due to a crush injury or rhabdomyolysis. Hypocalcaemia and hypophosphataemia are common and are attributed to impaired renal synthesis of 1, 25-dihydroxycholecalciferol.

During the recovery phase of ATN, glomerular function can outpace recovery of tubular function, so there may be massive polyuria with large losses of water and electrolytes that need to be measured and replaced. At the same time a transient but sometimes marked hypercalcaemia may develop as the recovering tubules respond to the secondary hyperparathyroidism caused by hypocalcaemia.

ENDOCRINE FUNCTION

Renin

The first part of the distal convoluted tubule of each nephron contains a region, the macula densa, whose cells are in contact on one side with the tubular lumen and on the other with the afferent arteriole of the glomerulus at a point where its endothelial cells contain secretory granules of renin. These tubular and arteriolar cells together with interstitial cells that resemble mesangial cells form an endocrine organ, the juxtaglomerular apparatus, that secretes renin both into the arteriole and into the interstitial space. Within the kidney the system is responsible for the regulation of afferent arteriolar tone and therefore individual nephron GFR, increasing it in response to a reduced rate of flow of sodium to the macula densa and a decreased mean arterial pressure, and vice versa; other intrarenal regulators of arteriolar tone include dopamine, catecholamines, prostaglandins and bradykinin. In the peripheral circulation, renin converts angiotensinogen to angiotensin I, which is converted to the active hormone angiotensin II by angiotensin-converting enzyme (ACE), largely during the first pass through the lungs.[22] Angiotensin II controls peripheral arteriolar tone and therefore blood pressure, and aldosterone secretion and therefore sodium reabsorption. Aldosterone production is also stimulated directly by hyperkalaemia and suppressed by hypokalaemia. Atrial natriuretic peptide (ANP) is released by increased cardiac atrial pressure and causes natriuresis and inhibits renin, angiotensin II and aldosterone production at physiological concentrations in normal man.

Chronic renal disease is a common cause of secondary hypertension. About 90% of patients with end-stage renal failure are hypertensive. In acute glomerulonephritis, hypertension is common and is usually but not always transient. Unilateral renal disease can cause hypertension that is cured by unilateral nephrectomy. In all these conditions the evidence that increased renin production by the diseased kidney is a major factor in the hypertension is said to be inconclusive.[23] The situation is different in hypertension secondary to unilateral renal vascular disease. Although 50% of such patients have peripheral venous renin activities that are within the reference range, a ratio of the renal-vein renin concentrations on the two sides that is greater than 1.6 predicts the success of vascular surgery with a 93% probability; however, 50% of patients with a normal ratio also improve following surgery.[23]

Treatment of a patient who has hypertension and associated renal disease with an ACE inhibitor to lower blood pressure commonly leads to a further reduction in GFR, underlining the role played by the renin–angiotensin system in maintaining glomerular perfusion.

The *syndrome of hyporeninaemic hypoaldosteronism* is being increasingly recognized. It is most commonly diagnosed following the unexpected discovery of hyperkalaemia, perhaps with an RTA, when plasma electrolytes are measured in the elderly. The patients usually have renal disease that has produced some reduction in GFR, and over half are diabetics. Presentation is much less commonly symptomatic, with muscle weakness or cardiac arrhythmias. The diagnostic features are normal basal and stimulated cortisol concentrations, an inappropriately low or low normal peripheral aldosterone concentration in the presence of hyperkalaemia, with subnormal responses of both aldosterone concentration and renin activity to sodium depletion. There is usually a good response to treatment with the mineralocorticoid fludrocortisone. The pathophysiology of the syndrome is uncertain.[24]

Erythropoietin

Erythropoietin (Epo) is a glycoprotein with a molecular weight of about 36 000. It is synthesized predominantly in the endothelial cells of the capillaries that surround the tubules in the renal cortex and outer medulla, but some Epo synthesis also takes place in the liver. It is released in response to impaired oxygen delivery to the cells because of either anaemia or a lowered Po_2. The receptors for the hormone are on erythroblasts, which mature and divide when stimulated.

Almost all patients with chronic renal failure have a normochromic normocytic anaemia, most untreated dialysis patients having a haematocrit of between 20 and 30%, although some are much lower. Plasma Epo concentrations can be measured and are commonly low or low normal—but are inappropriately low by a factor of more than 10 in the presence of anaemia. The anaemia is a significant cause of morbidity, and many dialysis patients receive blood transfusions from time to time. Recombinant human erythropoietin (rHuEpo) has been synthesized and is available, at some expense, for treatment.[25] The symptoms that improve following improvement of the anaemia are generalized coldness, anorexia, insom-

nia, depression and sexual disinterest and dysfunction; the cardiomegaly of anaemia is also reduced.

It is clearly important to exclude causes of anaemia other than Epo deficiency before embarking on treatment with rHuEpo. During treatment, haemoglobin, reticulocytes and plasma ferritin concentration may be monitored at 2-weekly intervals. If the haemoglobin response is poor, less than 10 g/L per month, a transferrin iron saturation of less than 20% suggests functional iron deficiency, even with a satisfactory ferritin concentration, and the patient may respond if rHuEpo is then supplemented with intravenous iron dextran.[26]

1,25-Dihydroxycholecalciferol

1,25-Dihydroxycholecalciferol (1,25-DHCC) is a renal hormone that is synthesized in the cells of the proximal convoluted tubule by the 1α-hydroxylation of 25-DHCC, itself derived from 25-hydroxylation of vitamin D in the liver. It regulates calcium absorption from the gut and is required for the normal mineralization of bone. Many tissues and organs other than the kidney appear to be able to synthesize some 1,25-DHCC; it acts as a local hormone in cell differentiation and intercellular communication but local 1,25-DHCC normally makes no contribution to calcium homeostasis. Synthesis of the renal hormone is stimulated by PTH and therefore indirectly by hypocalcaemia, and directly by hypophosphataemia. Phosphate depletion also impairs the catabolism of 1,25-DHCC. Increased circulating 1,25-DHCC produces feedback inhibition of the 1α-hydroxylase and the induction of a 'shunt' pathway to 24,25-DHCC. Hyperphosphataemia is a potent inhibitor of hormone synthesis.[27]

Bone disease is common in untreated, advanced renal disease. Impaired synthesis of 1,25-DHCC due to hyperphosphataemia and to loss of renal mass causes hypocalcaemia and secondary hyperparathyroidism. Increased PTH concentrations increase osteoclast resorption of bone, which is partly replaced by fibrous tissue—*osteitis fibrosa*. Deficiency of 1,25-DHCC impairs mineralization, leading to wide osteoid seams and an increased trabecular surface covered by osteoid—*osteomalacia*. Commonly osteitis fibrosa and osteomalacia coexist. The clinical manifestations include bone pain and proximal muscle weakness. Isolated osteomalacia and aplastic bone disease with decreased mineralization but no increase in osteoid is one of the metabolic effects of aluminium toxicity, deposition in osteoid inhibiting mineralization.[28] The condition has become less common now that aluminium accumulation as a result of aluminium contamination of dialysis fluids has been eliminated.

Biochemical features of *renal osteodystrophy* include the hyperphosphataemia of renal failure, an adjusted plasma calcium concentration that is low or low normal, and usually an increased plasma activity of the bone isoenzyme of alkaline phosphatase.

Plasma intact PTH is usually high and is always high in relation to the calcium concentration. Reduction of the plasma phosphate concentration by moderate dietary restriction and administration of oral aluminium hydroxide to reduce inhibition of 1α-hydroxylase used to be the mainstay of treatment. However, alfacalcidol and calcitriol (1, 25-DHCC) have become available to raise the plasma hormone concentration directly by oral administration and so avoid the danger of oral aluminium and the side-effects of the alternative phosphate binder, calcium carbonate. Failure of intact PTH concentrations to fall substantially after administration of alfacalcidol or calcitriol followed by the appearance of hypercalcaemia indicates the development of an autonomous parathyroid adenoma in one of the hyperplastic glands—*tertiary hyperparathyroidism*.

RENAL FUNCTION AFTER TRANSPLANTATION

A transplanted kidney that is going to function well starts to produce urine within 2–10 min of the anastomosis of its blood vessels to those in the recipient's iliac fossa. It has commonly been anoxic for some time before its blood supply is restored, so there is often a degree of tubular dysfunction. Recovery, as in ATN, tends to lag behind glomerular function with similar consequences—water and electrolyte losses that must be measured and replaced. The preoperative plasma hyperosmolality and sodium and water retention may contribute to this diuresis, which usually lasts for only 1 or 2 days.

Proteinuria from the transplanted kidney is common, with glomerular proteinuria lasting a day or two and a gradually diminishing low molecular-weight protein loss due to proximal tubule dysfunction thereafter. Transient glycosuria is also common.

Transient hyperkalaemia and a mild RTA are almost invariable, owing to distal renal tubule dysfunction, and hyperkalaemia persisting as long as 3 months after transplantation has been reported in up to one-third of patients. Occasionally, when tubular function has become normal, hypokalaemia due to potassium loss from the transplanted kidney may follow hyperaldosteronism caused by renin production from the patient's diseased kidneys.

Transient hypercalcaemia following transplantation due to secondary hyperparathyroidism used to be common but is less so now that secondary hyperparathyroidism can be suppressed before transplantation by oral treatment with alfacalcidol or calcitriol. Tertiary hyperparathyroidism may be revealed by persistent hypercalcaemia after transplantation.

The anaemia of chronic renal failure responds to Epo produced by the transplanted kidney and is usually corrected within 3 or 4 months of transplantation.

It is necessary to monitor the function of the transplanted kidney to detect early rejection. The excretion of some urinary enzymes including N-acetyl-β-D-glucosaminidase and alanine aminopeptidase have been followed for this purpose, as have some tissue-specific proteins.[29] A difficulty with this approach is that drugs used for immunosuppression can cause renal tubular damage. There is some evidence that the lymphocyte count of tissue fluid obtained by fine-needle aspiration from the upper pole of the kidney, when compared with the lymphocyte count in peripheral blood, can give the earliest warning of rejection. Monitoring for late rejection generally relies on sequential measurement of plasma creatinine concentration, together with measurement of either the excretion of protein in a 24-h urine specimen or the protein/creatinine ratio in the first urine specimen collected after discarding the overnight urine.

REFERENCES

1. Wesson L.G. (1969). *Physiology of the Human Kidney*, New York: Grune and Stratton.
2. Brenner B.M., Meyer T.W., Hostetter T.H. (1982). Dietary protein intake and the progressive nature of kidney disease: the role of hemodynamically mediated glomerular injury in the pathogenesis of progressive glomerular sclerosis in aging, renal ablation, and intrinsic renal disease. *N. Engl. J. Med.*, **307**, 652.
3. Morrison R.B.I., Davison J.M., Kerr D.N.S. (1987). Clinical physiology of the kidney: tests of renal function and structure. In *Oxford Textbook of Medicine*, 2nd edn (Weatherall D.J., Ledingham J.G.G., Warrell D.A. eds) Oxford University Press, pp. 18.1–18.17.
4. Mulligan J.S., Blue P.W., Hasbargen J.A. (1990). Methods for measuring GFR with technetium-99m-DTPA: an analysis of several common methods. *J. Nucl. Med.*, **31**, 1211.
5. Shemesh O., Golbetz H., Kriss J.P., Myers B.D. (1985). Limitations of creatinine as a filtration marker in glomerulopathic patients. *Kidney Int.*, **28**, 830.
6. Jacobsen F.K. et al. (1980). Evaluation of kidney function after meals. *Lancet*, i, 319.
7. Bauer J.H., Brooks C.S., Burch R.N. (1982). Clinical appraisal of creatinine clearance as a measurement of glomerular filtration rate. *Am. J. Kidney Dis.*, **2**, 337.
8. de Lauture H. et al. (1973). Concentrations of cholesterol, uric acid, urea, glucose and creatinine in a population of 50 000 active individuals. In *Reference Values in Human Chemistry* (Siest G. ed.) Basel: Karger, pp. 141–152.
9. Payne R.B. (1986). Creatinine clearance: a redundant clinical investigation. *Ann. Clin. Biochem.*, **23**, 243.
10. Savory D.J. (1990). Reference ranges for serum creatinine in infants, children and adolescents. *Ann. Clin. Biochem.*, **27**, 99.
11. Chennavasin P., Brater D.C. (1981). Nomograms for drug use in renal disease. *Clin. Pharmacokinet.*, **6**, 193.
12. Levey A.S. (1990). Nephrology forum. Measurement of renal function in chronic renal disease. *Kidney Int.*, **38**, 167.
13. de Wardener H.E. (1985). *The Kidney*, 5th edn, Edinburgh: Churchill Livingstone.
14. Bergeron M., Gougoux A. (1989). The renal Fanconi syndrome. In *The Metabolic Basis of Inherited Disease*,

6th edn (Scriver C.R., Beaudet A.L., Sly W.S., Valle D. eds) New York: McGraw-Hill, pp. 2569–2580.

15. Bijvoet O.L.M., Morgan D.B., Fourman P. (1969). The assessment of phosphate reabsorption. *Clin. Chim. Acta*, **26**, 15.

16. Kenny A.P., Glen A.C.A. (1973). Tests of phosphate reabsorption. *Lancet*, **ii**, 158.

17. Rasmussen H., Tenenhouse H.S. (1989). Hypophosphatemias. In *The Metabolic Basis of Inherited Disease*, 6th edn (Scriver C.R., Beaudet A.L., Sly W.S., Valle D. eds) New York: McGraw-Hill, pp. 2581–2604.

18. DuBose T.D., Alpern R.J. (1989). Renal tubular acidosis. In *The Metabolic Basis of Inherited Disease*, 6th edn (Scriver C.R., Beaudet A.L., Sly W.S., Valle D. eds) New York: McGraw-Hill, pp. 2539–2568.

19. Wrong O., Davies H.E.F. (1959). The excretion of acid in renal disease. *Q. J. Med.*, **28**, 259.

20. Oster J.R., Hotchkiss J.L., Carbon M., Farmer M., Vaamonde C.A. (1975). A short duration renal acidification test using calcium chloride. *Nephron*, **14**, 281.

21. Reeves W.B., Andreoli T.E. (1989). Nephrogenic diabetes insipidus. In *The Metabolic Basis of Inherited Disease*, 6th edn (Scriver C.R., Beaudet A.L., Sly W.S., Valle D. eds) New York: McGraw-Hill, pp. 1985–2011.

22. Hollenberg N.K., Dzau V.J. (1987). The renin–angiotensin system. In *Clinical Disorders of Fluid and Electrolyte Metabolism*, 4th edn (Maxwell M.H., Kleeman C.R., Narins R.G. eds) New York: McGraw-Hill, pp. 371–383.

23. Ledingham J.G.G. (1987). Secondary hypertension. In *Oxford Textbook of Medicine*, 2nd edn (Weatherall D.J., Ledingham J.G.G., Warrell D.A. eds) Oxford University Press, pp. 13.382–13.396.

24. Defronzo R.A. (1987). Hyperkalemic states. In *Clinical Disorders of Fluid and Electrolyte Metabolism*, 4th edn (Maxwell M.H., Kleeman C.R., Narins R.G. eds) New York: McGraw-Hill, pp. 547–584.

25. Eschbach J.W. (1989). Nephrology forum. The anemia of chronic renal failure: pathophysiology and the effects of recombinant erythropoietin. *Kidney Int.*, **35**, 134.

26. Mcdougall I.C., Hutton R.D., Cavill I., Coles G.A., Williams J.D. (1990). Treating renal anaemia with recombinant human erythropoietin: practical guidelines and a clinical algorithm. *Br. Med. J.*, **300**, 655.

27. DeLuca H.F., Krisinger J., Darwish H. (1990). The vitamin D system: 1990. *Kidney Int.*, **38** (suppl. 29), S2.

28. Starkey B.J. (1987). Aluminium in renal disease: current knowledge and future developments. *Ann. Clin. Biochem.*, **24**, 337.

29. Flynn F.V. (1990). Assessment of renal function: selected developments. *Clin. Biochem.*, **23**, 49.

20. Renal Stones

S. Hanson

Introduction
Theory of stone formation
   Chemical aspects
   Physiological derangements leading to
     formation of renal stones
   Pre-urinary risk factors
Clinical features
   Bladder stones
   Kidney and ureteric stones

INTRODUCTION

Urolithiasis (renal calculi) is an increasingly common disorder of modern times but calculi were found in Egyptian mummies from 6000 BC. The formation of stones in the renal tract is not a specific disease but arises as a complication of many different diseases. Thus, in spite of recent advances in the surgical treatment of stones such as extracorporeal shock-wave lithotripsy, the role of the laboratory has not diminished. It is important to determine the reason for the production of stones.

Soluble ions and waste products of metabolism are excreted into the urine by the kidneys. The urine passes down the renal tract to be voided in the act of micturition. Renal lithiasis is essentially a disorder arising from the precipitation of sparingly soluble salts and acids. These should obey the chemical laws of crystal nucleation, growth and aggregation. The mean transit time from the kidney to the bladder is 5–10 min. In order to allow a stone to grow these crystals or aggregations (100–200μm in size) become trapped or attached in the renal tract where further growth can occur until a calculus is formed. This can either be voided painlessly or give rise to painful clinical conditions associated with renal and urinary dysfunction.

THEORY OF STONE FORMATION

Chemical Aspects

Urine is a polyionic solution. For stones' formation the urine must be supersaturated from time to time to allow crystallization and precipitation to occur. The state of saturation is influenced by monovalent ions. As the concentration of these increases, the activity of divalent ions such as calcium and oxalate decrease, allowing more to remain in the soluble phase. The pH also influences the availability and solubility of substances.

Saturation concentration is the concentration of a solution at which the solid phase of the salt is in equilibrium with the liquid phase. Any solution with a concentration less than the saturation concentration is *undersaturated*, and any solution with a higher one is *supersaturated*.

Oversaturation is the concentration at which spontaneous precipitation occurs. The region between oversaturation and the saturation concentration is known as the *metastable region*. In this region, heterogeneous crystallization occurs and is much more common than crystallization in the oversaturation region.

Crystal nucleation is a process initiated by a crystal nidus or foreign material (e.g. protein) in a supersaturated urine. Whether the urine is in the metastable or oversaturated region will determine the composition of the resulting stone. Urine from stone and non-stone formers is often metastably saturated with respect to calcium oxalate but the growth of crystals and size of the aggregates are higher in stone formers.

Crystal retention is a requisite for stone disease. The renal papilla is an important site for crystal fixation.

Factors that modify stone formation are shown in Table 20.1.

The composition of the urine shows diurnal variation. The times associated with the highest supersaturation occur between 6 and 10 a.m. and between 6 and 10 p.m. Meals cause variations, especially in the concentration of calcium. The highest excretion of oxalate and urate occurs early in the morning. Examination of 24-h urine collections may not reveal these surges, accounting for the observation that some recurrent stone formers continue to make stones in spite of apparently low concentrations of risk factors in 24-h urine collections.

Measurements of the State of Saturation

There are many available but none is ideal. The best estimate is the activity product of the constituent ions. The concentration products and ionic concentrations are poorer indicators of the saturation for the reason given above.

$$\text{Activity of ion} = \text{concentration of ion} \times \text{activity coefficient.}$$

$$\text{Activity coefficient} = \frac{1}{\text{ionic strength}}.$$

Formulae are available to classify urines as high or low risk. Supersaturated urine that does not contain crystals means that, for example, the calcium oxalate is being held in solution above its saturation point. Occurrence of a seed crystal or a transient increase in concentration (e.g. a postprandial rise of calcium or oxalate excretion) can trigger crystallization.

Laboratory Analysis of Renal Calculi

Quantitative analysis of the renal stones is helpful in determination of their aetiology and in the rationalization of therapy. X-ray diffraction is the 'gold stand-

TABLE 20.1
MODIFIERS OF STONE FORMATION

Inhibitors

Ions: citrate, magnesium, pyrophosphate

Larger molecules:

(i) Glycosaminoglycans (GAGs)—urinary GAGs are polysaccharide chains of repeating disaccharides derived by degradation of high molecular-weight proteoglycans; renal excretion is by glomerular filtration; GAG excretion is greater in male subjects, rising postprandially and at night; excretion rises by 50% in the summer;

   GAGs inhibit calcium oxalate crystallization

(ii) Nephrocalcin is a recently isolated γ-carboxyglutamic acid-containing protein; it inhibits calcium oxalate crystallization and may be structurally abnormal or deficient in some stone patients

Complexers

Specific charged ions combine with potential crystalline components to form soluble complexes reducing the free ionic concentration:

(i) anions such as citrate, phosphate and sulphate complex calcium

(ii) cations such as magnesium complex oxalate

Promoters

Tamm–Horsfall protein and the organic matrix

TABLE 20.2
FREQUENCY AND PRESENTATION OF STONE

	%
Frequency of stone type (UK)	
Calcium oxalate	40
Calcium phosphate/calcium oxalate	14
Magnesium ammonium phosphate	15
Calcium phosphate	13
Mixed component	6
Uric acid	8
Cystine	1
Site of stone on presentation	
Passed spontaneously	40
Kidney	25
Ureter	20
Bladder	15

ard' of analysis but is only available at specialized centres. Infrared spectroscopy is useful to identify non-crystalline substances such as drug metabolites and amorphous material in the renal stone. Sample preparation is simple and small amounts of sample can be analysed. Optical crystallography also provides useful information.

In the UK, 80% of calculi are calcium salts, the most common being calcium oxalate, both the monohydrate and dihydrate being formed (Table 20.2). They are spiky and discoloured with altered blood. The phosphates occur as apatites ($Ca_{10}(OH)_2(PO_4)_6$) and struvite ($MgNH_4PO_4.6H_2O$). These tend to be larger, smoother and more friable. Most renal stones are a mixture of calcium oxalate

and phosphate. Pure calcium phosphate stones are found after recurrent urinary infections. Uric acid and cystine stones (soft and brownish yellow) are less common. Rare stones include xanthine, resulting from liver xanthine oxidase deficiency, silicates seen after prolonged administration of magnesium trisilicate, and 2,8-dihydroxyadenine due to a defect in adenine phosphoribosyltransferase. Uric acid and xanthine stones are radiolucent. Stone composition is altered by infection and dissolution.

Physiological Derangements Found in the Urine That Can Lead to the Formation of Renal Stones

Hypercalciuria

Normal urinary calcium excretion is between 0.1 and 4 mg/kg b.w. per 24h in men and women. Some 50–70% of patients with stone and 20% of non-stone formers show hypercalciuria. Most stones contain calcium and hypercalciuria is the most common disorder amongst these patients. The normal dietary intake of calcium is 500–1000 mg daily, the gut being the sole site of entry for calcium, which is regulated by the action of vitamin D. A high intake of refined carbohydrate, high protein intake and/or high salt intake increases the amount of calcium absorbed. Adults maintain zero balance, with 99% of the body's total calcium content (1 kg) in the bone. The kidneys filter 10 g daily but only about 200 mg appears in the urine, i.e 98% is reabsorbed under the control of parathyroid hormone (PTH).

Urinary calcium shows postprandial and diurnal variations. Long-term cyclic and seasonal variations also occur, as described below. These all affect the degree of saturation. The increased calcium and oxalate excretion seen in the summer months are not associated with variations in urinary pH, creatinine, phosphate or magnesium excretion. At this time, higher saturation levels of octo calcium phosphate and calcium oxalate in the urine reflect the increased vitamin D synthesis in the skin. Stone formers show an 50% rise in the recurrence rate of stones in the summer due entirely to the passage of small oxalate stones. No seasonal increase in the incidence of large stones is seen, suggesting that the increase of urinary saturation promotes formation of these small stones. Diurnal variations compound these changes and patients must be encouraged to maintain a water diuresis at this times of maximum concentration (i.e. 6–10 a.m. and 6–10 p.m.).

Hypercalciuria is important in stone formation because:

1. A rise in calcium concentration is as effective as oxalate in raising the activity product of calcium oxalate when using the stability constant of calcium oxalate at 37°C.
2. Continuing hypercalciuria is an important determinant of continuing stone formation during drug therapy.

Types of Hypercalciuria

1. Absorptive (AH). The basic abnormality is increased intestinal absorption of calcium, raising the circulating calcium load, which increases the renal filtered load. Parathyroid function is suppressed, causing a rise in urinary calcium concentration secondary to the reduced reabsorption of the load. The excess renal loss balances the increased absorption maintaining calcium homeostasis.

- **Type I** AH occurs with both high and low calcium intakes.
- **Type II** AH only occurs with high calcium intake.
- **Type III** AH is secondary to a renal leak of phosphate. The resulting hypophosphataemia stimulates synthesis of 1,25 dihydroxyvitamin D (1,25 (OH)$_2$D), leading to enhanced intestinal absorption of calcium.

The exaggerated calciuria following the calcium load test in patients from these groups demonstrates increased intestinal absorption. If the skeleton was the source of the urinary calcium the annual loss would be equivalent to 9% of the skeleton, leading to overt bone disease. This is plainly not so. Calcium kinetic studies in patients show increased exchangeable calcium pools with increased turnover rates implying accelerated bone remodelling.

2. Renal hypercalciuria (RH). There is impairment of tubular reabsorption of calcium leading to a lowering of the plasma calcium, thus stimulating the production of PTH. Calcium is mobilized from the bone; PTH stimulates 1,25 (OH)$_2$D synthesis, leading to increased intestinal absorption of calcium from the gut normalizing the plasma calcium. Calcium loading suppresses urinary cAMP (*see* hyperparathyroidism). RH can be treated with certain diuretics that reduce calcium excretion. The mechanism of this action is as follows:

(i) increases sodium loss by mildly contracting the extracellular space, stimulating the tubular reabsorption of sodium and the closely linked transport of calcium;
(ii) potentiates the action of PTH raising cAMP, stimulating the reabsorption of calcium;
(iii) decreases the recurrence rate of stones by increasing urinary magnesium output.

The term 'idiopathic hypercalciuria' is obsolete.

Are these conditions separate entities?

1. Parathyroid function is suppressed or normal in AH and should be enhanced in RH. Calcium studies show suppression of urinary cAMP in AH because the increased absorption of calcium suppresses PTH. RH patients show inappropriately high PTH with elevated urinary cAMP. This disturbance is corrected by an oral calcium load, and suppressed by thiazides, demonstrating the secondary nature of the PTH stimulation.

2. Renal calcium leak is demonstrated by a raised urinary calcium:creatinine ratio after a prolonged fast (12 h), suggesting that renal reabsorption of calcium is impaired in this condition.

However, not all patients fall into these clear-cut groups and some workers consider this classification somewhat arbitrary. At present we find this classification a useful basis on which to manage patients.

Hypercalcaemic States with Hypercalciuria

1. *Resorptive hypercalciuria* (*primary hyperparathyroidism*). The high PTH causes excessive bone resorption and increased intestinal absorption of calcium secondary to 1,25 (OH)$_2$D synthesis. The raised plasma calcium increases the renal filtered load. Hypercalciuria occurs in this condition, despite the action of PTH to increase the reabsorption of calcium. The filtered load is so high that the effectiveness of PTH is reduced. The raised plasma calcium suppresses renal calcium reabsorption.

2. *Vitamin D excess*. Excessive intake of vitamin D leads to calcium overload and renal stones. The role of vitamin D in urolithiasis is difficult to understand. The action of PTH will raise the level of vitamin D. Many hypercalciuric patients have high normal values. Difficulties in interpretation occur because vitamin D can upregulate its own receptors, leading to a greater response than is suggested by the plasma levels.

3. *Sarcoidosis*. Increased intestinal absorption and bone dissolution occur.

4. *Milk alkali syndrome.*

5. *Immobilization.*

6. *Multiple myeloma.*

The conditions leading to hypercalciuria may lead to deposits of calcium oxalate and hydroxyapatite in the kidney, a condition called *nephrocalcinosis*. This does not excite much inflammatory cell infiltration.

Correct identification of the type of calciuria avoids the misuse of therapeutic agents, e.g. thiazides, sodium cellulose phosphate and orthophosphate.

Hyperuricosuria

Uric acid is an end-product of purine metabolism. The kidney is a major site of disposal where secretion and reabsorption occur. If the serum concentration is raised, increasing the filtered load in the kidney, uricosuria will follow. No protein binding occurs so glomerular filtration is complete.

Normal excretion: < 4.5 mmol/24 h (women)
  < 4.7 mmol/24 h (men).

Uricosuria occurs as an isolated finding or associated with calcium oxalate stone formation (20%). Uric acid acts as a nidus on which calcium oxalate crystallization occurs or it decreases the activity of the crystal growth inhibitory factors.

At a pH of 5.75 (the pK_a of uric acid) only half the molecules are in the form of soluble sodium urate. If the pH is raised to 6.8 the solubility of the urate is increased 10-fold. When assessing the amount of urate excreted both the volume and pH must be taken into account, e.g. 750 mg in 1 L at pH 5 will produce crystals whereas the same amount is fully soluble in 2.5 L at pH 7.

Uric acid lithiasis occurs in the following conditions:

1. Low urinary pH even with *normal uricosuria*—
   - chronic diarrhoea,
   - ileostomy,
   - medication to acidify the urine.
2. *Hyperuricaemia*—20% of gouty patients make renal stones. Excess alcohol intake increases the plasma urate leading to hyperuricosuria
3. *Chronic dehydration.*
4. *Dietary protein excess*—purine-rich foods such as meat, fish or poultry provide increased substrate.
5. *Increased substrate production*—the treatment of the leukaemias or severe exfoliative dermatitis leads to hyperuricosuria due to the release of nucleic acids from increased cell turnover.
6. Disturbance of the *biosynthetic purine pathway* leading to increased endogenous production.
7. Disturbances in *renal tubular reabsorption* of uric acid. These are usually temporary following extracellular re-expansion and administration of uricosuric agents such as probenecid. The steady state is soon restored but the tubular impairment persists.

Hyperuricosuric Calcium Lithiasis. Ten per cent of calcium stone formers have hyperuricosuria as the only abnormal finding but uricosuria occurs with other physiological derangements. The uricosuria caused by the purine indulgent can be controlled by dietary restriction. Some patients on severe restriction still show hyperuricosuria due to increased endogenous urate production, the cause of which has not been elucidated.

Hypocitraturia

Citrate is a potent stone inhibitor because it forms a soluble complex with calcium, lowering the ionic concentration of calcium, and thus the saturation of stone-forming calcium salts.

Citrate:
- directly inhibits the agglomeration of calcium oxalate and nucleation of calcium oxalate;
- has a modest effect on calcium oxalate crystal growth;
- impairs urate-induced crystallization of calcium oxalate.

Thus in hypocitraturia there is increased urinary saturation, enhanced nucleation and aggregation of calcium oxalate.

Hypocitraturia is said to occur when citrate excretion is less than 1.7 mmol/24 h. It occurs in 12–25% of patients with stone as an isolated finding or with other risk factors. The amount of citrate in the urine is a function of filtration, reabsorption, peritubular transport and synthesis by the tubules. Secretion is unimportant in man. Peritubular transport and tubular synthesis affect the citrate excretion in the urine by altering renal tissue citrate content and the filtered load. Seventy-five per cent of the filtered load is reabsorbed in the proximal tubule. The physiology of the renal handling of citrate is not completely understood.

Citrate excretion is:
- enhanced by alkalosis, PTH, vitamin D, growth hormone and oestrogen;
- impaired by acidosis, hypokalaemia, androgens, urinary tract infection, high-protein diet with a high-acid ash content.

Acid–base status is most important in citrate balance. Acidosis enhances renal tubular reabsorption and reduces citrate synthesis. In intracellular alkalosis, citrate uptake by the mitochondria is decreased and accumulates in the cytosol. This leads to decreased uptake by the tubular cell, increasing the urinary citrate. Oral administration of any alkali increases citrate excretion.

In stone patients, hypocitraturia may occur as an isolated abnormality (thought to be due to increased tubular reabsorption of citrate) but is usually associated with the causes listed below.

Causes of Hypocitraturia. The principal causes are as follows:

1. *Renal tubular acidosis* (RTA): a group of disorders resulting from tubular damage without glomerular involvement—a hyperchloraemic metabolic acidosis, disordered potassium homeostasis and an inability to acidify the urine after an acid load to below a pH of 5.2 confirm the diagnosis, having excluded an identifiable cause of the acidaemia.
   (i) *type 1* (distal RTA) is associated with a high incidence of nephrolithiasis and nephrocalcinosis. It is a primary or acquired condition. It can be secondary to many conditions such as medullary sponge kidney, multiple myeloma or renal transplantation. Drugs such as analgesics and lithium and infective states as in chronic pyelonephritis can induce this complication.
   (ii) *type 2* (proximal RTA) in which there is failure of bicarbonate reabsorption. This is uncommon in the adult and is often associated with proximal tubular transport defects (Fanconi syndrome). Stone formation is rare.
   Management of these patients is to treat any underlying disease, hyper- or hypo-calcaemia and to give potasssium chloride to correct the metabolic defect.

2. *Intestinal malabsorption states*
- chronic diarrhoea states
- thiazide diuretics (secondary to potassium loss),
- diet high in acid-ash content as in a high intake of red meat,
- lactic acidosis from physical exercise,
- high sodium intake (intracellular acidosis),
- urinary tract infection due to the bacterial degradation of citrate,
- idiopathic—probably due to increased renal tubular reabsorption of citrate.

Management of these patients from the stone point of view is to treat any underlying disease, correct hyper- or hypokalaemia and prescribe potassium citrate to correct the metabolic defect.

Hyperoxaluria

The total amount of oxalate in the urine is derived from:

- endogenous production from glycine in the liver (50%);
- precursors such as ascorbic acid (40%);
- gastrointestinal absorption.

Oxalate intake in the Western diet is 100–900 mg/day, of which only 12% is absorbed in the normal subject. It is found in tea, decaffeinated or instant coffee, carbonated drinks, nuts, rhubarb, green leafy vegetables, haricot and kidney beans, etc. Chocolate and cocoa contain glycolate that is converted to oxalate in the body. Oxalate does not undergo further breakdown in the body. Normal urinary excretion is up to $450 \mu mol/24$ h ($60 mg/24$ h). It is very insoluble and a small increase in oxalate excretion has a marked effect on urinary crystallization. The normal ratio of calcium:oxalate in the urine is 5:1. The crystal habits of calcium oxalate require a ratio of 1:1. Thus modest rises in urinary oxalate are important in the genesis of oxalate stones.

Hyperoxaluric States. 1. Primary hyperoxaluria.

There is excess synthesis and excretion of oxalic acid; two types are distinguished:

- **Type I, glycolic aciduria**—inherited as an autosomal recessive gene. Most present before the age of 5 years. There is a deficiency of alanine:glyoxylate aminotransferase (AGT), leading to an accumulation of glyoxylate, which is oxidized to glycolate and oxalate. Patients present with nephrocalcinosis and urolithiasis. Oxalate deposits are found in many tissues (oxalosis). Untreated the condition is fatal by the age of 20 but liver transplantation corrects the enzyme defect in the liver.
- **Type II, L-glyceric aciduria**—D-glyceric dehydrogenase is defective leading to excessive synthesis of L-glyceric acid and oxalate. These patients present before the age of 4 years with calcium oxalate lithiasis.

2. *Secondary hyperoxaluria.* The secondary causes of hyperoxaluria are not associated with increases in other organic acids and are much more common in clinical practice:

(i) **Enteric hyperoxaluria**—diseases such as inflammatory bowel disease, chronic biliary or pancreatic disease or short bowel syndrome increase intestinal absorption (up to 40% dietary oxalate). The increased absorption is secondary to fat malabsorption. Excess free fatty acids bind intestinal calcium leaving unbound oxalate for absorption in the colon, the permeability of which is increased by excess of bile salts. Oxalate absorption may be reduced by increasing dietary calcium.

(ii) **Diet**—increased intake of precursors:

- protein (source of glycine),
- ascorbic acid,
- sugars,
- increased intake of oxalate.

(iii) **Ethylene glycol** ingestion causes extensive precipitation of calcium oxalate in the renal tubules.

(iv) **Methoxyflurane**—this anaesthetic agent can cause hyperoxaluria and nephrocalcinosis.

(v) **Pyridoxine deficiency**—this is a necessary cofactor for AGT. Deficiency leads to a syndrome akin to primary hyperoxaluria type I.

Cystinuria

This is an inheritable disorder characterized by excessive urinary excretion of cystine, lysine, ornithine and arginine (dibasic amino acids) in the urine. Amino acid transport in the cells of the gastrointestinal tract and renal tubules is defective. The only clinical condition this gives rise to is urolithiasis because of the insolubility of cystine. The aminoaciduria is of the 'leak' type rather than overflow, the plasma cystine being rather lower than normal. Little or no cystine is reabsorbed, as the clearance rate is nearly as high as the glomerular filtration rate.

The incidence in the UK is 1 in 20 000. The disorder presents in childhood or early adulthood. The stones can grow to fill the pelvicalyceal space (the 'staghorn calculus').

- Normal cystine excretion is 10–100 μmol (70 mg)/24 h.
- Heterozygotes excrete 20–600 μmol (250 mg)/24 h.
- Homozygotes excrete 1400–4200 μmol (1000 mg)/24 h.

The solubility of cystine in 0.9% saline within the pH range at 37°C is 1250 $\mu mol/L$. In most normal subjects and heterozygotes the urine is well undersaturated with respect to cystine and stones are unlikely. Homozygotes often have supersaturated urine, leading to crystalluria and stones. The management of the condition is directed to maintaining the urinary concentration of cystine below its equilibrium solubility in urine. A fluid intake greater than 3 L/day is required to maintain a good urine flow throughout the 24 h. The urine should be alkalinized and dietary protein restriction leads to some reduction in excretion of cystine. Drug treatment with penicillamine may be necessary in some patients but this can lead to proteinuria, which therefore must be frequently checked.

Hypomagnesuria

The magnesium in the urine complexes with the oxalate or phosphate ion, thus acting as an inhibitor of crystal growth of calcium oxalate and calcium phosphate. Long-term treatment with oral magnesium increases urinary excretion of citrate by decreasing tubular reabsorption. Hypomagnesuria is a risk factor in stone formation.

Pre-urinary Risk Factors

Intrinsic

1. Hereditary:
 (i) renal tubular acidosis—73% of these develop nephrocalcinosis or urolithiasis;
 (ii) primary hyperoxaluria;
 (iii) cystinuria;
 (iv) hyperuricosuria;
 (v) absorptive hypercalciuria—this is the most common finding in adults presenting with stone disease and appears to be a dominant trait.

2. Age: stones are rare in children, who have a high level of inhibitors and low levels of urinary calcium, and in the elderly, who have a low saturation of calcium salts. Men present with a peak in the third to fifth decade. Women show an early peak at 30 years of age and a second increase at the menopause associated with the increase in urinary calcium seen at this time.

3. Sex: urolithiasis is more common in men; the M:F ratio is 4:1. Men excrete more calcium oxalate and uric acid leading to higher urinary concentration of these salts. Oestrogens in women increase the concentrations of citrate, a stone inhibitor.

4. Mechanical factors:
 (i) anatomical, e.g. bifid ureters, horseshoe kidney;
 (ii) medullary sponge kidney—this is an abnormality of the renal pyramids stemming from the obstruction and cystic dilatation of the collecting ducts at the papillary tips; it is usually bilateral. Sixty per cent of patients make stones; the condition has a benign prognosis, but repeated infections may be a problem.

Extrinsic

1. Geography: the southern United States have the highest rate of upper urinary tract stones in affluent countries. In Europe the Mediterranean countries have a higher incidence than northern Europe. This may be partly due to climate.

2. Climate: the highest rates occur in the hottest parts of the high-incidence countries. In Britain there is a peak in stone episodes in the summer. Urinary calcium rises in the summer, and in stone formers is up by 4–5 mmol/24 h. Serum $25(OH)_3D$ concentrations rise, increasing and correlating with increased intestinal absorption of calcium. A less than adequate fluid intake may compound the problem.

3. Diet
- *Protein*. Affluence correlates with the **protein** intake of a population. Protein can increase the supersaturation of the urine in the following ways:
  (i) hypercalciuria is produced by the increased ammonium ion and sulphur-containing amino acids producing a degree of renal tubular acidosis;
  (ii) hyperphosphaturia results from the renal tubular acidosis;
  (iii) hyperuricosuria is produced from the high purine intake and the ammonium production forming ammonium acid urate;
  (iv) hyperoxaluria is caused by the increased synthesis of oxalate from the amino acids such as glycine, tyrosine, hydroxyproline, etc.

Thus four major urinary risk factors are increased by excessive protein intake.

- *Carbohydrate*. Administration of glucose or sucrose is accompanied by an exaggerated calciuresis among hypercalciuric patients and their relatives, owing to the calciuric effect of insulin.
- *Excess sodium intake*. A close relation exists between renal tubular calcium and sodium handling, most factors causing natriuresis increase calcium excretion. Sodium and calcium are reabsorbed at common sites in the tubule. Some stone patients appear more sensitive to the effect of a sodium load on the degree of calciuria, and a high dietary salt intake is a risk factor in these patients.

4. Occupation: there is a higher incidence of stones in sedentary workers (in the armed forces, office personnel have a higher incidence than active units such as the Royal Marines). Workers in hot temperatures produce more stones. The strenuous physical nature of some jobs may dislodge stones before they reach a size to cause clinical problems.

5. Water
- *Amount*:
  (i) chronic dehydration stone disease;
  (ii) hot climate;
  (iii) hot occupation;
  (iv) low fluid intake—patients whose 24-h urinary volumes are less than 1400 mL show an increased recurrence rate.
- *Composition*. Stone formation is higher in soft water areas than in hard water areas, the incidence is higher in the north and west of England (soft water) than in the east and south (hard water). Low levels of magnesium in soft water are more

important than the amount of calcium present in hard water.

6. Infection stones—chronic infection in the urinary tract can cause renal calculi that are composed of magnesium ammonium phosphate ($MgNH_4.6H_2O$; struvite) and carbonate apatite ($Ca_{10}PO_4.6CO_3$). The critical ingredient is infection with a urease producing organism:

$$3H_2O + (NH_2)_2CO \rightleftharpoons 2NH_4^+ + HCO_3^- + OH^-.$$

The pH of the urine rises and precipitation of the stone can occur at any pH over 7.2. The stones formed can be very large, filling the pelvicalyceal space (staghorn calculus). Forty-five different micro-organisms produce urease. The most common found in stone patients are *Proteus* and *Pseudomonas*. The stone material should be cultured to identify the causative organism (urine culture is not as specific). The condition is more common in female patients, after spinal cord injury and in patients with ileal loops. Unfortunately, long-term antibiotic therapy may lead to selection of antibiotic-resistant, urease-forming organisms.

● *Prevention*:
  (i) sterilize the urine with antimicrobials;
  (ii) urease inhibitors such as acetohydroxamic acid;
  (iii) substrate depletion with the use of intestinal phosphate binders to lower the urinary phosphate excretion;
  (iv) surgical removal of the stone.

7. Medication—ascorbic acid, acetazolamide and triamterene are but three of the therapeutic agents implicated in stone formation.

CLINICAL FEATURES

Small stones can be voided spontaneously and are usually calcium oxalate. Larger stones tend to contain more phosphate. Predominantly phosphate stones indicate past or present urinary tract infection. Patients with hyperparathyroidism and renal tubular acidosis pass oxalate stones containing some phosphate.

Urolithiasis is a curse of both deprivation and affluence. Bladder stones are associated with severe deprivation. Upper renal-tract calculi occur in affluent societies.

Bladder Stones

Vesical (bladder) calculi are common worldwide where there is poverty and malnutrition. In the eighteenth and nineteenth centuries they were rife in England, especially in East Anglia. Agricultural workers were very poor and the diet of the children deficient in protein. The infants were fed on 'pap'—a liquid preparation made from cereals. As living standards have improved in this century the incidence of bladder stones has fallen markedly.

Childhood vesical stones are still common in areas of the world such as China and northern India, with Thailand having the highest incidence. The affected children have hyperoxaluria with hypophosphaturia. They come from the poorest classes, most are boys under the age of 10 years. After surgical removal of the calcium oxalate stone, recurrence is rare (cf. adult stone disease). The condition is due to low dietary phosphate and protein, with a high consumption of oxalate-rich vegetables. A low fluid intake in a hot climate compounds the problem.

A rarer type of bladder stone occurs in Egypt associated with infection by schistosomiasis but the stones are magnesium ammonium urate and calcium phosphate.

Kidney and Ureteric Stones

Upper urinary-tract stones are 10 times more common than bladder stones in the UK. They vary between very large stones filling the pelvicalyceal space to stones of microscopic size. Most weigh less than 1 g. Both kidneys are equally affected and 40% of patients have bilateral stones. The recurrence rate is high and is about 75% within 10 years in an untreated population. Most stones are passed spontaneously, only 35% requiring surgical intervention. Although the composition and aetiology are very varied, all present in the same way, causing urinary tract dysfunction. Obstruction of the renal tract, bleeding or infection cause patients to seek help. Renal colic associated with obstruction is very painful and cannot be ignored by patient or doctor for long! X-ray examination usually confirms the diagnosis. Not all stones are radiopaque but their presence can be inferred by a filling defect seen on the intravenous urogram.

The annual incidence in the UK is 7/10 000. The prevalence is 1.5% in England (cf. the prevalence in the southern United States of 12%).

The causes of nephrolithiasis can be classified as follows.

● Absorptive hypercalciuria:
  type 1,
  type 2,
  type 3 (phosphate leak).
● Renal hypercalciuria.
● Resorptive hypercalciuria.
● Hyperuricosuric calcium nephrolithiasis.
● Hyperoxaluric calcium nephrolithiasis:
  enteric hyperoxaluria,
  primary hyperoxaluria,
  dietary hyperoxaluria.
● Hypocitraturic calcium nephrolithiasis:
  distal renal tubular acidosis,
  chronic diarrhoeal syndrome,
  idiopathic.
● Hypomagnesuric calcium nephrolithiasis.
● Gouty diathesis.

- Infection stones.
- Cystinuria.
- Low urine volume.
- No apparent cause.

The number of patients in each diagnostic group varies from centre to centre. Most can be classified. The diagnosis and separation into groups are important because a rational approach to therapy can lead to successful management and a reduction in stone episodes.

Should the single stone former be investigated? If not, conditions such as RTA, renal hypercalciuria with secondary hyperparathyroidism and other serious systemic diseases would be missed. A minimum protocol would entail making one 24-h urine collection on a free diet and a 2-h fasting urine collection to exclude RTA and hypercalciuria.

The investigations are time consuming and expensive. They must be done as an outpatient procedure. The aim of the metabolic evaluation is to identify the particular physiological and environmental defect in an individual to enable rational management of the stone disease. All effective treatments are designed to reduce the state of saturation of the urine and can be achieved by common sense, diet and drugs. Most stone clinics show a gratifying reduction in recurrence rate. Patients appreciate an explanation of their problem and are encouraged to self-monitor the specific gravity of the urine to minimize the risk of crystallization, this reducing the recurrence rate. Nephrolithiasis is a chronic illness requiring integrated surgical and medical care.

FURTHER READING

Pak C.Y.C. (1992). Kidney stones. In *William's Textbook of Endocrinology*, 8th edn (Wilson, J.D., Foster D.W. eds) Philadelphia: Saunders.

Nath R., Thun S. K., Murthy M., Talwar H., Farooqui S. (1984). *Molecular Aspects of Idiopathic Urolithiasis*, vol. 7:1 of *Molecular Aspects of Medicine*, Oxford: Pergamon.

Smith L. ed. (1991). *Renal stones*, vol. 19:4 of *Endocrinology and Metabolism Clinics of North America*, Philadelphia: Saunders.

Pak C. Y.C. (1988). Medical management of nephrolithiasis in Dallas—update 1987. *J. Urol.*, **140**, 461.

21. The Assessment of Gastrointestinal Function
M. H. Z. Labib and B. J. M. Jones

The oesophagus
  Ambulant oesophageal pH monitoring
  Oesophageal acid-perfusion test (Bernstein test)
The stomach
  Gastric digestion
  Gastric motility and gastric emptying
  Measurement of gastric emptying
  Acid secretion
  The control of acid secretion
  Gastric secretory tests
  Pepsinogen
  Gastrin
  Gastrinoma
  Gastrin stimulation tests
  Hypergastrinaemia and carcinogenesis
  Helicobacter pylori and acid-related disease
The small intestine
  Water and electrolyte absorption
  Digestion and absorption of carbohydrates
  Digestion and absorption of proteins
  Digestion and absorption of fats
  Absorption of vitamins, folates and iron
  Assessment of mucosal damage and intestinal permeability
  Assessment of carbohydrate absorption
  Assessment of fat absorption
  Assessment of bacterial overgrowth
  Assessment of dysfunction of the terminal ileum
  Assessment of orocaecal transit time
  Assessment of gastrointestinal protein loss
The colon
  Colonic motility
  Colonic absorption and secretion
  Diarrhoea
  Faecal occult blood and colorectal tumours
The pancreas
  Regulation of pancreatic secretion
  Clinical presentation of pancreatic disease
  Acute pancreatitis
  Chronic pancreatitis
Malabsorption
  Definition
  Symptoms
  Practical approach to the investigation of diarrhoea/steatorrhoea
  Disorders causing diarrhoea or steatorrhoea

THE OESOPHAGUS

Propulsive motility of the oesophagus conveys food and liquids to the stomach via the lower oesophageal sphincter or valve, which relaxes in response to swallowing. Failure of the sphincter to remain closed between swallows allows gastric contents, particularly acid, to reflux into the oesophagus. This may occur as a normal phenomenon but rapid clearance of acid by oesophageal peristalsis is usually sufficient to prevent acid-related symptoms or damage.

Reflux of acid into the oesophagus may give rise to symptoms typical of reflux dyspepsia or ulcerative oesophagitis, with progression to stricture formation. Some patients may present with atypical pain suggestive of a cardiac pathology. Others may experience nocturnal asthma provoked by acid regurgitation.

Whilst endoscopic and radiological findings often confirm the diagnosis, in some cases it is necessary to correlate symptoms with evidence of acid reflux over a period of time. Alternatively, an acid provocation test may reproduce symptoms convincingly.

Ambulant Oesophageal pH Monitoring

This technique is now well established in clinical practice.[1] A pH-measuring electrode or 'radio pill' is positioned 5 cm proximal to the lower oesophageal sphincter and continuous recording of pH is maintained for up to 24 h. A diary card to record all nutrient intake and symptoms is kept by the patient, who can also activate an event marker on the recording apparatus. Interpretation of results has been difficult because of the wide range of results quoted by various workers. In clinical practice, generally accepted normal values during 24-h monitoring are:

(i) the length of time pH is below 4 is less than 6% of total time supine;
(ii) the length of time pH is below 4 is less than 10.5% of total time erect;
(iii) time taken to clear a reflux episode (pH to return to above 4) is less than 5 min.

Using the percentage time that pH is below 4, a sensitivity of 87% and specificity of 97% have been achieved. In one study, the reproducibility over two consecutive 24-h periods was 77% and the level for distinguishing normals from pathological refluxers was pH below 4 for less than 3.5% of total time.[2] An alternative but complicated scoring system that gives 90.3% sensitivity and 90% specificity has also been devised.[3]

Oesophageal Acid-perfusion Test (Bernstein Test)

Although largely replaced by 24-h ambulant oesophageal pH monitoring, acid perfusion of the lower oseophagus is occasionally indicated to reproduce pain from the lower oesophagus.[4] This pain is often misconstrued by patient and physician as cardiac in origin. In the upright position, isotonic NaCl is perfused through a naso-oesophageal tube at 10 mL/min for 10 min, increasing to 20 mL/min for 5 min; then 0.1 mmol/L HCl at 10 mL/min is perfused for 15 min without the patient's knowledge. If pain occurs the acid infusion is stopped and 0.05 mmol/L sodium bicarbonate is infused. Electrocardiographic monitoring should also be done because oesophageal pain can lead to ECG changes and can also lower the threshold for angina. The test may be positive in normal subjects and a negative test does not exclude oesophageal disease as the cause of chest pain.

THE STOMACH

The stomach acts as a muscular reservoir for storage, maceration and initial digestion of food. The main anatomical regions of the stomach, the cardia, fundus, body, antrum and pylorus, have different physiological functions. The fundus and body contain columnar glandular epithelium with secretory glands emptying into pits within the epithelium. The glandular cells within the pits comprise oxyntic (parietal) cells secreting hydrochloric acid and intrinsic factor, chief cells secreting pepsinogen, and mucus-secreting cells. The glands in the antrum secrete pepsinogen and contain G cells (gastrin) and D cells (somatostatin), which release their hormones into the portal venous system.

A number of factors are involved in protecting the surface mucosa of the stomach from the effect of hydrochloric acid and pepsin. The cell membrane and tight intercellular junctions impede ionic movement and provide a physical barrier to hydrogen ion flux. The concept of a 'mucus-bicarbonate' barrier has excited much interest. The mucous layer has little buffering ability but acts by increasing the unstirred water-layer effect by a factor of 4, thus decreasing acid diffusion from lumen to mucosa. This alone would be insufficient to explain the pH of 6–8 at the epithelial cell surface. Secretion of bicarbonate directly into the submucous space allows maintenance of a pH gradient from lumen to mucosa. Thus, the mucous layer does not prevent secretion of acid into the lumen from the pits but appears to allow an alkaline microclimate adjacent to the mucosa. Pepsin is inactivated at high pH and the mucosa is therefore protected from proteolysis by the mucus–bicarbonate barrier. This barrier can be broken very easily by a variety of clinically relevant factors: aspirin, non-steroidal anti-inflammatory drugs, alcohol and stress have all been shown to decrease the mucous layer and are associated with an increased incidence of gastric erosions or ulcers. The alkaline microclimate adjacent to the mucosa also facilitates colonization of the submucous space by the clinically important bacteria *Helicobacter pylori* and *Gastrosporillium hominis*.

Gastric Digestion

Salivary amylase continues to hydrolyse starch until intraluminal pH falls too low. Acid or pepsin proteolysis commences in the stomach, but ceases on contact with alkaline duodenal contents. Lipase secreted by the tongue, soft palate and gastric mucosa can hydrolyse up to 30% of fats in the stomach. The lingual and gastric lipases are active at low pH and do not require bile salts to function. Water, alcohol and certain lipid-soluble drugs such as aspirin can be absorbed directly from the stomach. The stomach also contains some alcohol dehydrogenase activity and up to 20% of ethanol ingested may be oxidized in the stomach, thereby decreasing the bioavailability of alcohol. The locally produced acetaldehyde is thought to be the cause of alcoholic gastritis in chronic alcoholics. Interestingly, H_2-antagonists suppress the activity of gastric alcohol dehydrogenase thus increasing ethanol bioavailability.

Gastric Motility and Gastric Emptying

The integrated function of the stomach and pylorus depends upon vagal tone, pyloric integrity and negative feedback systems within the stomach and duodenum. The fundus and body do not exhibit phasic contractions but instead relax to accommodate a meal and contract in tonic fashion to propel food down towards the antrum. Several minutes after food enters the stomach, gentle peristaltic movements, called mixing waves, pass over the stomach every 15–25 s. These waves macerate food, mix it with gastric secretions, and reduce it to a thin liquid called chyme. As digestion proceeds in the stomach, more vigorous mixing waves begin at the body of the stomach and intensify as they reach the pylorus. As food reaches the pylorus, each mixing wave forces a small amount of the gastric contents into the duodenum through the pyloric sphincter.

Gastric emptying is determined by the volume and composition of gastric contents. Liquid meals empty faster than solid meals. Gastric emptying is somewhat slower for protein foods than for food rich in carbohydrate, and emptying is slowest after a meal containing large amounts of fat. Several factors, such as the osmolality, acidity and the amount of fat in duodenal contents, can influence gastric emptying via negative feedback mechanisms triggered by duodenal mucosal receptors. However, the dominant factor determining gastric emptying is nutritive density, the higher-density meals emptying more slowly. Despite this, higher-density meals may still deliver greater amounts of calories to the duodenum. The mediators of this negative feedback loop are the enterogastric reflex and hormones released in response to certain constituents in chyme; secretin, cholecystokinin (CCK) and gastric inhibitory peptide (GIP). These mediators inhibit both gastric secretion and motility so that the rate of stomach emptying is limited to the amount of chyme that the small intestine can process. Surgical vagotomy delays emptying of solids by inhibiting antral contractions but enhances emptying of liquids by increasing fundal tone. Proximal or highly selective vagotomy does not appear to affect antral function to the same extent as a truncal vagotomy.[5] Increased gastric emptying of triglycerides and starch also occurs in pancreatic exocrine insufficiency due to reduced production of osmotically active particles in the duodenum and hence reduced stimulation of the duodenal osmoreceptors.[6] A similar situation pertains with lactose in patients with hypolactasia.[6] Damage to the pylorus by peptic ulceration or surgery allows rapid uncontrolled gastric emptying, which may lead to 'dumping' or overwhelm residual small-bowel absorptive capacity in patients with short-bowel syndrome.

Measurement of Gastric Emptying

In clinical practice, techniques for assessing gastric emptying that involve intubation and sampling of gastric contents have now been superseded by the use of non-invasive, radiolabelled markers. An understanding of the mechanisms controlling gastric emptying is, however, essential for interpretation of many clinical conditions and biochemical tests of small-bowel or pancreatic function.

Acid Secretion

Hydrochloric acid is secreted by parietal cells at a concentration of approximately 155 mmol/L. The pH of parietal secretion is about 0.9 but as the secretion mixes with saliva, mucus and food the hydrogen ion concentration decreases to 40 mmol/L and the pH rises to 1.5–3.5. The hydrochloric acid secreted into the lumen is derived from the blood and is thought to involve active transport of hydrogen and chloride across the membrane of the parietal cells. Current interest in gastric acid has little to do with its role of initiating proteolysis with pepsin. It is the central role of acid in initiating and maintaining peptic ulceration of the oesophagus, stomach, duodenum and occasionally the jejunum or the isolated area of gastric epithelium in a Meckel's diverticulum that has led to a greater understanding of the control and mediation of acid secretion. Acid also provides a barrier to enteric infections acquired by the oral route.

The Control of Acid Secretion

Stimulation of acid secretion can be separated into cephalic, gastric and intestinal phases, which may occur simultaneously depending upon the stimulus. The cephalic phase begins with sight, smell, taste, mastication or thought of food and can be abolished by vagotomy. The gastric phase occurs as food enters the stomach and distends the fundus.[7] This phase is mediated by local and vagal reflexes and therefore cannot be completely abolished by vagotomy. Release of gastrin by antral G cells occurs in response to gastric luminal peptides or amino acids via receptors on the luminal microvillous G-cell border. The vagus also mediates a portion of its secretory activity via gastrin release, although recent studies have detected gastrin within the vagus nerve itself.[8] Gastrin stimulates acid release from parietal cells and also contracts the lower oesophageal sphincter and relaxes the pyloric sphincter. Curiously, antral distention only induces acid secretion in patients with duodenal ulcers.[7] Acid inhibition of gastrin occurs via somatostatin released from D cells adjacent to the G cells or by direct acid inhibition of G-cell secretion.[9]

The intestinal phase of gastric secretion is initiated when weakly acidic, partially digested proteins enter the duodenum. These stimulate the duodenal mucosa to release enteric gastrin, which in turn stimulates acid release from parietal cells. Infusion of peptides and amino acids into the duodenum, however, can produce some acid secretion without a rise in plasma gastrin concentration. This may be mediated by an unidentified hormone normally metabolized in the liver since portal blood not exposed to passage through the liver enhances this phase of gastric secretion.[10]

The parietal cell is the target of all the above stimuli (Fig. 21.1). Three main mediators of parietal cell activation are recognized: acetylcholine, gastrin and histamine.

The discovery of the H_2-receptor on the serosal surface of the parietal cell led to the development of the H_2-receptor antagonists and a new era of peptic ulcer therapy. Blockade of the H_2-receptor by antagonists such as cimetidine or ranitidine also blocks gastrin-induced acid release and vagal acid release, suggesting that histamine has a principal role in mediating stimulation of the Na:K ATPase pump on the luminal surface of the parietal cell. However, H_2-receptor blockers in clinical doses do not eliminate acid production, particularly that stimulated by meals, whereas the newer proton-pump inhibitors virtually eliminate acid secretion to all stimuli, though not sufficiently to mimic the achlorhydria of atrophic gastritis found in pernicious anaemia. In one study, the median integrated 24-h intragastric acidity decreased from 1148 to 490 mmol/h per litre and 36 mmol/h per litre during treatment with ranitidine and omeprazole, respectively, whilst the median 24-h plasma gastrin rose from 328 to 799 and 1519 pmol/h per litre, respectively. These increased rates of plasma gastrin secretion are, however, much lower than the median integrated 24-h plasma gastrin of 9886 pmol/h per litre found in pernicious anaemia.[11]

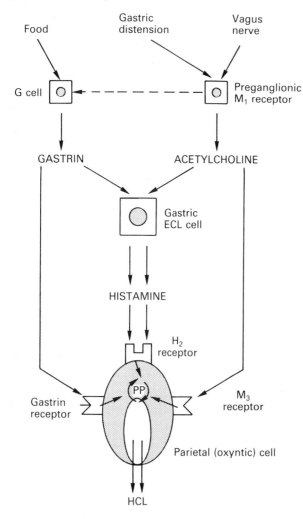

Figure 21.1 The control of gastric acid secretion in man. M, muscarinic; ECL, enterochromaffin-like cells; PP, proton pump.

These findings are important when considering the effect of long-term acid suppression on nitrosamine production by gastric luminal bacteria, which may play a part in gastric carcinogenesis. Also, enteric infections are more likely to occur the greater the loss of acid secretion.

Gastric Secretory Tests

Gastric secretion in the basal state and after stimulation can be assessed by a number of clinical laboratory tests.[12] These tests have been widely used in the past to detect hypersecretion and to assess patients after peptic ulcer surgery. The advent of fibreoptic endoscopy has, however, reduced the diagnostic utility of secretory tests, whilst the potent ulcer-healing agents now available have drastically reduced the number of patients undergoing elective peptic ulcer surgery or antireflux procedures.

Indications

- Diagnosis of pernicious anaemia

- Diagnosis of acid hypersecretion secondary to hypergastrinaemia in Zollinger–Ellison syndrome (gastrinoma), G-cell hyperplasia, hypercalcaemia and short-bowel syndrome

- To assess completeness of suppression of acid secretion following surgery for peptic ulcer

- To assess acid secretion in unresponsive patients on acid-suppressive therapy with H_2-receptor antagonists or proton-pump inhibitors

- To differentiate between benign and malignant ulceration

- To help in the selection of operative procedure for oesophageal reflux; hypersecretors do well with vagotomy alone without reconstruction of the cardia

Pentagastrin Test

Pentagastrin is a pentapeptide containing the same terminal sequence of four amino acids that is responsible for the physiological action of gastrin. The test is made after an overnight fast and cessation of all antisecretory drugs or antacids for 2–7 days. A nasogastric tube is passed and the patient positioned on the left side to avoid outflow of gastric juice into the duodenum. No saliva must be swallowed throughout the test and the overnight gastric secretions are discarded. For calculation of basal acid output (BAO), four 15-min samples are collected by aspiration before the pentagastrin injection and BAO is calculated from the sum of free acid concentration in the four portions and expressed in mmol/h. For maximum stimulation, pentagastrin, 6 μg/kg, is given subcutaneously. A dose of 12 μg/kg may be required after surgery but it is best to use the same dose pre- and postoperatively. After pentagastrin injection, the gastric juice is collected for four 15-min periods and the acid content is calculated from titration against NaOH. The peak acid output (PAO) is calculated by adding the two highest concentrations of free acid (mmol/15 min) and multiplying by 2 to give PAO/h. Alternatively, gastric secretion in the first 10 min after pentagastrin is discarded and all secretions from 10 to 30 min (20 min) are collected. The PAO is then calculated by multiplying the concentration of free acid (mmol/20 min) by 3 to give PAO/h. Intraindividual variation is small, with a coefficient of variation of 4.6%.[12]

Interpretation of BAO and PAO. Interpretation of the test is beset by difficulties caused by variations in the technique and the expression of results. In normal subjects, BAO is 0–5 mmol/h and PAO is 10–30 mmol/h in women and 15–40 mmol/h in men.[12] Younger subjects have higher values and the differences between sexes decrease over the age of 50.

Normal values exclude pernicious anaemia. Benign gastric ulcers are generally associated with normal PAO and those in the prepyloric or pyloric channel and duodenal ulcers may have high acid output. Sixty per cent of patients with prepyloric, pyloric or duodenal ulcers may, however, have a normal PAO. Duodenal ulcer patients characteristically fail to switch off acid secretion overnight, although the detection of this phenomenon requires 24-h intragastric pH monitoring, which has remained a research tool. Duodenal ulcer is virtually excluded by a PAO of less than 10 mmol/h in women and less than 15 mmol/h in men. BAO adds little to PAO in patients with duodenal ulcer but BAO is generally raised, although the BAO/PAO ratio is similar to normal. The level of PAO in such patients has proved to be an unreliable guide to the type of gastric operation or to prognosis for recurrence.

BAO and PAO are both zero in pernicious anaemia and achlorhydria. The latter is also found in asymptomatic normal subjects, in atrophic gastritis, and in 18% of patients with gastric cancers. Although gastric cancer is more common in achlorhydria, up to 80% of gastric cancer patients secrete acid. Few patients with benign gastric ulceration have zero BAO and PAO, so a gastric ulcer in the presence of achlorhydria should be assumed to be a cancer till proved otherwise.

The main use of the pentagastrin test apart from postoperative assessment is in the detection of Zollinger–Ellison syndrome due to a gastrin-secreting tumour. A raised BAO (more than 15 mmol/h) or PAO (more than 50 mmol/h) distinguishes the high gastrin level of Zollinger–Ellison syndrome from achlorhydria. It should be emphasized, however, that the incidence of Zollinger–Ellison syndrome is very low. A small number of patients with duodenal ulcers have hypergastrinaemia with a high PAO but with no evidence of a gastrinoma. In some of these, G-cell hyperplasia in the antrum is responsible and antrectomy is curative. The association of hypergastrinaemia and hyperacidity has also been recorded in some patients with the short-bowel syndrome.

Partial gastrectomy—antrectomy (Billroth I or II) for example—leaves much of the gastric parietal-cell area intact but removes G-cell gastrin secretion. Vagotomy reduces the stimulus to cholinergic receptors on the parietal cells, although the vagus also stimulates some gastrin secretion. Assessment of postoperative acid secretion is best accomplished with the pentagastrin test rather than with the Hollander insulin test (*see* below). Both tests are subject to technical problems relating to aspiration of gastric contents since pyloroplasty or gastroenterostomy may allow much of the secretions to escape collection. A successful vagotomy should reduce PAO to 30% of the preoperative level. A PAO that is 50% of the preoperative level suggests incomplete vagotomy. PAO of more than 20 mmol/h in men or more than 18 mmol/h in women, 10 days after vagotomy, indicates a 25% risk for recurrence of ulcer.

Sham-feeding Test

This is a physiological test of vagal function.[13] After an overnight fast, nasogastric intubation is done and BAO assessed. A standard meal is then given to the patient to chew and spit out. None must be swallowed. Acid output during the procedure allows assessment of residual vagal function.[12,13] Interpretation is as for the pentagastrin test. There is no doubt that this test is simpler and safer than the insulin test.

Insulin Test (Hollander Test)

Induction of hypoglycaemia by insulin stimulates acid secretion via the vagus nerve. A dose of 0.1–0.2 unit/kg soluble insulin is injected intravenously and 15-min collections of gastric secretions are made over 2 h. Blood glucose is also measured at frequent intervals. Adequate stimulation of gastric secretion requires the plasma glucose concentration to fall to less than 2.5 mmol/L (45 mg/dL), a concentration associated with unpleasant symptoms and potentially dangerous. Incomplete vagotomy is indicated by an increase in acidity of 20 mmol/L over BAO in two consecutive 15-min samples, a total acid output of more than 2 mmol/h, or detection of 10 mmol/L free acid in any sample, if there is no detectable BAO.[12] Alternatively, trebling of BAO in any sample has been used to indicate incomplete vagotomy. The premise that hypoglycaemia-induced acid secretion is mediated solely by the vagi is incorrect since adrenaline released during hypoglycaemia also stimulates gastrin. Moreover, the detection of acid secretion after surgery is a poor predictor of recurrent ulcer and the absence of secretion does not preclude recurrence. It seems doubtful whether insulin testing is justified when safer tests are available and relapses of ulcer disease after surgery can now be treated effectively by acid-suppressing drugs.

Alternative Methods of Assessing Gastric Secretion

Whilst there are obvious attractions in non-invasive tests, in practice they lack the accuracy of the invasive stimulation tests.

Diagnex Blue Test. This is a non-quantitative test for achlorhydria. The blue dye azure A bound to a cation-exchange resin (Diagnex blue) is taken orally. This dissociates in the presence of acid, releasing the dye, which is then absorbed in the small intestine. On excretion in the urine, it gives a blue colour indicating gastric acid secretion. This test is unreliable and is now rarely used.

^{99m}Technetium Colloid Scan. ^{99m}Technetium is taken up by acid-producing mucosa. Uptake of 1 μCi after pentagastrin 6 μg/kg subcutaneously is proportional to acid output or PAO and is also useful for the diagnosis of extragastric acid-secreting mucosa as in a Meckel's diverticulum in the ileum.

Pepsinogen

At least seven different fractions of pepsinogen in blood have been separated by electrophoresis. The five fractions that migrate toward the anode most rapidly are immunologically identical and have been termed group I pepsinogens. They are found only in chief cells and mucus-secreting cells in the fundus and body of the stomach. The other two fractions, which migrate behind the group I pepsinogens, are immunologically similar to each other and are called group II pepsinogens. They are found in the oxyntic mucosa, cardiac and pyloric glands and in duodenal Brunner's glands. Pepsinogen secretion responds to acid-stimulating factors and serum levels of pepsinogen I correlate well with PAO ($r = 0.74$) except in renal failure.

Gastrin

Gastrin is produced by G cells of the antrum and to a lesser extent by G cells in the proximal duodenum and δ cells of the pancreas but has also been located in the hypothalamus, pituitary and vagus.[8] Three molecular forms exist; big gastrin (G 34), little gastrin (G 17) and mini-gastrin (G 14). Other immunoreactive forms of gastrin have been identified, big-big gastrin for example, but are now believed to be artefacts that occur on gel filtration. Big gastrin (G 34) predominates during fasting, but modern assays concentrate on the measurement of little gastrin (G 17), which rises within 20 min of a meal and accounts for 75% of biologically active gastrin after meals. Gastrin is secreted in response to antral distention, meals and partially digested proteins in the stomach. Other stimuli of gastrin release include alcohol, caffeine, calcium and insulin-induced hypoglycaemia. Gastrin stimulates the secretion of acid, pepsinogen and intrinsic factor by the gastric mucosa. It also stimulates the release of secretin by small-intestinal mucosa and the secretion of bile and pancreatic bicarbonate and enzymes. Gastrin increases mucosal growth, gastric and intestinal motility, and blood flow to the stomach.

In healthy individuals, plasma gastrin concentrations after overnight fasting are usually less than 50 pmol/L (100 ng/L) but values may be higher in elderly subjects. The main use of plasma gastrin assays is in the diagnosis of gastrinoma (Zollinger–Ellison syndrome) and G-cell hyperplasia when hypergastrinaemia is associated with gastric hypersecretion. There are many other causes of hypergastrinaemia but these are usually associated with low or normal gastric acidity:

- gastrinoma (Zollinger–Ellison syndrome)
- G-cell hyperplasia
- pernicious anaemia
- achlorhydria
- pyloric obstruction
- vagotomy
- gastric carcinoma
- post proximal gastrectomy
- chronic renal failure
- H$_2$-receptor antagonists
- proton-pump inhibitors
- hypercalcaemia
- liver cirrhosis
- rheumatoid arthritis
- short-bowel syndrome.

Plasma gastrin is not usually elevated in duodenal ulcer disease and should be low in antrectomy patients. If a gastrinoma is suspected (or G-cell hyperplasia), the diagnosis can be confirmed if the fasting plasma gastrin concentration is more than 100 pmol/L (200 ng/L) and BAO is more than 15 mmol/L with a BAO/PAO ratio of more than 60%. The plasma gastrin in gastrinoma may, however, be less than 100 pmol/L (200 ng/L) and in this case a gastrin stimulation test should be undertaken (*see* below). A recent report showed that 11 out of 30 patients with Zollinger–Ellison syndrome had near-normal plasma gastrin concentrations but that serum from these patients stimulated acid secretion in rats and dogs, indicating the presence of a non-gastrin secretagogue that does not cross-react with G 17 or 34 on radioimmunoassays and is inactivated by trypsin.[14]

Gastrinoma

This is a rare condition affecting less than 0.1% of patients with duodenal ulcers and is the second most common neuroendocrine tumour after insulinoma. Eighty per cent of gastrinomas are multiple and 60% have metastasized by the time of diagnosis. The primary tumour is usually found in the pancreas. Therapeutic options include resection of the primary tumour, total or partial gastrectomy or use of H$_2$-receptor antagonists such as cimetidine, ranitidine or famotidine. More recently, omeprazole, a proton-pump inhibitor, has proved to be the most effective drug. G-cell hyperplasia can be cured by antrectomy or controlled by the drugs mentioned above.

Gastrin Stimulation Tests

Several stimulation tests have been developed to identify patients with gastrinoma. These have included measurements of plasma gastrin concentrations in response to a test meal or to an intravenous infusion or injection of secretin, calcium, magnesium, bombesin, glucagon or aminophylline. Of these, only the secretin and calcium stimulation tests have proved reliable.

Secretin Stimulation Test

The secretin challenge is the most useful stimulation test for gastrinoma. After an overnight fast, secretin (2 U/kg) is given as an intravenous bolus and blood is collected for the measurement of plasma gastrin concentration at 2.5, 5, 10, 15, 20, 25 and 30 min after the injection. Secretin suppresses plasma gastrin in normal subjects but stimulates gastrin release in patients with gastrinoma. Plasma gastrin increases by at least 50% 5 min after the injection. The test has a sensitivity of 90% and a specificity of nearly 100%.[15] The reduced sensitivity reported in some studies may have been due to the use of Boots secretin (Warren-Teed Laboratories, Inc., Columbus, OH), which is six to eight times less potent than the pure natural GIH secretin (Karolinska Institute, Stockholm, Sweden). The secretin test is quick, safe and reliable but false-positive and false-negative results may occur after partial gastrectomy.

Calcium Stimulation Test

After an overnight fast, calcium gluconate (5 mg/kg per hour) is given intravenously for 3 h and blood is collected at 30-min intervals for the measurement of plasma gastrin and serum calcium concentrations. In normal subjects and duodenal ulcer patients (without gastrinoma), the calcium infusion will produce modest increases in gastric acid and plasma gastrin (usually less than 50%). In patients with gastrinoma, basal acid output usually doubles and plasma gastrin rises by 100% or more. The test has some disadvantages, namely, it is lengthy, may be associated with side-effects, and may produce false-positive and false-negative responses.

Hypergastrinaemia and Carcinogenesis

With the advent of powerful acid-suppressing therapy such as cimetidine and omeprazole, long-term control of peptic ulceration is now possible. There is, however, considerable concern over the long-term safety of such drugs, which induce hypergastrinaemia.[16] The association between hypergastrinaemia, achlorhydria and gastric cancer has been recognized for many years. More recently the detection of benign gastric carcinoid tumours and enterochromaffin hyperplasia in rats on lifetime high doses of omeprazole or ranitidine has raised the possibility that prolonged acid suppression in man may also lead to similar tumours. Carcinoid tumours of the enterochromaffin-like cells have occasionally been identified in patients with Zollinger–Ellison syndrome or pernicious anaemia but the associated plasma gastrin concentrations have been much higher than those in patients on omeprazole. A more pertinent question, which remains to be answered, is whether long-term acid suppression by drugs may lead to an increased risk of adenocarcinoma as in patients with pernicious anaemia or many years after partial gastrectomy.

Helicobacter pylori and Acid-related Disease

Helicobacter pylori (*Campylobacter pylori*) is a spiral bacterium residing on the luminal surface of gastric epithelial cells and beneath the mucous layer, particularly in the gastric antrum. The observation that *H. pylori* was associated very strongly with antral gastritis and duodenal ulcer disease, and to a lesser extent with gastric ulcer, has led to extensive research. The concept of peptic ulcer disease having an infective origin is exciting because it opens up the possibility of therapeutic interference with its natural history.[17] Two mutually compatible theories for the link between *H. pylori*, gastritis and duodenal ulcer disease have been proposed:

1. Excess acid secretion noted in duodenal ulcer disease is secondary to increased G-cell gastrin secretion. G cells are found in close proximity to *H. pylori*, which is able to create an alkaline microclimate beneath the mucous layer, thus reducing the negative feedback on gastric acid secretion.[18]
2. Gastric metaplastic islands are found frequently in the duodenum and may be due to excess acid. *Helicobacter pylori* may colonize these islands and breach the mucosal defences, thereby allowing acid access to the mucosa.[17]

Clinical Biochemistry of *H. pylori*

Helicobacter pylori contains large quantities of urease, which allows its detection by a number of biochemical methods.

Urease Tests Various tests are now available for the rapid detection of *H. pylori* in gastric biopsy specimens. These tests are based on the addition of urea and phenol red. In infected specimens, the released ammonium ions produce a colour change from yellow to pink. The 'gold standard', however, remains culture of *H. pylori*, although fastidious conditions are required. Histological identification with special stains by an experienced histopathologist gives comparable results. Culture and histology are, however, both expensive and time consuming.

The CLO (Campylobacter-like Organisms) Test. Urea is incorporated in a small well of agar containing phenol red.[19] The endoscopic gastric antral biopsy is placed on the agar, sealed in place and incubated at 30°C. If *H. pylori* is present, a positive reaction can be seen within 20 min. This test has a sensitivity of 70% and a specificity of 100%.

Urea Broth Test. The biopsy specimen is incubated in 2% urea broth in the presence of an indicator such as phenol red, *m*-cresol purple or thymol blue. The original test, which uses 2% Christensen's urea broth, has a high rate of false-positive results.[20] Modified 2% urea broths have a sensitivity of 94–98% and a specificity of nearly 100%. In the UK this test costs as little as 5 p compared to £ 2.00 for a commercially available CLO slide test.

Rapid Urease Test. A 1-min test has been recently described using a freshly prepared solution of 1 mL 10% urea in deionized distilled water with two drops of 1% phenol red.[21]

Breath Tests for *H. pylori*

Two tests, the [14C]- and [13C]-urea breath tests, are currently available. Both are non-invasive but the measurement of 13C, a naturally occurring non-radioactive isotope, requires a mass spectrometer, whereas 14C, a radioactive isotope, can be counted using the more available liquid scintillograph. Production of 14CO$_2$ or 13CO$_2$ from a labelled dose of urea is proportional to the urease activity present in *H. pylori* within the stomach.

[14C]-Urea Breath Test. After an overnight fast, a 350-mL test meal is given followed immediately by 10 μCi (400 kBq)[14C]-urea (Amersham International) in 20 mL of water.[22] Breath samples are collected at frequent intervals up to 120 min following the ingestion of [14C]-urea by exhalation through a tube of anhydrous calcium chloride into a vial containing 2 mmol hyamine in 2 mL ethanol and phenolphthalein. Decolorization occurs when 2 mmol of exhaled CO$_2$ are collected. After the addition of 10 mL of scintillate, 14C activity is measured by liquid toluene scintillation. A single measurement at 40 min following ingestion of [14C]-urea gives an adequate assessment of the presence of *H. pylori*. A smaller dose of [14C]-urea (110 kBq) has been used by some workers, making repeated testing more acceptable; nevertheless the test should not be used in children and premenopausal women.

[13C]-Urea Breath Test. The rationale and method are similar to that for the [14C]-urea test but the measurement of 13C requires gas isotope-ratio mass spectrometry,[23] which limits the use of the [13C]-urea test, although postal services are now available in the UK commercially (Europa Scientific, Crewe and BSIA Ltd, Middlesex). A low-cost alternative to mass spectrometry may be available in the near future with infrared heterodyme ratiometry, which is currently being developed.

The sensitivity of the [13C]-urea test has been quoted to be 98.7% and correlation with the [14C]-urea test is very close. The advantage of the 13C test over the 14C test is that it can be repeated with no radioactive exposure.

Use of Urea Breath Tests in Clinical Practice. Whilst culture, histology and urease tests on endoscopic biopsies will remain natural adjuncts of an initial diagnostic endoscopy, there is a definite need for a reliable, cheap and non-invasive test to assess the progress of eradication of *H. pylori*. The [13C]- and [14C]-urea tests satisfy these criteria. Epidemiological data may also be obtained with these techniques but without the corresponding clinical information on gastroduodenal pathology. The [14C] and [13C]-urea tests can both be used quantitatively to provide evidence of the degree of infection.

H. pylori Antibodies

Colonization of the stomach with *H. pylori* elicits a systemic antibody response that may be of use in non-invasive epidemiological studies, bearing in mind that up to 60% of normal people over 60 years may be infected. Antibodies are invariably indicative of chronic infection (IgG) and remain present throughout the infection, declining over a 6-month period after elimination of the organism.[24] Reinfection leads to a rapid rise in titre. An enzyme-linked immunosorbent assay (ELISA) technique, which is based on CLO-specific urease antigen, has been used to detect infected patients. Positive ELISA tests are, however, of no value in diagnosing peptic ulcer disease or gastritis because of the high prevalence of *H. pylori* in the population at large. There is, however, a role for serum *H. pylori* antibody assays in following up treated patients.

THE SMALL INTESTINE

The small intestine, which is approximately 6 m long, begins at the pylorus and joins the large intestine at the ileocaecal valve. Its main function is the digestion and absorption of foodstuffs. The presence of folds, villi and microvilli vastly increases the surface area of epithelium available for digestion and absorption. Digestion mainly occurs in the lumen by pancreatic enzymes and is completed by intestinal mucosal enzymes (oligosaccharidases, disaccharidases, peptidases, ribonuclease and deoxyribonuclease) situated on the surface of the microvilli or the brush border.

Absorption through the villi and across the intestinal wall can occur by several mechanisms: diffusion, facilitated diffusion, osmosis and active transport (Fig. 21.2). The duodenum, jejunum, ileum and terminal ileum contribute differently to the function of the small intestine (Table 21.1).

Water and Electrolyte Absorption

The total volume of fluid absorbed each day by the gut is about 9 L, of which 1.5 L is derived from ingestion of liquids and 7.5 L is derived from gastrointestinal secretions. Approximately 8–8.5 L of the fluid are absorbed in the small intestine; most of the remainder is absorbed in the large intestine. Water is absorbed passively in response to the osmotic forces created by the active transport of sodium, monosaccharides and amino acids. The normal rate of absorption is about 200–400 mL/h. The mucosal intercellular junctions become progressively tighter and less leaky from duodenum to rectum so that water absorption becomes correspondingly more efficient.

Electrolytes can be absorbed passively, depending on concentration and electrical gradients, or actively.

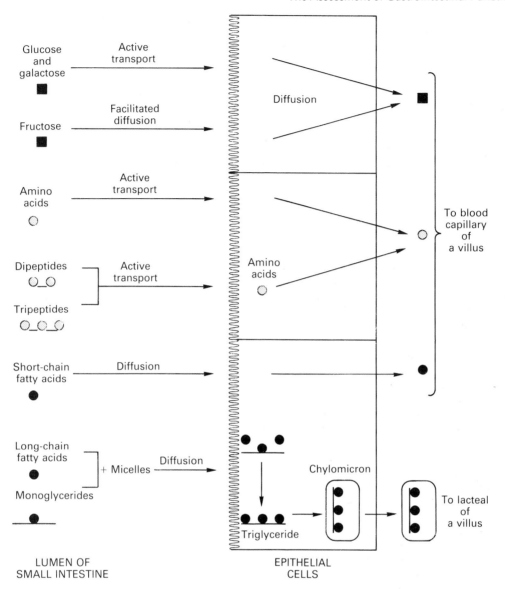

Figure 21.2 Mechanisms of absorption across the intestinal wall.

In the ileum, sodium is absorbed in exchange for hydrogen ions and chloride in exchange for bicarbonate. Calcium ions are absorbed in the jejunum either by passive diffusion or by an active transport mechanism which depends on 1,25-dihydroxy-vitamin D.

Digestion and Absorption of Carbohydrates

The daily intake of carbohydrate for a human adult consuming 2600 kCal/day consists mainly of: starch 200 g, sucrose 80 g, lactose 20 g, fructose 10 g and a variable amount of non-digestible polysaccharides such as cellulose and pectin. Essentially all carbohydrates are absorbed as monosaccharides. Dietary starch is broken down by salivary and pancreatic amylase to maltose, maltotriose and α-limit dextrins.

These, together with ingested disaccharides, are hydrolysed by brush-border oligosaccharidases to the monosaccharides glucose, galactose and fructose. Glucose and galactose are transported into epithelial cells of the villi by a carrier-mediated active process that is linked to sodium transport. Fructose is transported by facilitated diffusion. Absorbed monosaccharides diffuse out of the epithelial cells by sodium-independent carriers and are transported via the portal circulation to the liver and then to the general circulation. Whilst most carbohydrate in liquid enteral feeds can be absorbed very efficiently in the first 100 cm of the small intestine, some carbohydrate in the normal diet (about 15 g of dietary fibre and 5 g of soluble carbohydrate per day) reaches the colon undigested. It is then reclaimed as short-chain fatty acids following bacterial degradation.

TABLE 21.1
FUNCTION OF THE SMALL INTESTINE

Duodenum
Activation of pancreatic enzymes by enterokinase
Osmoreceptor feedback to stomach
Mixing of gastric, biliary and pancreatic juices
Absorption of carbohydrate and iron

Jejunum
Absorption of all macronutrients
Absorption of water-soluble vitamins
Absorption of fat-soluble vitamins
Absorption of trace elements and divalent cations
Absorption of bicarbonate

Ileum
Conservation of water and electrolytes
Higher affinity for monosaccharide absorption
Absorption of fat
Passive absorption of bile salts
Secretion of bicarbonate

Terminal ileum and ileocaecal valve
Prevention of bacterial contamination of small bowel
Negative feedback on proximal intestinal motility stimulated by fat (ileal break)
Absorption of vitamin B_{12}–intrinsic factor complex
Active absorption of conjugated bile salts

Digestion and Absorption of Proteins

The average daily dietary intake of protein is 90–100 g. Another 40–70 g of endogenous protein, derived from gastrointestinal secretions and shedding of mucosal cells, enter the intestine daily. Protein digestion is initiated by pepsin in the stomach, where the low pH denatures the protein, unfolding the polypeptide chains for better access by gastric, pancreatic and intestinal proteolytic enzymes. In the lumen of the duodenum and jejunum, protein is further digested by the pancreatic proteases trypsin, chymotrypsin, elastase, exopeptidases and carboxypeptidases to produce small peptides (2–6 amino-acid residues in length) and single amino acids. Some peptides are further broken down to single amino acids by the aminopeptidases of the brush border whereas others are absorbed intact and later hydrolysed by cytoplasmic peptidases. Amino acids are transported into the epithelial cells by an active transport process coupled with active sodium transport. At least seven carrier transport systems with overlapping specificities for different amino acids have been described. Following absorption, amino acids are transported to the liver via the portal circulation before entering the systemic circulation.

Digestion and Absorption of Fats

The average daily dietary intake of fat is 80–120 g, which is mainly in the form of triglycerides. Other lipid-soluble components form a much smaller pro-

portion of the total fat intake: cholesterol 0.5–1.0 g, phospholipids and fat-soluble vitamins. Absorption of dietary triglycerides is more than 95% whereas that of cholesterol is only 20–50%. In the stomach, triglycerides are emulsified by mechanical means and are hydrolysed by lingual and gastric lipases, which are active at a low pH and do not require bile salts. In the duodenum and jejunum, emulsion of triglycerides is further hydrolysed by pancreatic lipase in the presence of bile salts to produce fatty acids and monoglycerides. These products combine with bile acids and phospholipids to form water-soluble macromolecular complexes called micelles. On coming into contact with the surfaces of the epithelial cells, fatty acids and monoglycerides diffuse into the cells, leaving the bile acids behind to form further micelles. This diffusion is facilitated by a fatty acid-binding protein present in the cytosol of the cell. Within the epithelial cells, fatty acids containing more than 12 carbon atoms are re-esterified to triglycerides, which then aggregate with phospholipids, cholesterol and its esters, and a specific apolipoprotein (apo B-48) to form chylomicrons. The chylomicrons leave the epithelial cells by exocytosis and are transported by the lymphatic vessels to the thoracic duct and then to the systemic circulation. Fatty acids containing fewer than 10–12 carbon atoms pass directly, without re-esterification, from the mucosal cells into the portal circulation. Fat absorption is highly efficient so that in a person ingesting 100 g fat/day faecal fat excretion is less than 6 g/day.

Absorption of Vitamins, Folates and Iron

Fat-soluble vitamins A, D, E and K are absorbed along with ingested dietary fats in micelles and therefore their absorption is dependent on the presence of bile salts. Most water-soluble vitamins are absorbed by an active transport process that is probably carrier mediated.

Vitamin B_{12} requires combination with intrinsic factor (IF), produced by the gastric parietal cells, for its absorption. When the vitamin B_{12}–IF complex reaches the distal ileum, it is bound by receptors on the surface of mucosal epithelial cells, and then enters the cells. Within the cells, the vitamin B_{12}–IF complex is dissociated and vitamin B_{12} is transported via the portal circulation to the liver. Vitamin B_{12} also has a high affinity for glycoproteins secreted in saliva, gastric juice, bile and intestinal juice called R proteins. Pancreatic proteases split the R proteins from vitamin B_{12} in the duodenum to enable vitamin B_{12} to combine with IF. The vitamin B_{12}–R complex cannot be absorbed in the ileum.

Dietary folates, which are mainly present in the form of polyglutamates, are hydrolysed to monoglutamates by pteroylpolyglutamate hydrolase in the intestinal mucosa. Within the epithelial cells, most of the folate is reduced and methylated before entering the circulation as N_5-methyltetrahydrofolate.

TABLE 21.2

TESTS OF ASSESSMENT OF SMALL-INTESTINAL FUNCTION

Function assessed	Test	Specimen
Mucosal damage and intestinal permeability	D-Xylose absorption test	Urine *or* blood
	Cellobiose/mannitol test	Urine
	[^{51}Cr]-EDTA	Urine
	PEG	Urine
Carbohydrate absorption	Lactose tolerance test	Blood
	Breath hydrogen test	Breath
	Galactose	Urine *or* blood
Fat absorption	Faecal fat excretion	Faeces
	[^{14}C]-triolein	Faeces
	[^{125}I]-glycerol trioleate	Faeces
	[^{14}C]-triolein	Breath
	[^{14}C]-tripalmitin	Breath
	[^{14}C]-trioctanoin	Breath
	[^{13}C]-trioctanoin	Breath
Bacterial overgrowth	Lactulose	Breath
	Glucose	Breath
	[^{14}C]-cholylglycine	Breath
	[^{14}C]-D-xylose	Breath
	Bile acids	Intestinal aspirate
	Bile acids	Blood
	Indicans	Urine
	Fatty acids	Intestinal aspirate
Terminal ileum	^{75}SeHCAT	Faeces *or* total body counting
	[^{14}C]-cholylglycine	Breath
	[^{14}C]-cholyltaurine	Faeces
	Schilling test	Urine
Orocaecal transit time	Lactulose	Breath
	Sulphapyridine	Blood
Protein loss	[^{51}Cr]-albumin	Faeces
	[^{131}I]-albumin	Blood, urine *and* faeces
	α_1-antitrypsin	Faeces

The average daily intake of iron is 10–15 mg, mostly in the form of haem proteins, haemoglobin and myoglobin. Haem is absorbed intact, releasing the free iron inside the enterocyte. Inorganic iron must be in the ferrous state to be absorbed. Absorption occurs principally in the duodenum by a specific cellular mechanism regulated by the presence of ferritin and transferrin in the enterocytes.

Assessment of Small-intestinal Function

Various tests of the function of the small intestine are shown in Table 21.2 and now discussed in detail.

Assessment of Mucosal Damage and Intestinal Permeability

D-Xylose Absorption Test. D-Xylose is an aldopentose that is not normally found in significant amounts in the body. It does not require digestion and approximately 60% of an oral dose is absorbed in the upper small intestine (duodenum and jejunum). About one-half is metabolized and the remainder is subsequently excreted in the urine. The amount of xylose excreted in a timed urine collection or the concentration in blood at a specified time after ingestion of a standard dose has been used to assess the absorptive capacity of intestinal mucosa. Several modifications have been proposed: a 5-g dose, with a 5-h urine collection or a 1-h blood xylose measurement, is the most widely used in the UK. A total urinary excretion of 1.1 g (23% of the given dose) over 5 h or a blood xylose of 1.33 mmol/L (20 mg/dL) at 1h are considered to be the lower limit of normal.

Abnormally low results occur in many disorders of the small intestine such as coeliac disease, Crohn's disease (regional ileitis), radiation enteritis and resections. False-positive results can be due to:

- intestinal hurry
- bacterial overgrowth
- oedematous states
- impaired renal function
- incomplete urine collection.

Many drugs, such as aminosalicylic acid, aspirin,

colchicine, digoxin, indomethacin, monoamine oxidase inhibitors, metformin, nalidixic acid and neomycin can also give low results, mainly due to impaired absorption. Despite these limitations, the xylose test is useful in evaluating patients with malabsorption since it is essentially normal in patients with pancreatic insufficiency.

The xylose absorption test has been widely used as a screening test for coeliac disease, but in recent years its sensitivity and specificity have been questioned. Various investigators found false-positive rates ranging from 17% to 60% and false-negative rates ranging from 21% to 30%.[25,26] Measurement of serum xylose at 1h, corrected for surface area, was said to improve the predictive value of the test, but this was not confirmed and has led to the suggestion that the test should be abandoned as a screening test.[26] A parallel approach for screening patients with suspected coeliac disease, using the xylose test and erythrocyte folate, showed that the predictive accuracy for absence of coeliac disease was 100% when both tests were normal.[27] In another, an antigliadin antibody panel (IgG and IgA) and the xylose absorption test were used with similar findings.[28] Recently, various antibodies have been detected in the serum of patients with coeliac disease but their specificities and sensitivities have been variable (coeliac disease is further discussed in the section on malabsorption below).

Cellobiose/Mannitol Test. In disease states of the small intestine, there is decreased permeability to small polar molecules such as urea, polyethylene glycol, mannitol and D-xylose but an increase in the permeability of large molecules such as cellobiose and lactulose. The simultaneous administration of mannitol and cellobiose and the determination of their excretion ratios have shown good separation of healthy subjects and patients with untreated coeliac disease.[29] In one study, the sensitivity of the test was 96% compared with 67% for the xylose test and 46% for erythrocyte folate; the predictive value of a normal mannitol/cellobiose ratio for the absence of villous atrophy was 99% compared to 82% for erythrocyte folate and 76% for the xylose test.[30] In a more recent study involving 1010 unselected patients the sensitivity of the test was 96% for coeliac disease with a specificity of 70%.[31] The simultaneous administration of L-rhamnose and lactulose has also been used to detect small-intestinal damage with similarly good results.[32] Abnormal ratios of cellobiose/mannitol and L-rhamnose/lactulose are also found in patients with Crohn's disease, not only in the presence of overt small-bowel involvement but also when inflammation is apparently confined to the colon.[33]

Other Tests of Intestinal Permeability. The absorption of different polyethylene glycols (PEG) has been used to assess intestinal permeability but complex mathematical treatment is required before the urinary excretion of PEG reflects intestinal absorption.[34] Intestinal permeability can also be assessed by the urinary recovery of orally administered [51Cr]-EDTA. The urinary recovery is increased in untreated coeliac disease[35] and jejunal biopsy specimens show an increased uptake. [51Cr]-EDTA is easy to assay but some investigators have not been able to confirm its value in the diagnosis of coeliac disease.[36]

Assessment of Carbohydrate Absorption

Generalized carbohydrate malabsorption occurs only after extensive loss of mucosal surface—severe coeliac disease and extensive small-bowel resection for example. Specific carbohydrate malabsorption can occur as a result of deficiency of brush-border oligosaccharidases. The most common is lactase deficiency (hypolactasia) but sucrase-isomaltase or trehalase deficiency can also occur. Glucose-galactose malabsorption from a defect in sugar transport is a rare autosomal recessive disorder in which symptoms occur in affected neonates as soon as milk is introduced but also follow ingestion of foods containing glucose or galactose.

Tests for the Diagnosis of Disaccharidase Deficiency
The most reliable diagnostic test for disaccharidase deficiency is the measurement of the activity of the enzyme in jejunal biopsy specimens—lactase activity in hypolactasia for example. This test, however, is invasive and many indirect tests have been suggested as alternatives. The measurement of plasma glucose concentration or breath hydrogen following the ingestion of the disaccharide in question has been widely used to screen for specific disaccharidase deficiencies (*see* below).

Lactose Tolerance Test. This test is based on serial blood-glucose determinations after an oral load of lactose, usually 50 g or 1 g/kg body weight. A rise in blood glucose of less than 1.1 mmol/L over the fasting level is suggestive of lactase deficiency, especially if it is associated with abdominal pain and diarrhoea. Abnormal results may also be due to defective mucosal transport of monosaccharides and therefore any abnormal test must be followed by a control test in which the equivalent amounts of glucose and galactose to that of the lactose are given. A normal rise in blood glucose in the control test indicates normal transport of monosaccharides. The test has high false-positive and -negative rates and has been shown to correlate poorly with lactase activity in biopsy specimens.[37]

Breath Hydrogen Test for Lactose Absorption. Hydrogen is not normally produced by mammalian cells. Its presence in the breath indicates breakdown of carbohydrate in the intestine by anaerobic bacteria, usually in the colon. The detection of hydrogen in the breath has been used to demonstrate carbohydrate maldigestion or malabsorption (*see* Table 21.3).

TABLE 21.3

BREATH TESTS IN ASSESSMENT OF GASTROINTESTINAL
FUNCTION

Function assessed	Test	Gas measured
Carbohydrate absorption	Lactose	H_2
	Sucrose	H_2
Fat absorption	[14C]-triolein	$^{14}CO_2$
	[14C]-tripalmitin	$^{14}CO_2$
	[14C]-trioctanoin	$^{14}CO_2$
	[13C]-trioctanoin	$^{13}CO_2$
Bacterial overgrowth	Glucose	H_2
	Lactulose	H_2
	[14C]-cholylglycine	$^{14}CO_2$
	[14C]-D-xylose	$^{14}CO_2$
Terminal ileal function	[14C]-cholylglycine	$^{14}CO_2$
Orocaecal time	Lactulose	H_2

The breath hydrogen test is based on the rise in exhaled breath hydrogen that is formed from unabsorbed lactose in the colon. Serial samples at intervals of 15 min–1 h for 2–6 h are required. The rise in breath hydrogen following the oral administration of 50 g lactose has been shown to correlate well with the enzymatic assay of biopsy specimens.[37] False-negative results can occur in patients with colonic bacteria incapable of producing hydrogen and after antibiotic therapy. False-positive results can occur in small-intestinal bacterial overgrowth and in rapid transit time. Because of its simplicity, sensitivity, specificity and non-invasiveness, the breath hydrogen test has been recommended as the test of choice for the diagnosis of hypolactasia.[37]

Serum and Urinary Galactose. Galactose determination provides a simple way to assess lactase activity indirectly. After an overnight fast the patient is given a solution containing 50 g lactose and 150 mg ethanol/kg body weight orally at the same time. The ethanol is required to inhibit the rapid metabolism of galactose in the liver. After 40 min a capillary blood sample or a urinary sample are collected for the measurement of galactose concentration. A level of less than 0.3 mmol/L in the blood or less than 2.0 mmol/L in the urine indicates hypolactasia. A qualitative test-strip for galactose detection (Kabi-Vitrum, Stockholm, Sweden) has also been used.[38] In a recent study, the specificities of blood and urine galactose (96% and 98%, respectively) were similar to that of the breath hydrogen test (96%) but the sensitivities were much better (blood galactose 81%, urine galactose 94%, and breath hydrogen 69%).[39] Therefore, it would appear that galactose determinations either in blood or urine may provide a simple and convenient method for the diagnosis of hypolactasia but further confirmation of reliability is required.

Assessment of Fat Absorption

Faecal Fats

Most faecal fats are derived from non-absorbed dietary fats but a significant amount (about 2 g) is derived from sloughing of intestinal epithelial cells and intestinal bacteria. The measurement of faecal fat is still considered by some to be the best single test for evidence of maldigestion and malabsorption of fat, whether this is due to intestinal disease, pancreatic insufficiency or bacterial overgrowth. Collection should be made over a period of not less than 3–5 days. Ideally, fat intake should be controlled to between 80–100 g a day, at least 2 days before and during collection. The use of markers (chromium sesquioxide, radiopaque pellets or carmine) may improve the accuracy of timed collections. The stool is mixed with water, homogenized and a 10-ml portion is analysed by hydrolysis, extraction and titration of fatty acids. A daily fat excretion of more than 18 mmol (5 g) is considered abnormal and indicates steatorrhoea. Mild steatorrhoea may occur in thyrotoxicosis, untreated pernicious anaemia, Addison's disease, liver cirrhosis and intestinal hurry from any cause. The test suffers from the difficulties in obtaining accurate collections and is unpleasant for the patient and the laboratory staff.

Faecal Isotopic Tests of Fat Malabsorption

Several isotopic tests to assess fat absorption have been described.[40,41] In these, radiolabelled triglycerides are given orally and the amount of radioactivity is determined in the stools. Procedures using radio-iodinated triglycerides are unreliable because of the instability of the bond between the radio-iodine and the triglycerides in the gut. To distingish between pancreatic maldigestion and intestinal malabsorption radiolabelled triglycerides ([14C]-triolein) and fatty acids ([3H]-oleic acid) are given simultaneously and the ratio of the two isotopes is determined in the stools.[41] A dual isotope test using a labelled non-absorbable lipid-phase marker, [75Se]-glycerol triether, and [125I]-glycerol trioleate has recently been described.[42] The isotope ratio in a single stool sample was a reliable indicator of steatorrhoea, with a sensitivity of 87.5% and a specificity of 81.8%. The dual isotope test has an advantage over $^{14}CO_2$ breath tests (*see* below) as it can provide a quantitative measurement of fat absorption.

Breath Tests for Fat Malabsorption

In these tests, radioactive carbon (^{14}C) is incorporated into various organic compounds and the radioactive carbon dioxide ($^{14}CO_2$) resulting from their assimilation and metabolism is measured in breath samples. Several compounds have been used ([14C]-trioctanoin, [14C]-tripalmitin and [14C]-triolein) but the use of [14C]-triolein has been the most successful.[43] [13C]-labelled compounds such as [13C]-triolein can also be used. They have the advantage of avoid-

TABLE 21.4
CAUSES OF INTESTINAL BACTERIAL OVERGROWTH

Reduced gastric acid
Achlorhydria

Resection of ileocaecal valve

Structural abnormalities
Blind loops
Diverticula
Fistulae
Strictures

Impaired motility
Chronic intestinal pseudo-
obstruction
Diabetes mellitus
Radiation enteritis
Systemic sclerosis

Immune disorders
α-chain disease
IgA deficiency
Hypogammaglobulinaemia
Severe combined immunodeficiency

ing radioactivity but the released $^{13}CO_2$ requires a mass spectrometer for measurement.

$[^{14}C]$-Triolein Breath Test. In the simplest form of the test, 5 μCi (200 kBq)$[^{14}C]$-triolein mixed with 5 g of trioctanoin and 30 mL of cottonseed oil (20 g fat) are ingested after an overnight fast. Breath samples are collected before and hourly for 6 h after ingestion and the amount of exhaled $^{14}CO_2$ is determined in each sample and expressed as percentage dose excreted per hour. In normal subjects, at least 3.5% of the dose of $[^{14}C]$-triolein is detected in one or more of the breath samples. An accumulated value at 6 h of more than 9% of the administered dose is considered normal, whereas less than 6% is excreted in steatorrhoea. Low values indicate fat malabsorption but false-positive results may occur in obesity, diabetes, thyroid and pulmonary disease due to alteration of the metabolism of absorbed $[^{14}C]$-triolein or the excretion of $^{14}CO_2$ in breath. Data from four studies showed that the predictive value of a positive test (excluding obese subjects) is 89% and the predictive value of a negative test is 97%.[43–6]

Assessment of Bacterial Overgrowth

Gastric acid secretion and intestinal peristalsis normally prevent excessive bacterial proliferation in the proximal small intestine. Reduced gastric secretion or stasis from anatomical abnormalities (e.g. strictures) or impaired motility (e.g. diabetes mellitus) can result in bacterial overgrowth (Table 21.4). The presence of bacterial overgrowth in the small intestine may lead to malabsorption due to deconjugation of bile salts and also some degree of mucosal damage. Malabsorption of vitamin B_{12} also occurs through

binding and utilization by the bacteria in the proximal intestine, which reduce its availability for normal absorption in the distal ileum. The quantitative culture of upper intestinal aspirates has long been considered to be the most accurate diagnostic test for demonstrating bacterial overgrowth. However, this technique is complicated and time consuming, and its reliability has recently been questioned. To overcome these problems, indirect tests such as the hydrogen breath test, the bile-acid breath test and the $[^{14}C]$-D-xylose breath test have been developed.

Breath Tests for Bacterial Overgrowth

Breath Hydrogen Tests. Breath hydrogen is derived from the interaction between ingested carbohydrate and intestinal bacteria. Normally, ingestion of a well-absorbed carbohydrate such as glucose causes no increase in breath hydrogen, since little carbohydrate reaches the colonic bacteria. In bacterial overgrowth of the small intestine the interaction occurs in the proximal intestine resulting in a hydrogen peak before the carbohydrate reaches the caecum. A standardized dose of the test sugar (50 g glucose or 10 g lactulose) is given orally after an overnight fast, and end-expiratory breath samples are then collected at 15 or 30 min intervals for up to 3 h for the measurement of hydrogen by gas chromatography. In normal subjects, small but measurable amounts of hydrogen (5–25 parts/10^6) are produced in the fasting state, presumably due to degradation of sugar residues of gastrointestinal mucins. Following the ingestion of lactulose, a hydrogen peak appears between 45 and 120 min when the lactulose reaches the colon. In patients with small-intestinal bacterial overgrowth, an early peak of more than 20 parts/10^6 above baseline appears more than 15 min before the colonic peak. In some subjects, an early rise in breath hydrogen occurs at about 10 min and is probably due to fermentation by oral bacteria since it can be avoided by use of chlorhexidine antiseptic mouthwash.[47] The lactulose breath-hydrogen test is useful in detecting bacterial overgrowth but false-negative results can occur in patients with delayed gastric emptying, in those with a colonic flora incapable of producing hydrogen, and following antibiotic therapy. In addition, hydrogen-utilizing bacteria may produce methane in a significant number of patients and it has been suggested that both breath hydrogen and methane should be measured for adequate assessment of carbohydrate fermentation. False-positive results can occur with rapid transit time, which may need to be simultaneously assessed using a bolus of barium and fluoroscopy.

Bile-acid Breath Test. Bile acids in their conjugated forms are normally absorbed in the terminal ileum. A small fraction usually escapes to the colon where it is deconjugated by bacterial enzymes and excreted as free bile acids in stool. Increased deconjugation of bile acids can occur in bacterial overgrowth of the small intestine and forms the basis of the bile-acid breath test.[48] When a radiolabelled bile acid ([14C]-cholylglycine) is ingested, bacterial deconjugation releases [14C]-glycine, which is rapidly converted to $^{14}CO_2$ either by intestinal bacterial enzymes or tissue enzymes. The $^{14}CO_2$ is then transported in the blood and the amount expired in the breath is a direct reflection of bacterial deconjugation of bile salts. In this test, 5 μCi (200 kBq) [14C]-cholylglycine is given orally after an overnight fast. Breath samples are collected before and at hourly intervals for 6 h after ingestion of the isotope. Breath is collected in a liquid scintillation vial containing 1 mmol hyamine hydroxide to which thymolphthalein is added as an indicator. The radioactivity in each sample is measured by liquid scintillation and the results are expressed as the percentage of administered dose of radioactivity/mmol expired CO_2, corrected for body weight. In normal subjects, values are below 0.1% in each of the first three samples and should not exceed 0.3% in any sample throughout the test. In small-bowel bacterial overgrowth, values are raised from 2 h onwards with maximal values at 3–5 h.[11] The test is dependent on an intact terminal ileum and adequate absorption of bile acids, and therefore gives abnormal results in terminal ileal disease (*see* below). Intestinal hurry may give late-positive results due to deconjugation by normal colonic bacteria. The reliability of the test has been questioned recently in view of the high frequency of bile-acid malabsorption in patients with diarrhoea of unidentified aetiology.[49] In one study, the sensitivity of the test was only 34% in detecting patients with positive cultures from jejunal aspirates.[50] Antibiotic therapy and the inability of certain organisms to deconjugate bile acids may account for some of the false-negative results.

14C-D-Xylose Breath Test. D-Xylose is normally rapidly absorbed in the jejunum and excreted in the urine without being significantly metabolized. Intestinal bacteria can, however, metabolize D-xylose, releasing CO_2, and the measurement of $^{14}CO_2$ in the breath following oral administration of [14C]-D-xylose has been used to detect small-intestinal bacterial overgrowth. In this test, 5 μCi (200 kBq) [14C]-D-xylose and 1 g unlabelled D-xylose dissolved in 250 mL of water are given after an overnight fast. Breath samples are collected at 30, 60, 120, 180 and 240 min and the expired CO_2 is trapped in scintillation vials for the measurement of radioactivity. The results are expressed as the percentage $^{14}CO_2$ of the given dose of [14C]-D-xylose/mmol expired CO_2, corrected for endogenous CO_2 production. A peak value at 30 min exceeding 0.12% or an accumulated value at 2 h exceeding 3.3% is considered abnormal. The test is largely independent of ileal function and small-intestinal transit time and has been shown to have high specificity and sensitivity compared with the bile-acid breath test.[51]

Other Tests of Small-intestinal Bacterial overgrowth

High levels of unconjugated bile acids in intestinal-juice aspirates have been found in patients with bacterial overgrowth.[52] More recently, technological advances have allowed the measurement of unconjugated bile acids in serum. A preliminary study in a small number of patients showed increased serum deoxycholic acid in a patient with proven bacterial overgrowth whereas it was absent in patients with ileal resection.[53] The potential clinical value of measuring the serum unconjugated bile acids merits further assessment.

The concentrations of volatile fatty acids (acetate, propionate and butyrate) in jejunal aspirates have been shown to be increased in patients with bacterial overgrowth but there was a considerable overlap with results obtained from patients with gastrointestinal disorders who had no evidence of bacterial overgrowth.[54]

The measurement of urinary indoxyl sulphate or indican has been used to detect bacterial overgrowth in the intestine. The test is unreliable, showing unacceptable false-positive and -negative rates, and has been abandoned.

Assessment of Dysfunction of the Terminal Ileum

The terminal ileum is the principal site for the absorption of bile acids and vitamin B_{12}. The enterohepatic circulation of bile acids occurs five times per day, with a 95% reclamation per cycle. In disease of the terminal ileum or after ileal resection the unabsorbed bile salts reach the colon and cause excessive loss of water and electrolytes resulting in watery diarrhoea. Deconjugation by colonic bacteria leads to increased absorption of unconjugated bile acids. Although there is a compensatory increase in synthesis of bile salts by the liver, this may not compensate for the excessive faecal loss, resulting in a decreased body pool of bile salts, malabsorption of fat, and steatorrhoea. Disease of the terminal ileum also results in vitamin B_{12} deficiency, which may occur after months or years depending on the level of body stores.

[75Se]-Homocholic-tauro Acid Test (SeHCAT)

[75Se]-HCAT is the taurine conjugate of a synthetic bile acid that contains a γ-emitting isotope, selenium-75. [75Se]-HCAT is highly resistant to bacterial deconjugation and therefore its absorption reflects the ileal mucosal capacity for bile-acid absorption.[55] After an overnight fast, 10 μCi (400 kBQ) [75Se]-HCAT is given orally alone or with a liquid test meal containing 12 g glucose, 12 g maize oil and 21 g skimmed milk. Absorption of [75Se]-HCAT is then assessed either by whole-body counting or counting of unprocessed sealed containers of stool. Whole-body counting is done after 2, 24, 28, and 72 h and 1 week, or stools are collected for 5 days. A fall in bile-acid absorption as small as 2% per cycle can lead to a profound fall in

TABLE 21.5
CAUSES OF A POSITIVE [^{75}Se]-HCA SCAN

Terminal ileal resection
Terminal ileal disease
Crohn's
Tuberculosis
Lymphoma
Yersiniosis
Radiation enteritis

Previous enteric infection
Shigellae
Campylobacter jejuni

Cholecystectomy
Post-gastrectomy or *-vagotomy*
Non-steroidal anti-inflammatory drug therapy
Thyrotoxicosis

7-day retention and a value of less than 8% at 1 week is considered to be diagnostic of bile-acid malabsorption. Comparison of results for [^{75}Se]-HCAT retention between different centres of investigation is made difficult by the variation in counting techniques, test duration and cut-off levels for abnormalities. In one study, whole-body retention of under 8% at day 7 had a sensitivity of 97% for bile-acid malabsorption whereas a value in excess of 15% had a specificity of 99%.[49] Others suggest 50% retention on day 4 as the most accurate value to discriminate between normals and abnormals.[57] In our own unit, we have found that a retention in excess of 19% at day 7 indicates normal function of the terminal ileum and a value below 13% is associated with dysfunction.

The use of [^{75}Se]-HCAT scanning has opened up new areas of interest in the investigation of chronic idiopathic diarrhoea or steatorrhoea. There are many causes of an abnormal SeHCAT scan (Table 21.5) and in the majority of cases the cause is obvious from the history. In a number of cases, however, there is no obvious explanation for the bile-salt malabsorption demonstrated by the test. Investigation of chronic 'idiopathic' diarrhoea has led a number of researchers to detect bile-salt malabsorption.[58] Some believe this to be an epiphenomenon, however, caused by the diarrhoea rather than contributing to it. Thus, treatment with cholestyramine of patients with idiopathic diarrhoea was not beneficial in one study.[58] Furthermore, bile-salt malabsorption could be induced in normal subjects in whom diarrhoea was provoked by lactulose ingestion.[59] However, a very recent publication in this area confirms that many patients with idiopathic chronic diarrhoea have significant bile-salt malabsorption that responds to cholestyramine therapy.[60] We have recently identified a further subgroup of such patients in whom a prior enteric infection was the common initiating factor for the diarrhoea. All our patients had abnormal [^{75}Se]-HCAT 7-day retention ($< 13\%$) and all responded dramatically to cholestyramine.[61] The

mechanisms underlying these observations are the subjects of further research.

Bile-acid Breath Test
The bile-acid breath test (*see* Assessment of bacterial overgrowth above) has been used for several years to assess bile-acid malabsorption. As delineated above, bacterial overgrowth in the small intestine can also give abnormal results. Measurement of ^{14}C in a simultaneous faecal collection has been suggested to differentiate between ileal malabsorption and bacterial contamination.[48] Alternatively, the SeHCAT, which is a reliable test for identification of bile-acid malabsorption, can be used in combination with the bile-acid breath test to distinguish between bacterial contamination and bile-acid malabsorption.

Faecal Isotope Tests
The measurement of faecal radioactivity after oral or intravenous administration of a radiolabelled bile acid, [^{14}C]-cholyltaurine, has been used to assess bile-acid malabsorption. Faecal excretion of more than 50% of the bile-acid label in the first 24 h indicates bile-acid malabsorption. Increased excretion may also occur in accelerated transit time and idiopathic diarrhoea. Whether this is due to accelerated evacuation of unabsorbed bile acids from the colon or impaired ileal absorption consequent on rapid intestinal transit is not known.

Schilling Test
Malabsorption of vitamin B_{12} can be due to defective secretion of intrinsic factor by the stomach or, more commonly, to defective intestinal absorption. Lack of intrinsic factor is found in pernicious anaemia, after total gastrectomy, and in a significant number of patients who have undergone partial gastrectomy. Defective intestinal absorption may occur in Crohn's disease, ileal resection, bacterial overgrowth, severe pancreatic insufficiency and rarely in coeliac disease. Various drugs such as *p*-aminosalicylic acid, neomycin, colchicine, metformin and slow K can cause vitamin B_{12} malabsorption. Deficiency of vitamin B_{12} may itself impair its small-bowel absorption and therefore repletion of vitamin B_{12} stores is recommended before Schilling or Dicopac testing. The Schilling test has been widely used to assess vitamin B_{12} absorption and to differentiate between gastric and ileal forms of vitamin B_{12} malabsorption. In the classical Schilling test, an oral dose of labelled vitamin B_{12} is given after an overnight fast and urine is collected for 24 h for determination of radioactivity. An intramuscular 'flushing' dose of 1 mg of unlabelled vitamin B_{12} is given to saturate plasma and tissue binding sites so that the absorbed vitamin B_{12} is excreted in the urine. In normal subjects, 10% of the oral dose is excreted in the urine over 24 h. If excretion is less than 10%, the procedure is repeated with the simultaneous oral administration of labelled vitamin B_{12} and intrinsic factor. In patients with

intestinal malabsorption oral administration of intrinsic factor does not increase the percentage dose excreted. A dual isotope technique (the Dicopac test, Amersham International), which is a simplified procedure involving the simultaneous oral administration of [^{58}Co]-free cyanocobalamin and [^{57}Co]-cyanocobalamin bound to intrinsic factor, is now commonly used in UK. The percentage of each tracer dose and the ratio of ^{57}Co% to ^{58}Co% are determined in urine collected over the next 24 h. In normal subjects, the excretion of either isotope exceeds 14% and the ratio is 0.7 to 1.2. In intestinal malabsorption the excretion of both isotopes is usually less than 7%, with a normal ratio. Excretion values of more than 9% for ^{57}Co, less than 10% for ^{58}Co and a ratio exceeding 1.3 indicate lack of intrinsic factor. The Dicopac test is simple and rapid but its reliability has been questioned. A recent evaluation showed that using the two criteria (% urinary excretions and a ratio of ^{57}Co to ^{58}Co exceeding 1.3) identified only 44.3% whereas using the ratio as the only criterion identified 96.5% of patients with pernicious anaemia.[62]

Assessment of Orocaecal Transit Time

Abnormal motility and transit time can occur in many diseases, for example coeliac disease, giardiasis, Crohn's disease, hypolactasia, diabetes mellitus, irritable bowel syndrome, systemic sclerosis and thyroid disorders. Rapid movement of nutrients through the small intestine may lead to malabsorption and diarrhoea. Orocaecal transit time can be assessed radiologically by monitoring the passage of barium through the small intestine, isotopically by labelled test meals, or more simply by the lactulose breath-hydrogen test.

The Lactulose Breath-hydrogen Test

A standardized dose of lactulose (10 or 20 g) in 250 mL of water is given orally after an overnight fast. The end-expiratory breath samples are collected before and at 10-min intervals thereafter for 4 h. The orocaecal transit time is taken as the interval between finishing the lactulose drink and the beginning of sustained rise in breath hydrogen in three consecutive samples, where at least a 10 parts/10^6 incremental increase occurred between any two of the samples. This test, however, is not reproducible[63] and can give misleading results in patients with bacterial overgrowth (*see* above) and in subjects with a colonic flora incapable of producing hydrogen. It has also been suggested that lactulose itself, being a non-absorbable carbohydrate, has a laxative effect and may cause acceleration of transit time. More recently, the test has been shown to be more reproducible when the lactulose is given with a standard breakfast.[64]

Sulphasalazine/Sulphapyridine Test

A pharmacological method based on the measurement of plasma sulphapyridine after the oral administration of sulphasalazine has also been described to assess orocaecal time.[65] This method has been shown to give a longer orocaecal transit time than the lactulose breath-hydrogen test but when sulphasalazine was given with lactulose the transit time assessed by plasma sulphapyridine was much shorter, suggesting that lactulose itself alters the transit time.[66]

Assessment of Gastrointestinal Protein Loss

Excessive protein loss into the bowel lumen is a non-specific feature of many gastrointestinal diseases, as follows:

- allergic enteritis
- coeliac disease and tropical sprue
- colonic tumours
- Crohn's disease
- gastric tumours
- gastric ulcers (multiple)
- fistulae
- lymphoma
- lymphangiectasia
- Ménétrier's disease
- post-infection
- ulcerative colitis
- villous adenoma of the colon
- Whipple's disease.

This may result in hypoalbuminaemia and oedema, which may overshadow the intestinal symptoms. Assessment of protein loss can be made using a radiolabelled protein such as [^{51}Cr]-albumin or [^{67}Cu]-caeruloplasmin, or using a radiolabelled macromolecular substance such as [^{131}I]-polyvinylpyrrolidine.[11] Faecal clearance of an endogenous protein such as α_1-antitrypsin has also been used.

[^{51}Cr]-Albumin

In this test, 100 μCi [^{51}Cr]-albumin is given intravenously. Stools are collected for 5 days and after homogenization the total radioactivity is measured. In normal subjects, less than 1% of the injected dose appears in the stool each day. A modification in which [^{51}Cr]-chloride is injected to label the patient's own albumin has also been used.

[^{131}I]-Albumin and [^{125}I]-Albumin

Methods employing radio-iodinated proteins such as [^{131}I]- or [^{125}I]-albumin can be used to assess gastrointestinal protein loss. Accurate quantitation of protein loss, however, cannot be estimated because of the rapid reabsorption of ^{131}I or ^{125}I after protein catabolism in the gut and because of the secretion of the label in salivary secretions. The method is complex and lengthy, requiring blood and urine collection for 21 days, and is used only for research purposes.

α_1-Antitrypsin clearance

α_1-Antitrypsin, a protease inhibitor synthesized by

the liver, is resistant to digestion within the gut and can be measured in the stool, providing a reliable marker of gastrointestinal protein loss. This is of particular use in the assessment of Crohn's disease activity.[67]

THE COLON

The colon is approximately 1.5–2 m long and acts as a reservoir for the formation of faeces in addition to electrolyte and water reclamation. Its function is greatly influenced by its luminal contents, which contribute to a more recently recognized function—absorption of small molecular fragments of carbohydrate, protein and fat that have escaped small-bowel absorption. This almost certainly means a greater physiological role for colonic mucosa and in overall nutrition than was previously recognized.

Colonic Motility

The colon is a relatively inactive organ compared to the small bowel. Its contractions are non-propagative or segmented and tend to slow colonic flow. Loss of contractility results in rapid colonic transit and diarrhoea. Coordinated propulsive waves may occur after laxatives and in certain conditions may give rise to diarrhoea.[68] Both gastrin and the vagus exert a powerful influence on colonic motility, although the colon has no intrinsic pacemaker like the stomach.

Colonic Absorption and Secretion

The principal functions of the colon are the formation and dehydration of stools, absorption of electrolytes and water, and degradation of unabsorbed macronutrients.

Salt and Water Absorption

The colonic mucosa has tight intercellular junctions, which facilitate efficient extraction of sodium from small-bowel effluent and stools. The small-bowel effluent of 1500 mL that enters the colon every day contains 200 mmol Na^+, 100 mmol Cl^- and 10 mmol K^+. Normal stools contain 1–5 mmol Na^+, 1–2 mmol Cl^- and 5–15 mmol K^+ in 100–150 mL of water and a mass of 200 g. The colon is not physiologically homogeneous.[69] The proximal colon absorbs Na^+ better than the distal and Cl^- absorption is best in the transverse and sigmoid colon. The principal mechanisms of Na^+ absorption have been identified in man but they do not account for 100% of Na^+ absorbed:

(i) electrogenic Na^+ absorption not linked with another solute occurs more in the distal colon;

(ii) electroneutral Na^+ absorption, which appears to be indirectly linked with Cl^--absorption via parallel exchange mechanisms, Na^+–H^+ and Cl^-–HCO_3^-.

At equal concentrations of Na^+ and Cl^-, chloride absorption is greater than Na^+ and the difference is accounted for by HCO_3^- secretion. Failure of Cl^-–HCO_3^- exchange results in severe infantile diarrhoea in congenital chloridorrhoea. Unlike the small bowel, colonic NaCl absorption is not stimulated by glucose or amino acids.[69]

Water absorption occurs against a gradient of up to 50 mmol/L, unlike the isotonic absorption in the small bowel. The colon receives up to 1500 mL of fluid from the small bowel every day with peak flows of up to 5 mL/min, 2 h after a meal. Stool water is approximately 100–150 mL a day. Water absorption is stimulated by net NaCl absorption. The tight intercellular junctions prevent leakage back to the lumen. An increase in colonic water load by 4 L may lead to diarrhoea, but up to 80% of the total load may be absorbed and values of up to 7 L absorbed a day have been observed. The bolus size appears to be more critical; a 250-mL bolus does not alter faecal water output but 500 mL produces a liquid stool.[69] The control mechanisms for delivery of small-bowel effluent via the intact ileocaecal valve are therefore as important to colonic function as those that control gastric emptying via an intact pylorus.

Potassium Absorption

Potassium absorption is mainly passive and K^+ accumulates in the colonic lumen when luminal K^+ is less than 15 mmol/L. In dietary potassium excess or chronic renal failure, K^+ secretion is enhanced, thereby contributing to potassium homeostasis. K^+ is lost in faecal bacteria and colonic mucus, which contain up to 100 mmol/L.

Calcium, Magnesium and Zinc Absorption

Calcium, magnesium and zinc are absorbed mainly in the small bowel but absorption in the colon may occur under certain conditions, magnesium sulphate enemas for example. Failure of absorption, or secretion of these divalent cations, may occur in inflammatory bowel disease.[69]

Short-chain Fatty Acids

Although carbohydrate absorption is complete in the first 100 cm of the small bowel during liquid enteral feeding, this is not the case with normal diet. Complex carbohydrates, including fibre, reach the colon undigested in significant amounts and are degraded by bacteria to short-chain fatty acids (SCFA). Although SCFA are osmotically active, they are efficiently absorbed and are no longer thought to be a potent cause of osmotic diarrhoea.[69] SCFA also enhance colonic Na^+ absorption. In animals, up to 40% basal energy is derived from SCFA absorbed in the colon but in man it is not yet known how much SCFA contribute to energy intake. However, after jejunoileal bypass for obesity, up to 40% of unabsorbed carbohydrate is recovered via colonic SCFA absorption.[70] Moreover, subtotal resection of the colon does not influence SCFA concentration in stools.[71] Why starch should escape small-bowel absorption is of considerable interest since more starch may enter the colon than dietary fibre. Many cereals, potatoes and bananas contain amylase-resistant starch. For example, the baking of white bread alters starch to an amylase-resistant form. Raw starch granules in oats are amylase sensitive but 80% of banana starch is not because the crystal structure of this starch granule is in the resistant B form. Potato starch also has B-form crystal structure when raw but cooking renders this starch digestible, though 15% remains resistant. Some beans also contain amylase inhibitors. The physical form of carbohydrate is also important, particularly if the cellulose cell wall has not been broken down by cooking or chewing. Simple dietary sugars such as fructose (fruit), trehalose (mushrooms), stacchyose and raffinose (onions and legumes) may also be unabsorbed in the small intestine and contribute to colonic gas and SCFA production.

Protein and Fat Degradation
Protein degradation occurs in the colon, releasing ammonia, which is converted back to amino acids in the liver. Most ammonia, however, is derived from bacterial action on urea diffusing into the gut lumen. Fat may be absorbed intact but most is converted to poorly absorbed soaps or hydroxy-fatty acids, which contribute to diarrhoea.

Flatus Production
Hydrogen, CO_2 and methane are the main gases generated by bacterial degradation of starch in the colon but not all bacteria are capable of methane production. Some adaptation to fermentable carbohydrates may occur in man so that gas production diminishes, perhaps as a result of lactic acid production, which favours the growth of lactobacilli.[69,70] Only 30–50% of Western populations excrete methane in exhaled breath, although some produce methane without excretion in breath. In some subjects, sulphate-reducing bacteria produce sulphite and H_2S and such subjects do not produce methane. Explosions may occur during electrocautery procedures in the colon if the bowel has not been prepared or if mannitol preparations are used. Polyethylene glycol preparations are free from this hazard.

Diarrhoea

Diarrhoea is defined as a loose watery stool of greater than 200 g/day.

Mechanisms
Diarrhoea results from the failure of the small and/ or large bowel to absorb/reabsorb exogenous fluid intake or endogenous secretions. Approximately 9 L of fluid enter the gut each day (2 L from diet and 7 L of secretions) and all but 200 mL is absorbed under

normal conditions. The absorptive capacity for exogenous fluids is considerable, at least 8 L a day in the small bowel and 7 L a day in the colon. Absorptive capacity may be exceeded for the following reasons:

  (i) excessive fluid intake;
 (ii) diminished absorptive capacity;
(iii) decreased transit time;
 (iv) excessive endogenous secretion.

These four categories are not mutually exclusive causes of diarrhoea and in many conditions more than one process may account for it. For example, in coeliac disease, diminished absorptive capacity, increased small-bowel secretion and osmotic load due to malabsorbed carbohydrate and protein all contribute to diarrhoea. Paradoxically, small-bowel transit may be slow because of negative feedback from the terminal ileum, which is rarely affected in coeliac disease. Magnesium sulphate, which causes diarrhoea by an osmotic effect, also stimulates small-intestinal motility.

1. Excessive Fluid Intake. This is a rare cause of diarrhoea and may occur in polydipsic patients and with excessive beer intake. Patients with diseases or resections of small or large bowel are more susceptible to diarrhoea induced or exacerbated by excessive fluid intake. This may become critical in patients with short-bowel syndrome when bowel effluent not only may exceed input but also contains large quantities of electrolytes and trace elements.

2. Diminished Absorptive Capacity. This may relate either to specific reduction in digestion (e.g. hypolactasia) or generalized reduction in overall absorptive surface area (e.g. coeliac disease), or both. The diarrhoea associated with many conditions is often multifactorial, with diminished absorption, increased secretion and osmotic factors all contributing.

3. Decreased Transit Time (Diarrhoea Motrice). At one time, increased motility was thought to explain most causes of diarrhoea but the discovery of secretory diarrhoeas has altered this concept. All causes of increased luminal influx may lead to enhanced motility as a secondary phenomenon. Laxatives, including castor oil, phenolphthalein and magnesium sulphate, all cause an increase in small-intestinal motility for up to 72 h. Quinidine decreases bowel transit time to one-third and erythromycin, metaclopramide and domperidone enhance peristalsis. Gastric emptying is enhanced by pyloric damage and hypolactasia or exocrine pancreatic insufficiency. Small-bowel motility is much faster when the 'ileal break' is no longer active, as after surgery or in Crohn's disease.

4. Excessive Endogenous Secretion. Excessive salivary, pancreatic or biliary secretions have not been described. Gastric secretion may be excessive in Zollinger–Ellison syndrome but this is only one cause

TABLE 21.6
CAUSES OF SECRETORY DIARRHOEA

Infections
Viral:
  rotavirus, Norwalk agent
Bacterial:
  salmonellae, shigellae, staphylococci, campylobacter,
  yersiniae, enterotoxigenic *E. coli*, cholera
Protozoal:
  Giardia lamblia, Entamoeba histolytica

Inflammation
Ulcerative proctocolitis
Crohn's colitis

Drugs
Laxatives
Antibiotics (with or without *Clostridium difficile* toxin)
5-aminosalicylate

Hormonal
Polypeptide-secreting tumours:
  VIPoma, medullary carcinoma of thyroid, gastrinoma,
  carcinoid syndrome, somatostatinoma, glucagonoma
Thyrotoxicosis (motility more important)

of the diarrhoea seen in this condition. Small-bowel villous atrophy and acid destruction of pancreatic enzymes also occur. Fordtran suggested the terms 'osmotic' and 'secretory' diarrhoea to distinguish between decreased absorption and enhanced secretion, respectively. Net small or large bowel secretion is often the result of a combination of these two categories.

Osmotic and Secretory Diarrhoea
Differentiation between osmotic and secretory diarrhoea is sometimes important to identify the small group of patients with secretory diarrheoa in whom standard investigations failed to reveal a diagnosis (Table 21.6). The measurement of stool volume in response to fasting and the calculation of osmotic gap in stool may be useful.

1. *Response to Fasting.* Fasting over 1–3 days with simultaneous intravenous hydration has little influence on stool volume in pure secretory states. However, abolition of diarrhoea with fasting does not rule out a secretory diarrhoea. For example, bile-acid and fatty-acid malabsorption stimulates net colonic water and electrolyte secretion, which is eliminated by fasting.[72]

2. *Osmotic Gap.* The osmolality, sodium and potassium content of the stool supernatant after centrifugation are measured and the osmotic gap is calculated;

$$\text{osmotic gap} = \text{osmolality} - 2\,[\text{Na} + \text{K}].$$

A value in excess of 50 mosmol/kg indicates an osmotic diarrhoea but in some studies a value of up to 100 mosmol/kg has been used.[73] The response to fasting and calculation of osmotic gap are particu-

larly helpful in patients with large volume stools of greater than 500 mL/day but differentiation is more difficult with lesser volumes. Thus diarrhoea that responds to fasting (a reduction in volume to 200 g) and has an osmotic gap of more than 50 mosmol/kg is probably osmotic in origin.

Aetiological factors
Chronic secretory diarrhoea may be caused by salmonellae, campylobacter, yersiniae and *Giardia lamblia* via cytopathic effects on small-or large-bowel mucosa or via secretagogue enterotoxins. Drugs such as quinidine, certain antibiotics, diuretics and occasionally 5-aminosalicylates may cause secretory diarrhoea but the most important are the laxatives of the phenolphthalein and anthracene groups. Excessive ingestion of magnesium-containing medications (e.g. milk of magnesia, antacids or magnesium-containing mineral supplements) can cause an osmotic diarrhoea and can also stimulate small-bowel motility. Measurement of faecal magnesium concentration and output may be useful in identifying patients with surreptitious magnesium intake.[74]

Excessive ingestion of poorly absorbable sugars such as fructose in fruit juice, sorbitol in vitamin C supplements or chewing gum, and lactulose can cause osmotic diarrhoea and often goes unrecognized. Hormonal causes of secretory diarrhoea are uncommon or rare and should only be suspected after assessing the response to fasting and exclusion of other more common causes.

Faecal Occult Blood and Colorectal Tumours

Eighty per cent of all colorectal cancers and about 50% of all larger adenomas are characterized by intermittent minor bleeding. Such occult blood can be detected in the stools using chemical or immunological methods. The chemical methods depend upon the oxidation of a phenolic chromogen in gum guaiac by the peroxidase-like activity of haem to yield a blue-coloured end-product. A modified guaiac-based test (Haemoccult test), with a sensitivity that has been kept deliberately low to reduce the number of false-positive results, is the most commonly used test of faecal occult blood. False-negative reactions are, however, common if blood loss is less than 10 mL a day. False-negative results may also occur with dry faecal specimens. Rehydration of the Haemoccult slide has been attempted to avoid this problem but is not recommended as it has been shown to affect the sensitivity and specificity of the test.[75] The guaiac-based methods are liable to dietary interference from red meats and blood products and from naturally occurring peroxidases in uncooked vegetables and fruits such as cauliflower, turnip, broccoli, cucumber, mushrooms, courgette and melon. A positive Haemoccult test due to increased gastrointestinal blood loss may occur in patients taking aspirin and non-steroidal anti-inflammatory drugs. Several immunological tests specific for human haemoglobin have been developed.[76,77] They are more sensitive and less liable to interference from animal haemoglobin and vegetable peroxidases. The increase in sensitivity, however, is associated with a corresponding decrease in specificity.

Faecal occult-blood tests have been shown to be useful for screening patients with symptoms suggestive of colorectal disease. In one study of 742 patients, 19% had positive tests and of these 20% had a colorectal cancer. Of the 81% of patients with negative tests only 1.5% had a colorectal cancer.[78] The majority of patients with colorectal carcinoma, however, present with tumours that have already spread beyond the bowel, and despite improved diagnostic techniques in recent years the 5-year survival rate has remained unchanged at 50%. A significant improvement in the prognosis of colorectal carcinoma can only be expected if the tumour is detected in its early phase and therefore can only be achieved by screening asymptomatic populations over the age of 40 or 50. Results from three European randomized controlled trials of population screening using the Haemoccult test showed positive rates of 1.1–2.3%. The positive predictive values were 11–17% for cancer and 36–41% for adenomas.[79–81] In addition and of considerable significance is the rate of false-negative Haemoccult test results in patients with cancer, which has been reported at 20–44%, giving a sensitivity of 54–77%. A recent report by the United Kingdom Coordinating Committee on Cancer Research (UKCCCR) has recommended that Haemoccult, or other faecal occult-blood tests of equal or better performance, should be used in selecting symptomatic patients in general practice for referral for urgent investigation.[82] Screening for colorectal carcinoma by annual faecal occult-blood testing for all adults above the age of 50 years has been recommended in some countries. Although preliminary reports have produced encouraging results, controversy still exists over the cost and benefits of such a policy. Improvements in specificity and sensitivity of faecal occult-blood tests and proof of benefit in reducing cancer morbidity and mortality are required before screening programmes are generally adopted.

THE PANCREAS

The pancreas is a soft, oblong gland (12.5 cm long and 2.5 cm thick) that lies posterior to the greater curvature of the stomach. Its head is in the duodenal curve and its tail extends to the spleen. It is made up of small clusters of glandular epithelial cells. About 1% of the cells, the islets of Langerhans, form the endocrine portion of the pancreas and consist of α, β and δ cells that secrete glucagon, insulin and somatostatin, respectively. The remaining 99% of the cells, called acini, are the exocrine portion of the organ and secrete various digestive enzymes in a bicarbonate-rich juice. The pancreatic juice is drained via a system of ducts into the main pancreatic duct, which, in most people, unites with the common bile duct before opening into the duodenum at the ampulla of Vater.

Regulation of Pancreatic Secretion

Each day the pancreas produces about 1500 mL of pancreatic juice. It consists mostly of water, sodium, potassium, chloride, bicarbonate and enzymes. The sodium bicarbonate gives the pancreatic juice a slightly alkaline pH (7.1–8.2) that stops the action of pepsin from the stomach and creates the proper environment for the enzymes in the small intestine. The pancreatic enzymes are:

- a carbohydrate-digesting enzyme (amylase)
- several protein-digesting enzymes (trypsin, chymotrypsin and carboxypolypeptidase)
- a fat-digesting enzyme (pancreatic lipase)
- nucleic acid-digesting enzymes (ribonuclease and deoxyribonuclease).

Pancreatic secretion is regulated by both neural and hormonal mechanisms. When the cephalic and gastric phases of gastric secretion occur, parasympathetic impulses are simultaneously transmitted along the vagus nerve to the pancreas that result in the secretion of pancreatic enzymes. In response to chyme, the small intestine secretes secretin and cholecystokinin; the secretin stimulates the pancreas to produce a juice rich in sodium bicarbonate ions and the cholecystokinin produces a juice rich in digestive enzymes.

Clinical Presentation of Pancreatic Disease

Pancreatic disease can manifest as acute sudden parenchymal destruction (acute pancreatitis) or slowly progressive destruction (chronic pancreatitis) that may be accompanied by impaired islet-cell function giving rise to overt diabetes mellitus.

Acute Pancreatitis

Acute pancreatitis occurs most frequently in patients with disease of the biliary tract, alcoholism or both. It may occur during the course of infections such as mumps, coxsackie B virus and *Mycoplasma pneumoniae*. Metabolic abnormalities such as hypertriglyceridaemia and hyperparathyroidism are also associated with acute pancreatitis. The patient commonly presents with acute upper abdominal pain, which often radiates to the back. Nausea and vomiting occur in up to 90% of cases. Severe pancreatitis may present with hypovolaemic shock or coma. Metabolic complications include hypocalcaemia (in up to 30% of cases), which occurs 5–7 days after onset, hyperglycaemia (in 30–70%) and hyperlipidaemia. Non-metabolic complications include pseudocyst formation, hepatocellular and/or obstructive jaundice, haemorrhage, pleural effusion, ascites and, rarely, pancreatic abscess formation (in up to 5%).

TABLE 21.7

CAUSES OF HYPERAMYLASAEMIA

Gastrointestinal and abdominal disorders
Pancreatic disease (P):
    acute pancreatitis
    chronic pancreatitis
    pancreatic pseudocyst or abscess
    pancreatic carcinoma
    pancreatic trauma
Dissecting or ruptured aortic aneurysm (P)
Acute mesenteric infarction (P)
Perforated duodenal ulcer (P)
Intestinal obstruction (P)
Acute appendicitis
Peritonitis (P and S)
Liver metastasis (S)
Biliary-tract disease (P)
Ruptured tubal pregnancy (S)
Ovarian malignancy (S)
Pelvic inflammatory disease (S)
Prostatic malignancy (S)
Prostatitis (S)
Renal failure (S and P)
Renal transplantation (S)

Thoracic disorder
Congestive heart failure
Lung carcinoma (S)
Pulmonary infarction (S)
Cardiac surgery (S)

Miscellaneous
Acute alcohol intoxication (P and S)
Diabetic ketoacidosis (P and S)
Mumps (S)
Cystic fibrosis with normal pancreatic function (S)
Macroamylasaemia (S)
Septicaemia
Drugs:
    opiates (P), heroin (S), azathiaprine, chlorthiazides, oestrogens, valproate, frusemide, sulphonamides and tetracyclines

Predominant isoenzyme type: (P) pancreatic; (S) salivary.

Diagnosis

The only definitive way to diagnose acute pancreatitis is direct inspection of the pancreas at laparotomy. In practice, the diagnosis in the majority of cases is based on high clinical probabilities and is supported by indirect tests.

Serum and Urinary Amylase. The laboratory test most widely used to support the diagnosis of acute pancreatitis is the total serum amylase activity. This rises within 2–12 h of the onset, reaching a maximum at 12–72 h and returning to normal by the third or fourth day. There is usually a four- to six-fold increase in serum amylase activity and a value of around three times the upper limit of normal is widely used in the UK to support the diagnosis. The magnitude of the rise is not related to the severity of the attack but the greater the rise, the higher the probability of acute pancreatitis. A normal serum amylase activity is very rare in acute pancreatitis and may occur if the patient presents a few days after the onset of an attack or if serum is lipaemic. In these cases, measurement of urinary amylase activity may be useful since hyperamylasuria may persist for longer periods after serum amylase activity has returned to normal following acute pancreatitis. Increase in total serum or urinary amylase activity is not specific for acute pancreatitis and both may be increased in many other conditions (Table 21.7). Determination of isoenzymes (P-type or S-type) may sometimes help to identify the origin. Hyperamylasuria parallels hyperamylasaemia except in the rare condition macroamylasaemia. In this condition amylase is probably complexed with IgG, IgA or other plasma proteins and cannot be filtered through the glomeruli because of its large size (> 200 000 mol.wt.).

Increased renal clearance of amylase related to creatinine clearance (amylase clearance/creatinine clearance) has been suggested as a more specific test for the diagnosis of acute pancreatitis.[83] Raised values, however, have been observed in many other conditions and may simply be due to tubular proteinuria associated with acute severe illness.[83]

Total amylase activity in blood comprises two pancreatic isoamylases: isoP1 and isoP2 and four salivary isoamylases: isoS1–4. Determination of pancreatic isoamylase is now possible with a variety of techniques that include electrophoresis, chromatography, isoelectric focusing and radioimmunoassay. A test using an amylase inhibitor from wheat, which is 100 times more potent at inhibiting isoS than isoP, is now commercially available (Pharmacia Uppsala, Sweden). IsoP determination may be useful in differentiating between hyperamylasaemia caused by acute pancreatitis and other causes of hyperamylasaemia. An electrophoretically distinct isoamylase isoP3 has been isolated in the serum of patients with acute pancreatitis. In a comparative study, the diagnostic efficiency of isoP3 was 98%, 82% for total amylase and 91% for isoP2.[84]

Serum Lipase. Most of the lipase found in serum is produced in the pancreas but some is also secreted by gastric, pulmonary and intestinal mucosa. In acute pancreatitis, serum lipase activity rises within 2–12 h of the onset of the attack and may remain elevated for 10–14 days. The determination of serum lipase may therefore be useful in patients presenting late in the course of the disease when both serum and urinary amylase have returned to normal. Several methods are now available for measuring serum lipase activity, which include turbidimetric, colorimetric using a defined synthetic substrate, and enzyme immunoassay. In one study, serum lipase identified all patients with acute pancreatitis (sensitivity 100%) and was most useful in patients with a modest increase in total serum amylase.[85] In a more recent evaluation, the three pancreatic enzymes (immunoreactive trypsin, lipase and pancreatic isoamylase) showed similar sensitivities and specificities in the diagnosis of acute pancreatitis.[86]

Serum Immunoreactive Trypsin and Trypsinogen. The pancreas synthesizes two different trypsins (I and II) in the form of the inactive proenzymes (trypsinogens I and II). When these zymogens are secreted into the duodenum, the trypsinogens are converted to the active enzyme trypsin. The trypsin liberated is rapidly bound by protease inhibitors such as α_1-antitrypsin and α_2-macroglobulin. Catalytic assays give negative results with these forms of bound trypsin but recently radioimmunoassay methods capable of measuring most forms of the enzyme in serum have been developed. In acute pancreatitis, serum immunoreactive trypsin rises in parallel with serum amylase activity to peak values ranging from 2 to 400 times the upper reference range. Concentrations have, however, also been shown to be increased in 52% of patients with chronic pancreatitis, 19% in pancreatic carcinoma, 64% in common bile-duct stones and 100% in patients with chronic renal failure.[87]

Serum Elastase. Elastase is an endopeptidase found in pancreatic juice that occurs in the circulation of normal healthy individuals in the form of its zymogen, proelastase. In acute pancreatitis, free elastase, in addition to proelastase, escapes into the circulation and high serum concentrations persist for several days after amylase activities have returned to normal. In a recent study, the sensitivity of serum elastase-1 level for acute pancreatitis was 97% at the day of admission and 100% within 48 h after the onset of pain. The sensitivities at 48–96 h after the onset of pain compared with other enzymes were: elastase 93%, lipase 78%, trypsin 59% and amylase 17%.[88] The specificity is also high with respect to other gastrointestinal diseases but levels are raised in chronic pancreatitis and pancreatic carcinoma.[89]

Serum Phospholipase A_2. Phospholipase A_2 is produced in the pancreas in the form of its inactive precursor, prophospholipase A_2, which is activated to phospholipase A_2 by trypsin and other proteolytic enzymes when secreted into the duodenum. Phospholipase A_2 converts lecithin and cephalin in cell membranes and bile into their cytotoxic lysocompounds, which have detergent-like properties. Intrapancreatic activation and release of these lysocompounds in acute pancreatitis may lead to pancreatic necrosis. Patients with acute pancreatitis have marked elevations in serum phospholipase A_2 activity, which correlated with the severity of the disease.[90] In one study, serum phospholipase A_2 determinations, by an enzymatic method, discriminated clearly between patients with acute necrotizing pancreatitis and those with oedematous pancreatitis.[91] Others, however, found that serum phospholipase A_2 activities did not correlate with patients' survival and were not helpful in assessing prognosis.[92]

Assessment of Severity of Acute Pancreatitis
Several methods have been proposed for objectively assessing the severity of acute pancreatitis.[93] The four most valuable indicators are serum albumin less than 30 g/L, haematocrit less than 30%, serum creatinine more than 180 μmol/L and serum calcium (corrected for albumin) less than 2.0 mmol/L. Serum concentrations of C-reactive protein also have been recently shown to be useful in assessing the severity of acute pancreatitis.[94]

Chronic Pancreatitis

Chronic pancreatitis is the clinical manifestation of a continuing process of inflammation and fibrosis of the pancreas resulting in permanent loss of function. It is much less common than acute pancreatitis. Chronic pancreatitis is usually associated with ethanol abuse and sometimes with hyperparathyroidism or hyperlipidaemia but no cause is found in about half of the affected patients. The most common presenting feature is recurrent episodes of abdominal pain, which may be indistinguishable from that of acute pancreatitis. In a minority of patients (5–10%) the disease is painless and these may present with steatorrhoea, weight loss or diabetes mellitus.

Diagnosis
The diagnosis of chronic pancreatitis is usually suspected in a patient with a history of ethanol abuse and recurring attacks of abdominal pain. A plain radiograph of the abdomen may show pancreatic calcification. The diagnosis can be confirmed by demonstrating pancreatic exocrine hypofunction by direct intubation techniques or indirect tests.

Biochemical Assessment of Exocrine Pancreatic Function
Diagnostic tests of exocrine pancreatic function are summarized in Table 21.8.

A. Direct or Intubation Tests. These involve the collection of duodenal aspirate by intubation or of pure pancreatic juice by direct cannulation of the pancreatic duct using endoscopic retrograde cholangiopancreatography (ERCP). The total output of pancreatic juice, bicarbonate and enzymes (trypsin, lipase, amylase) are measured after stimulation either directly (secretin–cholecystokinin, caerulin or bombesin) or indirectly (Lundh meal).

(a) *Secretin–cholecystokinin Test.* In this test, a double-lumen gastroduodenal tube is positioned under fluoroscopic guidance so that the distal opening lies beyond the ampulla of Vater in the duodenum and the proximal opening in the stomach. Continuous suction of gastric juice is applied to avoid contamination. After two baseline 15-min aspirates have been obtained, secretin (0.25–1.0 Crick–Harper–Raper units/kg per hour) is given by continuous

TABLE 21.8
DIAGNOSTIC TESTS OF EXOCRINE PANCREATIC FUNCTION

A. *Direct tests*
a. Secretin–cholecystokinin, caerulin or bombesin test
b. Lundh test

B. *Indirect tests*
a. Tubeless tests:
   PABA test
   Pancreolauryl test
b. Faecal tests:
   Faecal fats
   Faecal nitrogen
   Faecal trypsin and chymotrypsin
   Faecal isotopic tests
c. Breath tests:
   $^{14}CO_2$ breath tests
d. Serum enzymes:
   Serum pancreatic isoamylase
   Serum lipase
   Serum immunoreactive trypsin
e. Sweat tests:
   Sweat sodium and chloride

infusion, followed 30 min later by cholecystokinin (1 Ivy–Hunde unit/kg). Aspiration of duodenal content is continued for 80 min. Other peptide hormones like caerulin and bombesin can be used instead of cholecystokinin.[95]

(b) *Lundh meal.* This is an artificial meal containing fat (6%), protein (5%), carbohydrate (15%) and a non-nutrient fibre (74%). It provides a physiological stimulus because it relies on endogenous release of secretin and cholecystokinin from the duodenal mucosa. Abnormal results, however, can be obtained in patients with mucosal diseases (e.g. coeliac disease). In addition, the test has many limitations. Water and bicarbonate output cannot be measured as these are affected by the contents of the meal. Total enzyme output, which is much more discriminatory than mean or maximum enzyme concentration, cannot be determined because duodenal contents can only be sampled intermittently.

Interpretation and Predictive Value of Direct Tests. In healthy individuals, the volume flow following stimulation is 2.0 mL/kg and the peak bicarbonate concentration is 80–90 mmol/L. Low concentrations of bicarbonate have been reported in patients with chronic pancreatitis, pancreatic carcinoma, cystic fibrosis and pancreatic calcification. Variations in the dosage, potency of secretin preparations and the technique used account for the significant overlap in results obtained by different investigators. A reduction in the output of water and bicarbonate seems to be more pronounced in chronic pancreatitis whereas a decrease in enzyme output is more affected in pancreatic carcinoma. Trypsin is the most frequently measured enzyme because it is less sensitive to pH

variations but at least two enzymes should be measured following stimulation because enzyme secretion may be divergent in different disease states. Low trypsin activities were found in 88% of patients with pancreatic insufficiency.[96]

Limitations of Direct (Intubation) Tests. Although the direct (intubation) tests are probably the most sensitive and specific tests for pancreatic insufficiency they suffer from several drawbacks. They are technically difficult and techniques have not been standardized in respect of dosage and potency of preparations, for example. They are invasive and unpleasant to the patient. Misleading results may be obtained due to contamination with gastric juice and incomplete collections.

A. Indirect Tests
(a) Tubeless tests. In these tests, the patient is orally given a substrate that upon hydrolysis by a pancreatic specific enzyme liberates a product. This product is readily absorbed from the gut, conjugated and excreted in the urine where it can be measured.

PABA Test. This uses a synthetic peptide, *N*-benzoyl-L-tyrosyl-*p*-aminobenzoic acid (**NBT-PABA**), which is hydrolysed by chymotrypsin to release *p*-aminobenzoic acid (**PABA**). The latter is readily absorbed, and after conjugation in the liver, is excreted in the urine. Its concentration in a timed urine collection can be determined spectrophotometrically or by high-performance liquid chromatography. The substrate is usually given in dosages between 0.15 g and 2 g, together with a test meal, a Lundh meal for example. The patient is encouraged to drink water to ensure adequate diuresis and the urine is collected for a period of 6 h. Alterations in intestinal absorption, hepatic function and renal excretion may affect the results. For these reasons, various modifications have been proposed. Free PABA can be given on a separate day and a 'PABA excretion index' is derived. Concurrent administration of [^{14}C]-PABA- or *p*-aminosalicylic acid with the NBT-PABA has also been used.[97,98] A number of drugs (e.g. paracetamol, diuretics, sulphonamides and chloramphenicol) and certain foodstuffs (e.g. prunes and cranberries) may interfere with the spectrophotometric assay.

Pancreolauryl Test. This uses the synthetic ester fluorescein dilaurate as a substrate, which is hydrolysed by pancreatic cholesterol ester hydrolase to release fluorescein.[99] This free water-soluble product is readily absorbed in the small intestine, partly conjugated in the liver and excreted in the urine as fluorescein glucuronide. This compound becomes orange-green and fluoresces at an alkaline pH and can easily be measured by spectrophotometry or fluirometry. Its concentration in a timed urine collection is directly proportional to the digestive capacity and hence the exocrine pancreatic function. In the test, 0.5 mmol of fluorescein dilaurate in capsules is given orally, together with a standard meal. Digestive aids and drugs such as sulphasalazine or vitamins should be avoided before and during the test. The patient is encouraged to drink at least 500 mL of water or dilute orange squash to ensure sufficient diuresis and the urine is collected for a period of 10 h. To allow for individual variations of intestinal absorption, hepatic conjugation and urinary excretion, the test is repeated on a separate day using 0.5 mmol of free fluorescein. The percentage of fluorescein excreted on the test day (T) and the control day (C) is calculated and the ratio of T/C is derived. A T/C ratio of 30 or more is considered normal and a ratio of less than 20 indicates pancreatic insufficiency. A T/C ratio between 20 and 30 is considered equivocal and the test should be repeated. False-positive results have been found in patients with gastric and gallbladder resections, coeliac disease and some cases of inflammatory bowel disease.[100] Bacterial overgrowth may influence the results as some bacteria (streptococci) are able to hydrolyse fluorescein dilaurate.

Predictive Value of Tubeless Test. Various reports indicate that the PABA test has a sensitivity ranging from 39% to 94% and specificity from 76% to 100%.[99,101] Compared with direct and other indirect tests of pancreatic function, the sensitivity of the pancreolauryl test varies from 63% to 100% and specificity from 39% to 100%.[102] In comparison with the PABA test, the pancreolauryl test is probably more sensitive and specific. In addition, it requires no complex hydrolytic conditions and is not subject to interference from drugs or serum compounds. Both tests, however, provide satisfactory simple screening tests of exocrine pancreatic function and can also be used in monitoring pancreatic enzyme replacement therapy.

(b) Faecal tests. Pancreatic function is essential for the digestion and absorption of dietary starch, fats and proteins. Increase in faecal fats and nitrogen occurs in significant pancreatic insufficiency and microscopic examination of the stool shows undigested cell nuclei and meat fibres and droplets of neutral fat.

Faecal Fat Excretion. Faecal fat concentration (*see* p. 359) is abnormal in up to 50% of patients with chronic pancreatitis. The major clinical limitation of faecal fat analysis is its inability to differentiate between intestinal and pancreatic causes of steatorrhoea. A normal fat excretion does not exclude pancreatic insufficiency since steatorrhoea may not develop until 90% of the acinar tissue is destroyed and when lipase and co-lipase activities are 1–2% of normal levels.

Faecal Isotopic Tests. Faecal isotopic tests to assess fat absorption (*see* Small intestine above) have been used to differentiate between pancreatic maldigestion and intestinal malabsorption (*see* Small intestine above). The differentiation is based on the assumption that radiolabelled fatty acids, but not radiolabelled triglycerides, should be absorbed normally in pancreatic steatorrhoea. In one study using [14C]-triolein and [3H]-oleic acid, separation was accomplished in 16 out of 17 patients with pancreatic and intestinal disease on the basis of the ratio of the two isotopes in the stool.[41]

Faecal Nitrogen. Faecal nitrogen excretion is also raised in pancreatic insufficiency but to a lesser extent than faecal fats and therefore is less widely used.

Faecal Trypsin and Chymotrypsin. The measurement of faecal trypsin or chymotrypsin activity has been used for the diagnosis of pancreatic insufficiency, especially in children with suspected cystic fibrosis. Faecal chymotrypsin is more stable and more sensitive in detecting pancreatic dysfunction.[103] Chymotrypsin, however, is firmly bound to stool particles and early attempts to solubilize the enzyme were unsuccessful. A simple photometric assay, which eliminates problems caused by debris-bound enzyme, has recently been introduced.[104] False-low results may occur in severe coeliac disease and partial gastrectomy due to inadequate stimulation of pancreatic secretion and false-normal results may occur in patients with mild pancreatic insufficiency.[96]

(c) Breath tests. The [14C]-triolein breath test (*see* Small intestine above) has been recommended as a preliminary screening test for fat malabsorption. Patients with suspected pancreatic insufficiency who have an abnormal [14C]-triolein test may be further investigated by repeating the test using equimolar amounts of 14C-labelled fatty acids. Normal results would then indicate that fat malabsorption is due to pancreatic insufficiency and not to intestinal malabsorption. In another modification, the [14C]-triolein was ingested with and without pancreatic enzyme supplements. This modified test clearly differentiated between patients with pancreatic insufficiency and those with steatorrhoea due to other causes.[105]

(d) Serum Pancreatic Enzymes. Random levels of total serum amylase or following stimulation by secretagogues are of no value in the diagnosis of pancreatic insufficiency. Serum isoP, lipase and immunoreactive trypsin were low, normal or high in patients with chronic pancreatitis or pancreatic cancer.[106] Low levels are only found in patients with severe pancreatic insufficiency and steatorrhoea but are too insensitive to detect early disease. Attempts have been made to increase the diagnostic value of serum enzyme measurements by stimulating pancreatic secretion. There was no increase in serum trypsin following a Lundh meal,[107] administration of cholecystokinin[108] or caerulin.[109] Secretin stimulation, however, produced a rise in serum trypsin in normal subjects and in patients with mild pancreatic insufficiency without steatorrhoea but no rise in patients with pancreatic steatorrhoea.[109,110] Administration of bombesin produces a marked increase in serum trypsin in healthy subjects; this response is significantly reduced in patients with chronic pancreatitis.[111]

Serum immunoreactive trypsin is a useful screening test for pancreatic insufficiency in cystic fibrosis.[112] In healthy newborn infants, concentrations of serum trypsin are usually within the reference range for older children but infants with cystic fibrosis have a high serum trypsin due to pancreatic ductular blockage.[113] Neonatal screening programmes for cystic fibrosis have demonstrated that the measurement of immunoreactive trypsin in blood collected on filter paper has a sensitivity close to 100% with a false-positive incidence of less than 1%.[114] False-negative results may, however, occur in patients without pancreatic involvement.

(e) Sweat tests. Cystic fibrosis is the most common genetic disorder in caucasian populations, with an average incidence of 1:2000 live births. Nearly 90% of patients with cystic fibrosis present with exocrine pancreatic insufficiency caused by obstruction of the small ducts by abnormal mucus secretion. Abnormal electrolytes' secretion is a characteristic and constant finding in cystic fibrosis and the diagnosis is usually based on clinical history together with the finding of elevated sodium and chloride concentrations in sweat. The test usually becomes positive between 3 and 5 weeks of age with levels above 60 mmol/L for sodium and above 70 mmol/L for chloride. Sweat is collected by iontophoresis into a preweighed filter paper or a Macroduct collector[115] (Wescor Macroduct System). A minimum acceptable weight of 100 mg of sweat or a volume of 10 μL is required. Very low sweat rates may occur in premature, malnourished or dehydrated infants and may lead to falsely low results. False-high levels may be obtained if the skin is contaminated and has not been cleaned properly. A retrospective analysis of 1183 sweat sodium and chloride results from two centres in the UK showed that in all 67 patients with cystic fibrosis the sweat chloride concentration was greater than 70 mmol/L and the sum of sodium and chloride was greater than 140 mmol/L but the sodium concentration was less than 60 mmol/L in seven patients.[116] It is therefore recommended that both sodium and chloride should be measured to minimize the possibility of misdiagnosis.

MALABSORPTION

Definition

Malabsorption is the failure of the small-bowel mucosa to absorb single or multiple nutrients, resulting in gastrointestinal symptoms and nutritional deficiencies. Malabsorption may result from inadequate luminal digestion, defective mucosal absorption, disturbance of lymphatic bowel drainage or various combinations of these (Table 21.9).

Symptoms

Although steatorrhoea is the most common manifestation of malabsorption and is defined as greater than 5 g (18 mmol/L) faecal fat excretion a day, malabsorption does not always lead to steatorrhoea. Watery diarrhoea may predominate and occasionally patients may be constipated. Non-specific abdominal symptoms such as pain, cramps, bloating, gurgling, nausea and flatulence are common. The combination of weight loss and voracious appetite occurs frequently, as in thyrotoxicosis, which is also a rare cause of steatorrhoea. Symptoms relating to malnutrition or to specific nutrient deficiencies may also be apparent, together with appropiate biochemical evidence such as low serum albumin, electrolyte disturbances, hypocalcaemia, hypophosphataemia, low serum zinc, magnesium, iron and vitamin D.

Practical Approach to the Investigation of Diarrhoea/ Steatorrhoea

We would suggest a practical approach to the investigation of diarrhoea or steatorrhoea that reflects hospital clinical practice and is based upon the concept that common pathologies occur commonly (Table 21.10).

Clinical Assessment

A clear and detailed history often points to the cause of the diarrhoea or steatorrhoea. A history of gastrectomy or pancreatic surgery would be sufficient to explain the cause of the diarrhoea. Assessment of alcohol intake or a history of acute pancreatitis would suggest pancreatic steatorrhoea. The onset of acute watery diarrhoea during or soon after returning from holiday points to an infective cause. A history of nocturnal diarrhoea always implies organic disease such as ulcerative colitis. Passage of liquid stools followed by formed stools on the same day may indicate a distal colitis with sparing of the proximal colon. Bitty stools mixed with watery stools, or hard stools alternating with loose stools, suggest irritable bowel syndrome or diverticular disease. Diarrhoea in the presence of demonstrable constipation is termed 'spurious' diarrhoea and is the result of constipation, whatever the cause. The presence of mucus or blood is also of great importance. The passage of blood *per rectum* may be mimicked by beetroot or intravenous bromsulphaline, which colour the stools red. In addition to melena, black stools may be caused by bismuth-containing drugs and iron preparations. Finally, it is important to identify whether the 'diarrhoea' is, in fact, steatorrhoea. The full description of stools is often elicited only with some difficulty from embarrassed patients. The pale, fatty, foamy,

TABLE 21.9

TABLE 21.9
AETIOLOGICAL CLASSIFICATION OF MALABSORPTION

I. Intestinal diseases
Mucosal
Coeliac disease
Cow's milk sensitivity in infants
Disaccharidase deficiences:
  hypolactasia
  sucrase-isomaltase deficiency
Tropical sprue
Whipple's disease
Intestinal lymphangiectasia
Glucose-galactose malabsorption
Enterokinase deficiency
Abetalipoproteinaemia
Structural
Gastrointestinal resection
Crohn's disease
Blind loops, fistulae, diverticula
Lymphoma
Idiopathic chromic ulcerative enteritis
Eosinophilic gastroenteropathy
Amyloidosis

II. Biliary insufficiency
Biliary obstruction
Parenchymal liver disease
Terminal ileal resection
Terminal ileal disease
Bacterial overgrowth

III. Pancreatic insufficiency
Pancreatic disease
Carcinoma of the pancreas
Chronic pancreatitis
Cystic fibrosis
Pancreatectomy
Pancreatic duct obstruction
Defective stimulation of pancreatic secretion
Gastric surgery
Intestinal disease
Malnutrition
Inactivation of pancreatic enzymes
Zollinger–Ellison syndrome

IV. Infection
Travellers' diarrhoea
Acute enteritis
Intestinal parasitic diseases
Intestinal tuberculosis
Small-intestinal bacterial overgrowth

V. Drugs
Antacids
Cholestyramine
Colchicine
Ethanol
Laxative abuse
Metformin
Methotrexate
Methyldopa
Neomycin
P-Aminosalicylic acid
Phenindione

VI. Systemic diseases
Addison's disease
Carcinoid syndrome
Collagen diseases
Diabetes mellitus
Hyperparathyroidism
Hyperthyroidism
Hypoparathyroidism
Hypothyroidism

TABLE 21.10
INVESTIGATIONS OF DIARRHOEA AND STEATORRHOEA

Initial investigations
Serum urea, creatinine and electrolytes
Serum bilirubin, liver enzymes and prothrombin time
Serum calcium, phosphate and magnesium
Serum albumin, total proteins and immunoglobulins
Serum α_1-acid glycoprotein and C-reactive protein
Thyroid function tests
Plasma glucose
Full blood count, red-cell folate and serum vitamin B_{12}
Faecal fat excretion
Microbiological stool analysis

Investigations to identify the cause of diarrhoea or steatorrhoea
Small- and large-bowel contrast radiography
Non-invasive tests of small-bowel mucosal damage and intestinal permeability
Histological examination of small- and large-bowel mucosa
Assessment of exocrine pancreatic function: PABA or pancreolauryl test
Assessment of terminal ileal function: ^{75}SeHCAT
Stool osmotic gap and response to fasting

offensive and floating stools requiring more than one flush are characteristic of steatorrhoea but often the history is inadequate. The presence of obvious free-fat globules in the stool is said to signify a pancreatic pathology and the so called 'silver' stool, pancreatic carcinoma.

Initial General Investigations
Serum Electrolytes, Urea and Creatinine. Diarrhoea can cause electrolyte disturbance and dehydration to a degree that will depend on the severity of the diarrhoea or extent of malabsorption.

Liver Enzymes, Bilirubin and Prothrombin Time. Raised serum alanine or aspartate aminotransferase and alkaline phosphatase activities, serum bilirubin and prolonged prothrombin time will point to common bile duct obstruction or parenchymal liver disease such as primary biliary cirrhosis as the cause of malabsorption.

Serum Calcium, Phosphate and Magnesium. Low or low-normal serum calcium concentration in the presence of low phosphate and raised serum alkaline phosphatase suggests vitamin D deficiency as a result of severe malabsorption. Hypomagnesaemia is not uncommon in malabsorption and should be recognized since correction of the hypocalcaemia may be difficult in the presence of hypomagnesaemia.

Total Protein, Albumin and Immunoglobulins. In the absence of liver disease, low serum albumin may reflect nutritional status but it may also be caused by protein-losing enteropathy. Raised total protein in the presence of low albumin may indicate raised

TABLE 21.11
CONDITIONS IDENTIFIED BY SMALL-BOWEL RADIOGRAPHS

Blind loops
Carcinoid
Carcinoma
Crohn's disease
Diverticulosis
Idiopathic chronic ulcerative enteritis
Intestinal resection
Lymphoma
Mesenteric ischaemia
Neuropathic or myopathic pseudo-obstruction
Radiation enteritis
Scleroderma/systemic sclerosis
Small-bowel fistula
Tuberculosis

concentrations of one or more of the globulins, which may occur in malabsorption, especially IgA. Serum IgM may be very high in primary biliary cirrhosis. However, low serum concentrations of all immunoglobulins (IgG, IgM and IgA) may be found in patients with malabsorption with hypogammaglobulinaemia or protein-losing enteropathy. Low serum IgA but normal IgG and IgM will identify patients with rare selective IgA deficiency. Hypogammaglobulinaemia with an abnormal band representing α-heavy chains is characteristic of α-chain disease.

Serum α_1-Acid Glycoprotein (Orosomucoid). Serum levels of α-acid glycoprotein and other acute-phase proteins are often raised in inflammatory bowel disease but may be misleadingly low in severe protein-losing enteropathy.

Thyroid Function Test. The assessment of thyroid function is important in excluding thyrotoxicosis as the cause of diarrhoea. Thyrotoxicosis may rarely cause malabsorption.

Plasma Glucose. Fasting or 2-h postprandial plasma glucose should be measured to exclude diabetes mellitus, which can cause variable combinations of diarrhoea and steatorrhoea due to autonomic neuropathy.

Full Blood Count. Anaemia due to iron, folate or vitamin B_{12} deficiency is a feature of malabsorption. Serum iron and total iron-binding capacity, serum ferritin, serum or preferably red cell folate and serum vitamin B_{12} should all be measured. Iron and folate deficiency may indicate proximal bowel disease whereas vitamin B_{12} deficiency may indicate terminal ileal disease or bacterial overgrowth.

Faecal Fat. The direction of clinical investigations depends initially on differentiating between diarrhoea and steatorrhoea. This may be accomplished by simply inspecting the stools, a 3-day faecal fat estimation or radioisotopic techniques such as the triolein breath test. Simple microscopy for fat globules is used in some laboratories as a qualitative screen for steatorrhoea, thereby avoiding the unpleasant quantitative analysis of stools. If steatorrhoea is confirmed, colonic disease as the primary cause is excluded. If steatorrhoea is absent, pancreatic exocrine insufficiency and cholestatic liver disease are excluded.

Microbiological Stool Analysis. It is mandatory to exclude infection as the first step in the investigation of a patient with diarrhoea or malabsorption. Multiple stool specimens may be required and obscure organisms including viruses, fungi and parasites should be sought vigorously, especially in immunocompromised patients as with the acquired immune deficiency syndrome (AIDS). Occasionally, invasive methods of obtaining small-bowel contents or mucosa for microbiological examination, for *Giardia lamblia* or *Strongyloides* for example, may be required. Infection may also be the mediator of malabsorption associated with structural abnormalities such as small-bowel diverticulosis, post-gastrectomy and blind-loop syndrome. Achlorhydria predisposes to colonization of the small bowel and this should be suspected if pernicious anaemia is present.

Investigations to Identify the Cause of Diarrhoea or Steatorrhoea

Small- and Large-bowel Contrast Radiography. A barium follow-through or small-bowel enema may provide evidence of structural pathology such as Crohn's disease or jejunal diverticulosis (Table 21.11). Diffuse mucosal causes such as coeliac disease may also be suspected. Large-bowel radiography may reveal diverticulosis, tumours, inflammatory bowel disease, ischaemic colitis, fistulae, pneumatosis coli and Cronkite Canada syndrome.

Non-invasive Tests of Small-bowel Function. Tests such as xylose absorption, cellobiose/mannitol test or [^{51}Cr]-EDTA may be used, especially in children, as screens for identifying patients who require a small-bowel biopsy. These tests, however, may give normal results in the presence of mild mucosal abnormalities and small-bowel biopsy remains the definitive test for excluding small-bowel pathology such as coeliac disease.

Histological Examination of Small- or Large-bowel Mucosa. If a diagnosis has not been reached using barium studies, a biopsy of small bowel either endoscopically or with a Crosby/Watson capsule should be done. Diseases with specific histological features by which a confident diagnosis can be made from this biopsy include coeliac disease, Whipple's disease, diffuse lymphoma, abetalipoproteinaemia, lymphangiectasia and giardiasis. Other conditions in which a presumptive diagnosis may be made include Crohn's disease and radiation enteritis. Specific stains may reveal amyloid infiltration and measurement of enzyme activity in biopsy material may be useful in identifying specific enzymes' deficiency, hypolactasia and sucrase-isomaltase deficiency for example.

Histological examination of terminal ileal mucosa obtained at colonoscopy may confirm Crohn's disease, lymphoma, yersiniosis, tuberculosis or radiation enteritis. Colonoscopic colorectal biopsies permit positive diagnosis of ulcerative colitis, ischaemic or radiation colitis, infective or pseudomembranous colitis and may reveal melanosis coli, which indicates long-term laxative usage.

Assessment of Exocrine Pancreatic Function. If barium studies and small-bowel biopsy do not identify the cause of malabsorption and steatorrhoea is present, exocrine pancreatic function should be assessed (*see* Pancreas above). In addition to pancreatic disease, pancreatic insufficiency may occur after gastrectomy and in severe pathologies of small-bowel mucosa (due to CCK-PZ and enterokinase deficiency) but this is unlikely in the presence of normal radiographic and biopsy features in the small bowel.

[75Se]-Homocholic-tauro Acid Test (SeHCAT). If all the above investigations do not reveal the cause of the diarrhoea, assessment of bile-acid absorption by SeHCAT should be made. Patients with bile-acid malabsorption may respond, often dramatically, to a therapeutic trial of cholestyramine, colestipol or aluminium hydroxide.

Stool Osmotic Gap and Response to Fasting. If steatorrhoea has been excluded and no cause for the diarrhoea has been disclosed, the distinction between osmotic and secretory diarrhoea may be useful in identifying patients with surreptitious laxative abuse or peptide-secreting tumours. In these cases, a laxative screen should be made and a search for a polypeptide-secreting tumour such as a VIPoma or somatostatinoma should be initiated.

Disorders Causing Diarrhoea or Steatorrhoea

Biliary Pathology

Loss of biliary secretion due to common bile-duct obstruction or liver pathology can cause steatorrhoea. The degree of steatorrhoea is usually mild and faecal fat concentration is about 50–70 mmol/day. The patient presents with jaundice that is associated with raised serum bilirubin and alkaline phosphatase and prolonged prothrombin time. The diagnosis of biliary obstruction is confirmed by abdominal ultrasound, supplemented by endoscopic retrograde cholangiography, or by other radiological techniques. The presence of antimitochondrial antibodies would suggest primary biliary cirrhosis, which should be confirmed by a liver biopsy. Biopsy may be also useful in the diagnosis of other causes of cholestatic jaundice such as sclerosing cholangitis.

Crohn's Disease

Crohn's disease is a chronic inflammatory disorder of the gastrointestinal tract of unknown aetiology. The ileocaecal region is the most commonly affected site but any part of the gut may be involved. The disease has a variable course and the inflammatory process may progress to ulceration, fibrosis and the formation of strictures and fistulae. Crohn's disease should be suspected in young adults and older patients with abdominal pain, vomiting, diarrhoea, steatorrhoea, weight loss, constitutional disturbance, rectal bleeding, anaemia and extra-alimentary manifestations such as erythema nodosum, pyoderma gangrenosum, iritis and sacroiliitis. Bacterial overgrowth in the small bowel and bile-acid malabsorption may contribute to the diarrhoea or steatorrhoea. Protein metabolism is affected by decreased nutritional intake, increased protein losses (protein-losing enteropathy) and increased catabolism. Protein-losing enteropathy may explain the often disproportionately low serum albumin and peripheral oedema.

Laboratory data show anaemia, often of mixed type due to iron, folate and vitamin B_{12} deficiency. Serum albumin may be suppressed and other nutritional measures impaired. The white count, platelets, erythrocyte sedimentation rate (ESR) and plasma viscosity are often elevated, together with acute-phase proteins including fibrinogen, C-reactive protein and α_1-acid glycoprotein (orosomucoid). The Schilling test or Dicopac often indicates terminal ileal disease, which is usually apparent radiographically but may require confirmation by [75Se]-HCAT scan or ileoscopy. The extent of intestinal protein loss can be assessed by faecal α_1-antitrypsin levels or [51Cr]-albumin loss in stools.[67] Rectocolonic biopsies, even in apparently normal mucosa, may detect characteristic histological changes.

Although laboratory indices of the activity of Crohn's disease are rarely used in isolation from clinical assessment, a number of newer tests are proving valuable in quantifying the severity of inflammation. For many years, clinical 'disease activity indices' have been the mainstay of objective assessment with only little help from laboratory data.[117] These methods are cumbersome to use, which has stimulated a search for a laboratory test capable of providing the same information. Serum C-reactive protein (CRP) and α_1-acid glycoprotein (orosomucoid) rise during exacerbations of disease and remain elevated with continuing disease activity. Persistent elevation of CRP[118] or orosomucoid[119] during an apparent clinical remission is thought to indicate a high probability of imminent relapse. In one study, serum orosomucoid and α_1-antitrypsin increased between 3 months and 1 month before relapse in Crohn's disease.[120] A laboratory index for the prediction of relapse in Crohn's disease using ESR, serum α_1-acid glycoprotein and α_2-globulin levels has been formulated:

$$(-3.5 + ESR \times 0.03) + (\alpha_1\text{-acid glycoprotein} \times 0.013) + (\alpha_2\text{-globulin} \times 2),$$

and a value in excess of 0.35 is predictive of relapse.[121] CRP and orosomucoid levels, however, correlate poorly with the linear extent of disease. Faecal α_1-antitrypsin levels provide a good measure of the intestinal activity and extent of Crohn's disease and they may be useful in monitoring the response to therapy or the presence of residual disease after surgery.[68] Serum fibrinopeptide-A levels have been shown to correlate strongly with the Crohn's disease activity index and persistent elevation of this protein, despite apparent clinical improvement, may predict a relapse within 3 months of steroid withdrawal.[122] Urinary neopterin, a metabolic product of the cellular immune system, also correlates well with clinical assessment of activity.[123]

[^{99m}Tc]-HMPAO (hexamethyl propylene amine oxime) labelling of white cells is used for both imaging and quantification of inflammatory activity. The latter is assessed by measuring stool ^{99m}Tc excretion after intravenous injection. Other methods include ^{111}In leucocyte scanning and faecal excretion but correlation with disease activity is not as reliable as with the technetium technique and the radiation dose is considerably higher.

In the absence of a 'gold standard' for measuring disease activity, faecal loss of ^{99m}Tc white cells and faecal α_1-antitrypsin levels are proving very useful. In daily clinical practice, laboratory measurements of haemoglobin, platelets, ESR, serum CRP and orosomucoid provide adequate information in the majority of cases of inflammatory bowel disease.

Ulcerative Colitis

Ulcerative colitis is a chronic inflammatory disease that most commonly affects the rectum and left colon but may involve the whole colon. Patients usually present with intermittent attacks of diarrhoea and rectal bleeding, often with pus and mucus. Systemic manifestations may include fever, tachycardia, erythema nodosum, pyoderma gangrenosum, arthritis, iritis and episcleritis. Pericholangitis, cirrhosis, chronic active hepatitis and sclerosing cholangitis may all complicate ulcerative colitis. Although the disease process is usually confined to the mucosa, in severe cases it may extend into the muscular wall of the colon, resulting in toxic megacolon. This can lead to severe disturbance of fluid and electrolytes, with shock, renal failure and cardiac arrhythmias. Sigmoidoscopy and rectal biopsy usually provide the diagnosis. Laboratory data may show low haemoglobin, leucocytosis, high ESR and electrolyte disturbance. Serum albumin may be low and acute-phase proteins such as α_1-acid glycoprotein and CRP are raised. Raised serum liver enzymes, especially alkaline phosphatase, may indicate pericholangitis or sclerosing cholangitis.

Irritable Bowel Syndrome

Irritable bowel syndrome is a condition in which patients have symptoms suggestive of bowel dysfunction but no organic pathology can be demonstrated.

The diagnosis is based on clinical grounds and should only be made after the exclusion of all other possible causes. It is a common condition and it has been estimated that the syndrome accounts for up to 50% of all patients referred to gastroenterology clinics. Patients commonly present with a history of abdominal pain, altered bowel habit with alternating diarrhoea and constipation, and abdominal distention. The type and extent of investigations required to confirm the clinical suspicion depend on the age of the patient and the type and severity of symptoms. Raised serum CRP and ESR are particularly useful in differentiating irritable bowel syndrome from inflammatory bowel disease.

Coeliac Disease (Gluten-sensitive Enteropathy)

Coeliac disease can present at any age and clinical features may include steatorrhoea, weight loss, anaemia, malaise, abdominal distension, growth retardation, late menarche, nutritional deficiencies and an itchy rash (dermatitis herpetiformis). The last may occur even in the absence of gastrointestinal symptoms. Laboratory findings include iron deficiency anaemia, folate deficiency and haematological evidence of hyposplenism. The presence of folate deficiency with normal serum vitamin B_{12} is strongly suggestive of coeliac disease, which rarely affects the terminal ileum. Biochemical assessment includes faecal fat estimation, nutritional indices (serum albumin, calcium, phosphate, magnesium, iron and zinc), gliadin antibodies, xylose absorption test or other tests of mucosal permeability (*see* Small intestine above). Exocrine pancreatic function tests may be abnormal but pancreatic insufficiency is usually reversible with recovery of small-bowel function. The definitive diagnosis can be achieved only by jejunal biopsy using endoscopy or the Crosby capsule and demonstration of mucosal abnormality. Recently, various antibodies have been detected in the serum of patients with coeliac disease; antigliadin antibodies (IgG-AGA and IgA-AGA), antireticulin (ARA), endomysin (EMA) and human jejunal antibodies (JAB).[124,125] Sensitivities and specificities for AGA and ARA vary widely but JAB was found in 93% of patients with untreated coeliac disease, in 90% of coeliac patients after gluten challenge but in none of the patients on gluten-free diet.[126] The clinical application of these antibodies awaits further assessment.

Hypolactasia

Absorption defects can be caused by a deficiency in brush-border oligosaccharidases. The most common defect is hypolactasia, which may occur as a congenital, autosomal recessive condition affecting neonates or as a milder form in adult primary hypolactasia. It affects up to 15% of the population in the UK but may reach 100% in certain African races and others not of north-west European origin. Lactase is very sensitive to disturbances of villous integrity such as starvation, coeliac disease, Crohn's disease, giardia-

TABLE 21.12

CAUSES OF PANCREATIC EXOCRINE INSUFFICIENCY

Pancreatic
Chronic pancreatitis
Carcinoma of the pancreas
Pancreatic fistula
Cystic fibrosis
Pancreatic resection
Congenital lipase or colipase deficiency
Malnutrition

Non-pancreatic
Post-gastrectomy and Roux en Y anastomosis
Zollinger–Ellison syndrome
Severe small-bowel mucosal pathology (e.g. coeliac disease):
    decreased CCK-PZ release
    enterokinase deficiency

---

sis, tropical sprue, rotavirus, cholera and bacterial overgrowth. Acid pH in the stools of children may suggest disaccharidase deficiency but this is seldom useful in adults. The inability to split lactose results in its malabsorption and its passage to the colon, causing increase in osmotic load and diarrhoea. Fermentation by colonic bacteria results in gaseous distention and abdominal discomfort. The short-chain fatty acids released by colonic fermentation are absorbed, thus compensating for the small-bowel malabsorption of lactose. Most patients with this condition, however, do not develop diarrhoea without a considerable milk intake. The diagnosis of hypolactasia is discussed elsewhere (*see* Small intestine above).

Short-bowel Syndrome and Intestinal Failure

Short-bowel syndrome may result from massive resection of the small bowel, usually for Crohn's disease, mesenteric infarction or trauma. Intestinal failure is not synonymous with short-bowel syndrome since the bowel may be completely intact but functionally inadequate for maintenance of adequate nutrition.[127] Resection of the jejunum leads to folic acid deficiency and hypolactasia but has surprisingly little effect on macronutrient absorption or salt and water homeostasis. This is because of the marked adaptive capability of the ileum and the progressively tighter intercellular junctions of the ileum and colon. However, loss of the pylorus, ileocaecal valve or colon may prove disastrous if residual small-bowel length is barely sufficient.[5]

Pancreaticobiliary function may be impaired after duodenal or jejunal resection due to removal of the sites of CCK and secretin production. Pancreatic exocrine insufficiency may thus coexist. Vitamin B_{12} and bile-salt malabsorption are inevitable consequences of terminal ileal resection. Steatorrhoea may be reduced by pancreatic supplements or a switch from long-chain to medium-chain triglycerides in the diet. Bile-salt malabsorption enhances oxalate absorption, leading to hyperoxaluria and renal oxalate

stones. Gallstones are also more frequent, owing to disturbance in cholesterol metabolism.

Salt and water losses may be critical and may result in electrolyte disturbances; chloride losses may lead to hypochloraemic alkalosis and bicarbonate losses to acidosis. Biochemical monitoring is essential for adequate supervision of patients with short-bowel syndrome. Frequent monitoring of serum electrolytes and renal function is required and urinary sodium excretion should be assessed to determine whether there is any reserve capacity for renal compensation for gut Na losses. Serum concentrations of divalent cations (e.g calcium, magnesium) and trace elements (e.g. zinc) should be determined and these substances replaced appropriately.[128] Biochemical assessment of patients with short-bowel syndrome may indicate whether long-term nutritional support is necessary.

Exocrine Pancreatic Insufficiency

Loss of pancreatic secretion, either due to a primary defect in the pancreas or secondary to non-pancreatic causes, is an important cause of malabsorption (Table 21.12). Chronic pancreatitis is the most common cause of pancreatic exocrine insufficiency. Steatorrhoea is the presenting feature in 5–10% of patients. Patients with chronic pancreatitis often have abnormal gastric secretory and motor function and rapid emptying of gastric contents.[6] As a consequence, the acidity of duodenal contents denatures the small amount of pancreatic enzymes still being secreted by the damaged pancreas and results in worsening of the steatorrhoea. Glucose intolerance is common and overt diabetes mellitus occurs in more than 10% of patients. The combination of steatorrhoea with diabetes mellitus is therefore characteristic, but not diagnostic, of pancreatic steatorrhoea. The diagnosis can be confirmed radiologically by the presence of characteristic pancreatic calcification or by endoscopic retrograde pancreatography showing specific ductal abnormalities in 80% of patients. The assessment of pancreatic exocrine insufficiency has already been discussed above.

The Contaminated Small-bowel Syndrome

The normal gastric acid helps to minimize the entry of organisms into the small intestine and the jejunum is normally relatively sterile. Organisms become more abundant further down the small intestine and at the terminal ileum the flora resembles that of the proximal colon but in much lower concentrations. In conditions that can lead to stasis, stagnation of intestinal contents and proliferation of colonic-type bacteria occur (*see* Table 21.4). Deconjugation of bile salts and mucosal damage by bacteria can lead to malabsorption, particularly of fat, but malabsorption of carbohydrates, proteins and micronutrients may also occur. Malabsorption of vitamin B_{12} can occur due to binding and utilization by bacteria. In many cases, the diagnosis is suspected from the history—diabetes mellitus, previous surgery or radiotherapy for example. In others, features of systemic sclerosis may be obvious on examination. Tests of mucosal damage such as the xylose absorption test and cellobiose/mannitol test are usually abnormal. Cultures of upper-intestinal aspirates or breath tests confirm the diagnosis (*see* Small intestine above). Small-bowel radiographs may identify anatomical abnormalities or disordered motility. If no cause is found, serum immunoglobulins may reveal hypogammaglobulinaemia or IgA deficiency.

Radiation Enterocolitis

Intestinal damage may occur in 3–25% of patients treated with radiation for abdominal or pelvic malignancy. Extensive damage to mucosa can occur within hours of radiation exposure and can lead to fluid and electrolyte disturbances. Chronic intestinal damage may develop within a few months to many years following radiation. Intestinal ischaemia can lead to strictures and fistulae, resulting in malabsorption. Bile-salt malabsorption may follow damage to the terminal ileum. History of previous exposure to radiation is suggestive and small-bowel radiographs may reveal anatomical abnormalities such as strictures and fistulae. Tests of mucosal damage and malabsorption are abnormal.

Post-gastroduodenal Resection

Although such surgery is declining in popularity with the advent of antisecretory drugs for peptic ulcer, there are many patients who underwent gastric surgery for peptic ulcer or neoplastic disease who are now developing complications. The causes of steatorrhoea following gastric surgery (Billroth II or Polya gastrectomy) are:

- rapid gastric emptying due to loss of pyloric control or osmoreceptor feedback from the bypassed duodenum and pancreatic secretions;
- poor mixing of gastric effluent with pancreatic and biliary secretions;[6]
- small-bowel bacterial overgrowth due to achlorhydria;
- blind afferent-loop bacterial overgrowth;
- pancreatic atrophy;
- lack of stimulation of biliary and pancreatic secretions.

Patients may present with dumping syndrome, diarrhoea, weight loss, anaemia and bone disease. Biochemical investigations may show low serum iron, vitamin B_{12}, folate, calcium, vitamin D and raised alkaline phosphatase. Occasionally, small-bowel disease such as coeliac disease may be unmasked by partial gastrectomy.

Malabsorption due to Drugs

Many drugs, such as cholestyramine, neomycin, colchicine, biguanides, para-aminosalicylic acid, laxatives, methyldopa, and cytotoxic drugs (e.g. methotrexate), may all cause malabsorption (*see* Table 21.9). The mechanisms involved are mucosal damage, inhibition of brush-border enzymes, precipitation of bile acids and alteration of bowel flora. The malabsorption, of macro- and micronutrients, is dose related and reversible with withdrawal of the offending drug.

Phenytoin may lead to folate and vitamin D deficiency. Acute and chronic alcohol ingestion may result in marked diarrhoea and intestinal malabsorption. Direct effects of alcohol on the intestine include rapid intestinal transit, decreased activity of mucosal disaccharidases, and increased permeability to water and solutes. Steatorrhoea has been attributed to reversible functional pancreatic insufficiency and, in alcoholic liver disease, to diminished bile secretion.

Laxative Abuse

Surreptitious laxative abuse is a common cause of secretory diarrhoea. The presence of hypokalaemia and melanosis coli are strongly suggestive. Melanosis coli is specific for anthraquinolone laxatives, occurring within 4 months and is reversible.[129] If suspected, a search in the patient's locker and a laxative screen must be made. Detection of laxatives in the urine may be possible some time after intake has ceased as a result of the enterohepatic circulation of such drugs. Chronic abuse of irritant purgatives may also cause malabsorption. Measurement of faecal magnesium concentration may be useful in detecting patients with magnesium-induced diarrhoea, which has been recently shown to be an important cause of chronic diarrhoea.[74]

Lymphomas, Small-bowel Tumours and Carcinoids

Whilst relatively rare, lymphoma and small-bowel carcinomas may supervene in long-standing coeliac disease, particularly if adherence to a gluten-free diet has been inadequate. Secretory diarrhoea can be the main symptom in some patients with carcinoid tumours and other classical symptoms may not neccessarily be present. Raised urinary 5-hydroxyindole acetic acid usually confirms the diagnosis but slightly elevated levels may be found in untreated coeliac disease, tropical sprue and Whipple's disease.

Polypeptide-secreting Tumours

Polypeptide-secreting tumours are rare causes of secretory diarrhoea.[14] The Werner–Morrison syndrome (pancreatic cholera), a condition characterized by watery diarrhoea, hypokalaemia and gastric hypo- or achlorhydria, is due to overproduction of vasoactive intestinal polypeptide by a pancreatic tumour (VIPoma) and is associated with increased plasma concentration of VIP. Although VIP is thought to be responsible for the diarrhoea, other hormones found in association with a VIPoma as part of multiple endocrine neoplasia may also influence secretion—prostaglandins, secretin, glucagon, gastric inhibitory peptide (GIP), somatostatin, calcitonin and serotonin, for example. It should be emphasized that plasma VIP concentrations similar to those found in VIPomas can also be found in cases of extrapancreatic tumours associated with diarrhoea, for example in medullary carcinoma of the thyroid and ganglioneuroblastomas, and also as a 'secondary phenomenon' in a number of other unrelated causes of diarrhoea such as coeliac disease.

Gastrin-secreting tumours may also cause diarrhoea and malabsorption by producing excessive gastric secretion, leading to destruction of small-bowel villi and pancreatic enzymes and also having a direct secretory effect on jejunal water and electrolyte handling. Diagnosis of this condition has already been discussed.

In medullary carcinoma of the thyroid, calcitonin stimulates jejunoileal secretion but production of prostaglandins may be a more important cause of the diarrhoea in this condition.

Other gut hormones such as secretin, cholecystokinin, glucagon, somatostatin and GIP have all been shown to reduce ionic and water absorption. Somatostatin-producing tumours associated with secretory diarrhoea have been described but, paradoxically, somatostatin has been shown to reduce gut effluent in the short-bowel syndrome.

Miscellaneous Conditions

Several rare inherited metabolic disorders, for example cystinuria and Hartnup disease, are associated with specific absorption defects. The manifestations and diagnoses of these conditions are covered in Chapter 16.

REFERENCES

1. Atkinson M. (1987). Monitoring oesophageal pH. *Gut*, **28**, 509.
2. Johnsson F., Joelsson B. (1988). Reproducibility of ambulatory oesophageal pH monitoring. *Gut*, **29**, 886.
3. De Meester T.R. et al. (1980). Technique, indications and clinical use of 24 hour oesophageal pH monitoring. *J. Thorac. Cardiovasc. Surg.*, **79**, 656.
4. Winnan G.R., Meyer C.T., McCallum R.W. (1982). Interpretation of the Bernstein test: a reappraisal of criteria. *Ann. Int. Med.*, **96**, 320.
5. MacGregor I.L., Parent J., Meyer J.H. (1977). Gastric emptying of liquid meals and pancreatic and biliary secretion after subtotal gastrectomy or truncal vagotomy and pyloroplasty in man. *Gastroenterology*, **72**, 195.
   and
   MacGregor I.L., Martin M.S., Meyer J.H. (1977). Gastric emptying of solid food in normal man and after subtotal gastrectomy and truncal vagotomy with pyloroplasty. *Gastroenterology*, **72**. 206.
6. Mallinson C.N. (1968). Effect of pancreatic insufficiency and intestinal lactase deficiency on the gastric emptying of starch and lactose. *Gut*, **9**, 737.
7. Bergegardh S., Nilsson G., Olbe L. (1976). The effect of gastric distension on acid secretion and plasma gastrin in duodenal ulcer patients. *Scand. J. Gastroenterology*, **11**, 475.
8. Uvnas-Wallensten K., Rehfeld J.H., Larsson L.I., Uvnas A.S. (1977). Heptadecapeptide gastrin in the vagal nerve. *Proc. Natl. Acad. Sci. (USA)*, **74**, 5705.
9. Adrian T.E., Bloom S.R., Polak J.M. (1981). Regulatory peptides of the foregut. In *Gastroenterology 1: Foregut* (Baron J.H., Moody F.G. eds.) *Butterworths International Medical Reviews*, London: Butterworths, pp. 67–107.
10. Orloff M.J., Chandler J.G., Alderman S.J., Keiter J.E., Rosen, H. (1969). Gastric secretion and peptic ulcer following portacaval shunt in man. *Ann. Surg.*, **170**, 515.
11. Lanzon-Miller S. et al. (1987). Twenty four hour intragastric acidity and plasma gastrin concentration in healthy subjects and patients with duodenal or gastric ulcer or pernicious anaemia. *Aliment. Pharmacol. Ther.*, **1**, 225.
12. Bateson M.C., Bouchier I.A. (1988). Chapter in *Clinical Investigations in Gastroenterology*, London: Kluwer pp. 36–39.
13. Fieldman M., Richardson C.T., Fordtran J.S. (1980). Experience with sham-feeding as a test for vagotomy. *Gastroenterology*, **79**, 792.
14. Chey W.Y. et al. (1989). Ulcerogenic tumour syndrome of the pancreas associated with non-gastrin secretagogue. *Ann. Surg.*, **210**, 140.
15. McGuigan J.E., Wolfe M.M. (1980). Secretin injection test in the diagnosis of gastrinoma. *Gastroenterology*, **79**, 1324.
16. Koop H., Klein M., Arnold R. (1990). Serum gastrin levels during long-term omeprazole treatment. *Aliment. Pharmacol. Ther.*, **4**, 131.
17. Axon A.T.R. (1988). *Campylobacter pylori*. In *Recent Advances in Gastroenterology* (Pounder R. ed.) Edinburgh: Churchill Livingstone, pp. 225–244.
18. Levi S., Beardshall K., Haddad G., Playford R., Gosh P., Calam J. (1989). *Campylobacter pylori* and duodenal ulcers: the gastrin link. *Lancet*, **ii**, 1167.
19. Marshall B.J., Warren J.R., Francis G.J., Langton S.R., Goodwin C.S., Blincow E.D. (1987). Rapid urease test in the management of *Campylobacter pyloridis* associated gastritis *Am. J. Gastroenterology*, **82**, 200.
20. McNulty C.A.M. (1989). Detection of *Campylobacter pylori* by the biopsy urease test. In *Campylobacter pylori and Gastroduodenal Disease* (Rathbone B.J., Healley R.V. eds.) Oxford: Blackwell, pp. 69–73.
21. Thillainayagam A.V., Arvind A.S., Cook R.S., Harrison I.G., Tabaqchali S., Farthing M.J.G. (1991). Diagnostic efficiency of an ultrarapid endoscopy room test for *Helicobacter pylori*. *Gut*, **32**, 467.
22. Weil J., Bell G.D. (1989). Detection of *Campylobacter pylori* by the ^{14}C urea breath test. In *Campylobacter pylori and Gastroduodenal Disease* (Rathbone B.J., Healley R.V. eds.) Oxford: Blackwell, pp. 83–93.
23. Klein P.D., Graham D.Y. (1989). Detection of *Campylobacter pylori* by the ^{13}C urea breath test. In *Campylobacter pylori and Gastroduodenal Disease* (Rathbone B.J., Healley R.V. eds.) Oxford: Blackwell, pp. 94–105.
24. Newell D.G., Stacey A.R. (1989). The serology of *Campylobacter pylori* infections. In *Campylobacter pylori and Gastroduodenal Disease* (Rathbone B.J., Healley R.V. eds.) Oxford: Blackwell, pp. 74–82.
25. Sladen G., Kumar P. (1973). Is the xylose test still a worthwhile investigation? *Br. Med. J.*, **3**, 223.
26. Bode S., Gudmand-Hoyer E. (1987). The diagnostic

value of the D-xylose absorption test in adult coeliac disease. *Scand. J. Gastroenterology*, **22**, 1217.

27. Labib M., Gama R., Marks V. (1990). The predictive value of D-xylose absorption test and erythrocyte folate in adult coeliac disease: a parallel approach. *Ann. Clin. Biochem.*, **27**, 75–77

28. Rich E.J., Christie D.L. (1990). Anti-gliadin antibody panel and xylose absorption test in screening for celiac disease. *J. Pediatr. Gastroenterology Nutr.*, **10**, 174.

29. Cobden I., Dickinson R.J., Rothwell J., Axon A.T.R. (1978). Intestinal permeability assessed by excretion ratios of two molecules: results in coeliac disease. *Br. Med. J.*, **2**, 1060.

30. Cobden I., Rothwell J., Axon A.T.R. (1980). Intestinal permeability and screening tests for coeliac disease. *Gut*, **21**, 512.

31. Juby L.D., Rothwell J., Axon A.T.R. (1989). Cellobiose/mannitol sugar test—a sensitive tubeless test for coeliac disease: results on 1010 unselected patients. *Gut*, **30**, 476.

32. Menzies I.S., Pounder R., Heyer S., Laker M., Bull J., Wheeler P. (1979). Abnormal intestinal permeability to sugars in villous atrophy. *Lancet*, **ii**, 1107.

33. Ukabam S.O., Clamp J.R., Cooper B.T. (1982). Abnormal small intestinal permeability to sugars in patients with Crohn's disease of the terminal ileum and colon. *Digestion*, **27**, 70.

34. Sundquist T., Sjodahl R., Magnusson K.E., Jernstrom I., Tagesson C. (1980). Passage of molecules through the wall of the intestinal tract. II. Application of low molecular weight polyethylene glycol and a deterministic mathematical filter function for determining the intestinal permeability in man. *Gut*, **21**, 208.

35. Bjarnason I., Peters T.J., Veall N. (1983). A persistent defect in intestinal permeability in coeliac disease demonstrated by a ^{51}Cr-labelled EDTA absorption test. *Lancet*, **i**, 323.

36. O'Mahoney C.P., Stevens F.M., Bourke M., McCarthy C.F., Weir D.G., Feighery C.F. (1984). ^{51}Cr-EDTA test for coeliac disease. *Lancet*, **i**, 1354.

37. Newcomer A.D., McGill D.B., Thomas P.J., Hofmann A.F. (1975). Prospective comparison of indirect methods for detecting lactase deficiency. *N. Engl. J. Med.*, **293**, 1232.

38. Arola H., Koivula T., Jokela H., Isokoski M. (1982). Simple urinary test for lactose malabsorption. *Lancet*, **ii**, 524.

39. Arola H. et al. (1988). Comparison of indirect diagnostic methods for hypolactasia. *Scand. J. Gastronterology*, **23**, 351.

40. Adlung J., Grazikowske H. (1979). Diagnosis of fat absorption with ^{14}C-tripalmitate/^{3}H-palmitic acid. *Scand. J. Gastroenterology*, **14**, 587.

41. Thorsgaard Pederson N. (1984). Estimation of assimilation of simultaneously ingested ^{14}C-triolein and ^{3}H-oleic acid as a test of pancreatic digestive function. *Scand. J. Gastroenterology*, **19**, 161.

42. Lembeke B., Lösler A., Caspary W.F., Schürnbrand P., Emrich D., Creutzfeldt W. (1986). Clinical value of dual-isotope trioleate and glycerol ^{75}Se-triether. *Dig. Dis. Sci.*, **31**, 822.

43. Newcomer A.D. et al. (1979). Triolein breath test. *Gastroenterology*, **76**, 6.

44. West P.S., Levin G.E., Griffin G.E., Maxwell J.D. (1981). Comparison of simple screening tests for fat malabsorption. *Br. Med. J.*, **282**, 1501.

45. Einarsson K., Bjorkhem I., Eklof R., Blomstrand R. (1983). ^{14}C-triolein breath test as a rapid and convenient screening test for fat malabsorption. *Scand. J. Gastroenterology*, **18**, 9.

46. Turner J.M. Lawrence S., Fellows I.W., Johnson I., Hill P.G., Holmes G.K.T. (1987). ^{14}C-triolein absorption: a useful test in the diagnosis of malabsorption. *Gut*, **28**, 694.

47. Mastropaolo, G., Rees W.D.W. (1987). Evaluation of the hydrogen breath test in man: definition and elimination of the early hydrogen peak. *Gut*, **28**, 721.

48. Lauterburg B.H., Newcomer A.D., Hofmann A.F. (1978). Clinical value of the bile acid breath test. *Mayo Clin. Proc.*, **53**, 227.

49. Merrick M.V., Eastwood M.A., Ford M.J. (1985). Is bile acid malabsorption underdiagnosed? An evaluation of accuracy of diagnosis by measurement of SeHCAT. *Br. Med. J.*, **290**, 665.

50. Watson W.S., McKenzie I., Holden R.J., Craig L., Sleigf J.V., Crear G.P. (1980). An evaluation of the ^{14}C-glycocholic acid breath test in the diagnosis of bacterial colonisation of the jejunum. *Scott. Med. J.*, **25**, 23.

51. King C.E., Toskes P.P., Guilarte T.R., Lorenz E., Welkos S.L. (1980). Comparison of the one-gram D-[^{14}C] xylose breath test to the [^{14}C] bile acid breath test in patients with small intestine bacterial overgrowth. *Dig. Dis. Sci.*, **25**, 53.

52. Northfield T.C., Drasar B.S., Wright J.T. (1973). Value of the small intestinal bile acid analysis in the diagnosis of stagnant loop syndrome. *Gut*, **14**, 341.

53. Setchell K.D.R., Harrison D.L., Gilbert J.M., Murphy G.M. (1985). Serum unconjugated bile acids: qualitative and quantitative profile in ileal resection and bacterial overgrowth. *Clin. Chim. Acta*, **152**, 297.

54. Chernov A.J., Doe W.F., Gompertz D. (1972). Intrajejunal volatile fatty acids in the stagnant loop syndrome. *Gut*, **13**, 103.

55. Delhez H., Van den Berg J.W.O., Van Blankenstein M., Meerwaldt J.H. (1982). A new method for the determination of bile acid turnover using ^{75}Se-homocholic taurine. *Eur. J. Nucl. Med.*, **7**, 269.

57. Bjarnason I. et al. (1987). Non-steroidal anti-inflammatory drug induced intestinal inflammation in humans. *Gastroenterology*, **93**, 480.

58. Schiller L.R. et al. (1987). Studies of the prevalence and significance of radio-labelled bile acid malabsorption in a group of patients with idiopathic chronic diarrhoea. *Gastroenterology*, **92**, 151.

59. Schiller L.R., Bilhartz L.E., Santa-Ana C.A., Fordtran J.S. (1990). Comparison of endogenous and radiolabelled bile acid excretion in patients with idiopathic chronic diarrhoea. *Gastroenterology*, **98**, 1036.

60. Williams A.J.K., Merrick M.V., Eastwood M.A. (1991). Idiopathic bile acid malabsorption—a review of clinical presentation, diagnosis, and response to treatment. *Gut*, **32**, 1004.

61. Sandregesaran K., Jones B.J.M. (1991). Chronic diarrhoea, bile salt malabsorption and previous enteric infection. *Gut*, **32**, A566.

62. Atrah H.I., Davidson R.J.L. (1989). A survey and critical evaluation of a dual isotope [Dicopac] vitamin B$_{12}$ absorption test. *Eur. J. Nucl. Med.*, **15**, 57.

63. La Broy J.L.A., Male P.-J., Beavis A.K., Misiewicz J.J. (1983). Assessment of the reproducibility of the lactulose H$_2$ breath test as a measure of mouth to caecum transit time. *Gut*, **24**, 893.

64. Ladas S.D., Latoufis C., Giannopoulou H., Hatziioannou J., Raptis S.A. (1989). Reproducible lactulose hydrogen breath test as a measure of mouth to caecum transit time. *Dig. Dis. Sci.*, **34**, 919.

65. Kennedy M., Chinwah P., Wade D.N. (1979). A pharmacological method of measuring mouth-caecal transit time in man. *Br. J. Clin. Pharmacol.*, **8**, 372.

66. Staniforth D.H. (1989). Comparison of orocaecal transit times assessed by the lactulose/breath hydrogen and the sulphasalazine/sulphapyridine methods. *Gut*, **30**, 978.

67. Meyers S., Wolke A., Field S.P., Fever E.J., Johnson J.W., Janowitz H.D. (1985). Fecal alpha-1-antitrypsin measurement: an indicator of Crohn's disease activity. *Gastroenterology*, **89**, 13.

68. Vantrappen G., Janssens J., Hellemans J. (1981). Intestinal motility: its role in diarrhoea. In *Diarrhoea in Disorders of Intestinal Transport* (Ruppin H., Domschke W., Soergel K.H. eds.) Stuttgart: Georg Thieme Verlag, pp. 22–29.

69. Steadman C., Phillips S.F. (1990). Absorption of fluids and electrolytes by the colon: relevance to inflammatory bowel disease. In *Inflammatory Bowel Diseases*, 2nd edn (Allan R.N., Keighley M.R.B., Alexander-Williams J., Hawfins C. eds.) Edinburgh: Churchill Livingstone, pp.55–69.

70. Bond J.H., Currier B.E., Buchwald H., Levitt M.D. (1980). Colonic conservation of malabsorbed carbohydrate. *Gastroenterology*, **78**, 444.

71. Mortensen P.B., Hegnjoj J., Rannen T., Rasmussen H.S., Holtug K. (1989). Short chain fatty acids in bowel contents after intestinal surgery. *Gastroenterology*, **97**, 1090.

72. Shian Y.F., Feldman G.M., Resnick M.A., Coff P.M. (1985). Stool electrolyte and osmolality measurements in the evaluation of diarrhoeal disorders. *Ann. Int. Med.*, **102**, 773.

73. Ladefoged K., Schaffalitzky de Muckadek O.B., Jarnum S. (1987). Faecal osmolality and electrolyte concentrations in chronic diarrhoea: do they provide diagnostic clues? *Scand. J. Gastroenterology*, **22**, 813.

74. Fine K.D., Santa Ana C., Fordtran J.S. (1991). Diagnosis of magnesium-induced diarrhoea. *N. Engl. J. Med.*, **324**, 1012.

75. Winawer S.J. (1980). Screening for colorectal cancer—an overview. *Cancer*, **45**, 1095.

76. Saito H. et al. (1985). An immunological test for faecal occult blood by counter immunoelectrophoresis. *Cancer*, **56**, 1549.

77. Turunen M.J., Liewendah L.K., Partanen P., Aldercreutz H. (1984). Immunological detection of faecal occult blood in colorectal cancer. *Br. J. Cancer*, **49**, 141.

78. Leicester R.J., Lightfoot A., Miller J., Colin-Jones D., Hunt R. (1983). Accuracy and value of the Haemoccult test in symptomatic patients. *Br. Med. J.*, **286**, 673.

79. Kewenter J., Bjork S., Haglind E., Smith L., Svanvik J., Ahren C. (1988). Screening and rescreening for colorectal cancer: a controlled trial of faecal occult blood testing in 27 700 subjects. *Cancer*, **62**, 645.

80. Kronberg O., Fenger C., Sondergaard O., Pedersen K.M., Olsen J. (1987). Initial mass screening for colorectal cancer with fecal occult blood test. A prospective randomised study at Funen in Denmark. *Scand. J. Gastroenterology*, **22**, 677.

81. Hardcastle J.D. et al. (1989). Randomised, controlled trial of faecal occult blood screening for colorectal cancer: results for first 107 349 subjects. *Lancet*, **i**, 1160.

82. UKCCCR (1989). *Faecal Occult Blood Testing: Report of United Kingdom Co-ordinating Committee on Cancer Research Working Party* (September, 1989). UKCCR, Room 1, 2nd Floor, Africa House, 64–78 Kingsway, London WC2B 6BG, UK.

83. Warshaw A.L., Fuller A.F. (1975). Specificity of increased renal clearance of amylase in diagnosis of acute pancreatitis. *N. Engl. J. Med.*, **292**, 325.

84. Massey T.H. (1985). Efficiency in the diagnosis of acute pancreatitis increased by improved electrophoresis of amylase P3 on cellulose acetate. *Clin. Chem.*, **31**, 70.

85. Thomson H.J., Obekpa P.O., Smith A.N., Brydon W.G. (1987). Diagnosis of acute pancreatitis: a proposed sequence of biochemical investigations. *Scand. J. Gastroenterology*, **22**, 719.

86. Moller-Peterson J., Klaerke M., Dati F. (1986). Evaluation and comparison of cathodic trypsin-like immunoreactivity, pancreatic lipase and pancreatic isoamylase in the diagnosis of acute pancreatitis in 849 consecutive patients with acute abdominal pain. *Clin. Chim. Acta*, **157**, 151.

87. Elias E., Redshaw M., Wood T. (1977). Diagnostic importance of changes in circulating concentrations of immunoreactive trypsin. *Lancet*, **ii**, 66.

88. Büchler M., Malfertheimer P., Uhle W., Beger H.G. (1986). Elastase-1 in acute pancreatitis. *Proceedings: Second International Meeting of Pancreatology, Sao Paulo, Brazil*, A72.

89. Hamano H., Hayakawa T., Kondo T. (1987). Serum immunoreactive elastase in diagnosis of pancreatic cancer, a sensitive marker for pancreatic cancer. *Dig. Dis. Sci.*, **32**, 50.

90. Hoffman G.E., Schmidt D., Bastian B. (1985). Bestimmung der Phospholipase A in Serum bei akuter Pankreatitis. *J. Clin. Chem. Clin. Biochem.*, **23**, 582.

91. Büchler M., Malfertheiner P., Schdlich H., Nevalainen T., Mavromatis T., Beger H.G. (1989). Prognostic value of serum phospholipase A in acute pancreatitis. *Klin. Wochenschr.*, **67**, 186.

92. Kazmierczak S.C., Van Lente F., Hodges E.D. (1991). Diagnostic and prognostic utility of phospholipase A activity in patients with acute pancreatitis: comparison with amylase and lipase. *Clin. Chem.*, **37**, 356.

93. Ranson J.H.C., Pasternack B.S. (1977). Statistical methods for quantifying the severity of clinical acute pancreatitis. *J. Surg. Res.*, **22**, 79.

95. Basso N. et al. (1975). External pancreatic secretion after bombesin infusion in man. *Gut*, **16**, 944.

96. Otte M. (1979). Pankreasfunktionsdiagnostik. *Der Internist*, **20**, 331.

97. Tetlow V.A., Lobley R.W., Herman K., Braganza J.M. (1981). A one-day oral pancreatic function test using a chymotrypsin-labile peptide and a radioactive marker. *Clin. Trials J.*, **17**, 121.

98. Berg J., Chesner I., Allen-Narker R., Buckley B., Lawson N. (1986). Exocrine pancreatic function as determined in a same-day test with use of bentiromide and *p*-aminosalicyclic acid. *Clin. Chem.*, **32**, 1010.

99. Cavallini G. et al. (1983). Reliability of the Bz-Ty-PABA and the pancreolauryl test in the assessment of exocrine pancreatic function. *Digestion*, **27**, 129.

100. Boyd E.J., Cumming J.G.R., Cushieri A., Wood R.A., Wormsley K.G. (1982). Prospective comparison of the fluorescein-dilaurate test with the secretin-cholecystokinin test for pancreatic exocrine function. *J. Clin. Pathol.*, **35**, 1240.

101. Cobden I., et al. (1984). Prospective comparison of three non-invasive tests for pancreatitic disease. (Letter.) *Br. Med. J.*, **289**, 830.

102. Freise J., Ranft V., Fricke K., Schmidt F.W. (1984). Chronic pancreatitis: sensitivity, specificity and predictive value of the pancrelauryl test. *Z. Gastroenterologie*, **22**, 705.

103. Sale J.K. et al. (1974). Trypsin and chymotrypsin in duodenal aspirate and faeces in response to secretin and cholecystokinin-pancreozymin. *Gut*, **15**, 132.

104. Kasper P., Möller G., Wahlefeld A. (1984). A new photometric assay for chymotrypsin in stool. *Clin. Chem.* **30**, 1753.

105. Goff J.S. (1982). Two-stage triolein breath test differentiates pancreatic insufficiency from other causes of malabsorption. *Gastroenterology*, **83**, 44.

106. Ventrucci M. et al. (1983). Comparative study of serum pancreatic isoamylase, lipase and trypsin-like immunoreactivity in pancreatic disease. *Digestion*, **28**, 114.

107. Lake-Bakaar G., McKavanagh S., Redshaw M., Wood T., Summerfield J.A., Elias E. (1979). Serum immunoreactive trypsin concentration after a Lundh meal: its value in the diagnosis of pancreatic disease. *J. Clin. Pathol.*, **32**, 1003.

108. Koop H., Lankish P.G., Stockmann F., Arnold R. (1980). Trypsin radio-immunoassay in the diagnosis of chronic pancreatitis. *Digestion*, **20**, 151.

109. Adrian T.E. (1980). Plasma trypsin-like immunoreactivity in normal subjects and in patients with pancreatic disease. *Scand. J. Gastroenterology*, **16** (suppl. 60), 15.

110. Vezzadinni P., Gullo L., Sternini L., Bonora G., Ferri G.L., Labo G. (1984). Serum immunoreactive trypsin response to secretin injection in patients with chronic pancreatitis. *Am. J. Gastroenterology*, **79**, 213.

111. Hafkenscheid J.C.M., Hessels M., Jansen J.B.M.J., Lamers C.B.H.W. (1984). Serum trypsin, α-amylase and lipase during bombesin stimulation in normal subjects and patients with pancreatic insufficiency. *Clin. Chim. Acta*, **136**, 235.

112. Masoero G., Andriulli A., Santini B., Benitti V., Ansaldi N., Verme G. (1983). Serum trypsin-like immunoreactivity in cystic fibrosis. *Am. J. Dis. Child.*, **137**, 167.

113. Crossley J.R., Smith P.A., Edgar B.W., Gluckman P.D., Elliott R.B. (1981). Neonatal screening for cystic fibrosis, using immunoreactive trypsin assay in dried blood spots. *Clin. Chim. Acta*, **113**, 111.

114. Wilcken, B., Brown A.R.D., Urwin R., Brown D.A. (1983). Cystic fibrosis screening by dried blood spot trypsin assay: results in 75 000 newborn infants. *J. Pediatr.*, **102**, 383.

115. Kirk J.M., Adams A., Westwood A., McCrae W.M. (1983). Measurement of osmolality and sodium concentration in heated cup sweat collections for the investigation of cystic fibrosis. *Ann. Clin. Biochem.*, **20**, 369.

116. Green A., Dodds P., Pennock C. (1985). A study of sweat sodium and chloride: criteria for the diagnosis of cystic fibrosis. *Ann. Clin. Biochem.*, **22**, 171.

117. Best W.R., Becktel J.M., Singleton J.W., Kern F. (1976). Development of Crohn's disease activity index. *Gastroenterology*, **70**, 439.

118. Bourivant M., Leoni M., Tariciotti D., Fais S., Squarcia O., Pallone F. (1988). The clinical significance of serum C-reactive protein levels in Crohn's disease. *J. Clin. Gastroenterology*, **10**, 401.

119. Andre C., Descos L., Landais P., Fermian J. (1981). Assessment of appropriate laboratory measurements to supplement the Crohn's disease activity index. *Gut*, **22**, 571.

120. Wright J.P., Alp M.N., Young G.O., Tigler-Wybrandi N. (1987). Predictors of acute relapse of Crohn's disease—a laboratory and clinical study. *Dig. Dis. Sci.*, **32**, 164.

121. Brignola C., Campieri M., Bazzocchi G., Farrugia P., Tragnone A., Lanfranchi G.A. (1986). A laboratory index for predicting relapse in asymptomatic patients with Crohn's disease. *Gastroenterology*, **91**, 1490.

122. Edwards R.L. et al. (1987). Activation of blood coagulation in Crohn's disease. *Gastroenterology*, **92**, 329.

123. Riebnegger G. et al. (1986). A simple index relating clinical activity in Crohn's disease with T-cell activation: haematocrit; frequency of liquid stools and urinary neopterin as parameters. *Immunobiology*, **173**, 1.

124. Elewant A., Dacremont G., Robberecht E., Leroy J., De-Bacts M. (1989). IgA isotyping of antigliadin antibodies: a possible clue for a less invasive diagnosis of coeliac disease. *Clin. Chim. Acta*, **183**, 285.

125. Rossi T.M. et al. (1988). Relationship of endomysial antibodies to jejunal mucosal pathology: specificity towards both symptomatic and asymptomatic celiacs. *J. Pediatr. Gastroenterology Nutr.*, **7**, 858.

126. Kapati S., Bürgin-Wolff A., Krieg T., Meurer M., Stolz W., Braun-Falco O. (1990). Binding to human jejunum of serum IgA antibody from children with coeliac disease. *Lancet*, **336**, 1335.

127. Scott N.A., Leinhardt D.J., O'Hanrahan T., Finnegan S., Shaffer J. L., Irving M.H. (1991). Spectrum of intestinal failure in a specialised unit. *Lancet*, **337**, 471.

128. Jones B.J.M. (1987). Nutritional management of the short bowel syndrome. *J. Clin. Nutr. Gastroenterology*, **2**, 99.

129. Ewe K., Arbach U. (1986). Factitious diarrhoea. *Clin. Gastroenterology*, **15**, 723.

22. Tests of the Functions of the Liver

N. McIntyre and S. Rosalki

'Liver function tests'
    Serum bilirubin (total and conjugated, bili-alb and bili-proteins)
    Urinary bilirubin
    Urinary urobilinogen
    Aspartate and alanine aminotransferases
    Alkaline phosphatase
    γ-Glutamyl transferase
    Plasma proteins
Tests other than the routine profile that may be of value
    Serum bile acids
    Glutathione-*S*-transferase
    Cholinesterase
    5'-Nucleotidase
    Serum protein electrophoresis
    Specific protein measurements
    Clearance tests
    Miscellaneous tests sometimes used in the investigations of liver disease
The use of liver function tests
    Applications of liver function tests

'LIVER FUNCTION TESTS'

The tests used by clinical laboratories and designated 'liver function tests' detect the biochemical consequences of impaired hepatocellular function, loss of hepatocellular integrity, or biliary obstruction (cholestasis). *Dynamic tests* (clearance tests) can be used to examine and provide quantitative data on selected aspects of the numerous liver functions, but these 'true' liver function tests are infrequently employed. Additional tests, not necessarily of liver function, may be used to define a specific aetiological agent causing liver damage.

Laboratories use a battery of tests ('liver profile') to examine liver function and tend to select tests with whose performance and interpretation they are familiar, and which they believe will be of the greatest clinical use in the detection and subsequent management of liver disease.

Most laboratories include serum (or plasma) total bilirubin (as an indicator of cholestasis), aspartate and/or alanine aminotransferase (hepatocellular integrity), alkaline phosphatase (cholestasis), and serum albumin (hepatocellular synthetic function); some add serum γ-glutamyltransferase (γGT), bile acids, and/or other tests listed in Table 22.1, the indications for which are discussed below. In addition

TABLE 22.1

SOME TESTS USED AS 'LIVER FUNCTION TESTS'

Tests used as indices of uptake, conjugation and excretion of anionic compounds
Serum total bilirubin (and direct and indirect)
Urinary bilirubin (and urobilinogen)
Bile acids

Tests reflecting hepatocellular damage
Aspartate and/or alanine aminotransferase
Glutathione-*S*-transferase
Clearance tests
Serum ferritin
Vitamin B_{12}

Tests used to indicate obstruction to bile flow
Alkaline phosphatase
γ-glutamyltransferase
5'-nucleotidase
Lipoprotein X

Tests of synthetic function
Serum albumin
Prealbumin
Cholinesterase
Lecithin–cholesterol acyltransferase
Serum proteins—electrophoresis
Prothrombin and partial thromboplastin times

to these, tests for urinary bilirubin and urobilinogen are usually made in the ward or clinic. Prothrombin and partial thromboplastin times and factor V assay, which are altered from impaired hepatic synthesis of coagulation factors and are useful markers of the severity of liver disease, will not be considered here as 'liver function tests'; they are discussed fully in Chapter 29.

None of these tests, except perhaps serum bile-acid measurements, is specific for liver disease. Increased levels of plasma total bilirubin, aspartate and alanine aminotransferase, alkaline phosphatase and γGT, and low levels of albumin and clotting factors, may all occur with other diseases.

If the best use is to be made of liver function tests, there must be an understanding of how to interpret them, when they are useful, and their limitations in clinical practice. In this chapter the most frequently measured individual tests will first be considered, followed by the ways in which they and less frequent tests should be used.

Serum Bilirubin (Total and Conjugated, Bili-alb and Bili-proteins)

As early as 1916 it was established that there were two types of bilirubin in jaundiced serum; one reacted directly with Ehrlich's diazo reagent ('direct' bilirubin), the other required addition of alcohol for colour development ('indirect' bilirubin).[1] Direct-reacting bilirubin was found with large bile-duct obstruction and some other types of liver disease, but not with haemolytic jaundice.

TABLE 22.2
CAUSES OF HYPERBILIRUBINAEMIA[57]

Unconjugated (premicrosomal)
Excessive bilirubin production (haemolytic)
Ineffective haemopoiesis
Haemolytic disorders
Abnormal bilirubin metabolism (congenital)
Immaturity of enzyme systems:
   physiological jaundice of newborn
   jaundice of prematurity
Inherited defects:
   Gilbert's syndrome
   Crigler–Najjar syndrome
Drug effects

Conjugated and unconjugated (postmicrosomal)
Hepatocellular abnormality (hepatocellular)
Primary hepatocyte disease:
   hepatitis, cirrhosis, neoplasm, drugs
Intrahepatic cholestasis:
   drugs, pregnancy
Benign postoperative jaundice
Congenital conjugated hyperbilirubinaemia:
   Dubin–Johnson syndrome
   Rotor syndrome
Mechanical obstruction of bile ducts (obstructive)
Extrahepatic:
   calculus, neoplasm, stricture, atresia
Intrahepatic:
   infantile obstructive cholangiopathy, sclerosing cholangitis, primary biliary cirrhosis

It was later established that bilirubin itself was the indirect-reacting material and that direct-reacting bilirubin was a mixture of bilirubin mono- and diglucuronides (i.e. bilirubin esters).[2] It was soon realized that bilirubin is conjugated in the liver and that the glucuronides are efficiently excreted in bile, little normally appearing in blood. Impaired excretion of conjugated bilirubin by hepatocytes explained the jaundice of hepatobiliary disorders.

Bilirubin is insoluble in water, is bound to albumin, and does not appear in urine. Bilirubin glucuronides are water soluble and appear in urine when their plasma level is increased (*see* Urinary bilirubin below). But when serum bilirubin glucuronides are elevated, some of the bilirubin may be covalently bound to serum albumin and other proteins;[3] this fraction (bili-alb or bili-protein) is often a major component of serum total bilirubin, particularly during recovery from jaundice. It is not filtered by the glomerulus, and so bilirubinuria is absent in many patients with 'direct' hyperbilirubinuria. Therefore a negative test for urinary bilirubin does not exclude the presence of conjugated hyperbilirubinaemia.

Methods
In most laboratories, total serum bilirubin is measured by adding a diazo reagent (e.g. diazotized sulphanilic acid) to serum in the presence of methanol,

caffeine or other accelerator. The depth of the violet colour produced is proportional to the total bilirubin concentration. Without accelerator the colour development is less intense and the reading is taken as the amount of 'direct' bilirubin; 'indirect' bilirubin is the difference between total and 'direct' measurements.

'Direct' and 'indirect' bilirubin results are not accurate measurements of bilirubin and bilirubin esters, as some free bilirubin appears to react directly with the reagent. 'Direct' bilirubin is an overestimate of bilirubin esters at low bilirubin levels, but an underestimate at high concentrations. The former is especially undesirable, as the measurement of bilirubin and bilirubin esters at relatively low levels of total bilirubin allows identification of 'unconjugated hyperbilirubinaemia', as in Gilbert's syndrome and haemolysis. The upper reference limit for 'direct-reacting' bilirubin is usually taken as about 3 μmol/L; concentrations above 5 μmol/L, in the presence of normal total bilirubin, suggest hepatobiliary disease, but this is only true if the reliability of the analysis can be assured.

New methods give accurate measurements of bilirubin and its mono- and diconjugates, but they are rarely employed in routine laboratories. They show that conjugated bilirubins normally constitute only about 4–5% (< 1 μmol/L) of total bilirubin. Accurate measurement of bilirubin conjugates (e.g. by alkaline methanolysis and high-performance liquid chromatography) is the most sensitive marker of hepatobiliary disease; it even allows the distinction to be made between the 'unconjugated hyperbilirubinaemia' of Gilbert's syndrome and that of haemolysis; the proportion of bilirubin conjugates (as a percentage of total bilirubin) is normal in patients with haemolysis but low (< 1.7%) in Gilbert's syndrome.

Interpretation of bilirubin levels (Table 22.2)
The reference interval for the total bilirubin concentration in serum or plasma is between about 3 and 15 μmol/L though many laboratories use an upper limit of 17 μmol/L. It is about 3–4 μmol/L higher in men than in women; as Gilbert's syndrome is often 'diagnosed' when the plasma bilirubin is only just over 17 μmol/L, this explains, in part, why this disorder appears more prevalent in men.

Bilirubin concentrations of between 17 and 70 μmol/L are seen without increased conjugated bilirubin or other abnormal liver function tests in benign unconjugated hyperbilirubinaemias and with haemolysis. Haematological investigations usually confirm the presence of haemolysis and often give the cause. When haemolysis occurs together with underlying liver damage, bilirubin concentrations tend to be much higher.

When other liver function tests are also abnormal, bilirubin above 17 μmol/L usually results from liver disease; then bilirubin esters are elevated. Elevated serum total bilirubin reflects increased production, reduced hepatic uptake and/or conjugation, or decreased biliary excretion of the pigment.

The actual concentration of total bilirubin is of little diagnostic value. With complete bile-duct obstruction the bilirubin tends to reach a plateau between 170 and 500 μmol/L; urinary excretion then appears to be the major factor in removal, but it is also broken down to unidentified compounds. Extreme hyperbilirubinuria (up to 1250 μmol/L) is usually due to severe parenchymal liver disease, often in association with renal failure and/or with haemolysis, as in sickle-cell disease, with glucose-6-phosphate dehydrogenase deficiency or with blood transfusion, for example.

In uncomplicated acute liver diseases, such as viral hepatitis, the serum bilirubin is of poor prognostic value; even after deep jaundice, complete recovery can occur with resolution of the underlying condition. However, in fulminant liver failure the peak bilirubin is a prognostic sign; and in chronic liver diseases, a gradual and pronounced increase in serum bilirubin, without obvious cause (such as blood transfusion or administration of certain drugs), is an ominous prognostic sign.

Urinary Bilirubin

When bilirubinuria is present the urine is usually a dark-brown colour. Other compounds also cause dark urine, and bilirubinuria should be confirmed with test strips impregnated with a diazo reagent, for example, which can detect as little as 1–2 μmol/L of bilirubin. This test is underused. Bilirubinuria establishes the presence of liver damage, and it occurs even with small increases in plasma conjugated bilirubin (if it is not bound to protein). It usually precedes jaundice, often being found when the total plasma bilirubin is normal or only slightly elevated. When frank jaundice is present, bilirubinuria is less important; it simply confirms that the plasma level of bilirubin esters (not bound to protein) is increased.

In jaundiced patients the absence of bilirubinuria is important, particularly if other liver function tests are normal, as it suggests an unconjugated hyperbilirubinaemia or haemolysis. However, in patients with jaundice of some duration, bilirubinuria may be absent if conjugated pigment is present in plasma mainly as bili-alb; this can occur during recovery from acute viral hepatitis when there may be no bilirubin in the urine even at serum bilirubin concentrations as high as 170 μmol/L; at the onset of acute viral hepatitis, however, bilirubinuria is common before jaundice appears.

Urinary Urobilinogen

Bilirubin esters undergo bacterial hydrolysis and degradation in the ileum and colon with the production of 'urobilinogen' (a mixture of isomers). Urobilinogen is excreted in the faeces, but some is absorbed and travels in the portal vein to the liver, where most is removed and excreted in bile. A small amount escapes hepatic uptake and is excreted in the urine.

The urinary excretion of urobilinogen is markedly dependent on urine pH, tubular reabsorption increasing with urinary acidity, which also renders urobilinogen unstable. The peak urinary output of urobilinogen tends to occur between 12.00 h and 16.00 h, probably in association with the 'alkaline tide'.

Urinary urobilinogens give a purple reaction with Ehrlich's aldehyde reagent. A test strip impregnated with this reagent allows rough and ready quantification. The test should be done on freshly voided urine.

Increased amounts of urobilinogen may result from overproduction of bilirubin, as with haemolysis, or from constipation or bacterial contamination of the small bowel. With liver damage, more urobilinogen escapes hepatic uptake and biliary excretion, and is excreted in urine. With complete or nearly complete biliary obstruction, urinary levels fall as less bilirubin enters the intestine for conversion to urobilinogen and less urobilinogen is absorbed. Urobilinogen production and urinary excretion are also reduced with diarrhoeal states and after treatment with antibiotics. Thus, increases and decreases in urinary urobilinogen may occur that are unrelated to changes in hepatic function. For these reasons, urobilinogen measurement is of limited clinical value.

Aspartate and Alanine Aminotransferases[4]

The aspartate and alanine aminotransferases are enzymes present in liver, and increased in plasma in hepatocellular injury, which catalyse the reversible transfer of an amino group from aspartate or alanine to α-oxoglutarate to yield oxaloacetate or pyruvate, respectively, and glutamate. Their value for the recognition of liver-cell injury has been recognized for more than 35 years.

Both enzymes are released from damaged liver cells, due to increased permeability of the cell membrane or to cell necrosis. Aspartate aminotransferase (AsT) is present in high concentrations in liver, heart muscle, skeletal muscle, kidney, pancreas and red cells. These release AsT into the blood when they are damaged, and the serum level rises. It is not, however, possible to identify the organ source of raised serum AsT from the properties of the serum enzyme. Haemolysis also causes a small but definite increase in serum AsT. Plasma or serum should be separated quickly to avoid release of erythrocyte enzyme, which may occur with storage even without obvious haemolysis.

Two AsT isoenzymes are found in liver, one in cytoplasm, the other in mitochondria, and they can be measured individually in serum.

Release of mitochondrial AsT from hepatocytes is thought to imply more severe cellular damage than release of the cytoplasmic isoenzyme or of alanine aminotransferase. The ratio of the mitochondrial to cytoplasmic or total AsT is especially increased in severe cell necrosis and in alcoholic liver disease, but its value as a differential diagnostic test is not established.

Alanine aminotransferase (AlT) is present in low concentration in tissues other than liver, in which it is confined to the cytoplasm; high serum levels of this enzyme are therefore considered relatively specific for hepatic damage, but the concentration often rises in muscle diseases also, such as Duchenne dystrophy or active polymyositis. In liver diseases, AlT tends to rise and fall in parallel with AsT, but a small elevation of AlT is often found without an increase of AsT.

Some laboratories measure both AsT and AlT, others only one. Their relative diagnostic value is discussed below. AlT is more specific for liver disease, but it is rarely difficult on clinical grounds to decide that an increased AsT is due to hepatic damage.

Aminotransferases in Liver Disease

Aminotransferase measurements are useful for detecting hepatocellular damage, and for monitoring subsequent progress; return to normal suggests resolution. For this purpose, AlT activity is generally more sensitive; it is more often elevated than AsT, and is slower to return to normal with resolution.

Aminotransferase levels are of only limited value in differential diagnosis. They assist differentiation of 'hepatocellular' (high enzyme levels) from 'obstructive' jaundice (minor increase). But there are many exceptions to this 'rule' (*see* below), and the classification of jaundice into hepatocellular and obstructive causes on this basis is unhelpful.

Very high concentrations of aminotransferase are of diagnostic value. A level in excess of 20 times the upper reference limit (i.e. above about 1000 units/L) is strongly suggestive of acute hepatitis, due to a virus or a drug, and normal or low levels early in an illness virtually exclude acute hepatitis as a cause. However, these very high levels tend to fall rapidly, and blood must be taken early in the illness. A marked elevation is also seen when there is a profound fall in blood pressure, as in shock, and with acute heart failure; both diagnoses are usually obvious clinically. In viral hepatitis, and with some drugs, there is a gradual rise in aminotransferase levels for a week or two before the onset of jaundice. In shock and acute heart failure there is usually an abrupt rise, and a rapid fall if the underlying problem can be treated effectively.

Occasionally, striking elevations are seen with extrahepatic obstruction, chronic active hepatitis, and with ascending cholangitis, and an erroneous diagnosis of acute hepatitis is often made. Rarely, a marked elevation of serum AsT has been reported due to the presence of 'macro AsT', a complex of the enzyme with large molecular-weight immunoglobulin, usually IgG.[5]

In uncomplicated viral hepatitis, despite very high initial concentrations, aminotransferase levels approach normal within 5 weeks of onset of illness,

normal values being achieved in 75% of cases within 8 weeks. In hepatitis B, C and D infections, more persistent elevations suggest the development of chronic liver disease. Even in hepatitis A, which has no long-term sequelae, aminotransferase levels may take many months to return to normal, and exacerbations may occur in which they rise again. Fluctuating aminotransferases are a particular feature of hepatitis C.

More modest increases in aminotransferase, up to about eight times normal, are seen in many liver diseases—chronic hepatocellular disease, cirrhosis, hepatic infiltration, neoplasia or cholestatic jaundice, for example—as well as in the later stages of acute hepatitis. AlT is more frequently increased, except in alcoholic cirrhosis and infiltrative disease. Minor increases, generally below twice the upper reference limit, are occasionally found without evidence of significant disease on liver biopsy. This is particularly true for AlT, which rises in many conditions (e.g. in obese patients), and for AsT after short periods of heavy 'binge' drinking in healthy subjects.

Aminotransferase concentrations may be normal in patients with established but well-compensated cirrhosis, and in patients with chronic and incomplete biliary obstruction. While they usually rise in acute liver diseases, relatively small increases are sometimes encountered, even in fulminant hepatitis. AsT levels may appear disproportionately low in Wilson's disease, even when the illness is very severe, presenting as fulminant hepatitis or subacute hepatic necrosis.

Many workers have tried to use the AsT:AlT ratio to differentiate various types of liver disease. In general, AlT activity exceeds that of AsT in toxic and viral hepatitis, chronic active hepatitis and cholestatic jaundice, but this is only a guide in the individual case. AsT is the higher of the two in alcoholic liver disease, neoplastic and infiltrative liver disease and in non-biliary cirrhosis. An AsT:AlT ratio greater than 2 has been considered evidence of alcoholic hepatitis and/or cirrhosis, distinguishing these conditions from extrahepatic obstruction and viral hepatitis, in which the ratio is normally less than 2.[6] But this distinction is rarely difficult on clinical grounds, and the sensitivity and specificity of this ratio are only about 70%; values in excess of 2 are seen in a significant proportion of patients with postnecrotic cirrhosis and chronic hepatitis, with Wilson's disease,[7] and occasionally with viral hepatitis. Low hepatic AlT has been suggested as the reason for the high AsT:AlT ratio seen in plasma in alcoholics.

It has been claimed that an increase in the AsT:AlT ratio suggests development of cirrhosis in patients with chronic viral hepatitis (B, δ and C) and 'primary biliary cirrhosis'[8] but there is considerable overlap in individual cases.

Not surprisingly, attempts have also been made to use the degree of abnormality, and change in aspartate aminotransferase relative to the change in bilirubin, alkaline phosphatase, and other biochemical markers, in order to identify different hepatobiliary diseases. By and large, the results of these attempts have been disappointing.[9]

The serum AsT increases in many other diseases. It rises with myocardial infarction and myocarditis, with pulmonary embolism, with disease of skeletal muscle and with trauma (even with intramuscular injections); measurement of serum creatine kinase is of great value in identifying aminotransferase elevations due to muscle disease. Confusion may arise when these conditions coincide with liver disease, and then AlT estimations are helpful, although severe muscle disease can cause an increase in this enzyme. In chronic alcoholics, painless chronic myopathy is frequent and acute myopathy may follow a drinking bout. This may contribute to the serum aminotransferase elevation seen in such patients.

Alkaline Phosphatase[4,10]

Alkaline phosphatases are zinc metalloenzymes that release inorganic phosphate from several organic orthophosphates. They are present in nearly all tissues. Their natural substrates may include pyrophosphate, phosphoserine and phosphoethanolamine: intestinal alkaline phosphatase may act as a Ca^{2+}-dependent ATPase. In the liver, alkaline phosphatase can be found histochemically in the microvilli of the bile canaliculus and on the sinusoidal surface of hepatocytes. Alkaline phosphatase exists in tissue-specific isoforms, some of which are true isoenzymes in that they are the products of separate genes. The alkaline phosphatases from liver, bone and kidney are thought to be coded for by the same ('tissue-unspecific') gene, while the alkaline phosphatases from intestine and placenta have different genes.

Alkaline phosphatase activity in normal serum is due mainly to the isoforms from bone and liver, with near equal proportions of each in adults; intestinal alkaline phosphatase may also contribute up to 20% of total activity; placental enzyme may appear in mid-pregnancy.

Measurement

Fresh, unhaemolysed serum or heparinized plasma should be used for alkaline phosphatase estimation, but not plasma for which citrate, oxalate or EDTA were used as anticoagulants, as these form a complex with the zinc in the alkaline phosphatase, causing irreversible enzyme inactivation.

The reference range (and units) for total alkaline phosphatase activity vary with the method used. The internationally recommended 'reference' method uses *p*-nitrophenol phosphate as substrate, in an alkaline transphosphorylating buffer such as 2-amino-2-methyl-1-propanol.[11] Activity also varies with age and sex, and with several other factors. The alkaline phosphatase is above the normal adult range until about 20 years of age; there are two peaks, one in the neonatal period and the other in adolescence (i.e.

during periods of increased bone growth). Levels also tend to rise in older subjects, with increased amounts of liver alkaline phosphatase in elderly men and bone alkaline phosphatase in postmenopausal women.[12] A postprandial increase in the intestinal alkaline phosphatase isoenzyme is seen after a fatty meal in some normal subjects, usually those from blood groups A and O who also carry the ABH red-cell antigen and are Lewis-antigen negative.

In pregnancy the plasma alkaline phosphatase activity increases during the third month, reaches up to three times the usual adult female level in late pregnancy, and may remain elevated for a few weeks after delivery. This is mainly placental phosphatase, together with some increase of the bone isoform.

The various alkaline phosphatase isoenzymes in serum can be identified and measured by several methods, and an elevation of one of them may be found even when the total alkaline phosphatase is normal.

Electrophoresis (usually on cellulose acetate or agarose gel) identifies two liver fractions, a major fraction of α_2-globulin mobility ('slow' liver band), sometimes accompanied by a fraction of α_1-globulin mobility ('fast' liver), together with bone isoenzymes. Liver and bone alkaline phosphatase may be difficult to separate from each other but can be easily distinguished, and quantified, using wheatgerm-lectin affinity electrophoresis;[13] intestinal isoenzyme is easily identified by its β-globulin mobility.

Non-electrophoretic methods may also be used to distinguish between the alkaline phosphatase isoenzymes. Liver alkaline phosphatase is more heat stable than bone, but heat-sensitivity assays are tedious and inaccurate unless done scrupulously. Monoclonal antibodies can distinguish between bone and liver isoenzymes, with some cross-reactions but without interference from alkaline phosphatase from other tissues. However, convenient clinical assays are not yet available. Measurement of bone and non-bone (mainly liver) enzyme using wheatgerm-lectin precipitation[13] provides a convenient and increasingly popular procedure for distinguishing the contribution of these fractions to plasma total alkaline phosphatase.

Alkaline Phosphatase and Liver Disease

The serum alkaline phosphatase activity rises in many liver diseases, the highest levels occurring with obstruction to the flow of bile, either intrahepatic or extrahepatic, or with intrahepatic space-occupying lesions such as primary or metastatic liver tumours. The elevated plasma alkaline phosphatase seen with liver disease does not result from failure of the liver to excrete the enzyme. The phosphatase is produced in the liver, and in animal studies hepatic synthesis of alkaline phosphatase increases after biliary ligation. There appear to be two hepatic isoenzymes, one from hepatocytes ('slow' liver) and a high molecular-mass biliary or 'fast' liver alkaline phosphatase, which originates from the plasma membrane. With biliary obstruction, canalicular membrane alkaline phosphatase, solubilized by retained bile salts or shed as fragments, reaches the plasma by paracellular regurgitation or via transcellular endocytosis. 'Biliary' enzyme seems a better marker of biliary obstruction than total serum alkaline phosphatase activity.

In acute viral hepatitis, alkaline phosphatase is usually either normal or moderately raised, but up to 40% of patients have levels two-and-a-half times the upper reference limit. Hepatitis A infection may cause a cholestatic picture, with pruritus and elevation of alkaline phosphatase, and cholestatic features may also be seen with hepatitis A and B infection. Very high alkaline phosphatase may be found in Epstein–Barr virus infection ('glandular fever'), even with normal bilirubin levels, though this is uncommon.

The serum alkaline phosphatase is increased by drugs that cause cholestatic liver disease; elevation was also reportedly caused by cimetidine,[14] frusemide,[15] phenobarbitone,[16] and phenytoin.[17]

Elevation of a serum alkaline phosphatase having the properties of hepatic alkaline phosphatase has been described in Hodgkin's disease, congestive heart failure, and in infectious and inflammatory diseases not primarily involving the liver, such as polymyalgia rheumatica.[18] The origin of the phosphatase in the latter is not clear; but the alkaline phosphatase may be acting as an acute-phase reactant.[19]

High alkaline phosphatase activity is not always found in 'cholestatic' liver disease. Even with a confirmed extrahepatic block, due to tumour or stones, the alkaline phosphatase may be normal or only slightly raised in a small proportion of cases. A normal alkaline phosphatase has also been seen in patients with primary biliary cirrhosis,[20] and in primary sclerosing cholangitis.[21] This may cause diagnostic confusion.

A low serum alkaline phosphatase has been found in Wilson's disease presenting with haemolytic anaemia and evidence of severe liver dysfunction.[22]

Increased serum intestinal alkaline phosphatase activity may be found in cirrhosis and may result from diminished hepatic uptake, perhaps due to destruction of receptors for intestinal alkaline phosphatase on the liver-cell surface, or to diminished hepatic excretion or catabolism. In some jaundiced patients, increased amounts of the bone isoenzyme can be detected, with increased osteoblastic activity in hepatic osteodystrophy for example, or when osteomalacia complicates liver disease.

Tumours may secrete alkaline phosphatase into plasma. Some tumours produce specific isoenzymes—for example the Regan, Nagao and Kasahara isoenzymes. The Regan isoenzyme (a heat-stable placental-type isoenzyme) may be found in patients with carcinoma of the bile duct. The Kasahara isoenzyme (a fetal intestinal-type phosphatase) has been found in the serum of about 30% of patients with primary liver-cell carcinoma.[23] Patients with hepatocellular carcinoma may also have another,

heat-labile alkaline phosphatase, which differs from the other three tumour-produced enzymes. These isoenzymes are of relatively little diagnostic value in liver disease, since they are present in a relatively small proportion of patients with the tumours, and their activity is generally at a low level, so that sensitive immunological methods are generally required for their identification. When detected they may be of value for monitoring antitumour therapy; successful treatment is associated with a fall or with disappearance of the isoenzyme from the plasma.

Alkaline phosphatase isoenzymes are of limited value in the differential diagnosis of liver disease; the 'biliary' enzyme rises more frequently in cholestatic and neoplastic disorders, and intestinal alkaline phosphatase in parenchymal disease, but there is considerable overlap. Isoenzyme studies do help to decide whether an elevated alkaline phosphatase activity is due to liver disease or bone disease. If separation of alkaline phosphatase isoenzymes is not available, other markers of biliary obstruction, such as γGT or sometimes 5'-nucleotidase, are used to confirm a hepatic origin for raised alkaline phosphatase levels. The measurement of γGT has 90% sensitivity and specificity for this purpose, as it is normal in bone disease. When a large alkaline phosphatase elevation is accompanied by a modest γGT elevation the possibility of concomitant bone and liver disease should be considered (but *see* below).

Occasionally there is a high liver phosphatase in serum due to binding with serum immunoglobulins. This occurs particularly in association with autoimmune disease[24] and ulcerative colitis.[25] Binding interferes with the normal clearance of the enzyme from plasma. Rarely the plasma concentration of liver alkaline phosphatase is found increased in families with no evidence of another disease to account for this finding.[26,27] A liver-like enzyme has been reported as being transiently increased in plasma in association with gastrointestinal infection in the condition of transient hyperphosphatasaemia of infancy.[28]

Elevation of alkaline phosphatase occurs in many diseases other than those involving the liver. A list of causes of an isolated increase in serum alkaline phosphatase is given in Table 22.3 (and in[10]).

γ-Glutamyltransferase (γGT)[29,30]

γGT is a membrane-bound glycoprotein that catalyses the transfer of γ-glutamyl groups from γ-glutamyl peptides, particularly glutathione, to other peptides, to aminoacids and to water. It is found mainly in the membranes of cells with a high rate of secretory or absorptive activity. Large amounts are present in the kidneys, pancreas, liver, intestine and prostate, and it is also found in many other tissues. The γGT activity in bile is approximately 100 times greater than in normal serum.

Several isoforms of γGT have been described, but

TABLE 22.3

CAUSES OF 'ISOLATED' SERUM ALKALINE PHOSPHATASE INCREASE

Increased liver isoenzyme
Hepatic metastases of infiltrative disease
Primary biliary cirrhosis
Cholelithiasis
(NB: usually accompanied by γ-glutamyltransferase increase)
Minor increase with age
Increased bone isoenzyme
Physiological—childhood, puberty, postmenopausal (minor)
Osteoblastic bone disease, e.g. Paget's, osteomalacia, metastases etc.
Increased intestinal isoenzyme
Liver disease (cirrhosis)
Diabetes mellitus
Chronic renal failure
Intestinal disease (lymphoma, α-chain disease)
Physiological (minor) increase after fat ingestion especially in H-substance secretors of blood group O and B
Placental isoenzyme
Physiological—pregnancy
Malignant disease (minor activity increase)
Indian childhood cirrhosis
Variant or unusual forms
Immunoglobulin-bound—autoimmune disease, inflammatory bowel disease
Tumour-derived—ovarian, testicular, hepatocellular cancer (minor activity increase)
Liver-like + bone—benign transient hyperphosphatasaemia (massive increase)
Genetically determined increase
Any or all isoenzyme form(s)

there is no clear evidence of tissue specificity. The heterogeneity is related to the number of sialic acid residues, to the degree of glycosylation and to binding to lipoproteins.[31]

Measurement

The reference interval for serum γGT is higher in men than in women. Serum γGT is very high in neonates and infants up to 1 year, and levels increase above the age of 60. Reference levels are lower in lifelong abstainers from alcohol than in the general population.

Serum γGT concentrations rise in almost all kinds of liver disease and so they are of little value in differentiating between them. It is a very sensitive indicator of the presence of liver disease (sensitivity 0.87–0.95) especially of cholestastis (intra- or extra-hepatic type), but specificity is limited by the many other conditions that cause an increase of γGT due to mild, clinically insignificant hepatic involvement. The highest levels of γGT (averaging 10–20 times the upper limit of normal) occur with intrahepatic biliary obstruction or with primary or secondary hepatic malignancies. However, normal or low γGT may be seen occasionally in patients with intrahepatic

cholestasis, even with very high bilirubin and alkaline phosphatase,[32] and values are usually normal in cholestasis of pregnancy. In infants with idiopathic cholestasis the presence of normal γGT has been found to be of poor prognostic significance.[33]

In acute viral hepatitis, serum γGT concentrations reach a peak in the second or third week of the illness but in some the γGT is still up at 6 weeks. Levels remain high with the development of chronic active hepatitis or cirrhosis.

γGT levels are of definite, though limited, value in the management of alcoholic patients in whom concentrations may rise, presumably due to enzyme induction, even when there is no significant underlying liver disease; but there is a poor correlation between alcohol intake and serum γGT activity. On cessation of drinking γGT falls to normal over 2–5 weeks; if it remains high, continued alcohol intake is likely, liver damage may have occurred, or there may be another reason for the high γGT. Unfortunately, about one-third to one-half of heavy drinkers show no elevation of γGT in the absence of liver disease, so it is not a sensitive screening test for alcohol excess. γGT levels do not rise as the result of an alcoholic binge in healthy subjects, but may do so in alcoholics and patients with other liver disorders.

An increase in γGT activity is seen in several conditions other than liver disease and alcoholism (e.g. acute pancreatitis), and in 50–70% of cases of acute myocardial infarction. The source of the increased γGT with myocardial infarction is not clear, as there is no measurable activity in cardiac or skeletal muscle; it is probably due to secondary effects on the liver, as high concentrations are also found in congestive cardiac failure.

Serum γGT activity increases with the administration of enzyme-inducing drugs. Moderate increases occur with phenobarbitone, phenytoin and other anticonvulsant drugs, paracetamol, tricyclic antidepressants, and glutethimide. Smaller increases are seen with anticoagulants, oral contraceptives and antihyperlipidaemic drugs.[34]

Elevated serum γGT activity is found in about 20% of patients with uncomplicated diabetes mellitus; levels are rarely more than twice the upper limit of normal. The liver is thought to be the source but other clinical or biochemical evidence of liver disease is rarely found. Some dispute the association with diabetes mellitus, arguing that the raised γGT seen in diabetic patients is due to associated conditions.[35]

Causes of an isolated increase of γGT are presented in Table 22.4. Sometimes very high concentrations of serum γGT are found (*c.* 1000 u/L) with no obvious cause.

Plasma Proteins

The liver secretes many circulating plasma proteins. Liver disease may affect their plasma concentration, but the effects are complex and depend not only on

TABLE 22.4
CAUSES OF INCREASED PLASMA GGT

Hepatobiliary disease
Pancreatic disease
Alcohol
Drugs (especially enzyme inducers)
Non-hepatobiliary disease with liver involvement (slight γGT increase):
  Anorexia nervosa
  Dystrophia myotonica
  Guillain–Barré syndrome
  Hyperthyroidism
  Obesity-hyperlipidaemia/diabetes mellitus
  Porphyria cutanae tarda
  Postmyocardial infarction
Neurological disease (slight γGT increase)
Malignant disease/radiotherapy (γGT possibly from shedding of enzyme-containing plasma membrane fragments)

TABLE 22.5
CAUSES OF LOW PLASMA ALBUMIN CONCENTRATION

Impaired albumin synthesis
Malnutrition
Malabsorption
Liver disease
Malignant disease
Increased albumin loss
Proteinuria, e.g. nephrotic syndrome
Protein-losing enteropathy—inflammatory bowel disease
Burns
Exudative skin disease
Increased albumin catabolism
Hypercatabolic states—injury, post–operative
Altered distribution between intra-extravascular compartments from increased vascular permeability
Inflammatory states—acute-phase reaction
Overhydration
Genetic variation
Analbuminaemia
Interrupted synthesis
Acute (and chronic) inflammatory conditions

changes in protein synthesis but also on effects on the volume and distribution of extracellular fluids, and on the half-life of individual proteins. There may also be changes in the metabolism of proteins produced outside the liver. The estimation of 'total plasma protein' alone is of relatively little value. It may be normal despite gross disturbances of the individual components. The significance of a high or low total level can be interpreted only after measurement of the major fractions. Measurement of total protein together with albumin is used to calculate 'globulin' by difference; serum protein electrophoresis is often done in conjunction with these measurements.

Serum or Plasma Albumin[36]

Albumin is the most abundant circulating protein. The plasma albumin concentration is normally between 35 and 50 g/L. Albumin accounts for the colloid osmotic pressure of plasma, and it has binding sites with great affinity for many naturally occurring compounds, including bilirubin, and for many drugs. The liver is the only site of synthesis, producing about 15 g/day in a normal 70-kg person. About 1 g daily is lost into the gastrointestinal tract; most of the remainder is degraded by a mechanism that appears to be under metabolic control. When synthesis falls, the reduction in plasma albumin is minimized by a decrease in the fractional catabolic rate for albumin. The total exchangeable pool of albumin is normally about 3.5–5.0 g/kg body weight; 38–45% of it is within the intravascular space.

Because the plasma albumin concentration reflects hepatic protein synthesis it has been regarded as a valuable test of liver function. But hepatic synthesis is only one of several factors lowering plasma albumin, which also results from increased gastrointestinal or renal loss, increased catabolism, altered vascular permeability or overhydration. Even with markedly reduced synthesis the effect on plasma albumin may take many days to become apparent because of its long half-life (about 20 days). Patients without pre-existing liver disease suffering fever or trauma may have an albumin half-life reduced to about 7 days, albumin concentrations falling rapidly to below 30 g/L;[37] this suggests a marked increase in albumin removal as well as inhibition of albumin synthesis.

The low serum albumin often found with severe chronic liver disease is probably due to reduced synthesis. But in patients with ascites and hypoalbuminaemia, plasma levels may also be low because the plasma volume is large and more albumin than normal is present in the extravascular space. Although the fractional catabolic rate is low, the absolute rate of degradation, and synthesis, may be normal or even high. In cirrhotics with ascites, hepatic secretion of albumin is disturbed; while some enters the bloodstream directly via the sinusoids, much of it is released directly into the ascites.

Alterations in the concentration of plasma albumin must be interpreted with caution because of the many conditions other than liver disease that may result in low plasma albumin levels. These are listed in Table 22.5.

TESTS OTHER THAN THE ROUTINE PROFILE THAT MAY BE OF VALUE

These include bile-acid determination, additional enzyme indicators of hepatocellular injury (glutathione-*S*-transferase, cholinesterase) or cholestasis (5′nucleotidase), protein electrophoresis, and specific protein measurement and clearance tests.

Serum Bile Acids

Bile acids result from catabolism of cholesterol. The two main primary bile acids, cholic and chenodeoxycholic acids, are produced in the liver, conjugated with glycine or taurine, and excreted in bile. They play an important part in the digestion and absorption of fat and fat-soluble compounds. They are reabsorbed in the terminal ileum by a very efficient active transport mechanism, but some escape into the colon where bacteria cause deconjugation, and/or dehydroxylation of the molecule at the 7-α position. The latter reaction converts cholic acid to deoxycholic acid, and chenodeoxycholic to lithocholic acid. These secondary bile acids are absorbed from the colon and travel to the liver via the portal vein. The normal liver removes primary and secondary bile acids very efficiently from portal blood and excretes them rapidly into bile. This completes the enterohepatic circulation of bile acids (i.e. liver–bile–intestine–portal vein–liver).

With liver disease there may be a reduction in primary bile-acid synthesis, or a change in the relative proportions of cholic and deoxycholic acids (normally about twice as much cholic acid is produced); unusual bile acids may be produced. The amount of bile acid conjugated may alter or there may be a change in the taurine:glycine ratio. If less primary bile acid enters the intestine there may be less secondary bile acid, and a reduction in plasma levels of deoxycholate. Impaired liver function, or diversion of portal blood, impairs hepatic bile-acid removal from portal blood, causing increased levels of plasma bile acids, particularly after meals. Biliary obstruction increases plasma bile acids, owing to their regurgitation from the bile ducts into the bloodstream. High plasma bile-acid concentrations increase urinary excretion of bile acids.

Few of these effects are of value in the clinical assessment of patients. The simplest bile-acid measurement is the total bile-acid concentration, either fasting or after a meal, but even this test is rarely available in routine laboratories. The normal fasting serum bile-acid concentration is up to about 15 μmol/L (depending on the method, which varies with the laboratory). The fasting serum bile acid is elevated in only about two-thirds of patients with various types of liver disease, and it is of limited value in screening for patients with liver disease.

After a meal, concentrations remain high in almost all patients with significant liver disease and the 2-h postprandial bile-acid level is therefore a valuable screening test for liver disease.

Should serum bile-acid measurements be added to the conventional battery of 'liver function tests'? The finding of a high serum bile-acid concentration has high specificity for the detection of liver disease (when compared with other individual tests), but its sensitivity is limited. Adding a bile-acid test would be unlikely to improve the specificity already obtained with a battery of tests.

Glutathione-S-transferase (GST)[38]

Glutathione-S-transferases are widely distributed detoxification enzymes. A cationic B form occurs in liver as a bilirubin-binding protein (ligandin), whereas anionic forms are present in lungs, muscle and erythrocytes. Serum GST-B has attracted recent interest as a highly sensitive index of hepatocellular integrity. It is especially elevated in acute hepatitis of viral or drug origin, with increases five- to ten-fold higher than of aminotransferases. Massive increases have been observed with paracetamol toxicity and with fulminant hepatitis. It has a short plasma half-life, which facilitates the recognition of cessation of active cellular damage. GST is more frequently elevated than AsT in chronic active hepatitis. High values have been observed with hepatic metastases and in untreated hyperthyroidism—the latter presumably due to subclinical liver damage, and in alcoholic liver disease, particularly in response to 'binge' drinking. While measurement of GST enzymes has considerable potential, this is offset by the limited availability and inconvenience of the radioimmunoassay used.

Cholinesterase[39,40]

Cholinesterase is a plasma enzyme, produced by the liver, which is capable of hydrolysing a variety of choline esters. Plasma activity falls with decreased protein synthesis in liver disease. Enzyme levels generally follow a path similar to that of plasma albumin. Low activity occasionally results from genetic polymorphism, when there may be altered inhibition characteristics of the plasma enzyme.

In acute hepatitis, of infective or toxic origin, plasma cholinesterase activity falls modestly within a few days of onset, returning gradually to normal with recovery. Chronic hepatitis, cirrhosis, neoplastic and other infiltrative diseases of the liver also result in low activity. In obstructive jaundice, normal values are the rule, unless there is concomitant liver disease or the obstruction is due to malignancy, when reduced values are found. Malignant disease, even when localized and not involving the liver, can give low enzyme activity due to impaired enzyme synthesis. With fatty liver, levels are normal or increased. Cholinesterase is best studied serially and is of greatest value as a prognostic tool. A sudden or marked fall to a quarter of the usual activity indicates ominous deterioration. A large number of drugs have been reported as causing a reduction in cholinesterase activity.

5'-Nucleotidase[4]

5'-Nucleotidase, an alkaline phosphatase that attacks nucleotides with a phosphate at the 5' position of the pentose, is present in all human tissues but only liver disease appears to cause significant elevation of 5'-nucleotidase activity. The normal range of activity in plasma is from 1 to 15 iu/L (measured at 37°C).

The highest activity occurs with either intrahepatic or extrahepatic obstruction to bile flow, but it also increases in chronic active hepatitis, cirrhosis, hepatitis and other hepatocellular disorders. The use of measurement of 5'-nucleotidase activity to confirm that liver disease is the cause of elevated alkaline phosphatase has been largely superseded by measurement of γGT. It may still be useful in infancy and in pregnancy. Bone alkaline phosphatase and γGT levels are both high for physiological reasons in infancy. In pregnancy the placental isoenzyme causes elevated alkaline phosphatase in the third trimester, but γGT activity may fall; γGT activity may remain unaltered in pregnancy cholestasis.[41] However, in both circumstances, studies of alkaline phosphatase isoenzymes are a better method of establishing the presence of obstructive liver disease than 5'-nucleotidase activity.

Serum Protein Electrophoresis

Certain types of electrophoretic pattern are characteristic, but not diagnostic, of certain types of liver disease. Considering the globulins in order from the anode, the following comments apply. α_1-Globulin is principally composed of α_1-antitrypsin and α_1-acid glycoprotein (orosomucoid); both are acute-phase proteins, increasing in many inflammatory disorders. α_1-Antitrypsin deficiency should be suspected if there is a weak α_1 band. Within the α_2-globulin complex, haptoglobin is also an acute-phase protein. Increased clearance of haptoglobin–haemoglobin complexes causes the reduced haptoglobin level seen with intravascular or severe extravascular haemolysis. Biliary obstruction may be associated with an excess of α_2- and β-globulins, owing to accumulation of abnormal lipoproteins. In cirrhosis in addition, the β-globulin iron-binding protein, transferrin, may be reduced; it also shows a non-specific reduction in inflammatory disorders. The immunoglobulins (principally IgG, IgA and IgM) are located within the γ-globulin fraction and extend anodally therefrom. A diffuse (polyclonal) increase of staining in this region is often observed in chronic liver disease (especially chronic active hepatitis), and in chronic inflammatory and autoimmune disorders. In non-biliary cirrhosis (especially alcoholic) there may be increased IgA. This immunoglobulin runs in the β–γ region, and an increase in IgA gives rise to increased staining at this site, an appearance known as β–γ 'fusion' or bridging.

Specific Protein Measurements

Changes in specific proteins are best defined by quantitative immunological measurement. Those whose determination is of particular interest in liver disease include prealbumin, α_1-antitrypsin, α-fetoprotein, caeruloplasmin and the immunoglobulins.

Prealbumin (Transthyretin)

This is a tetramer of four identical subunits that binds iodothyronines, plus one molecule of retinol-binding protein (RBP); it probably helps to reduce urinary excretion of RBP. The plasma prealbumin concentration is 0.2–0.3 g/L; that of RBP 0.04–0.05 g/L. Measurement of prealbumin has been proposed as a liver function test.[42] Its concentration tends to fall in liver disease, presumably due to impaired synthesis. Because its half-life is only about 2 days, changes may precede alterations in the level of plasma albumin. Plasma prealbumin determinations have been considered of particular value in the identification of drug-induced hepatotoxicity.[43]

α_1-Antitrypsin[44]

α_1-Antitrypsin is a glycoprotein of approximately 54 000 Da, synthesized by the liver. It acts as an inhibitor of serine proteinases, especially elastase. It is present in serum at a concentration of 1–1.6 g/L and is an acute-phase protein, serum concentrations being increased with inflammatory disorders; they also increase in pregnancy and in women receiving oral contraceptives. Liver disease occurs with α_1-antitrypsin deficiency, an inherited disorder sometimes identifiable by a reduced α_1 band on electrophoresis; deficiency should be confirmed by quantitative measurement. α_1-Antitrypsin shows genetic polymorphism. Approximately 90% of caucasian populations are homozygous for the M allele (i.e. MM phenotype); other alleles coded at this locus include F, S, Z and null forms. α_1-Antitrypsin phenotype is best determined by isoelectric focusing; allelic variation may be associated with both low plasma concentration and deficient functional (inhibitory) capacity. Plasma levels of α_1-antitrypsin vary with phenotype; they are approximately 15% of normal with ZZ; 38% with SZ; about 60% with MZ and FZ.

The presence of the Z allele, particularly in the homozygous form, is associated with defective processing of the protein in the liver. The precursor protein, deficient in sialic acid, is poorly secreted by the hepatocytes; its intrahepatic accumulation may be a factor in the genesis of liver damage. Neonatal hepatitis is seen in Pi ZZ homozygotes, and less frequently with MZ and SZ phenotypes. Cirrhosis in adults has been found with ZZ, MZ, SZ and FZ phenotypes.

α-Fetoprotein (AFP)[45]

This protein, the principal fetal protein in plasma in early gestation, is subsequently present at very low levels (reference limit 25 μg/L or ng/mL); it can be measured by radio- or enzyme immunoassay. It increases with hepatocellular carcinoma, and more than 90% of such patients have increased serum levels. Elevations are also observed in up to 15% of cirrhosis without hepatocellular carcinoma, in chronic hepatitis, in the regeneration phase of viral hepatitis, and with hepatic metastases, but they are generally minor and transient compared to those observed in hepatocellular carcinoma. To improve specificity for hepatocellular carcinoma (with some loss of sensitivity) high AFP levels (above 400 μg/L) are generally regarded as a diagnostic prerequisite; at such levels, 70% or more patients with hepatocellular carcinoma show abnormality with less than 5% false positives, many of which are transient; high AFP levels are more often found with hepatocellular carcinoma in blacks and in Chinese, and less often in white Europeans.

Elevation of AFP is less frequent when hepatocellular carcinoma arises in the non-cirrhotic liver, and may be lacking in hepatocellular carcinoma associated with oral contraceptive therapy. Serial determination of AFP is valuable for monitoring patients with cirrhosis; increasing levels should lead to a search for an hepatocellular carcinoma. It is also valuable in monitoring the treatment of hepatocellular carcinoma as levels may become low after successful therapy.

Caeruloplasmin

Caeruloplasmin is an intensely blue α_2-globulin, normally present in plasma at a concentration of 0.2 to 0.4 g/L. It is synthesized in liver and is an acute-phase protein. It is an oxidase for certain aromatic amines and phenols, for cysteine, Fe^{2+} ions and ascorbic acid, but its physiological function is unknown. The plasma concentration rises in pregnancy and with oestrogens, with infections, rheumatoid arthritis, some malignancies, with active non-Wilson's liver disease and in obstructive jaundice.

Serum caeruloplasmin is an important diagnostic marker in Wilson's disease, in which the plasma level is usually reduced. Low caeruloplasmin is also seen in neonates, Menkes' disease, kwashiorkor and marasmus, protein-losing enteropathy, nephrotic syndrome, severe hepatic insufficiency, copper deficiency, and in hereditary hypocaeruloplasminaemia.[46]

Clearance Tests[47]

Clearance tests can provide a quantitative estimate of hepatic functional reserve, disease severity and progression, though they are not widely used for the investigation of liver disease. Galactose clearance, aminopyrine clearance and bromosulphthalein and indocyanine-green clearance have been most frequently studied. Two recently introduced procedures, caffeine clearance and lignocaine clearance, also merit mention.

Galactose Elimination Capacity

After absorption, galactose is removed from blood only by the liver and kidneys. At high plasma galactose concentrations there is a constant rate of removal of galactose by the liver consequent upon its hepatic conversion to galactose-1-phosphate.

Hepatic galactose uptake can be measured by intravenous injection of galactose 0.5 g/kg body weight over about 5 min, with measurement of plasma galactose levels at 5-min intervals for 60 min; urinary galactose elimination is also measured. From 20 to 40 min after injection the disappearance of galactose from the blood is linear with time and one can calculate the galactose elimination capacity. In normal subjects it

is approximately 270 ± 40 (SD) mg/min per m^2 of body surface area or 6.7 ± 1.0 mg/min per kg body mass.

The galactose elimination capacity correlates well with other indices of hepatocellular function—prothrombin time, plasma albumin concentration and aminopyrine clearance for example—and has the advantage that it measures a single aspect of hepatocellular function. It is affected only by the number of individual hepatocytes and by their functional capacity, that is it provides a measure of functioning cell mass. There is considerable overlap between normal subjects and patients with several kinds of liver disease and the test is most useful for repeated studies done on individual subjects.

Aminopyrine Removal and Breath Test

Aminopyrine is removed from plasma by hepatic demethylation, and the clearance of labelled aminopyrine ([^{14}C]-dimethyl aminoantipyrine) has been used particularly to study the hepatic effects of drugs. Its disappearance rate from plasma can be measured after intravenous injection, but the main attraction of this compound lies in its use in simple breath tests. If [^{14}C]-aminopyrine is given orally to non-ambulant subjects, CO_2 can be collected from the breath. The specific activity of the breath CO_2 is measured and, assuming constant endogenous production of CO_2, the amount of labelled $^{14}CO_2$ produced by demethylation of aminopyrine can be calculated.

The disappearance of $^{14}CO_2$ over about 12 h correlates well with bromosulphthalein disappearance (see below) and with the galactose elimination capacity. It is, however, rather tedious to sample the breath over many hours, and similar results may be obtained by taking the mean value for CO_2 specific activity during the first 2 h after the ingestion of the drug, or by sampling the breath at 2 h. Specific activity values obtained from normal subjects have been compared with those obtained from patients with various kinds of liver disease. Values for patients with hepatocellular dysfunction are generally lower than those found in normal subjects. The more severe the dysfunction the lower the clearance, so that aminopyrine clearance is generally lower in chronic active hepatitis than in chronic persistent hepatitis. Normal values may be found in patients with biliary obstruction. Increased values may be found with hepatic enzyme induction from drugs or alcohol.

The aminopyrine 2-h breath test is not a useful differential diagnostic test but it does allow serial measurements of one aspect of hepatic function to be made in the same patient. There is, of course, some reluctance to use radioactive material with a long half-life for repeated studies in man, but the radiation dosage of the test is small.

Hepatic Removal of Bromosulphthalein and Indocyanine Green

Bromosulphthalein (BSP) is removed from blood by hepatic parenchymal cells, bound by intracellular proteins such as ligandin and Z protein, and excreted in bile either unconjugated (approximately 30%) or after conjugation with glutathione. It is easy to measure in blood and bile. In the past a simple test of BSP excretion was widely used to detect hepatobiliary disease in non-jaundiced subjects. For this, 5 mg of BSP/kg body weight is injected intravenously over 30 s. The plasma concentration of BSP is measured in a single blood specimen taken 45 min later, and the retention of BSP at 45 min calculated. In normal subjects this is up to 7% of the original dose. Higher values are found with many types of liver disease. In the familial conjugated hyperbilirubinaemia of the Dubin–Johnson syndrome, retention at 45 min is usually normal but a secondary rise at 90 min is usual. This contrasts with Rotor's syndrome in which BSP retention is normal at 45 min with no secondary rise. Kinetic analysis of plasma disappearance curves has demonstrated abnormalities of hepatic BSP uptake in 30–50% of patients with Gilbert's disease.

The conventional BSP removal test has never been popular in Britain, because it provides very limited information and it is a potentially dangerous test. Local damage results if BSP extravasates at the site of injection: anaphylaxis has been reported, and if the BSP is not properly prepared for injection there may be neurological problems associated with the injection of microcrystals.

Indocyanine green (ICG) is rapidly removed by the liver, and is excreted into the bile without conjugation. It is much safer than BSP, is simple to measure, and can also be used to study hepatic uptake, storage and transport of an exogenous dye. ICG retention at 20 min can be measured and plasma disappearance curves can be analysed. The chief disadvantages of using ICG are that it costs much more than BSP and is unstable in plasma, which means that plasma levels have to be measured soon after withdrawal of the sample.

Both BSP and ICG have been used in research studies to measure hepatic blood flow on the basis of the Fick principle. Plasma levels of either BSP or ICG are held constant during a continuous infusion of the dye; hepatic blood flow can then be calculated by dividing the rate of infusion by the difference in concentration of dye between arterial and hepatic venous plasma. It is unfortunate that this measurement involves hepatic venous catheterization, since the blood flow through the liver is clearly an important functional characteristic.

Caffeine Clearance[48]
The clearance of caffeine provides a quantitative measure of hepatic microsomal demethylation mediated by cytochrome P-448, and measurement of caffeine levels in saliva after oral caffeine provides a simple, non-invasive, harmless means of investigating hepatocellular function. Clearance is markedly decreased in cirrhosis and mildly reduced in non-cirrhotic disease. Caffeine clearance correlates with other clearance tests (e.g. aminopyrine breath test and galactose elimination capacity) but appears more sensitive.

Lignocaine Clearance[49]
In this test, the metabolite of lignocaine, monoethylglycine xylidine, formed by hepatic de-ethylation is measured in serum 15 min after intravenous lignocaine. A high level indicates good hepatocellular function. The procedure has been recommended as a rapid method of assessing liver function in potential liver transplant donors and in their recipients, and for post-transplant follow up.

Miscellaneous Tests Sometimes Used in the Investigations of Liver Disease

Plasma Vitamin B_{12}
Levels of this vitamin increase with various kinds of liver disease; it is released from damaged hepatocytes, more is bound to transcobalamin I, the major B_{12} carrier in normal blood, and there is a more striking rise in the amount bound to transcobalamin II. Dialysable B_{12} levels increase markedly and urinary B_{12} excretion rises. Serum B_{12}-binding proteins may be increased in cases of hepatocellular carcinoma, and there is a particular association with the fibrolamellar form of the tumour.[50]

Serum Ferritin
This is increased in patients with hepatocellular damage, from almost any cause, and also rises in patients with iron overload.

Arterial Ammonia
This tends to be raised in patients with chronic liver disease, particularly if they show hepatic encephalopathy or if there is a significant degree of portal–systemic shunting; it also increases in severe acute hepatitis and with fulminant hepatic failure. But the correlation between the ammonia level and the degree of encephalopathy is poor.

High blood ammonia concentrations are also seen in hereditary disorders in which there are deficiencies of urea-cycle enzymes; in these conditions the blood ammonia is usually higher than that seen with acquired liver diseases and other liver function tests tend to be normal.

Lipoprotein X (LP-X)
An abnormal lipoprotein, LP-X, was once considered of diagnostic value in liver disease because it was present in 99% of patients with histological cholestasis, and absent in 97% of those without cholestasis.[51] This is, however, of little differential value as 'cholestasis' is sometimes found in hepatitis and cirrhosis as well as in extrahepatic obstruction and with intrahepatic cholestases. Furthermore, LP-X may be

undetectable in patients with clear evidence of surgical or other forms of obstruction to the biliary tree. This limits the value of LP-X, even for screening.

Lecithin–cholesterol acyltransferase (LCAT)
LCAT is a glycoprotein produced in the liver for secretion into plasma, where it catalyses the formation of cholesteryl ester. Reduced plasma LCAT activity is an important determinant of the plasma lipid and lipoprotein changes found in liver disease. It has a short plasma half-life and some believe that, as a single test, it is the most sensitive index of hepatocellular dysfunction.[52,53]

THE USE OF LIVER FUNCTION TESTS

Most standard liver function tests are simple to do, relatively inexpensive and easily automated for use in multichannel automatic analysers. Physicians may therefore receive the results of liver function tests without requesting them, or may ask for them without apparent reason. Often liver function tests are requested because the doctor suspects liver disease and hopes that they will confirm this suspicion and give a clue to the nature of the underlying hepatic pathology. If the results are normal, no further action will result in most cases, and little harm will be done. Problems may arise if the results are abnormal. The requesting doctor may not look at the results; s/he may ignore them (if they do not fit within the clinical preconceptions); or s/he may be stung into inappropriate action!

Applications of Liver Function Tests

Like all special investigations, liver function tests can be used for:

- screening (or profiling), to detect unsuspected liver disease;
- confirmation of liver disease when it is suspected clinically;
- differential diagnosis;
- prognosis;
- monitoring progress and assessing response to therapy;
- clinical research.

Unfortunately no investigation is equally useful for all of these purposes.

Screening and Profiling
'Screening' is the routine performance of investigations on an apparently healthy population; 'profiling' may be defined as the routine use of tests on patients, regardless of the clinical presentation. Both are done to detect unsuspected conditions that might be helped by treatment. Profiling may shed light on the cause of the patient's symptoms or, if the results are negative, it may allow exclusion of some conditions; it also provides background data that may subsequently help in assessing new clinical events, or in predicting or evaluating complications of therapy.

For screening or profiling, the main concern is to detect unsuspected disease and we want to be confident that a negative test excludes the disease (true negative). If there are a relatively large number of false-positive results, the position can be clarified by further diagnostic tests; false-positive results are a major problem only if further diagnostic tests are costly or potentially hazardous to the patient. For screening or profiling, therefore, a test must have high sensitivity, sensitivity being defined as the number of true-positive results divided by the total number of subjects who have the disease (that is, true positives plus false negatives).

Screening and profiling tests are done on very large numbers of patients. Such tests must therefore be cheap to do, and they must not cause patients discomfort or inconvenience.

'Batteries' of Liver Function Tests. A single liver-function test is of little value for screening for liver disease because serious liver diseases may be associated with normal serum levels of either bilirubin, AsT or AlT, alkaline phosphatase, albumin, or γGT. With any of these tests, employed individually, the number of false negatives would be unacceptably high. Furthermore, a positive result for only one of these tests has limited value in indicating the presence of liver disease, since many other diseases cause an increase in the level bilirubin or the activities of ASt, alkaline phosphatase or γGT, or a reduction in albumin concentration.

The use of a battery of liver function tests, however, is a highly sensitive procedure; the number of false negatives is minimized by this strategy. Few subjects with significant liver disease have a complete set of normal results with the commonly used batteries of liver function tests, although this does occur (e.g. in well-compensated cirrhosis), and if such patients are missed it is unlikely that there would be any untoward clinical consequences; they tolerate drugs, surgical procedures, and other treatments far better than those in whom there is clear evidence of liver damage.

The use of a battery of liver function tests is also associated with high specificity. Specificity is calculated by dividing the true negatives by the number of subjects without the disease (that is, true negatives plus false positives). A test is specific to the extent that it identifies those who do not have the disease, particularly in that it minimizes false positives. When more than one liver function test is abnormal, the probability of liver disease is very high. False positives are uncommon. They do however occur: for example, a patient with chronic malabsorption may have high serum alkaline phosphatase (from bone) and low serum albumin; with myocardial infarction there may be high AsT (from cardiac muscle) and elevated bilirubin, due perhaps to a functional and relatively trivial hepatic disturbance.

It may be appropriate to perform a battery of liver function tests routinely on hospital inpatients and outpatients. In a hospital population about 4% have raised AsT and a greater proportion have increased AlT. Alcoholic liver disease (often just a fatty liver) is the major cause, and mild elevations may fall with cessation of drinking; obesity is also an important factor.[54] Another 4–5% show increased alkaline phosphatase; bone disease, such as Paget's disease, is an important cause in the elderly. Only in a small number of patients does the finding of high alkaline phosphatase lead to a new diagnosis of liver disease. Similar results have been found in a 'healthy' outpatient population.[55] Most of these abnormalities (c.90%) had not been previously recognized but a new diagnosis was established in only about 10% of those with the abnormal results.

Although there does not appear to be a high diagnostic yield from profiling, other advantages have been pointed out—reassurance for the patient, data that make other tests unnecessary, and baseline investigations against which to compare future test results. The last is a particularly valuable feature in the hospital setting.

In a 'normal' (but not necessarily unselected) population studied at the British United Provident Association (BUPA) Centre, unsuspected liver disease, usually due to excessive alcohol intake, was found in about 1% of the subjects studied. Individual liver-function tests were found to be abnormal in a larger proportion of subjects.[56] Total bilirubin above 17 μmol/L was found in about 5% of those attending; approximately 2% of men had a level greater than 25 μmol/L, but only 0.5% of women. Bilirubin was usually absent from the urine and other liver function tests were normal. This hyperbilirubinaemia is almost always benign and due to Gilbert's syndrome. The consequences of finding this high bilirubin may be deleterious, as the patients may then be subjected to unnecessary, expensive and potentially hazardous medical or surgical intervention. However, knowledge of the presence of Gilbert's syndrome may explain the jaundice that is sometimes seen in patients with abdominal pain, who may reduce their food intake and thus put up their bilirubin level.

The value of γGT as a screening test is controversial. Levels of γGT exceeding the usually accepted upper limit of normal (50 mu/L in men, 30 mu/L in women) were found in about 15% of those screened at the BUPA Centre and as a result the upper limit of their normal range was readjusted to 80 in men, and 50 in women. Even then, 6% of men had an abnormal level and in 4% the level was greater than 100 mu/L. γGT is a very sensitive indicator of liver disease (0.87–0.95) but lacks specificity, since many conditions with only minimal liver disturbance cause an increase of γGT. However, sensitivity and specificity are of restricted value to the practising clinician, whose main need is to know the predictive value (i.e. the probability) that a positive test indicates the presence of disease (true positives divided by true positives plus false positives) or that a negative test indicates the absence of disease (true negatives divided by true negatives plus false negatives). Unfortunately, the predictive value of a test is markedly dependent on the type of population studied and the proportion of those who have the disease. γGT has a very poor predictive accuracy in a population where the majority are disease free.

Role of Liver Function Tests in Diagnosis[57]
Standard liver-function tests have only limited differential diagnostic value. They allow patients to be categorized as having simple unconjugated hyperbilirubinaemia (i.e. an elevation of serum total bilirubin with little or no increase in conjugated bilirubin, absence of bilirubinuria, and no abnormality of other liver function tests). Also, when the aminotransferases are very high (in the thousands) the patient is almost certainly suffering from an acute hepatitis, due to a virus or drugs, or an acute reduction in hepatic blood flow.

Liver function tests have been used to classify jaundice for diagnostic purposes, for example as 'haemolytic jaundice' when jaundice is acholuric (i.e. urinary bilirubin is absent) and the serum bilirubin is predominantly unconjugated; as 'hepatocellular jaundice' when there is an increase in both unconjugated bilirubin and bilirubin esters, with normal or only slightly increased alkaline phosphatase and a marked increase in aminotransferases; or as 'obstructive jaundice' (or 'cholestasis') when most of the serum bilirubin is conjugated (although this is rarely confirmed), aminotransferase levels are only moderately elevated, and there is a more marked increase in alkaline phosphatase (more than 2.5 times the upper reference limit). This clarification is undesirable, however, because if used in this way, many conditions generally considered 'hepatocellular' (e.g. viral hepatitis, drug-induced hepatitis, alcoholic liver disease, chronic active hepatitis, and cirrhosis) might be classified as obstructive or cholestatic jaundice because they may all present with biochemical (and clinical) features that are 'typical' of extrahepatic biliary obstruction. Differential diagnosis must therefore depend on other evidence also, such as viral markers, autoantibodies, history of alcohol abuse or drug intake, cholangiography, ultrasound or computerized tomographic scanning, or liver biopsy.

To assess the ability of any liver function test to effect diagnostic discrimination it is essential that a variety of well-characterized hepatobiliary disorders with both typical and atypical clinical features be studied in adequate numbers of patients and that attention is paid to the degree of overlap in results between disease categories. Furthermore, it is essential to consider sensitivity, specificity, predictive value and efficiency, and the effect of disease prevalence when the diagnostic usefulness of any test or combination of tests is being assessed.

Monitoring

Much of the work of chemical pathology and haematology laboratories involves repetition of tests done to monitor progress. With repeated measurements on a single patient, clinically significant trends may be detected, even if all the results remain within the conventional normal range. Clinicians should therefore be aware of the precision of the laboratory tests they use and of normal biological variations, so that the significance of a change between consecutive tests can be estimated. Tests for monitoring tend to be repeated on many occasions. They should therefore be cheap; expensive tests would be justified only if they were to be used to make important clinical decisions.

Conventional liver-function tests are satisfactory for monitoring progress. They are quantitative, precise and cheap. When results are abnormal due to liver disease, they tend to change only in one direction, that is, increasing in the case of bilirubin, aminotransferases, alkaline phosphatase and γGT, and decreasing in the case of albumin. The degree of change of aminotransferases and alkaline phosphatase may be of little prognostic significance, but high levels of bilirubin and low levels of albumin (or clotting factors) tend to indicate severe liver damage. Improvement in hepatic status is usually, but not invariably, accompanied by a return of all tests towards normal values. The results of individual tests often change in opposite directions; for example, in acute hepatitis the aminotransferases may fall from a very high level while the bilirubin continues to rise.

Hepatology has made striking advances since the introduction of tests to measure serum bilirubin, alkaline phosphatase, and aminotransferases. Much of the effort that has been expended has gone into the search for improved diagnostic techniques other than biochemical and in many instances the results have been outstandingly successful. There are now excellent methods that allow us to delineate gross alterations in the biliary tree, to localize intrahepatic lesions, and to biopsy or aspirate these lesions. Advances in histopathology allow precise diagnosis of many types of hepatic disorder. New immunological techniques, some of which can be applied to biopsy samples, have revolutionized diagnosis, particularly in the field of viral disease of the liver. But when the effort has been to search for new biochemical tests to replace or supplement the long-established tests of liver function, or to look for aetiological clues in patterns of test responses, the results have been disappointing.

The diagnostic limitations of conventional liver function tests, and their general limitations when employed individually, do not mean that these tests are without value. As we have indicated, the commonly used batteries of liver function tests are of considerable value for screening and profiling, are helpful in monitoring the progress of liver disease, and aid in predicting prognosis. For these purposes, they are tried and tested. They will continue to play an important part in the detection and management of liver disease.

REFERENCES

1. van den Bergh A.H.H., Muller R. (1916). Ueber eine direkte und eine indirekte Diazoreaktion auf Bilirubin. *Biochem. Z.*, **77**, 90.
2. Billing B.H., Lathe G.H. (1956). The excretion of bilirubin as an ester glucuronide, giving the direct van den Bergh reaction. *Biochem. J.*, **63**, 6P.
3. Lauff J.J., Kasper M.E., Wu T.W. Ambrose R.T. (1982). Isolation and preliminary characterization of a fraction of bilirubin in serum that is firmly bound to protein. *Clin. Chem.*, **28**, 629.
4. Rosalki S.B. (1976). Enzyme tests in disease of the liver and biliary tract. In *Principles and Practice of Diagnostic Enzymology* (Wilkinson S.H. ed) London: Edward Arnold.
5. Konttinen A., Murros J., Ojala K., Salaspuro M., Somer H., Rasanen J. (1978). A new cause of increased serum aspartate aminotransferase activity. *Clin. Chim. Acta*, **84**, 145.
6. Cohen J.A., Kaplan M.M. (1979). The SGOT/SGPT ratio—an indicator of alcoholic liver disease. *Dig. Dis. Sci.*, **24**, 835.
7. Shaver W.A. (1987). Correspondence: Reply to letter entitled 'Unmeasurable serum alkaline phosphatase activity in Wilson's disease associated with fulminant hepatic failure and hemolysis' by Wilson R.A., Clayson K.J., Leon S. *Hepatology*, **7**, 615.
8. Williams A.L.B., Hoofnagle J.A. (1988). Ratio of serum aspartate to alanine aminotransferase in chronic hepatitis: relationship to cirrhosis. *Gastroenterology*, **95**, 734.
9. Clermont R.J., Chalmers T.C. (1967). The transaminase tests in liver disease. *Medicine*, **46**, 197.
10. Nemesanszky E. (1986). Alkaline phosphatase. In *Clinical Enzymology* (Lott J. A., Wolf P. L. eds.) New York: Field Rich.
11. Tietz N. W., Rinker A. D., Shaw L. M., (1983). IFCC methods for the measurement of catalytic concentration of enzymes, Part 5. *Clin. Chim. Acta*, **135**, 339F.
12. Kuwana T., Sugita O., Yakata M. (1988). Reference limits of bone and liver alkaline phosphatase isoenzymes in the serum of healthy subjects according to age and sex as determined by wheat germ lectin affinity electrophoresis. *Clin. Chim. Acta*, **173**, 273.
13. Rosalki S. B., Foo A. Y. (1984). Two new methods for separating and quantifying bone and liver alkaline phosphatase isoenzymes in plasma. *Clin. Chem.*, **30**, 1182.
14. Payne C. R., Ackrill P., Ralston A. J. (1982). Acute renal failure and rise in alkaline phosphatase activity caused by cimetidine. *Br. Med. J.*, **285**, 100.
15. Math M. V. (1982). Furosemide and increased serum alkaline phosphatase (hepatic isoenzyme). *Clin. Chem.*, **28**, 1812.
16. Balazs T., Farber T. M., Feuer A. (1978). Drug-induced changes in serum alkaline phosphatase and alanine aminotransferase activities not related to hepatic injuries. *Arch. Toxicol.*, **1** (suppl.), 159.
17. Moss D. W. (1975). Alkaline phosphatase isoenzymes: technical and clinical aspects. *Enzyme*, **20**, 20.

18. Brensilver H. L., Kaplan M. M. (1975). Significance of elevated liver alkaline phosphatase in serum. *Gastroenterology*, **68**, 1156.

19. Parker S. G., Agius L., James O. F. W. (1989). Induction of hepatic alkaline phosphatase activity by the acute phase protein response *in vitro*. *Clin. Sci.*, **76** (suppl. 20), 19P.

20. Sherlock S., Scheuer P. J. (1973). The presentation and diagnosis of 100 patients with primary biliary cirrhosis. *N. Engl. J. Med.*, **289**, 674.

21. Cooper J. F., Brand E. J. (1988). Symptomatic sclerosing cholangitis in patients with a normal alkaline phosphatase: two case reports and a review of the literature. *Am. J. Gastroenterol.*, **83**, 308.

22. Shaver W. A. Bhatt H., Combes B. (1986). Low serum alkaline phosphatase activity in Wilson's disease. *Hepatology*, **6**, 859.

23. Higashino K. et al. (1975). Hepatocellular carcinoma and a variant alkaline phosphatase. *Ann. Int. Med.*, **83**, 74.

24. Crofton P. M., Kilpatrick D. C., Leitch A. G. (1981). Complexes in serum between alkaline phosphatase and immunoglobulin G: immunological and clinical aspects. *Clin. Chim. Acta*, **111**, 257.

25. Leroux-Roels G. G., Wieme R. J., de Broe M. E. (1981). Occurrence of enzyme-immunoglobulin complexes in chronic inflammatory bowel disease. *J. Lab. Clin. Med.*, **97**, 316.

26. Wilson J. W. (1979). Inherited elevation of alkaline phosphatase activity in the absence of disease. *N. Engl. J. Med.*, **301**, 983.

27. McEvoy M., Skrabanek P., Wright E., Powell D. (1987). Family with raised serum alkaline phosphatase activity in the absence of disease. *Br. Med. J.*, **282**, 1272.

28. Stein P., Rosalki S. B., Foo A. Y., Hjelm M. (1987). Transient hyperphosphatasemia of infancy and early childhood: clinical and biochemical features of 21 cases and literature review. *Clin. Chem.*, **33**, 313.

29. Rosalki S. B. (1975). Gamma-glutamyl transpeptidase. *Adv. Clin. Chem.*, **17**, 53.

30. Nemesanszky E. (1986). Gammaglutamyltransferase (GGT). In *Clinical Enzymology* (Lott J. A., Wolf P. L. eds) New York: Field Rich.

31. Nemesanszky E., Lott J. A. (1985). Gamma-glutamyltransferase and its isoenzymes: progress and problems. *Clin. Chem.*, **31**, 797.

32. Kajiwara E. et al. (1983). Low gamma-glutamyltranspeptidase activity in patients with acute intrahepatic cholestasis. (In Japanese) *Jpn. J. Gastroenterology*, **80**, 2224.

33. Maggiore G., Bernard O., Riely C. A., Hadchouel M., Lemonnier A., Alagille D. (1987). Normal serum gamma-glutamyl-transpeptidase activity identifies groups of infants with idiopathic cholestasis with poor prognosis. *J. Pediatr.*, **111**, 251.

34. Henny J. et al. (1982). Use of the reference state concept for interpretation of laboratory tests: drug effects on gamma-glutamyltransferase. *Adv. Biochem. Pharmacol.*, **3**, 209.

35. Joubaud F. et al. (1987). Etude de la gamma-glutamyltransferase chez les diabetiques. *Semin. Hôp. Paris*, **63**, 1851.

36. Rothschild M.A., Oratz M., Schreiber S.S. (1988). Serum albumin. *Hepatology*, **8**, 385.

37. Rayner B.L., Willcox P.A. (1988). Community-acquired bacteraemia; a prospective survey of 239 cases. *Q. J. Med.*, **69**, 907.

38. Beckett G.J., Hayes J.D. (1987). Plasma glutathione-*S*-transferase measurements and liver disease in man. *J. Clin. Biochem. Nutr.*, **2**, 1.

39. Brown S.S., Kalow W., Pilz W., Whittaker M., Woronick C.L. (1981). The plasma cholinesterases: a new perspective. *Adv. Clin. Chem.*, **22**, 1.

40. Sawhney A.K., Lott J.A. (1986). Acetylcholinesterase and cholinesterase. In *Clinical Enzymology* (Lott J.A., Wolf P.L. eds) New York: Field Rich.

41. Bertrand L., Arnefaux J. (1973). Valeur de la gamma-glutamyl transpeptidase dans les maladies du foie et des oies biliaires. Confrontations cliniques, essais experimentaux. *Ann. Med. Interne*, **124**, 173.

42. Rondana M., Milani L., Merkel C., Caregaro L., Gatta A. (1987). Value of prealbumin plasma levels as liver test. *Digestion*, **37**, 72.

43. Hutchinson D.R., Smith M.G., Parke D.V. (1980). Prealbumin as an index of liver function after acute paracetamol poisoning. *Lancet*, **ii**, 121.

44. Feld R.D. (1989). Heterozygosity of α_1-antitrypsin: a health risk. *Crit. Rev. Clin. Lab. Sci.*, **27**, 461.

45. Kew M.C. (1975). Alpha-fetoprotein. In *Modern Trends in Gastroenterology*, vol. 5 (Read A. ed.) London: Butterworth.

46. Edwards C.Q., Williams D.M., Cartwright G.E. (1979). Hereditary hypoceruloplasminemia. *Clin. Genetics*, **15**, 311.

47. Larrey D., Branch R.A. (1983). Clearance by the liver: current concepts in understanding the hepatic disposition of drugs. *Semin. Liver Dis.*, **3**, 285.

48. Jost G., Wahllander A., von Mandach U., Preisig R. (1987). Overnight salivary caffeine clearance: a liver function test suitable for routine use. *Hepatology*, **7**, 338.

49. Oellerich M. et al. (1989). Lignocaine metabolite formation as a measure of pre-transplant liver function. *Lancet*, **i**, 640.

50. Paradinas F.J. et al. (1982). High serum vitamin B_{12} binding capacity as a marker of the fibrolamellar variant of hepatocellular carcinoma. *Br. Med. J.*, **285**, 840.

51. Seidel D., Gretz H., Ruppert C. (1973). Significance of the LP-X test in differential diagnosis of jaundice. *Clin. Chem.*, **19**, 86.

52. De Martiis M., Barlattani A., Parenzi A., Sebastiani F. (1983). Pattern of lecithin–cholesterol-acyl-transferase (L-CAT) activity in the course of liver cirrhosis. *J. Int. Med. Res.*, **11**, 232.

53. Simko V., Kelley R.E., Dincsoy H.P. (1985). Predicting severity of liver disease: twelve laboratory tests evaluated by multiple regression. *J. Int. Med. Res.*, **13**, 249.

54. Friedman L.S. et al. (1987). Evaluation of blood donors with elevated serum alanine aminotransferase levels. *Ann. Int. Med.*, **107**, 137.

55. Whitehead T.P., Wootton I.D.P. (1974). Biochemical profiles for hospital patients. *Lancet*, **ii**, 1439.

56. Wilding P., Rollason, J.G., Robinson D. (1972). Patterns of change for various biochemical constituents detected in well population screening. *Clin. Chim. Acta*, **41**, 375.

57. Rosoff L., Rosoff L. (1977). Biochemical tests for hepatobiliary disease. *Surg. Clin. North Am.*, **57**, 257.

23. Clinical Diagnosis and the Acute Abdomen

H. Ellis

Introduction
Steps in diagnosis
  The history
  Clinical examination
  Differential diagnosis
  Special investigations—an overview
Acute appendicitis
  Differential diagnosis
  Special investigations
Acute intestinal obstruction
  Special investigations
  Perforated peptic ulcer
  Special investigations
Acute pancreatitis
  Clinical features
  Special investigations
Medical conditions that may simulate the
  acute abdomen
  Chest diseases
  Diabetes
  Sickle-cell anaemia
  Other medical conditions

INTRODUCTION

The patient with acute abdominal pain remains one of the last bastions of clinical medicine. There are three reasons for this statement. First, in no other common situation is reliance on clinical features, immediate decision and accurate diagnosis of such paramount importance. Second, it is the clinical diagnosis that counts, since ancillary investigations, both from the laboratory and the X-ray department, are rarely diagnostic, often misleading and can never be used for more than confirmation of the clinical diagnosis. Third, in no other condition commonly encountered is there such a wide differential diagnosis, which, indeed, covers the whole of medical practice.

In most other fields an initially tentative or even incorrect clinical diagnosis is not necessarily harmful; we can wait until it is confirmed or refuted by laboratory and radiological investigations and even await the progression of the natural history of the disease. Provided we take sensible and appropriate measures, a misdiagnosis at our first clinical consultation is readily corrected. For example, a woman is seen by her general practitioner because she has a lump in the breast. Initial diagnosis is that the lump is malignant; her doctor takes the wise appropriate step and arranges an urgent consultation with a surgical col-league. The surgeon agrees that this tentative diagnosis may indeed be true and makes urgent provision to admit the patient to hospital for excision and histological examination of the lump. When the lump is put under the microscope it proves to be completely benign. The diagnostic process may be reversed; that is to say, an initial diagnosis of a benign breast lump is replaced, after histological examination, with the diagnosis of malignant disease of the breast. Once again, as long as appropriate sensible steps have been taken, no harm has come to the patient. But in acute abdominal conditions, delays of even a few hours in initiating the correct line of treatment may make the difference between a smooth or stormy course; indeed, may even place the patient's life in danger. For example, the general practitioner who labels a child with acute appendicitis as a case of gastroenteritis and prescribes a kaolin mixture and a sedative overnight may be faced, the next morning, with a desperately ill patient suffering from a generalized peritonitis. The Casualty Officer who sends an abdominal injury home labelled 'slight bruising of the abdominal wall' may be confronted, a few hours later, with a moribund example of haemoperitoneum due to a ruptured spleen. Sir Heneage Ogilvie, of Guy's Hospital, summed this up perfectly years ago when he wrote that 'in the acute abdominal emergencies the difference between the best and the worst surgery is infinitely less than that between early and late surgery, and the greatest sacrifice of all is the sacrifice of time'. Put into less elegant but more practical English, this can be paraphrased 'it is better for you to have your inflamed appendix removed a few hours after the onset of your illness by the House Surgeon than to have your gangrenous perforated appendix removed a couple of days later by the Professor of Surgery'.

In dealing with the patient with acute abdominal pain, clinicians must steel themselves to realize that they must rely almost entirely on clinical features rather than laboratory and radiological investigations. These days clinicians have become so used to being able to skimp on history and examination that it comes as a severe shock to realize that, in the middle of the night, in the patient's home or in the casualty department, they are going to be forced to rely on their own five senses. It is a very good aphorism that, in the diagnosis of the acute abdomen, the special investigations can only be used to reinforce a clinical diagnosis; seldom if ever can they refute it. We shall be developing this theme as we consider specific examples of acute abdominal pain but a few examples may now be used to underline this statement. Thus, if the clinical diagnosis is one of acute appendicitis it is common practice to ask for a white blood count. Indeed, in the USA, the textbooks list a leucocytosis as one of the cardinal features of this condition. Certainly, one is used to seeing a raised white count in such cases but every clinician will have also encountered many examples of classical acute appendicitis, confirmed at operation, where the white-cell count was within normal limits. It is true that many cases of perforated peptic ulcer are associated, radiologically, with the presence of free gas under the diaphragm on a plain radiograph of the abdomen in the erect position. Yet in about a quarter of the cases X-rays fail to reveal free gas, particularly when the perforation has sealed or when fluid rather than gas has principally escaped into the peritoneal cavity through the perforation. It is true that most cases of intestinal obstruction are associated with distended loops of intestine and with the presence of multiple fluid levels on the radiograph of the abdomen. However, once again, it is well known that, in some 10% of cases, intestinal obstruction, indeed strangulation of the bowel, may be associated with perfectly normal radiographic appearances. This occurs when a closed loop of intestine containing fluid and free from gas becomes obstructed. Failure to observe our cardinal principle of relying on clinical features and being prepared to discount special investigations may put the patient into the gravest peril.

Acute abdominal pain is not only a vitally important diagnostic problem but it is also often a difficult one, and therefore of particular fascination to the clinician. It is no exaggeration to say that abdominal pain may result from disease of almost any organ in the body. Apart from the abdominal and the retroperitoneal viscera themselves, and these include, of course, the pelvic organs, one must also consider the chest, the central nervous system, and even the ears and the throat. Basal pneumonia, acute cardiac ischaemia and spinal root irritation can all mimic the acute abdomen. We have recently transferred a patient admitted to the Coronary Unit as a case of massive myocardial infarction to the operating theatre to deal with his ruptured aortic aneurysm; many a patient with prodromal herpes zoster has been labelled 'biliary colic' or 'pain of renal origin' before the typical rash appears, and children with otitis media are notorious for complaining of belly-ache. Metabolic disorders, particularly diabetes, but also acute porphyria, may give acute abdominal symptoms. Finally, those extraordinary individuals suffering from the Munchausen syndrome provide us with teasing diagnostic difficulties and manage to simulate a wide variety of acute abdominal catastrophes to perfection.

It is a good discipline, therefore, when approaching any patient with abdominal pain to consider its anatomical source; is it intra-abdominal? is it arising from a retroperitoneal structure (pancreas, kidney, aorta)? or is it of extra-abdominal origin, neurological or functional?

STEPS IN DIAGNOSIS

The essence of clinical diagnosis is, of course, a careful history and full examination; neither is easy when the patient has acute abdominal pain.[1]

The History

Great skill and a fine economy must be employed in taking a history from a patient with acute abdominal symptoms. There is nothing to gain and much to lose by exhausting and exasperating an ill patient with irrelevant questions. However, such valuable gems of information as a missed menstrual period, which suggests ectopic pregnancy, or shoulder-tip pain of diaphragmatic irritation in a perforated peptic ulcer or in haemoperitoneum following abdominal trauma, may only be revealed by direct questioning. We need to know about the speed of onset, the severity, the exact duration of the pain and its accompaniments. Most serious intra-abdominal conditions stop the patient from sleeping and make it impossible for him or her to continue at work. Of course there are always exceptions to any rule; I shall never forget as a house surgeon being called to the admission ward to see an obese lady admitted with acute abdominal pain. On arrival, I found that she was in a deep sleep and had a mind to going back to bed myself. However, I roused her, elicited rigidity and exquisite tenderness in the right iliac fossa and assisted at the removal of her gangrenous and perforated appendix.

Perforation, torsion and stone impaction all have a sudden acute onset and indeed the patient can describe the exact moment at which the agony commenced. Inflammatory conditions and intestinal obstruction, in contrast, tend to come on more insidiously.

Sometimes it is difficult to be sure whether the patient's symptoms represent some quite minor abdominal upset or warrant more serious consideration. This is a problem that particularly confronts the general practitioner when called to the patient's home. Here I have always found Sir Zachary Cope's aphorism most helpful; that a previously healthy patient who complains of severe abdominal pain for more than about 6 h duration is *usually* suffering from an acute surgical condition. The description of pain given by the patient is rarely diagnostic. Since it is usually a unique experience for the patient, he or she can only describe it as 'severe' or 'agony' or 'not too bad'. A very florid clinical description—'like a piece of barbed wire heated to a dull red heat and slowly tightened up around my abdomen'—is very likely to be functional in origin. It is the accompaniments of the pain that are far more valuable than any description by the patient of the pain itself. A patient with renal or biliary colic, or with an intestinal obstruction, can usually hardly hold still with the pain and may develop all sorts of strange contortions in an effort to find a position of relief. In contrast, the patient with peritonitis finds the slightest movement agonizing and usually simply wants to be left alone with knees drawn up, clutching the abdomen and keeping as still as possible. Jaundice or haematuria during the present or a previous attack of pain are important pointers to gallstones or to renal calculi, respectively. While on this topic it is worth remembering the important clinical observation by French and Robb,[2] who found that, unlike the usual textbook description, biliary and renal colics are only very rarely intermittent in nature. Usually the pain in these conditions is constant and continuous or else continuous with exacerbations. In contrast, intestinal colic does indeed come on with waves of intermittent pain.

One last point in the history; most patients are more than anxious to tell the doctor about their bowel actions but they will usually only discuss passage of flatus on direct questioning. In spite of the layman's views to the contrary, a few days of constipation are of no great relevance. However, 24 h without the passage of wind denotes either complete intestinal obstruction or paralytic ileus.

Clinical Examination

The clinical examination requires particular skill. The sick, anxious patient is apprehensive that the doctor is going to produce still more pain and yet it is vital to get the patient to cooperate and to relax. The problem is particularly difficult, of course, with a small child where, in addition, there is the presence of tense anxious parents, hoping for reassurance and yet fearing the worst.

The common mistake in an emergency situation is to rush ahead and palpate the abdomen at once. Time spent in careful observation of the patient as a whole and of the abdomen in particular is time well spent indeed. It is a good plan to start by taking the temperature and pulse rate; useful in themselves, they also give the clinician useful time for general observation. One should be suspicious of the diagnosis of acute appendicitis without pyrexia; it does occur, but it is unusual. In contrast, a pyrexia is rare with a perforated peptic ulcer. Atrial fibrillation in a patient with acute abdominal pain with the features of ileus will suggest a mesenteric embolism. A coated tongue is certainly a common finding in peritonitis and acute appendicitis but it is not an invariable finding; indeed it is a very good rule that there is no such thing as 'always' or 'never' in the acute abdomen. Look at the patient's posture. The restlessness of colic is in sharp contrast to the fear of movement which is so typical of peritoneal irritation. The girl sent into hospital as a case of acute appendicitis who is pale and fainting is more likely to have a ruptured ectopic pregnancy with haemoperitoneum.

Attention is now turned to the abdomen itself. It should be carefully inspected for distension (either local or generalized), for visible peristalsis or for the presence of previous laparotomy scars. A previous abdominal operation, carried out no matter how many years previously, always raises the suspicion of intra-abdominal adhesions or bands. It is a good rule that this should be the first diagnosis in a patient with intestinal obstruction who has a scar on the abdominal wall. Although the anatomical boundaries of the abdomen are the xiphoid above to the pubis below, the wise clinician will extend these borders to the nipples above and the knees below and will ensure that all the territory between is laid bare for inspection. Perhaps the most common sign to be missed is a small strangulated inguinal, or particularly, femoral hernia, especially in an obese female patient. It may seem unbelievable that a patient with intestinal obstruction does not know that he has an irreducible hernia but this is certainly the case. Indeed, I have known of a distinguished doctor who correctly diagnosed himself as having intestinal obstruction but who realized he had a strangulated inguinal hernia only when his surgical colleague pointed this out to him.

An absolute rule, therefore, is always to inspect and palpate the hernial orifices in every patient with acute abdominal pain. At the same time take this opportunity to feel the femoral pulses; their absence is a good clue to the rare dissecting aortic aneurysm.

Palpation is a delicate art which requires constant practice to perfect. The heavy-handed tyro may think that the abdomen is rigid, yet the more experienced clinician will find the muscles to be relaxed under his or her gentler touch. There is all the difference between voluntary and protective guarding against rough palpation and the involuntary and reflex rigidity of muscles due to underlying peritoneal irritation or inflammation, which can be detected with the lightest touch. An abdomen that will relax completely and will allow the posterior abdominal wall to be massaged under the examiner's hand rarely harbours any acute abdominal disorder. However, constant localized tenderness and muscle spasm and the presence of release tenderness are signs that can be trusted and that almost invariably indicate serious mischief beneath. The same applies to tenderness in the pelvic peritoneal pouch on rectal or vaginal examination, which naturally must never be omitted. Digital examination of the pelvis may also reveal such important features as faecal impaction or the presence of a tender pelvic mass. Finally, auscultation may reveal the typical noisy bowel sounds of mechanical intestinal obstruction, the transmitted heart sounds of free fluid in the peritoneal cavity or the ominous silence of peritonitis.

Particular skill is required in the examination of the abdomen in children. Once the patient is hurt or frightened, he or she cries, the abdominal muscles are voluntarily contracted into iron bands and any opportunity of further examination is lost. Utmost gentleness is essential. The young child is best held in the mother's arms and the examiner's warmed hand then insinuated beneath the blanket and under the cover of soothing words. If all this fails, the young patient must be examined again after suitable sedation.

Having finished clinical examination, a specimen of urine is obtained and examined, especially for blood, pus, bile and sugar.

Differential Diagnosis

It may not, and indeed often cannot, be possible to make an exact pathological diagnosis in a case of acute abdominal pain but at least the clinician should attempt to diagnose the type of disease process that is going on. The clinician must consider whether the lesion is situated within the abdomen (including the retroperitoneum and pelvis) or whether possibly the pain is referred from the chest or is of neurological or functional origin. It is useful to consider the following check-list of the causes of acute intra-abdominal pain:

(1) inflammation (for example, appendicitis, chole-cystitis or sigmoid diverticulitis);
(2) obstruction of a hollow viscus—the intestine (which may or may not be strangulated), the bile duct or the ureter;
(3) perforation of a hollow viscus;
(4) haemoperitoneum (for example, ruptured spleen or ruptured ectopic pregnancy);
(5) torsion of a viscus;
(6) a vascular catastrophe (mesenteric occlusion or dissecting aortic aneurysm).

An especial difficulty in late cases is that one pathological process may by now have merged into another. In particular, an inflamed or strangulated viscus may by now have ruptured so that the immediate features are those of acute peritonitis. Here reliance must be placed quite heavily on the history of the events leading up to the patient's present clinical condition. A rigid abdomen with all the features of peritonitis within a few hours of onset suggests a primary perforation, of which the most common cause is a perforated peptic ulcer. However, generalized rigidity in a patient seen at 48 h who gives a typical history of central abdominal pain that moves to the right iliac fossa and is now generalized suggests that a gangrenous appendix has by now ruptured.

Having determined the type of abdominal emergency, we then usually have to rely on the laws of probability to guess at the underlying disease. For example, there is nothing at all on history or examination to distinguish between an acutely inflamed appendix and an acute Meckel's diverticulitis, and certainly no laboratory investigation will distinguish between the two. The only difference is that the first is extremely common and the second rather rare. Of course, occasionally good luck or experience will allow the clinician the satisfaction of correctly diagnosing the uncommon, often because some small extra fact in the history or an additional physical sign has been elicited. Thus, pigment spots on the lips and buccal mucosa might suggest that a young patient with intestinal obstruction may have an intussusception of small intestine produced by a Peutz–Jegher polyp.

Special Investigations—an Overview

What help can we obtain from the laboratory and from the radiological department in the diagnosis and the differential diagnosis of acute abdominal pain? Unfortunately, although occasionally invaluable, these special investigations often yield little, if any, more information than that obtained by careful history and examination and, indeed, every now and then they may be frankly misleading. Both the clinician and colleagues in the ancillary departments should have the following aphorism written in capital letters of gold in the ward and the laboratory: 'If the special investigations fit in with the diagnosis made after careful clinical study, then they provide useful confirmatory evidence of the diagnosis. If, however, there is total disagreement between a laboratory or radiological test and the carefully elicited clinical features in an acute abdominal emergency, then it is wise to side with the clinical diagnosis rather than that obtained on laboratory findings.' Let us take a very common clinical example. A man is admitted with all the clinical features of acute appendicitis; he has a typical history, a raised temperature and the signs of local peritoneal inflammation. If a white-cell count is now obtained and is found to be raised with a marked polymorph leucocytosis, then this is an interesting finding and reinforces the diagnosis. If, however, the white-cell count is normal, the doctor should certainly not budge from the clinical diagnosis of acute appendicitis, which can occur, of course, in the presence of an entirely normal white-cell count. Another example is a raised serum amylase, which is extremely good supporting evidence to the clinical diagnosis of acute pancreatitis, but an elevation of the amylase may occur in perforated peptic ulcer and after morphine; moreover an overwhelming pancreatitis may be associated with a perfectly normal amylase level, which is often normal, in addition in acute pancreatitis following abdominal trauma.

The electrocardiogram and the estimation of the serum transaminases are certainly helpful in making the differential diagnosis between the pain of myocardial ischaemia and an acute upper abdominal crisis such as cholecystitis. However, one must bear in mind that a patient with a recent ischaemic episode may have thrown off an embolism and now be suffering from a mesenteric arterial embolus.

Urine examination, we have already noted, hardly falls into the ambit of a 'special investigation' and is perhaps better regarded merely as an extension of the clinical evaluation of the patient presenting as an acute abdominal emergency. It should certainly never be omitted but, once again, needs cautious interpretation. Pyuria at microscopic level may be seen in patients with acute appendicitis, particularly in a low-lying pelvic appendix that is abutting against the bladder or in a retrocolic inflamed appendix lying against the ureter or even on the renal pelvis. The differential diagnosis between appendicitis and right-sided pyelitis under such circumstances requires very careful clinical judgement. The presence of sugar in the urine is, of course, a vital finding and will need to be followed up by blood-sugar estimation. Hyperglycaemia may well mimic an acute abdominal episode but equally well one must remember that the diabetic patient is not immune from any of the common abdominal emergencies.

X-ray films of the chest and abdomen, the latter preferably taken with the patient in both the errect and lying position, may yield considerable information. The presence of free gas beneath the diaphragm is pathognomonic of perforation of a hollow viscus, except in the postoperative period following laparotomy when the air that has been admitted into the opened abdomen remains visible for some days. However, once again, one must not rely too heavily on this radiological sign; in perhaps 25% of perforations, especially those that have sealed rapidly or where fluid rather than gas has escaped into the peritoneum, the radiographs appear perfectly normal. Intestinal obstruction on X-ray examination of the abdomen usually demonstrates one or more distended loops of bowel with fluid levels seen on the erect films. In theory it would appear to be easy enough to distinguish these findings from the generalized gaseous distension of the intestine in peritonitis or in paralytic ileus (and the latter often accompanies ureteric colic); in practice, however, the two are confused with surprising ease. Furthermore, if the obstructed loop of bowel happens to be distended entirely with fluid, the characteristic air distension is absent and the involved segment of intestine, which may even be entirely gangrenous, is radiologically invisible. Fortunately renal and ureteric stones are usually radiopaque and can often be identified on plain abdominal radiographs. Yet about 10% of these are radiolucent and in other cases they may be confused with calcified phleboliths or faecal debris. Unfortunately only about 10% of gallstones are radiopaque and, again, they may be confused with other opaque intra-abdominal shadows. X-rays are certainly helpful in acute abdominal emergencies but the quality of films that can be obtained in patients who are seriously ill and restless often leaves much to be desired, particularly when taken in the middle of the night or at the weekend by junior radiographers. One must really weigh up the value likely to accrue from these investigations against the delay they cause in initiating treatment and the disturbance necessary to an already exhausted patient.

Modern imaging techniques are being introduced into the investigation of the acute abdomen. Ultrasonography can demonstrate the presence of gallstones and delineate the thickened wall of an inflamed gallbladder, visualize the pancreas and define an aortic aneurysm and pelvic masses; HIDA scanning can demonstrate the biliary tree in the presence of a non-functioning gallbladder; laparoscopy is being applied more and more to the diagnosis of the acute abdomen, especially in suspected gynaecological emergencies. These and other methods all depend, of course, on the availability of sophisticated equipment and perhaps more importantly, of skilled operatives.

Having now considered the special investigations in general terms, we will now turn to specific entities presenting as acute abdominal pain and consider the laboratory tests in these instances.

ACUTE APPENDICITIS

Acute appendicitis is the most common cause of the acute abdomen in the UK. The exact incidence is not known because the disease is not notifiable, but it is estimated that about 125 000 patients are treated yearly in the UK for appendicitis. In 1985 the annual deaths from acute appendicitis amounted to 147 cases in the UK; 10 of these occurred in children between the ages of 1 and 14 years. When deaths do occur these are usually in infants and the elderly, and associated with delay in diagnosis and the presence of advanced peritonitis. Also associated with mortality are concomitant serious medical conditions, especially myocardial and pulmonary disease.

The vast majority of patients present with localized pain and tenderness in the right iliac fossa. Nausea and vomiting usually follow the onset of the attack and anorexia is almost invariable. Typically the pain starts centrally and shifts to the right iliac fossa after about 6 h; more accurately, the pain moves to the site of the inflamed appendix, so that it may be experienced in the suprapubic region if the appendix lies in the pelvic position, or in the right loin if the appendix is tucked away behind the ascending colon. Usually the pain is aggravated by movement. When the appendix perforates, the pain may temporarily remit, only to return in a more severe and generalized form with profuse vomiting as general peritonitis develops.

On examination the patient is flushed and in pain; usually the temperature and pulse are elevated. It is uncommon for the tongue to be clean and for there not to be foetor oris. In the region of the inflamed appendix there is usually guarding with localized tenderness on palpation and on sudden release of pressure of the examiner's hand. On rectal examination, tenderness is only found when the appendix is in the pelvic position or when there is pus in the pelvic cul-de-sac. In late cases with generalized peritonitis the abdomen is diffusely tender and rigid, the bowel sounds are absent and the patient is obviously very ill. Later still the abdomen is distended and the patient shows the features of advanced peritonitis. If, however, the perforated appendix becomes walled off by surrounding structures into an appendix mass, the examiner can palpate the tender swelling in the right iliac fossa but the rest of the abdomen is soft with no evidence of a generalized peritonitis.

Nothing can be as easy, nor as difficult, as the

diagnosis of acute appendicitis. The straightforward case is obvious but difficulties are especially likely to be encountered in young children, the elderly, the pregnant, those with an appendix in an unusual site, those who are poor historians and the obese. Even today many children do not reach hospital until the appendix has perforated and gangrene and perforation occur five times more commonly in the elderly than in the young adult with appendicitis.

Appendicitis in children is particularly worrying. Because in the infant the appendix has a relatively wide lumen, appendicitis is rare below the age of 12 months but after this the incidence increases quite rapidly. Both the mortality and the morbidity of appendicitis are higher in preschool children than in those over the age of five and this undoubtedly reflects delays in diagnosis. The picture is often not the classical one seen in older age groups. There may not be the early central abdominal colic and the shift of pain to the right iliac fossa; the child frequently only complains of generalized abdominal pain. Vomiting is usual but is by no means inevitable. There may be diarrhoea, constipation, or the bowels may remain perfectly normal. Extreme patience is required when it comes to examining the abdomen of the ill child. If there is localized tenderness and muscle guarding in the right iliac fossa in a previously healthy child, then the chances are very strong indeed that the appendix is acutely inflamed.

Differential Diagnosis

Other intra-abdominal conditions that commonly mimic appendicitis are perforated peptic ulcer, acute cholecystitis, acute intestinal obstruction (especially in the elderly), acute diverticulitis of the colon, acute regional ileitis and, in children, acute Meckel's diverticulitis and mesenteric adenitis. Renal colic and acute pyelonephritis may also be confused with acute appendicitis and in women one includes the common pitfalls of acute salpingitis, ruptured ectopic pregnancy and a ruptured cyst of the corpus luteum.

Other conditions outside the abdomen may mimic acute appendicitis. It is well known that pneumonia may produce acute abdominal pain in children. Jona and Belin[3] found that 12 of 250 children who presented with acute abdominal pain had a basal pneumonia as the only cause. It is interesting that of these 12 children, eight had only mild respiratory symptoms, four had none at all and only two had abnormal physical findings when the chest was examined. However, the abdominal pain was severe, sustained and was associated with abdominal tenderness and even, on occasion, with absent bowel sounds. These authors point out that a chest radiograph is valuable and should include a good lateral film because consolidation may be hidden by the diaphragm in the usual posteroanterior film. However, any experienced surgeon will remember a case of acute appendicitis occur-

ring in a child who has a respiratory tract infection or even pneumonia. Other conditions include diabetes mellitus, infectious hepatitis, gastroenteritis and sickle-cell crisis (which should always be thought of in black children).

An important paper by Valerio[4] describes three children with acute abdominal pain that was the presenting feature of their undiagnosed diabetes. He stresses three important clinical clues: first, a history of polyuria, polydipsia and anorexia, which precede the abdominal pain; second, deep sighing rapid respirations; and third, severe dehydration. The abdominal pain is usually generalized in contrast to the localized right iliac fossa pain and tenderness of acute appendicitis. It may be difficult to get a urine specimen to test for sugar because of the dehydration and an important step in confirming the suspected diagnosis is to arrange an immediate blood-sugar estimation. The abdomen will become pain free and soft within a few hours of appropriate treatment for the diabetes but obviously very close observation is required during this crucial period.

Special Investigations

Acute appendicitis is essentially a clinical diagnosis and there is no laboratory or radiological test that is diagnostic of the condition.

White Blood Count

This is raised above 12 000 in about three-quarters of patients and is only slightly raised or normal in the remainder. Smith[5] in a study of 100 consecutive cases of confirmed acute appendicitis, found that six had entirely normal white-cell counts.

Urine Examination

This should of course be routine in every case of acute abdominal pain. Graham[6] quantitatively analysed midstream urine samples in 71 patients operated on with a diagnosis of appendicitis. Of these, 62 had acute appendicitis and the remaining 9 had a normal appendix removed; 3 of these had mesenteric adenitis, the other 6 had no abnormality detected. In the whole group of patients, microscopic pyuria was found in 9, all female, one of whom also had haematuria. One male with acute appendicitis had microscopic haematuria also. The distribution of microscopic pyuria, this author points out, was about that expected in the normal population. Significant haematuria should point to a urinary tract lesion, but, as indicated in this study, the presence of unequivocal clinical features should not deter the surgeon from proceeding to appendicectomy.

Radiography of the Abdomen

There are a number of radiological signs which have been described in plain radiographs of the abdomen in patients with acute appendicitis.[7] These include:

1. Fluid levels localized to the caecum and to the terminal ileum, indicating localized inflammation in the right lower quadrant of the abdomen.
2. Localized ileus, with gas in the caecum, ascending colon or terminal ileum.
3. Increased soft-tissue density in the right lower quadrant.
4. Blurring of the right flank stripe, the radiolucent line produced by fat between peritoneum and transversus abdominis.
5. A faecolith in the right iliac fossa (which may be confused with a ureteric calculus or a calcified mesenteric lymph node and which may also be found in a normal subject).
6. Blurring of the psoas shadow on the right side.
7. A gas-filled appendix.
8. Free intraperitoneal gas (extremely rare).
9. Deformity of caecal gas due to an adjacent inflammatory mass. This is difficult to interpret because there may be disturbance of caecal gas from intraluminal fluid or faeces.

In a review of 200 patients undergoing laparotomy for acute appendicitis, 54% of patients with acute non-perforated appendicitis had one or more of these signs positive and the incidence rose to 80% in patients with advanced appendicitis.[7] Fifteen out of 41 patients who did not have acute appendicitis showed one or more of these radiographic appearances. Eight of these had another acute lesion in the right iliac fossa and three had no abnormality discovered at the time of operation.

Ultrasonography and Laparoscopy

Both may be used to differentiate appendicitis from gynaecological emergencies. Recently, skilled ultrasonographists have been able to visualize the thickened, inflamed and non-compressible appendix, but the accuracy and value of this first specific test for acute appendicitis await further evaluation.[8]

ACUTE INTESTINAL OBSTRUCTION[9]

Acute intestinal obstruction is subdivided into simple and strangulated. In the first, there is purely obstruction to the passage of intestinal contents, but in the second there is, in addition, an obstruction to the blood supply of the involved segment of the gut, which, left untreated, will inevitably lead to gangrene and perforation of the infarcted bowel. Strangulation may be produced by a band or adhesion, strangulated hernia, volvulus or intussusception.

Intestinal obstruction is characterized by a classical quartet of pain, vomiting, constipation and distension. They may all exist in a particular case or occur in any combination. The pain is a typical colic, cramp-like and intermittent, but may have been disguised by morphia. The vomit, which typically becomes dark brown and faeculent, may be late or even absent in colonic obstruction. Distension of the abdomen is more marked the lower the obstruction and may be imperceptible in a high small-bowel obstruction. If the occlusion is incomplete, flatus may still pass and in any case a loaded colon below an obstruction may still provide one or two bowel actions before constipation becomes total. Examination of the abdomen may reveal distension and the presence of visible peristalsis. Careful inspection should be made for the presence of an abdominal scar, which always suggests an underlying band or adhesion, and a specific search should be made for a strangulated external hernia. Palpation of the abdomen usually reveals tenderness and release tenderness and these, together with muscle guarding, tend to be more marked in the strangulated case. A mass may be detected on palpation that might be a carcinoma of the colon, diverticulitis of the sigmoid or an intussusception. Typically in an intestinal obstruction the rectum is ballooned and occasionally a low-lying obstructive tumour or an impacted mass of faeces may be found on rectal examination. Auscultation of the abdomen often reveals characteristic noisy sounds that accompany each wave of colicky peristalsis.

Special Investigations

There are no specific laboratory tests for intestinal obstruction. Leucocytosis is suggestive of strangulation but is not at all a reliable sign. The laboratory may, however, give valuable help in the important task of fluid replacement in these often dehydrated patients. Elevation of the haemoglobin and of the packed cell volume indicate haemoconcentration and act as guides to fluid replacement. Severe electrolyte depletion owing to loss of gastrointestinal fluid will be reflected by lowered serum sodium, potassium, chloride and bicarbonate concentrations with a raised blood urea.

Plain X-ray films of the abdomen are helpful in cases of intestinal obstruction but it must be stressed that the radiographs may be entirely negative in some 5–10% of cases. The physical basis of the radiological signs is that gas and fluid accumulate in the bowel above the obstruction, so that, with the patient in the erect position, the association of gas and fluid gives rise to a series of fluid levels. When the patient is in the supine position, the radiographs show the amount and distribution of gas in the gut. The distended loops of small intestine generally lie transversely in a step-ladder fashion across the central abdomen. The distribution of gas may enable the surgeon to differentiate between an obstruction in the small or large bowel.

Two specific forms of intestinal obstruction may give quite typical radiographic appearances on the plain films. An obstruction due to a gallstone lodged in the small intestine may show air in the biliary system (as a result of a cholecyst–duodenal fistula) together with direct visualization of the stone and radiographic evidence of small-bowel occlusion. Volvulus of the sigmoid colon usually demonstrates a tremendously distended sigmoid loop, which may extend up to the diaphragm and may even fill the right side of the abdomen.

In some cases, radiographs may be taken with radiopaque material. A micropaque, barium sulphate suspension can be given as a barium meal and follow-through study. There is little danger of its impaction above a small-bowel obstruction because the considerable fluid accumulation above the block rapidly dilutes the medium. A barium enema radiograph is particularly helpful in cases of suspected colonic obstruction due to carcinoma or diverticular disease. It is also useful in differentiating organic large-bowel obstruction from pseudo-obstruction of the colon.

PERFORATED PEPTIC ULCER

This is yet another example of a common acute abdominal emergency where clinical features are all-important and where laboratory investigations have virtually no part to play in diagnosis. The clinical presentation in the great majority of patients will present no serious difficulty in diagnosis. The sudden onset of the pain is very characteristic. It is agonizing, and involves the whole abdomen. Radiation of the pain to one or other shoulder (referred via the phrenic nerve) is highly characteristic, but is so often masked by the intense abdominal pain that it may not be revealed unless sought by direct questioning. About 70% of patients will give a history of previous symptoms suggestive of peptic ulcer and, indeed, there may have been an actual previous perforation.

The clinical findings are typical; the patient is cold and clammy, in obvious pain and does not wish to move. Respirations are rapid and shallow but, certainly in the early hours after perforation, the pulse is only slightly raised and the blood pressure normal. The rigid abdomen is quite typical—beautifully described by Moynihan as 'every part offers the most inflexible opposition to pressure, the rigidity is obdurate, persistent and unyielding'. Bowel sounds are usually absent and diminution of liver dullness can sometimes be demonstrated by percussion over the lower chest. However, this is not a sign to be relied upon.

Special Investigations

Haematological and other laboratory tests are of no value in the diagnosis of perforated peptic ulcer, although they may be needed to help in the differential diagnosis in some obscure cases.

The radiographic appearances, however, can be helpful although it is important to remember that the radiographs may be entirely negative in about a third of the patients.[10] The characteristic appearance is of free gas between the liver and the right side of the diaphragm. Gas beneath the left leaf of the diaphragm may be confused with gas within the stomach fundus but this may be resolved by inspecting a lateral decubitus film. A generalized 'ground glass' appearance suggests excessive free peritoneal fluid.

The differential diagnosis of the causes of free gas beneath the diaphragm includes perforation of any other part of the gut (for example, perforation of an acutely inflamed diverticulum of the colon), laparotomy within the previous couple of weeks, spontaneous rupture of a gas cyst of the intestine, subphrenic abscess, tubal insufflation within the previous 24 h and introduction of gas at peritoneal dialysis.

ACUTE PANCREATITIS

Acute pancreatitis is interesting in that its aetiology (or, more probably, aetiologies) remains the subject of debate. It is well recognized that there is an association with the presence of gallstones, acute alcoholism, and also a large number of rarer causes, although in many cases no precipitating factor can be identified.

Among the less common associations may be mentioned hyperparathyroidism,[11] mumps, pregnancy, trauma to the pancreas or surgery on the biliary or upper gastrointestinal tract, and a large number of drugs, particularly steroids (well reviewed by Nakashima and Howard[12]).

Trapnell and Duncan[13] in a 20-year review of 590 cases of acute pancreatitis in the Bristol area, found 54% were associated with biliary-tract disease, and 4.4% with chronic alcoholism; however, no less than 34.4% were idiopathic. However, in areas where alcohol consumption is far greater (e.g. Glasgow, New York and Sweden), between a quarter and two-thirds of cases are associated with high alcohol consumption. The reasons for these associations remain conjectural but at least suggest that clinical pancreatitis is the end-result of a number of quite different precipitating factors.

The importance of accurate diagnosis in acute pancreatitis is that the majority of these cases can be treated non-operatively. However, in a proportion of cases neither the clinical features nor the laboratory investigations make the diagnosis certain and, under such circumstances, it may be necessary to perform a diagnostic laparotomy.

Clinical Features

Although pancreatitis is occasionally seen in children and more often in young adults, it only becomes common after the age of 50. Onset is usually sudden and severe, situated in the upper abdomen and radiating, in some 65% of cases, into the thoracolumbar region of the spine. The great majority of patients also have repeated vomiting.

On examination, the severe case is pale and

shocked. The local examination of the abdomen is characterized by rather less marked physical signs than would be expected by the severity of the pain. The pancreas, being retroperitoneal, produces less peritoneal irritation than a ruptured or inflamed intra-abdominal viscus. Usually, therefore, although there is quite marked upper abdominal tenderness, rigidity and guarding are not usually marked features. However, these may be present and may closely mimic a perforated peptic ulcer.

Special Investigations

Acute pancreatitis is unique among the common acute abdominal emergencies in that there is a fairly reliable laboratory confirmatory investigation, the serum amylase.

Serum Amylase

The normal value of the serum amylase activity ranges from 80 to 150 Somogyi units. In the majority of cases of acute pancreatitis this level rises to 1000 units or more. However, in a small number of cases the amylase activity may be normal, and this is particularly so when blood is taken 2 or 3 days after the onset of the pancreatitis by which time, in the majority of patients, the level has fallen to normal. Serum amylase activity may also be increased in other conditions associated with severe abdominal pain. These include a perforated peptic ulcer, acute cholecystitis, and intestinal obstruction. The amylase level may also be elevated in renal failure and following the administration of morphia and its derivatives which may cause spasm of the sphincter of Oddi. Although raised in these various conditions, the amylase activity very rarely reaches the high level seen in acute pancreatitis.

A number of other biochemical abnormalities may be found in this condition:

- *Plasma calcium* concentration may fall and the degree of hypocalcaemia is related to the severity of the pancreatitis. Occasionally there may be clinical tetany and in such cases the prognosis is poor.
- *Blood sugar* concentration may be elevated transiently in acute pancreatitis, with associated glycosuria.
- The *plasma bilirubin* concentration may be elevated due to oedema of the pancreatic head; indeed there may be mild clinical jaundice.
- The *serum methaemalbumin* level may be raised in severe pancreatitis and indicates a severe degree of inflammation of the gland.
- *Plain radiographs of the abdomen* are not diagnostic. There may be a C-shaped loop of gas-filled duodenum due to localized ileus, absence of the psoas shadows due to retroperitoneal oedema and small fluid levels due to a generalized ileus. The frequent association with biliary disease may be demonstrated by the presence of radiopaque gall-

stones. A chest radiograph occasionally shows small left pleural effusion.
- *Ultrasonography and computerized tomagraphic scanning* are useful in the diagnosis of peripancreatic collections of fluid or pus and are helpful in delineating the swollen and oedematous or necrotic pancreas. In many cases, however, the gaseous distension of the gut makes ultrasonography difficult.

Although these special investigations are undoubtedly of value, the surgeon, faced with the patient in whom the possibility of a ruptured abdominal viscus is suspected, will be wise to submit the patient to laparotomy, even in the face of a raised serum amylase. The biochemical tests are, however, of considerable value in reinforcing a clinical diagnosis of acute pancreatitis and will encourage the surgeon, under these circumstances, to manage the patient conservatively.

MEDICAL CONDITIONS THAT MAY SIMULATE THE ACUTE ABDOMEN

Although many essentially medical diseases may be associated with, or present as, acute abdominal pain, it is equally important to remember that a patient under treatment with some medical condition may develop an acute abdominal emergency. Indeed, it is a well-known aphorism that the most dangerous place to perforate is in a medical ward! I have personally operated upon a child with acute appendicitis who was under treatment with pneumonia, dealt with another who was in a plaster bed with severe spinal tuberculosis and seen a perforated peptic ulcer in a patient with post-traumatic paraplegia. Patients may develop a mesenteric embolism while recovering from a myocardial infarct and, much more commonly, get faecal impaction or acute retention of urine while on strict bedrest with this condition.

In clinical practice, a careful history combined with meticulous clinical examination will usually enable the practitioner to decide whether the situation represents an acute abdominal emergency in a patient with an associated medical condition, or whether the acute abdominal pain is due to the medical disease itself. For example, a known diabetic patient, who is well stabilized, develops an acute abdominal pain with classical features of intra-abdominal pathology. His stable diabetic condition should not give rise to any confusion. In contrast, a patient with uncontrolled diabetes in precoma with marked ketonuria who is also complaining of abdominal pain should alert the clinician to a diagnosis of prediabetic coma with associated abdominal symptoms. In this latter case, the rapid disappearance of the abdominal pain over the next few hours as the diabetes comes under control will clinch the diagnosis. Perhaps the most important thing to bear in mind is to beware of a 'label' attached to a patient; just because he has had several attacks of pain in the past due to cardiac ischaemia does not mean that his present attack may not be one of acute cholecystitis. It is always best to bring quite a fresh mind to the problem and consider each patient and each painful episode on its own merit.

Chest Diseases

Upper abdominal pain, tenderness and guarding may be associated with acute pulmonary or pleural infection (*see above* under Acute appendicitis). The local abdominal tenderness secondary to pulmonary disease is not usually increased by abdominal palpation, the respiratory rate is usually increased, associated with shallow breathing and the pain is frequently aggravated by taking a deep breath. Chest radiography is valuable and a lateral film should also be taken since basal shadowing may be hidden behind the diaphragm on the posteroanterior film.

Upper abdominal pain is not unusual in an acute coronary thrombosis but there is seldom associated rigidity or tenderness and there are the other clinical features suggesting cardiac origin of the pain. The electrocardiogram and serum transaminase estimations are certainly valuable confirmatory aids in this condition.

Diabetes

We have already discussed the abdominal pain and vomiting that may accompany prediabetic coma. The increasing thirst, polyuria, drowsiness and dehydration should alert the surgeon. A vital requirement is to test the urine as a routine and to make a blood-sugar estimation. Even if there is an associated abdominal condition, the first necessity is to correct the diabetes. If the abdominal features clear over the next 2 or 3 has the diabetes comes under control then obviously they were due to the medical condition. If they do not improve, the possibility of some surgical lesion must be further considered.

Sickle-cell Anaemia

This is more or less confined to the black races and is not uncommon in the West Indian community in this country. Abdominal pain with associated tenderness and guarding may occur during an acute haemolytic episode; the nature of the pain is not known. The blood film is characteristic and having determined that the patient has sickle-cell anaemia, close observation must be initiated to decide whether or not the pain is due to a haemolytic crisis or whether there is an associated abdominal catastrophe. It is important to remember that patients with any haemolytic anaemia have a raised incidence of gallstones.

Other Medical Conditions

Among other conditions listed as being associated with abdominal pain one can mention herpes zoster affecting the lower thoracic segments, epidemic myalgia (Bornholm disease), the abdominal crises of tabes dorsalis, acute lead poisoning and acute porphyria, but these are all extremely rare. Perhaps under the heading of medical conditions is a convenient place to mention the *Munchausen syndrome*; patients who are either mentally abnormal or who are drug addicts and who can mimic to perfection many diseases including acute abdominal emergencies. Ureteric colic is a favourite and the patient is often shrewd enough to explain to the doctor that he cannot undergo intravenous pyelography because he is iodine sensitive! A bizarre previous history, no fixed address, antecubital injection marks and the long memory of the Casualty Sister are all helpful in making the diagnosis.

REFERENCES

1. Ellis H. (1968). Diagnosis of the acute abdomen. *Br. Med. J.*, **1**, 491.
2. French E.B., Robb W.A.T. (1963). Biliary and renal colic. *Br. Med. J.*, **2**, 135.
3. Jona J.Z., Belin R.P. (1976). Basal pneumonia simulating acute appendicitis in children. *Arch. Surg.*, **III**, 552.
4. Valerio D. (1976). Acute diabetic abdomen in children. *Lancet*, **i**, 66.
5. Smith P.H. (1965). The diagnosis of appendicitis. *Postgrad. Med. J.*, **41**,2.
6. Graham J.A. (1965). Urinary cell counts in appendicitis. *Scott. Med. J.*, **10**, 126.
7. Brooks D.W., Killen D.A. (1965). Roentgenographic findings in acute appendicitis. *Surgery*, **57**, 377.
8. Pearson R.H. (1988). Ultrasonography for diagnosing appendicitis. *Br. Med. J.*, **297**, 308.
9. Ellis H. (1989). *Maingot's Abdominal Operations*, 9th edn, vol. 2. New York: Appleton Lange, pp. 885–904.
10. Gough M.H., Gear M.W.L. (1971). *The Plain X-ray in the Diagnosis of the Acute Abdomen*. Oxford: Blackwell Scientific.
11. Rosin R.D. (1976). Pancreatitis and hyperparathyroidism. *Postgrad. Med. J.*, **52**, 95.
12. Nakashima Y., Howard J.M. (1977). Drug induced acute pancreatitis. *Surg. Gynecol. Obstet.*, **145**, 105.
13. Trapnell J.E., Duncan E.H.L. (1975). Patterns of incidence of acute pancreatitis. *Br. Med. J.*, **2**, 179.

SECTION 6
DISORDERS OF THE BLOOD CONSTITUENTS

24. Haem Synthesis and the Porphyrias
G. H. Elder

Haem biosynthesis
  Pathway
  Regulation
Excretion of haem precursors
Determination of porphyrins and their precursors
  Clinical chemistry
  Specimen collection
  Measurement of PBG and ALA in urine
  Measurement of porphyrins in urine, faeces, plasma and erythrocytes
  Measurement of total porphyrin concentrations
  Measurement of individual porphyrins
  Enzyme measurements
Enzyme defects in the porphyrias
  Molecular pathology
Clinical features of the porphyrias
  Porphyrias associated with acute attacks
  Porphyrias associated with skin lesions
Laboratory diagnosis of the porphyrias
  Patients with symptoms that suggest acute porphyria
  Patients who present with skin lesions
  Detection of asymptomatic carriers of genes for the autosomal dominant porphyrias

The porphyrias are a group of disorders of haem biosynthesis in which characteristic clinical features are associated with increased formation of porphyrins and porphyrin precursors (Table 24.1).[1-3] The pri-mary abnormality in each type of porphyria is a decrease in the activity of a particular enzyme of the biosynthetic pathway. Each type is defined by a specific pattern of accumulation and excretion of haem precursors that reflects an increase in the intracellular concentration of the substrate of the defective enzyme. Recognition of these patterns by the selection and correct interpretation of appropriate biochemical investigations is essential for the accurate diagnosis and the proper management of the porphyrias since the clinical features alone are not sufficiently distinctive.

HAEM BIOSYNTHESIS

Haem biosynthesis takes place in all cells that contain functioning mitochondria. Adult human subjects synthesize about 0.45 mmol of haem each day. Some 70–80% of this is produced in erythroid cells for the formation of haemoglobin. Most of the remaining 20–30% is synthesized in the liver where a major fraction is used for the assembly of microsomal haemo-proteins of the cytochrome P-450 series, which act as catalysts for the oxidative metabolism of many drugs, chemicals and endogenous compounds.

Pathway

The pathway of haem synthesis is outlined in Fig. 24.1. The enzymology of each reaction has been reviewed.[2] Although most of the reactions take place in the cytosol fraction of the cell, the first and three final stages take place in the mitochondrion and the enzymes catalysing these reactions are not present in mature erythrocytes. The first stages consist of a series of irreversible condensation reactions, initiated by the formation of 5-aminolaevulinate (ALA) from glycine and succinyl CoA, which is catalysed by ALA-synthase (Fig. 24.1). Two molecules of ALA then combine under the influence of the enzyme ALA-dehydratase to form the pyrrole porphobilino-gen (PBG). These reactions lead to the formation of the linear tetrapyrrole, hydroxymethylbilane, which undergoes cyclization with rotation of one of the pyrrole units to form the asymmetrical porphyrino-

TABLE 24.1
THE MAIN TYPES OF PORPHYRIA

Disorder	Acute attacks	Skin lesions	Estimated prevalence of overt cases
PBG-synthase-deficiency porphyria	+	−	
Acute intermittent porphyria	+	−	1–2 : 100 000
Congenital erythropoietic porphyria	−	+	Less than 1 : 10⁶
Porphyria cutanea tarda	−	+	1 : 25 000
Hereditary coproporphyria	+	+	Less than 1 : 250 000
Variegate porphyria	+	+	1 : 250 000
Erythropoietic protoporphyria	−	+	1 : 200 000

Estimated prevalences are for the UK.

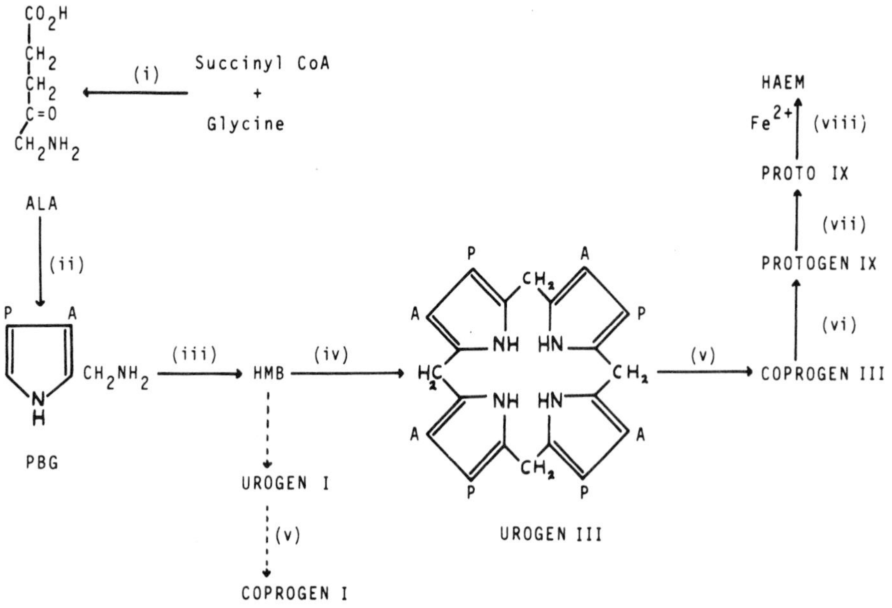

Figure 24.1 The pathway of haem biosynthesis. Reactions are catalysed by (i) ALA-synthase, (ii) PBG-synthase, (iii) PBG-deaminase, (iv) uroporphyrinogen III synthase, (v) uroporphyrinogen decarboxylase, (vi) coproporphyrinogen oxidase, (vii) protoporphyrinogen oxidase, (viii) ferrochelatase. HMB, hydroxymethylbilane; A, P, acetic acid and propionic acid substituents.

gen, uroporphyrinogen III. Hydroxymethylbilane is unstable and readily undergoes non-enzymatic cyclization to uroporphyrinogen I. Except in pathological conditions where hydroxymethylbilane accumulates, this chemical reaction accounts for less than 1% of the porphyrin that is formed each day.

In the second part of the pathway a series of side-chain modifications produces protoporphyrinogen IX, which then undergoes aromatization to protoporphyrin IX, with final insertion of ferrous iron to form haem (Fig. 24.1).

The porphyrinogens that are the intermediates in the conversion of PBG to protoporphyrin IX are unstable, colourless compounds that readily oxidize to porphyrins, which are not metabolized. Thus increased formation of porphyrinogens leads to accumulation in tissues and increased excretion of both porphyrinogens and porphyrins. Because most techniques for the determination of porphyrins in urine and faeces include procedures that oxidize porphyrinogens, these compounds are included in the values that are obtained for porphyrin excretion.

Regulation

The supply of haem and protein for haemoprotein is closely coordinated so that neither component persists in excess to any extent. The rate of haem synthesis is determined by the activity of the first enzyme of the pathway, ALA-synthase, which in differentiated cells has a lower activity than subsequent enzymes. ALA-synthases from the two main sites of haem

synthesis, hepatocytes and erythroid cells, have different properties and are encoded by separate genes on chromosomes 3 and X, respectively. Mechanisms for the regulation of ALA-synthase activity, and the coordination of haem and protein supply, are also different.[4]

In liver, ALA-synthase is under negative feedback control by haem. Haem decreases the synthesis of mature enzyme by a complex mechanism that includes repression of transcription and inhibition of the translocation of precursor ALA-synthase into mitochondria. This mechanism allows effective short-term control because the turnover of ALA-synthase is rapid, the half-life in rat liver being about 60 min. Hepatic ALA-synthase is induced by a wide variety of lipophilic drugs, such as barbiturates, and foreign chemicals, many of which are metabolized by the cytochrome P450-mediated mono-oxygenase system. These compounds appear to act mainly by stimulating the synthesis of apocytochrome P450s, which then combine with preformed haem and thus, by depleting the intracellular concentration of 'regulatory' haem, derepress the synthesis of ALA-synthase. However mRNA measurements have suggested that they may also directly induce ALA-synthase.

Induction of ALA-synthase and the other enzymes of the haem biosynthetic pathway is an early event during erythroid differentiation. Once the pathway is fully induced, ALA-synthase activity appears to determine the rate of haem formation. In contrast to the liver enzyme, erythroid ALA-synthase is not induced by drugs or xenobiotics. However, activity appears

TABLE 24.2
REFERENCE RANGES FOR HAEM PRECURSORS IN URINE, FAECES AND ERYTHROCYTES

Haem precursor	Urine	Faeces	Erythrocytes
ALA	0–34 μmol/L		
PBG	0–8.8 μmol/L		
Total porphyrin	20–320 nmol/L	10–200 nmol/g dry wt.[1]	0.4–1.7μmol/L[2]
Porphyrin fractions			
Uroporphyrin	0–40 nmol/day		
Coproporphyrin	0–280 nmol/day	0–46 nmol/g dry wt.	
Protoporphyrin		0–220 nmol/g dry wt.	
Ether-insoluble porphyrin[3]		0–24 nmol/g dry wt.	
Individual porphyrins			
Uroporphyrin	0–24 nmol/L	<2% total	
Hepta (7CO$_2$H)	0–4 nmol/L	<2% total	
Hexa (6CO$_2$H)	0–3 nmol/L	<2% total	
Penta (5CO$_2$H)	0–5 nmol/L	<2% total	
Isocoproporphyrin		<0.5% total	
Coproporphyrin	23–115 nmol/L (60–70%)	2–33% total (10–20%)	
Protoporphyrin		60–98% total	

Figures in parentheses give per cent isomer type III.
[1]Ether-soluble porphyrin only; [2] more than 90% of total porphyrin in erythrocytes is zinc-protoporphyrin; [3] includes uroporphyrin, heptacarboxylic porphyrin, X-porphyrin.
Data from Elder et al. (1990).[6]

to be influenced by controls that act at a post-transcriptional level. One may serve to coordinate ALA-synthase activity with iron supply, while another appears to involve negative feedback regulation of enzyme activity by haem. The latter effect, in conjunction with regulation by haem of the activity of the specific protein kinase that phosphorylates the α subunit of the eukaryotic initiation factor eIF2, regulates the coordination of haem and globin synthesis.[4]

EXCRETION OF HAEM PRECURSORS

In relation to the quantities required for haem synthesis, only small amounts of haem precursors accumulate in tissues and are excreted in the urine and faeces (Table 24.2).

ALA and PBG are excreted exclusively in the urine. The distribution of porphyrins between urine and faeces is determined by their chemical structure and the excretory capacity of the liver. In general, urinary excretion becomes increasingly favoured as the number of carboxyl groups increases. Thus uroporphyrin is excreted mainly in the urine, while protoporphyrin excretion is restricted to the bile. Coproporphyrin I is taken up and excreted by the liver in preference to the series III isomer. Thus faecal coproporphyrin is mainly coproporphyrin I while both isomers are present in about equal amounts in urine. When the excretory function of the liver is impaired, coproporphyrin is diverted from the biliary route and both the total amount of coproporphyrin and

TABLE 24.3
CAUSES OF COPROPORPHYRINURIA OTHER THAN PORPHYRIA

Toxic conditions
Alcoholism
Lead poisoning

Impaired biliary excretion
Hepatocellular disease
Cholestasis
Pregnancy
Oestrogen therapy, oral contraceptives

Others (?impaired biliary excretion)
Dubin–Johnson syndrome
Miscellaneous systemic diseases:
  severe infections
  rheumatic fever
  reticuloses

the percentage of the series I isomer increases in the urine (Table 24.3). The only exception to this finding is in the Dubin–Johnson syndrome where a characteristic decrease in the urinary excretion of coproporphyrin III is found.[5]

Normal faeces contain more protoporphyrin and other dicarboxylic porphyrins than can be accounted for by biliary excretion. It is probable that much of this dicarboxylic porphyrin comes from the action of bacteria on haem derived from the lining of the alimentary tract and from the diet.

TABLE 24.4
COMPOUNDS IN URINE THAT GIVE A RED COLOUR WITH
EHRLICH'S REAGENT

Compounds that react with p-*dimethylaminobenzaldehyde*
Urobilinogen
Porphobilinogen
Unidentified metabolites of:
   methyldopa
   levomepromazine
   Cascara sagrada bark extract

Compounds that give a red colour with 7M–*HCl*
Food additives: methyl red
Phenazopyridine HCl (pyridium)
Indoles: indoleacetic acid

DETERMINATION OF PORPHYRINS AND THEIR PRECURSORS

Clinical Chemistry

Laboratory investigation of the porphyrias requires measurement of PBG and ALA in urine, and porphyrins in urine, faeces, erythrocytes and plasma.[6] Because methods for the measurement of individual porphyrins are complex, it is customary to investigate porphyrin overproduction in two stages. First, the total porphyrin concentration is measured to select samples for further investigation. Methods for this purpose need to be simple and reliable so that they can be used widely to screen for porphyria. Second, individual porphyrins are measured in order to define the pattern of porphyrin overproduction and thus identify the type of porphyria.

Specimen Collection

Porphyrins are reasonably stable in solution, provided they are protected from light and oxidants. PBG is less stable and, particularly in acid solution, rapidly polymerizes to uroporphyrin and a brownish-red pigment, porphobilin.

Fresh random samples of urine (about 25 mL) are more suitable than 24-h collections for the diagnosis of porphyria. Urine should be analysed for PBG and porphyrins as soon as practicable, though concentrations are unlikely to change sufficiently within 36 h to produce an incorrect diagnosis, particularly if the urine is kept at neutral pH in the dark at 4°C.[6] Longer storage is best carried out at −20°C, if necessary after adjusting the pH to 7.0–7.5 with sodium bicarbonate.

About 5 g wet weight of faeces is adequate for determination of porphyrin concentrations. Ideally, porphyrins in faeces should be analysed within a few hours of collection. However, if delay is unavoidable, diagnostically significant changes are unlikely to occur within 36 h at room temperature and samples are stable for many months at −20°C.

Blood samples, anticoagulated with EDTA and kept in the dark, show no loss of protoporphyrin for up to 8 days at room temperature and for up to 8 weeks at 8°C or lower.

Measurement of PBG and ALA in urine

Detection and measurement of PBG is based on its reaction with *p*-dimethylaminobenzaldehyde in HCl (Ehrlich's reagents) to give a red compound that, unlike the compound formed with urobilinogen, is not extracted by organic solvents from aqueous solution. This reaction forms the basis of the Watson–Schwartz and Hoesch tests that are widely used to screen for excess PBG in urine.

A modified Watson–Schwartz test that has a lower limit of detection of about 35–50 μmol/L for PBG is made as follows. Equal volumes of fresh urine and Ehrlich's reagent (0.24% in 7MHCl) are mixed, allowed to stand for 2 min, mixed with an equal volume of saturated sodium acetate and shaken with a volume of butanol or amyl alcohol–benzyl alcohol (3:1, v/v) about equal to the original volume of urine. The red colour formed by PBG appears on addition of Ehrlich's reagent and is not extracted into the organic phase. Extraction must be repeated until the organic phase is colourless before the test can be regarded as positive. Urobilinogen and some other compounds also react with Ehrlich's reagent but are extracted into the organic phase (Table 24.4). A positive test must always be confirmed by quantitative determination of PBG after purification by anion-exchange chromatography.[6]

Methods for the measurement of ALA depend on condensation with acetylacetone or ethylacetoacetate to form a pyrrole that reacts with Ehrlich's reagent. They require chromatography to separate ALA from PBG and to concentrate ALA.[6]

Measurement of Porphyrins in Urine, Faeces, Plasma and Erythrocytes

Porphyrins have characteristic electronic absorption spectra with an intense maximum around 400 nm that is known as the Soret peak.[7] For porphyrins of clinical significance, Soret maxima in acid solution range from 398 to 407 nm and have molar absorption coefficients of 262–541 × 10^3 L/mol per cm. Irradiation at wavelengths around 400 nm produces an intense red fluorescence with emission maxima around 600 nm, the exact wavelength depending on the type of porphyrin and solvent.[7] This property enables porphyrins to be detected in solution and on chromatograms by direct inspection in long-wavelength ultraviolet light.

All clinically important porphyrins are readily extracted into polar organic solvents (butan-1-ol, amyl alcohol) from aqueous solutions at the pH of their isoelectric points (around pH 3.5). Solubility in less polar solvents, such as ether or ethylacetate, is inversely proportional to the number of acidic side-chains, with uroporphyrin being insoluble in ether.

Measurement of Total Porphyrin Concentrations

The total porphyrin concentration can be measured directly in diluted, acidified urine by derivative spectroscopy or by spectrofluorimetry. If equipment for these techniques is not available, direct spectrophotometry of acidified urine[6] is a reliable, if less accurate, method of screening for increased urinary porphyrin concentration. Total ether-soluble porphyrins in faeces may also be measured after separation of red-fluorescent chlorophyll derivatives by solvent partition spectrophotometry, the technique described by Lockwood et al.[8] being sufficiently simple to serve as a screening test. Qualitative screening tests for increased urinary and faecal porphyrin excretion based on solvent extraction require experience in interpretation, are subject to interference, are insensitive[9] and should be replaced by one of the methods described above.

In recent years, a number of fluorimetric micromethods that measure total porphyrins in whole blood, washed erythrocytes or plasma have been introduced.[6] These are sufficiently simple and rapid to be used as screening tests and have largely replaced methods based on solvent extraction or fluorescence microscopy, both of which may produce false-negative results. The fluorimetric micromethods involve extraction of porphyrins into acid, which removes zinc from zinc-protoporphyrin. As distinction between zinc-protoporphyrin and free protoporphyrin is important for the diagnosis of erythropoietic protoporphyia, all samples with an increased porphyrin concentration should be investigated further using a neutral extractant, such as ethanol.[6] Increased concentrations of porphyrin in plasma can be detected rapidly by fluorescence-emission spectroscopy of plasma. This technique is particularly useful for the diagnosis of variegate porphyria because the plasma in this condition contains a protein-bound porphyrin with a characteristic emission peak around 625 nm.[10]

Measurement of Individual Porphyrins

Fractionation of the mixtures of porphyrins that occur in urine, faeces and plasma is readily achieved by high-performance liquid chromatography (HPLC) or thin-layer chromatography (TLC). HPLC enables the individual porphyrins to be measured directly by spectrophotometry or fluorimetry. Porphyrins separated by TLC may be measured after elution from the plate or by reflectance methods. However, patterns are usually so distinctive as to make measurement unnecessary.[6]

Porphyrins as their methyl esters are readily separated by TLC according to the nature and number of their acidic side-chains, but position isomers and some dicarboxylic porphyrins are not resolved. Simple methods for the extraction and methyl esterification of porphyrins from biological samples have been described.[6]

A large number of methods have now been developed for the separation of porphyrin methyl esters by HPLC and of porphyrins by reverse-phase (RP) HPLC. Ammonium acetate buffer:organic modified RP-HPLC systems[11] are robust and provide complete resolution of all porphyrins derived from haem biosynthesis, including separation of type I and III isomers.

Enzyme Measurements

A number of methods for the measurement of PBG deaminase and other enzymes of the haem biosynthetic pathway have been described.[3,6] Most are complex and restricted to specialized laboratories. Enzyme measurements are rarely essential for the diagnosis of porphyria. Their main use is for the detection of latent porphyria in families and, less commonly, for the investigation of atypical forms of the main types of porphyria.

ENZYME DEFECTS IN THE PORPHYRIAS

Each of the main types of porphyria results from partial deficiency of one of the enzymes of the pathway of haem biosynthesis (Table 24.5).[2,3] Each enzyme deficiency is compensated by a mechanism that involves derepression of ALA-synthase and a consequent increase in the intracellular concentration of the substrate of the defective enzyme.[2,3] This mechanism is able effectively to maintain haem synthesis, except in the liver during an attack of acute porphyria, but leads to the specific patterns of overproduction of haem precursors that characterize each type of porphyria (Table 24.6) and are associated with symptoms.

PBG-synthase-deficiency porphyria and congenital erythropoietic porphyria are inherited as autosomal recessive conditions. The other enzyme deficiencies, with the exception of that which produces type I porphyria cutanea tarda (PCT), are inherited in an autosomal dominant fashion. Enzyme activities in all the autosomal dominant porphyrias, except erythropoietic protoporphyria, are about 50% of normal, reflecting expression of the normal gene allelic to the mutant gene. In erythropoietic protoporphyria, ferrochelatase activity is decreased by 70% or more in those with overt disease and by about 60% in asymptomatic carriers.[3] In recent years, rare homozygous variants have been described for each of the autosomal dominant porphyrias.[3,12] Enzyme activities tend to be decreased by at least 80%, leading to sustained overproduction of haem precursors and clinical presentation during childhood.[13]

Although the enzyme defects of the porphyrias, with the exception of one form of PCT and a rare

TABLE 24.5
THE PORPHYRIAS: ENZYME DEFICIENCIES AND INHERITANCE

Disorder	Enzyme deficiency	Inheritance	Chromosomal	Human cDNA or gDNA cloned
PBG-synthase deficiency	PBG-synthase	Autosomal recessive	9q34	+
Acute intermittent porphyria	PBG-deaminase[1]	Autosomal dominant	11q23-ter	+
Congenital erythropoietic porphyria	Uroporphyrinogen III synthase	Autosomal recessive	10q25.2–26.3	+
Porphyria cutanea tarda:				
Type I (sporadic)	Uroporphyrinogen decarboxylase			
Type II (familial)	Uroporphyrinogen decarboxylase	Autosomal dominant	1p34	+
Hereditary coproporphyria	Coproporphyrinogen oxidase	Autosomal dominant	9	
Variegate porphyria	Protoporphyrinogen oxidase	Autosomal dominant		
Erythropoietic protoporphyria	Ferrochelatase	Autosomal dominant	18q22	+

[1]Synonyms: hydroxymethylbilane synthase, uroporphyrinogen-I-synthase.

TABLE 24.6
LABORATORY DIFFERENTIATION OF THE PORPHYRIAS

| Disorder | Urine | | Faeces | Erythrocytes |
	PBG/ALA	Porphyrins	Porphyrins	Porphyrins
PGB-synthase deficiency[1]	ALA	Copro III	Not increased	Zn-proto
Acute intermittent porphyria	PBG > ALA	(porphyrin mainly from PBG)	Normal, occasionally slight increase (copro, proto)	Not increased
Congenital erythropoietic porphyria	Not increased	Uro I > copro I	Copro I	Zn-proto, copro, uro
Porphyria cutanea tarda	Not increased	Uro > hepta[3]	Isocopro, hepta[3]	Not increased
Hereditary coproporphyria	PBG > ALA[2]	Copro III (porphyrin from PBG)	Copro III	Not increased
Variegate porphyria	PBG > ALA	Copro III (porphyrin from PBG)	Proto IX > copro III X-porphyrin	Not increased
Erythropoietic protoporphyria	Not increased	Not increased	± Protoporphyrin	Protoporphyrin

[1]Lead poisoning produces an identical overproduction pattern.
[2]PBG and ALA excretion may be normal when only skin lesions are present.
[3]Hexa- and pentacarboxylic porphyrins and coproporphyrin are increased to a smaller extent.

subtype of acute intermittent porphyria, are present in all nucleated cells, the compensatory changes are restricted to certain tissues. Thus, in the hepatic porphyrias (see Table 24.1) they are evident only in the liver and there is no detectable increase in the concentration of porphyrins or porphyrin precursors in erythroid cells. In practice, measurement of erythrocyte porphyrin concentration enables the main porphyrias to be divided into two groups that show important clinical differences and have been used as the basis of the simple classification shown in Table 24.1. This classification does not include PBG-synthase-deficiency porphyria, which has been described in only four patients,[3] or the rare homozygous variants, in all of which erythrocyte porphyrin concentrations are increased, nor porphyria

caused by production of porphyrins by hepatic tumours, a syndrome that is clinically indistinguishable from PCT.[14] In addition, more than one type of porphyria may be present in the same individual.[15]

Although enzyme activities are similar in all individuals who inherit the gene for one of the autosomal dominant types of porphyria, the consequences vary. Thus the majority are likely to remain asymptomatic throughout life (latent porphyria) and a substantial porportion of these will have no detectable evidence of haem precursor overproduction; the rest will be asymptomatic but have increased concentrations of haem precursors in their tissues, urine or faeces (latent or subclinical porphyria). In the minority (less than 20%) that develop clinically overt porphyria, symptoms are always associated with increased production of haem precursors: PBG or ALA during acute neurovisceral attacks, and porphyrins when skin lesions are present. During remission, overproduction of haem precursors will decrease and, in the hepatic porphyrias, may occasionally return to normal, although this process usually takes many months or years.

The reason for the low clinical penetrance of the autosomal dominant porphyrias is not understood. Acquired factors, such as certain drugs in the acute hepatic porphyrias and iron overload in type II PCT, are important contributors but do not provide a full explanation.

Molecular Pathology

cDNAs have now been obtained for all but two of the enzymes that are defective in the porphyrias (see Table 24.5) and several of the corresponding genes have been cloned.[16] Recent enzymatic and molecular genetic investigations have revealed extensive molecular heterogeneity in several types of porphyria.[16]

Acute Intermittent Porphyria

There are two isoenzymes of PBG-deaminase, the enzyme that is defective in AIP. The erythroid isoenzyme is restricted to erythroid tissues whereas the non-erythroid, or ubiquitous form, is present at low concentrations in all tissues. The amino-acid sequences of the two isoenzymes are identical, except that the ubiquitous enzyme has 17 additional amino acids at the NH_2-terminus. Both isoenzymes are generated from a single gene on chromosome 11 by a mechanism that uses tissue-specific promoters and alternative splicing of pre-mRNA.[16]

As decreased activity of PBG-deaminase in the liver is the fundamental defect in AIP, mutations that produce this condition would be expected to decrease either the ubiquitous isoenzyme alone or to occur in that section of the gene that encodes both isoenzymes. Both types have been identified. Although greater than 95% of AIP families have decreased PBG-deaminase in all tissues, rare families in which erythroid enzyme activity is preserved have been described. Mutations that lead to abnormal splicing of exon 1 have been identified in two of these families.[16]

In the usual form of AIP in which all tissues are affected, immunochemical measurements of erythrocyte PBG-deaminase allow two main types to be identified. About 85% of families have cross-reacting immunological material (CRIM)-negative mutations, in which the product of the mutant gene cannot be detected by cross-reaction with antiserum raised to normal enzyme, while the remainder have CRIM-positive mutations. Molecular genetic investigation of CRIM-negative and CRIM-positive AIP has revealed a large number of different mutations. Of these, only two of those that produce the less common CRIM-positive form and the mutation responsible for the

founder effect that explains the high frequency of AIP in northern Sweden have been found in more than one family.[16,17]

Porphyria Cutanea Tarda and Related Disorders

PCT results from a decrease in the activity of uroporphyrinogen decarboxylase in the liver. It is a heterogeneous disorder and it is probable that in most cases a number of inherited and acquired factors interact to produce the hepatic enzyme defect.[18]

There are two main types of PCT:

- sporadic or type I, in which erythrocyte uroporphyrinogen decarboxylase activity is normal and there is no family history of porphyria;
- familial or type II, where decreased uroporphyrinogen decarboxylase activity in all tissues is inherited as an autosomal dominant trait.

The clinical penetrance of the type II defect is low so that the majority of gene carriers are asymptomatic. Type I PCT is more common than type II and accounts for 70–80% of patients in most countries. In addition, familial PCT with normal erythrocyte enzyme activity has been described and PCT may also be produced by poisoning with polyhalogenated aromatic hydrocarbons. A number of different mutations have been identified in type II PCT and in the putative homozygous form of this condition, hepatoerythropoietic porphyria.[19,20]

In sporadic and familial PCT, hepatic uroporphyrinogen decarboxylase activity appears to be iron dependent. Thus depletion of hepatic iron stores leads to clinical remission and may, in type I PCT, restore enzyme activity to normal while replenishment of iron stores produces relapse. The mechanism of this effect is uncertain but recent studies in animal models of PCT suggest that a catalytic site-directed inhibitor of uroporphyrinogen decarboxylase may be produced in the liver when uroporphyrinogen is oxidized by a cytochrome P450-dependent reaction in the presence of iron.[18]

CLINICAL FEATURES OF THE PORPHYRIAS

Patients with porphyria present in three different ways: with an acute attack of porphyria, with skin lesions alone, or with an acute attack accompanied by skin lesions (see Table 24.1). In variegate porphyria and hereditary coproporphyria, acute attacks and skin lesions may occur together or separately.

Porphyrias Associated with Acute Attacks

Clinically identical attacks of acute porphyria occur in AIP, variegate porphyria, hereditary coproporphyria (see Table 24.1) and in PBG-synthase-deficiency porphyria.[1-3] They are accompanied by skin lesions in about half of the patients with variegate porphyria and in about a third of those with hereditary coproporphyria.[1,2]

TABLE 24.7

SOME FACTORS THAT MAY PRECIPITATE ACUTE ATTACKS OF
PORPHYRIA

Drugs[1]
Barbiturates, sulphonamides, oestrogens, progestogens, griseofulvin, sulphonylureas, methyldopa, nikethemide, dichloralphenazone, glutethimide, diazepam, carbamazepine, ethosuximide, phenytoin, phenylbutazone, chloramphenicol

Other factors
Low-calorie diet
Cyclic—menstrual
Alcohol
Infection
Emotional stress

[1]More complete lists are given in references 1–3.

The clinical features of acute porphyria have been reviewed.[1,2] The most common symptom is severe abdominal pain, which may be accompanied by neurological and mental disturbances. About two-thirds of patients develop muscular weakness, which may progress to quadriparesis and respiratory paralysis. Acute attacks are more common in women and are most frequent in the third and fourth decades, being very uncommon before puberty.

Hyponatraemia is common, when vomiting is severe or renal function deteriorates. Occasionally it may be caused by inappropriate secretion of arginine vasopressin (antidiuretic hormone). Hypothalamic neuroendocrine dysfunction has been postulated to explain this finding and asymptomatic abnormalities of growth hormone and ACTH control.[1,2] Various abnormalities of thyroid function have also been described but patients are usually euthyroid, although transient hyperthyroidism has been reported.[1,2]

Most acute attacks are precipitated by drugs, especially barbiturates and anticonvulsants, alcohol, endocrine factors or calorie restriction (Table 24.7). Many of the drugs that provoke acute attacks stimulate the synthesis of, and are metabolized by, cytochrome P450. The increase in hepatic ALA-synthase activity and PBG formation that accompanies acute porphyria suggests that the short-term demand for increased haem synthesis imposed by these drugs cannot be met because the rate of haem synthesis becomes limited by PBG-deaminase activity. Thus, during the acute attack, there appears to be hepatic haem deficiency with sustained depression of ALA-synthase.[1–3]

The relation between these biochemical changes and the neurological disturbance that underlies all the clinical features of the acute attack has not been defined. Possible mechanisms have been reviewed.[1,2] In general, theories have focused on either the direct effects of haem deficiency in the nervous system, for which at present there is little evidence, or the secondary effects on the nervous system of metabolic disturbances in the liver. Current views tend to favour a toxic effect of ALA on the nervous system, largely because attacks occur only in association with increased production of ALA and are seen only in those conditions in which this occurs: PBG-synthase deficiency porphyria, other acute porphyrias and hereditary tyrosinaemia.[21] In addition, ALA is known to cross the blood–brain barrier. However, neurotoxicity of ALA has not been demonstrated convincingly in animals. Hepatic haem deficiency decreases the activity of tryptophan pyrrolase and it has also been suggested that alterations in the metabolism of neuroactive tryptophan metabolites may be important in the pathogenesis of acute porphyria.[22] Again, experimental evidence of neurotoxicity is lacking, although it seems possible that such changes may contribute to the mental disturbances that are a feature of the acute attack.

Manoeuvres that are known to prevent the induction of ALA-synthase in laboratory animals appear to be effective in the treatment of acute porphyria in man. Thus, there are several reports that loading with carbohydrate or intravenous administration of haem decrease PBG and ALA formation and may produce clinical remission.[23]

Porphyrias Associated with Skin Lesions

Porphyria Cutanea Tarda, Variegate Porphyria, Hereditary Coproporphyria, Congenital Erythropoietic Porphyria

The skin lesions in these disorders occur in sun-exposed areas and are fundamentally similar, although their severity varies. The most prominent abnormality is increased mechanical fragility with displacement of the epidermis and the formation of erosions in response to trivial injury. Subepidermal bullae are frequent and are the usual presenting feature. Pigmentation and hirsutism are common, and sclerodermatous changes may also occur.

The most common disorder in this group is PCT. The clinical features have been described by Grossman et al.[24] Most cases occur in association with liver-cell damage, particularly when caused by alcohol, but oestrogens are also important precipitating factors.[18] Biochemical evidence of liver dysfunction, especially minor increases in serum aspartate transaminase and ferritin levels, is common but does not normally include jaundice or severe liver disease. Needle biopsy of the liver usually reveals inflammatory changes, often with some fatty infiltration, with cirrhosis being present in less than one-third of patients.[18] The liver contains an increased concentration of uroporphyrin and biopsy cores frequently show red fluorescence when viewed in long-wave ultraviolet light. PCT increases the risk of hepatocellular carcinoma in patients with chronic liver disease.[18]

Almost all patients have hepatic siderosis and total

body-iron stores are increased in about two-thirds of European patients, although rarely to the extent found in haemochromatosis. Possible causes of the hepatic siderosis, including heterozygosity for the haemochromatosis gene, have been reviewed.[18] Depletion of iron stores by repeated venesection leads to clinical and biochemical remission in the majority of patients, as does treatment with chloroquine.[25] Acute attacks of porphyria do not occur in PCT.

When variegate porphyria presents with skin lesions alone, it cannot be distinguished clinically from PCT. Neither the family history nor the usual absence of liver disease provides reliable means of differentiation. The proportion of patients that present in this way is probably of the order of 70% in the UK. In contrast, hereditary coproporphyria almost always presents as acute porphyria, and is accompanied by skin involvement in about one-third of cases.

Congenital erythropoietic porphyria is a very rare disorder in which severe skin lesions caused by photosensitization by porphyrins usually develop in infancy and may be accompanied by haemolytic anaemia. A milder form of this condition, with onset in adult life, has been described and may be mistaken for PCT.[26]

Erythropoietic Protoporphyria

The characteristic clinical features of this form of cutaneous porphyria have been described.[27] Onset is usually during childhood. Photosensitivity with an oedematous reaction in sun-exposed skin is the most prominent feature. Bullae are unusual and increased mechanical fragility is not present. Residual scarring from healed lesions is much less prominent than in the other cutaneous porphyrias. Patients may develop cholelithiasis, with gallstones that contain protoporphyrin. The most important complication is liver disease, which develops in a small proportion of patients and usually progresses rapidly to death in liver failure with massive accumulation of protoporphyrin in the liver.[28] This complication is difficult to predict or prevent and the only effective treatment appears to be liver transplantation.

LABORATORY DIAGNOSIS OF THE PORPHYRIAS

Patients with Symptoms that Suggest Acute Porphyria

Acute attacks of porphyria are associated with increased excretion of PBG. The urine may be dark reddish-brown, due to polymerization of PBG to porphyrins and other compounds, or normal in colour, perhaps darkening later on standing.

In this group, therefore, the essential first test is examination of the urine for PBG. A negative screening test does not exclude increased PBG excretion. However, if the abdominal pain of a patient is severe enough to require admission to hospital and is caused by acute porphyria, it is unlikely that the screening

test will be negative, provided fresh urine is examined. On occasions, particularly in variegate porphyria and heriditary coproporphyria, PBG excretion may decrease rapidly after the onset of the attack so that the screening test becomes negative. Thus, quantitative measurement is essential if clinical suspicion of acute porphyria persists. Measurement of urinary porphyrins is of little diagnostic value in this group of patients.[6] In practice, tests for excess PBG and porphyrins are often done together. Provided the sample is fresh, an increased porphyrin concentration with a normal PBG concentration in urine from a patient with abdominal pain is almost always due to secondary coproporphyrinuria (*see* Table 24.3).

The other essential investigation for this group of patients is measurement of faecal porphyrins. This test enables AIP, variegate porphyria and hereditary coproporphyria to be differentiated (*see* Table 24.6) and also identifies those patients with variegate porphyria or hereditary coproporphyria who are investigated after urinary PBG excretion has returned to normal. Occult gastrointestinal bleeding may increase the faecal porphyrin concentration but can be distinguished from variegate porphyria and hereditary coproporphyria showing that only dicarboxylic-acid porphyrins are increased.[6]

Patients who Present with Skin Lesions

The full investigation of a patient who presents with skin lesions that might be due to porphyria entails measurement of porphyrins in blood, faeces and urine (*see* Table 24.6). In practice, the order in which these investigations are carried out is determined by the clinical presentation. If erythropoietic protoporphyria (EPP) is suspected, erythrocyte porphyrin measurement is the first and most important investigation, whereas for skin lesions of the type seen in PCT, determination of urinary and faecal porphyrins takes precedence.

EPP can be differentiated from other causes of acute photosensitivity by measurement of erythrocyte porphyrins[6]. An increased concentration suggests EPP but the diagnosis needs to be confirmed by showing that the increase is caused by protoporphyrin and not by its zinc chelate (Fig. 24.2), which is increased in all other conditions in which erythrocyte porphyrin levels are raised, such as lead poisoning, iron deficiency, some other anaemias, and rare types of porphyria.[6]

In all other types of porphyria that present with skin lesions, except congenital erythropoietic porphyria (CEP) and the rare homozygous variants, the red-cell porphyrin concentration is normal (*see* Table 24.1). Their presence can be confirmed or excluded by measurement of the total porphyrin concentration in urine and faeces.[6] If either is increased, individual urinary and faecal porphyrins should be separated by TLC or HPLC to identify the type of porphyria (*see* Table 24.6). In addition, isomer-type analysis is

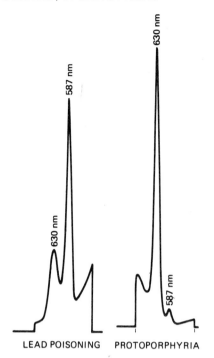

Figure 24.2 Fluorescence emission spectra of ethanol extracts of whole blood. Excitation wavelength, 415 nm.

required to confirm a diagnosis of CEP (*see* Table 24.6). Fluorescence emission spectroscopy of plasma is useful for the rapid diagnosis of variegate porphyria.[10] Secondary coproporphyrinuria (*see* Table 24.3) can be distinguished from all types of porphyria with increased urinary coproporphyrin excretion by showing that the faecal porphyrin composition is normal.[6] Both the urinary and faecal porphyrin concentrations may be normal in PCT during remission but measurement of individual porphyrins will usually enable the diagnosis to be made.

Detection of Asymptomatic Carriers of Genes for the Autosomal Dominant Porphyrias

Measurement of erythrocyte PBG-deaminase activity is widely used for the detection of carriers of the AIP gene. It has two important advantages over determination of urinary PBG. First, it enables gene carriers to be identified before puberty, when PBG excretion is rarely abnormal and acute attacks are very uncommon. Second, it allows the substantial percentage of adult latent porphyrics with normal PBG excretion to be detected. However, it does not enable carrier status to be determined in all relatives of affected individuals because, apart from those rare families in which the enzyme defect is absent from red cells, there is some overlap between AIP and normal ranges.[1–3,6,29] In addition, erythrocyte PBG-deaminase activity may be altered by various non-porphyric illnesses[3] and is increased by even small increases in the proportion of young erythrocytes in the incuba-

tion, so the test is unsuitable for carrier detection before the age of 6–8 months and in those with haematological abnormalities.

In suitable familes, analysis of DNA is a better method for detecting gene carriers than enzyme measurement. Two approaches are possible. In families where the mutation has been identified, direct detection of the mutation can be done.[16] Alternatively, intragenic restriction fragment length polymorphisms can be used for gene tracking.[6,16] Both approaches have some disadvantages. The extensive molecular heterogeneity of AIP[29] means that the mutation is unknown in many families and identification using current techniques is often difficult and time-consuming. Gene tracking is more generally applicable but is restricted to families with potentially informative probands and requires sufficient affected relatives to establish linkage, usually with PBG-deaminase deficiency, as clinical penetrance is low and most families contain few symptomatic individuals.

Detection of carriers of the variegate porphyria gene depends on measurement of plasma and faecal porphyrin concentrations, as excretion of urinary haem precursors is usually normal. In suspected adult gene carriers with normal or equivocal porphyrin concentrations and in prepubertal children, measurement of protoporphyrinogen oxidase is required. Adults with latent hereditary coproporphyria can be detected by measuring faecal coproporphyrin excretion, with assay of coproporphyrinogen oxidase being reserved for those in whom this measurement is normal, including all children before puberty.

Detection of asymptomatic carriers of the genes for type II PCT and EPP is less important for the management of these conditions but may be required, particularly when patients are anxious to know whether their children have inherited porphyria. For type II PCT, measurement of erythrocyte uroporphyrinogen decarboxylase is required.[3,18] Some asymptomatic carriers of the gene for EPP may have unequivocally increased erythrocyte protoporphyrin concentrations but, in many, determinations of carrier status can be made only by measurement of ferrochelatase activity in lymphocytes or skin fibroblasts. However, recombinant DNA methods are likely to become available in the near future now that cDNA for human ferrochelatase has been cloned.[30]

REFERENCES

1. Moore M.R., McColl K.E., Rimington C., Goldberg A. (1987). *Disorders of Porphyrin Metabolism.* New York: Plenum Press.
2. Kappas A., Sassa S., Galbraith R.A., Nordmann Y. (1989). The porphyrias. In *The Metabolic Basis of Inherited Disease,* 6th edn (Scriver C.R., Beaudet A.L., Sly W.S., Valle D. eds.) New York: McGraw-Hill, pp.1305–1366.
3. Nordmann Y., Deybach J.-C. (1990). Human hereditary porphyrias. In *Biosynthesis of Heme and Chlorophylls* (Dailey H.A. ed.) New York: McGraw-Hill, pp.491–542.

4. Dierks P. (1990). Molecular biology of eukaryotic 5-amino-laevulinate synthase. In *Biosynthesis of Heme and Chlorophylls* (Dailey H.A. ed.) New York: McGraw-Hill, pp.201–234.

5. Frank M., Doss M. (1989) Relevance of urinary coproporphyrin isomers in hereditary hyperbilirubinaemias. *Clin. Biochem.*, **22**, 221.

6. Elder G.H., Smith S.G., Smyth S.J. (1990). Laboratory investigation of the porphyrias. *Ann. Clin. Biochem.*, **27**, 395.

7. Smith K.M. (1975). *Porphyrins and Metalloporphyrins.* Amsterdam: Elsevier.

8. Lockwood W.H., Poulos V., Rossi E., Curnow D.H. (1985). Rapid procedure for faecal porphyrin assay. *Clin. Chem.*, **31**, 1163.

9. Deacon A.C. (1988). Performance of screening tests for porphyria. *Ann. Clin. Biochem.*, **25**, 392.

10. Poh-Fitzpatrick M.B. (1986). A plasma porphyrin fluorescence marker for variegate porphyria. *Arch. Dermatol.*, **116**, 543.

11. Rossi E., Curnow D.H. (1986). Porphyrins. In *HPLC of Small Molecules: A Practical Approach* (Lim C.K. ed.) Oxford and Washington DC: IRL Press, pp.261–303.

12. Llewellyn D.H. et al. (1992). Homozygous acute intermittent porphyria: compound heterozygosity for adjacent base transitions in the same codon of the porphobilinogen deaminase gene. *Hum. Genetics,* **87**, 97.

13. Elder G.H. (1992) Disorders of porphyrin metabolism. In *The Biochemical Basis of Pediatric Diseases* (Soldin S.J., Rifai N., Hicks J.M. eds.) Washington DC: American Association for Clinical Chemistry Press.

14. O'Reilly K., Snape J., Moore M.R. (1988). Porphyria cutanea tarda resulting from primary hepatocellular carcinoma. *Clin. Exp. Dermatol.*, **13**, 44.

15. Doss M. (1988). New dual form of porphyria. *Lancet,* **i**, 945.

16. Elder G.H. (1993) Molecular genetics of disorders of haem biosynthesis, *J. Clin. Pathol.*, **46**, 977.

17. Lee J.-S., Anvret M. (1991). Identification of the most common major mutation within the human porphobilinogen deaminase gene in Swedish patients with acute intermittent porphyria. *Proc. Nat. Acad. Sci. USA*, **88**, 10912.

18. Elder G.H. (1990). Porphyria cutanea tarda: a multifactorial disease. In *Recent Advances in Dermatology*, no.8 (Champion R.H., Pye R.J. eds.) Edinburgh: Churchill Livingstone, pp.55–70.

19. Garey J.R. et al. (1990). Uroporphyrinogen decarboxylase: a splice site mutation causes the deletion of exon 6 in multiple families with porphyria cutanea tarda. *J. Clin. Invest.*, **86**, 1416.

20. Koszo F., Elder G.H., Roberts A., Simon N. (1990). Uroporphyrinogen decarboxylase deficiency in hepatoerythropoietic porphyria: further evidence for genetic heterogeneity. *Br. J. Dermatol.*, **122**, 365.

21. Mitchell G. et al. (1990). Neurologic crises in hereditary tyrosinemia. *N. Engl. J. Med.*, **322**, 432.

22. Litman D.A., Correia M.A. (1985) L-Tryptophan: a common denominator of biochemical and neurological events of acute hepatic porphyria. *Science*, **222**, 1031.

23. Mustajoki P., Tenunen R., Pierach C., Volin L. (1989). Heme in the treatment of porphyrias and haematological disorders. *Semin. Hematol.*, **26**, 1.

24. Grossman M.E. et al. (1979). Clinical features and laboratory findings in 40 patients. *Am. J. Med.*, **67**, 277.

25. Ashton R.E., Hawk J.L.M., Magnus I.A. (1984). Low-dose oral chloroquine in the treatment of porphyria cutanea tarda. *Br. J. Dermatol.*, **111**, 609.

26. Nordmann Y., Deybach J.-C. (1986). Congenital erythropoietic porphyria. *Semin. Dermatol.*, **5**, 106.

27. De Leo V.A., Poh-Fitpatrick M.B., Matthews-Roth M.M., Harberg L.C. (1976). Erythropoietic protoporphyria. Ten years experience. *Am. J. Med.*, **60**, 8.

28. Rank J.M., Straka, J.G., Bloomer J.R. (1990). Liver in disorders of porphyrin metabolism. *J. Gastroenterol. Hepatol.*, **5**, 573.

29. Pierach C.A. et al. (1987). Red blood cell porphobilinogen deaminase in the evaluation of acute intermittent porphyria. *J. Am. Med. Assoc.*, **257**, 60.

30. Taketani, S., Nakahashi Y., Osumi T., Tokunage R. (1990). Molecular cloning, sequencing and expression of mouse ferrochelatase. *J. Biol. Chem.*, **265**, 19377.

25. Haemoglobin-opathies

D. Williamson, R. W. Carrell and H. Lehmann [†]

Introduction
Haemoglobin structure and function
  Haem and the haem pocket
  Globin structure: solubility and stability
  Cooperativity and the haemoglobin
    tetramer
  Modifiers of oxygen transport
Haemoglobin genetics and expression
  Haemoglobin of embryo, fetus and adult
  α-Gene duplication
  Globin gene structure
Haemoglobin variation and disease
  The abnormal haemoglobins
  Non-genetic variation: the glycosylated
    haemoglobins
  The haemoglobinopathies
  The thalassaemias
Laboratory diagnosis
  Routine screening
  Variant identification

INTRODUCTION

The structure of haemoglobin is typified by the adult human haemoglobin, HbA. This is formed of four globin polypeptide chains each with its own haem group, the globin chains being in the form of two unlike pairs, i.e. $\alpha_2 \beta_2$.

The term *haemoglobinopathies* is a collective one for the genetic defects affecting haemoglobin structure or synthesis. These have been intensively studied and a major conclusion has been the truth of the familiar laboratory law, that everything that can go wrong will go wrong! The defects can be divided into two categories: (i) those that affect the structure of the haemoglobin, usually due to the substitution of one amino acid by another, i.e. the *abnormal haemoglobins*, and (ii) those that primarily affect the rate of synthesis of one of the globin chains causing an imbalanced production of the haemoglobin subunits, the *thalassaemias*. There are many different types of thalassaemias, but there are two major classifications: (i) the α-thalassaemias, in which there is a defect in synthesis of the α-chain with consequent excess of β-chains, and (ii) the β-thalassaemias, in which there is a deficit in β-chain synthesis and hence an excess of α-chains.

The structural variants of haemoglobin, the abnormal haemoglobins, are each individually character-

ized and may be accompanied by functional alterations to give disease as in sickle-cell anaemia, where there is a substitution of the sixth amino acid of the β-chain, glutamic acid, by valine, i.e. HbS $\alpha_2 \beta_2^{6Glu \rightarrow Val}$. Many other abnormal haemoglobins, however, are just chance mutations that do not noticeably affect function or the health of the carrier.

Although the distinction between the thalassaemias and the abnormal haemoglobins is quite clear in terms of their definitions, it is not nearly so clear at the level of laboratory-bench diagnosis. The haemoglobinopathies usually present to the clinical biochemist in the form of a blood sample accompanied by some sketchy clinical details ending with '. . . ? haemoglobinopathy'. If this question is to be answered competently two things are required of the clinical biochemist. The first is a clear understanding of the basic principles of the structure, function and genetics of haemoglobin; the second is a systematic diagnostic approach that will cover the likely possibilities. These topics and an approach to diagnosis are reviewed in this chapter at a level relevant to the general clinical laboratory; more detailed background and reference information is given in the sources appended under Further Reading.

HAEMOGLOBIN STRUCTURE AND FUNCTION

Barcroft[1] pointed out in 1928 that, physiologically, haemoglobin was required to be:

(i) capable of transporting large quantities of oxygen;
(ii) very soluble;
(iii) capable of taking up oxygen at suitable velocity and in sufficient amounts in the blood and of releasing it to the tissues;
(iv) able to buffer a bicarbonate solution.

This list is still relevant, though now it could be restated to give a greater emphasis on structure, that is:

(i) haem and the haem pocket: oxygenation;
(ii) globin structure: solubility and instability;
(iii) the haemoglobin tetramer: cooperativity;
(iv) modifiers of oxygen transport.

Haem and the Haem Pocket

Haem

Oxygenation occurs at the haem group, which is a coordinate of iron and protoporphyrin. The full structure of protoporphyrin is given in Chapter 24; essential features are its near-planar nature and its highly mobile electron flux. This flux is readily excited by light in the 400-nm range to give the characteristic red (Soret) absorption spectrum. Free protoporphyrin will emit light to give fluorescence but this fluorescence is quenched in haem by the coordinated iron. However, haemoglobin fluorescence may exception-

---

[†] Deceased.

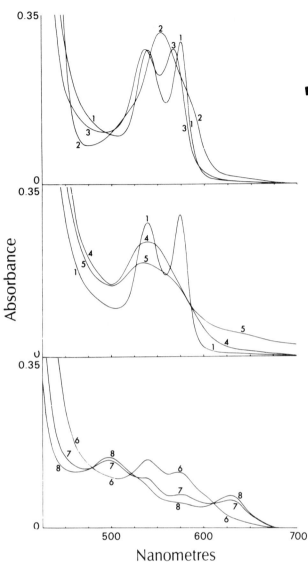

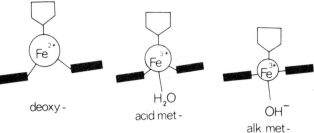

Figure 25.2 Deoxyhaemoglobin and acid and alkaline methaemoglobins showing the changes in charge and relation of iron to the haem plane that produce changes in the adsorption spectra. Note how the iron shrinks and moves into the plane of the haem with linked movement of the proximal histidine (see Fig. 25.3). (Reproduced with permission from Carell and Lehmann.[3])

from the iron to the oxygen so the iron is in a transition state between Fe^{2+} and Fe^{3+}. The oxygen of oxyhaemoglobin can be readily displaced by small anions such as Cl^- or OH^- (water) to give the ferric methaemoglobin. The changes in charge distribution that result are reflected by characteristic changes in absorption spectra (Fig. 25.1).

As well as changes in charge distribution there are also changes in the spin state of the iron; these are of significance in triggering the cooperative changes in haemoglobin on oxygenation, as well as resulting in spectral modifications. Both ferrous and ferric iron can exist in high- or low-spin states according to the pairing of their outer orbital electrons. The radius of the iron atom increases in the high-spin state with a consequent lengthening of iron–porphyrin bonds. This causes a movement of iron out of the plane of the haem when the low-spin oxyhaemoglobin is converted to high-spin deoxyhaemoglobin (Fig. 25.2). This movement of the iron will be transmitted to the linked histidine with resultant distortion of the globin and triggering of changes in the other globin subunits of the haemoglobin molecule.

Figure 25.1 Absorption spectra of haemoglobin derivatives measured in phosphate buffer, pH 7.4, except as indicated below. 1, oxyhaemoglobin; 2, deoxyhaemoglobin; 3, carboxyhaemoglobin; 4, cyanmethaemoglobin; 5, haemichrome; 6, methaemoglobin pH 6.0 phosphate buffer; 7, methaemoglobin; 8, methaemoglobin in pH 11.0 glycine buffer. (Reproduced with permission from Carell and Lehmann.[3])

Haem Pocket

The partial transfer to oxygen of an electron from the haem iron makes it very susceptible to displacement by OH^- or Cl^-. This is highly disadvantageous as it results in the physiologically inert methaemoglobin, $Fe^{3+}OH^-$, and the release of the toxic superoxide radical, O_2^-. A consequent priority for reversible oxygenation is that the haem should be buried in a non-polar, hydrophobic environment, which prevents access of polar ligands such as water. This is achieved by placing the haem in a hydrophobic pocket in the globin, in a position structurally comparable to that of a coin pushed deep into a soft bun.

The 20 amino acids lining the pocket form a close steric fit with the haem group, limiting access to the iron and contributing to the overall stability of the globin. The structure of the haem pocket was tightly

ally occur when iron is prevented from coordinating with the protoporphyrin and is replaced by zinc. This forms the basis of a simple and useful screening test[2] for iron deficiency or lead poisoning, by measurement of whole-blood fluorescence.

The electron flux of the protoporphyrin readily allows transfer of charge to the haem iron. This iron has four coordinate bonds to the porphyrin, a fifth bond to a histidine of the globin and a sixth bond to various ligands such as oxygen. The iron is in the ferrous (Fe^{2+}) form in deoxyhaemoglobin but in oxyhaemoglobin there is a partial transfer of an electron

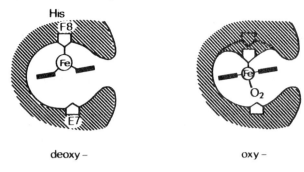

deoxy –   oxy –

Figure 25.3 Schematic representation of the haem pockets of deoxy- and oxyhaemoglobin. The porphyrin ring with its four bonds is shown in planar section. The proximal histidine (F8) forms the fifth coordinate, the sixth coordinate being formed by the ligand, oxygen in this case, which lies between the iron and the distal histidine (E7). Note the linked movement of the globin and the iron as changes in the radius of the iron cause it to move into and out of the haem plane. (Reproduced with permission from Carell and Lehmann.[3])

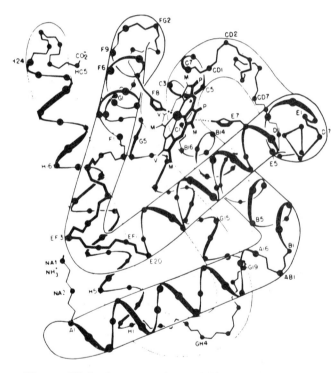

Figure 25.4 Structure of myoglobin, which exemplifies those of all the globins: 80% of the molecule is in the helical form, each helix being designated by a letter and number, and non-helical portions by two letters and a number according to their position (thus A1–A16, helical; CD1–CD7, non-helical). (Reproduced by courtesy of Dr R. E. Dickerson; published in *The Proteins*, vol. II (Neurath H. ed.) New York: Academic Press, Fig. 15, p. 634.)

defined by evolution several hundred million years ago; since then it has remained relatively static whereas the rest of the molecule has changed to meet the requirements of different species. Consequently, chance mutations that occur to haem-pocket residues are likely to produce pathology; either by allowing globin bonding to the sixth ligand position, i.e. abnormal methaemoglobins, or due to a distortion of globin structure to give instability of the molecule with consequent red-cell haemolysis.

Two of the amino acid residues lining the haem pocket are of particular importance; these are the two haem-linked histidines illustrated in Fig. 25.3. The proximal histidine (F8) forms the fifth coordinate of the iron and the distal histidine (E7) occupies a position where it can form a polar bond with the partially negative oxygen of oxyhaemoglobin. Distortion of the globin, as occurs in partial denaturation, may allow the distal histidine close enough to the iron to bond to it to form the unstable globin haemichromes, initially haemichrome I. If further distortion occurs, other side-chains in the globin may displace the histidine to form the irreversible globin haemichrome II, with resultant denaturation and precipitation.

Globin Structure: Solubility and Stability

If one prime task of the globin molecule is to provide a hydrophobic environment for the haem group, the other is the need to give solubility to the molecule as a whole. This need for solubility is a demanding requirement as the red cell is packed with haemoglobin, which forms a third of its net weight. Some idea of the packing can be given by comparison of the red cell and the molecules to a football stadium filled with tennis balls, with only the interstices available for the water of the solution. It is not surprising, then, that one of the likely consequences of globin mutations is a change in solubility, or stability, that results in intracellular precipitation of haemoglobin with consequent haemolysis.

The globin molecule is highly soluble because it is folded in such a way that its ionized and polar amino-acid side-chains are externally situated. As shown in Fig. 25.4, globin is formed of eight helices (A–H) linked by short interhelical segments (AB, CD, etc.). The non-polar aspect of each helix points internally to provide a hydrophobic environment for the haem, the polar aspect of each helix is externally orientated to provide solubility.

Cooperativity and the Haemoglobin Tetramer

Cooperativity

The globin monomer, as in myoglobin or in an isolated haemoglobin subunit, has a hyperbolic oxygen dissociation curve (Fig. 25.5). Oxygen is bound with high affinity and is released only at very low oxygen tension. The requirement for a physiological oxygen carrier is that it should release a substantial proportion of its oxygen at the tissue tension of 40 mmHg and the rest well before reaching zero

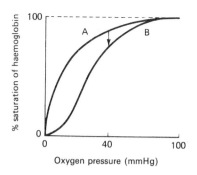

Figure 25.5 Comparison of the hyperbolic oxygen dissociation curve of myoglobin (A) with the sigmoid curve of haemoglobin (B). Note the increased efficiency of the release of oxygen of the sigmoid curve at the mean venous tension of 40 mmHg. (Reproduced with permission from Lehmann and Casey.[4])

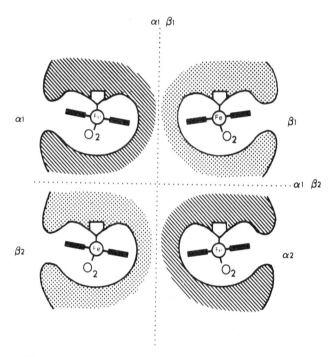

Figure 25.6 The haemoglobin tetramer diagrammatically represented in the oxy-, R, state to show the nomenclature of the $\alpha\beta$ interfaces. The change to the deoxy-, T, state involves a sliding movement of the $\alpha_1\beta_2$ junction, the α-chains moving close together and a gap opening between the β-chains that allows entry of 2,3-biphosphoglycerate. (Reproduced with permission from Carrell and Lehmann.[3])

oxygen tension. This need for a sigmoid oxygen-dissociation curve is met by cooperativity, the term used to describe the way in which the deoxygenation of one globin subunit of haemoglobin decreases the oxygen affinity of the other subunits. This cooperative interaction of subunits involves a change in structural conformation of the haemoglobin molecule: the R–T transformation.

The affinity of fully oxygenated haemoglobin for oxygen is the same as that of its isolated subunits and for this reason oxyhaemoglobin is said to be in the relaxed, R, state. However, on deoxygenation, cooperative effects between the globin subunits constrain the molecule in a low-affinity, tense, T state. A simple analogy is to that of a sponge which in its relaxed (R) form will readily take up water but if held in the tense (T) form will readily lose, and less readily take up, water.

Hill Equation

Cooperativity can be treated quantitatively. The oxygenation of myoglobin or of a single haemoglobin subunit follows first-order kinetics:

$$Mb + O_2 \rightleftharpoons MbO_2$$
$$[1 - Y] \quad [O_2] \quad [Y]$$

where Y is the fractional saturation and $[O_2]$ the partial pressure of oxygen. If K is the equilibrium constant, then the fractional (percentage) saturation is the hyperbolic function

$$Y = \frac{K[O_2]}{1 + K[O_2]}$$

Hill showed that, for the haemoglobin tetramer, the oxygen dissociation could be represented by the sigmoid function

$$Y = \frac{K[O_2]^n}{1 + K[O_2]^n}$$

where n, the Hill number, indicates the degree of subunit interaction. Normally its value is 2.8 but it will be lower in mutant haemoglobins with decreased cooperativity. In myoglobin and the isolated haemoglobin subunits, n has a value of 1, i.e. no cooperativity.

Haemoglobin Tetramer

The cooperativity of haemoglobin requires a tetramer formed of two pairs of unlike globins, as in HbA, $\alpha_2\beta_2$, adult human haemoglobin. Together the four subunits form an ellipsoid with a molecular weight of 67 000 and dimensions of 64 × 55 × 50 Å. Cooperativity occurs due to small changes in subunit shape, i.e. tertiary changes, that result in much larger changes in the overall molecular shape, i.e. quaternary changes. The detailed molecular changes have been elucidated and reviewed by Perutz.[5,6] He points out that the molecule undergoes 'paradoxical breathing', decreasing in size on oxygenation and increasing on deoxygenation.

Oxyhaemoglobin is in the relaxed, R, state with each of its subunits having the same conformation as they would in the free state. The loss of oxygen from one or more subunits results in a change of conformation of the molecule as a whole to the tense, T, state with consequent further loss of oxygen. The R–T transformation involves a sliding rotation of one $\alpha\beta$

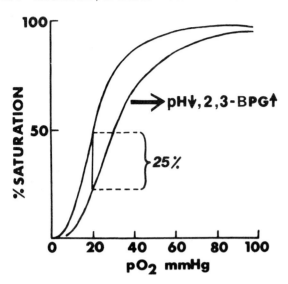

Figure 25.7 The oxygen dissociation curve of haemoglobin moves to the right (decreased affinity) with a drop in the pH or a rise in the 2,3-biphosphoglycerate. As shown, even with a small shift, as in a pH change from 7.6–7.2, will result in a large increase (25%) in oxygen delivery at the partial pressure of the working tissues.

pair about the other; the movement taking place at the $\alpha_1\beta_2$ junction (Fig. 25.6). This movement, on partial deoxygenation, allows ionic and hydrogen bonds to form between subunits, which in turn induce a change in shape of the individual subunits. This tertiary change, although small, results in a movement of the F-helix away from the haem; in doing so the haem-linked histidine pulls the iron out of the plane of the haem with a change to the high-spin state, with consequent release of any bound oxygen (*see* Fig. 25.3). This is a reciprocal process; loss of oxygen from one subunit will cause tertiary changes that favour ionic bonding with other subunits and hence the overall R–T transformation. Similarly, the change to the quaternary T conformation will induce each subunit to take up the tertiary T conformation, with loss of oxygen from individual globin subunits.

An important conclusion for the clinical biochemist is that mutations which cause gross changes in oxygen affinity are likely to involve only a few residues; those of the $\alpha_1\beta_2$ interface, those forming stabilizing bonds between subunits and those directly involved in the tertiary, T, change.

Modifiers of Oxygen Transport

It is a mistake to think of oxygen delivery primarily in terms of haemoglobin concentration. It is true that gross anaemia will affect peripheral oxygenation but, in most situations, changes in the oxygen affinity of haemoglobin are of much greater importance. Normally only 25% of the oxygen carried in the blood is released to the tissues, but this can be greatly in-

creased by small alterations in the shape of the oxygen dissociation curve (Fig. 25.7). This comes about by the action of small molecules that provide additional ionic bonds to stabilize the T quaternary structure of deoxyhaemoglobin.

An appreciable decrease in oxygen affinity, with consequent release of oxygen, occurs in working tissues due to accumulation of carbon dioxide and lactic acid. The decrease in affinity that occurs with increased acidity, in the physiological range, is known as the alkaline Bohr effect. The release of lactic acid in the periphery gives increased hydrogen ion concentration; this causes protonation of key basic residues in haemoglobin, which then form ionic bridges to stabilize the deoxy configuration. This results in both the release of oxygen to the tissues and the buffering of pH, as hydrogen ions are taken up at the periphery and released to the lungs where they are neutralized by combination with bicarbonate ions.

Similarly, carbon dioxide can combine with the N-terminal amines of globin subunits to give carbamino groups, which can form stabilizing bridges in deoxy- but not oxyhaemoglobin. The overall result is that haemoglobin acts as a transport agent that selectively releases oxygen to working tissues and removes hydrogen ions and carbon dioxide for excretion in the lungs.

As well as adaptions that influence the release of oxygen to specific tissues there is also an overall control of oxygen dissociation by the red-cell metabolite, 2,3-diphosphoglycerate. This binds stoichiometrically to haemoglobin forming ionic bonds with groups in a pocket between the β-chains in the deoxy-, T, conformation. This stabilizes the deoxy-conformation to give a decrease in oxygen affinity. Consequently the red cell can partially compensate for the decrease in oxygen transport that would otherwise occur in anaemia or with reduced environmental oxygen as occurs at high altitudes. It also explains the difference between the oxygen affinities of fetal and adult blood that facilitates placental exchange of oxygen. Both HbF and HbA have the same dissociation curves in simple solution, but in the red cell the affinity of HbA is decreased because of the 2,3-diphosphoglycerate effect. However, the γ-chains of HbF lack one of the 2,3-diphosphoglycerate binding sites and consequently fetal red-cell haemoglobin has a higher affinity for oxygen than that of the adult.

2,3-Diphosphoglycerate is a side-product of the glycolytic pathway, formed in the Rapoport–Leubering cycle, which bypasses the phosphoglycerate-kinase step of the main pathway (Fig. 25.8). The synthesis of 2,3-diphosphoglycerate is controlled by a number of factors that compensate for any changes in oxygen delivery.[7] For example, the decrease in oxygen affinity that occurs with increased acidity will be compensated by an equivalent increase in affinity due to inhibition of 2,3-diphosphoglycerate synthesis by lowered pH. This gives an automatic correction of oxygen dissociation in acid–base disturbances, but

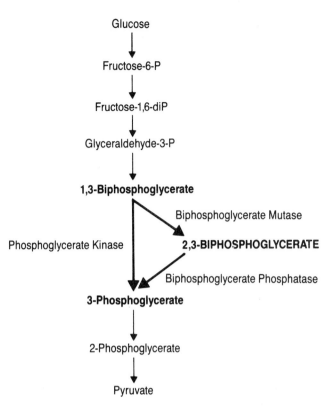

Glucose

↓

Fructose-6-P

↓

Fructose-1,6-diP

↓

Glyceraldehyde-3-P

↓

1,3-Biphosphoglycerate

Biphosphoglycerate Mutase

Phosphoglycerate Kinase   **2,3-BIPHOSPHOGLYCERATE**

Biphosphoglycerate Phosphatase

3-Phosphoglycerate

↓

2-Phosphoglycerate

↓

Pyruvate

Figure 25.8 The Rapoport–Luebering pathway for the production of 2,3-diphosphoglycerate.

whereas the Bohr effect acts immediately, adjustment of the 2,3-diphosphoglycerate concentration takes place over some 8 h. For this reason the correction of acid–base disturbances is best made over a period of hours rather than precipitately. In prolonged acidosis, 2,3-diphosphoglycerate concentration will be low and a sudden correction of the blood pH will cause a drastic increase in the oxygen affinity of the haemoglobin, with decreased oxygen release. The only way

the body can meet the oxygen demand is by increasing cardiac output; thus cardiac failure may be the end-result of a sudden correction of acidosis in an elderly or debilitated diabetic.

HAEMOGLOBIN GENETICS AND EXPRESSION

Haemoglobin of Embryo, Fetus and Adult

Human haemoglobins can be divided into three groups, each designed to meet a different physiological requirement for oxygen: the first are those required for the uptake of oxygen in the free-floating embryo, the second are those required for the uptake of oxygen against the placenta, and the third are those required in the mature human for atmospheric respiration. These haemoglobins are summarized in Fig. 25.9 and their chronological appearance is shown in Fig. 25.10. Diagnostically, the important haemoglobins are HbF, $\alpha_2\gamma_2$; HbA, $\alpha_2\beta_2$; and HbA$_2$, $\alpha_2\delta_2$. All of these are present in the mature human: HbA forming 97% of haemoglobin of the adult and HbA$_2$ some 3%. HbF, which forms about 60% of the haemoglobin of the newborn, comprises less than 1% of that of the normal adult. Synthesis of this trace amount of fetal haemoglobin in the adult appears to reside in a distinct population of cells known as F-cells, with the adult level of HbF and F-cells remaining relatively constant. Disorders that increase the amount of HbF can do so by both increasing the number of F-cells and the amount of HbF per F-cell. Usually the bone marrow is dominated by mature cell lines but stressed erythropoiesis, as in the leukaemias or severe congenital anaemias, will give a large increase in *de novo* synthesis with significant increases in HbF production. In these situations, the HbF is predominantly found in those cells that have arisen from new lines.

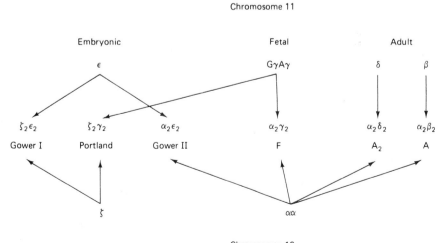

Figure 25.9 Human haemoglobins and the genetic control of their production.

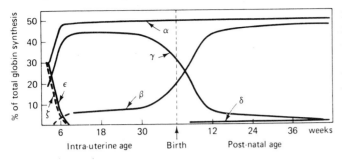

Figure 25.10 Changes in globin-chain synthesis during human development. (Adapted from Wood.[8])

As shown in Fig. 25.9, there are two fetal haemoglobins, which differ, almost imperceptibly, in the structure of their γ-chains; one having alanine at position 136, the other glycine. This slight structural difference is diagnostically useful as it enables a better definition of the various genetic abnormalities that lead to persistence of fetal haemoglobin into adult life; these may result in persistent expression of one, or both, of the γ-genes.

α-Gene Duplication

The duplication that has occurred with the γ-globin genes has also occurred with the α-globin; in this last instance to give identical duplicates. The presence of paired α-chain genes means that an abnormal α-globin will involve approximately one-quarter of the total haemoglobin, i.e. one of the four α-chain alleles; an abnormal β-globin will involve 50% of the HbA, i.e. one of the two β-chain alleles. In fact the α_1- and α_2-globin genes are not equivalent, but the α_2-gene has a greater contribution to α-globin production than the α_1-gene. The normal levels of α-globin variants consequently range between 15 and 25%. The presence of identical duplicates also opens the possibility of unequal crossing over to give chromosomes with either three or one α-chain genes.[9] The loss of one gene will decrease, by about half, the α-globin produced from that chromosome to give, overall, a small deficit of α-chains; this is a mild α^+-thalassaemia, also known as α-thalassaemia-2 trait. This deletion of a single α-globin gene provides a slight compensatory advantage in malarial areas.[10] As a consequence, a significant proportion of individuals who originate from Africa, South Asia or the Mediterranean areas have only three, or even two, α-chain alleles compared with the four alleles present in most of the human population.

The frequency of variations in the numbers of α-genes is one factor in the variability observed in the relative proportions of α-chain variants. The same variant may form less than 20% of the total HbA in an individual, with five α-globin alleles, whereas in another individual, with two alleles, it will form 50% of the total haemoglobin. A similar variation is seen in the proportion of β-chain variants for the same reason. A heterozygote for HbE will have some 30% of the abnormal haemoglobin (less than the expected 50%, primarily because the mutation also causes decreased synthesis of the abnormal β-chain). However, if synthesis of α-chains is decreased due to the loss of one α-gene then the proportion of HbE further decreases to around 24%, with the loss of two α-genes the proportion of HbE falls to around 17%. Careful measurement of variant proportions may, in this way, provide evidence of the α-thalassaemic carrier states that can otherwise be detected only by DNA analysis techniques.

Globin Gene Structure

The duplication of the α-chain genes is, in terms of geological time, a relatively recent event but it illustrates the way in which the globin genes evolved; by the process of duplication, mutation and then specialization.

The globin genes are closely linked, although at some time the α-globin genes on chromosome 16 have segregated from the non-α-globins on chromosome 11. The structures of the α- and β-globin gene clusters are extremely well characterized and a schematic representation is shown in Fig. 25.11.

The order of the genes on each of the chromosomes represents the order of their expression during development. The pattern of gene duplication is clearly evident, but as well as the formation of the functional duplicates (α_2 and α_1, $^G\gamma$ and $^A\gamma$, δ and β) there has also been the formation of non-functional 'pseudo' genes from duplicated loci which have undergone mutations that prevent their expression (β_1, α_1, α_2, δ_1). These pseudogenes do not seem to be of significance to normal haemoglobin expression but appear to be dormant remnants of globin gene evolution.

The genes that code for globin structure are overwhelmed in size by massive amounts of non-coding flanking sequences. Within these flanking sequences there are a number of essential regulatory elements that control the appropriate expression of the genes, that is, sequences involved in the initiation and control of gene transcription, which include the so-called TATA and CCAAT box sequences that lie upstream of the site for initiation of transcription. The function of most of the flanking DNA, however, is not known. When these regulatory sequences are taken into consideration, the gene complex extends over a much larger region of chromosomal DNA than that immediately occupied by the structural coding sequences illustrated in Fig. 25.11.

As well as the non-coding flanking sequences there are also non-coding intervening sequences, or introns, that interrupt the structural coding of the globin genes. These introns, although of variable length, are consistently found in globin genes, homologously placed between codons (amino acids) 30 and 31, and 104 and 105, of the β-globin messenger. The introns

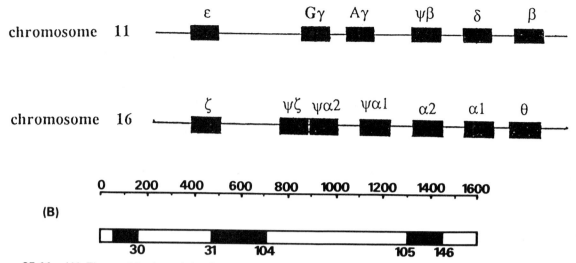

Figure 25.11 (A) The positioning of the functional and non-functional globin genes; non-α on chromosome 11 and α on chromosome 16. The exact status of the θ gene is not known—no protein product has yet been indentified. (B) A magnified depiction of the β-globin gene showing how the structural gene is interrupted by large, non-coding introns. The structural sequences are in black.

are transcribed into nascent mRNA but are excised to give the messenger ready for ribosomal translation. This splicing of the introns is dependent on specific 'donor' and 'acceptor' sequences in the DNA, which define the splice junctions. Splicing errors can and do occur through mutations inactivating these sequences or activating alternative splicing sequences. These mutations account for a significant proportion of thalassaemias.

An important practical observation is that although there is absolute conservation of the structural portion of the gene, there is considerable variation in flanking and intron sequences, even within a single species. The degree of this non-expressed polymorphism within man is sufficient to allow precise gene-linkage studies using DNA from non-specific sources such as amniotic fibroblasts or white cells. Specific polymorphisms that affect the recognition sequences of restriction enzymes have been shown to occur in both the α- and β-globin clusters in specific and relatively stable patterns (haplotypes) on different chromosomes. These therefore provide linkage markers that can be used to trace the inheritance of globin genes. These are useful for the construction of family pedigrees in prenatal diagnosis and have also been used in population studies to trace the origins of various haemoglobin mutations. A further example of this variability within the α-globin cluster is the existence of hypervariable regions (HVRs), which consist of multiple repeat sequences. These are highly polymorphic but are again genetically stable elements that can be used in gene-linkage studies along with restriction enzyme site polymorphisms.

HAEMOGLOBIN VARIATION AND DISEASE

Haemoglobin is the best studied of all proteins in terms of its structure and its variant forms in man. The study of these abnormal haemoglobins has greatly increased our knowledge of the relation of structure to function in proteins; it has also provided a model of protein variation that is being rediscovered again and again in other genetic diseases. The adage of the turn of the century with respect to pathology—'Know syphilis and you will know disease'—could now be restated with respect to molecular pathology—'Know the haemoglobinopathies and you will know genetic disease'.

The Abnormal Haemoglobins

Over 500 abnormal haemoglobins have now been identified and named after their place of discovery.[11] Initially, the majority of these were found as the result of electrophoretic screening of population samples. Most examples found by this approach turned out to be relatively harmless substitutions of one amino acid for another on the exterior of the molecule where a change in charge alters electrophoretic mobility but is not likely to produce gross molecular pathology. More recently, most new variants have been found as a result of an elective investigation of individuals with evidence of haemoglobin malfunction, usually haemolysis or dysfunction of oxygen transport. These malfunctions mainly arise from lesions that affect the internal amino acids of the globin or involve gross changes such as deletions or insertions of sections of the sequence. A third category of variants has also been recently identified;

First Base	Second Base: U	Second Base: C	Second Base: A	Second Base: G	Third Base
U	UUU Phe UUC Phe UUA Leu UUG Leu	UCU Ser UCC Ser UCA Ser UCG Ser	UAU Tyr UAC Tyr UAA Stop UAG Stop	UGU Cys UGC Cys UGA Stop UGG Trp	U C A G
C	CUU Leu CUC Leu CUA Leu CUG Leu	CCU Pro CCC Pro CCA Pro CCG Pro	CAU His CAC His CAA Gln CAG Gln	CGU Arg CGC Arg CGA Arg CGG Arg	U C A G
A	AUU Ile AUC Ile AUA Ile AUG Met	ACU Thr ACC Thr ACA Thr ACG Thr	AAU Asn AAC Asn AAA Lys AAG Lys	AGU Ser AGC Ser AGA Arg AGG Arg	U C A G
G	GUU Val GUC Val GUA Val GUG Val	GCU Ala GCC Ala GCA Ala GCG Ala	GAU Asp GAC Asp GAA Glu GAG Glu	GGU Gly GGC Gly GGA Gly GGG Gly	U C A G

Figure 25.12 The messenger RNA triplet code for amino acids. The code for mitochondrial RNA differs slightly. UGA codes for tryptophan and AUA for methionine.

these are the structural variants that result in diminished synthesis to give a thalassaemic-like picture[12] as seen in the chain-elongation mutants. Together all these abnormalities illustrate the complexity of variation that can occur in the amino acid sequence of the globins[13] and in the nucleotide sequence of the globin mRNA.[14]

Point Mutations

Most abnormal haemoglobins have single amino-acid substitutions due to a point mutation, the substitution of a single base in a triplet codon (*see* genetic code, Fig. 25.12). For example, the codon GGU, which codes for β24 glycine, has been substituted: by CGU (arginine) in Hb Riverdale–Bronx, by GUU (valine) in Hb Savannah and by GAU (aspartic acid) in Hb Moscva. It is now clear from sequencing of many individual globin genes that there is a degree of polymorphism in the nucleotide sequence so that in some individuals a different codon may be used to code for the same amino acid; for example, the codon for valine β67 is GUG, which is compatible with two substitutions found at this position, alanine (GCG) in Hb Sydney and glutamic acid (GAG) in Hb Milwaukee. However, a third variant, Hb Bristol, has an aspartic acid at position β67, which requires a codon GAU or GAC, incompatible with a single mutation from that of valine GUG. In other words, some individuals exist with either GUC or GUU as the alternative codons for valine to GUG, at position β67.

Deletions and Insertions

A number of variants have been identified that have lost or gained small portions of their amino acid sequence. Usually deletions occur between small areas of repetitive sequence as in Hb Gun Hill where there is a deletion between two Leu-His sequences in the β-chain:

Leu-	His-	Cys-	Asp-	Lys-	Leu-	His.
91	92	93	94	95	96	97

An example of an insertion is the α-chain variant, Hb Grady, in which the tripeptide sequence Glu-Phe-Thr is repeated. It is likely that these deletions and insertions have arisen from unequal crossing over during meiosis, though it is possible that they could result from a defect in DNA repair or replication.

Fusion Variants

These variants have formed by non-homologous cross-overs between adjacent genes to give $\delta\beta$ or $\gamma\beta$ hybrid or fusion forms. The identification of these fusion variants allowed the deduction of the arrangement of the globin genes on chromosome 11 even before it was confirmed by genomic mapping (Fig. 25.11).

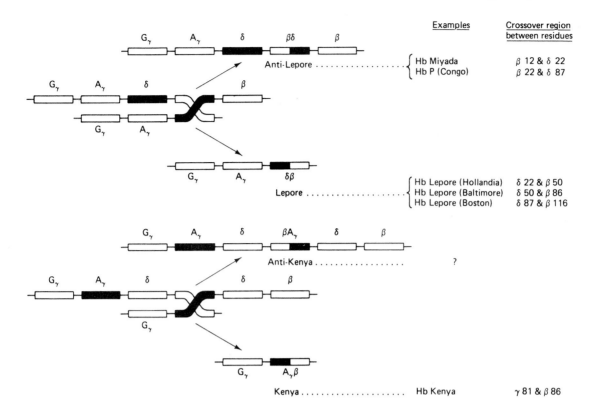

Figure 25.13 Mechanism of production of the crossover variants Hb Lepore and Hb Kenya. There are three different forms of Hb Lepore resulting from crossovers between the δ- and β-chain loci at different sites. (Reproduced, with permission, from Weatherall D.J. and Clegg J.B. (1979). *Cell*, **16**, 467.)

The most important of the fusion variants are the Hbs Lepore, illustrated in Fig. 25.13. These arise from a fusion of the δ- and the β-chains to give several varieties of $\delta\beta$ products, depending on the level of junction of the δ- and β-fragments. The $\delta\beta$ product is produced at only one-fifth the rate of that of the β-chain it replaces and this leads to a surplus of α-chains with mild thalassaemic findings. As a consequence, the Hbs Lepore have a similar distribution to the thalassaemias and are a relatively common finding in Mediterranean and other populations from endemic malarial areas. The other fusion globins, the converse antiLepore variants (Fig. 25.13) and the $\gamma\beta$ Hb Kenya, are less frequently found.

Termination, Frame-shift and Nonsense Errors
A mutation affecting a single base in a globin gene may produce effects other than a simple amino-acid substitution. A mutation in the codon that signals termination of the globin polypeptide may result in elongation products. For example, the α-chain termination mutants (Hb Constant Spring, Icaria and Koya Dora) have an elongation of some 30 residues, which represents translation of the normally untranslated 3' mRNA up to the next termination codon. The most common example, present in many South-East Asians, is Hb Constant Spring: an α-chain variant in which the stop codon UAA has mutated to

CAA, the codon for glutamine. The resultant globin is synthesized at a decreased rate and results in a mild thalassaemia.

Another type of variation is the frame-shift error in which one or two nucleotides are inserted into, or lost, from the structural gene. These frame-shift mutations will result in an alteration of the sequence beyond the mutation and are unlikely to produce a viable globin unless they occur near the C-terminus of the globin gene. An example is the α-chain of Hb Wayne, which is unchanged up to position 138 but then has a sequence of eight new amino acids. As shown, this is explicable by the loss of adenine from the codon for α139 Lys.

α-A	137	138	139	140	141	142	143
	Thr	Ser	Lys	Tyr	Arg	Stop	
	ACC	UCC	AAA	UAC	CGU	UAA	GCU

α-Wayne	137	138	139	140	141	142
	Thr	Ser	Asn	Thr	Val	Lys
	ACC	UCC	AAU	ACC	GUU	AAG

Similarly, Hb Tak and Hb Cranston have elongated β-chains that are explicable by frame-shift mutations.

Yet another type of mutation is the nonsense error in which there is a conversion of the codon for an amino acid to a stop or nonsense codon. An example is Hb McKees Rock where the two C-terminal β-chain residues, β145–146, are absent. This can be explained by the mutation of the β145 tyrosine codon, UAU, to a termination-nonsense codon UAA or UAG. Once again these mutations will only produce a viable globin product if they are near the COOH-terminus. Nonsense or frame-shift mutations earlier in the nucleotide sequence will produce a non-viable product to give, phenotypically, a thalassaemia.

Distribution of Variants in Man

Some of the abnormal haemoglobins, such as Hbs S, C, D and E, affect hundreds of thousands of people while others, such as G-Philadelphia and O-Arab, have an increased frequency within relatively limited groups. Knowledge of the distribution of variants[4] is useful both diagnostically and anthropologically. Diagnostically, the knowledge that HbE is common in South-East Asians will usually allow its provisional differentiation from HbC, a variant with similar electrophoretic mobility but a distribution largely confined to West Africans. Anthropologically, the variants are of interest as they illustrate the migration and mixture of peoples; for example, the not infrequent finding of HbD Punjab in Europeans is likely to be one of the longest-lasting reminders of the British Empire.

However, there needs to be caution in plotting of migrations on the basis of variants as undoubtedly many examples arise from new mutations. It would be a bold anthropologist who could link the first three observations of HbM Hyde Park in a Japanese, a black American and a European New Zealander!

The establishment of chance mutations within a population is much more likely when there is a balanced polymorphism, that is where the disadvantages of the mutant are balanced by other advantages. An example is HbS or sickle-cell haemoglobin (β6 Glu→Val) where the heterozygote has the advantage of protection against malignant malaria. HbS is mostly associated with tropical Africa where it may affect up to 40% of some East African tribes. It is present at a lesser frequency in non-tropical Africa and is found in North, but not South, Africa. There are foci of sickling in Italy, the Middle East and in India. Sickle-cell anaemia has become an important public health problem in a much wider area due to African settlement in the USA, the West Indies, tropical Latin America and, more recently, in Europe.

Haemoglobin C (β6 Glu→Lys) is a West African genetic marker with its highest incidence in Northern Ghana and Upper Volta. As mentioned previously, HbE (β26 Glu→Lys), which has the same electrophoretic charge as HbC, is frequently found in South East Asia including Vietnam and also in South-West China. Haemoglobin D (β121 Glu→Gln) is present in 3% of Punjabis and is a not uncommon finding in the increasingly mixed populations of some countries. This relatively common haemoglobin is of diagnostic

importance as it moves on electrophoresis with HbS and consequently the HbSD mixed heterozygote can easily be mislabelled as a HbS homozygote.

Two other, less frequent, West African haemoglobins are Hb Korle-Bu (β73 Asp→Asn), found predominantly in Ghana, and HbG Philadelphia, found predominantly in Nigeria. HbO Arab (β121 Glu→Lys), first found in Arabs, is in fact at its highest incidence in Macedonia; it occurs occasionally in the Middle East and in the Northern Sudan. Hb Hasharon (α47 Asp→His) at first found occasionally in Ashkenazi Jews is now also seen with some regularity in Italy, particularly the Ferrara region.

Non-Genetic Variation: The Glycosylated Haemoglobins

Haemoglobin can undergo several types of modification subsequent to its synthesis. One example is the minor HbF fraction that results from acetylation of the amino-terminus of some of the circulating γ-chains. Another example is the proteolytic loss from the α-chains of the terminal arginine that takes place when haemoglobin is released into the plasma to give a fast electrophoretic component, but by far the most important of the modified forms are the glycosylated haemoglobins, a series of glucose adducts to haemoglobin. Early studies showed that ion-exchange chromatography of HbA yielded several minor fractions with increased negative charge, the most significant of which were HbA_{1a}, HbA_{1b} and HbA_{1c}, the group being collectively labelled HbA_1. Rahbar[15] in 1968 showed that the amount of these fast components was considerably increased in diabetic subjects and later work showed that the increase was primarily due to an increase in HbA_{1c}. This is produced by the formation of a Schiff base between the aldehyde of glucose and the terminal amino acid of the β-chain to give a ketoamine linkage.[16,17] The level of HbA_{1c} was shown to correlate with the degree of hyperglycaemia to which the haemoglobin has been exposed over its average life of 1–3 months. Thus the HbA_{1c} gives a potential measure of the efficiency of long-term control of diabetes; the normal individual has some 7–8% of haemoglobin in glycosylated form, of which approximately 40% is HbA_{1c}, whereas a diabetic with bouts of hyperglycaemia may have a level of 14% or more. This enables an assessment of overall control of blood-glucose levels as opposed to the intermittent levels available from individual blood-glucose analyses. The potential value of the measurements is enhanced by the demonstration that a similar glycosylation is occurring in other proteins including those of basement membranes and crystallin, the principal protein of the lens. The inference is that protein glycosylation is at least a contributory factor to the long-term degenerative changes associated with poorly controlled diabetes.

Some earlier methods for determination of HbA_{1c} in effect measured 'fast' haemoglobin, a mixture of glycosylated haemoglobin components, but also included other modified forms of haemoglobin that increased on storage and could result in falsely elevated measurements. This situation has improved with the development of a number of techniques that measure glycated haemoglobin or specifically HbA_{1c}, including colorimetric, electrophoretic and chromatographic methods using affinity- or ion-exchange resins. Automated high-performance liquid chromatography (HPLC) using ion-exchange separations is now available, enabling quick and precise determination of HbA_{1c} in clinical laboratories.

The Haemoglobinopathies

Used in its strictest sense, the term 'haemoglobinopathies' covers those variants that result in clinically apparent disease. The identification of their abnormalities enabled the correlation of the molecular defect with the disease process and helped open up the new field of molecular pathology.[18]

Sickle-Cell Disease

This is due to the enhanced tendency of HbS (β6 Glu→Val) to become insoluble in deoxygenated solutions due to the formation of unidirectional crystals.[16] These crystals are apparently formed in a transitory manner by HbA but the replacement of the hydrophilic glutamic acid at position β6 in HbA by the hydrophobic valine in HbS stabilizes the crystals. Crystallization is due to the formation of strands by end-to-end association of haemoglobin molecules, which are then wound around a central core to form tubular fibrils.

The unidirectional haemoglobin crystals form spikes that deform the shape of the red cells and make them unduly rigid. These rigid, sickle-shaped cells are susceptible to haemolysis and have a shortened half-life. They are also liable to form plugs in the microcirculation causing ischaemia and further sickling, with local infarction. Initially the cells are reversibly sickled and, on oxygenation, can revert to their normal shape. However, after several bouts of sickling, the red cell develops membrane damage and becomes an irreversibly sickled cell, giving rise to an increased viscosity even in fully oxygenated blood.

Sickling is primarily a problem that affects homozygotes and it rarely causes difficulties for the AS heterozygote. The severity of the disease may be greatly modified by interaction with other haemoglobins.[16,19] Haemoglobins C and O Arab (β121 Glu→Lys) will copolymerize with HbS. Similarly, the double mutant HbS Oman,[20] containing the O Arab and S mutations on the same β-globin chains, shows enhanced sickling properties. Conversely, Hb Korle-Bu (β73 Asp→Asn) is a protective agent against sickling, either by itself or as the double mutant Hb Harlem (β6 Glu→Val, β73 Asp→Asn). Such mutants, which increase or decrease the sickling tendency of HbS, have helped in identifying some of the interactions involved in the stabilization of the HbS polymer.[16]

Haemoglobin F does not readily take part in filament crystallization and is therefore a powerful anti-sickling agent. Even in homozygous HbS disease, a fetal haemoglobin level above 10% usually ensures a mild clinical course and a value above 20% protects against most symptoms.

The important point for the clinical biochemist is that diagnostically the task is not completed by the identification of the presence of HbS along with a positive sickle-cell test. Is there a coincidental HbD? Is there also β- or α-thalassaemia? Is there another haemoglobin such as O Arab or C Harlem? What is the HbF level? All of these factors are important in the assessment of apparent sickle-cell disease and their significance should be recognized and reported to the clinician.

The Unstable Haemoglobins

Abnormalities that disrupt the shape of the globin molecule will decrease its solubility and cause precipitation of the haemoglobin within the red cell to give particulate inclusions—Heinz bodies. Some 80 of these unstable haemoglobins have been identified,[11,13] almost always as the result of the investigation of the accompanying Heinz-body haemolytic anaemia.[21,22] A similar number of haemoglobins has been described with subclinical degrees of instability.

Most of the unstable haemoglobins have amino acid abnormalities that cause either spatial disruption of the haem pocket or of the α_1–β_1 interface, or produce a major lesion, such as deletion, that grossly distorts globin conformation. The largest proportion is due to substitutions within the haem pocket (Fig. 25.14), where even minor steric alterations will allow entry of anions to give methaemoglobin formation. The associated distortion allows bonding with globin side-chains to give haemichrome formation with irreversible denaturation and precipitation. The other lesions of the unstable haemoglobins will also produce haem-pocket disruption, with the consequent course of events summarized[23] in Fig. 25.15.

The haemolytic anaemias occur in the heterozygous carriers of unstable haemoglobins, the most common and severe forms being due to β-chain abnormalities. These give rise to initial symptoms in early infancy following the disappearance of HbF. Globin instability has two main effects, one in the bone marrow, the other in the circulation. The newly formed, unstable globin is liable to misfold in shape and be eliminated in the red-cell precursors of the bone marrow by proteolysis. With major instability this may cause a gross disturbance of erythropoiesis to give a dyserythropoietic bone-marrow picture. Usually some half of the unstable globin survives to give circulating levels of 10–30% of the total haemoglobin. This circulating, unstable haemoglobin is readily precipitable either by drugs or by the increased temperature that accompanies even minor childhood

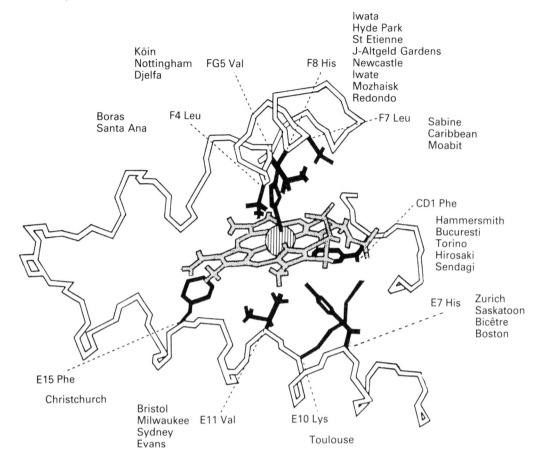

Figure 25.14 The haem group (shaded) with some of the amino acid residues in contact with it in the haem pocket. Substitutions of the nine residues shown account for a third of the unstable haemoglobins, as indicated by the associated names.

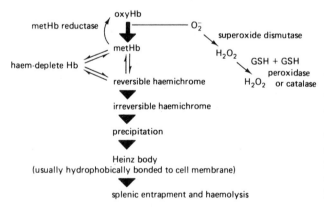

Figure 25.15 Sequence of events leading to precipitation and Heinz-body formation by the unstable haemoglobins.

infections.[24] The result is precipitation of the haemoglobin as Heinz bodies, which are removed by the spleen. This removal, descriptively called pitting (Fig. 25.16), results in loss of cell membrane, distortion of the red cell and haemolysis.

The diagnosis of the unstable haemoglobins is almost entirely dependent on the demonstration of their presence by a positive stability test. The details of these tests are discussed later, but they are simple to do and the important point is that they should be routinely used in the work-up of any suspected haemoglobinopathy or unexplained congenital anaemia. Many of the abnormalities do not cause a readily discernible change in mobility on electrophoresis or chromatography, and the use of stress tests for stability is the only means of demonstrating the presence of an abnormal component and of isolating it for further investigation.

Oxygen-affinity Variants

As discussed, the R–T transformation in haemoglobin primarily involves residues in the α_1–β_2 interface, the haem pocket and the 2,3-diphosphoglycerate-binding site. Mutations at these sites are likely to alter cooperativity,[25] usually to decrease it to give increased oxygen affinity. Increased affinity will result in a lessened release of oxygen at the periphery and the body will respond to

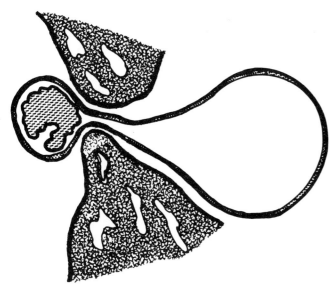

Figure 25.16 Inclusion, or Heinz, bodies are removed from the red cell by the process of pitting, a plucking of the rigid body and associated red-cell membrane as the erythrocyte moves through the interstices of the splenic sinusoids.

this by increasing red-cell production to give an erythraemia that may present as a polycythaemia, but the haematocrit is often within the upper limit of normal. Less frequently, mutations may result in a partial locking of the molecule in the deoxy-, T form, to give decreased affinity and an apparent cyanosis.

The possibility of an abnormal haemoglobin should always be considered in the investigation of polycythaemia or cyanosis, particularly if there is a family history of the condition or if it has been present from an early age. It is not excluded by the absence of any electrophoretic abnormality since, as with the unstable haemoglobins, the mutations may not involve any change in charge, e.g. the high-affinity variant Hb Heathrow (β103 Phe→Leu). Similarly, although it was thought that a normal white-cell count with erythraemia indicated the likelihood of a high-affinity variant, experience has shown that the white-cell count may well be raised.

The lesson is that wherever there is a suspicion of an abnormality of oxygen affinity it should be checked by measurement of the P_{50} of the whole cells along with that of a normal control. A deviation of the P_{50} by more than 3 mmHg from that of the control is of significance and should be checked. This requires measurement of the dissociation curve of haemolysates, both in the presence of 2,3-diphosphoglycerate and when stripped of phosphate.[26,27] The demonstration of a consistent change in oxygen affinity confirms the presence of an abnormal haemoglobin. A stability test should always be done, as lesions gross enough to cause a change in oxygen affinity will also usually produce a decrease in stability. The corollary is also true; the unstable haemoglobins usually have some alteration in oxygen affinity. Clinically the combination of the two effects may be apparent with evidence of haemolysis, owing to the instability, and an unexpectedly high haemoglobin concentration due to increased oxygen affinity.

Over 100 abnormalities producing clinically evident changes of oxygen affinity have been identified.[11,25] The majority have occurred at the α_1–β_2 interface. Examples are the substitutions that occur at position β99, which is normally occupied by an aspartic acid residue that forms a hydrogen bond important in stabilizing the deoxy- conformation. This aspartic acid is replaced in six variants associated with polycythaemia; Hb Yakima (β99 His), Kempsey (β99 Asn), Radcliffe (β99 Ala), Ypsilante (β99 Tyr), Hotel Dieu (Gly) and Chemilly (Val). An increase in affinity also results from the replacement of the penultimate tyrosine (β145), which is responsible for the locking of the tertiary structure in the T form. This occurs with Hb Bethesda (β145 Tyr→His), Rainier (β145 Tyr→Cys), Fort Gordon (Tyr→Asp) and McKees Rock (Tyr→Term). Alteration at a 2,3–diphosphoglycerate-binding site will also give increased affinity as in Hb Rahere (β82 Lys→Thr) or Helsinki (β82 Lys→Met).

Methaemoglobinaemia

The iron of the haem group is maintained in its ferrous state by the protective environment of the globin haem pocket. Fluctuations in the conformation of this pocket will occur from time to time and, even with normal HbA, this is sufficient to allow a daily conversion of some 3% of red-cell haemoglobin to the ferric methaemoglobin. Several reductive mechanisms exist in the red cell, the most important of which is the NADH-linked methaemoglobin reductase. This enzyme is more correctly labelled as cytochrome b_5, which then directly reduces the ferric iron or methaemoglobin.[28]

An increased level of methaemoglobin may result[3] from increased oxidation, as in nitrite-induced methaemoglobinaemia; or from decreased reduction, as in methaemoglobin-reductase deficiency; or from globin abnormalities that result in internal oxidation as in the Hbs M.

It is also useful to remember that the reductive mechanisms are confined to the red cell and consequently haemolysates stored for more than a day or two will contain appreciable levels of methaemoglobin. For this reason, blood samples for haemoglobin investigations should always be transported as red cells and haemolysed just before testing.

The presence of methaemoglobin A can be demonstrated using a lysate divided into two samples. To one is added a few crystals of sodium dithionite. After mixing and a wait of 5 min this sample is used as a blank for a scanned spectrum of the other sample. The appearance of a peak at 632 nm confirms the presence of methaemoglobin and allows its quantitation.

Acquired Methaemoglobinaemia

Methaemoglobin formation can occur as a result of exposure to a number of drugs and chemicals such as aromatic amines. It is interesting that many of the initial studies on the drug-induced methaemoglobinaemias were made in Germany during the 1939–45 war. This was prompted by the occurrence of methaemoglobinaemia in workers in the explosives industry, a serious problem that resulted from the need in Germany to use benzene-based derivatives rather than the toluene-based explosives produced in other countries. Nowadays the biochemist is more likely to see acquired methaemoglobinaemia or resulting from nitrate contamination of water supplies or as a side-effect of therapeutic drugs.[29,30] These are particular problems in the newborn, whose red-cell reductive capacity is not fully developed.

The diagnosis of acquired methaemoglobinaemia can usually be made from the history of exposure along with a demonstration *in vitro* of a normal rate of reduction by the red cells of nitrite-induced methaemoglobin. Red cells are oxidized with nitrite, any excess being removed by further washing. The cells are then incubated in the presence of lactate along with similarly treated cells from two normal controls. In the acquired, as opposed to the congenital methaemoglobinaemia, about 10% of the methaemoglobin will be reduced each hour.

Congenital Methaemoglobinaemia

This arises from a deficiency of the NADH-linked cytochrome b_5 reductase. The result, in the homozygote, is an accumulation of some 10–20% methaemoglobin in the blood. The problem presents in the infant as cyanosis but, unfortunately, methaemoglobinaemia is frequently not thought of until after extensive cardiac investigations, including catheterization, have proved negative.

The enzyme cytochrome b_5 reductase exists in two forms. The full-sized molecule consists of the enzyme portion plus a hydrophobic tail that binds to the microsomal membrane. This form is found in all cells of the body except the red cell, which has no microsomes and consequently its cytochrome b_5 has lost the hydrophobic tail and is soluble in the cytoplasm. A defect that prevents loss of the tail will result in a simple red-cell deficiency, i.e. methaemoglobinaemia, whereas a defect that affects the enzymic portion will affect other cells as well as the red cell. Consequently, some of the congenital methaemoglobinaemias are accompanied by general changes, notably mental retardation.

The presence of a congenital methaemoglobinaemia can be confirmed by the nitrite-reduction test described in the previous section, which differentiates it from an acquired methaemoglobinaemia. Enzymic methaemoglobinaemia can be differentiated from an abnormal HbM by the oral administration of methylene blue (1–3 mg/kg body weight) or ascorbic acid (0.25–0.5 g/day). This will decrease methaemoglobin levels to near normal in individuals with the reductase deficiency since ascorbate gives direct reduction of methaemoglobin A and methylene blue gives reduction utilizing NADPH, thus bypassing the cytochrome b_5 reductase system. There will be no appreciable improvement in patients whose methaemoglobinaemia is due to an abnormal haemoglobin.

The Haemoglobins M

Cyanosis may be due to the presence of an abnormal haemoglobin with a substitution in the haem pocket that allows ligand formation to the ferric iron. This will occur if a negatively charged group can closely approach the haem iron. The replacement of either the proximal or distal histidine by tyrosine allows binding by the hydroxyl of the tyrosine to give a stable ferric haemoglobin as in HbM Saskatoon ($\beta 63$ His→Tyr), HbM Boston ($\alpha 58$ His→Tyr), HbM Hyde Park ($\beta 92$ His→Tyr) and HbM Iwate ($\alpha 87$ His→Tyr). It also occurs with HbM Milwaukee, in which a glutamic acid is substituted for valine $\beta 67$ in a position that allows direct binding of the carboxylic groups to the iron, again converting it to the ferric form.

Cyanosis will be apparent from birth in the case of an α-chain HbM and from about 6 months in the case of a β-chain HbM. The condition is dominant, in that all known cases have been heterozygotes. This may help in its differentiation from a methaemoglobin reductase deficiency which gives rise to cyanosis only in the homozygote. However, caution has to be used with this guideline, as an appreciable proportion of observed cases of HbM, as with unstable haemoglobins and oxygen-affinity variants, have arisen as new mutations and can be absent in both parents. Electrophoresis at pH 6.5–7.0 will identify the Hbs M, which have a different mobility from HbA at this pH. Additional evidence may be provided by the spectrum of a dilute haemolysate, as the Hbs M have characteristically altered spectra, though this may be most evident if a preliminary purification of the abnormal component can be made. The electrophoretic demonstration of HbM can often be facilitated by prior reaction of the haemolysate with potassium ferricyanide, which converts the normal HbA to methaemoglobin.

The Thalassaemias

Pathology and Haematology

The stability of normal haemoglobin is dependent on the presence of an equal number of α- and β-subunits to give stable $\alpha_2\beta_2$ tetramers. The underproduction of one subunit will result in an excess of the other with consequent instability and red-cell pathology. This imbalance in globin-chain production is the basic defect present in the very heterogeneous group of diseases, the thalassaemias.[31] Each type of thalassaemia is named according to the subunit whose synthesis is suppressed and is further classified as to

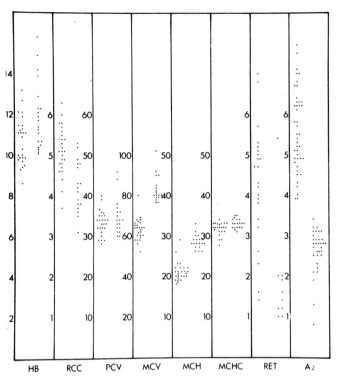

Figure 25.17 Red-cell indices in β-thalassaemia minor (left) and in non-thalassaemic individuals (right) as obtained from one laboratory. The ordinates are as follows: haemoglobin (Hb), g/dL; red-cell count (RCC), ×10^{12}/L; packed-cell volume (PVC), %; mean corpuscular volume (MVC), fL; mean corpuscular haemoglobin (MCH), pg; mean corpuscular haemoglobin concentration (MCHC), g/dL; reticulocyte count (RET), %; haemoglobin A$_2$. (Reproduced, with permission, from Cauchi and Tauro.[32])

whether it is a heterozygous or homozygous suppression. Thus β-thalassaemia is the suppression of β-chain synthesis; β-thalassaemia minor or trait is the heterozygous suppression of one β-allele; β-thalassaemia major is the homozygous suppression of both β-alleles.

There are two factors involved in the pathology of the thalassaemias: the consequences of the presence of an excess of one of the subunits and the effect on the cell of an overall reduction of haemoglobin.

The presence of excess globin subunits, particularly in the homozygous thalassaemias, causes considerable disruption of marrow red-cell synthesis. This is due to precipitation of the excess chains with consequent intramedullary haemolysis and distortion of red-cell morphology. Peripheral haemolysis occurs, partly due to pitting of inclusions by the spleen (Fig 25.16), with this in turn leading to splenomegaly. There is a considerable increase in erythropoiesis, to give marrow overgrowth with bone malformation. The accompanying increased haemolysis combined with intermittent transfusion may lead to iron overload. Assessment of iron stores provides one means

of differentiating the thalassaemia traits from the morphologically similar iron deficiency anaemias: the thalassaemias will characteristically have a normal or raised iron-binding saturation and plasma ferritin concentration.

The underproduction of total haemoglobin in the heterozygous thalassaemias results in a decrease in mean cell volume (MCV < 80 fL) and a decrease in mean cell haemoglobin (MCH < 27 pg). There is usually a compensatory increase in red-cell numbers (RBC > 5 × 10^{12}/L) so that anaemia is not usually a striking feature of thalassaemia minor. In the β-thalassaemias there may be an increase in synthesis of HbF, as γ-chain production attempts to compensate for β-chain suppression. In β-thalassaemia trait the HbF level is usually 0.6–3.0% (normal < 0.8%); in homozygous β-thalassaemia, HbF forms 10–90% of the total haemoglobin. The other compensatory increase is in the level of HbA$_2$ ($\alpha_2\delta_2$). This provides the single most useful laboratory test for β-thalassaemia heterozygotes (Fig. 25.17), who usually have a raised proportion of HbA$_2$ greater than 3.5% (normal < 3.3%).

The pathology of the α-thalassaemias is somewhat different from the β-thalassaemias because whereas free α-chains are highly unstable and predominantly precipitate in the red-cell precursors of the bone marrow, β- and γ-chains are able to form tetramers capable of surviving for some time in the peripheral circulation. These tetramers, β_4 (HbH) and γ_4 (Hb Barts), provide diagnostic evidence of the presence of α-thalassaemia. The tetramers are not efficient oxygen carriers but otherwise they behave like a moderately unstable haemoglobin, halfway in stability between HbE and a grossly unstable variant, e.g. Hb Köln.

The two types of thalassaemia therefore each have a characteristically different pathophysiology. In the β-thalassaemias the main problem is a disruption of bone marrow synthesis due to the early precipitation of the grossly unstable free α-chains. In the α-thalassaemias the pathology is that of a typical unstable haemoglobin with peripheral inclusion-body formation and haemolysis. Of course, in the severe α-thalassaemias, i.e. HbH disease, the primary problem is the gross underproduction of haemoglobin with a consequent failure in oxygen transport.

Molecular Defects

The introduction of the techniques of genomic mapping, DNA amplification and sequencing, have allowed definition of many of the molecular lesions involved in the thalassaemias.[33–35] These have proved to be extraordinarily diverse and it is clear that many independent mutations have become established at a population level, all resulting in decreased expression of globin genes. These deleterious mutations have been preserved because of their balancing protective advantage in malarial areas. Thus multiple thalassaemic lesions must be added to the already

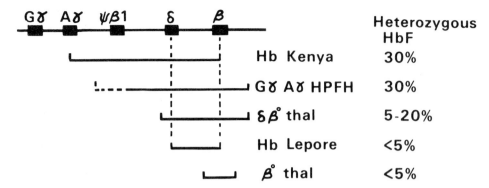

Figure 25.18 A diagrammatic representation of the size of deletions responsible for the thalassaemia-like lesions of the non-α globin. Note that the further the deletion extends toward the γ-genes the greater is the derepression of the HbF synthesis. HPFH, hereditary persistence of fetal haemoglobin. (Adapted from Jackson and Williamson.[33])

diverse range of other genetic red-cell defects that have arisen in malarial regions (*see* below).

The lesions producing thalassaemia are of the three types:

- structural globin variants,
- structural gene deletions,
- mutations of the DNA that controls expression of the structural genes.

The best example of a globin structural variant causing thalassaemia is Hb Constant Spring, the α-chain elongation variant commonly found in South-East Asians. Other examples exist of mutations within the structural gene that result in a non-viable and therefore non-expressed globin.

A few gene deletions have been described in a minority of the β-thalassaemias, whereas gene deletions are the most common cause of α-thalassaemia; the loss of one α-gene being a common finding in Africans and Southern Asians. Deletions may be extensive, affecting not only a single structural gene, but also multiple genes and areas of DNA controlling gene expression, as seen in some of the $(\delta\beta)^0$-, $(\beta)^0$-thalassaemias and heriditary persistence of fetal haemoglobin (HPFH) disorders (Fig. 25.18). This illustrates why a deletion of the δ- and β-genes if limited may result in a δβ-thalassaemia with a poorly compensated increase in HbF. If, however, the deletion extends in the 5′ direction towards the γ-genes, it may remove areas of sequence preventing their expression resulting in full expression of HbF to give a harmless HPFH.

β-Thalassaemia

There is considerable heterogeneity in the β-thalassaemias. Though in some instances there have been deletions of portions of the β-gene, in most instances the gene is intact. The problem in most cases appears to be due to a failure in expression, either transcription or processing of the β-globin mRNA. If this failure is complete, and no β-globin is produced, then there is a β^0-thalassaemia. In some cases there is only a partial reduction in mRNA to give the less

severe β^+-thalassaemia. There have now been more than 90 different mutations identified[34] that result in either β^0- or β^+-thalassaemia.

So far only three deletional forms of β-thalassaemia have been found and only one of these occurs with significant frequency, although it is localized to parts of India and Pakistan.

δβ-Thalassaemia

In δβ-thalassaemia there is a complete lack of HbA and HbA_2. These have been shown to be due to a variety of different deletions, some more extensive than others, removing part of the β-globin gene cluster and resulting in a typical thalassaemic phenotype with hypochromic microcytic red cells.

Hb Lepore

Here there is a deletion of part of the β- and part of the δ-globin genes. The area controlling δ-gene expression is unaffected and the fused δβ globin, Hb Lepore, is consequently expressed and synthesized similarly to δ-globin. The result is a mild thalassaemia.

Hereditary Persistence of Fetal Haemoglobin

This term covers a variety of conditions, all associated with increased HbF production beyond infancy.[36] The level of HbF production in the various HPFH disorders ranges from 2 to 20% in heterozygotes. The distribution of the HbF is also variable. In a few of the HPFH disorders with the higher levels of HbF (10–20%), single-base mutations have been described in the promoter regions of one of the γ-genes, important in the control of its transcription.[37] Other HPFH disorders involve deletions similar to the $(\delta\beta)^0$ thalassaemias but which display normal red-cell morphology.

α-Thalassaemias

The presence of four α-globin genes results in the α-thalassaemias having a graded severity, from the clinically insignificant suppression of one gene to the invariably fatal suppression of four genes. These

α-Genes		Deleted	Name	Clinical	Endemic	Cord Bart's
‖	‖	1 gene	α-thal-2 heterozygote	Minimal effect	Africa Asia	1–2%
✳	‖					
✳	‖	2 cis	α-thal-1 heterozygote	α-thal minor	S-E Asia	1–5%
✳	‖					
‖	‖	2 trans	α-thal-2 homozygote	α-thal minor	Africa Asia	1–5%
✳	✳					
✳	‖	2 cis	mixed	Hb H	S-E Asia	15%
✳	✳	1 trans	α-thal-1 α-thal-2	disease		
✳	✳	4	α-thal-1 homozygote	Hydrops foetalis	S-E Asia	90%
✳	✳					

Figure 25.19 α-Thalassaemia classification according to the number of non-functioning (✳) genes. The crossed genes will usually be due to a deletion but virtually the same phenotypic result would follow if the cross indicated a Constant Spring α-globin gene.

phenotypes and their rather confusing terminology are illustrated in Fig. 25.19. The terminology α^0-and α^+-thalassaemia has been more recently adopted to conform with that of the β-thalassaemias. These terms refer to chromosomes with no (α^0) or reduced (α^+) α-globin production. Thus, α-thal-2 is equivalent to α^+-thalassaemia and α-thal-1 to α^0-thalassaemia. The vast majority of the α-thalassaemias are caused by gene deletions, although to date there have been 14 point mutations defined causing α-thalassaemias.[9,35] As with the β-thalassaemias, these cause mRNA processing and translational defects. The most common non-deletional form of α-thalassaemia, however, is the structural variant Hb Constant Spring. To all practical purposes this last can be equated in effects with a gene deletion and can be substituted as such in Fig. 25.19 in order to determine its clinical effect.

As shown in the figure, each chromosome can have either a single or double α-gene deletion. The single gene deletion by itself causes no clinically evident changes, though an increased (1–2%) amount of Hb Barts (γ_4) is present in cord blood. This mild loss of α-globin production is termed α-thalassaemia-2 trait (α^+-thal). Its combination with a similar (*trans*) deletion on the other chromosome will give a clinically evident, but still mild, α-thalassaemia minor. At the molecular level, there are two main deletions producing α^+-thalassaemia, the $-\alpha^{3.7}$ and $-\alpha^{4.2}$ deletions, which involve the deletion of 3.7 kb and 4.2 kb of DNA, respectively. The $-\alpha^{3.7}$ deletion is the most common and is found in all populations, whereas the $^-\alpha^{4.2}$ deletion is mostly found in Asians, but also in Pacific, Mediterranean and black populations.

The two most common deletions producing α^0-thalassaemia (α-thal-1), $^{--SEA}$ (South-East Asian) and $^{--MED}$ (Mediterranean) are both extensive deletions removing 20 to 30 kb of DNA including both α-loci.

The South-East Asian races therefore can have two genotypically distinct but phenotypically similar forms of α-thalassaemia trait (two-gene deletions, *cis* or *trans*). It also follows that the combination of lesions may lead in these Asian races, but not in the black races, to a three-gene deletion, i.e. HbH disease, or the fatal four-gene deletion, hydrops foetalis.

Diagnostically, the main problem is the recognition of α-thalassaemia minor, or trait, with two-gene deletion. The red-cell indices are those of a typical thalassaemia minor and the diagnosis is often made by exclusion. In blood films incubated with brilliant cresyl blue a careful search will demonstrate the presence of an occasional red cell containing inclusions, the golf-ball like HbH cell. The diagnosis can be confirmed by DNA analysis or prospectively, but less reliably, by examination of cord blood for Hb Barts.

Malaria and Red-cell Abnormalities
An attempt has been made here to show the heterogeneity of the thalassaemias, but these diseases are only a part of an extraordinarily heterogeneous group of genetic defects that have accumulated as protective devices against malaria.[38,39] The clinical biochemist should be aware of the range of red-cell defects involved, as they must all be considered in the differential diagnosis of individuals with suspected haemoglobinopathies; particularly those with family links to the malarial areas of the world. The range of defects is best illustrated by an outline of the common mechanisms by which they all provide a defence against fatal malarial infection.

Part of the malarial parasite's life-cycle occurs within the red cell and, true to its parasitic nature, it utilizes the red cell's metabolism to reduce released oxidants. The parasite produces H_2O_2, which is reduced by NADPH produced by the red cell's hexose monophosphate shunt. A defect of the major enzyme of this shunt, glucose-6-phosphate dehydrogenase (G-6-PD), will result in inadequate reduction with oxidation and elimination of the affected cell.

Even in the presence of fully active red-cell reductive mechanisms the production of oxidants by the malarial parasite is liable to oxidize the red-cell haemoglobin to methaemoglobin. Normally this is a reversible process, but mildly unstable haemoglobins such as HbE, HbF, HbH and Hb Bart's will more readily form insoluble haemichromes to give inclusion-body formation and, again, preferential elimination of infected cells. The sensitivity of HbF to oxidation explains one reason for the protection afforded by the thalassaemias but the main reason for the protection is probably the inherently increased susceptibility of the thalassaemic cell to oxidative haemolysis. Thalassaemic cells are exposed to oxidative damage by superoxide release from isolated haemoglobin subunits and due to the presence of free iron. The additional oxidative load of an intracellular parasite appears *in vitro* to lead to membrane changes that are incompatible with parasite multiplication. *In vivo* there will again be an increased elimination of affected cells.

The range of red-cell defects therefore can be seen as mechanisms that give preferential elimination of cells exposed to the additional oxidative stress of the malarial parasite. The defects include G-6-PD deficiency, HbE, the thalassaemias, the Hbs Lepore, and HPFH. Two factors that could also be included under this heading are the external protective mechanisms of the antimalarial drugs and extreme pyrexia—both of these will similarly give additional oxidative stresses favouring elimination of infected cells.

The other outstanding protective mechanism, HbS, probably, though not certainly, functions through a different mechanism. The maturation of *Plasmodium falciparum* into schizonts takes place in the latter part of the intraerythrocytic stage of parasite development. At this stage the red cell moves into deeper tissues with a lower oxygen tension. Under these circumstances, initial crystallization of HbS occurs, but not sickling. This initial presickling stage is incompatible with parasite survival, possibly because of membrane electrolyte leakage similar to that occurring in the oxidized thalassaemic cell. It is this protective advantage against *P. falciparum* malaria in the HbS heterozygote that has balanced the gross disadvantage to the homozygote of sickle-cell disease.

LABORATORY DIAGNOSIS

Routine Screening

Approach
The possibility of a haemoglobinopathy usually arises from haematological findings and it is desirable that there should be cooperation between the haematologist and biochemist in its further investigation. It is useful to have a preliminary screen established covering both the haematological and biochemical aspects of the investigations. Often the diagnosis seems obvious, sickle-cell disease for example, and it is tempting to haemolyse all the sample and move directly to electrophoretic confirmation of the presence of HbS. However, subsequently the possibility of more subtle complications can often arise, such as HbS/β-thalassaemia or HbS/HPFH, that require studies on fresh whole cells.

To avoid these problems a full screen should be done wherever possible on each sample. This would routinely consist of: haematological studies (red-cell indices, prolonged incubation for inclusion bodies, iron studies); HbA$_2$, HbF, sickling test, stability test and electrophoresis at alkaline pH. This provides a good general screen for the haemoglobinopathies, though other tests may be added such as staining of red cells for HbF, acid gel electrophoresis, globin-chain electrophoresis, isoelectric focusing, G-6-PD screening test, and spectrophotometric scanning for

methaemoglobin or other derivatives. Details of the techniques involved are given in the standard texts in the bibliography.

Specimen Collection
A sample of 5–10 mL of anticoagulated blood is adequate for almost all investigations. Haemoglobin rapidly deteriorates in haemolysates and it is preferable to transport the sample as whole blood. If a few mg of a 99:1 mixture of glucose and chloramphenicol is added this should keep the sample in a condition to survive a week of airmail transport or 2 weeks of storage in the refrigerator. Red-cell indices and morphological examination should be done on a fresh EDTA sample.

Haematology
Accurate red-cell indices are available from automated equipment. Iron studies should be made, as iron deficiency gives a haematological picture similar to that of the thalassaemias minor and concomitant iron deficiency may also distort the findings in other haemoglobinopathies.

A test for red-cell inclusions[26] should be routinely made to help in the diagnosis of α-thalassaemia and the unstable haemoglobin diseases. The inclusions, or Heinz bodies may already be present in the cells and can be seen by staining with methyl violet. However, they are removed by the spleen and in the unsplenectomized patient they are best demonstrated by prolonged incubation of the red cells with a redox dye such as brilliant cresyl blue. The inclusions can vary from the large, round, Heinz body to the multiple punctuate inclusions of the HbH cell.

Tests for Sickle-cell Anaemia
The presence of HbS can be demonstrated by either a microscopic sickling test or a solubility screening test. The latter is the most suitable for the biochemical laboratory, but either should be confirmed by subsequent electrophoresis. The solubility screening test is based on the comparative insolubility of reduced HbS in concentrated phosphate buffer. It is best done[26] with haemolysate or washed cells, since misleading results may be obtained with whole blood; increased γ-globulins can give rise to false positives, and false-negative results may be obtained when there are reduced red cell:plasma ratios, as in severe anaemia.

Haemolysate Preparation
Haemoglobin studies are best made with a carefully prepared 10% (10 g/dL) haemolysate. The red cells are washed to remove plasma proteins and at this stage the buffy coat can be removed for DNA extraction if desired. Red cells are lysed with a detergent or, more usually, hypotonically by addition of water. Cell debris can be removed by vigorous shaking with carbon tetrachloride.

Haemolysates can be stored indefinitely in liquid nitrogen but long-term refrigerated storage is best[40] in the form of carbon monoxyhaemoglobin with addition of cyanide and EDTA.

Measurement of HbA₂

The careful measurement of HbA_2, as a percentage of the total haemoglobin is a key part of the diagnostic screen.[40] It is the single most useful criterion for the diagnosis of β-thalassaemia minor, where it is raised above the normal range (1.8–3.3%), usually being above 3.6%. Normal or low values are obtained with $\delta\beta$-thalassaemia, Hb Lepore and the α-thalassaemias.

The difference between the upper limit of normal and the level diagnostic of β-thalassaemia minor is slight and there are few laboratory tests that require greater precision and accuracy in their performance. Measurement can be made either by cellulose acetate electrophoresis with elution and comparison of the A and A_2 bands, or by column chromatography. The cellulose acetate technique has the advantage that it will detect HbH and also other abnormal haemoglobins that may give false results with the column technique. On the other hand, the column technique is more suitable for handling large numbers of samples. Automated HPLC methods have now been developed for quantitation of HbA_2 using ion-exchange separations and will be particularly suitable for diagnostic laboratories making large numbers of estimations. HPLC procedure with ion-exchange chromatography allow the combination of haemoglobin quantitation with variant detection and will provide a useful initial means of screening samples for the presence of electrophoretic variants. In all cases, standards ought to be utilized to calibrate the accuracy of the measurements.

Measurement of HbF

The presence of a raised HbF level indicates a life-long anaemia and is a characteristic finding in the β- and $\delta\beta$-thalassaemias. It also occurs in the defects of γ-chain switching, i.e. HPFH, and the measurement of HbF levels is a prerequisite for the assessment of the severity of sickle-cell disease.

Measurement of the total fetal haemoglobin is based on the γ-chain lacking an internal cysteine present in the β-chain. This cysteine in the β-globin is ionized at alkaline pH, causing instability and precipitation. The γ-chain, lacking this cysteine, is stable at alkaline pH and is said to be alkali resistant. Haemolysate is added to an alkaline ammonium sulphate solution and, after a fixed period to allow the precipitation of adult haemoglobin, a filtrate is prepared, the concentration of which gives a measure of HbF. The normal adult HbF level is less than 0.8% of the total haemoglobin; a result above 1.5% indicates haematological disease.

The procedures for the estimation most commonly in use[26] are modifications based on the Betke method, which gives precise results in the important decision range of 0.2–4% but can continue to give reliable results up to 10–15%. Radial immunodiffusion is a useful technique for measuring higher levels of HbF but lacks precision in the range of 2% and below.

In disorders leading to increased HbF production it can be useful to determine whether the HbF is distributed heterogeneously or homogeneously throughout the red cells, which can help differentiate between some of the forms of HPFH and $\delta\beta$-thalassaemias. The determination of the distribution[41] is based on the work of Kleihauer, who showed that an acid buffer adjusted to the pK of HbF will wash out all the non-fetal haemoglobin from an alkali-fixed form, allowing staining of the remaining HbF. Alternatively, the HbF may be more sensitively visualized with fluorescence-labelled antiHbF antibody.

Stability Test

As with the measurements of HbA_2 and HbF, a stability test should be routinely done on all samples being assessed for a haemoglobinopathy. Unless this is done, unstable haemoglobin variants may go undetected as there is often no associated change in electrophoretic mobility. Furthermore, the finding of a mild instability is a valuable aid in the detection and identification of other variants, particularly HbE and HbH.

The most commonly performed is the isopropanol test[42] in which fresh haemolysate is incubated at 37° with a 17% isopropanol solution for 30 min. The change in polarity of the solvent provides a denaturation stress that causes precipitation, with obvious flocculation, of unstable variants. An apparent positive result may be given in the presence of HbF levels above 5% (HbF is mildly unstable compared to HbA). For this reason positive results should be checked by the less sensitive 50°C heat-stress test. Methaemoglobin A is also unstable and it is important that any of the stability tests should be made with freshly prepared haemolysate, though the red cells can be stored for up to 10 days in the refrigerator before preparation of the haemolysate.

A positive stability screening test may be further investigated and an index of the degree of instability of a particular haemoglobin given by the measurement of methaemoglobin precipitation curves.[23] The haemolysate is first oxidized to methaemoglobin by reaction with potassium ferricyanide. The methaemoglobin solution is buffered and portions incubated for 10 min over a range of temperatures. The degree of precipitation is determined by recording the turbidity of the solution in a spectrophotometer at 750 nm. The plot of turbidity against temperature gives a precipitation curve that allows a comparison between unstable haemoglobins; the precipitation temperature of a haemoglobin is taken as that where the turbidity reaches 0.2, which for normal HbA is close to 56°C. Some examples of unstable haemoglobins were illustrated in Fig. 25.14.

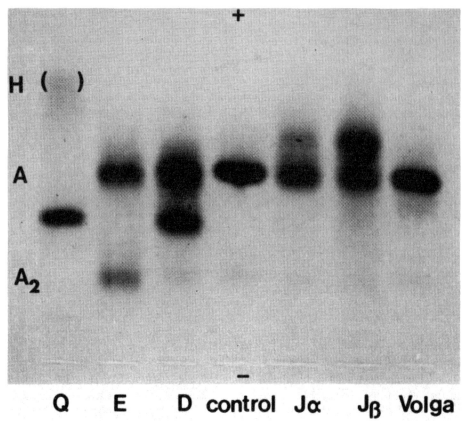

Figure 25.20 Starch gel electrophoresis (pH 8.6) of haemoglobin. Note (1) that HbQ, an α-variant, is linked to α-thalassaemic gene; (ii) HbE in conjunction with α-thalassaemia may mimic a raised HbA_2; (iii) HbD moves in the same position as HbS; (iv) the Jα and Jβ variants show the typical difference in proportions between α- and β-variants; (v) Hb Volga, an unstable variant, shows no change in charge (*see* Fig. 25.21) but there is a noticeable HbF band.

Oxygen Affinity

One of the most important, but difficult, groups of haemoglobinopathies to diagnose is the group of variants with altered oxygen affinity. These are mostly high-affinity variants that are suspected because of a polycythaemia, present from youth, and often with a family history. The identification of the underlying abnormality is usually a time-consuming and expensive task. The first priority is to establish if there really is an inherent change in oxygen affinity. The P_{50}, the oxygen partial pressure at half saturation, should be determined on whole blood and stripped (phosphate-free) haemolysate. The Hill coefficient should be calculated and the effect of added 2,3-diphosphoglycerate to the stripped haemolysate should be assessed. Commercial oxygen-electrode equipment designed for plotting continuous oxygen dissociation curves is available and is useful for screening samples. The approach to screening for changes in oxygen affinity has been summarized elsewhere[27] but in practice it is difficult unequivocally to exclude a change in affinity and if there is a real suspicion of an abnormality the sample should be sent to a reference laboratory for full oxygenation studies.

Electrophoresis

Electrophoresis of freshly haemolysed blood at alkaline pH should be part of the routine haemoglobinopathy screen (Fig. 25.20). Cellulose acetate[43] is now most commonly used, but for a full examination electrophoresis should also be done at acid pH, in citrate agar, and also in dissociating buffers containing 6M-urea to visualize the isolated globin chains (Fig. 25.21). Isoelectric focusing provides an additional approach, though its great selectivity may be confusing to the worker who is not familiar with the mobility of the various derivatives of normal haemoglobin.

Interpretation of Results

The investigation of suspected haemoglobinopathies is seldom routine as there are usually multiple factors to consider. Nevertheless, the scheme[44] outlined in Fig. 25.22 allows the categorization of the majority of the diagnostically confusing thalassaemia traits. It brings together the haematological indices[32] and individual tests outlined in the preceding sections. The diagnosis of the thalassaemias major is usually self-evident on morphological evidence plus altered

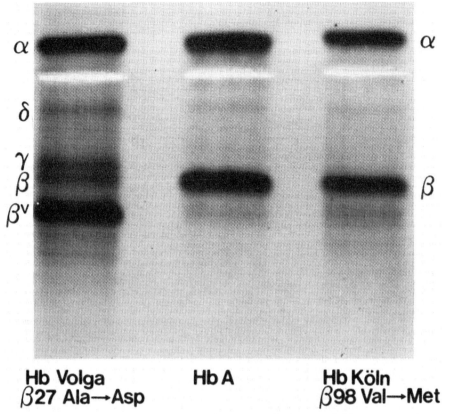

Figure 25.21 Starch gel electrophoresis in 6M-urea of two unstable haemoglobins compared to a control HbA. The true charge change is revealed in the unfolded globin of Hb Volga (*see* Fig. 25.20).

haemoglobin composition, HbH in three-gene α-thalassaemia for example.

It should be remembered that the haematological findings of a thalassaemia trait can also be due to a heterozygous HbE or Hb Lepore. Both should, how-ever, be readily identifiable by electrophoresis: HbE giving a fraction of some 30% of the total haemoglobin in the position of HbA_2, plus a mildly positive isopropanol stability test; Hb Lepore giving a fraction of some 10% of the total that moves in a position

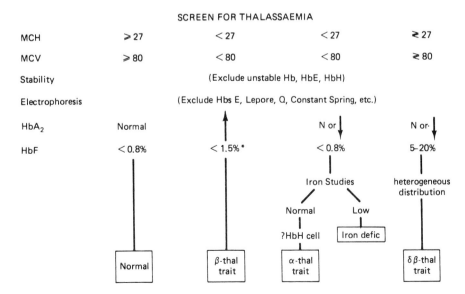

Figure 25.22 A summarized screen to give initial differentiation of the thalassaemia traits. *The level of HbF in *β*-thalassaemia trait is usually normal but 30% are raised level, usually below 1.5% and seldom more than 3%. HbF levels quoted are measured by the Betke technique[41] (normal < 0.8%).

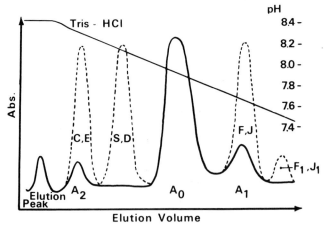

Figure 25.23 DEAE–Sephadex column chromatography of a normal haemolysate using a tris–HCl pH elution gradient. The positions of some common variants are superimposed; note that all will have an 'A₁' artefact as shown in the F_1 or J_1 of the last peak.

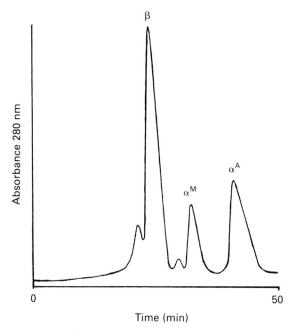

Figure 25.24 Cation-exchange chromatography (Mono-S) of the globin chains from a heterozygote for HbM Boston, showing normal β-chains and the normal and variant α-chains.

between HbA and HbA$_2$ close to that of HbS or HbD. An α-thalassaemia may be indicated by the finding of HbQ (*see* Fig. 25.20) or, more commonly, by Hb Constant Spring, which can be seen on electrophoresis as minor bands running between HbA$_2$ and the origin.

HbS will be readily diagnosable because of the associated sickling but beware of a concomitant HbD; the SD heterozygote will mimic electrophoretically the SS homozygote. HbC, which runs in the same position as HbE, can usually be distinguished from it on the

basis of racial background but an additional differentiation is the stability of HbC to isopropanol stress.

This outline covers the major, clinically associated haemoglobin abnormalities that can be readily handled by the non-specialist in the laboratory. The finding of a grossly positive stability test or of a change in oxygen affinity requires the more detailed investigations available in reference laboratories.

Variant Identification

Isolation of Variants

The standard method of preparative isolation of abnormal haemoglobins is by anion-exchange column chromatography as illustrated in Fig. 25.23. The column is equilibrated and the haemoglobin is applied in alkaline buffer. As the pH is decreased the more positively charged components such as A$_2$, C and E are eluted, followed by Hbs S and D, the main HbA$_0$ peak and then its derivative HbA$_1$ peak along with HbF. It is a useful practice routinely to pool each peak to allow calculation of their relative proportions from the Soret-band absorbance (420 nm).

The high sensitivity of current HPLC peptide mapping, amino acid analysis and sequencing methods can allow identification of mutants from relatively small quantities of protein (several mg), which can be readily isolated using small-scale, fast chromatographic separations on ion-exchange columns.

The isolation of unstable haemoglobins is most readily achieved by isopropanol precipitation, using a scaled-up modification of the diagnostic technique.

Chain Separation and Labelling

The development of the technique for preparative globin chain separation by Clegg, Naughton and Weatherall[45] represented a major advance both in the isolation of abnormal components and in the diagnosis of thalassaemia. Freshly prepared globin is applied to a carboxymethylcellulose column and equilibrated with an alkaline buffer in 8M-urea with added SH-reducing agent. As the pH is lowered to below 7 there is a precisely reproducible elution of the β-chain followed by the α-chain; the presence of a mutant chain being shown by an extra peak whose position is directly related to the magnitude of charge change involved in the mutation. The technique provides preparative yields but can also be used diagnostically[31] to measure synthesis ratios of α- and β-globins. Globin is prepared from reticulocyte-rich preparations that have been incubated with [¹⁴C]-labelled amino acids. Counting of the separated globin peaks allows calculation of the relative $\alpha:\beta$ synthesis rates. In the normal, the ratio is usually close to 1.00 but it is proportionally altered in the α- and β-thalassaemias. Several milligrams of globin, sufficient in most cases for mutant characterization, can be isolated using fast chromatographic procedures based on the above procedure on small columns of cation-exchange materials (Fig. 25.24).

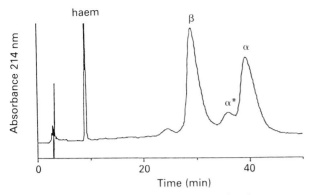

Figure 25.25 Separation of globin chains by reverse-phase HPLC (Vydac C4 column). The normal α- and β-globin chains are indicated as well as the abnormal α^*-chain, which carries the substitution α32 Met→Thr.

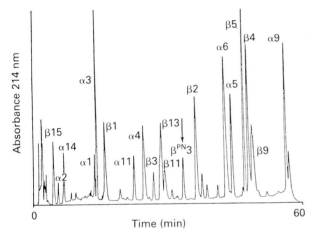

Figure 25.26 A reverse-phase HPLC separation of tryptic peptides from the unstable and high oxygen-affinity variant, Hb Palmerston North. The position of the abnormal peptide is indicated by the arrow.

Reverse-phase HPLC is a useful analytical technique, particularly for the detection of abnormal globin chains[46] carrying electrophoretically neutral mutations, as this provides a separation of globin chains based on their relative hydrophobic properties. Figure 25.25 shows the separation of an abnormal α-globin chain that has a methionine→threonine substitution, silent on all purely charge-based separation procedures. This is a sensitive procedure analytically that requires less than a milligram of protein but may also be used preparatively to isolate globin chains for further characterization.

Peptide Mapping

The identification of the amino acid abnormality in a haemoglobin is made by the process of peptide mapping. The whole globin or isolated globin chain is broken down into a limited number of peptides using a specific enzyme, usually trypsin. Cleavage occurs at lysine residues to give some 15 tryptic peptides from

each globin chain. These peptides can be analysed in one of a number of ways. Most commonly, this is done with (HPLC).[47] This is a high-resolution technique that gives excellent separations of tryptic peptides with high sensitivity and good recovery yields. A separation of the tryptic digest into discrete peptide peaks is achieved (Fig. 25.26), which is dependent on peptide size and amino acid composition (particularly hydrophobicity). The only peptides that should be altered in their retention on the column are therefore those with a change in their amino acid composition.

Previously, two-dimensional peptide mapping (fingerprinting)[48] on paper or thin-layer plates using electrophoresis in one dimension, followed by chromatography in the second dimension, was the standard adopted approach. This can still be a useful technique, its advantage being the ability to use chemical staining for some specific amino acid residues that can allow the ready identification of the substitution involved in many variants. With either of these approaches, peptides may be isolated for subsequent amino acid analysis and sequence determination.

DNA Analysis

The development of the techniques of molecular biology have allowed a comparable approach[33] to the mapping of genomic DNA to that used for the peptide mapping of proteins. A major difference is that the DNA relating to globin synthesis is present in every cell and is capable of amplification; thus globin-gene analysis can be potentially made on cells from limited sources and independent of the chronology of expression. For example, DNA from chorionic villi or amniotic fibroblasts can be utilized to obtain information about the genes for adult, embryonic and fetal globin.

The basis of gene mapping is the availability of specific enzymes, the restriction endonucleases, that give precisely defined cleavage of DNA sequences to yield, from the total DNA, a large, but finite, number of fragments. These DNA fragments can be separated by agarose gel electrophoresis and then transferred by blotting to membranes, hybridized with a radio-labelled globin probe sequence, and an autoradiograph prepared. This will show only the DNA fragments containing the globin genes of interest. This approach is most commonly used to characterize gene deletions such as in α-thalassaemias, by detecting size variations in the DNA fragments generated. For example, digestion of normal DNA with the restriction enzyme *Bam*HI, followed by electrophoretic separation of the fragments and hybridization with an α-globin specific probe, detects a single DNA band 14 kb in size. In the common $-\alpha^{3.7}$ deletion form of α^+-thalassaemia, two fragments are detected; a shorter 10.5-kb fragment arising from the thalassaemic chromosome and the 14-kb fragment from the normal chromosome.

The non-deletional forms of thalassaemia and the abnormal haemoglobins cannot be analysed in this

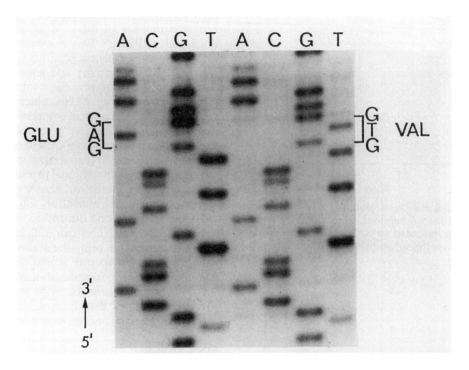

Figure 25.27 DNA sequencing autoradiograph demonstrating the HbS, $\beta6$ Glu→Val, mutation. The left-hand four lanes (A,C,G,T) correspond to the nucleotide sequence of a DNA fragment containing exons 1 and 2 of β-globin from a normal individual and right-hand four lanes from a homozygote for HbS.

way. Because they are mainly single-base mutations, they can only be characterized by sequencing of the globin DNA, although known mutations may be tested for by restriction enzyme digestion of DNA if the mutation itself affects a restriction-enzyme recognition site, or by hybridization with mutant-specific oligonucleotide probes. DNA amplification using the polymerase chain reaction[49] has facilitated the investigation of these mutations. Using specific oligonucleotide primers flanking the relevant DNA sequence, a fragment of DNA can be amplified. This DNA can then be directly sequenced (Fig. 25.27) or digested with a restriction enzyme and the resulting fragments separated according to size on an agarose gel and viewed directly by ethidium bromide staining. Indeed, this approach has been used in the diagnosis of a number of the clinically important haemoglobinopathies including HbS,[50] HbE and β-thalassaemia. Amplification of genomic DNA and sequencing of the amplified product is a useful alternative approach to protein-sequencing techniques for the characterization of unknown mutations.

REFERENCES

1. Barcroft J. (1928). *The Respiratory Function of the Blood*, Cambridge University Press.
2. Lamola A.A., Yamane T. (1974). Zinc protoporphyrin in the erythrocytes of patients with lead intoxication and iron deficiency anaemia. *Science*, **186**, 936.
3. Carrell R.W., Lehmann H. (1979). Abnormal haemoglobins. In *Chemical Diagnosis of Disease* (Brown S.S., Mitchell F.L., Young D.S., eds.) Amsterdam: Elsevier North Holland, pp.879–966.
4. Lehmann H., Casey R. (1982). Human haemoglobin. In *Comprehensive Biochemistry*, **19b Part II** (Neuberger A., van Deenan L.L.M. eds.) Amsterdam: Elsevier, pp.347–417.
5. Perutz M.F. (1978), Hemoglobin structure and respiratory function. *Sci. Am.*, **239**, 66.
6. Perutz M.F. (1987), Molecular anatomy, physiology and pathology of hemoglobin. In *The Molecular Basis of Blood Diseases* (Stamatoyannopoulos *et al.* eds.) Philadelphia: Saunders.
7. Bellingham A.J. (1974). The red cell in adaption to anemic hypoxia. *Clin. Hematol.*, **3**, 577.
8. Wood W.G. (1976). Haemoglobin synthesis during human fetal development. *Br. Med. Bull.*, **32**, 282.
9. Higgs D.R., Vickers M.A., Wilkie A.O.M., Pretorius I.M., Jarman A.P., Weatherall D.J. (1989). A review of the molecular genetics of human α-globin gene cluster. *Blood*, **73**.
10. Flint J. et al. (1986). High frequencies of α-thalassaemia are the result of natural selection by malaria. *Nature*, **321**, 744.
11. International Haemoglobin Information Centre (1991). *Hemoglobin*, **15**, 139.
12. Adams J.G., Coleman M.B. (1990). Structural hemoglobin variants that produce the phenotype of thalassaemia. *Semin. Hematol.*, **27**, 229.
13. Lehmann H., Kynoch P.A.M. (1976). *Human Haemoglobin Variants and Their Characteristics*, Amsterdam: North Holland.

14. Forget B.G. (1977). Nucleotide sequence of human β-globin messenger DNA. *Hemoglobin*, **1**, 879.

15. Rahbar S. (1968). An abnormal hemoglobin in the red cells of diabetics. *Clin. Chim. Acta*, **22**, 296.

16. Bunn H.F., Forget B.G. (1986). *Hemoglobin: Molecular, Genetic and Clinical Aspects*, Philadelphia: Saunders.

17. Bunn H.F. et al. (1979). Structural heterogeneity of human haemoglobin A due to non-enzymatic glycosylation. *J. Biol. Chem.*, **254**, 3892.

18. Perutz M.F., Lehmann H. (1968). Molecular pathology of human haemoglobin. *Nature*, **219**, 902.

19. Milner P.F. (1974), The sickling disorders. *Clin. Hematol.*, **3**, 289.

20. Langdown J.V. et al. (1989). A new doubly substituted sickling haemoglobin: HbS-Oman. *Br. J. Haematol.*, **71**, 443.

21. White J.M., Dacie J.V. (1971), The unstable hemoglobins—molecular and clinical features. *Prog. Hematol.*, **III**, 69.

22. Winterbourn C.C. (1990). Oxidative denaturation in congenital haemolytic anemias: the unstable hemoglobins. *Semin. Hematol.*, **27**, 41.

23. Carrell R.W., Winterbourn C.C. (1981), The unstable haemoglobins. In *Human Haemoglobin and Hemoglobinopathies: a Current Review to 1981* (Schneider R.G., Charache S., Schroeder W. eds.) *Texas Rep. Biol. Med.*, **40**, 431.

24. Winterbourn C.C., Williamson D., Vissers M.C., Carrell R.W. (1981). Unstable haemoglobin haemolytic crises: contribution of pyrexia and neutrophil oxidants. *Br. J. Haematol.*, **49**, 111.

25. Jones R.T., Shih T-B. (1980). Haemoglobin variants with altered oxygen affinity. *Hemoglobin*, **4**, 243.

26. Dacie J.V., Lewis S.M. (1991). In *Practical Haematology*, 7th edn, Edinburgh: Churchill Livingstone.

27. Rosa J. et al. (1975). Testing for hemoglobins with abnormal oxygen affinity curves. In *Abnormal Hemoglobins and Thalassaemia. Diagnostic Aspects* (Schmidt R.M. ed.) New York: Academic Press, pp.79–116.

28. Hultquist D.E., Douglas R.H., Dean R.T. (1975). The methaemoglobin reduction system of erythrocytes. In *Erythrocyte Structure and Function* (Brewer G.J. ed.) New York: Liss, pp.297–300.

29. Stern A. (1989). Drug-induced oxidative denaturation in red blood cells. *Semin. Hematol.*, **26**, 301.

30. Winterbourn C.C. (1985). Free-radical production and oxidative reactions of hemoglobin. *Environ. Health Perspect.*, **64**, 321.

31. Weatherall D.J., Clegg J.B. (1981). *The Thalassaemia Syndromes*, 3rd edn, Oxford: Blackwell.

32. Cauchi M.N., Tauro G. (1979). The quantitation of haemoglobin A₂ and F. Report of the techniques review group to the Thalassaemia Society of Victoria. *Pathology*, **11**, 175.

33. Jackson I.J., Williamson R. (1980). Annotation: mapping of the human globin genes. *Br. J. Haematol.*, **46**, 341.

34. Kazazian H.H. (1990). The thalassaemia syndromes: molecular basis and prenatal diagnosis in 1990. *Semin. Hematol.*, **27**, 209.

35. Liebhaber S.A. (1989). α Thalassaemia. *Hemoglobin*, **13**, 658.

36. Stamatoyannopoulos G., Nienhuis A.W. (1987). Hemoglobin switching. In *The Molecular Basis of Blood Diseases* (Stamatoyannopoulos G. et al. eds.) Philadelphia: Saunders.

37. Ottolenghi S., Mantovani R., Nicolis S., Ronchi A., Giglioni B. (1989). DNA sequences regulating human globin gene transcription in non-deletional hereditary persistence of fetal hemoglobin. *Hemoglobin*, **13**, 523.

38. Etkin N.L., Eaton J.W. (1975). Malaria-induced erythrocyte oxidant sensivity. In *Erythrocyte Structure and Function* (Brewer G.J. ed.) New York: Liss, pp.219–320.

39. Nagel R.L., Roth E.F., Jnr. (1989). Malaria and red cell genetics defects. *Blood*, **74**, 1213.

40. Huntsman R.G., Carrell R.W., White J.M. (1978). Recommendation for selected methods for quantitative estimation of HbA₂ and HbA₂ reference preparation. *Br. J. Haematol.*, **38**, 573.

41. Efremov G.D., Huisman T.H.J. (1974). The laboratory diagnosis of the hemoglobinopathies. *Clin. Hematol.*, **3**, 527.

42. Carrell R.W., Kay R. (1972). A simple method for the detection of unstable hemoglobins. *Br. J. Haematol.*, **23**, 615.

43. Schneider R.G. (1980). Electrophoretic methods in hemoglobin identification. *Hemoglobin*, **4**, 521.

44. Galanello R. et al. (1979). β⁰ thalassaemia trait in Sardinia. *Hemoglobin*, **3**, 33.

45. Clegg J.B., Naughton M.A., Weatherall D.I. (1966), Abnormal human haemoglobin. Separation and characterization of the α and β chains by chromatography. *J. Mol. Biol.*, **19**, 91.

46. Schroeder W.A. (1986). HPLC of globin chains and of peptides in the identification of hemoglobin variants. In *Methods in Hematology 15: The Hemoglobinopathies* (Huisman T.H.J. ed.) New York: Churchill Livingstone.

47. Shimizu K., Wilson J.B., Huisman T.H.J. (1980). The distribution of the percentages of G and A chains in human hemoglobin by HPLC. *Hemoglobin*, **4**, 487.

48. Lehmann H., Huntsman R.G. (1974). *Man's Haemoglobin*, 2nd edn, Amsterdam: North Holland, pp.431–451.

49. Saiki R.K. et al. (1988). Primer-directed enzymatic amplification of DNA with a thermostable DNA polymerase. *Science*, **239**, 487.

50. Saiki R. et al. (1985). Enzymatic amplification of β-globin genomic sequences and restriction site analysis for diagnosis of sickle-cell anaemia. *Science*, **230**, 1350.

51. Grosveld F., Dillon N., Higgs D. (1993) The regulation of human gene expression. In *Clinical Haematology— International Practice and Research. The Haemoglobinopathies*. London: Ballière Tindall, pp. 31–55.

FURTHER READING

Bunn H.F., Forget B.G. (1986). *Hemoglobin: Molecular, Genetic and Clinical Aspects*, Philadelphia: Saunders.

Higgs D.R., Weatherall D.J. (1993) *Clinical Haematology— International Practice and Research. The Haemoglobinopathies*. London: Ballière Tindall.

Huisman T.H.J. (1986). *Methods in Hematology. The Hemoglobinopathies*, New York: Churchill Livingstone.

Lehmann H., Huntsman R.G. (1974). *Man's Haemoglobins*, Amsterdam: North Holland.

Schneider R.G., Charache S., Schroeder W. (1981). Human hemoglobin and hemoglobinopathies: a current review to 1981. *Texas Rep. Biol. Med.*, **40**.

Weatherall D.J., Clegg J.B. (1981). *The Thalassaemia Syndromes*, 3rd edn, Oxford: Blackwell Scientific.

26. Disorders of Iron Metabolism

M. Worwood

Introduction
Proteins of iron metabolism
  Transferrin
  Ferritin and haemosiderin
Iron turnover within the body
Diagnosis of iron deficiency and iron overload
  Serum iron, total iron-binding capacity and
    percentage saturation
  Erythrocyte protoporphyrin
  Serum ferritin
Iron-deficiency anaemia
Haemochromatosis
  Idiopathic haemochromatosis
  Secondary iron overload

INTRODUCTION

Respiration in mammals depends on iron both for the carriage of oxygen by haemoglobin in the red cells of the blood and in the use of oxygen in the tissues. Despite its essential nature and high abundance in the earth's crust, its bioavailability is poor.

Iron is a transition metal and therefore has the ability both to exist in several oxidation states and to form stable complexes. It is these properties that have made the transition elements important components of electron- and oxygen-carrying proteins. The most common valency states for iron are Fe^{2+} and Fe^{3+}. In acid solution these ions exist as the free ion surrounded by six molecules of water, but neutralization of such solutions results in progressive hydrolysis with eventual precipitation of ferric hydroxide. If the water molecules are replaced by appropriate ligands a stable complex can be formed, which is soluble at neutral pH. Both Fe^{2+} and Fe^{3+} generally form octahedral complexes in which the central metal ion is surrounded by six ligands. The biological chemistry of iron is the chemistry of these complexes. Although many sugars, amino acids and nucleotides will form complexes with iron, almost all the iron in the body is found in very specific protein complexes.

The body of a normal, well-fed man contains about 4 g of iron, most of which is found in haemoglobin, the oxygen-carrying protein of the red blood cell (Table 26.1). About 10% of body iron is found in myoglobin in muscle, but the many iron-containing proteins or enzymes,[1] such as the cytochromes and iron–sulphur proteins, which take part in redox reactions throughout the body, account for only a small percentage of total iron. Another small fraction is transferrin-bound iron in plasma and extravascular fluids.

The remaining iron is the so-called storage iron, which represents the balance between intake and loss. Men may have up to 2 g of storage iron, although about 1 g is usual, but women of child-bearing age may have little or none. Continual net loss of iron leads to exhaustion of iron stores and then to iron-deficiency anaemia.

Iron-deficiency anaemia is widespread in the poorer countries of the world, especially in women, whose iron losses are greater than those of men due to menstruation and childbirth. In the developed world, iron-deficiency anaemia in men is usually the result of pathological blood loss. Iron overload is comparatively rare but is found in patients with idiopathic haemochromatosis, who have a genetically determined abnormality of iron absorption, and in patients with refractory anaemia, who require regular blood transfusions in order to remain alive (500 mL of blood contains about 250 mg of iron). In either case, the body's limited ability to excrete iron causes a gradual accumulation of storage iron that eventually leads to tissue damage.

TABLE 26.1
DISTRIBUTION OF IRON IN THE BODY (70-KG MAN)

Protein	Location	Iron content (mg)
Haemoglobin	Red blood cells	2600
Myoglobin	Muscle	400
Cytochromes, other haem-containing enzymes, and iron–sulphur proteins	All tissues	50
Transferrin	Plasma and extravascular fluid	5
Storage iron (ferritin and haemosiderin)	Largely in liver, spleen, and bone marrow	Up to 1000

PROTEINS OF IRON METABOLISM

Transferrin

The iron-binding protein of the plasma is transferrin, which is very similar to lactoferrin found in granulocytes and milk (for a recent review, *see* de Jong et al.[2]). Both are monomeric glycoproteins of about 80 kDa. The polypeptide chain of transferrin has 679 amino acids organized in two homologous domains. The protein contains about 6% carbohydrate on two identical and nearly symmetrical branched heterosaccharide chains, both of which are in the C-terminal domain. Each domain has a single iron-binding site that requires both Fe^{3+} and an anion (usually carbonate or bicarbonate). The affinity of transferrin for iron is very high; at pH 7.4 in the presence of bicarbonate, the affinity constant for the binding of one iron atom is approximately 10^{20}/mol.

The plasma concentration of transferrin is normally about 2.4 g/L and each milligram of transferrin can bind 1.4 μg of iron. The protein is normally 20–40% saturated with iron. Iron is released from transferrin on acidification, but delivery of transferrin iron to cells (particularly to immature red cells for haemoglobin synthesis) takes place by interaction with specific receptors,[3] followed by removal of iron and release of apotransferrin within the cell. The transferrin receptor is a transmembrane glycoprotein consisting of two identical subunits of 95 kDa joined by a disulphide bond.[4] The genes for both transferrin and its receptor[5] are found on the long arm of chromosome 3. Although there are structural differences between the two iron-binding sites of the transferrin molecule, there do not appear to be significant differences in the way in which each site delivers iron to the red cell.[3]

Ferritin and Haemosiderin

Iron is stored in cells as ferritin and haemosiderin. Ferritin is a soluble, spherical protein enclosing a core of iron. Ferritin is found in all cells and in low concentrations in plasma and urine.[6] Particularly high concentrations are present in the liver, spleen, and bone marrow. Human apoferritin (approx. 480 kDa) is composed of 24 subunits (each of about 20 kDa). The subunits are roughly cylindrical in shape and form a nearly spherical shell that encloses a central core containing up to 4500 atoms of iron in the form of ferric hydroxyphosphate.

The amino acid sequences of human spleen and liver ferritin are known and X-ray crystallographic analysis at 2.8 Å resolution has demonstrated the arrangement of the subunits within the molecule, as well as channels between the subunits through which iron enter and leave (for a review, *see* Theil[7]).

Human ferritins are made up of two types of subunit in varying proportions. In liver and spleen ferritin, the 'L' subunit predominates and has an apparent molecular mass of 19 kDa on denaturing polyacrylamide gel in electrophoresis. In the more acidic isoferritins found in the heart, in red cells, and elsewhere, the 'H' subunit predominates, with an apparent molecular mass of about 21 kDa. The H subunit has a molecular mass slightly greater than that of the L subunit (182 instead of 174 amino acids). DNA sequencing has demonstrated about 55% homology between the two subunit sequences. The gene for the L subunit is located on chromosome 19q13.3–q13.4 and the gene for the H subunit is found on chromosome 11q13.[8]

In vitro, ferritin can be shown to have all the qualifications required of an iron-storage protein. Apoferritin will bind and oxidize Fe^{2+} and deposit Fe^{3+} within the protein. Release of iron may be effected by reducing agents. Studies in both animals and cultured cells show that apoferritin is synthesized in response to iron administration. This control is largely exercised at the level of translation.[8] The 5'-untranslated region of the ferritin mRNA contains a 28-base sequence that forms a 'stem-loop' structure. This has been termed an 'iron response element' (IRE). A cytoplasmic protein that binds to this sequence and prevents translation has also been identified. In the presence of iron, this protein is unable to bind to the mRNA, polysomes form and translation proceeds. A related mechanism operates in reverse for the transferrin receptor. Here there are stem-loop sequences in the 3'-untranslated region and protein binding prevents degradation of mRNA. Hence iron deficiency enhances transferrin-receptor synthesis.

Haemosiderin is a degraded form of ferritin in which the protein shells have partly disintegrated, allowing the iron cores to aggregate. It is usually found in lysosomes and may be seen under the light microscope after tissue sections have been stained with potassium ferroxyanide in the presence of hydrochloric acid (Prussian blue or Perls' reaction). Normally most of the storage iron is present in ferritin, but with increasing iron accumulation, the proportion present as haemosiderin increases.

IRON TURNOVER WITHIN THE BODY

Quantitatively, iron metabolism is largely the synthesis and breakdown of haemoglobin (Fig. 26.1). The exchange of iron between cells and tissues through the plasma and extravascular fluids is carried out by transferrin. The plasma iron pool (transferrin-bound iron) is about 4 mg, although the daily turnover is over 30 mg. Transferrin circulates through interstitial spaces in liver, spleen and bone marrow and more slowly in muscle and skin; it returns to the blood via the lymphatics. Most of the iron leaving the plasma is taken up by erythroblasts in the bone marrow for incorporation into haem. Some of the immature red cells are destroyed by phagocytic cells in the marrow ('ineffective erythropoiesis') but most of the iron re-

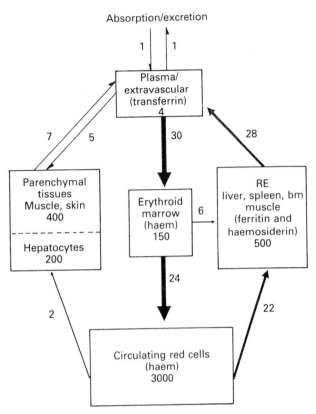

Absorption/excretion

Figure 26.1 Major pathways of iron metabolism. Figures within boxes give the approximate size of the compartments with the form of iron in brackets. The amounts of iron exchanging between the different compartments are given in mg/day. RE, reticuloendothelial cells; bm, bone marrow. (Data taken from [10].)

T ABLE 26.2

ESTIMATION OF STORAGE IRON LEVELS

Direct
Phlebotomy
Measurement of tissue iron concentration[31]
Dual-energy computed tomography[a]
Magnetic susceptibility[a]
Magnetic resonance imaging[a]

Indirect
Serum iron/total iron-binding capacity
Serum ferritin
Erythrocyte protophorphyrin
Urinary iron excretion after administration of chelating agents

Therapeutic
Response to iron administration

[a]These 'non-invasive' methods are at present only applicable to the detection of iron overloads.[32]

enters the blood as haemoglobin in the erythrocytes. These are eventually destroyed in the reticuloendothelial system, where iron is released from haem by

haem oxygenase[9] and is returned to the plasma. This cycle of iron metabolism may be investigated with radioactive iron.[10] In addition there is exchange of iron between all other cells and tissues and the plasma but the amounts involved are small.

Iron losses are limited and there is no physiological mechanism for increasing the rate of loss when there is excess iron. The major site of loss in men is the gastrointestinal tract, with blood loss, biliary excretion and loss of exfoliated epithelial cells giving a total of about 1 mg/day. Less than 100 μg Fe daily is lost in the urine. In women, blood losses in menstruation increase the average daily iron loss to 2–3 mg, and pregnancy causes an overall net loss of about 500 mg Fe.[10]

The iron content of the body is normally regulated closely by variation in the amount of iron absorbed.[11] Iron is absorbed primarily in the duodenum and upper jejunum. The amount absorbed depends both on the availability of the iron in the diet for absorption and on the iron requirements of the body. In general, iron in meat and fish is well absorbed (availability of in excess of 10%), whereas iron in vegetables is much less available (below 1%). The relation between iron retention and body iron stores is well established but the way in which this control is exercised remains unknown.

DIAGNOSIS OF IRON DEFICIENCY AND IRON OVERLOAD

There are three types of disorder of iron metabolism:

- deficiency
- overload
- maldistribution within the body.

To identify such disorders it is necessary to measure haemoglobin concentration (as an indication of total haemoglobin iron) and the level of storage iron. Sometimes further investigations into iron loss or into flow rates within the body are also required.

The methods that may be used to estimate the level of iron stores are summarized in Table 26.2. Only the blood assays are of general application in the hospital laboratory, and these will be considered here.

Serum Iron, Total Iron-binding Capacity and Percentage Saturation

The principles and practice of measuring the amount of iron bound to circulating transferrin are well established.[12] Iron is released from transferrin by acidification, reduced to the ferrous form, and detected by adding a chromagen, which forms an intensely coloured complex. Many automated laboratory analysers include serum iron determination and there is a standard method recommended by the ICSH (Expert Panel on Iron).[13]

Measurement of the serum iron concentration provides little useful clinical information because of the considerable variation from hour to hour and day to day in normal individuals.[14] Transferrin iron is only 0.1% of the total body iron, and the transferrin iron pool turns over 10–20 times each day. Changes in supply and demand due to infection, inflammation, or surgery therefore cause rapid changes in serum iron concentration. The serum iron concentration is normally within the range of 10–35 μmol/L. Concentrations below the normal range are found in patients with iron-deficiency anaemia, and those above the normal range are found in some patients with iron overload. Many hospital patients have a low serum iron concentration, however, which is a response to inflammation, infection, surgery, or chronic disease. Low serum iron concentrations do not necessarily indicate an absence of storage iron.

More information may be obtained by measuring both the serum iron concentration and the total iron-binding capacity (TIBC), from which the percentage of transferrin saturation with iron may be calculated.[12] The TIBC is a measurement of transferrin concentration; often this is measured directly by immunological techniques. A transferrin saturation of 16% is usually considered to indicate an inadequate iron supply for erythropoiesis. Low transferrin saturation, however, is also noted in inflammation, infection, etc., as mentioned above. Of more significance is a raised TIBC (greater than 70 μmol/L or 390 μg/dL), which is a characteristic of a deficiency of storage iron. High transferrin saturations (60%) are found in cases of iron overload, hypoplastic anaemia, haemolytic anaemia, and acute leukaemia.

These measurements of serum iron, which for many years formed the basis of much clinical investigation of iron metabolism, are now seen to provide an inadequate index of storage iron and have been to a large extent replaced by the assay of serum ferritin. In screening for idiopathic haemochromatosis, however, it is essential to measure both the serum iron concentration and the TIBC (or transferrin concentration) and to calculate the percentage of saturation (*see* below).

Erythrocyte Protoporphyrin

This assay has been used for some years as a screening test for lead poisoning. More recently, there has been considerable interest in its use in evaluating iron supply to the bone marrow. The protoporphyrin concentration of red blood cells increases in iron deficiency. A widely used technique directly measures the fluorescence of zinc protoporphyrin (μmol/mol haem) in an instrument called a haematofluorometer.[15] The small sample size (about 20 μL of venous or skin-puncture blood), simplicity, rapidity, and reproducibility within a laboratory are advantages. Furthermore, the test has an interesting retrospective application. Because it takes some weeks for a significant proportion of the circulating red blood cells to

be replaced with new cells, it is possible to make a diagnosis of iron-deficiency anaemia some time after iron therapy has commenced. Chronic diseases that reduce serum iron concentration, but do not reduce iron stores, also increase protoporphyrin levels.

The measurement of erythrocyte protoporphyrin levels as an indicator of iron deficiency has particular advantages in paediatric haematology and in large-scale surveys in which the small sample size and simplicity of the test are important. The normal range in adults is less than 80 μmol/mol haem. In the general clinical laboratory, however, it provides less information about iron storage levels in anaemic patients than the serum ferritin assay and provides no help in the diagnosis of iron overload.

Serum Ferritin

The small amounts of ferritin that circulate in the plasma may be measured by immunoassay.[6] In most normal adults, serum ferritin concentrations lie within the range of 15–300 μg/L. Mean concentrations are lower in children than adults, and from puberty to middle age mean concentrations are higher in men than in women. In older men and women, mean concentrations are similar. Good correlations have been found between serum ferritin concentrations and storage iron mobilized by phlebotomy, stainable iron in the bone marrow, and the concentration of both non-haem iron and ferritin in the bone marrow. This suggests a close relation between the total amount of storage iron and serum ferritin concentration in normal individuals. Serum ferritin concentrations are relatively stable in healthy persons.[14] In patients with iron-deficiency anaemia, serum ferritin concentrations are less than 15 μg/L, and, as far as is known, a reduction in the level of reticuloendothelial stores is the only cause of a low serum ferritin concentration. This is the key to the use of the serum ferritin assay in clinical practice.[6]

In infection, inflammation and chronic disease in which iron is transferred from haemoglobin to the reticuloendothelial stores, the increased level of storage iron is reflected in the serum ferritin concentration (compare this response to that of serum iron). The serum ferritin concentration can be used in these circumstances to assess the adequacy of the iron stores. If a normal haemoglobin concentration is to be regained once the underlying cause of the disease has been removed, sufficient iron will have to be available to synthesize the haemoglobin required. The lower the haemoglobin the higher the serum ferritin concentration should be. Thus, a patient with rheumatoid arthritis and a haemoglobin concentration of 11 g/dL should have a serum ferritin concentration of more than 70 μg/L.

Unfortunately, interpretation of serum ferritin concentrations in patients with chronic disease is not quite as straightforward as this. Some patients with an absence of storage iron in bone marrow may have serum ferritin concentrations of up to 100 μg/L. The reason may lie in the unreliability of the assessment of stainable iron in the bone marrow or in the direct response of ferritin protein synthesis to infection or inflammation ('the acute-phase response'). Mean serum ferritin concentrations, therefore, are somewhat higher in patients with inflammation than in those with similar levels of stainable iron in the bone marrow but without inflammation. Nevertheless, a useful rule may be stated: in patients with anaemia secondary to acute or chronic disease, a serum ferritin concentration less than 100 μg/L indicates that the level of storage iron is probably inadequate for haemoglobin regeneration.

Iron overload causes high concentrations of serum ferritin, but so may liver disease and some forms of cancer. High concentrations of serum ferritin can only be ascribed to iron overload after careful consideration of the clinical situation; a normal serum ferritin concentration, however, provides good evidence against iron overload. Serum ferritin concentrations are always high in patients with advanced idiopathic haemochromatosis, but the serum ferritin assay alone should not be used for screening for the disorder (*see* below).

IRON-DEFICIENCY ANAEMIA

A diagnosis of iron-deficiency anaemia can usually be made after consideration of the clinical picture and the full blood count, or after examination of the blood film. To establish the diagnosis may require the assay of serum ferritin and final confirmation is provided by a response to oral iron therapy. This topic is covered in Chapter 27, but the non-haematological consequences of iron deficiency should also be remembered.[16] Iron-deficiency anaemia has been shown to be associated with a reduction in work output but there is also evidence that iron deficiency in the absence of anaemia (i.e absent iron stores) also reduces work output. Iron deficiency has complex effects on immunity—low levels of plasma iron deny iron to the invading micro-organism but may also reduce the efficiency of the immune response. Finally, iron deficiency, even in the absence of anaemia, may be associated with lower score in tests of development, learning and scholastic achievement (recent studies have been reported and analysed by Haas and Fairchild[17]).

All these topics are still under debate but the answers are important and are necessary for deciding on issues such as the advisability of routine supplementation with iron during pregnancy,[18,19] and of the benefits and dangers of fortification of foodstuffs.

One further development of the concept of iron deficiency is 'functional iron deficiency'. Recombinant human erythropoietin is now commonly used to treat anaemia in patients with renal failure undergoing dialysis. MacDougall et al.[20] have shown that some patients (with apparently adequate levels of storage iron) show a poor response unless they are given intravenous iron. It seems that, despite serum ferritin concentrations in the normal range and stainable iron in the bone marrow, these patients are unable to supply iron at a sufficient rate to regenerate haemoglobin rapidly. Usually this is associated with a transferrin saturation of less than 20%.

HAEMOCHROMATOSIS

There are both primary and secondary forms of iron overload. The primary form is idiopathic (familial, hereditary) haemochromatosis. Secondary iron overload is most commonly encountered in patients with thalassaemia or other refractory anaemia who require regular blood transfusions.[21]

Idiopathic Haemochromatosis
Inheritance
In 1935, Sheldon[22] reviewed more than 300 published cases and suggested that the disease was inherited. Simon and colleagues[23] subsequently reported an association between the HLA isoantigens A3, B7, and B14 and haemochromatosis, confirming the inherited nature of the disease. These studies led to the finding that the disease was determined by a locus closely linked to the HLA loci with a recessive transmission.[24]

Haemochromatosis was thought to be rare, with an incidence of about 1 in 10 000. Some autopsy studies have revealed an incidence of 1–2/1000, however. Recent population studies, with the assumption of an autosomal recessive inheritance, have indicated that the gene frequency is as high as 1 in 20 to 1 in 10 in populations of European origin (*see*, for example, Leggett et al.[25]). The high frequency of the haemochromatosis allele in some populations means that homozygote/heterozygote matings are to be expected, thereby causing the disease to appear in successive generations—a characteristic of dominant inheritance.

Clinical Features of Advanced Disease[26]
Hepatomegaly and skin pigmentation are almost always found. The pigmentation is due to increased amounts of melanin and iron. Diabetes develops in about 60% of patients, and hypogonadism is common. Arthropathy is now frequently recognized. Relatively few patients present with heart disease. Iron is deposited most heavily in the liver and pancreas but also accumulates in the pituitary, adrenal, thyroid and parathyroid glands. The iron is present primarily as haemosiderin rather than ferritin and at tissue concentrations of up to 100 times normal. Relatively little iron is deposited in the reticuloendothelial system, and the grade of stainable iron in the bone marrow may be within the normal range

TABLE 26.3
DIAGNOSIS OF HEREDITARY HAEMOCHROMATOSIS

Indicators of iron status (*normal ranges*)	
Serum iron	10–35 μmol/L
Transferrin saturation	16–60%
Serum ferritin	15–300 μg/L (men)
	15–200 μg/L (women)
Urinary iron	0.5–2.0 mg/24 h
Parenchymal cell iron (grade 0–4)	0–1
Hepatic iron concentration	up to 1.0 mg/g wet wt.
Mobilizable iron (iron removed by phlebotomy)	0–1.5 g

despite a total body iron content considerably in excess of normal.

Diagnosis

In advanced disease all indicators of iron storage levels will be abnormal (Table 26.3). It is generally agreed, however, that the earliest indication of iron overload may be obtained by measuring the transferrin saturation. Those who have not yet accumulated much iron and have serum ferritin concentrations within the normal range may have elevated transferrin saturations. It should be noted that, because of their greater iron losses, women tend to develop iron overload later in life than men (often not until after the menopause).

The measurement of transferrin saturation should be repeated to ensure that it is consistently elevated. The finding of elevated transferrin saturation, elevated serum ferritin concentration, and some of the clinical features of the disease may be sufficient for a diagnosis. Some physicians, however, regard a liver biopsy as essential. This makes possible the histochemical estimation of liver iron concentration, chemical estimation of liver iron concentration, and a direct assessment of liver damage. Heterozygotes do not develop massive iron overload or the physical signs of the disease, but in about 25% of heterozygotes either raised transferrin saturation or raised serum ferritin concentration may be observed.

Detection of homozygotes makes it possible to prevent iron accumulation and tissue damage. For this reason, family members should be examined once haemochromatosis is diagnosed. HLA typing should be done in order to identify those carrying two, one, or no genes for haemochromatosis.[26] Measurements of transferrin saturation and serum ferritin concentration are made to identify individuals with iron overload so that treatment may be instituted. Although measurement of transferrin saturation and serum ferritin concentration will always identify a patient with a major iron overload, the early stages of iron accumulation may be missed in some family members if HLA typing is not performed.

Treatment

The most effective treatment is phlebotomy. Up to 1 L of blood (500 mg of iron) may be removed each week, although 500 mL is usual. The blood iron and haemoglobin concentrations remain steady during phlebotomy, but the ferritin concentration falls. When the ferritin concentration falls below 15 μg/L and the haemoglobin concentration is less than 12 g/dL, it may be assumed that the iron stores are exhausted. Occasional additional phlebotomy is required to maintain iron stores within the normal range. Chelation therapy is expensive and less effective than bleeding.

The Molecular Lesion

Iron accumulates because there is excessive iron absorption across the small intestine with no compensatory increase in iron excretion. From the amount of iron accumulated, it can be calculated that there is a net iron retention of 1–3 mg/day. The abnormality at the molecular level remains a mystery.[26] Recent genetic studies indicate that the genes for transferrin and its receptor are on chromosome 3 and that ferritin H and L subunit genes are found on chromosomes 11 and 19, respectively. This seems to rule out mutations in these proteins as the primary cause of haemochromatosis.

Association of Idiopathic Haemochromatosis with Other Disorders[26]

Iron may accumulate in some patients with thalassaemia or hereditary spherocytosis even in the absence of transfusions. It has been assumed that anaemia itself, or increased plasma iron turnover, somehow increases the amount of iron absorbed. There is now evidence, however, that some patients with major iron overload may have inherited at least one gene for idiopathic haemochromatosis. This has been described in thalassaemia minor, hereditary spherocytosis, and idiopathic refractory sideroblastic anaemia.

Secondary Iron Overload

Patients with aplastic anaemia and homozygous β-thalassaemia (as well as other refractory anaemias) may require 10–50 units (500 mL) of blood per year. As 500 mL of whole blood contains about 250 mg Fe and excess iron is not excreted, iron overload develops rapidly.[21]

In addition to any transfusional iron load, patients with a marked expansion of the erythroid marrow (β-thalassaemia, congenital dyserythropoietic anaemia, and sideroblastic anaemia) also demonstrate enhanced absorption of dietary iron, which either causes, or contributes to, iron overload. There is increasing evidence that patients with β-thalassaemia minor, hereditary spherocytosis and sideroblastic anaemia who are also heterozygous for the haemochromatosis gene may also develop iron overload.[26]

Treatment

It is sometimes possible to use phlebotomy to reduce the iron overload, particularly in cases of sideroblastic anaemia when the degree of anaemia is not great but the usual form of treatment is chelation by parenteral desferrioxamine.[21]

In homozygous β-thalassaemia, desferrioxamine is usually given subcutaneously at 40–50 mg/kg over a 12-h infusion on 5 or 6 nights a week from the age of about 3 years. Automatic electric infusion pumps are available for this. Modest doses of vitamin C are usually given to enhance chelation, although there has been concern about toxicity.

There are problems caused by toxicity of desferrioxamine, particularly visual abnormalities and hearing loss.[27] Most symptoms occur in patients receiving high doses of desferrioxamine but with normal or only slightly raised iron stores and are reversible if detected early. The difficulty in ensuring compliance with the treatment regimen and the very high cost of chelation with desferrioxamine are major drawbacks. There has therefore been considerable interest in the last 10 years in developing effective and safe oral chelators.[28,29] Most experience has so far been obtained with the 1,2 dimethyl derivative of 3-hydroxypyrid-4-one (L_1) but there have been reports of toxicity and further commercial development of the drug has been suspended.[30,31].

REFERENCES

1. Worwood M. (1977). The clinical biochemistry of iron. *Semin. Hematol.*, **14**, 3.
2. de Jong G., van Dijk J.P., van Eijk H.G. (1990). The biology of transferrin. *Clin. Chim. Acta*, **190**, 1.
3. Huebers H.A., Finch C.A. (1987). The physiology of transferrin and transferrin receptors. *Physiol. Res.*, **67**, 520.
4. Trowbridge I.S., Shackelford D.A. (1986). Structure and function of transferrin receptors and their relationship to cell growth. *Biochem. Soc. Symp.*, **51**, 117.
5. Bowman B.H. (1988). Transferrin—evolution and genetic regulation of expression. *Adv. Genetics*, **25**, 1.
6. Worwood M. (1986). Serum ferritin. *Clin. Sci.*, **70**, 215.
7. Theil E.C. (1990). The ferritin family of iron storage proteins. *Adv. Enzymol.*, **63**, 421.
8. Worwood M. (1990). Ferritin. *Blood Rev.*, **4**, 259.
9. Schacker B.A. (1988). Heme catabolism by heme oxygenase: physiology, regulation and mechanism of action. *Semin. Hematol.*, **25**, 349.
10. Jacobs A., Worwood M. (1980). Iron metabolism, iron deficiency and iron overload. In *Blood and its Disorders* (Hardisty, R.M., Weatherall, D.J. eds.) Oxford: Blackwell Scientific, pp.149–197.
11. Cook J.D., Skikne B.S. (1987). Intestinal regulation of body iron. *Blood Rev.*, **1**, 267.
12. Dawson D.W., Hoffbrand A.V., Worwood M. (1990). Investigation of megaloblastic and iron-deficiency anaemias. In *Practical Haematology*, 7th edn. (Dacie J.V., Lewis S.M. eds.) Edinburgh: Churchill Livingstone, pp.397–420.
13. ICSH (1990). Revised recommendations for the meas-urements of the serum iron in human blood. *Br. J. Haematol.*, **75**, 615.
14. Dallman P.R. (1984). Diagnosis of anemia and iron deficiency: analytic and biological variations of laboratory tests. *Am. J. Clin. Nutr.*, **39**, 937.
15. Labbe R.F., Labbe R.L. (1989). Zinc protoporphyrin: a product of iron-deficient erythropoiesis. *Semin. Hematol.*, **26**, 40.
16. Cook J.D., Lynch S.R. (1986). The liabilities of iron deficiency. *Blood*, **68**, 803.
17. Haas J.D., Fairchild M.W. (1989). Summary and conclusions of the International Conference on Iron Deficiency and Behavioral Development. *Am. J. Clin. Nutr.*, **50**, 703.
18. Hibbard B.M. (1988). Iron and folate supplements during pregnancy: supplementation is valuable only in selected patients. *Br. Med. J.*, **297**, 1324.
19. Horn E. (1988). Iron and folate supplements during pregnancy: supplementing everyone treats those at risk and is cost effective. *Br. Med. J.*, **297**, 1325.
20. MacDougall I.C., Hutton R.D., Cavill I., Coles G.A., Williams J.D. (1989). Poor response to treatment of renal anaemia with erythropoietin corrected by iron given intravenously. *Br. Med. J.*, **299**, 157.
21. Pippard M.J. (1989). Desferrioxamine-induced iron excretion in humans. *Baillières Clin. Haematol.*, **2**, 323.
22. Sheldon J.H. (1935). *Haemochromatosis*, Oxford University Press.
23. Simon M., Bourel M., Fauchet R., Genetet B. (1976). Association of HLA-A3 and HLA1B14 antigens with idiopathic haemochromatosis. *Gut*, **17**, 332.
24. Simon M., Alexandre J-L., Fauchet R., Genetet B., Bourel M. (1980). The genetics of hemochromatosis. In *Progress in Medical Genetics* (New Series) vol.4, *Genetics of Gastrointestinal Disease* (Steinberg A.G., Bearn A.G., Motulsky A.G., Childs B. eds.) Philadelphia: Saunders, pp.135–168.
25. Leggett B.A., Halliday J.W., Brown N.N., Bryant S., Powell L.W. (1990). Prevalence of haemochromatosis amongst asymptomatic Australians. *Br. J. Haematol.*, **74**, 25.
26. Bothwell T.H., Charlton R.W., Motulsky A.G. (1989) Hemochromatosis. In *The Metabolic Basis of Inherited Disease* (Scriver C.R., Beaudet A.L., Sly W.S., Valle D. eds) 6th edn, New York: McGraw-Hill, pp.1433–1462.
27. Porter J.B., Huehns E.R. (1989). The toxic effects of desferrioxamine. *Baillières Clin. Haematol.*, **2**, 459.
28. Nathan D.G., Piomelli S. (1990). Introduction: oral iron chelators. *Semin. Hematol.*, **27**, 83.
29. Kontoghiorghes G.J., Hoffbrand A.V. (1988). Proposals for effective and oral chelation in transfusional iron overload. In *Recent Advances in Haematology* (Hoffbrand A.V. ed.) Edinburgh: Churchill Livingstone, pp.75–98.
30. Berdoukas V., Bentley P., Frost H., Schnebli H. (1993) Toxicity of oral iron chelator L1. *Lancet*, **341**, 1088.
31. Torrance, T.D., Bothwell, T.H. (1980). Tissue iron stores. In *Iron* (Cook J.D. ed.) *Methods in Hematology*, vol.I, New York: Churchill Livingstone, pp.90–115.
32. Stark, D.D. (1991). Hepatic iron overload: paramagnetic pathology. *Radiology*, **179**, 333.
33. Hershko C. (1993) Development of oral iron chelator L1. *Lancet*, **341**, 1088.

27. Anaemias
C. Barton

Introduction
Erythropoiesis
    Erythropoietin
    Other required factors
The anaemias
    Iron-deficiency anaemia
    Megaloblastic anaemias
    Acute blood loss
    Haemolytic anaemias
    Anaemia in systemic disease
    Blood dyscrasias
Aids to diagnosis
    Clinical
    Laboratory

INTRODUCTION

Other chapters relevant to this section include:

- Haemoglobinothpathies (Ch. 25)
- Disorders of iron metabolism (Ch. 26)
- Abnormalities of plasma proteins (Ch. 28).

ERYTHROPOIESIS

During fetal development, normal red blood-cell production (erythropoiesis) begins in the yolk sac, but by the sixth week of life the liver is the primary site, to be succeeded by the bone marrow after 20 weeks' gestation (Fig. 27.1). Different haemoglobins are present in the red cells at each stage, with properties relevant to the particular oxygen requirements of the fetal tissues at that point. The bone marrow cavity provides the microenvironment necessary for long-term cellular development. Progenitor cells for the requisite cell lines develop next to the marrow sinuses, through which the mature cells can enter the circulation. The cells and signals controlling this process at the cellular level are not fully understood, but are thought important in the pathogenesis of some anaemias (e.g. aplastic anaemia) and in the recovery of haemopoiesis following bone marrow failure or engraftment.

Progenitor cells are pluripotent, and *in vitro* can give rise to all marrow cell lines (Fig. 27.2). When committed to a certain cell line they are responsive to a humoral feedback mechanism. Red-cell maturation results in each stem cell forming 16 daughter cells. The process takes about a week, as more haemoglobin forms in the cytoplasm and there is less nuclear material. If this process is in balance, the nucleus eventually becomes pyknotic and is extruded in the marrow, and the mature red cell containing some RNA (a reticulocyte) is released into the circulation.

If there is asynchrony between nuclear and cytoplasmic maturation, so that nuclear maturation takes longer than normal, macrocytes result; if insufficient haemoglobin forms in the cytoplasm as in iron deficiency, microcytes result.

Erythropoietin

In the adult, the red-cell mass is normally constant, but increases in response to anoxia, and is depressed when the required haemoglobin level is regained. A glycoprotein, called erythropoietin, which only affects

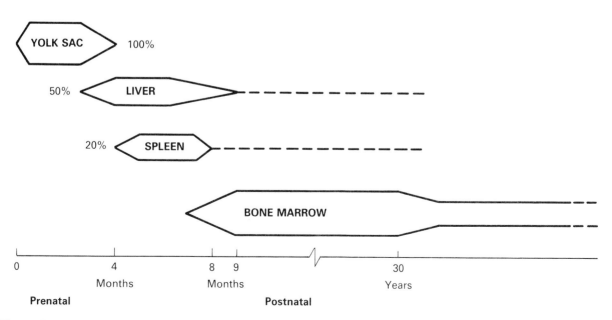

Figure 27.1 Sites of erythropoiesis throughout life.

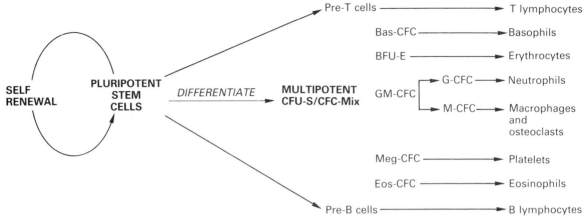

Figure 27.2 Scheme of haemopoiesis. Bas, basophil; BFU, burst-forming unit; CFC, committed cells; CFU, colony-forming unit; E, erythrocyte; Eos, eosinophil; G, granulocyte; M, macrophage; Meg, megakaryocyte.

red-cell maturation, was discovered in the 1950s. It is produced primarily by the kidney. The gene for this glycoprotein has been cloned and recombinent erythropoietin is now available for therapeutic purposes. The molecular mass of erythropoietin is 29 900 Da. Assays for erythropoietin are made by either biological or immunological methods. Radioimmunoassays (RIAs), which use recombinant human erythropoietin, can be used to measure normal plasma levels, but may need to be checked by a biological assay as in some instances the immunological protein may be biologically inactive.

Erythropoietin mRNA can be shown in renal and hepatic tissue using gene probes. In the kidney, erythropoietin is produced in peritubular interstitial cells, and hepatic production in the adult is really only of any importance when there is renal failure.

The action of erythropoietin on committed red-cell precursors is by rapid stimulation of RNA synthesis, especially globin mRNA. Specific erythropoietin receptors are present on the erythroid precursors. Lack of erythropoietin, and also direct suppression of erythroid precursors by certain classes of thymocytes, stops erythropoiesis. This is seen in the red-cell aplasia associated with thymoma.

In patients, recombinant human erythropoietin has been shown to reverse the anaemia of end-stage renal failure. The increase in red-cell mass is dose dependent; side-effects include a tendency to thrombosis and hypertension, but the benefits to the patient are considerable. The expense of erythropoietin therapy precludes, as yet, its routine use.

Excess erythropoietin, resulting in an increased red-cell mass (*polycythaemia*) can be found in patients with renal tumours, and in those suffering from chronic hypoxia, as in congenital cyanotic heart disease for example.

Other Required Factors (Fig. 27.3)

Other hormones that affect red-cell production include corticosteroids, androgens, thyroxine and growth hormone. The marrow also needs other essential substances such as iron, folic acid, vitamin B_{12}, pyridoxine, ascorbic acid, riboflavin and vitamin E. Trace elements, for instance zinc, cobalt, manganese and copper, may also be necessary as anaemia results when animals are experimentally fed diets deficient in these substances.

Severe protein malnutrition in *kwashiorkor* or the combined protein–calorie malnutrition state of *marasmus* also results in anaemia, and is mirrored in developed countries by the anaemia of anorexia nervosa.

Correct assembly of DNA, RNA and protein in the red cell together with iron to produce structurally normal haemoglobin, and an ability for the mature red cell to stabilize an intact membrane and function by enzymatic metabolism of glucose, are also necessary. Genetic abnormalities in membrane cytoskeleton, haemoglobin and enzyme properties can also cause anaemia: worldwide these are almost as important as the deficiencies of vitamins, trace elements and the essential substances detailed above.

Iron

Disorders of iron metabolism are described in Chapter 26. Normal iron requirements in adults are approximately 1 mg/day. Two μg of vitamin B_{12} and 100 μg of folic acid are necessary for daily adult requirements, while children and pregnant women have higher requirements.

Vitamin B_{12} and Folate

A macrocytic anaemia results from deficiencies of vitamin B_{12} and folate, with the marrow aspirate showing a characteristic megaloblastic appearance in both red- and white-cell precursors, owing to delayed nuclear maturation. DNA synthesis is impaired when the enzymes acting in the synthesis of purines or pyrimidines are deficient, or when DNA polymerization is defective. Vitamin B_{12} deficiency probably inhibits DNA synthesis by its effect on folate metabo-

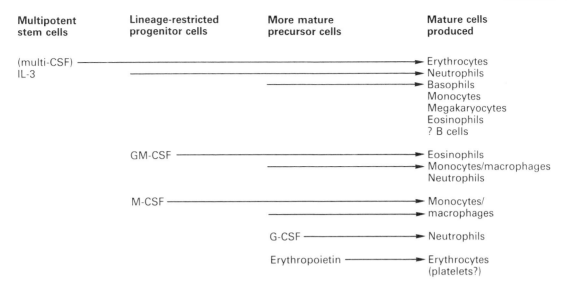

Multipotent stem cells	Lineage-restricted progenitor cells	More mature precursor cells	Mature cells produced

Figure 27.3 Growth factors in haemopoiesis. CSF, colony-stimulating factor; G, granulocyte; GM, granulocyte/ macrophage; IL-3, interleukin 3; M, monocyte.

lism; folate deficiency produces an inadequate supply of 5, 10 methylene tetrahydrofolate reductase, inhibiting the synthesis of thymidilate. This is a rate-limiting reaction in DNA synthesis.

Patients with severe B_{12} deficiency can respond haematologically to large doses of folic acid, although the B_{12} neuropathy is not alleviated. Thymidine given parenterally corrects deficiencies of both vitamins. People on regular folic acid supplements should have vitamin B_{12} levels checked to pre-empt the development of B_{12} deficiency neuropathy. As B_{12} stores last for several years this check does not need to be done more than annually.

With vitamin B_{12} and folate deficiency, intracellular folate is low, while forminoglutamic acid (FIGLU) and 5-amino-4-imidazole carboxamide (AICAR) excretion is raised, and serine–glycine interconversion reduced. Cellular uptake of methyl tetrahydrofolate is reduced and serum folate increased in severe B_{12} deficiency. An explanation for this is supplied by the 'methyl folate trap' hypothesis, but the exact mechanism is still subject to debate. The hypothesis suggests that in the absence of B_{12}, homocystine cannot be metabolized to methionine, and methyl tetrahydrofolate gives rise to tetrahydrofolate.

Vitamin B_{12} is generated by micro-organisms, and is found in animal products; liver is a rich source. Absorption from the gastrointestinal tract involves the vitamin being carried by a glycoprotein (intrinsic factor) produced by gastric parietal cells. The complex is absorbed in the terminal ileum, and the vitamin combines with transcobalamin II, a β-globulin present in plasma, to be distributed to the tissues. Other transcobalamins can carry the B_{12} in the circulation. Transcobalamin II deficiency results in severe functional B_{12} deficiency, although serum levels appear normal: this can occur as a congenital abnormality.

Assays for vitamin B_{12} can be microbiological using the protozoon *Euglena gracilis* or the bacterium *Lactobacillus leishmanii*. These assays are subject to the problems of all biological assays and RIA provides a quicker and more reliable method, the normal kit assaying folic acid and B_{12} simultaneously. Rigorous quality control of any assay is essential.

Folic acid is present in most foodstuffs, but inactivated by cooking at high temperatures. Vegetarians are unlikely to become folic acid deficient but are at risk of B_{12} deficiency. The stores of folate may be depleted within weeks (average stores last 4 months) so that any chronically ill patient may need folate supplements. Absorption occurs in the upper small intestine. Folic acid is absorbed more easily than polyglutamates, which need to be broken down to monoglutamates before absorption and transport to the liver for storage.

THE ANAEMIAS

The life-span of a red cell in the peripheral blood is 120 days. The cell is then normally destroyed in the reticuloendothelial system. Inadequate production, excess cellular destruction or blood loss can all lead to anaemia and mixtures of these features are often found in blood disorders.

Iron-deficiency Anaemia

The main features associated with iron deficiency are described in Chapter 26.

Megaloblastic Anaemias

Megaloblastic anaemias due to vitamin B_{12} or folate deficiency have similar presenting complaints.

Vitamin B_{12} Deficiency

The most important cause of B_{12} deficiency is *pernicious anaemia*, although this is rare as a world problem. Deficiency of intrinsic factor leads to malabsorption of vitamin B_{12} and the insidious onset of progressive anaemia. When anaemia develops slowly, adaptation to the low level of haemoglobin occurs and the patient can be severely anaemic at presentation. The patient may complain of tiredness and breathlessness on exertion, a sore tongue or mouth, loss of appetite and loss of weight. With the tendency to pancytopenia, bruising due to the low platelet count may bring the patient to medical attention. In B_{12} deficiency, a peripheral neuropathy can occur, even in the absence of anaemia; the patient has pins and needles in the extremities and sometimes difficulty in walking, together with unsteadiness. Some patients have optic atrophy and mild psychiatric problems. It is thought that B_{12} may be necessary either for fatty acid metabolism in myelin, or that the lack of methionine may cause central problems.

Because of ineffective erythropoiesis and increased breakdown of red-cell precursors, mild jaundice due to unconjugated hyperbilirubinaemia is present, and laboratory tests also show raised lactate dehydrogenase (LDH) and hydroxybutyrate dehydrogenase (HBD).

The blood test shows anaemia and often pancytopenia. A blood film shows macrocytic red cells, with considerable size variations. Megaloblasts may be present in the peripheral blood, and are helpful in confirming that megaloblastic anaemia is the problem, rather than another cause of macrocytosis where the marrow is not affected, as for instance in hypothyroidism or scurvy. The neutrophils show marked hypersegmentation and increased peroxidase content. This may be shown by some of the automated differential counters. The platelet count may be low. The megaloblastic nature of the disorder can be confirmed by a marrow aspirate.

There is a strong autoimmune flavour to the development of pernicious anaemia. Family members may have thyroid disorders, and vitiligo. The HLA types B8, B12 and DW15 are associated if myxoedema or thyrotoxicosis coexists with the anaemia. Antibodies to gastric parietal cells are present in 90% of patients, and strongly associated with gastric atrophy. If antibodies to intrinsic factor are present, this is pathognomonic of pernicious anaemia. Two types of antibody exist. Type 1 (blocking) antibodies are present in half the cases of pernicious anaemia, directed against the B_{12}-binding site of the intrinsic factor. Type 2 antibodies bind to the ileal absorption sites. They are present in about one-third of those who have type 1 antibodies.

Although pernicious anaemia is often associated with infertility, pregnancy can occur and intrinsic-factor antibodies may then cross the placenta to cause transient intrinsic-factor deficiency in the newborn. These cases are distinct from those of true juvenile pernicious anaemia or congenital intrinsic-factor deficiency.

In addition to the tests for vitamin B_{12} in the patient's serum, the *Schilling test* of B_{12} absorption, with or without intrinsic factor, is a useful adjunct for diagnostic completeness. The patient, who is fasting, is given an oral dose of radioactively labelled B_{12}, often simultaneously with one of radioactive B_{12} attached to intrinsic factor. A flushing dose of non-radioactive B_{12} is given parenterally. The amount of B_{12} excretion can be estimated in faeces, or more usually urine, and the results distinguish between pernicious anaemia or malabsorption, as in pernicious anaemia more of the isotope bound to intrinsic factor is absorbed and excreted than the non-bound isotope.

There is an increased incidence of gastric carcinoma in those with pernicious anaemia (4%) so that gastroscopy or barium studies need to be considered if a history of indigestion is obtained.

Any gastric surgery can interfere with the mechanism of intrinsic-factor secretion, and patients with ileal disease (e.g. Crohn's) may also have B_{12} malabsorption. Other disorders of the small intestine—diverticular disease, fistulae or blind-loop syndrome for example—can also lead to problems of B_{12} absorption. The fish tapeworm (*Diphyllobothrium latum*) is a well known if almost apocryphal cause. Infestation with this parasite is now rare outside parts of Russia and Finland. It is thought that the mechanism of B_{12} deficiency in such cases is destruction of intrinsic factor by bacterial overgrowth or the tapeworm.

Vitamin B_{12} deficiency is treated by hydroxycobalamin, usually given parenterally when malabsorption or pernicious anaemia is the root cause. Response is rapid, with a reticulocytosis that peaks within 4 days. Potassium supplements are often necessary to cope with the rapid demands of cell synthesis. Care should be taken in the elderly patient who may have coexistent cardiac problems. There is some recent work to suggest that B_{12} supplements are satisfactory when given orally but this route is not suitable if there is a problem with patient compliance.

Folate Deficiency

Surgical removal of the stomach or small bowel can also lead to folate deficiency, as do the malabsorption disorders such as coeliac disease and tropical sprue.

Serum and red-cell vitamin levels are helpful for diagnosis. The red-cell folate reflects the body state more accurately, and is less affected by transient dietary change. A histidine loading test leading to increased urinary excretion of FIGLU in folic acid deficiency is now used only infrequently as confirmation.

Folic acid supplements are often given as part of planned treatment in inflammatory bowel disorders, or in coeliac disease with a gluten-free diet, until the small-bowel mucosa has returned to normal.

Recurrent folate deficiency in this circumstance can be a sign of non-compliance with the diet or recurrence of an inflammatory bowel problem.

People who have extra requirements—pregnant women, or those with inherited red-cell disorders leading to increased red-cell turnover for example (hereditary spherocytosis, sickle-cell disease, etc.)—should have folic acid supplements. There is evidence that in those with folate deficiency, bone marrow arrest is more likely when another insult ensues, for instance infection, alcohol, or antifolate drugs such as trimethoprim. Other antifolate drugs include methotrexate (used to treat psoriasis and malignant disease) and the antiepileptics primidone (mysoline) and diphenylhydantoin sodium (epanutin).

Acute Blood Loss

After acute blood loss, the patient's symptoms are mainly due to volume depletion, so that the initial picture is one of shock. The patient is collapsed and short of breath, with low blood pressure, fast heart rate but thin and thready pulse and a cold clammy periphery. If resuscitation is with fluids, the missing blood volume is replaced and the haemoglobin level equilibrates after 24 h. The marrow can compensate for acute blood loss by increasing red-cell production. If anaemia becomes established more gradually, compensation may be more complete and the patient will complain of a variety of problems—for example tinnitus, palpitations, cramp, loss of appetite or angina. Those adults who object to blood transfusion on religious grounds have survived blood loss or haemolysis resulting in haemoglobin levels of 30–50 g/L (3–5 g/dL). Full supportive care with oxygenation, and proactive replacement with vitamins such as folic acid may help recovery. An understanding approach to support the patient in their beliefs is desirable. In some countries the courts may order transfusions for minors in life-threatening situations.

Haemolytic Anaemias

When the life-span of the red cell is shortened, any extra blood loss can produce rapid and profound anaemia. The red-cell mass, volume and life-span can be measured with chromium-51. The half-life of normal red cells is 30 days. In haemolytic states (e.g. sickle-cell disorders), the cell life-span may be 10–15 days. In haemolytic anaemia the bone marrow activity is normally higher than average, as evinced by the reticulocyte count, which represents the newly released red cells. Normally this is 1–2%, but a patient with a sickling disorder (see Chapter 25) will have a steady-state reticulocyte count of 20% for instance. A high reticulocyte count in the absence of blood loss is useful confirmation of haemolysis. A base-line reticulocyte level in compensated haemolytic states is useful to help decide when the patient is under extra haemolytic stress; reticulocytes, LDH or HBD can

supply evidence in the steady-state, for comparison in an acute haemolytic episode.

Biochemical estimation of red-cell breakdown products is useful in confirming haemolysis. Normally, red cells are broken down in the reticuloendothelial system, and bilirubin is released into the plasma. Here it is bound to albumin and is conjugated for excretion into bile by the liver. A high concentration of unconjugated bilirubin can be found in haemolysis and this is important in neonates, where the unconjugated bilirubin can cause kernicterus. Lipid-soluble bilirubin, although entering all cerebral tissue, tends to damage the basal ganglia and cerebellum. Mildly affected babies have high-tone hearing loss. Half of the severely affected children may die, the remainder survive with problems such as choreo-athetoid cerebral palsy.

In adults, the liver can usually cope with excreting increased amounts of bilirubin, which is eliminated as stercobilinogen in the faeces.

If red cells are destroyed intravascularly, haemoglobin is released directly into the plasma and is bound to haptoglobins. When these become saturated, free haemoglobin is passed through the kidneys into the urine, where it will test as blood on dipsticks but the urine will show no red cells on microscopy. In chronic haemoglobinuria, haemoglobin is absorbed into the renal tubules, and free iron released into the urine as haemosiderin. If acute intravascular haemolysis is suspected, then the globin breakdown product, methaemalbumin, can be detected spectroscopically in Schumm's test. Massive intravascular haemolysis, for example following an incompatible blood transfusion, can result in renal failure. Chronic haemolysis with iron loss through the kidneys will damage the renal tubules.

A blood film can sometimes be the basis of the diagnosis, since red-cell morphology in the haemolytic anaemias is often characteristic. Sickle cells, target cells, spherocytes and elliptocytes, as well as fragmented red cells, can be recognized by the experienced morphologist, while the automated cell counters can provide useful clues when they recognize spherocytes and other abnormal red-cell features.

Congenital Haemolytic Anaemias

These can arise as the result of disorders of the red-cell membrane, disorders of energy production in the red cell, or problems with the oxidation and reduction mechanisms. Disorders causing haemolysis due to abnormalities in the plasma are usually acquired rather than inherited. Many of the disorders can be inherited; those affecting the *milieu intérieur* being X-linked or autosomal recessive, while those affecting the red-cell membrane are often autosomal dominant.

Red-cell Membrane Defects. *1. Hereditary spherocytosis.* Autosomal dominant hereditary spherocytosis is the most common haemolytic anaemia among indi-

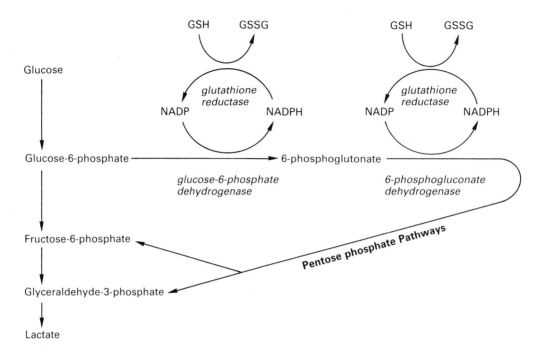

Figure 27.4 Oxidation of glutathione in the initial steps of the pentose phosphate pathway. GSH, reduced glutathione; GSSG, oxidized glutathione; NADP, oxidized nicotinamide-adenine-dinucleotide phosphate; NADPH, reduced nicotinamide-adenine-dinucleotide phosphate.

viduals from northern Europe, with an incidence of 1 in 5000; 75% of the cases are inherited with a dominant pattern. Clinical severity varies from case to case and family to family. Sporadic cases also occur. There is some linkage of dominant hereditary spherocytosis to chromosome 8.

The cause of the condition is thought to be a primary cell-membrane defect. There is a mild increase in glycolysis and ATP turnover to support increased cation (sodium and potassium) pumping through the leaky membrane. All patients with hereditary spherocytosis seem to have red-cell membranes deficient in spectrin, the major, highly flexible, cytoskeletal protein of the red cell, which accounts for half the skeletal mass of the cell.

Deficiency in the cytoskeleton can be measured by RIA to calculate the amount of spectrin. This is proportional to the amount of haemolysis observed in red cells subject to osmotic pressure. The abnormal red cells are normally destroyed in the spleen, and splenectomy both corrects the anaemia and reduces the tendency to gallstones. Gallstones can be found in children as young as 3 years old as the result of chronic haemolysis with extra bilirubin formation, and half of the affected adults have gallstones by middle age. As these are pigment stones they are most easily diagnosed by ultrasonograpy.

Before splenectomy the blood film is characteristic, with many small, dense spherocytes; after operation the blood film shows post-splenectomy changes with more spherocytes than usual, Howell–Jolly bodies, target cells and acanthocytes. Anaemia and jaundice improve and the reticulocyte count falls to near normal.

2. Hereditary elliptocytosis. Hereditary elliptocytosis, again diagnosed by looking at a blood film, is another red-cell membrane disorder, in which the interactions of spectrin with other membrane proteins are abnormal. Haemolysis is variable; the more deformed the red cells, the more affected the patient. Splenectomy can be clinically helpful.

Red-cell Metabolic Defects. *1. Glucose-6-phosphate dehydrogenase (G6PD) deficiency* (Fig. 27.4). This is probably the most common cause of haemolytic anaemia in the world (about 100 million affected individuals). There are many isoenzymes, some of which are functionally abnormal, and some present in less than adequate quantity. The net result is inadequate reduction of glutathione, and the tendency for cells to break down under oxidative distress. The distribution of the enzyme abnormalities in populations throughout the world suggests a link with the incidence of malaria, so that the heterozygous affected female is partially protected against this illness. Inheritance is sex linked, the gene being on the X chromosome. Males express little enzyme activity; carrier females, according to the Lyon hypothesis, can express either the normal or the abnormal chromosome, so their individual red cells can have normal or abnormal enzyme levels, although many have average activities between the normal and affected range. In some areas of the world the condition is so common that females can inherit two abnormal X chromosomes.

This enzyme marker became of great use in studies of malignancies to determine whether diseases were monoclonal in origin; both polycythaemia rubra vera and chronic myeloid leukaemia were shown to have originated from single stem-cell abnormalities by G6PD studies in females hemizygous for this enzyme.

Clinically, G6PD deficiency is an important cause of neonatal jaundice, particularly in the Far East and in the Mediterranean. Screening at birth is routine in such countries (e.g. Greece) so that affected individuals can avoid oxidant drugs (aminoquinilones, analgesics, sulphonamides, nitrofurantoin, vitamin K, etc.) In the Mediterranean, the bean *Vicia fava* can cause severe haemolysis in sensitive individuals exposed to its pollen. A few days after exposure, acute haemolysis occurs, which is intravascular. It may be preceded by shivering, abdominal pain, backache, and haemoglobinuria. The blood film shows all the hallmarks of haemolysis; Heinz bodies (oxidized, denatured haemoglobin) can be seen in reticulocyte preparations. Diagnosis is confirmed by measuring the enzyme level after the haemolytic episode is over. Unstable haemoglobin can also produce haemolysis after oxidant drug use (*see* Chapter 25).

2. Glycolytic pathway defects (Fig. 27.5). The blood film in these deficiencies, which are rare, gives a picture of a non-spherocytic haemolytic anaemia. These conditions are again more common in northern European populations. Clinical severity is variable, from the asymptomatic to the continually jaundiced. The reticulocyte count is often very high (50% or more). Diagnosis is confirmed by measuring the red-cell enzyme levels. Pyruvate kinase is the most commonly deficient enzyme.

Acquired Haemolytic Anaemias
Autoimmune haemolytic anaemia is due to antibodies directed against the red cell. Antihuman globulin reacting with immunoglobulin attached to the red cell gives a positive direct Coombs' test. If the antibody works best at 37°C, the haemolytic process is classified as 'warm'; if at 4°C, 'cold'. The antibody may well be suspected initially during blood cross-matching procedures for an anaemic patient.

Cold antibody types. The antibody attaches to red cells in the cold, and exposure to cold produces haemolysis; clinically this can be as paroxysmal cold haemoglobinuria with a patient having rigors, back and abdominal pain rather as described above under enzyme deficiencies, before passing red urine. This often follows a viral infection in children, particularly measles, mumps or chicken pox. In the laboratory, the Donath–Landsteiner test reveals an antibody that attaches to red cells at 4°C, fixing complement and causing red-cell lysis as the temperature increases.

Chronic cold haemagglutinin disease is associated with a high-titre antibody (often of IgM-κ light-chain type) that affects red cells in those parts of the body exposed to low temperatures. The fingers, toes and nose may become cyanosed (acrocyanosis) as agglutinates of red cells interfere with the circulation. The blood samples may show a characteristic clumpy appearance, and agglutinates are obvious on the blood film. A lymphoproliferative disorder may underlie the problem. Treatment is symptomatic, although gentle chemotherapy with alkylating agents can help. Wintering in a warm climate is recommended.

Both these conditions are rare; a cold antibody is much more likely to be found associated with glandular fever, or during an infection with *Mycoplasma pneumoniae*. Severe symptomatic anaemia can result, but is usually self-limiting. Transfusion should be reserved for severe clinical problems, as the transfused red cells will also be destroyed.

Warm antibody type. Drugs can produce an antibody-mediated haemolytic anaemia; some drugs (e.g. penicillin) bind to the membrane forming a complex that initiates a specific antibody; others (e.g. methyldopa) provoke an antibody that cross-reacts with red-cell components. Haemolysis is extravascular, and stops reasonably rapidly after the drug is withdrawn.

Idiosyncratic reactions to individual drugs that result in acute vascular haemolysis are less common but more severe. The antibodies produced are IgM and activate complement. Haemolysis occurs on the second exposure to the drug, but may be life threatening. Antibodies can be found that lyse red cells in the presence of the drug.

Similar extravascular haemolysis due to an autoimmune process can be idiopathic or secondary to another problem such as ulcerative colitis, systemic lupus erythematosus, chronic lymphatic leukaemia or a similar lymphoproliferative disorder, or other malignancy. Urgent treatment with steroids, splenectomy or immunosuppressive drugs may be necessary to control the haemolysis. The blood film shows spherocytes and a raised reticulocyte count; a reduction in these can be used to monitor response to therapy, but the direct Coombs' test can remain positive for many months even when active haemolysis has ceased.

Infections. Malaria, particularly *Plasmodium falci-*

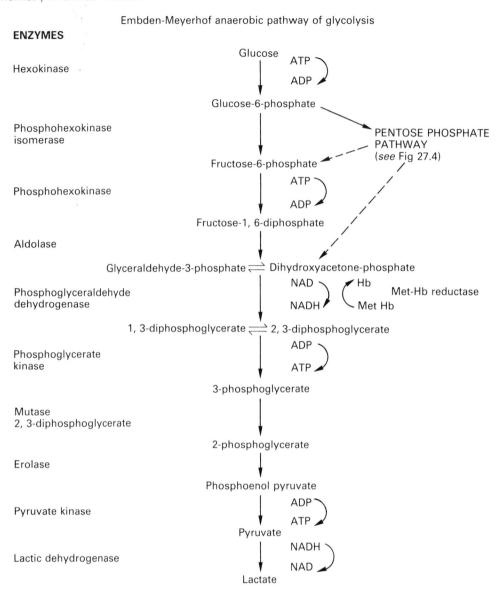

Embden-Meyerhof anaerobic pathway of glycolysis

ENZYMES

Hexokinase

Phosphohexokinase isomerase

Phosphohexokinase

Aldolase

Phosphoglyceraldehyde dehydrogenase

Phosphoglycerate kinase

Mutase
2, 3-diphosphoglycerate

Erolase

Pyruvate kinase

Lactic dehydrogenase

Figure 27.5 Embder–Meyerhof anaerobic pathway of glycolysis. ADP, adenosine diphosphatase; ATP, adenosine triphosphatase; NAD, oxidized nicotinamide-adenine-dinucleotide phosphate; NADH, reduced nicotinamide-adenine-dinucleotide phosphate.

parum, can cause marked intravascular haemolysis and haemoglobinuria (blackwater fever). People who are G6PD deficient can also suffer from haemolysis when given antimalarial treatment.

Severe bacterial infections, especially with Gram-negative organisms, release endotoxin which causes disseminated intravascular coagulation (DIC) and a mechanical haemolytic anaemia. *Clostridium welchii* septicaemia is associated with intravascular haemolysis, marked spherocytosis and fragmentation of red cells and renal failure. This used to be seen after septic abortions, and now needs consideration in victims of modern warfare.

Microangiopathic haemolytic anaemia. A blood film

showing microspherocytes, red-cell fragments and distorted red cells is produced when red cells have been broken down by fibrin strands in small blood vessels or by damaged endothelium. Severe burns produce such a picture; heat damage to the red cells may be partly responsible. The degree of red-cell breakdown, and whether it is predominantly intravascular or extravascular, affect the severity of the clinical picture.

Similar clinical problems can be produced by such disparate conditions as pre-eclampsia of pregnancy, DIC or, in children, haemolytic uraemic syndrome, which follows a febrile diarrhoeal illness.

In adults, thrombotic thrombocytopenic purpura, with haemolysis, thrombocytopenia, deranged coagulation tests, bizarre neurological episodes and renal impairment, runs a fluctuating but occasionally life-threatening course.

Management of these disorders depends on standard measures as far as the renal dysfunction is concerned, but other therapy with fresh frozen plasma or prostacyclin infusions may help in certain circumstances.

Other situations, such as mechanical haemolysis on artificial valves, direct red-cell trauma in march haemoglobinuria or in the pathological circulation around disseminated carcinoma metastases, can give rise to identical blood films.

Paroxysmal Nocturnal Haemoglobinuria. The red-cell membrane in this condition shows an acquired defect that makes it sensitive to complement lysis. Platelets and leucocytes are also abnormal; the clonality of the disorder has been confirmed by G6PD studies and the gene has been characterized. Haemolysis is intravascular, lysis occurring due to the activation of the alternative complement pathway, particularly during sleep, which accounts for the matinal haemoglobinuria. Diagnosis depends on thinking of the condition, as the blood film is not particularly helpful. Associated clinical features such as recurrent abdominal pain, headaches and recurrent episodes of thromboembolic disease may be helpful. Haemosiderin is found in the urine, reflecting the chronic haemolytic process. Low leucocyte alkaline phosphatase activity is a useful pointer, but the definitive laboratory test is the 'Ham's test' (acidified serum lysis). Red cells from the patient are suspended in fresh (complement source) normal ABO-compatible serum acidified to pH 6.5. At 37°C the cells will lyse, if sensitive, in 1 h, while normal control cells are unaffected. Paroxysmal nocturnal haemoglobinuria can follow an episode of aplasia. In a few patients, recovery can be spontaneous but marrow transplantation is considered for young patients if a suitable donor can be found. Otherwise the anaemia may require regular blood transfusions.

Anaemia in Systemic Disease

Any long-term chronic disease can be responsible for causing a mild anaemia, with normal-sized red cells containing normal amounts of haemoglobin. The serum iron level is low but so is the iron-binding capacity. A marrow aspirate stained for iron shows plentiful iron stores in the reticuloendothelial cells, but little in developing normoblasts. The cause is multifactorial, and not corrected more than partially by iron alone, as the underlying chronic disease needs to be remedied before the anaemia disappears. This anaemia is characteristic of disorders such as rheumatoid arthritis, chronic osteomyelitis or any other disease where the erythrocyte sedimentation rate (ESR) is high.

Blood Dyscrasias

Any disease process that affects the bone marrow environment and cell production can produce an anaemia as part and parcel of the main disorder. In malignant disorders, the biological advantage possessed by the predominant cellular expansion prevents normal cell-line maturation at some stage.

Leukaemia

An uncontrolled proliferation of any of the cell lines can produce a leukaemia; which is therefore myeloid, lymphoid, monocytic, megakaryocytic or erythroid leukaemia. These are further classified into chronic or acute according to the speed of onset and cell growth pattern. Clinically, symptoms are produced by absence of the normal cell lines. Anaemia is due to the lack of red cells, bruising or bleeding due to the lack of platelets, and infections due to absent or poorly functioning neutrophils. Leukaemic cells can form tissue deposits in the reticuloendothelial system, skin, central nervous system, etc.

Examination of the blood film and bone marrow yields enough information for a firm diagnosis. The morphology of the abnormal cell gives a working diagnosis, and the cell characteristics have been classified according to a collaborative French-American-British (FAB) scheme. The cell-surface receptor molecules are delineated by monoclonal antibody techniques, and intracellular enzymes (e.g. terminal deoxynucleotidyl transferase), so that a picture of the cell builds up that can be used to compare cases and therapy.

Malignant clones can also be detected by looking for evidence of monoclonality. In plasma cells and T-lymphoid cells, the gene rearrangements for immunoglobulin or the T-cell receptor, respectively, can help demonstrate this, although with plasma cells the gene product, or immunoglobulin, can also be clonal and more easily detected.

The chromosome pattern in the cells provides further information; structural changes can mean a poor prognosis while some help diagnosis. A translocation from chromosome 22 to chromosome 9 produces the short 22 known as the Philadelphia chromosome. This translocation produces a new gene on chromosome 22, which is transcribed as a protein kinase differing from the normal gene product and acting as a growth factor for the malignant clone.

Although anaemia develops quickly in the acute leukaemias and is usually the last cytopenia to resolve after successful chemotherapy, the onset is much more gradual in the chronic leukaemias.

Chronic lymphatic leukaemia presents less commonly with anaemia but more usually because the patient has noticed the enlarged lymph nodes associated with this disorder. An enlarged spleen is also often present, but marked splenomegaly is more common in other disorders such as prolymphocytic leukaemia or hairy-cell leukaemia. Cell markers and blood-film analysis confirm the diagnosis.

Splenomegaly is also marked in chronic myeloid leukaemia, where the blood film and the presence of the Philadelphia chromosome in blood or marrow culture confirm the diagnosis.

Treatment for the leukaemias has advanced apace and at the time of writing childhood leukaemia can be cured in 50% of cases, with better rates for acute lymphoblastic leukaemia than for acute myeloid leukaemia. Cures in adults can also be expected. Bone marrow transplantation from an HLA-identical sibling is a curative procedure in those young enough to endure an exhaustive treatment regimen and survive without emotional or psychological scars. For chronic myeloid leukaemia, bone marrow transplants are a treatment of choice.

The advent of interferon made from lymphoblastoid cell lines in large quantities or by recombinant DNA technology is an exciting new therapeutic concept. Interferons are a group of glycoproteins with molecular mass of 20 000 Da. Interferon is normally produced in response to viral infections, and when given intramuscularly reproduces many of the symptoms associated with a viral infection such as aching limbs, fever and headache. It also shows antitumour growth activity, however, and produces long response rates in patients suffering from hairy-cell leukaemia, where it is a strong therapeutic option and reverses the anaemia and pancytopenia caused by the accumulation of the abnormal hairy cells.

In chronic myeloid leukaemia, some patients given interferon have then lost the Philadelphia chromosome-bearing clone; a consummation previously only achieved by bone marrow transplantation.

Interferon may also have a part to play in extending disease-free intervals or in disease control in non-Hodgkin's lymphomas and myeloma.

The idea that tumours can be cured by specific environmental modulation rather than 'blunderbuss' chemotherapy is very encouraging; however, the long-term effects of immune-modulating agents are not known, and the use of these products is being monitored carefully.

Myeloma

Unlike leukaemia, myeloma, which is a malignant disorder of plasma cells, has not been conquered by standard chemotherapy protocols. For younger patients, bone marrow transplants are a hopeful option, and the role of interferon is being evaluated. The abnormal monoclonal immunoglobulin (paraprotein) produced by the tumour provides a useful biological marker of disease activity, and is often picked up by the biochemistry laboratory discovering an abnormal band on protein electrophoresis (*see* Chapter 28).

Anaemia is a common clinical finding; bone pain can be intractable and pathological fractures are common. The paraprotein can cause hyperviscosity, with a tendency to haemorrhage or thrombosis, and visual problems. The light chains of the immunoglobulin molecule (Bence–Jones protein) are excreted in the urine and cause tubular damage. Light chains are often associated with amyloid deposition. Bone marrow aspirates confirm the excess abnormal plasma cells, and radiographs show lytic lesions where plasma cells have accumulated in the long bones or skull.

The blood film shows a pancytopenia, with primitive white and red-cell precursors (a leucoerythroblastic film). This can also be caused by any bone marrow infiltrative process, for example with metastatic tumour, but in myeloma there may be a background blue staining of the abnormal protein present on the film.

Myelofibrosis

This is a myeloproliferative disorder where the fibrous element of the bone marrow predominates. There is compensatory extramedullary haematopoiesis in the areas where blood is made earlier in fetal life (the liver and spleen), and these organs, especially the spleen, become enlarged. Anaemia is due to both faulty red cell production and excess splenic destruction.

Myelodysplasia

In older patients, anaemia may reflect an abnormal marrow function, which is increasingly becoming recognized and classified as dysplasia. The anaemia is refractory to haematinics, and there may be disordered iron metabolism (sideroblasts; *see* Chapter 26), excess blasts, or excess monocytes. Eventually most of these disorders evolve into a more frankly leukaemic picture. During the chronic phase, transfusions relieve symptoms, and may help the patient for many years. Chemotherapy for either the chronic or acute phases is disappointing. Useful information is being found from chromosomal studies. There are often abnormal patterns, the evolution of which precedes clinical deterioration. In those young enough, a bone marrow transplant should be considered.

These disorders may be associated with environmental insults such as drug exposure, or occupational exposure to noxious agents, and registers of occupational associations are being established.

AIDS TO DIAGNOSIS

Clinical

The symptoms described by the patient, the speed of onset of the anaemia, and the presence of associated problems are important to note, to establish whether the anaemia is acute or chronic. Jaundice and haemoglobinuria are useful clinical pointers.

Examination of the patient for specific signs such as enlarged glands, spleen or liver, evidence of bruising or infection, and bone tenderness will help with further clues.

Laboratory

In the laboratory, modern cell counters can provide a quick and reliable full blood picture, with a white-cell differential, haemoglobin, red-cell count, platelet count, reticulocyte count, packed cell volume and red-cell indices. In many cases, the blood film is used to confirm the cell-counter information, adding extra information about red-cell shape, size and inclusions such as Howell–Jolly bodies or malaria parasites.

If the red-cell indices suggest iron deficiency with a low mean cell volume (MCV) and mean corpuscular haemoglobin (MCH), the presence of a high red-cell count may suggest the patient is a carrier for thalassaemia (*see* Chapter 25). Haemoglobin electrophoresis will show a characteristic pattern with raised levels of minor haemoglobins (A$_2$ and sometimes F). The iron levels, which should be abnormal in iron deficiency, are normal in β-thalassaemia trait, the carrier state. Serum ferritin levels to confirm the iron status may be helpful, especially if the patient has already started iron therapy.

A high MCV suggesting megaloblastic anaemia will be confirmed with a bone marrow aspirate. Vitamin levels, and a Schilling test, will help decide on vitamin B$_{12}$ or folate deficiency as the root cause, and also whether malabsorption is responsible. Immunological back-up can confirm pernicious anaemia, but malabsorption may need further gastroenterological investigation with radiological and endoscopic tests.

The haemolytic anaemias are classified according to the evidence of red-cell breakdown and pigment dissipation. Biochemical measurements of bilirubin, liver enzymes, red-cell enzymes and the presence of free haemoglobin or methaemalbumin are helpful. Haptoglobins are lowered in haemolytic states, but the normal range is wide, and may be altered by coexisting disease, so that this is not a very useful first-line investigation.

The reticulocyte count is important. This is a subjective test, as normally there are low levels (1% reticulocytes in a normal individual) so it is subject to statistical errors unless assessed by automated counter. It is, however, helpful to monitor marrow activity. A bone marrow examination may also be helpful if an aplastic crisis is suspected in a patient, but the blood film is of particular value for showing red-cell abnormalities.

If an antibody-mediated haemolytic state is suspected, a direct Coombs' test and cold agglutinin assay, together with a quantitation of which immunoglobin class or complement fraction is present on the red cell, are helpful for classification.

Coagulation studies are useful in suspected DIC, to monitor disease progression as well as the effect of blood-product therapy if fresh frozen plasma or cryoprecipitate is used.

A bone marrow aspirate and trephine histology are more useful for anaemias where underlying malignancy is suspected; and repeat tests to monitor therapy may also be necessary.

The elucidation of the cause of anaemia depends, as in all diseases, on close liaison between the clinician and the laboratory, so that information can be transferred to the maximum benefit and minimum inconvenience of the patient.

FURTHER READING

Weatherall D., Ledingham J., Warrell D. (1993). *Oxford Textbook of Medicine*, 2nd edn, Oxford Medical.

Hoffbrand A.V., Pettit J.E. (1993). *Essential Haematology*, 3rd edn, Oxford: Blackwell Scientific.

Nathan D.G., Oski F.A. (1993). *Hematology of Infancy and Childhood*, 4th edn, Philadelphia: Saunders.

Schrier S.L. ed. (1985) The red blood cell membrane. *Clinics in Haematol.*, **14** (1).

Cavill I. ed (1990) Advancing haematological techniques. *Clinical Haematol.*, **3** (4).

28. Abnormalities of Plasma Proteins

J. T. Whicher

Introduction
    History
    Clinical applications of protein studies
Metabolism of plasma proteins
    Synthesis
    Distribution
    Catabolism
Functions of plasma proteins
    Proteins of immune defence
    Proteins associated with inflammation
    Transport proteins
    Signal proteins
    Proteins of blood clotting
    Tissue-derived proteins and oncofetal
      proteins
The proteins of immune defence
    Immunoglobulins
Proteins associated with inflammation
    Acute-phase reactant proteins
    Protease inhibitors
    Haptoglobin
    Orosomucoid (44 kDa)
    Other proteins of inflammation
Transport proteins
    Albumin (68 kDa)
    Transferrin (77 kDa)
    Caeruloplasmin (130 kDa)
    Other transport proteins
Oncofetal and tissue proteins
    β_2-microglobulin (11 kDa)
    α-fetoprotein (69 kDa)
Plasma precursors of amyloid
Interpretation of electrophoresis
    Serum and plasma
    Cerebrospinal fluid
    Urine (CSF)
Specific protein measurements in disease
    Inflammation
    Immune-complex disease
    Infectious disease
    Liver disease
    Gastrointestinal disease
    Renal disease
    Neoplasia
    Skin disease

INTRODUCTION

Plasma contains a large number of different proteins of very varying structural characteristics. The function of only a relatively small proportion of them is known but it must be presumed that they are present either with a specific role in the plasma or that they represent cellular proteins shed into the circulation as a result of degradative processes. Many plasma proteins show characteristic changes in concentration or structure either due to genetic defects that may give rise to disease or as a result of secondary changes reflecting pathological or physiological processes.

All the transcellular fluids, such as cerebrospinal fluid (CSF), urine, synovial fluid and saliva, contain a considerable number of proteins, many of them derived from plasma but some secreted specifically into the fluid.

History

Plasma has always provided biochemists with an easily available material for the study of proteins, some of which are present in extremely high concentration. Detailed study of proteins did not really start until a series of workers between 1853 and 1869 studied the insolubility of some serum components upon acidification and the addition of water. It was in 1862 that Schmidt instituted the term globulin for the substances from serum that formed a precipitate of tiny spheres on the addition of water. The idea of salt fractionation then appeared and gave rise to a series of separation techniques still widely used today and upon which much of the subsequent work has depended. Thus in 1894 Gurber used ammonium sulphate to purify one of the first proteins ever to be crystallized—horse albumin.

Despite the advent of such techniques, little real advance was made as methods were not available to study the structure of proteins separated in this way. However, it was appreciated that the albumin/globulin ratio showed characteristic changes in disease.

It was not until the advent of analytical ultracentrifugation and moving boundary electrophoresis in the 1930s that the real characterization of serum proteins started. The electrophoretic pattern of human serum comprising albumin and the alpha, beta and gamma globulins was described by Tiselius, and in 1939 Tiselius and Kabat showed that antibody was a γ-globulin. In 1950, paper electrophoresis was described and by the late 1950s had spread into many laboratories giving rise to innumerable clinical studies. In 1953 Grabar and Williams described the use of antibody raised against human serum to characterize the proteins present after electrophoresis. Thus the essential facets of protein biochemistry had now been discovered; techniques for fractionation, separation and identification. The measurement of protein concentrations using specific antibody raised against a single purified protein appeared some 10 years later with the work of Mancini and of Laurell.

Clinical Applications of Protein Studies

Changes in proteins in plasma or other body fluids may be genetically determined and result directly in

TABLE 28.1
THE EFFECT OF STEROIDS ON PLASMA PROTEIN
CONCENTRATIONS

Protein	Corticoid	Androgen	Oestrogen
Prealbumin	−	+	−
Albumin	−	N	−
α_1-Lipoprotein	N	−	+ +
Orosomucoid	+	+	−
α_1-Antitrypsin	N	+	+ +
Haptoglobin	+	+ +	−
Caeruloplasmin	N	N	+ + +
Transferrin	N	+	+
β-Lipoprotein	+ +	+	N
IgG	−	N	−

These changes are due to a combination of changes in
volume of distribution and changes in the rate of synthesis

+ denotes increase; −, decrease; N, no change.

disease due to an abnormality or deficiency in a
specific protein. More commonly changes are secondary to a disease process affecting either protein synthesis, distribution or catabolism.

Genetic variants, though not common individually,
form an important group for the clinical laboratory
to investigate as they may be the diagnostic key to a
disease process. Secondary changes vary enormously
in clinical usefulness; they may be important to the
diagnosis such as the finding of a paraprotein in
myeloma, or simply be a part of the jigsaw of diagnostic information that allows us to assess the probability
of a particular disease. More recently we are beginning to appreciate the value of sequential protein
measurements in the monitoring of disease activity
and response to treatment.

The characteristics of plasma proteins that are
used in clinical practice are changes in their
concentration, function or structure. It is thus important that both qualitative and quantitative techniques
are available in the laboratory. Simple electrophoresis
on cellulose acetate or agarose is a most useful initial
investigation providing a considerable amount of information upon which the choice of specific protein
measurements can be made. It also allows the identification of a number of genetic variants that result in
changes in electrophoretic mobility. The identification of proteins separated by electrophoresis by the
use of immunofixation or immunoelectrophoresis further increases the discrimination of qualitative
examination.

For proteins present in plasma at concentrations
above 1 mg/L, quantitation may be done by gel
diffusion, electroimmunodiffusion, nephelometry and
turbidimetry. Below this concentration radioimmunoassay and enzyme immunoassay are the most widely
used techniques. Functional assays are essential for
proteins that are present in normal concentrations
but whose function may be defective.

METABOLISM OF PLASMA PROTEINS

Synthesis

Many plasma proteins, including albumin, are synthesized in the liver, although there is increasing evidence
for the production of some plasma proteins in peripheral tissues. Thus we know that immunoglobulins are
only synthesized by B-cells while cell-surface proteins
such as β-microglobulin are made by many different
cells.

The general mechanism of protein synthesis is
common to all cells. Intracellular proteins are usually
translated on cytoplasmic polyribosomes whereas proteins destined for the cell membrane or for secretion
are translated on the membrane-bound ribosomes of
the rough endoplasmic reticulum. After synthesis,
most proteins probably contain two additional peptides at the N-terminus. A hydrophobic prepeptide
acts as a 'leader' directing the molecule through the
membrane of the endoplasmic reticulum. This is
cleaved almost immediately leaving the protein with
a propeptide, which is not removed until maturation
occurs in the Golgi vesicles or in storage granules
immediately prior to secretion. Glycoproteins have
carbohydrate residues added by sugar transferases in
the lumen of the endoplasmic reticulum and these
may control folding of the polypeptide chain and act
as recognition sites for subsequent metabolism. For
example, it is probable that the carbohydrate moiety
of the glycoprotein hormones may be the key for
interaction with target cell-membrane receptors. Control of protein synthesis may be exerted on the rate
of transcription of mRNA from DNA or at the level
of translation. Both mechanisms have been described
for a number of proteins (Fig. 28.1).

Factors affecting plasma protein synthesis have
been studied in the liver. Many factors influence
hepatic plasma protein synthesis from specific regulatory factors to amino acid availability. Toxic factors
such as ethanol may inhibit synthesis and hormones
have an important but complex effect. In clinical
practice the effects of androgens and oestrogens are
the most important (Table 28.1). The synthesis of
several proteins by the liver is increased in protein-
losing states when the plasma albumin level is
decreased.

Specific synthetic regulatory mechanisms are also
being increasingly recognized. It is notable that the
synthesis of acute-phase proteins, most of which have
specific functions in the inflammatory reaction, is
increased in the liver during inflammation of many
tissues due to the action of cytokines.

Distribution

Plasma proteins pass continuously from the vascular
to the extravascular space. The passage across capillary walls is both through interendothelial junctions
(especially in the choroid plexus) and by pinocytic

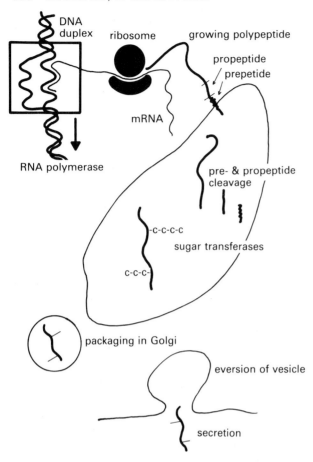

Figure 28.1 Protein synthesis. The gene for a polypeptide may exist as a number of separate segments on the chromosome. mRNA transcription skips intervening segments resulting in a single strand of message for an individual peptide chain. Most proteins probably possess two additional N-terminal peptides, the prepeptide, responsible for insertion into, and passage across, the membrane of the endoplasmic reticulum and the propeptide for maturation and transport to the Golgi apparatus. The prepeptide is probably cleaved shortly after entry into the lumen of the endoplasmic reticulum while the propeptide may be retained until just prior to secretion from the cell. Carbohydrate side-chains may be added by sugar transferases within the endoplasmic reticulum.

transport across endothelial cells. In both cases, proteins must pass across the basement membrane. It is probable that some of the pinocytic vesicles fuse with lysosomes, resulting in enzymatic degradation, and it is in this way that many plasma proteins are catabolized by the capillary endothelium. The protein content of the transcellular fluids and extracellular fluid is thus dictated by a combination of these two non-specific mechanisms as well as by specific transport mechanisms that may apply to some of the proteins crossing the endothelial cells in pinocytic vesicles. In all such fluids, low molecular-weight proteins predominate, owing to the molecular sieving

effect of the capillary basement membrane. It is important to appreciate that the protein content of such transudates will vary from tissue to tissue according to the nature of the capillary interendothelial junctions and also that the fluid, once formed, may be rapidly changed by subsequent metabolic processes. For example, the protein content of urine is very different from that of the glomerular filtrate, owing to the reabsorption of proteins in the proximal tubule. Ventricular CSF is very different from lumbar CSF due to the progressive equilibration of the fluid with plasma during its passage down the spinal column. The effect of changes in posture in altering the concentration of proteins in plasma is also of practical importance.

Catabolism

Plasma protein breakdown probably occurs to a greater or lesser extent in most cells of the body, and degraded plasma proteins may provide an important source of amino acids for cellular protein synthesis. In particular, degradation occurs in the capillary endothelial cell during the process of pinocytic transfer from lumen to basement membrane. Capillary endothelial cells have few lysosomes and while their catabolic activity is limited it is worth noting that the muscles of an adult man contain some 60 000 miles of capillaries with an area of about 6000 square metres. Thus even if only a small proportion of the proteins pinocytosed by each endothelial cell is catabolized, the catabolic potential is still enormous.

Proteins that have passed through the endothelium may then be catabolized by the tissue cells they come into contact with, again by pinocytosis and lysosomal degradation.

The role of the liver in protein catabolism has been extensively studied and a number of interesting ideas have emerged. The hepatic sinusoids lack a continuous basement membrane, the endothelial cells have marked intercellular fenestrations and the pericapillary cellular covering is far from complete. This has led to the proposal that the space of Disse and the hepatic sinusoid form a single mixing pool of proteins; plasma proteins thus enter and leave the hepatocyte without hindrance. This of course explains how high molecular-weight proteins and particles synthesized in liver cells, such as α_2-macroglobulin (725 kDa), and very low-density lipoprotein, enter the plasma. Most plasma proteins are glycoproteins and the evidence suggests that the carbohydrate side-chains may have a key role in controlling degradation. Desialation of many glycoproteins results in increased catabolism and it is possible that an intact carbohydrate moiety protects circulating proteins from hepatic catabolism. Removal of carbohydrate residues as a result of the action of circulating or membrane-bound enzymes may act as the catabolic initiating process for binding of the protein to hepatocyte membrane receptors, with subsequent pinocytosis and intracellular degradation by lysosomal enzymes. It is possible that other molecular changes such as polymerization or complex formation may also act as catabolic initiators.

The kidney has long been known to be the site of breakdown of low molecular-weight proteins such as immunoglobulin light chains. Between 2 and 4 g of plasma proteins are filtered by the glomerular capilliaries each day but only about 100 mg appear in the urine. Proteins pass through the glomerular filter in inverse proportion to their molecular size and are largely reabsorbed in the proximal tubule by pinocytosis and degraded by lysosomal enzymes. Pinocytosis by tubular cells is probably competitive and there may be selective mechanisms for some types of proteins.

We are thus left with the concept that plasma proteins may be taken up by various cells either by bulk pinocytosis or by receptor-mediated selective uptake and subsequently catabolized by lysosomal enzymes. This process probably occurs in most tissues but the capillary endothelial cell, the hepatocyte and the proximal tubule are of considerable importance.

FUNCTIONS OF PLASMA PROTEINS

Despite the enormous expansion in knowledge about plasma proteins in the last 10 years, many proteins still have no known biological function. A functional classification of plasma proteins is, however, useful in understanding the changes that occur in disease as proteins of similar function often form interacting systems (e.g. immunoglobulins and complement). It is probable that most of the plasma proteins present at relatively high concentrations have a functional role to play in circulating blood but it is clear that many of those present in trace amounts represent cell-surface or intracellular proteins that have been shed into the bloodstream.

Proteins of Immune Defence

Immunoglobulins provide the adaptive immune response of higher animals for the elimination of antigen. *Complement* provides both effector mechanisms for antibody and an additional non-adaptive defence mechanism. *C-reactive protein* may represent a primitive, non-adaptive mechanism activating complement.

Proteins Associated with Inflammation

A number of plasma proteins increase in concentration during inflammation in many tissues. The so-called 'acute-phase response' represents the switching on, by specific messengers known as cytokines, of synthetic mechanisms for proteins that are involved in the inflammatory process either as mediators, participants or inhibitors.

Transport Proteins

Plasma proteins are concerned in the transport of a wide range of substances from the site of production to their site either of action or of catabolism. Another important aspect of their role is the maintenance of a pool of biologically inactive substance in equilibrium with the pool of free active substance. It is being increasingly recognized that the carrier proteins may have a complex role in the metabolism of the molecules with which they are associated, such as interacting with enzymes or cellular receptors.

Signal Proteins

It is clear that many plasma proteins are in fact messengers of one sort or another. Most of the classical protein hormones are present at low concentrations but some such as human placental lactogen and the placental protein Sp 1 are present at high enough concentrations to have been classed as 'plasma proteins'.

Proteins of Blood Clotting

The interacting proteins of the blood clotting system form a quantitatively important part of the plasma proteins. It is important to realize that the inhibitors and active proteolytic enzymes of this system interact closely with the complement and kallikrein–kinin systems, and thus with inflammation. They will not be further considered in this review.

Tissue-derived Proteins and Oncofetal Proteins

Some of the proteins present in low concentrations in plasma are cell-membrane proteins shed into the blood during cell-membrane turnover or as a result of cell death. A number of other trace proteins, the oncofetal proteins, are produced by tumours as a result of derepression of genes coding for fetal proteins or proteins not normally produced by the tissue of origin of the tumour.

THE PROTEINS OF IMMUNE DEFENCE

Immunoglobulins

The immune system can be conveniently divided into two functionally cooperative but developmentally independent pathways of lymphoid differentiation. T lymphocytes derived from the thymus represent a functionally heterogeneous group of cells concerned with immune regulation and antigen elimination while B lymphocytes synthesize and secrete antibody.

The immunoglobulin molecules that mediate antibody activity are so far unique among proteins both in their remarkable structural heterogeneity and in that their synthesis is an adaptive response triggered by the antigenic configuration with which they will

TABLE 28.2
BIOLOGICAL PROPERTIES OF HUMAN IMMUNOGLOBULINS

Class	Subclass	Complement activation	Binding to macrophage Fc receptors	Transport across placenta	Transport into secretions	Fixation to mast cells and basophils
IgG	1	+				
	2	±				
	3	+	+	+	–	–
	4	–				
IgA	1 and 2	–	–	–	+	–
IgM		+	–	–	–	–
IgD		–	–	–	–	–
IgE		–	–	–	–	+

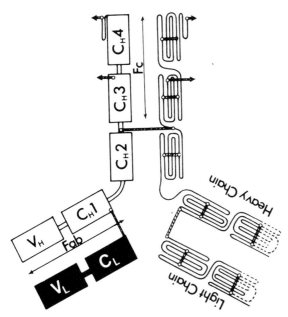

Figure 28.2 Diagram of one IgM subunit. The discontinuous lines in the V domains in the lower half of the diagram mark the hypervariable regions. The thick cross-hatched bars represent disulphide bonds, those with arrows interconnect the IgM subunits in the J chain. (Reproduced with permission from Pumphrey R.S.J. (1978). Structure and function of the immunoglobulins in *Immunochemistry in Clinical Laboratory Medicine* (Milford Ward A., Whicher J.T. eds.) Lancaster: MTP Press.)

TABLE 28.3
ANTIGENIC HETEROGENEITY OF IMMUNOGLOBULINS

Immunoglobulin class	Subclass	Allotype
IgA	α_1	
	α_2	Am$^+$, Am$^-$
IgG	γ^1	Gm1, 2, 3, 4, 17
	γ^2	Gm 23
	γ^3	Gm 5, 10, 13, 21, 6, 11, 14
	γ^4	
IgM		Mm
IgD		
IgE		

bonds. Each polypeptide chain falls into a series of globular regions called domains, which have considerable amino acid sequence homology (Fig. 28.2). The N-terminal domains of both H and L chains contain the variable amino acid sequence (V region), which determines antigenic specificity, thus allowing each molecule to have two antigen-combining sites. The remaining domains of the H chains (constant or C region) have certain structural and thus antigenic differences that allow their classification into five classes and a number of subclasses (Table 28.3). They also contain the effector sites, which allow the molecules to interact with cells and complement.

Immunoglobulin synthesis
Each immunoglobulin-producing cell (B lymphocyte) has some 10^5 immunoglobulin molecules embedded in the phospholipid bilayer of the cell membrane by a terminal hydrophobic peptide attached to the Fc region. There is strong evidence that the surface immunoglobulin acts as the receptor with which antigen interacts to trigger B-lymphocyte proliferation and maturation to the immunoglobulin-producing plasma cell (Fig. 28.3). H and L chains are synthesized on different polyribosomes present on the rough endoplasmic reticulum and molecular assembly occurs within the lumen of the endoplasmic reticulum. Plasma cells synthesize a slight excess of L chains,

interact. Functionally they have the capacity to complex with specific antigens and interact with both cells and other circulatory plasma proteins to give rise to a series of biological effector functions that result in the elimination of antigen (Table 28.2).

Immunoglobulin Structure
All immunoglobulins consist of one or more basic units comprised of two identical heavy (H) chains, each of molecular mass about 50 kDa, and two identical light (L) chains, each of about 20 kDa, joined together by a variable number of disulphide

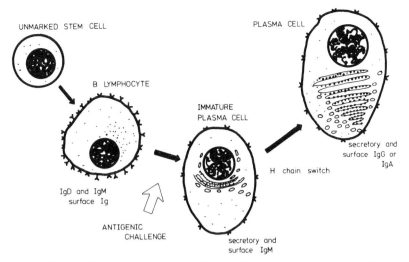

UNMARKED STEM CELL

B LYMPHOCYTE

IgD and IgM
surface Ig

ANTIGENIC
CHALLENGE

IMMATURE
PLASMA CELL

secretory and
surface IgM

H chain switch

PLASMA CELL

secretory and
surface IgG or
IgA

Figure 28.3 Maturation of B cell following antigenic challenge. The mature unstimulated B lymphocyte synthesizes surface IgM and IgD with variable-region sequence specificity for a specific antigen for which they act as the receptor. Differentiation to form the immature plasma cells results in switching off IgD H-chain synthesis with increasing production of secretory IgM with the same variable-region specificity as the surface IgM and IgD. Later in maturation H-chain constant-region synthesis switches from IgM to either IgG or IgA with transcription of the same V-region gene. In this way the type of immunoglobulin produced by a maturing clone of B cells changes from low-affinity IgM to high-affinity IgG or IgA. It is important to appreciate that the gene segments for the H-chain constant region and V-region sequences may be repeated on the chromosome. Similarly the V-region gene is probably made up of a number of segments, which are combined at random to form the heterogeneity of V-region sequences necessary for all the antibody specificities that occur.

most of which are normally catabolized within the lysosomes though a small amount of free L chains is secreted by the cells. Being of low molecular weight these are filtered at the glomerulus and predominantly reabsorbed in the proximal tubule. It is, however, normal to find some 10–20 mg/L of polyclonal free L chains in urine.

Functions of the Immunoglobulin Classes
A classification of the immunoglobulins is summarized in Table 28.3.

IgG (150 kDa)
IgG is a monomer of the basic immunglobulin unit and is present in high concentrations in plasma and in low concentrations in all extracellular fluids. It accounts for 75% of the plasma immunoglobulins and may be thought of as the antibody that protects the tissue spaces and, in particular, aggregates or coats small soluble proteins such as bacterial toxins. IgG is pumped across the placenta by an active transport process and provides protection for the fetus and for the newborn infant in the first few months of life before its own antibody synthesis is adequate.

IgA (160 kDa)
Most plasma IgA molecules are monomeric, though a small proportion form polymers and complex with other plasma proteins, especially albumin. The bulk of IgA synthesis occurs in plasma cells located be-neath the mucosa of the gastrointestinal tract, the respiratory tract, the skin and in exocrine glands, where it is produced as a dimer. IgA enters the epithelial cells of the mucosa, which synthesize and attach a secretory piece that binds to the two IgA molecules, forming a dimer that is secreted onto the luminal surface of the mucosa. This secretory IgA protects mucosal surfaces against bacterial invasion and is resistant to proteolysis in the gut. It is present in colostrum, where it protects the newborn infant from gastrointestinal infection.

IgM (950 kDa)
Plasma IgM consists of a pentamer of basic immunoglobulin units and because of its very high molecular weight is largely confined to the vascular space. IgM is present with IgD as one of the surface receptor immunoglobulins of the mature unstimulated B lymphocyte. IgM is the first immunoglobulin to be secreted after stimulation of the B lymphocyte to differentiate to form the plasma cell. Later in differentiation, H-chain C-region transcription switches to either IgG or IgA but with the same variable region gene and hence the same antibody specificity. This is why IgM is the first immunoglobulin to be synthesized following antigenic challenge. IgM synthesis is, however, maintained in response to certain antigens, in particular organisms present in the vascular space. The blood-group isohaemagglutinins belong to this immunoglobulin class.

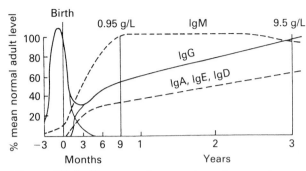

Figure 28.4 The normal maturation of serum immunoglobulin levels. IgM reaches adult levels by 9 months, IgG by 3 years and IgA, IgD and IgE by puberty, salivary IgA matures by about 6 weeks. (Reproduced with permission from Hobbs J.R. (1969). *Developmental Immunology* (Adinolfi A. ed.) London: Spastics International Press, p. 114 as modified by Keyser J. (1979). *Human Plasma Proteins*, Chichester: John Wiley, p. 2.)

IgE (190 kDa)

IgE is a monomeric immunoglobulin synthesized by plasma cells throughout the lymphoid system but in particular under the mucosae of the gut and respiratory tract. Plasma IgE is rapidly bound to the cell membranes of mast cells and basophils, and circulating levels are low. The combination of antigen with this cytophilic antibody causes degranulation of these cells with release of kinins, histamine and prostaglandins, which cause vascular permeability and smooth muscle contraction. Such phenomena are responsible for asthma and hay fever. The beneficial effect of this interaction remains to be convincingly elucidated.

IgD (175 kDa)

IgD together with IgM constitutes the membrane receptor of the B lymphocyte. Occasionally cells go on to synthesize IgD but the function of the plasma IgD is unknown.

Immunoglobulin Normal Ranges

Normal ranges for immunoglobulins are not distributed in a Gaussian fashion and the shape of the distribution differs for each immunoglobulin class. The levels of IgG and IgM and the rates at which they mature to adult levels from childhood are dependent on antigen challenge. In the tropics, mean IgG and IgM levels are often 200% of levels in England. If Africans are domiciled in England, IgM levels usually fall but IgG levels often remain elevated, reflecting a genetic influence. IgA levels are unaffected by environmental factors.

The newborn child has a high level of IgG of maternal origin, which declines to a very low level by about 6 months *post partum*. The child's own immunoglobulin synthesis begins with IgM and is followed by IgG at about three months after birth (Fig. 28.4). IgM reaches adult levels at about 9 months, IgG at 3 years and IgA, IgE and IgD at about 14 years. IgA in saliva reaches adult levels at about 6 weeks after birth.

Immunoglobulin Deficiency

Genetic Deficiencies. Primary genetic immunoglobulin deficiencies are rarer than secondary deficiencies. They are most often sought in children with recurrent infections or a combination of infections with allergy. They are, however, occasionally fortuitously recognized in the laboratory during electrophoresis done for other purposes. A number of classifications have been proposed but the WHO classification[1] is to be recommended. In view of their complexity it is not proposed to discuss them in detail (Table 28.4).

Decreased synthesis of most or all immunoglobulin classes has been described in a number of the familial syndromes, the most well known of which are infantile X-linked agammaglobulinaemia (Bruton form) and the severe combined immunodeficiencies (SCID). SCID is a combined B- and T-lymphocyte deficiency and patients usually die of viral infections. Agammaglobulinaemia is usually associated with pyogenic bacterial infections.

Selective immunoglobulin deficiency may affect all classes but primary IgA deficiency is by far the most common, with an incidence of about 1/500 of the population. It is usually symptomless but may be associated with gastrointestinal, respiratory or renal infections. Affected people have a higher incidence of immune complex disease.

The early diagnosis of immune deficiency is important if adequate treatment is to be instituted. Simple electrophoresis is inadequate as selective immunoglobulin deficiencies may be difficult to recognize; quantitative immunoglobulin measurements are essential. In newborn infants the low levels of serum immunoglobulins make the diagnosis difficult and if panhypogammaglobulinaemia or IgA deficiency are suspected salivary IgA measurements are very useful after 6 weeks of age when this immunoglobulin matures to adult levels.

Secondary Deficiencies. Secondary deficiencies are 10–100 times more common than primary deficiencies and may occur in about 4% of hospital patients.

Transient immunoglobulin deficiency in the newborn is important in premature babies. As can be seen from Fig. 28.4 the majority of maternal IgG crosses the placenta in the last trimester of pregnancy and the baby's own IgG does not reach acceptable levels until 6 months after birth. Those babies born before 22 weeks will have severe hypogammaglobulinaemia and those born before 34 weeks may develop it within 2 months. Some 4% of full-term infants show delayed maturation of IgG synthesis and may have a temporary hypogammaglobulinaemia lasting several months. The maturation of salivary IgA to normal levels by 6 weeks after birth and a rising serum IgM is a good indication that a baby will eventually acquire normal immunoglobulin synthesis. Careful

TABLE 28.4
THE PRIMARY IMMUNOGLOBULIN DEFICIENCIES

Deficiency	Immunoglobulins affected	T cells affected	Comments
Severe combined immunodeficiency Swiss type Sex-linked form	All classes	+	Die of severe fungal and viral infections in infancy
Combined immunodeficiency With thymoma With achondroplasia With thrombocytopenia and eczema	All classes Variable	+ Deficient response	Severe viral and fungal infections ?Defect in afferent limb of immunity
Hypogammaglobulinaemia X-linked, Bruton type Common and variable type	All classes	Normal	Pyogenic infections
Selective immunoglobulin deficiency Selective IgA and IgM deficiency (type I) Selective IgG and IgA deficiency (type II) Selective IgG deficiency (type III) Selective IgA deficiency (type IV) Selective IgM deficiency (type V) IgG subclass deficiency	IgA and IgM IgG and IgA IgG IgA IgM IgG subclasses	Normal Normal Normal Normal Normal Normal	Giardiasis common Respiratory tract infections Pyogenic infections Common—1/500 of the population Septicaemia occurs after splenectomy Pyogenic infections

TABLE 28.5
SECONDARY IMMUNOGLOBULIN DEFICIENCIES

Disorders of immunoglobulin synthesis (IgM ↓ ↓, IgA ↓, IgG N or ↓)
Lymphoid neoplasia—especially myelomatosis; chronic lymphatic leukaemia; lymphosarcoma
Toxic factors:
  uraemia
  corticosteroid therapy
  coeliac disease
  diabetes mellitus
Delayed maturation of immunoglobulin production in the neonate (all immunoglobulins affected)

Excessive immunoglobulin catabolism (IgG ↓ ↓, IgA ↓, IgM N or ↓)
Exogenous loss:
  nephrotic syndrome
  protein-losing enteropathy
  burns
Endogenous hypercatabolism:
  most causes of exogenous protein-loss malnutrition
  dystrophia myotonica (IgG only affected)

Decreased IgG transfer to the fetus
Prematurity

follow-up and treatment of infection are essential during the first year of life.

IgG has the longest half-life of the plasma immunoglobulins (22 days) and thus any factors increasing immunoglobulin catabolism will affect IgG most. Protein loss results in an increased endogenous catabolism of most plasma proteins and while proteins synthesized in the liver also show a marked increase in synthesis, immunoglobulins do not. The result is a progressive decrease in IgG, which may be reduced to levels of 1 g/L even despite small external losses, as for example in a selective glomerular proteinuria. Conditions giving rise to catabolic hypogammaglobulinaemia are shown in Table 28.5. This type of hypogammaglobulinaemia rarely gives rise to serious infection because the adaptive immune response is still intact with normal production of IgM and IgG in response to antigenic challenge.

Suppressed synthesis of immunoglobulins affects IgM most, then IgA and IgG least. The most

TABLE 28.6
SOME DISORDERS ASSOCIATED WITH POLYCLONAL
HYPERGAMMAGLOBULINAEMIA

Predominant increase in IgM
Congenital toxoplasma, rubella, syphilis
Primary biliary cirrhosis: marked ↑ in IgM
Q-fever endocarditis
Brucellosis
Malaria, trypanosomiasis, filariasis
Most primary viral infections

Predominant increase in IgG
Systemic lupus erythematosus: IgM often also ↑
Hypergammaglobulinaemic purpura
Chronic aggressive hepatitis: IgM often also ↑
Kala azar
Leprosy: IgM often also ↑

Predominant increase in IgA
Liver cirrhosis: may be associated with ↑ IgG
Crohn's disease
Ulcerative colitis
Fibrocystic disease
Bronchiectasis
Pulmonary tuberculosis
Sarcoidosis
Dermatomyositis
Rheumatoid arthritis
Pyelonephritis

common cause is lymphoid neoplasia, which may take months or years to manifest its effect. 'Toxic' factors may give rise to a similar picture (Table 28.5). There is a very real risk of infection in this type of immune deficiency as B-cell proliferation is suppressed and the immune response to antigenic challenge is progressively lost.

Polyclonal Hypergammaglobulinaemia
In most situations where an immune response is occurring, whether they are infections, immune-complex diseases, or autoimmune conditions, a polyclonal increase in immunoglobulins is seen. In certain conditions the immunoglobulin classes respond in a selective manner and may provide some clinically useful information. In general, however, immunoglobulin measurements provide little more information than is available on examination of the electrophoretic strip. For a detailed discussion see Hobbs.[2] An example of the patterns that are seen is shown in Table 28.6. In general terms autoimmune and immune-complex diseases give rise to a selective increase in IgG; skin, gut, respiratory and renal disease, particularly if associated with infection, stimulate the mucosal IgA system with increased serum IgA; organisms invading the bloodstream give rise to an increase in IgM.

Immunoglobulin measurements are useful in diagnosing infection *in utero* and in the first 6 months of life. The rise in normal IgM after birth is due to the first antigenic challenges met by the infant. Intrauterine infection may give rise to IgM production before birth, with high levels of cord blood IgM. This is particularly useful in aiding the diagnosis of congenital toxoplasmosis, rubella, cytomegalovirus, herpes simplex and syphilis, the so-called TORCH agents.

One of the areas in which the differential pattern of immunoglobulin response may be useful is in liver disease. A dominant and often very high level of IgM is typical of primary biliary cirrhosis. A mild IgM response is also seen early on in acute infective hepatitis, where it represents the response to primary antigenic challenge. It is also seen in infectious mononucleosis with or without liver involvement as this is usually a primary infection. IgG is raised in chronic aggressive hepatitis, while IgA is typically high in the macronodular Laennec type of cirrhosis, regardless of the cause.

IgE measurement has a role in the management of asthma and allergy, particularly in children, where high IgE levels are associated with extrinsic asthma and a good response to certain therapeutic regimens. The measurement of antigen-specific IgE by radioallergoabsorption techniques (RAST) or enzyme-linked immunosorbent assay (ELISA) gives similar information to skin tests in the identification of substances to which a patient is allergic. It is, however, useful in situations where skin testing is difficult (e.g. eczema) or dangerous (e.g. allergy to bee or wasp venom).

Oligoclonal Hypergammaglobulinaemia
Not infrequently a raised γ-globulin may be of restricted heterogeneity due to the response of relatively few B-cell clones to antigenic challenge. Such oligoclonal gammopathies show faint bands or zones in the γ-region on electrophoresis (*see* Fig. 28.17). These are often multiple and are usually distinguishable from true paraproteins (the product of a single clone of B cells) by the presence in different bands of both types of light chain on immunoelectrophoresis or immunofixation. Such restricted heterogeneity of immune response is a characteristic of chronic immune stimulation, where there is progressive switching-off of B-cell clones leaving only those with the highest-affinity receptors for the antigen still producing immunoglobulin. It is seen in chronic active hepatitis, chronic infections, immune-complex disease, and in viral infections in young children, particularly in the presence of partial immune deficiency where fewer B-cell clones are available to respond.

Monoclonal Hypergammaglobulinaemia
Immune stimulation usually results in a more or less heterogeneous population of B lymphocytes undergoing multiplication and differentiation to form plasma cells producing immunoglobulin directed against a wide range of antigenic configurations. This is because almost all macromolecular antigens have multiple antigenic sites. Under special conditions a restricted number of clones or a single clone may

TABLE 28.7
MALIGNANT B-CELL TUMOURS RESULTING IN MONOCLONAL COMPONENT

Disease	MC type	Incidence of MC (%)	Incidence of Bence–Jones (%)
Myelomatosis	IgG	50.0	60
	IgA	25.0	70
	IgM	0.5	100
	IgD	1.5	100
	IgE	0.1	Most
	Bence–Jones protein only	20.0	All
Soft-tissue plasmacytoma	Similar distribution to myelomatosis		
Waldenström's macroglobulinaemia	IgM	All	80
Non-Hodgkin's lymphoma	IgM, occasionally IgG or IgA	20.0	20
Chronic lymphatic leukaemia	IgM, occasionally IgG or IgA	15.0	15

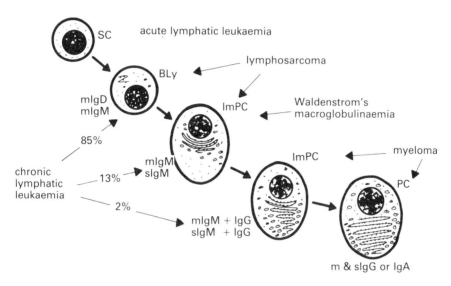

Figure 28.5 B-cell tumours classified according to their immunoglobulin production and cell type in relation to the normal maturation pathway of B lymphocytes: SC, lymphocyte stem cell; BLy, mature B lymphocyte; ImPC, immature plasma cell; PC, plasma cell; m, membrane-bound immunoglobulin; s, secretory immunoglobulin.

respond, provoking an oligoclonal gammopathy or occasionally monoclonal immunoglobulin production. Malignant proliferation of a single clone of immunoglobulin-producing B cells may also result in the production of a homogeneous population of immunoglobulin molecules with reference to class, subclass, light-chain type and charge. Such 'paraproteins' form discrete bands on electrophoresis. In recent years the term *monoclonal component* (MC) has been widely accepted to describe the serum immunoglobulin. The underlying B-cell proliferation is known as a *monoclonal gammopathy* (MG).

Aetiology and Incidence. The incidence of MC depends both on age and on the population under consideration. In a healthy population under the age of 60 years the incidence is about 0.2% and most of these are apparently benign and presumably reflect restric-

ted clonal response to antigenic challenge. In the age group over 90 years the incidence becomes something of the order of 17–19%, with a higher incidence of malignant B-cell tumours. Hospital populations show a majority of cases of malignant origin.[3]

The causes of malignant MC are listed in Table 28.7.

The malignant proliferation of B lymphocytes may be thought of as representing populations of cells that have undergone neoplastic transformation at various stages during the maturation process (Fig. 28.5). The B-cell lymphomas and chronic lymphatic leukaemias are typified by small lymphocytes with little capacity for immunoglobulin synthesis except for small quantities of IgM. Some 15% of such tumours produce detectable amounts of immunoglobulin. Waldenström's macroglobulinaemia is a lymphoma comprising intermediate B lymphocytes with the capacity to synthesize considerable quanti-

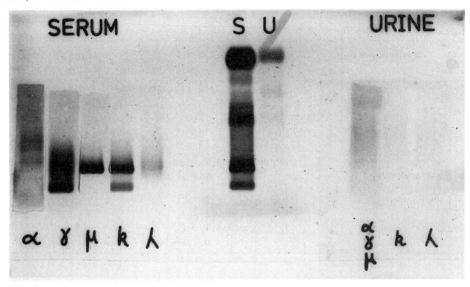

Figure 28.6 Immunofixation of a biclonal MC, S and U represent simple agarose electrophoresis of serum and urine: two MC are present in the serum. Immunofixation of the serum with antisera to immunoglobulin H chains (α, γ and μ) and κ and λ light chains reveals an IgM-κ, and IgG-κ MC. This probably represents a 'switch cell clone' transcribing both IgM and IgG H chains with the same V-region and L-chain segments. There is no Bence-Jones protein in the urine.

ties of IgM, producing high serum levels, which often give rise to the hyperviscosity syndrome. Skeletal manifestations are rare and like the lymphomas and chronic lymphatic leukaemia there is anaemia and lymphadenopathy. Myeloma is a malignant proliferation of more or less mature plasma cells, which most often secrete IgG and less commonly IgA and rarely IgD, IgM or IgE. IgA and IgG_3 may polymerize to cause hypercosity but the disease usually presents with bone involvement, pain or fracture, infection due to immune paresis and renal failure.

MC not associated with malignant MG may be associated with the conditions that give rise to the oligoclonal gammopathies. Such disorders are known as *monoclonal gammopathies of undetermined significance* (MGUS).

Laboratory Investigations. The investigation of MC is one of the most important protein studies carried out in laboratories.[4] The aim of the investigation is to establish the monoclonal nature and type of the MC, provide biochemical evidence of the likelihood of a malignant origin, and perform precise estimation of MC concentration for monitoring therapy.

1. *Establishment of monoclonality.* The existence of an MC must first be established by simple electrophoresis. If it is not detectable by these means then there is little likelihood of detection by immuno-elec-trophoresis unless it is hidden beneath another fraction on the electrophoretic separation. Immunofixation, however, increases the sensitivity of electrophoretic detection and may reveal MC not discernible

by simple electrophoresis; this is particularly true of Bence–Jones protein in serum or urine. Immunofixation or immunoelectrophoresis against monospecific antisera to H and L chains will enable identification and confirmation of monoclonality by the presence of a single class of H chain and one type of L chain. Immunofixation (Fig. 28.6) is by far the most reliable technique and will rapidly replace immunoelectrophoresis for these purposes.

The H-chain type of paraprotein is clinically very relevant as its nature may allow a search for the appropriate type of B-cell tumour in a previously undiagnosed case. For example, an IgM MC is most unlikely to be due to myeloma so that skeletal radiographs are unimportant but examining for enlarged lymph nodes is essential. In established myeloma the complications of the disease are very different with different immunoglobulin classes (Table 28.8).

2. *The presence of immunoglobulin fragments* is one of the most important criteria of malignancy (Table 28.9).[4] Their production by a B-cell clone suggests dedifferentiation and failure of normal immunoglobulin synthesis. Such fragments include free immunoglobulin L chains (Bence–Jones protein), IgM monomer, half-molecules and molecules with deletions.

Bence–Jones protein (BJP), monoclonal free light chain, is by far the most important of the fragments and its presence in urine is a strong but not invariable indication of a malignant B-cell tumour. However, it is important to remember that all plasma cells produce a slight excess of light chains, which are released from

TABLE 28.8
COMPLICATIONS ASSOCIATED WITH DIFFERENT IMMUNO-
GLOBULIN CLASSES IN MYELOMA

IgG myeloma
Mean half-life of MC 13 days, therefore MC reaches high
   levels
If MC level exceeds 80 g/L polymerization and hyperviscos-
   ity is likely, especially if IgG3
Immune paresis common
Amyloid less common than other types
Cryoglobulinaemia in about 2% of cases

IgA myeloma
Mean half-life of MC 5 days; lower levels reflect the same
   tumour mass as higher levels of IgG
Hypercalcaemia is common
Amyloid occurs in 5–10% of cases
Renal failure common even in the absence of Bence–Jones
   protein

Bence–Jones protein myeloma
Probably faster-growing tumour
Amyloid most common
Renal failure and hypercalcaemia more common than
   other types

the cells and pass through the renal glomerulus to be
largely reabsorbed in the proximal tubule. Increased
amounts of polyclonal light chain may be detectable
in the urine in conditions associated with polyclonal
hypergammaglobulinaemia or renal tubular damage.
It is thus essential to establish the monoclonality of
the light chains by immunofixation of adequately
concentrated (usually 300×) urine. It is important to
look for BJP not only as an indication of malignancy
but also in the investigation of a suspected B-cell
tumour in the absence of a serum MC, as some 20%
of myelomas have only BJP production from the
tumour. Such tumours may be more dedifferentiated
and aggressive.

Bence–Jones protein is usually found in the plasma
only in the presence of glomerular failure. It may
damage the renal tubule causing obstruction and
'myeloma kidney' and it may be responsible for amyloid formation.

3. *MC measurement* is important for a number of
reasons. The absolute level provides some indication
of the probability of malignancy, while a rising level is
a strong indicator of a proliferating malignant clone.
The MC is of course a tumour marker *par excellence*
and the level is useful for monitoring therapy of all
types of B-cell tumour. Immunochemical quantitation
is unsatisfactory as it may provide inaccurate results,
which vary enormously between batches and between
manufacturers of antisera. In addition, some turbidimetric arrays may pass into antigen excess. The most
satisfactory method is to quantitate on the basis of
densitometric scanning of an electrophoretic strip.

4. *Measurement of the immunoglobulins other than
the MC* is also useful in assessing the probability of

malignancy (Table 28.9) and in anticipating the complication of immune deficiency in known B-cell
tumours.

The Heavy-chain Diseases. Some monoclonal B-cell
tumours may produce only immunoglobulin H
chains. The most important of these, α-heavy chain
disease, is associated with gut lymphomas in people
predominantly of Mediterranean and Middle Eastern
origin. The diagnosis depends upon the demonstration of free H chains by immunoselection techniques.
An obvious MC may be absent due to postsynthetic
heterogenecity of the heavy chains.

Cryoglobulins. These may be simple monoclonal immunoglobulins that precipitate in the cold (type I).
Many MC have this characteristic when cooled to
4°C but are likely to be clinically significant only if
they precipitate above 22°C (Figs. 28.7 and 28.8).
Their presence is hence an important reason for
failing to detect a MC because it has precipitated in
transit to the laboratory and has been spun down
with the cells when the sample has been separated!

Cryoglobulins may also comprise immunoglobulin–anti-immunoglobulin complexes. These are
most often monoclonal IgM with antiIgG activity
complexed to IgG (monoclonal rheumatoid factor,
type II) but may be polyclonal, type II (polyclonal
rheumatoid factor). In all types of cryoglobulin the
aggregated immunoglobulin may activate complement and give rise to vasculitis.

If the diagnosis is suspected the blood must be
collected and separated at 37°C. If a precipitate then
appears on cooling it may be washed in saline at 4°C
and subjected to immunofixation to establish whether
it is monoclonal or polyclonal. Monoclonal rheumatoid factors may be dissociated from their IgG antigens by treatment with mercaptoethanol or dithioth-
reitol prior to electrophoresis. The immunoglobulin
present in the cryoprecipitate may be quantitated.

The Complement System
Physiology. The complement system comprises a
group of proteins which, following activation, interact with each other in a sequential fashion to produce
biological effector molecules that facilitate the elimination of antigens by lysis and phagocytosis. The
sequence of events may be summarized as follows
(Fig. 28.9).

1. Tissue is invaded by antigen, which is bound by
   specific antibody with activation of C1 by the
   Fc region of the immunoglobulin molecule.
   Complement may also be activated directly via
   the alternative pathway by bacterial lipopolysac-
   charide and at various points in both pathways
   by proteolytic enzymes released from leucocytes.
   Complement effector molecules are produced
   (the anaphylatoxins C3a and C5a), which cause
   histamine release from mast cells and result in
   smooth muscle contraction and vascular permeability. Oedema and stasis result, with passage

Criterion	Benign	Malignant
Immunoglobulin fragments:		
Bence–Jones protein	Trace amounts detectable occasionally	Often present
Monomeric IgM	Rarely present	Often present
Heavy-chain fragments	May occur due to degradation	Present in certain conditions
Suppression of normal immunoglobulins	Rare—unless MC associated with immune deficiency	Common and progressive— especially IgM
MC level	IgG usually not > 20 g/L IgA usually not > 10 g/L	High concentrations common
Progressive increase in MC concentration	Transient increase may occur	Almost invariable

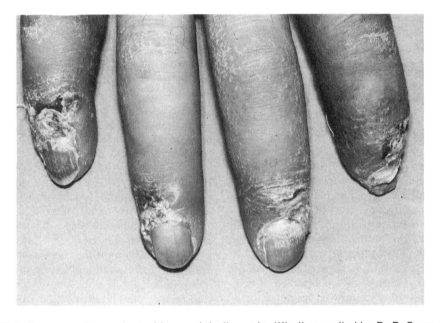

Figure 28.7 Digital gangrene in a patient with cryoglobulinaemia. (Kindly supplied by Dr P. Copeman.)

of further antibody and complement into the infected extravascular space.

2. The spread of infection is limited by thrombosis of surrounding blood vessels due to complement-induced platelet aggregation and intravascular coagulation.

3. Complement-derived chemotaxins (C3a, C5a and C567) result in migration of phagocytes into the area.

4. Phagocytes and killer cells adhere to the antigen by receptors for immunoglobulin Fc and complement (C3b, C3d and C4b) with phagocytosis and proteolytic destruction of the foreign material.

5. Cellular antigens may be lysed by complement (C5–9 complex).

The proteins of the system share a number of important properties. Proteolytic cleavage of some components by the ones preceding them in the path-way results in sequential activation producing low molecular-weight activation or conversion products that possess biological activities. Such cleavage may also result in the formation of binding sites for other components, allowing assembly of component complexes, and binding sites for cell membranes, resulting in transfer from the fluid phase to the cell surface. Control is exerted by the short half-life of active sites and by the presence of inhibitors at various points in the pathway.

A simple view of the classical and alternative pathways is presented in Fig. 28.10. It is probable that the alternative pathway is continuously cycling at a low level and that input either results from the generation of C423b by classical pathway activation or by protection of spontaneously generated C3bB from inactivation by C3b inactivator (C3b INA) and β_1H; alternative pathway activation. In both cases the feedback loop accelerates and C5 activation occurs. This pathway thus acts as a positive feedback loop.

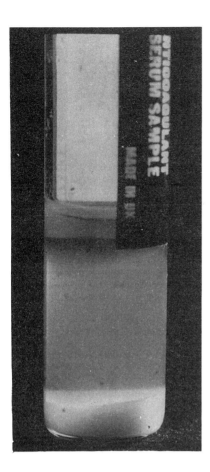

Figure 28.8 Serum from a patient with cryoglobulinaemia as seen after standing at 4°C. (Kindly supplied by Professor J.R. Hobbs.)

The Value of Complement Measurements in Disease. The complement pathway is thus an important part of the antibody-mediated immune defence mechanism. It is also able to interact directly, via the alternative pathway, with certain antigens resulting in effector mechanisms causing phagocytosis, inflammation and antigen elimination. This may in fact be the more important aspect of complement function, resulting in the immediate non-adaptive elimination of antigens.

Genetic deficiencies or defects in complement proteins may result in decreased resistance to infection and possibly to persistence in the host of viruses that may be responsible for chronic immune-complex disease. Deficiencies of inhibitors in the complement pathway may result in spontaneous activation of complement with the production of effector molecules causing disease. In these conditions, laboratory investigations are aimed at measuring the concentration or function of the affected proteins. Complement may also be the mediator of tissue damage in diseases associated with the deposition of antibody–antigen complexes within the vascular system. Complement is activated by the Fc region of antibody molecules within complexes that have adhered to vascular endothelium. Effector molecules are produced, which cause vascular permeability and chemotaxis of phagocytes that damage endothelial cells by releasing lysosomal and granule enzymes. The involvement of complement in the disease process results in consumption of some components whose concentration in the plasma falls with the production of detectable breakdown products. Labo-

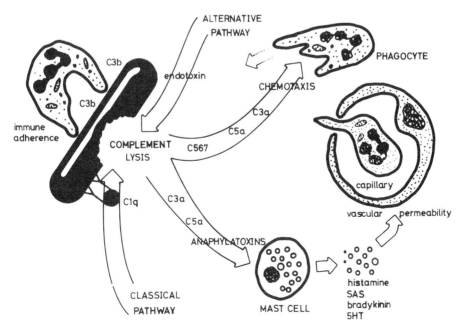

Figure 28.9 The role of complement in the defence against micro-organisms. Only the most important functions are shown.

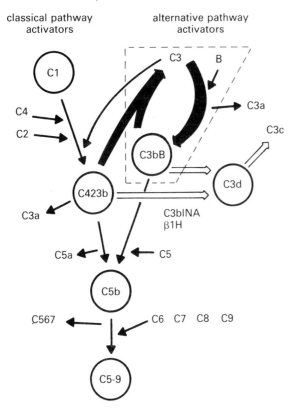

classical pathway
activators

alternative pathway
activators

Figure 28.10 Complement may be activated by either the classical or alternative pathways. Classical pathway activation usually results from antibody–antigen complexes activating C1. This initiates a proteolytic cascade generating C5b on to which C6–C9 assemble to form the lytic complex. The alternative pathway is a cycle that is activated directly by the protection of C3bB from the inhibitors C3INA and β1H (signified by a broken line) allowing the positive feedback loop to accelerate. The cycle is maintained by the low-level spontaneous generation of C3bB from C3 and B in the presence of Mg^{++} and factor D. C423b will also activate the cycle, thus amplifying classical pathway activation. Both pathways produce the lytic complex, the opsonins C3b and C3d, the chemotoxins C3a, C5a and C567, and the anaphylatoxins C3a and C5a.

ratory investigation may use both of these characteristics to indicate the presence of active immune-complex deposition in the vascular system and to monitor therapy for such immune-complex disease.

Inherited deficiencies of complement components. Genetic deficiencies of most of the complement components have now been described and fall into a number of clinically defined groups.

1. Deficiencies of the early part of the classical pathway, C1, C4 and C2, are associated with immune-complex diseases, especially systemic lupus erythematosus (SLE)-like syndromes. It would seem that the early classical pathway while being unimportant in the defence against bacteria may be important in the case of viruses that may be implicated in such immune-complex diseases as SLE. C2 deficiency is by far the most common and immunochemical assays for this protein are available.

2. Deficiencies of the alternative pathway have been identified and are associated with severe bacterial infections.

3. Deficiencies of the C5–C9 sequence have shown a striking association with Neisserial infections, suggesting that lysis is important in the elimination of these organisms. Some of these defects are functional in nature with normal immunochemically measured component concentrations.

4. Inherited deficiency of the inhibitor of activated C1, C1-esterase inhibitor (C1 INA), or hereditary angioneurotic oedema, is the most common, clinically important inherited deficiency within the complement system. Patients suffer from recurrent attacks of peripheral, bronchial and gastrointestinal oedema (Fig. 28.11). Spontaneous activation of C1 occurs with consumption of C4 and C2 but not of C3 or later components. It is probable that C1 activation is caused by proteolytic digestion of C1 by plasmin for which C1 INA is also an important inhibitor. A peptide that induces vascular permeability, released from C2, causes the oedema. Eighty per cent of patients have low levels (10–20% of normal) of C1 INA and are probably heterozygotes for a dominant gene. Twenty per cent have normal immunochemically measured levels of C1 INA but with a nonfunctional protein. A functional inhibitor assay is thus essential in investigating this disease. A low serum level of C4 is almost invariable and may be used as a screening test. The diagnosis is particularly important as there is a high mortality untreated and treatment with the anabolic steroids stanozolol and danazol is very effective.

Complement as an indicator system in immune-complex disease. Immune complexes in plasma may be measured directly by a number of methods varying enormously in their sensitivity and specificity. Evidence of complement activation may be used to infer the active deposition of immune complexes.

During the process of complement activation by immune complexes, several complement components are consumed, lowering their plasma levels, and activation products are produced, which may be detected in plasma. Either or both of these facets of complement activation may be used to infer immune-complex deposition but a number of factors must be taken into consideration.

1. Many complement components are acute-phase reactive proteins, their plasma levels rising in

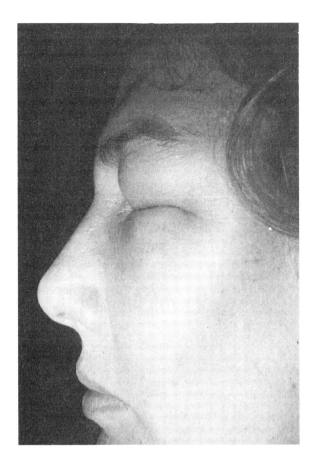

Figure 28.11 The typical features of facial oedema due to C1-esterase inhibitor deficiency. (Kindly supplied by Dr R.P. Warin.)

inflammatory conditions and perhaps masking the decrease caused by consumption.

2. Proteolytic enzymes from damaged tissue may give rise to complement breakdown products similar to those of immune activation.

3. Immune complexes may be produced in showers of short duration, the clinical features of vascular damage appearing after complement has returned to normal.

4. The low molecular-weight complement-activation products may result in overestimation of some components by radial immunodiffusion and Laurell rocket immunoelectrophoresis.

5. Activation of complement occurs easily *in vitro* and in the presence of Ca^{2+} and Mg^{2+}. This can be largely avoided by simple precautions including the use of EDTA in samples.

With these provisos, complement measurement is useful in investigating symptoms which could be due to immune-complex deposition. It is also of value in

the diagnosis and management of a few diseases where the changes are clear-cut (Table 28.10).

Bacterial Shock. Complement activation occurs during bacteraemia especially with Gram-negative organisms that activate the alternative pathway. Complement effector molecules may be implicated in the shock syndrome and the detection of breakdown fragments has been used in the rapid diagnosis of this condition.[5]

Laboratory Measurement of Complement Components. Immunochemical assays for many components are now widely available and useful, but some techniques such as radial immunodiffusion suffer severe inaccuracy in the presence of breakdown products. Overestimation, especially of C3, may thus occur in the situation where low levels are being sought as an indication of immune-complex disease.

Function assays for the enzymatic activity of individual complement components are essential when investigating genetic defects in the complement pathway as some of them are of a functional nature with normal component concentrations. All components may be assayed by using the end-product of complement activation, lysis, as the indicator system.

The activation or breakdown products of C3 and factor B are separable from the native molecules on the basis of their different sizes and charges and may thus be detected by immunoelectrophoresis, crossed immunoelectrophoresis or immunofixation. In some cases, for example C3a and C3d, antisera that are specific for the fragments are available allowing immunochemical analysis.

PROTEINS ASSOCIATED WITH INFLAMMATION

Acute-phase Reactant Proteins

The acute-phase reactants are a group of proteins whose concentration increases in plasma as a result of tissue damage and inflammation (Table 28.11). They are mainly glycoproteins, synthesized in the liver, and the evidence suggests that they have roles to play as mediators and inhibitors of inflammation. In addition some members of the family may act as scavengers of toxic products released by phagocytosis or tissue damage.

Liver synthesis of this group of proteins is regulated in a complex way by the cytokines interleukin 1, interleukin 6, tumour necrosis factor and leukaemia inhibitory factor released from macrophages and other cells at the site of inflammation. Some proteins show a decreased synthesis in inflammation. These negative acute-phase reactants are comprised mainly of transport proteins such as albumin and transferrin.

Clinically their measurement is of considerable value in the detection, prognosis and therapeutic

TABLE 28.10

DISEASES IN WHICH COMPLEMENT ASSAYS ARE OF VALUE IN DIAGNOSIS OR TREATMENT IN EUROPE*

	Disease	*Investigations*
Inborn errors of complement metabolism	C1 esterase-inhibitor deficiency	Functional and immunochemical assay of C1 inhibitor
	Monocomponent deficiencies	Total haemolytic complement; functional and immuno-chemical assays of components
Systemic immune-complex disease	Systemic lupus erythematosus	Decreased C4 level with C3 conversion products present are the most reliable tests
	Rheumatoid vasculitis	Decreased C3 with C3 conversion
	Polymyalgia rheumatica	C3 conversion products
	Mixed cryoglobulinaemia	C3 conversion products
	Subacute bacterial endocarditis	Decreased total C3 and C4 with conversion products
	'Shunt' nephritis	Decreased total C3 and C4 with conversion products
Glomerulonephritis	Post-streptococcal	C3 decreased with conversion products; returns to normal in 2 months
	Mesangiocapillary	Persistent low C3 with conversion products and normal C4; factor B conversion products may be found
Shock syndromes	Gram-negative bacteraemia	Decreased total C3. C3 conversion products present; normal C4 level
		Decreased factor B with conversion products

*Complement assays may be very useful in a number of tropical diseases with immune-complex deposition or alternative pathway activation. (Reproduced with permission from Whicher J.T. (1978). The complement system: In *Immunochemistry in Clinical Laboratory Medicine* (A. Milford Ward, J.T. Whicher eds.) Lancaster: MTP Press.)

TABLE 28.11

ACUTE-PHASE PROTEINS

Protein	*Possible role in inflammation*	*Response time*
C-reactive protein	Opsonin	6–10 h
C3		
C4		
Factor B	Antigen elimination	2–4 days
C1 INA		
α_1-Antichymotrypsin	Protease inhibition	10 h
α_1-Antitrypsin		24 h
Orosomucoid	?	24 h
Haptoglobin	? protease inhibition	24 h
Caeruloplasmin	? Free-radical elimination	2–4 days
Fibrinogen	Coagulation	24 h
Serum amyloid A protein	?	6–10 h

monitoring of patients with tissue damage. Elevation will occur in almost any disease that involves tissue damage, in particular infections, trauma, burns, immune-complex and autoimmune diseases, and malignancy. Most commonly the concentration of all the acute-phase proteins changes roughly in parallel but in some conditions selective increases in certain proteins are seen. Acute-phase protein changes are often more sensitive indicators of disease activity than ESR, viscosity or leucocyte count. For example, C-reactive protein levels correlate better with joint damage than other variables in rheumatoid arthritis.[6] Caeruloplasmin reflects disease activity in Hodgkin's disease where other indices may be normal. C1 INA

levels are a sensitive indicator of response to therapy in some lymphomas.

Protease Inhibitors

Plasma contains a number of protease inhibitors. They have varying degrees of specificity and their function is to inhibit circulating proteases, such as those involved in the complement and clotting systems, or lysozomal proteases, which may be released during phagocytosis or cell damage and death. Most but not all of these proteins are acute-phase reactants. It is also clear that a number of interactions between cells such as macrophages depend upon tissue fluid

	%
PiM	80.5
PiMS	9.0
PiFM	5.0
PiMZ	3.0
PiFS	0.3
PiS	0.25
PiSZ	0.17
PiFZ	0.10
PiF	0.09
PiZ	0.03

All other phenotypes have a frequency of 0.01% or less

(Reproduced with permission from A. Milford Ward, (1978) 'α_1-Antitrypsin' in *Immunochemistry in Clinical Laboratory Medicine.* A. Milford Ward, J.T. Whicher eds. Lancaster, MTP Press.)

or membrane-bound proteases. This has led to the suggestion that the acute-phase reactive protease inhibitors may have an important role in immune regulation.

α_1-Antitrypsin (54 kDa)

It seems clear that while antithrombin III and C1 INA are mainly concerned with specific inhibition of circulating proteases involved in the dynamic systems of the coagulation, complement and kinin pathways, α_1-antitrypsin, α_1-antichymotrypsin and α_2-macro-globulin inhibit lysozomal proteases. They perform an important role in neutralizing these enzymes, which are released in particular during phagocytosis of particulate material by polymorphonuclear leucocytes. In this way tissue damage in areas of inflammation is limited. The consequences of failure of this inhibition are seen in α_1-antitrypsin deficiency (*see* below).

α_1-Antitrypsin is a protein with relatively low molecular weight, which is able to pass into all body fluids. It is most active against serine proteases such as trypsin and elastase but is known to bind and inactivate a number of lysozomal proteases such as collagenase (metal protease), cathepsin B1 (thiol protease) and cathepsin D (carboxyl protease).

A small peptide is cleaved from the molecule upon binding to the protease. It seems probable that α_1-antitrypsin scavenges proteases in the tissue fluids and returns to the plasma where the protease is handed on to α_2-macroglobulin, which traps proteases by enfolding them. The α_2-macroglobulin–protease complex has a very much shorter half-life than the α_1-antitrypsin–protease complex, being rapidly catabolized in the reticuloendothelial system.

Genetic Variation.

α_1-Antitrypsin shows marked genetic polymorphism, more than 30 distinct allotypes having now been described in this protease inhibitor (Pi) system. The genotypes are designated by the prefix Pi and letters such as B, C, D, E, E_2, F, G, I, L, M, M_2, M_3, M^{Malton}, N, P, S, V, W, W_z, C, Y, Y_2, Z and null. However, it is important to appreciate that this is simply an electrophoretic classification and several structural variants may give rise to the same 'electrophoretic allotype'. Thus other evidence such as disease association and population distribution is required to indicate genetic homogeneity. The various phenotypes may be identified by separating the different α_1-antitrypsins by electrophoretic techniques, of which isoelectric focusing is the most widely used. The protein shows considerable microheterogeneity on isoelectric focusing, which probably reflects post-transcriptional differences in the carbohydrate moiety of the molecule. Differences between allotypes may reflect the carbohydrate microheterogeneity superimposed upon charge differences caused by inherited amino-acid substitutions in the polypeptide backbone.

The enormous clinical interest in α_1-antitrypsin polymorphism has centred around genetic variants associated with disease. Certain allotypes, notably those that are clearly established as polymorphisms, result in decreased secretion of α_1-antitrypsin from the liver. The PiW gene has 80% of the production of PiM, PiS 60%, PiP 25%, PiZ 15% and Pi null 0%. If normal mean plasma levels for the genotype PiMM are taken as 100%, then levels for PiZZ are 15%, PiSS 60%, PiMZ 57.5% and PiMS 80%. The incidence of these phenotypes in the population is shown in Table 28.12.

The reason for the decreased liver secretion of these variants is unclear. It is, however, known that the Z variant, which accumulates in the liver cells, has a substitution of a glutamic acid residue by glycine. It is probable that this gives rise to a failure of maturation of the protein within the endoplasmic reticulum, as there is some evidence that the protein in the liver cells has a retained propeptide and has incomplete addition of carbohydrate side-chains.

Despite the disease associations the gene frequencies for S and Z variants are higher than would be expected for random mutation. It is possible that heterozygotes have a higher fertility due to the decreased inhibition of sperm acrosine and cervical mucolytic enzymes.

Association with Disease. Pulmonary emphysema is associated with phenotypes giving rise to severe deficiencies of α_1-antitrypsin, namely PiZZ and PiSZ, though recent evidence suggests an increased incidence of lower-lobe emphysema occurring late in life even in PiMS individuals. The normal elastic tissue of the lungs is dependent on elastic fibrils and the ground substance between the alveolar cells. The lung is continually exposed to inhaled particles such as dust and cigarette smoke, together with occasional bouts of bacterial infection. All these insults result in phagocytic activity with release of macrophage lysosomal enzymes and oxygen radicals, which further reduce α_1-antitrypsin activity by damaging a methionine residue at the active centre of the molecule. In the presence of adequate tissue-fluid concentrations of α_1-antitrypsin, the delicate elastic tissue of the lung is protected against such enzymes as elastase. In α_1-antitrypsin deficiency, proteolytic damage results in distension of air sacs and loss of elastic recoil—emphysema. Diagnosis is important as the incidence and severity of lung disease can be greatly reduced by avoiding smoking and air-polluted atmosphere. Respiratory tract infection should be treated vigorously.

Some 10–20% of PiZZ infants develop neonatal hepatitis and about one-third of these progress to fatal cirrhosis. A small proportion of PiZZ adults develop cirrhosis. All PiZZ individuals have PAS-positive inclusions in the hepatocyte, which can be shown by immunofluorescence to be α_1-antitrypsin. It is probable that such liver cells accumulate the protein, which they are unable to secrete, and are more susceptible to injury, succumbing to what could otherwise be mild viral infections. It is also probable that proteolytic damage occurs in the liver as a result of inflammation secondary to infection and, in the absence of α_1-antitrypsin, damage to the collagen and elastic framework of the liver lobule results in the disorganized regeneration typical of cirrhosis.

In the investigation of such cases and their families it is important to realize that simple measurement of α_1-antitrypsin may be inadequate, owing to the fact that concomitant infection may give rise to an acute-phase increase in α_1-antitrypsin which masks the deficiencies associated with the phenotypes PiMZ and PiSS. Even in acute illness it is unlikely that PiZZ or PiSZ individuals will attain normal levels. It is possible to use quantitative α_1-antitrypsin measurements as a screening test only if another acute-phase protein such as orosomucoid is measured in parallel.

Simple serum protein electrophoresis is quite adequate for the detection of the severe deficiency phenotypes PiZZ and PiSZ. Agarose electrophoresis gives better resolution of the α_1-region. Phenotyping is now best done by isoelectric focusing in polyacrylamide or agarose gel.

α_1-Antichymotrypsin (68 kDa)

This protein has a high inhibitory specificity for chymotrypsins *in vitro*. It does not show strong inhibition of any known lysosomal proteases and its role *in vivo* is unclear though it may inhibit cathepsin G. It is found in high concentrations in bronchial secretions and it has been suggested that it has a role in protecting mucosal surfaces from proteolytic damage. It is a very rapidly reacting and sensitive acute-phase reactant, only C-reactive protein showing a faster response. It is in this capacity that it is most often measured.

α_2-Macroglobulin (725 kDa)

α_2-Macroglobulin is a very important protease inhibitor, synthesized by liver and reticuloendothelial cells, which binds all known proteases. It is of great interest

that protease–α_2-macroglobulin complexes still retain proteolytic activity for small substrates and the evidence suggests that these may have a role to play in the inactivation of low molecular-weight lymphokines and complement chemotactic factors.[7] α_2-Macroglobulin is a large molecule mainly confined to the vascular compartment and experimental evidence suggests that protease may be transferred from α_1-antitrypsin to α_2-macroglobulin.

α_2-Macroglobulin does not behave as an acute-phase reactant. Its level is raised in children before adolescence and gives a characteristic appearance to the juvenile electrophoretic strip (*see* below). Levels increase in pregnancy and in women taking oral contraceptives and may be very raised in nephrotic syndrome (*see* below). Measurement has no established role in clinical practice.

C1-esterase Inhibitor (104 kDa)

This protein has already been mentioned in the section on complement. Besides inhibition of activated C1 it inhibits plasmin, thrombin and kallikrein. It is an acute phase reactant showing a marked increase in active lymphoid malignancy and it may be useful as a monitor of disease activity. Paradoxically a secondary deficiency may occur in association with the same types of tumour. This can result in the clinical picture of angioneurotic oedema.

Antithrombin III (65 kDa)

Antithrombin III is an inhibitor of thrombin and in particular of activated factor X. Low levels may be associated with a thrombotic tendency and a genetic deficiency is known. The contraceptive pill causes a reduction in plasma level of about 40%. There has been some interest in the measurement of this protein in users of oral contraceptive to indicate those who may develop thrombosis.[8]

Haptoglobin

The haptoglobins are a family of haemoglobin-binding glycoproteins present in plasma. The haptoglobin molecule binds two molecules of oxyhaemoglobin, the complex being rapidly removed from the circulation by reticuloendothelial cells. This prevents undue loss of iron by urinary excretion. Haemoglobin is continually released from red cells due to damage as they circulate through small vessels. This is illustrated by the drop in haptoglobin concentration that occurs following severe exercise such as cross-country running. Haemoglobin is also released in areas of inflammation due to capillary damage, stasis and rupture of red cells.

Structurally, haptoglobin comprises a four-chain molecule with two small α-chains and two larger β-chains that contain the carbohydrate moiety. It shows marked genetic polymorphism and the known mutations fall into three groups. Chromosomal rearrangement with an internal gene duplication has probably resulted in the formation of the α^2-chain from the smaller α^1-chain. Single point mutations at amino acid 54 on the α^1-chain result in two variant chains α^{1S} and α^{1F}. Alteration in control of the rate of synthesis of either the α- or β-chains results in reduced haptoglobin synthesis in a manner analogous to the thalassaemias. Such hypohaptoglobinaemia occurs in up to 12% of children among American blacks. The common allotypes are the α^1- and α^2-variants of the α-chain, which show marked differences in different populations. In Europe the haptoglobin α^1-allotype has a frequency of 0.31–0.45 while it is 0.77 in the Congo and 0.10 in certain areas of India. The result of this is that in Europe the phenotype incidences are Hp 1–1 < Hp 1–2 < Hp 2–2. The presence of the α^2-heavy chain in Hp 1–2 and Hp 2–2 allows polymerization of the molecule to occur with an increase in molecular weight from 85 000 for Hp 1–1 to over 220 000 for Hp 2–2 complexes. The mean plasma level for Hp 1–1 individuals is higher than for Hp 2–2. Hp 2–2 occurs with a higher overall population frequency than Hp 1–1 and as it has been derived from Hp 1–1 it is probable that it confers an evolutionary advantage.

Haemolytic anaemia and liver disease both result in decreased haptoglobin levels and some clinical value may be obtained from detecting these changes. In the absence of inflammation the plasma haptoglobin level is as sensitive as radiochromium-labelled red-cell survival in detecting haemolysis. Haptoglobin is an acute-phase reactant and its level is usually elevated in the plasma in trauma, burns, infection, allergic tissue damage, cancer and leukaemia.

Laboratory measurement is beset by the problem that the polymorphic forms Hp1–2, Hp2–2 are underestimated by gel techniques by as much as 20%. Nephelometry is more satisfactory.

Orosomucoid (44 kDa)

Orosomucoid or α_1-acid glycoprotein is a strong acute-phase reactant present at fairly high concentrations in human plasma. It has a very high carbohydrate content comprising a large number of sialic acid residues, which show microheterogeneity due to different sialyl–galactosyl linkages. The protein is synthesized in the liver and the nature of the carbohydrate side-chains is affected by circulating oestrogen levels. Plasma orosomucoid shows remarkable heterogeneity due to multiple amino-acid substitutions, a property shared only by the immunoglobulins. It is also clear that it shows considerable homology with the variable region of the immunoglobulin light chain, a part of the IgG H-chain and the haptoglobin α-chain, which is itself related to the immunoglobulins. This has led to the suggestion that orosomucoid evolved from the immunoglobulin lineage probably after the duplication of the primitive L-chain but before the formation of the H-chain.

The acute-phase responsiveness of orosomucoid

suggests a role in inflammation though as yet no convincing hypothesis for its function has been proposed. It is known to bind propranolol and various Δ^4-3-keto-steroids, particularly progesterone. It is found on platelet membranes and may mediate their adherence to collagen. In clinical practice it is a valuable acute-phase protein to measure in the monitoring of inflammatory disease.

Other Proteins of Inflammation

Blood coagulation is clearly an important part of the inflammatory reaction and it is not surprising that a number of clotting proteins, in particular fibrinogen, are acute-phase reactants. Little is known of the changes that occur in plasma kinins such as prekallikrein.

C-reactive Protein

C-reactive protein is a complex molecule of molecular weight about 140 000 composed of six identical subunits. It is normally present in plasma with a concentration of about 6 mg/L but rises to high levels in inflammation. It is in this capacity as an acute-phase reactive protein (*see* below) that it is widely measured in clinical practice. Little is known of its function but it is known to bind strongly to the C-polysaccharide of the pneumococcus and other glycopeptides containing N-acetylgalactosamine 6-phosphate as a terminal sugar residue. After complexing with the polysaccharide it is able to activate complement via C1 with the production of effector molecules, which could encourage phagocytosis. This has led to the suggestion that its function is that of a non-adaptive defence protein. It is also able to bind to DNA and may be responsible for clearing DNA released from damaged cells.

TRANSPORT PROTEINS

A number of proteins exist for the purpose of carrying biologically active molecules in the plasma (Table 28.13). Such transport subserves a number of roles. Molecules may be transported that would otherwise be relatively insoluble in plasma, such as bilirubin, lipids and fatty acids. Many substances are biologically inactive when bound to plasma proteins and the bound molecules, being in equilibrium with the free, provide a pool to buffer changes in the free fraction. Toxic substances may also be rendered inactive by protein binding. There is an increasing realization that binding proteins may interact with receptors or enzymes affecting the metabolism of those molecules they carry. For example, apolipoprotein C interacts with lipoprotein lipase, and transferrin binds to membrane receptors in facilitating the uptake of the iron which it carries.

Albumin (68 kDa)

Function
Albumin, along with C-reactive protein, is unique among the major plasma proteins in containing no

TABLE 28.13
TRANSPORT PROTEINS

Protein	Mol. mass (Da)	Mean concentration (g/L)	Substance transported
Albumin	68 000	40.0	(see Table 28.14)
Transferrin	77 000	2.8	Iron
Caeruloplasmin	130 000	0.35	(Copper)
Haptoglobin	100 000–400 000	2.0	Haemoglobin
Haemopexin	57 000	0.75	Haem
Prealbumin	55 000	0.3	Vitamin A, thyroxine
Retinol-binding protein	21 000	0.045	Vitamin A
Thyroxine-binding globulin	57 000	0.035	Thyroxine
Transcortin	55 700	0.030	Corticosteroids
Sex hormone-binding globulin	94 000	0.020	Androgens and oestrogens
Group component (Gc globulin)	51 000	0.55	Vitamin D
Transcobalamin I	60 000–70 000	0.00003	
II	38 000	0.000015	Vitamin B_{12}
III	60 000–70 000	0.000025	
Apolipoproteins		See Chapter 35	

carbohydrate residues. It is a single polypeptide chain containing a solitary thiol group, which, binding a half-cystine, results in the formation of albumin polymers *in vitro*.

Albumin binds a very wide range of substances, in particular lipid-soluble anions. Most of the circulating long-chain fatty acids in plasma are albumin bound to a hydrophobic site with a normal level of 1–2 molecules per molecule of albumin. The same two sites bind bilirubin and drugs such as salicylate, warfarin, phenylbutazone and clofibrate. They may displace each other, giving rise to dangerous increases of drug activity since only the free drug is active. Calcium is very weakly bound at 16 sites.

Albumin is also important as an intravascular colloid, maintaining the slightly higher oncotic pressure of plasma over tissue fluid, but this role may be largely taken on by other proteins in the absence of albumin. Many cells are able to use albumin as a source of amino acids and take it up by pinocytosis.

Genetic Variation
Twenty-three structural variants of albumin have been described. They are inherited in an autosomal codominant fashion and in the heterozygote give rise to a bisalbuminaemia on electrophoresis. Both albumin bands are usually of equal staining density as they represent the product of two genes. A number of variants, however, give rise to dimerization *in vivo* and may give rise to wide albumin bands or double bands of unequal density. None of these 'para-albumins' is associated with disease.

Analbuminaemia is rare. Small amounts of albumin are usually present and affected people suffer no symptoms or at most mild oedema.

Variation in Disease
The factors affecting normal albumin level are its volume of distribution, synthetic rate and catabolic rate. In most disease processes a change in more than one of these factors is operating (Table 28.14). Changes in albumin level during the menstrual cycle and in pregnancy reflect alterations in the volume of distribution. In inflammation a rapid increase in volume of distribution due to vascular permeability is followed by a cytokine-mediated fall in synthesis.

Hypoalbuminaemia is a remarkably reliable indication of illness but has little diagnostic specificity. In many diseases decreased albumin synthesis results from malnutrition, and the increased endogenous catabolism associated with injury and pyrexia may decrease the half-life of albumin from the normal 21 days to as little as 7.

Liver disease commonly results in hypoalbuminaemia. This is usually mild but may become severe if recovery is delayed. In cirrhosis the actual rate of hepatic albumin synthesis may be normal or even increased but much of the new albumin enters the hepatic lymph and leaks across the liver capsule directly into the ascitic fluid. Plasma albumin level is thus not a reliable indicator of synthetic route or functional hepatocellular mass.

Increased glomerular permeability results in urinary albumin loss and the nephrotic syndrome. Plasma concentrates below 20 g/L usually result in oedema. The amount of albuminuria is not a reliable prognostic indicator in nephrotic syndrome, especially in children where 'benign' minimal change nephritis often gives rise to the most severe albuminuria.

Gastrointestinal protein loss is a common and important cause of hypoalbuminaemia and may result from either inflammatory or neoplastic disease. Protein loss into the gut can be readily estimated by measuring α_1-antitrypsin clearance into the faeces or, less reliably but more simply, the faecal α_1-antitrypsin

TABLE 28.14
ALBUMIN CHANGES IN DISEASE

Disease	Synthesis	Loss	Degradation rate	Exchangeable pool
Liver disease	↓		↓	↑
Nephrotic syndrome	↑	↑	↑	↓
Protein-losing enteropathy	↑	↑	↑	↓
Malnutrition	↑		↓	↓
Acute burn	↑ ↓	↑	↑	
Cushing's syndrome	↑ ↑		↑ ↑	↑
Thyrotoxicosis	↑ ↑		↑ ↑	↑

level. This is possible because α_1-antitrypsin is not degraded by proteases in the gut.[9]

Transferrin (77 kDa)

Transferrin is the major iron-transport protein of plasma. It is synthesized both in the liver and some other tissues such as the reticuloendothelial system. It has two binding sites for iron, probably with different affinities, one at the N-terminal and one at the C-terminal end of the molecule.[10] This protein has a central role in iron metabolism, returning iron derived from the catabolism of haemoglobin and other proteins to haemopoietic tissue. Unlike some other transport proteins it is returned to the circulation after unloading its iron at the cell membrane.

The concentration of transferrin in the blood is increased in pregnancy when levels in the last trimester may be higher than those seen in any other condition. Elevated levels are also seen with oral contraceptive use. Iron deficiency results in increased hepatic synthesis with raised serum levels. The more severe and prolonged the iron deficiency, the higher the transferrin level will be.

Transferrin concentration is decreased in malnutrition, liver disease and inflammatory diseases such as rheumatoid arthritis. In this latter group the transferrin level, showing a negative acute-phase response, reflects the severity and chronicity of the disease.

In clinical practice transferrin measurement, either immunochemically or as iron-binding capacity, has a role in assessing the differential diagnosis of anaemia. Iron is usually measured in association with transferrin and the saturation of the protein calculated. Simple iron-deficiency anaemia is usually associated with a raised serum transferrin level with a low saturation whereas anaemia due to failure to incorporate iron into red cells has a normal or low transferrin level with a high saturation.

A high level of saturation with a normal transferrin is seen in haemochromatosis and other forms of iron overload, and is a useful measure for diagnosing and monitoring therapy. It has, however, been to some extent superseded by the measurement of serum ferritin.

As with most serum proteins a number of allotypes have been described, all of which are rare. Atransferrinaemia is a rare cause of iron-deficiency anaemia that is unresponsive to iron therapy.

Caeruloplasmin (130 kDa)

Caeruloplasmin is an exquisitely coloured sky-blue protein that carries 8 atoms of copper per molecule. It is synthesized in the liver and binds some 95% of plasma copper, the remainder being attached to albumin.

The function of the protein is very much under debate.[11] Studies with labelled copper show negligible *in vivo* turnover, suggesting that caeruloplasmin does not act as a physiological transport protein. Copper is probably transported from the gut to the liver on albumin. It is also clear that copper is attached to caeruloplasmin before its secretion from the liver cell and that an increased hepatic copper pool increases caeruloplasmin synthesis. Caeruloplasmin acts as a weak oxidant in plasma and it has been suggested that it has a physiological role in the oxidation of ferrous ions at the cell surface to the ferric form for binding to apotransferrin. *In vitro* studies have shown that caeruloplasmin has antioxidant activity inhibiting peroxidation by important catalysts such as iron. It is also possible that the protein may inactivate free radicals produced by phagocytosis, thus having a role in inflammation, a suggestion supported by its acute-phase behaviour.

The majority of patients with Wilson's disease have low plasma concentrations of copper and caeruloplasmin. The disease is characterized by copper deposition in tissues, especially the liver, leading to cirrhosis, and the brain, with damage to the basal ganglia. The disease is probably genetically heterogeneus but the defect appears to result in a failure of biliary copper excretion with subsequent accumulation in tissues. The evidence suggests that an intracellular copper-binding protein may be at fault, preventing copper from reaching the intracellular pool necessary for biliary excretion and attachment to caeruloplasmin. The low plasma caeruloplasmin is thus a result of decreased intracellular copper availability.

Low plasma concentrations of copper or caeruloplasmin are thus an important guide in the diagnosis of Wilson's disease; the demonstration of high levels of copper in the liver by biopsy is also important.

Plasma caeruloplasmin concentration is decreased in severe liver disease, notably in primary biliary cirrhosis and primary biliary atresia, and also in malabsorption. Caeruloplasmin concentrations are raised two-to threefold in the last trimester of pregnancy and during therapy with oestrogen-containing drugs. It is a slow acute-phase reactant showing increases especially in diseases involving the reticuloendothelial system, such as Hodgkin's disease where it may be used as an indication of disease activity. Concentrations are increased in infective and obstructive diseases of the biliary tract, probably due to decreased biliary excretion resulting in an increased hepatocellular copper pool with consequent induction of caeruloplasmin synthesis.

Other Transport Proteins

Plasma lipids are transported in macromolecular micellar structures solubized by specific transport proteins.

The hormone carrier proteins are listed in Table 28.13 above. In general their measurement is of importance in that it allows an assessment of the level of free, and thus biologically active, hormone present in plasma. The role of the retinol-binding protein–prealbumin complex in the transport of vitamin A is of interest.

Haemopexin (70 kDa) binds free haem entering the plasma from the breakdown of haemoglobin released by intravascular haemolysis. The haemopexin–haem complex is taken up by the liver where the iron is bound to intracellular ferritin and the remainder of the haem is converted by haem oxygenase to bilirubin. Decreased serum levels are seen in haemolysis, and, as this protein unlike haptoglobin is not an acute-phase reactant, the low levels persist even when those of haptoglobin are normal or raised due to inflammation.

ONCOFETAL AND TISSUE PROTEINS

It seems probable that many tissue proteins are shed into the plasma as a result of cell turnover. This is true for a number of enzymes and some cell membrane proteins such as β_2-microglobulin. It is also clear that some malignant tumours are able to re-express genes normally repressed in mature cells of that tissue. This results in the synthesis, and often the appearance in the plasma, of proteins typical of other adult tissues or fetal cells. Some of the tumour proteins of fetal type, oncofetal proteins, are related to the major histocompatibility antigens and thus to β_2-microglobulin. β_2-Microglobulin, α-fetoprotein and the placental proteins will be briefly described here.

β_2-Microglobulin (11 kDa)

β_2-microglobulin is a single polypeptide chain of 100 amino acids devoid of carbohydrate with one intrachain disulphide bridge. It is the light or β-chain of the cell-surface HLA antigen. The heavy chain is attached to the cell membrane and bears the allotypic determinants that denote HLA specificity.[12] The HLA complex is important in cell recognition and it is probable that β_2-microglobulin controls biosynthesis of the intact molecule in the same way that the immunoglobulin light chain controls biosynthesis of the intact immunoglobulin molecule. Many tumour-specific antigens have been shown to be immunologically cross-reactive with β_2-microglobulin and it has been suggested that they might be regarded as modified histocompatibility antigens.

β_2-Microglobulin is synthesized by almost all human cells; tumour cells and lymphocytes have particularly high production rates. The molecule is released from the cell surface and stimulation of lymphocytes has been shown to result in increased release. It is freely filtered at the glomerulus and reabsorbed in the proximal tubule, where it is degraded in lysosomes. Excretion thus depends on glomerular filtration rate and high plasma levels are seen in renal failure.

Urinary β_2-microglobulin excretion is a widely used means of assessing renal tubular damage. It has proved valuable in evaluating damage due to nephrotoxic drugs and industrial pollutants such as cadmium. It is probably no more useful than creatinine clearance in predicting transplant rejection. Recently it has become apparent that it is very unstable in acid urine.

Plasma concentrations of β_2-microglobulin closely reflect creatinine clearance but are also affected by increased production rates occurring in some malignant tumours. Measurement may have a role in monitoring tumours particularly those of B-cell origin. Chronic lymphatic leukaemia, B-cell lymphomas and myeloma usually have raised levels. Interestingly, MGUS have normal levels, suggesting a possible diagnostic role in differentiating these two important conditions. Several inflammatory conditions involving B-cell stimulation have raised plasma β_2-microglobulin concentrations, such as rheumatoid arthritis, systemic lupus erythematosus and Crohn's disease. Plasma β_2-microglobulin levels may be a marker of disease activity in hepatitis, when a fall to normal suggests healing and a persistent high level forebodes the development of chronic hepatitis. In all such β_2-microglobulin measurements it is important to relate blood concentrations to the creatinine concentration to eliminate changes due to variation in glomerular function.

α-fetoprotein (69 kDa)

α-Fetoprotein is present in trace amounts in normal human serum.[13] In the fetus it is produced by the

TABLE 28.15

CLASSIFICATION OF AMYLOID ON THE BASIS OF THE MAJOR PROTEIN COMPONENT

Pathological type	Protein component
Amyloid associated with B-cell tumour	AL protein
Amyloid secondary to infections and immune stimulation	Amyloid A protein (AA protein)
Amyloid associated with renal failure	β_2-microglobulin fragment
Senile amyloid	Amyloid S protein (AS protein)
Familial forms:	
Familial Mediterranean fever	AA protein
Portuguese amyloid	Fragment derived from prealbumin
Localized amyloid:	
Thyroid	Fragment of thyrocalcitonin
Pancreas	Fragment of ? insulin or glucagon?
Skin	

yolk sac, liver and to some extent by the gut. The fetal plasma level is highest at 13 weeks of gestation when it accounts for almost one-third of the total plasma proteins and is about one million times higher than the adult level. It falls rapidly towards birth, adult levels being achieved in the first 2 weeks of life.

The majority of pregnancies affected by open neural-tube defects are associated with raised levels of α-fetoprotein in amniotic fluid. Determination of amniotic fluid and maternal serum levels in the 15th–25th week of gestation have proved valuable in screening for such defects (*see* Chapter 13). Some 30–70% of patients with germ-cell tumours and 80% of patients with hepatocellular carcinoma have an elevated serum α-fetoprotein and this has proved useful in the diagnosis and monitoring of such tumours.

Little is known about the function of this protein. It has a number of albumin-like properties, which suggest that it may be a transport protein. It also has well-established immunosuppressive effects suggesting a role in maternal–fetal immune regulation.

PLASMA PRECURSORS OF AMYLOID

Amyloid is an amorphous extracellular substance composed of non-branching linear fibrils. It is found in association with a number of conditions (Table 28.15) and may result in extensive damage to the tissues in which it is deposited. Analysis of the protein content of fibrils has revealed the presence of a number of different proteins that characteristically occur in certain types of amyloid. Precursor proteins for all forms of amyloid have been found circulating in the plasma and the evidence suggests that amyloid deposition occurs as a result of the proteolytic degradation of circulating proteins producing fragments capable of polymerization and deposition in tissue. It is probable that for amyloid to persist there must also be defects in the enzymatic degradation and phagocytic removal of such fibrils. It is thus clear that, biochemically, amyloid represents a heterogeneous collection of diseases giving rise to fibril deposition in tissues.

P-component is a protein invariably present as a minor constitutent in the fibrils of all types of amyloid. It has been identified in plasma as an acute-phase reactant closely related in amino-acid sequence to C-reactive protein. The major component of amyloid associated with B-cell dyscrasias is a proteolytically derived fragment of the variable region of the immunoglobulin light chain. In secondary amyloid, on the other hand, AA protein of molecular weight 10 000 is found in the fibrils. This protein is a proteolytic fragment of circulating plasma AA protein, which is an acute-phase reactant also showing an increase in concentration with increasing age.

Other proteins have been found in specific forms of amyloid such as a fragment derived from prealbumin in Portuguese amyloid. Amyloid may thus be thought of as a disease resulting from the deposition in tissues of a heterogeneous group of proteins derived by proteolysis from circulating serum proteins. There is also evidence in the case of AA protein and IgG light chains that certain amino-acid sequences present in the precursor protein may produce fragments particularly likely to polymerize in tissue, thus giving some basis for the observed genetic nature of some forms of amyloid.

The measurement of serum amyloid components is of some clinical value in particular for the detection of monoclonal light chains (Bence-Jones protein) in the diagnosis of AL-type amyloid. This is best carried out by electrophoresis and immunofixation of the patient's urine and is, of course, of considerable importance as it allows diagnosis and thus treatment of the underlying B-cell neoplasm, often resulting in considerable clinical improvement. Prognosis in AA amyloid is related to serum levels of amyloid A protein and C-reactive protein.

INTERPRETATION OF ELECTROPHORESIS

Serum and Plasma

Electrophoresis, whether done on cellulose acetate or agarose, is of immense value in the preliminary investigation of plasma proteins. Many important abnor-

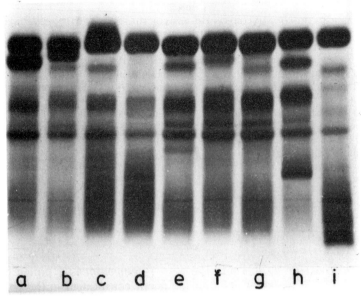

Figure 28.12 Examples of serum and plasma electrophoresis. Note the absence of the β_2-band due to C3 activation by freezing and thawing in all samples except (e). Samples (d) and (h) are plasma and contain a fibrinogen band.

(a) Bisalbuminaemia.

(b) Bisalbuminaemia, polymeric variant.

(c) Fast albumin due to bilirubin binding, slightly raised gammaglobulin (polyclonal IgG increase) with $\beta-\gamma$ fusion (IgA increase) in a patient with cirrhosis.

(d) Plasma from a patient with α_1-antitrypsin deficiency (PiZZ) with early cirrhosis resulting in a polyclonal increase in IgG.

(e) Mild acute-phase response with increased α_1 and α_2 zones in a patient with immune-complex disease. The β_2 band (C3) is visible but fainter than normal due to a low C3 (compare with Fig. 28.13 (e) and (f)).

(f) Fast α_1-antitrypsin variant in a patient with a slight acute-phase response.

(g) Slow α_1-antitrypsin variant (PiSS) in a child with an acute-phase response.

(h) Raised α_1, α_2 and fibrinogen in a patient with inflammation. Hp 1-1 phenotype resulting in a slightly fast α_2 zone.

(i) Low albumin, slow α_1-antitrypsin variant, decreased α_2 and increased gammaglobulin with oligoclonal IgG response in a patient with chronic aggressive hepatitis.

Reproduced with permission from Whicher J.T. (1980). The interpretation of electrophoresis. *Br. J. Hosp. Med.*, **24**, 348.

malities, such as genetic variants and MC may not be detected by specific protein quantitation alone. Agarose electrophoresis with amido-black staining will reveal proteins present in concentrations above 0.1 g/L. Some 10–13 components are usually clearly visible on the electrophoretic separation of serum or plasma (Figs. 28.12 and 28.13).

Prealbumin

This protein is usually faintly visible in normal individuals, particularly on cellulose acetate separations. Its disappearance is typical of liver cirrhosis, inflammation and malnutrition. High levels are seen in alcoholics.

Albumin

The albumin band shows an increased anodal mobility as a result of the binding of bilirubin, penicillin and acetylsalicylic acid and occasionally due to tryptic activity in acute pancreatitis. Certain variants may give rise to slow or fast bands usually seen in

the heterozygote as bisalbuminaemia. Albumin must be decreased by about 30% before a decrease in staining intensity is seen.

Albumin–α_1 Interzone

The staining intensity of this pale area is due to α_1-lipoprotein. A decrease is not easily recognized but occurs in severe inflammation, particularly of the liver while an increase is often seen in alcoholics, and women during puberty and pregnancy. Very high levels of α-fetoprotein such as occur occasionally in hepatoma may result in a band between the albumin and α_1-bands.

α_1-Zone

Orosomucoid and α_1-antitrypsin both migrate together but as orosomucoid stains poorly α_1-antitrypsin constitutes the great majority of the α_1-band. Greatly raised levels of orosomucoid do, however, give rise to an anodal broadening of the band. The acute-phase response is characterized by an increase in α_1-antitrypsin and thus of the α_1-band. A selective

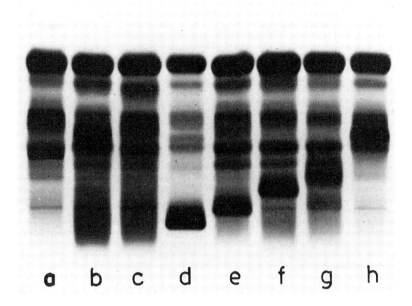

Figure 28.13 Examples of serum electrophoresis.

(a) Nephrotic syndrome. Prealbumin is visible; albumin is not noticeably decreased. There is a marked increase in the α_2 zone and in β-lipoprotein. The gammaglobulin reflects a hypercatabolic decrease in IgG secondary to the protein-losing state.
(b) Cathodal position and increased density of haptoglobin in a haemolysed sample or as a result of haptoglobin–haemoglobin complexes. Note clearly discernible α_2-macroglobin at the front of the α_2 zone where it normally fuses with haptoglobin.
(c) Simple acute-phase response with increased α_1 and α_2 zones.
(d) MC in a patient with myeloma. There is immune suppression with a pale γ-area and a decreased albumin. The split β is due to heterozygosity for a transferrin variant.
(e) IgG MC.
(f) IgG MC.
(g) IgA MC.
(h) IgA MC in the α_2 region.

Reproduced with permission from Whicher J.T. (1980). The interpretation of electrophoresis. *Br. J. Hosp. Med.*, **24**, 348.

increase of α_1 is a good indication of liver injury or increased oestrogen levels. An absence of increase with evidence of an acute-phase response in other proteins suggests the presence of a deficient α_1-antitrypsin allotype. Allotypes with altered electrophoretic mobility may be recognizable and homozygous PiZ individuals usually have virtually no visible α_1-band unless there is a marked acute-phase response. Children have lower α_1-antitrypsin levels than adults.

α_1–α_2-Interzone

Two very faint bands are usually seen just preceding the main α_2-band on agarose electrophoresis. These represent α_1-antichymotrypsin, inter-α-trypsin inhibitor and Gc globulin. They increase in intensity and coalesce in early acute inflammation as a result of a strong increase in α_1-antichymotrypsin.

α_2-Zone

This broad band is made up principally of α_2-macro-

globulin and haptoglobin. The genetic variants of haptoglobin possess different electrophoretic mobility. Haptoglobin 1–1, which is present in 15% of the population, has a faster mobility than α_2-macroglobulin and in fact covers the faint Gc-globulin and α_1-antichymotrypsin bands. Haptoglobin 1–2 and 2–2 migrate to the cathode side of α_2-macroglobulin, which is seen as the sharp leading edge of the α_2-zone. Haptoglobin is usually increased as part of the acute-phase response but a normal α_2-zone in the face of a raised α_1-band suggests enhanced haptoglobin catabolism as a result of haemolysis. This is often seen in malignancy and liver disease. Haptoglobin–haemoglobin complexes have a more cathodal mobility than haptoglobin and migrate in the α_2–β_1-interzone, where they are frequently seen in samples haemolysed *in vitro*. An increase in the sharp leading edge of the α_2-zone results from a high level of α_2-macroglobulin such as is often seen in normal children, in women either in pregnancy or taking oral contraceptives, and in the nephrotic syndrome.

$\alpha_2-\beta_1$-Interzone

Cold insoluble globulin (fibronectin) forms a sharp faint band between the α_2- and β_1-zones. It is precipitated by heparin and is thus not present in heparinized plasma. It is increased in pregnancy. β-Lipoprotein forms an irregular crenated band anywhere from the α_2 to the β_2-zones. The mobility is affected by concentration and by electrophoretic conditions. It is often visible on agarose but not usually on cellulose acetate when it overlays the α_2-band. An abnormal lipoprotein (lipoprotein $\times$) with low mobility is sometimes seen in the $\beta_1-\beta_2$-region in association with cholestasis.

β-Zone

Transferrin comprises the β_1-band seen in fresh samples, while native C3 forms the β_2-band. C3 breakdown whether *in vivo* or *in vitro* results in decreased intensity of the β_2-band with an increased intensity of the β_1-band owing to the more anodal mobility of C3c. Occasional splitting of the β_1-band is due to genetic variants of transferrin, which are not uncommon. An increased β_1-band is typical of iron-deficiency anaemia, while decreased levels are seen in malnutrition and liver disease. β_2-Intensity reflects native C3 levels and is therefore often decreased in serum samples and absent in frozen samples where *in vitro* C3 breakdown has occurred. Increased levels occur in the acute-phase response.

Fibrinogen

Plasma samples show a fibrinogen band in the $\beta-\gamma$-region, while a faint band in serum samples may be due to the presence of fibrinogen breakdown products formed as a result of allowing the serum to stand on the clot. Increased fibrinogen levels occur as part of the acute-phase response.

γ-Zone

In the normal γ-zone only the immunoglobulins are visible, though in pathological conditions other proteins may be seen. IgA has the most anodal mobility of the immunoglobulins and migrates in the $\beta-\gamma$ area. IgA deficiency is suggested by pallor in this area and high levels of IgA such as are commonly seen in cirrhosis and rheumatoid arthritis result in increased staining density, the so-called $\beta-\gamma$ fusion. Polyclonal IgM increases are difficult to recognize, while increase in IgG may involve all subclasses giving rise to a generalized increase in the γ-band, or may involve only fast or slow subclasses. Zones or faint bands in the γ-region are commonly seen in conditions giving rise to oligoclonal immunoglobulin responses; these suggest chronic immune stimulation and are commonly seen in chronic hepatitis and chronic viral infections.

MC are of immense importance and while usually present in the γ-region may fall anywhere on the separation, especially if they complexed with other proteins. Substances that may be mistaken for MC are occasionally seen. IgG aggregates produced by freezing and thawing samples and immune complexes produce diffuse bands at the origin. C-reactive protein typically forms a very narrow faint band in the mid-γ region. Lysozyme very rarely reaches high enough concentration in the plasma to be seen as a band cathodal to the slowest γ-band.

Infected Samples

Neuraminidase-producing bacteria contaminating samples may result in desialation of glycoproteins with all fractions except albumin and IgG running more cathodally than usual.

Cerebrospinal Fluid (CSF)

The investigation of CSF and urine proteins will be described in other sections of the book but brief mention will be made here of the electrophoretic appearances (Fig. 28.14). Ventricular and lumbar CSF differ enormously in protein content as the CSF reaching the lumbar cord has had time to equilibrate with plasma and consequently has a much higher content of plasma proteins. One of the most striking aspects of CSF electrophoresis is the strong prealbumin band. The α_1-zone is more cathodal than serum as a result of desialation of α_1-antitrypsin by brain neuraminidase. The α_2-zone is faint as high molecular-weight α_2-macroglobulin and haptoglobin polymers do not easily enter the CSF. Transferrin is present as two bands, in the native form in the β_1-position and as the desialated 'Tau protein' in the β_2. C3 is not visible in CSF and in fact has a slightly faster mobility than the Tau protein. The γ-region often contains a faint band in the mid-zone but the presence of multiple γ-bands is typical of intrathecal IgG synthesis such as occurs in disseminated sclerosis.

Urine

Glomerular proteinuria results in the passage of increased amounts of proteins with molecular weights above 60 000 into the urine. Thus in nephrotic syndrome albumin and transferrin are usually seen. Tubular damage results in the appearance of proteins not seen on serum electrophoresis such as the α_2-microglobulins and β_2-microglobulin. Bence–Jones protein may appear as a band *anywhere* on the electrophoretic separation; it is particularly prone to complex with albumin or α_1-antitrypsin. The acute-phase response often results in the appearance of increased amounts of α_1-proteins in the urine, as these low molecular-weight proteins easily pass the renal glomerulus and may saturate their tubular reabsorptive mechanisms (Fig. 28.15).

SPECIFIC PROTEIN MEASUREMENTS IN DISEASE

A combination of electrophoresis and specific protein measurements is of considerable value in the diagnosis and management of many diseases. Limited profiles of groups of proteins such as immunoglobulins

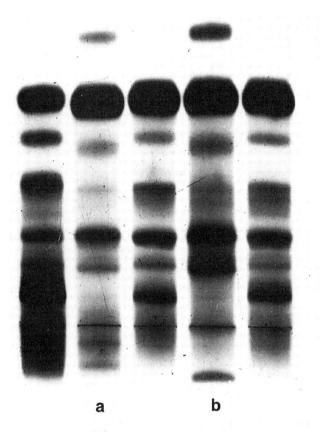

a   b

Figure 28.14 Electrophoresis of concentrated CSF. Intervening plasma separations have been placed on the plate for comparison. The prealbumin is prominent; the α_1 is slow due to desialation; the α_2 is faint; transferrin is in the normal β_1 position; the 'Tau' protein can be seen slightly cathodal to the position of C3 in plasma.

(a) Shows multiple γ-bands due to an oligoclonal IgG response in a patient with disseminated sclerosis.
(b) Shows a single γ-band in a patient with disseminated sclerosis.

Reproduced with permission from Whicher J.T. (1980). The interpretation of electrophoresis. *Br. J. Hosp. Med.*, **24**, 348.

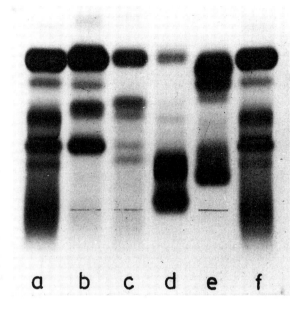

Figure 28.15 Electrophoresis of concentrated urine compared with normal serum.

(a) Normal serum.
(b) Glomerular proteinuria with albumin, α_1, α_2 and transferrin. Note the fast α_2 resulting from the passage of non-polymerized haptoglobin molecules into the urine in a patient with the Hp1-1 phenotype. Less α_2 is seen in nephrotics with the polymerizing phenotypes Hp1-2 and Hp2-2.
(c) Tubular proteinuria. Relatively small albumin band. Split α_2 due to the presence of α_2-microglobulins. Trace of transferrin with β_2-microglobulin in the β_2 position, just anodal to the serum C3.
(d) Bence-Jones proteinuria. Two dense bands of Bence-Jones protein in the γ-region.
(e) Factitious proteinuria due to the addition, by the patient, of egg white to the urine. Note that none of the bands has the same mobility as the bands in the serum (f). This expression of the Munchausen syndrome has been seen in a number of cases.
(f) Normal serum.

Reproduced with permission from Whicher J.T. (1980). The interpretation of electrophoresis. *Br. J. Hosp. Med.*, **24**, 348.

and complement components or acute-phase proteins are widely used in clinical laboratories. Some workers recommend the use of more comprehensive profiles, particularly in investigating non-specific symptoms.

Inflammation

Acute-phase protein measurements are useful in the differential diagnosis and management of inflammatory diseases. On electrophoresis the acute-phase reaction is seen as an increase in the α_1- and α_2-zones.

In acute generalized inflammation or tissue damage, C-reactive protein and antichymotrypsin rise rapidly within the first 12 h and are often associated with a fall in albumin and transferrin of about 10%. This is probably due to loss into inflammatory exu-

date. Orosomucoid, haptoglobin, fibrinogen and α_1-antitrypsin levels rise 24–48 h after the onset of inflammation. These are followed by a moderate rise in C3, C4, prothrombin, caeruloplasmin and plasminogen 4 or 5 days later. If an immune reaction is associated with the inflammation, immunoglobulin levels rise 10–14 days later. C-reactive protein has a short half-life and its concentration changes more rapidly than those of other proteins.

The level of some acute-phase proteins may be used as an indication of the severity of inflammation in chronic inflammatory disease with certain provisos. α_1-Antitrypsin and antichymotrypsin show little increase in disease associated with vasculitis such as rheumatoid arthritis, possibly due to catabolism of α_1-antitrypsin–protease complexes. Chronic inflammation involving the liver is often associated with high levels of α_1-antitrypsin with no orosomucoid increase. A similar pattern is produced by oestrogens or pregnancy. Failure of haptoglobin concentration to increase in chronic inflammation suggests increased intravascular haemolysis such as may occur with hepatic or bone marrow metastases, severe sepsis or autoimmune haemolysis. Children under 10 years of age often do not show a haptoglobin response. Normal or decreased fibrinogen levels in inflammation suggest active fibrinolysis such as occurs in disseminated intravascular coagulation. These changes are all reflected in the appearance of the electrophoretic strip. The ESR is useful in chronic disease as it integrates the effects of changes in several proteins and the red cell.

Immune-complex Disease

The diagnosis of immune-complex disease may be considerably aided by evidence of complement activation or consumption, which suggests active intravascular complex deposition. Direct measurements of immune complexes may be useful occasionally. Protein changes such as cryoglobulins, the raised IgA of rheumatoid arthritis or the presence of complement deficiency may give important clues about the aetiology. Disease activity and response to therapy may be monitored by measuring complement breakdown products and acute-phase proteins such as C-reactive protein. There is evidence that C-reactive protein levels reflect the probability of joint destruction in rheumatoid arthritis.

Infectious Disease

Infectious diseases are usually diagnosed and monitored by identification of the offending organisms. However, some diseases that may prove difficult to diagnose are associated with useful protein changes. For example, brucellosis, Q fever and kala azar are associated with marked increases in IgM whereas most chronic infections produce an IgG response. Immune deficiency and complement deficiencies are important, though rare, causes of chronic or recurrent infection, particularly in childhood. The important immune-complex deposition associated with many infections, such as the glomerulonephritis of subacute bacterial endocarditis, may be diagnosed and monitored by complement measurement. C3 breakdown is occasionally a vital clue in the differential diagnosis of bacterial shock in the surgical patient. The rapid diagnosis of infection complicating burns, leukaemia or the postoperative period can be very successfully made by serial measurement of C-reactive protein in such patients.

A raised IgM level in cord blood or in the neonate is a useful indication of intrauterine or early postnatal infection. It is useful to preserve a sample of cord blood frozen so that in the event of failure to thrive this can then be compared with a sample taken at the time.

Liver Disease

Protein changes may provide useful information in liver disease. Those which commonly occur are shown in Table 28.16. Electrophoresis is a helpful initial investigation in suspected cirrhosis. The albumin, α_1- and α_2-globulin levels are often decreased while the high IgA and IgG concentrations result in an increased γ-globulin band with β–γ fusion. Primary biliary cirrhosis often shows very high levels of IgM and chronic aggressive hepatitis of IgG; β–γ fusion is often not evident. Alcoholism is associated with high levels of α_1-lipoprotein with increased density of the albumin–α_1 interzone.

Gastrointestinal Disease

Protein changes in gastrointestinal disease are of little use diagnostically but may be of considerable value for assessing complications and monitoring therapy. α-Chain disease is one of the few conditions in which a specific marker protein is of considerable importance in establishing the diagnosis. The disappearance of free α-chains is strong evidence of a successful response to treatment. Carcinoembryonic antigen, while by no means specific for gut tumours, is nevertheless very useful for monitoring the effect of surgery, chemotherapy and radiotherapy.

Excessive protein loss from the gut characterizes many diseases diffusely involving the mucosa. Protein changes in the serum resemble those of the nephrotic syndrome without raised levels of α_2-macroglobulin and β-lipoprotein but with decreased albumin and transferrin. The clearance of α_1-antitrypsin into the faeces may be used to assess this loss.

Many inflammatory gut diseases show changes in acute-phase proteins but these are of limited use in management except in Crohn's disease.

IgA is raised in a number of conditions and a persistent high level in coeliac disease, despite treatment, suggests the possibility of lymphoma or progressive reticular hyperplasia. It is also worth noting that gut disease is common in IgA deficiency and that C1 INA deficiency often results in abdominal pain due to mucosal oedema with a history of recurrent laparotomies.

Renal Disease

Glomerular protein loss in renal disease results in characteristic serum changes, with increased levels of α_2-macroglobulin and β-lipoprotein and low levels of albumin, transferrin and IgG. Synthesis of α_2-macroglobulin and β-lipoprotein is switched on, possibly

TABLE 28.16
PROTEIN CHANGES IN LIVER DISEASE

Disease	Immunoglobulins	Acute phase proteins	Complement	Other proteins
Hepatitis A	IgM ↑ IgG ↑	↑ α_1-AT		
Hepatitis B	IgG ↑	↑ α_1-AT		
Alcoholic cirrhosis	Dominant IgA ↑	Haptoglobin ↓	Activation common	α-Lipoprotein ↑
Chronic aggressive hepatitis	Dominant IgG ↑			
Primary biliary cirrhosis	Dominant IgM ↑	Caeruloplasmin ↑ or ↓		Lipoprotein X
Liver secondaries		Haptoglobin ↓		CEA ↑
Hepatoma				α_1-Fetoprotein
Biliary obstruction		Caeruloplasmin ↑		Lipoprotein X
Decreased liver-cell mass				Prealbumin ↓
				Prothrombin ↓

due to albumin loss, and increased levels are attained because these proteins have high molecular weights and are not lost in the urine. The raised β-lipoprotein is the reason for the increased level of plasma cholesterol seen in the nephrotic syndrome. These changes result in the characteristic electrophoretic pattern of decreased albumin and γ-globulin with increased α_2-globulin. Selective protein clearances into the urine are of value in the prognosis and assessment of likely response to steroids in renal disease.[20] This is particularly true of children, where the differential diagnosis is simple and renal biopsy is undesirable. An IgG: albumin clearance of less than 0.16 suggests minimal-change nephropathy with an excellent steroid response. In adults a selective clearance may be misleading as, for example, in amyloidosis, where steroid treatment is disastrous.

A greater clearance of IgM than would be expected from albumin and IgG measurement is seen in pyelonephritis. The clearance of low molecular-weight proteins such as β_2-microglobulin into the urine is of considerable value in the assessment of tubular damage. Serum immunoglobulin changes are not particularly useful owing to a number of complicating factors. Proteinuria results in a catabolic decrease in IgG while uraemia causes a toxic inhibition of immunoglobulin synthesis that affects IgM most. IgA is often raised in pyelonephritis and glomerulonephritis.

Complement measurement is of great importance in distinguishing the serious membrano-proliferative glomerulonephritis from other milder forms.

Neoplasia

A wide range of tumours are now known to produce proteins that can be used with varying degrees of specificity for diagnosis and monitoring.

Secondary host responses to malignant tumours are now of some value in monitoring therapy. Most tumours elicit acute-phase responses. Measurement of serum caeruloplasmin or copper levels is widely used to monitor therapy and detect relapse in Hodg-

kin's disease. C1-esterase inhibitor and β_2-microglobulin are useful in other lymphoid neoplasms; β_2-microglobulin may be as useful in myeloma as the MC level. Acute-phase proteins are of some value in carcinoma of kidney, bronchus and ovary. Serial measurements are important in the management of malignant disease.

Skin Disease

Many skin diseases are associated with either generalized or localized vasculitis. The detection of immune-complex deposition is clinically important in terms of both aetiology and therapy. Eczema may be associated with IgA deficiency and raised IgE levels are commonly seen in atopic forms. Antigen-specific IgE measurement may be of value in assessing the possibility of desentitization. Raised IgA levels are common in many skin diseases but are of little value.

REFERENCES

1. Fudenberg H.H. et al. (1971). Primary immunodeficiencies, *Bull. WHO.*, **45**, 125.
2. Hobbs, J.R. (1971). Immunoglobulins in clinical chemistry. *Adv. Clin. Chem.*, **14**, 219.
3. Kohn J. (1979). Monoclonal proteins. In *Immunochemistry in Clinical Laboratory Medicine* (Milford-Ward, A., Whicher, J.T. eds.) Lancaster: MTP Press, pp.115–126.
4. Whicher J.T., Calvin J., Riches, P., Warren, C. (1987). The laboratory investigation of paraproteinaemia. *Ann. Clin. Biochem.*, **24**, 119.
5. Fearon D.T., Ruddy, S., Schur P.H., McCabe W.R. (1975). Activation of the properdin pathway of complement in patients with gram-negative bacteraemia. *N. Engl. J. Med.*, **292**, 937.
6. Scott D.L. et al. (1985). Anti-rheumatic drugs and joint damage in rheumatoid arthritis. *Q.J.Med.*, **54**, 49.
7. Banks, R.E., Evans, S.W., Van Leuven, F., Alexander D., McMahon M.J., Whicher J.T. (1990). Measurement of the fast or complexed form of α_2 macroglobulin in biological fluids using a sandwich enzyme immunoassay. *J. Immunol. Methods*, **126**, 13.
8. Fagerhol, M.K., Abildgaard U. (1970). Immunological

studies on human antithrombin III. Influence of age, sex and use of oral contraceptives on serum concentrations. *Scand. J. Haematol.*, **7**, 10.

9. Quigley E.M.M., Ross I.N., Haeney M.R., Holbrook I.B., Marsh M.N. (1987). Reassessment of faecal α-1-antitrypsin excretion for use as screening test for intestinal protein loss. *J. Clin. Pathol.*, **40**, 61.

10. Leibman A., Aisen P. (1979). Distribution of iron between the binding sites of transferrin in serum. Methods and results in normal human subjects. *Blood*, **53**, 1058.

11. Gutteridge J.M.C. (1978). Caeruloplasmin: a plasma protein, enzyme and antioxidant. *Ann. Clin. Biochem.*, **15**, 293.

12. Thompson O.M. et al. (1978). Isolation of human tumour-specific antigens associated with β_2-microglobulin. *Br. J. Cancer*, **37**, 753.

13. Norgaard-Pedersen B. (1976). Human alpha-fetoprotein, *Scand. J. Immunol.*, Suppl. 4.

FURTHER READING

Protein Metabolism

Mariani G. ed. (1984). *Pathophysiology of Plasma Protein Metabolism*, London: Macmillan.

Immunoglobulins

Hobbs J.R. (1971). Immunoglobulins in clinical chemistry. *Adv. Clin. Chem.*, **14**, 219.

Putnam F.W. (1977). Immunoglobulins I. Structure *and* Immunoglobulins II. Antibody specificity and genetic control. In *The Plasma Proteins*, vol. 3 (Putnam F.W. ed.) New York: Academic Press.

Whicher J.T. (1984). The role of immunoglobulin assays in clinical medicine. *Ann. Clin. Biochem.*, **21**, 461.

Complement

Whaley K. ed. (1985). *Methods in Complement for Clinical Immunologists*, Edinburgh: Churchill Livingstone.

Whaley K. ed. (1987). *Complement in Health and Disease*, Lancaster: MTP Press.

Acute-phase Proteins

Carrell R.W. (1986). α_1-Antitrypsin: molecular pathology, leucocytes, and tissue damage. *J. Clin. Invest.*, **78**, 1427.

Mackieuicz A., Kushner I. Baumann H. eds. (1993). *Acute Phase Proteins: Molecular Biology, Biochemistry and Clinical Applications*. London: CRC Press.

Whicher J.T., Dieppe P.A. (1983). Acute phase proteins. *Clin. Immunol. Allergy*, **5**, 425.

Transport Proteins

Putnam, F.W. (1975). Transferrin. In *The Plasma Proteins*, vol. 1 (Putnam F.W. ed.) New York: Academic Press.

Whicher J.T., Spence C.E. (1987). When is serum albumin worth measuring? *Ann. Clin. Biochem.*, **24**, 572.

Oncofoetal Proteins

Bagshawe, K.D., Searle, F. (1977). Tumour markers. *Essays Med. Biochem.*, **3**, 25.

Norgaard-Pedersen B., Axelsen N.H. eds. (1978). Carcinoembryonic proteins: recent progress. *Scand. J. Immunol.*, **8** (suppl.8).

Amyloid

Hind C.V.R., Collini P.M., Caspi D., Baltz M.L., Pepys M.B. (1984). Specific chemical dissociation of fibrillar and non-fibrillar comments of amyloid deposits. *Lancet*, **ii**, 376.

Rosenthal C.J., Franklin E.C. (1977). Amyloidosis and amyloid proteins. *Recent Adv. Clin. Immunol.*, **I**, 41.

Electrophoresis

Thompson E.J. (1979). Immunochemistry of CSF proteins. In *Immunochemistry in Clinical Laboratory Medicine* (Milford Ward A., Whicher J.T. eds.) Lancaster: MTP Press.

Whicher J.T., Spence C.E. (1987). Serum protein zone electrophoresis—an outmoded test. *Ann. Clin. Biochem.*, **24**, 133.

Specific Protein Measurement in Disease

Keyser J.W. (1987). *Human Plasma Proteins: Their Investigation in Pathological Conditions*, Chichester: Wiley.

29. Clinical Biochemistry of Blood Coagulation

D. E. G. Austen

Introduction
General haemostatic mechanism
  General clotting mechanism
  General fibrinolytic mechanism
Diseases of haemostasis
  Haemophilia
  Von Willebrand's disease
  Deficiencies of factor V, VII, X and
    prothrombin (factor II)
  Fibrinogen deficiency
  Factor XI deficiency
  Factor XII deficiency and kinin
    deficiency
  Factor XIII deficiency
  Antithrombin III deficiency
  Deficiencies of protein C, protein S and
    protein C inhibitor
  Platelet deficiencies
  Defects in fibrinolysis
  Acquired bleeding disorders
  Diseases not predominantly associated with
    defects of clotting factors, platelets or
    fibrinolysis
Biochemistry of factors and components
  Factor XII
  Kallikrein and prekallikrein
  High molecular-weight kininogen
  Factor XI
  Factor IX
  Factor VIII
  von Willebrand factor
  Factor VII
  Factor X
  Factor V
  Prothrombin (factor II) and thrombin
  Fibrinogen and fibrin
  Factor XIII
  Antithrombin III
  Protein C
  Protein S
  Thrombomodulin
  Thrombospondin
  Plasmin, plasminogen and antiplasmin
  Platelets
Assays of Factors and Components
  Principles
  Preliminary tests on the patient
  Preliminary tests on whole blood
  Preliminary tests on plasma
  One-stage assays
  Two-stage assays
  Assay of von Willebrand factor and its
    antigen
  Assay of prothrombin
  Assay of fibrinogen
  Assay of factor XIII
  Assay of antithrombin III
  Assay of inhibitors and antibodies
  Assay of protein C, protein S and
    thrombomodulin
  Tests on platelets
  Tests of fibrinolysis
  Carrier detection

INTRODUCTION

There has been so much work published on the subject of blood coagulation that it would be impossible to do justice to it all in one chapter. Inevitable selection has been made on the basis of including that which is most important in the treatment of patients. As a result, somewhat less space has been allotted to platelets and fibrinolysis, which constitute a relatively modest proportion of the daily routine in a coagulation laboratory.

GENERAL HAEMOSTATIC MECHANISM

General Clotting Mechanism

At the mechanical level, haemostasis involves the constriction of damaged vessels together with blockage of leaks by deposited fibrin and aggregated platelets. Thus both clotting factors (Table 29.1) and platelet reactions combine in carrying out this task. Platelets have several functions to perform. They need to aggregate, adhere to damaged tissue and to release essential chemicals, including ADP which promotes further aggregation.

Fibrin in the clot is formed as a result of sequential chemical reactions, illustrated in Fig. 29.1. As will be seen, the overall mechanism is one in which a clotting factor becomes activated and is then able to activate the next factor in line. Two pathways lead to the activation of factor X and thereafter a single path proceeds until finally fibrin is produced to form the clot. The two initial routes retain their old names of 'intrinsic' and 'extrinsic' pathways. Tissue juices from the wound initiate the extrinsic route while the intrinsic pathway starts with surface activation of factor XII.

The sequential reactions of clotting factors are catalysed at several points by phospholipid release from platelets; at the same time, thrombin produced in these reactions gives rise to further aggregation of platelets. The reactions represent an amplification whereby a small initial stimulus is converted into a large deposition of fibrin. At the same time, clotting is subject to precise regulation as individual reaction

TABLE 29.1

BASIC PROPERTIES OF THE CLOTTING FACTORS

Factor	Synonyms	Present in human serum	Present in Cohn's fraction	Easily adsorbed by alumina and barium sulphate	Precipitated by ammonium sulphate % saturation
I	Fibrinogen	No	I	No	25
II	Prothrombin	No	III & IV	Yes	50
III	Thromboplastin: tissue factor				
IV	Calcium				
V	Labile factor: proaccelerin Accelerator globulin	No	III	No	50
VII	Preconvertin: stable factor Autoprothrombin I Serum prothrombin conversion accelerator (SPCA) Serum accelerator globulin	Yes	III & IV	Yes	50
VIII	Antihaemophilic globulin (AHG) Antihaemophilic factor A Thromboplastinogen A Platelet cofactor I	No	I	No	33
IX	Christmas factor Plasma thromboplastin component (PTC) Antihaemophilic factor B: platelet cofactor II Thromboplastinogen B: autoprothrombin II	Yes	III & IV	Yes	50
X	Stuart Prower factor Autoprothrombin III	Yes	III	Yes	50
XI	Plasma thromboplastin antecedent (PTA) Antihaemophilic factor C	Yes	III & IV	Partly	33
XII	Hageman factor Surface factor	Yes	III & IV	Partly	50
XIII	Fibrin stabilizing factor (FSF) Fibrinase; Laki–Lorand factor	Yes	I	No	33

steps are controlled by the action of natural inhibitors.

The reaction chains shown in Fig. 29.1 are a somewhat simplified representation of the complete process. Increasingly, bypass loops are being discovered along the chain. Nevertheless, the simplified scheme is extremely useful in devising assays and interpreting results. Exciting work is now being reported on the participation of surfaces in clotting-factor reactions and on the existence of surface receptors for factors on the endothelium. There are probably important advances to be made here. It appears unlikely that clotting factors react entirely in the liquid phase. If they did then the products and intermediates would be swept along in the blood flow away from the place where they were needed.

General Fibrinolytic Mechanism

When bleeding stops and the clot is no longer required, another set of reactions comes into play. Plasminogen, an inactive precursor of plasmin that circulates in the blood, adsorbs on to fibrin. Plasminogen activators also adsorb on to fibrin and activate the plasminogen *in situ*. In this way, plasmin is formed in the adsorbed state and is largely protected from attack by its inhibitor, α-antiplasmin. As the clot is solubilized, plasmin is released into the circulation where it is rapidly neutralized by the inhibitor. Plasminogen activators that bring about the activation circulate in the blood at a low concentration but larger quantities can be released from tissues or vessel walls in response to stress or exercise.

DISEASES OF HAEMOSTASIS

Haemophilia

Haemophilia A and haemophilia B are severe hereditary bleeding disorders caused by deficiency in the blood of factors VIII and IX, respectively.

Haemophilia A is the most common hereditary bleeding disorder, von Willebrand's disease is the second and haemophilia B (sometimes called Christmas disease) is the third. Haemophilia A and B are clinically indistinguishable and laboratory assays are necessary to differentiate between them. Both are inherited by an X-linked recessive mechanism, which means that it is males who are predominantly affected but females can be carriers of the complaint. In

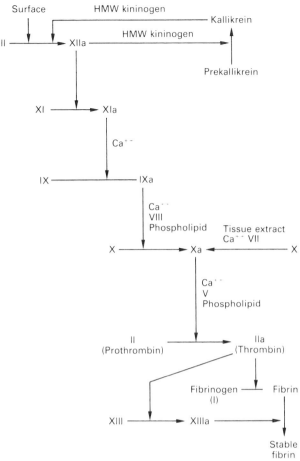

Figure 29.1 Sequential clotting reactions; HMW = high molecular weight.

affected individuals, bleeding can follow even minor trauma and can also be apparently spontaneous. Bleeding may be severe and prolonged, and is typically into muscles and joints. It may occur several hours after the trauma. Repeated episodes of bleeding into a particular joint can lead to crippling.

The two diseases are seen in a range of severities, fairly well correlated with the level of relevant factor in the blood. Complete absence of either factor gives rise to a condition in which minor trauma can lead to life-threatening bleeds. On the other hand, a small amount of factor decreases the severity enormously and at 5% of the normal concentration the patient experiences only occasional bleeds and then usually only after noticeable trauma.

Treatment requires replacement therapy involving intravenous injection of factor VIII or factor IX concentrate.[1] At present, these are fractionated from donated blood but materials produced by recombinant DNA techniques are becoming available in experimental amounts. Once it has been injected, factor VIII or IX has a half-life of approximately 12 h in the bloodstream and for this reason haemophiliacs are usually only treated when they have an actual bleeding problem. However, many haemophiliacs can now treat themselves at home if the episode is relatively minor. Factor replacement is required for surgery, including tooth extraction.

A very serious problem still remains in the treatment of haemophilia when a patient develops an antibody to the injected factor. This occurs in about 6% of haemophiliacs. Sometimes these antibodies can be so potent as to almost nullify the effect of treatment.

As a gross average, a female carrier of haemophilia will have 50% of the normal concentration of the relevant factor in her blood and this is more than enough for a problem-free life. However, the individual variation can be very wide and so some carriers have normal concentrations while others have low amounts. If the concentration is low, then they can experience bleeding problems, particularly menorrhagia and at childbirth. There are two reasons for this variation in factor level. First, there is a range of concentrations in the normal population and in the case of factor VIII the spread is particularly wide. Secondly, there is variation caused by the so-called Lyonization process whereby, in a female, one of her two X chromosomes predominates over the other. Therefore, in the carrier, the factor is low if the affected gene predominates and vice versa.

In very rare cases, haemophilia (usually haemophilia A) may develop in a patient without a previous bleeding history. Usually they have an underlying complaint such as rheumatoid arthritis, ulcerative colitis or penicillin allergy. It can also develop, though extremely rarely, in childbirth. The problem is caused by development of an antibody to the clotting factor and should the antibody disappear then the bleeding problem ceases. A bleeding problem can also disappear in a very rare form of haemophilia B called haemophilia B Leyden, where the patient becomes normal after puberty. It is believed this is caused by a defect in the promoter region of the gene that codes for factor IX and that something happens after puberty which can override the defect and switch on the gene.[2]

Von Willebrand's Disease

Von Willebrand's disease is a bleeding disorder that affects both sexes.[3] Factor VIII activity and von Willebrand factor are both reduced (in haemophilia A only factor VIII is reduced). The disease has been divided into three groups termed type I, type II and type III. Types I and II are the more common and represent an autosomal dominant condition. Originally, the perceived distinction between the two types was that type II had abnormalities in the multimeric structure of the von Willebrand-factor molecule but it was then discovered that some of the patients designated type I also had abnormalities. As a result the distinctions have become somewhat blurred. Each of the two types has been further subdivided into type Ia, type Ib, etc., but they represent a range of different characteristics within a very heterogeneous disease and should be considered more as a list than a classification. Type III, however, is different. It is an autosomal recessive condition in which the patient has low concentrations of both factor VIII and von Willebrand factor and bleeds severely. Their parents typically have no symptoms of the disease. Bleeding in von Willebrand's disease is different from that in haemophilia, although the muscle bleeds and haemarthroses, typical of haemophilia, are seen in the type III condition. Bleeding is from the mucous membranes. Epistaxis is common and can be sometimes difficult to control or even life-threatening. Gastrointestinal bleeding is fairly common and female patients can suffer from menorrhagia.

Treatment for all types of von Willebrand's disease consists of replacement therapy with plasma, cryoprecipitate or factor concentrates; it is given when the patient has a bleeding problem or when surgery or manipulation is required.

Deficiencies of Factor V, VII, X and Prothrombin (Factor II)

These factor deficiencies have been grouped together because of their relative rarity. Added together they make up only 1% of the patients with hereditary coagulation disorders and, as a result, it is more difficult to report a consensus of the types of bleeding experienced. In general there is excessive bruising, epistaxis and gastrointestinal bleeding. Female patients suffer from menorrhagia. Haemarthroses are not common but do occasionally occur. Naturally, as with all bleeding complaints, there is a potential problem with surgery and treatment would normally be given in advance of this. Treatment is by replacement therapy using intravenous infusion of plasma or, in the case of factor VII, X, and prothrombin,[4] concentrates are available. Deficiencies of factors VII, IX, X and prothrombin are seen in liver disease and in vitamin K deficiency (discussed in Factor VII below). Factor X deficiency is sometimes experienced in amyloidosis due to the amyloid deposits adsorbing the factor.[5]

Fibrinogen Deficiency

Deficiency of fibrinogen is rare as a congenital abnormality and, surprisingly, is a relatively less severe condition than haemophilia.[6] Bruising, gastrointestinal bleeding and bleeding from mucous membranes are fairly common; haemarthroses and menorrhagia sometimes occur. It is inherited by an autosomal recessive mechanism and treatment consists of infusion of plasma or of fibrinogen concentrate.

Dysfibrinogenaemia, which represents a qualitative defect in the fibrinogen molecule, is also rare. Some families with the defect will suffer from a mild bleeding disorder; others will have a tendency to thrombosis; or possibly have no clinical bleeding problems at all.

Fibrinogen deficiency is also seen as an acquired disorder during intravascular coagulation. This arises when clotting is triggered by entry of a material, probably tissue thromboplastin, into the circulation. Usually, there is an associated reduction of platelet numbers and a reduction in the concentrations of factors II, V and VIII. Profuse bleeding ensues, with epistaxis, melaena, haematemesis and massive bruising. Typical causes would be premature separation of the placenta, septicaemia, prostatectomy, carcinoma, snake bite or reaction to a drug. Treatment involves blood replacement, possibly intravenous infusion of clotting factors, and occasionally administration of heparin. If the prime cause of the problem can be removed, then rapid improvement is possible and this is seen when the uterus is emptied following premature separation of the placenta.

Factor XI Deficiency

Deficiency of factor XI usually gives rise to a mild bleeding complaint and patients suffer from excessive bruising, menorrhagia and epistaxis. Often the severity of bleeding does not correlate well with the concentration of the factor in the blood. The inheritance is by an autosomal mechanism and most of the patients are of Jewish origin. Treatment consists of intravenous infusion of plasma.

Factor XII Deficiency and Kinin Deficiency

Individuals who have a deficiency of factor XII, prekallikrein or high molecular-weight kininogen show prolonged clotting times in the preliminary tests of the intrinsic pathway.[7] However, they do not bleed abnormally. Levels of these clotting factors can be measured in the same way as with other factors but the main reason for making the measurements is to find a reason for the apparently abnormal preliminary tests and to avoid confusion with other clotting deficiencies.

Factor XIII Deficiency

Deficiency of factor XIII is a rare condition that gives rise to severe bleeding.[8] Classically, the first signs are seen with bleeding from the umbilical stump of a newborn child. Wound healing is slow, causing irregular and retracted scars. Intracranial bleeding is a very significant risk. Replacement therapy uses plasma or factor XIII concentrates and after infusion the half-life of the factor in the blood is several days. Only a small proportion of the normal amount of factor is necessary for adequate haemostasis and, therefore, intravenous transfusions are required relatively infrequently and prophylactic treatment is perfectly feasible. Factor XIII deficiency is inherited by an autosomal mechanism.

TABLE 29.2
PLATELET DISORDERS

Disorder	Platelet abnormality affecting coagulation
Thrombocytopenia	Reduced number of platelets
Thromboasthenia (Glanzmann's disease)	Abnormal ADP aggregation
Storage-pool deficiency:	
(i) Hermansky–Pudlak syndrome	Defective release reaction;
(ii) Wiskott–Aldrich syndrome	((ii) and (iii) also have
(iii) Chediak–Higashi syndrome	thrombocytopenia)
Cyclo-oxygenase deficiency	Defective release reaction
Defective nucleotide metabolism	Defective release reaction
Bernard–Soulier syndrome	Defective adhesion to subendothelium
Myeloproliferative disorders	Variable
Renal disease	Variable
Macroglobulinaemia	Variable
Administration of aspirin	Defective release reaction
Gray platelet syndrome	α-Granule deficiency

Antithrombin III Deficiency

Antithrombin III deficiency[9] is seen both as a quantitative deficiency and also as one in which the antithrombin is present as a defective molecular variant. In either case, patients show a marked tendency to develop venous thromboses. These can be controlled by conventional anticoagulant therapy, warfarin for example, or else by replacement therapy using antithrombin III concentrates. Reduced levels of antithrombin are seen in liver disease, hepatitis, myocardial infarction, postoperative states and with the use of oral contraceptives of high oestrogen content.

Deficiencies of Protein C, Protein S and Protein C Inhibitor

Protein C and protein S form part of the regulatory mechanism in clotting, their role being to neutralize activated factors V and VIII and dampen down the sequential reactions. Accordingly, a deficiency of either protein results in a thrombotic condition[10] and treatment is based on anticoagulant therapy using a vitamin K antagonist such as warfarin. Protein C is normally kept in check by protein C inhibitor and therefore when there is a deficiency of this inhibitor a bleeding state is induced due to an excess of protein C. In this disorder, concentrations of factor V and factor VIII are found to be decreased and it is clinically similar to an isolated deficiency of factor V. Treatment consists of intravenous infusion of plasma.

Platelet Deficiencies

Platelet abnormalities can be quantitative or qualitative. Platelets can be too few or too many in number.[11] They can fail to adhere to the subendothelium or they can fail to aggregate to form a platelet plug. A list of platelet disorders is given in Table 29.2.

Thrombocytopenia, the condition where platelets are too few in number, is the most common deficiency and most cases are of secondary thrombocytopenia, which results from the action of drugs, poisons, acute infection, radiation or as a consequence of malignancy or leukaemia. Hereditary thrombocytopenia is very rare.

Excessive bleeding can be associated with an increased number of platelets, as seen in *polycythaemia* or *thrombocythaemia*. Haemorrhagic disorders also arise where platelets are present in normal numbers but where they have diminished functional ability. These are discussed later.

Bleeding in platelet disorders is typically from mucous membranes. Epistaxis, intestinal or uterine bleeding are common, and petechiae or small, diffuse bruises are often seen in the skin. The diseases affect both sexes. Treatment may include intravenous infusions of platelet-rich plasma or platelet concentrates, in addition to the treatment of any underlying complaint.

Defects in Fibrinolysis

In 1978, the first cases of α_2-antiplasmin deficiency were described, characterized by prolonged bleeding after trauma, easy bruising and bleeding into joints. It is an autosomal recessive condition. This disease clearly represents a deficiency in the fibrinolytic system but other examples of apparent fibrinolytic deficiency are not so clear.[12] This is because the effects of excessive fibrinolysis are difficult to distinguish from those of *diffuse intravascular coagulation* (DIC), and a further complication is that increased fibrinolysis would be a natural outcome in DIC. Treatment for increased fibrinolysis would be a fibrinolytic inhibitor such as ε-aminocaproic acid or tranexamic acid but these would be contraindicated for DIC.

Bleeding as a result of increased fibrinolysis, which is not secondary to DIC, has been observed in liver disease, leukaemia and after surgery. A familial disease caused by excessive plasminogen activator has also been reported.

Acquired Bleeding Disorders

An important category of bleeding problems is seen with the development of antibodies to a specific clotting factor. Most numerous are those directed towards factor VIII or XI, particularly factor VIII, and these have already been discussed with haemophilia above. A less specific inhibitor can develop in *systemic lupus erythematosus*, when prolonged clotting times are recorded in preliminary tests. Excessive bleeding is not often encountered unless there is an associated thrombocytopenia or a deficiency in prothrombin. However, the development of thromboses can present a problem, even when the patient has this apparently anticoagulant antibody.

Another acquired bleeding disorder is seen in *vitamin K deficiency*, which can arise through inadequate diet, malabsorption syndrome or when there is insufficient flora in the gut for normal production of vitamin K. An example of the latter is in 'haemorrhagic disease of the newborn' caused by a delay in the development of gut flora in the child. Bleeding is due to a qualitative deficiency of factors II, VII, IX and X. In the absence of vitamin K these factors do not obtain the essential post-translation γ-carboxylation of their glutamic acid constituents. As a treatment, vitamin K is given and in severe cases, plasma or even factor concentrates.

Certain diseases can also give rise to a factor deficiency. In *amyloidosis*, factor IX and X can be reduced and this is believed to be caused by amyloid deposits binding the factor. In liver disease, the concentrations of factors II, VII, IX and X are decreased and when the disease is severe there can be additional deficiencies of factor V, factor XIII, plasminogen, antithrombin III and α$_2$-antiplasmin.

Diseases not Predominantly Associated with Defects of Clotting Factors, Platelets or Fibrinolysis

There is a series of diseases that have not been fully categorized, although, in a proportion of them, there does appear to be a defect in the connective tissues in and around the blood vessels that can give rise to a bleeding tendency. The chief conditions of this type are considered in the next seven subsections.

Henoch–Schönlein purpura

A condition that, in rare cases, can follow an infection, or possibly arise as a reaction to certain foods or sometimes have no obvious cause at all. The rash is usually below the waist and on the arms and face. Other manifestations are colic, bloody diarrhoea and swollen, tender joints, particularly the knees and ankles. The disease usually resolves but renal involvement is occasionally a serious side-effect.

Ehlers–Danlos syndrome

This is characterized by hyperextensibility of the joints and hyperelasticity of the skin. Sometimes the eyes reveal blue sclerae. If a bleeding problem is present it is usually mild and consists of easy bruising, bleeding from mucous membranes and bleeding at surgery. Investigation in some patients reveals abnormal collagen, which would result in defective platelet adhesion.

Pseudoxanthoma elasticum

This involves a loss of skin elasticity with the appearance of skin thickening and nodules. When there is excessive bleeding it is usually from the mucous membranes.

Osteogenesis imperfecta

This is marked by brittle bones and blue sclerae. Bleeding is not common but sometimes occurs in the form of easy bruising and bleeding from the mucous membranes. It has been suggested that platelets are sometimes abnormal as well.

Telangiectasia

This is characterized by vascular lesions that are also sites where bleeding can occur. These can arise in different areas of the body, developing during late childhood, and can produce serious bleeding or little at all, depending on their position. Haemorrhage is typically from the mucous membranes and epistaxis is the most common symptom.

Scurvy

Bleeding is encountered in scurvy, particularly from the mucous membranes. In patients old enough to have teeth, there is swelling and bleeding of the gums and, in adults, petechiae begin, particularly around the hair follicles.

Autoerythrocyte sensitization

This is a little understood condition found in adult women, usually with an emotional disturbance, who exhibit painful, raised bruises. It has been proposed that they become sensitized to their own red cells, presumably just in the skin area. There is no specific treatment but the disease does tend to become less severe over the years.

BIOCHEMISTRY OF FACTORS AND COMPONENTS

Factor XII

A deficiency of factor XII, previously known as

Hageman factor, does not result in excessive bleeding. Its action is in the initial stages of clotting when it becomes activated to factor XIIa, after which it activates factor XI. These reactions are illustrated in Fig. 29.1, where it will be seen that factor XIIa also activates prekallikrein, in the presence of high molecular-weight kininogen. To a limited extent it can also make factor VII active, which would not be predicted from the diagram since factor VII is in the other, so-called extrinsic pathway.

Factor XII is a single-chain glycoprotein with a molecular weight of approximately 80 000 and is present in the blood at a concentration of 30 μg/mL.[13] Limited proteolysis activates it by cleavage within a disulphide loop to generate the two-chain structure of factor XIIa. The two chains have molecular weights of approximately 52 000 and 28 000. Sometimes, the product of activation is called α-factor XIIa to distinguish it from β-factor XIIa, which is the product of a second proteolytic cleavage. β-Factor XIIa has only 1% of the ability to activate factor XI when compared with α-factor XIIa but it is still a potent activator of prekallikrein. How factor XIIa is regulated in the body is not clearly understood but several inhibitors are effective *in vitro*. These include C1-inhibitor and antithrombin III.

Kallikrein and Prekallikrein

Prekallikrein, previously called Fletcher factor, also acts in the initial stages of coagulation and, as with factor XII, a deficiency does not result in excessive bleeding. It is converted into the active protease, kallikrein, by the action of factor XIIa, but there is a circular aspect to this, because kallikrein activates factor XII (*see* Fig. 29.1). Both of these reciprocal activations are accelerated by the presence of high molecular-weight kininogen.

Prekallikrein is a single-chain glycoprotein with a molecular weight of approximately 80 000 and its concentration in blood is about 50 μg/mL.[14] Kallikrein has two chains. The major inhibitor of kallikrein appears to be C1-inhibitor but some inhibition has been reported for α_2-macroglobulin and antithrombin III.

High molecular-weight Kininogen

High molecular-weight kininogen (HMW kininogen) has also been known as Fitzgerald factor, Flaujeac factor and Williams factor. It acts as a cofactor in the reactions of factor XII and kallikrein as reported in the previous section (*see* Fig. 29.1). Additionally, it is cleaved by kallikrein to yield a kinin-free molecule (which still has coagulant activity) plus bradykinin.

Blood contains two distinct kininogens but the low molecular-weight one (approx. 60 000) has no coagulant activity, as far as is known. HMW kininogen is present at about 70 μg/mL and has a molecular weight of approximately 110 000.[15] Its cofactor activity is thought to be surface dependent and, *in vitro*, negatively charged surfaces have been shown to enhance this activity.

Factor XI

In the clotting sequence, factor XI is activated by factor XIIa to factor XIa and this protease in its turn, activates factor IX (*see* Fig. 29.1). Conversion to factor XIa does not require the presence of calcium ions but calcium is required for the subsequent reaction with factor IX.

Factor XI is a glycoprotein present at about 6 μg/mL in the blood.[14] It has a molecular weight of approximately 160 000 and consists of two chains, each of approximately 80 000. During activation, cleavage occurs within a disulphide group on each of the two chains to yield four disulphide-linked chains, two with a molecular weight of approximately 48 000 and two of approximately 33 000. *In vitro*, factor XIa is inhibited by C1-inhibitor and antithrombin III but its regulation in the body is not properly understood.

Factor IX

Factor IX is a single-chain glycoprotein with a molecular weight of approximately 57 000 and is present in the blood at a concentration of 5 μg/mL.[16] It is the clotting factor that is deficient in haemophilia B. Factor IX is activated by factor XIa (*see* Fig. 29.1) in the presence of calcium ions; in the laboratory, limited activation can be achieved in the presence of strontium, cupric or zinc ions. The role of factor IXa is to activate factor X in a reaction that also requires phospholipid and calcium ions. During this process there are two proteolytic cleavages. The first is within a disulphide link, yielding a two-chain molecule. In the second cleavage, part of the heavy chain is removed.

Factor IX has been produced by recombinant DNA techniques[17] and this work has shown that it consists of approximately 415 amino acids. The mRNA that codes for factor IX was shown to contain about 34 kb, which includes the coding for a 40 amino-acid signal peptide that is lost in transport out of the cell. Factor IX is formed in the liver and is reduced in liver disease. It is also decreased in vitamin K deficiency and exhibits some similarities to factors II, VII and X, as discussed for factor VII below.

Factor VIII

Factor VIII is synthesized in the liver and is deficient in the blood of patients in haemophilia A. It is found in close association with von Willebrand factor and it is believed that by being attached to that factor it acquires additional stability.[18] In early experimental work, before this association was understood, some of the physical properties of von Willebrand factor were wrongly attributed to factor VIII. The easiest way to separate them is to subject the material to high ionic strength or else to reducing conditions and then to separate the two by gel-filtration chromatography run under identical conditions. Some separation is also possible with ion-exchange chromatography but this is often associated with low yields. Factor VIII seems to attach itself to chromatographic materials but reagents that are strong enough for elution purposes usually result in degradation. It is therefore necessary to find column packings of just the right binding strength and the most successful are amino-hexyl sepharose[19] or certain polyelectrolyte polymers.

In the clotting sequence, factor VIII acts as cofactor in the activation of factor X by factor IXa, in the presence of phospholipid and calcium ions. In common with factor V, it is activated by thrombin and this increases its catalytic efficiency. Factor VIII is a glycoprotein of approximately 330 000 mol. wt., and is present in the blood at a concentration of approximately 0.2 μg/mL. It is relatively labile and is inactivated by chelating agents such as EDTA. It is destroyed by excess thrombin and therefore is not present in clotted blood or serum. Factor VIII can now be produced by recombinant DNA procedures and sufficient has been made to allow experimental trials in the treatment of patients. This work has also shown that factor VIII has approximately 2332 amino acids.[20] The mRNA that codes for the protein contains about 186 kb, which includes coding for a 19 amino-acid signal peptide that is lost during transport out of the cell. Using recombinant DNA techniques, it has also been possible to construct a variant factor VIII molecule in which a 909 amino-acid portion is missing and which has clotting activity.

von Willebrand Factor

In von Willebrand's disease there is a deficiency of both factor VIII and of von Willebrand factor. The latter is synthesized by endothelial cells and by megakaryocytes. It is present in the β-granules of platelets as well as in plasma. The factor has no known enzymatic activity but mediates in adhesion of platelets to exposed subendothelium at the site of a wound and promotes aggregation of platelets to form a thrombus. Von Willebrand factor appears to possess a multiplicity of adhesive functions, such as binding to cells, platelets, circulating protein or to subendothelium. On the platelet, glycoprotein IB and glycoprotein IIB/IIIA act as receptors for von Willebrand factor.

In the past, von Willebrand factor was known by other names. The molecule detected by immunological means was called factor VIII-related antigen, while the molecule detected by its biological activity towards platelets was termed ristocetin cofactor. The latter name arose because ristocetin aggregates platelets in the presence of von Willebrand factor and is used in its assay, as will be seen later. Factor VIII adheres to von Willebrand factor and, in so doing, it

appears to acquire significant stabilization. However, it should be noted that the concentration of von Willebrand factor in the blood is approximately 10 μg/mL, which exceeds that of factor VIII. Therefore, many of its molecules will circulate in the blood without factor VIII attached. The separation of factor VIII from von Willebrand factor is typically achieved by elevated ionic strength or by a reducing medium followed by gel-filtration chromatography run under identical conditions. Specialized ion-exchange chromatography can also be used, as discussed for factor VIII.

Von Willebrand factor is relatively more stable than factor VIII and, for example, it survives the clotting process to remain in clotted blood or serum. It is made up of subunits[21] whose individual molecular weight has been measured as 220 000, although amino-acid analysis has suggested a somewhat higher figure of 270 000. Subunits are joined together to form molecules with molecular weights that range between about 800 000–20 million and the factor can be chemically dissociated into a series of multimers with a wide range of sizes. A pattern of these displayed by electrophoresis is used as a means of detecting variant molecules.

Factor VII

Factor VII acts with tissue thromboplastin, presumably from the wound, together with phospholipid and calcium ions to bring about the activation of factor X. As seen in Fig. 29.1, this represents one of the two routes by which factor X is activated and is called the *extrinsic pathway*. Factor VII itself becomes activated in the process, which gives considerable enhancement to its reactions.[22] In addition to this well-established process, it has now been shown that factor VII and thromboplastin activate factor IX,[23] which would not be predicted from the simple scheme given in Fig. 29.1. This finding has also prompted a suggestion that perhaps this reaction in the extrinsic pathway is the main initiating stimulus to clotting, giving rise to reaction in both pathways and bypassing the contribution from factor XII and factor XI.

Factor VII is a single-chain glycoprotein of approximately 48 kD present in the blood at a concentration of about 0.6 μg/mL. Proteolysis within a disulphide loop generates the two-chain molecule of factor VIIa. Factor VII is synthesized in the liver and vitamin K is vital for post-translational γ-carboxylation of glutamic acid residues in the molecule. Without these modifications the factor is unable to participate in calcium-dependent binding to phospholipid and has no coagulant activity. Factors II, IX and X and protein C also require this modification. Factor VII has several physicochemical similarities to factors II, IX and X, and the four factors can be difficult to separate unless sophisticated techniques such as affinity chromatography are used. Moreover, factor VII is very sensitive to proteolytic degradation, which adds to the problems of purification. In general, it is easier to separate the four factors from bovine blood and this is one reason why so much of the experimental work has been done on the bovine factors.

Factor X

Factor X can be activated by both the intrinsic and the extrinsic pathways, as seen in Fig. 29.1. It is activated by factor IX in the presence of factor VIII, phospholipid and calcium ions as part of the intrinsic train and by tissue thromboplastin plus factor VII in the extrinsic route. Factor X can also be activated by venom from the Russell's viper, a feature that is utilized in assay methods. After activation, the role of factor X is to convert prothrombin (factor II) into thrombin in a reaction that also requires factor V plus phospholipid and calcium ions.

Factor X is produced in the liver and is reduced in liver disease. It is also decreased in vitamin K deficiency[24] and shows similarities to factors II, VII and IX as discussed for factor VII. It is a glycoprotein of approximately 55 kD, and is composed of two chains. It is present in blood at a concentration of approximately 10 μg/mL. Since much of the experimental work on factor X has been done with bovine blood, information on the two-chain structure of the human material is somewhat limited.

Factor V

Factor V is the necessary cofactor in the activation of prothrombin to thrombin by factor Xa (see Fig. 29.1).[25] Phospholipid and calcium ions are also required. In the blood it circulates as an inactive precursor and it must be activated by thrombin before it can effectively participate in its cofactor role. Thus once a little thrombin is formed these reciprocal activation steps provide rapid amplification of the process. Human factor V is destroyed by excess thrombin, although the bovine material is rather more stable. As a result, factor V is found in bovine but not in human serum. Calcium and other metal ions are necessary for the stability of factor V and as a result it is inactivated by chelating agents such as EDTA.

Protein C destroys factor V and factor VIII but in the body it is kept in check by protein C inhibitor. Accordingly, a bleeding disorder arises when there is a deficiency of protein C inhibitor. Factor V is a single-chain glycoprotein of approximately 340 000 mol. wt., and it circulates at a concentration of about 7 μg/mL in the blood.[26] It is activated by thrombin to form factor Va, which has two chains with molecular weights of approximately 94 000 and 74 000.

Prothrombin (Factor II) and Thrombin

Prothrombin is an inactive precursor that is converted to thrombin by the action of factor Xa in the presence of factor V, phospholipid and calcium ions (see Fig. 29.1).[27] It is produced in the liver and shows similarities to factors VII, IX and X. Like these factors, the levels of prothrombin are decreased in liver disease and in vitamin K deficiency. More details were given in the section on factor VII above. Prothrombin has a molecular weight of approximately 72 000 and is present in blood at a concentration of about 100 μg/mL.[28] In the first stage of its activation to thrombin, it is cleaved into two molecules of approximately the same size called prethrombin-2 and fragment 1–2. This is followed by a second proteolytic cleavage within a disulphide link of the prethrombin-2 yielding the two-chain molecule of thrombin. Thrombin has a molecular weight of approximately 37 000. In the simplified clotting sequence shown in Fig. 29.1, the role of thrombin is to clot fibrinogen and produce fibrin. However, it also activates factors V, VIII and XIII, as well as activating protein C and aggregating platelets. Antithrombin is responsible for regulating thrombin and its action is augmented because, as the concentration of thrombin is reduced, there is less available to activate factor V. This leads to a further dampening of the reactions.

Fibrinogen and Fibrin

Fibrin forms the network of a haemostatic plug and is produced by the action of thrombin on fibrinogen.[29] The latter is formed in the liver and is present in normal blood at a concentration of 2500–3500 μg/mL. It has a molecular weight of approximately 340 000 and under the electron microscope appears to consist of three spheres linked in a line. Controversy has arisen over this shape but opinion now appears to have returned to favour the three-sphere model. Fibrinogen consists of three pairs of non-identical polypeptide chains whose amine terminals are all held together by disulphide bridges in what has been termed the 'disulphide knot'. The three different pairs of chains are designated as Aα, Bβ and γ, and these consist of 610, 461 and 411 amino-acid residues, respectively. Since there is a pair of each type, this makes 2964 amino acids for the protein portion of the molecule, equivalent to a molecular weight of 329 840. This figure needs to be increased by about 10 000 to take account of the carbohydrate clusters which exist, one on each of the two β- and the two γ-chains. This gives a figure in agreement with the value of 340 000 quoted above. The reason for the slightly complicated designation of the chains is so that after the clotting process in which fibrinopeptides A and B are lost from chains Aα and Bβ, the remaining portions will be simply α, β and γ. When fibrinogen is clotted by thrombin, the first action is the release of these fibrinopeptides plus fibrin monomer. Monomers then aggregate, while being reinforced by the cross-linking caused by factor XIII, forming a gel composed of fibres around 1 μm in diameter. Incorporated in the gel are red cells, white cells and especially platelets.

Factor XIII

Factor XIII is a calcium-dependent transglutaminase.[30] Its role in clotting is to stitch together neighbouring molecules in the fibrin plug by forming bonds between suitably disposed lysines and glutamines, producing $\varepsilon(\gamma$-glutamyl)-lysine links. In this way, it brings about a vital stabilization of the clot. Factor XIII circulates in the blood as an inactive precursor with a molecular weight of approximately 320 000. It contains four subunits, two of type 'a' and two of type 'b', which have molecular weights of approximately 72 000 and 88 000. However, an intracellular form of factor XIII also exists, which consists of just two of the type 'a' subunit and which has a molecular weight of approximately 144 000.

Factor XIII becomes activated by the action of thrombin in the presence of calcium ions. Both types of factor XIII are effective because activity is associated with the 'a' subunit. Under the influence of thrombin and calcium, it releases a peptide of approximately 4000 mol. wt. The molecule dissociates and the active centre of the subunit is revealed.

Antithrombin III

Several antithrombins were originally described but much of the terminology is now redundant. Antithrombin I represented the ability of surfaces to adsorb thrombin; antithrombin V was the anticoagulant action of fibrin degradation products. The remaining three antithrombins, II, III and IV, were eventually considered to be synonymous and were combined under the single name of antithrombin III. This single-chain glycoprotein with a molecular weight between 56 000 and 65 000 is present in the blood at about 150–250 μg/mL.[31] It is the most important inhibitor of thrombin and of factor Xa, and it can also inactivate factors IXa, XIa and XIIa. Its activity is greatly enhanced by heparin, which, it has been suggested, introduces a spatial configuration change in the molecule. A deficiency of antithrombin III in a patient gives rise to a thrombotic condition.

Protein C

Protein C is a glycoprotein that circulates as an inactive zymogen at a concentration of about 4–5 μg/mL.[32] It is activated in a reaction that is slow in itself but dramatically accelerated by the presence of *thrombomodulin*, a membrane protein present on endothelial cells. Protein C is a two-chain glycoprotein with a molecular weight of approximately 62 000. It inhibits coagulation by degrading factors V and VIII in a proteolytic reaction accelerated by protein S, which additionally requires phospholipid and calcium

ions. Thus a deficiency of protein C gives rise to a thrombotic condition while a deficiency of protein C inhibitor leads to a bleeding state due to destruction of factors V and VIII. Protein C is produced in the liver and is reduced in liver disease and vitamin K deficiency as discussed for factor VII.

Protein S

Protein S circulates in two ways in the blood. Some is free and active while the remainder is complexed to C4b-binding protein and is inactive. It has a molecular weight of approximately 80 000 and is present in blood at 25 μg/mL. Protein S does not have proteolytic activitity in itself but acts as the cofactor for protein C.[33] Cofactor activity is destroyed by thrombin but calcium ions and thrombomodulin appear to limit destruction.

Thrombomodulin

Thrombomodulin is a membrane protein present on endothelial cells with a reported molecular weight of approximately 75 000. Binding to thrombin, it greatly enhances thrombin activation of protein C.[34] Moreover, in this bound state, thrombin is less effective in clotting fibrinogen or activating platelets, factor V and factor VIII. It is also less effective in inactivating protein S. Hence, thrombomodulin is able to endow thrombin with anticoagulant properties and thereby provide a feedback mechanism to limit sequential clotting reactions.

Thrombospondin

Thrombospondin is released from the α-granules of aggregating platelets and becomes enmeshed in the fibrin clot. It is a glycoprotein present at very low concentrations in plasma (0.02–0.2 μg/mL) but in serum there is a concentration of about 20 μg/mL because of the platelet release. It is synthesized by a variety of cells in culture and has a molecular weight of approximately 450 000. It has been suggested that thrombospondin potentiates platelet–platelet and platelet–protein interactions and may take part in cellular adhesion. It also binds to complex carbohydrates such as heparin.

Plasmin, Plasminogen and Antiplasmin

Plasmin is a proteolytic enzyme responsible for dissolving fibrin clots and plasminogen is its inactive precursor.[35] Plasminogen is a single-chain glycoprotein with a molecular weight of approximately 92 000, circulating in the blood at a concentration of about 75 μg/mL. As molecular contact of fibrin strands is limited to the nodular bodies, open channels are available for plasminogen and plasminogen activators to enter. There they both adsorb on to the fibrin and plasminogen is activated *in situ*. Plasmin is therefore produced where it is needed and where it is protected from attack by plasmin inhibitors. As fibrin dissolves, plasmin is released into the circulation and is rapidly consumed by the inhibitor.

Plasmin activators circulate in the blood at a low level but, following stress or exercise, the concentration markedly increases. The released material has a higher molecular weight of 67 000 compared to that of the circulating activator, which is of approximately 54 000. Active plasmin has a molecular weight of approximately 85 000 and is composed of two chains of 60 000 and 25 000. The major inhibitor of plasmin is α_2-antiplasmin, which circulates at a concentration of about 70 μg/mL and has a molecular weight of approximately 70 000. The next most important one is α_2-macroglobulin.

Platelets

Platelets are small cells, devoid of a nucleus and discoid in shape, measuring about 2–4 μm in diameter and about 1 μm thick.[36] Most are produced from megakaryocytes in the bone marrow, and have a lifespan of about 10 days. They are the smallest elements present in blood, negatively charged, and their normal concentration is between 150 000 and 300 000/mm³. A third of their total mass is concentrated in the spleen from where they circulate and exchange freely with the rest in circulation throughout the body. Newly formed platelets are larger than those that have aged in circulation.

The platelet is surrounded by a plasma membrane composed of mainly protein, phospholipid, cholesterol and some carbohydrate. Small channels connect the platelet interior to the surface and presumably these act as a pathway for platelet excretions to emerge. The plasma membrane is supported by bundles of microtubules and smaller microfilaments are present as well as a dense tubular system.

Within the platelet are different varieties of organelle, including several types of granules, mitochondria and dense bodies that are smaller and more electron-dense than the granules. Various materials are stored in both the granules and the dense bodies and these include 5-hydroxytryptamine, ADP, ATP, thrombasthenin, lysosomal enzyme, β-thromboglobulin, clotting factors, platelet factor 3 and platelet factor 4. In addition, clotting factors are adsorbed on to the plasma membrane and coagulation reactions that occur on the membrane appear to be strongly catalysed. On the exterior of platelets there are carbohydrate-rich domains incorporating many glycoproteins.[37] Some of these (glycoprotein Ib and glycoprotein IIb/IIIa) have been shown to be the receptors for von Willebrand factor. When exposed to aggregating agents, platelets change shape to a more spherical form and begin to aggregate. Release reactions then occur, yielding essential chemicals, including ADP, which presumably participates in the second and irreversible phase of aggregation. Platelets also have other functions such as participating in phagocytosis, inflammation reactions, immunological reactions and in interactions with tumour cells.

ASSAYS OF FACTORS AND COMPONENTS

Principles

In most coagulation assays, reagents are added to a diluted sample of blood plasma and the time taken for the solution to gel is recorded. Measurement is still commonly done manually with a stopwatch, being started as the last reagent is added to a mixture in a test-tube. After this the tube is moved gently in front of a lamp and the watch stopped when visible signs of a clot appear. Machines are now available that can perform the same task. They seem to be accurate and reliable, and as a result they are becoming more popular.

Clotting tests nearly always rely on comparing a patient's sample with a normal standard and the results are expressed either in units/mL or else as a percentage of an average normal level. National and international standards are available for most factors but the amounts are such that a large laboratory could not use them as a daily routine standard. Instead, they would be used to calibrate a freeze-dried plasma or concentrate that has been stored in vials at low temperature and these vials would be used as the working standard. If the clotting factor in question is stable, then an alternative standard can be prepared by making a pool of normal plasmas and storing this at $-40°C$ in small portions.

As an alternative to evaluating clotting time, it is now possible to employ a colorimetric substrate, which will produce a colour change. Typically, it would detect the presence of thrombin or activated factor X and would be the *p*-nitroanilide of a peptide. In the presence of one of the proteolytic enzymes that develop with clotting, the highly coloured *p*-nitroaniline is released. Colorimetric substrates are not yet common in coagulation laboratories except for use in certain specialized assays or where large numbers of an individual assay are required.

As well as studying clotting activity of a sample, it is also possible to measure the *antigen level* associated with a particular clotting factor. Such tests record the presence of the molecules of a clotting factor whether they have biological activity or not and so must be regarded as complementing biological tests rather than replacing them. Methods employed are discussed below, with the assays of von Willebrand factor, where they are particularly useful.

Results of coagulation assays are usually calculated by obtaining results at several different dilutions of both the sample and a standard. Graphs are plotted of the logarithm of the dilution against either the clotting time or the logarithm of the clotting time. Alternatively a simple program for a calculator or computer can be devised, which will make the same

TABLE 29.3
BLEEDING TIME TESTS AND TOURNIQUET TESTS

Disorders that give abnormal results in the bleeding time test
Thrombocytopenia
Qualitative platelet disorders
Uraemia
von Willebrand's disease
Afibrinogenaemia
Telangiectasia (if an abnormal vessel is punctured)

Disorders that give abnormal results in the tourniquet test
Thrombocytopenia
Qualitative platelet disorders
Scurvy

---

evaluation. It is best to test the sample and standard each at three different dilutions so that results appear on the graph paper as two parallel lines. In addition, each of those experimental points needs to be duplicated. In this way the sample can be expressed as a percentage of the standard with an accuracy of about 20% of the value obtained.

Preliminary Tests on the Patient

The first action in investigating a person with a suspected bleeding problem is to make an accurate record of the bleeding and family histories, which can only be done by an experienced clinical specialist. This is of vital importance because occasions do still arise where the battery of biological tests fails to find an abnormality and yet the clinical history provides clear evidence that a bleeding problem does exist. There are two tests that are routinely made directly on patients. One is the *bleeding time test*[38] in which a record is made of the time taken for a standard skin puncture to stop bleeding. The second is the *tourniquet test* where a sphygmomanometer cuff is applied to the upper arm at a pressure that restricts venous flow. The number of petechiae seen to develop is used as a measure of capillary fragility. Diseases that could give abnormal results in the two tests are listed in Table 29.3.

Preliminary Tests on Whole Blood

If whole blood devoid of anticoagulant is placed in a glass test-tube at 37°C it will clot in about 3–5 min for a normal person. This is the *whole-blood clotting time test*, which is still used but, in practice, prolongation of this clotting time would detect only the grossest of abnormalities. However, it does have some extra value because the serum which is produced can be used in a test that measures residual prothrombin. This is called the *prothrombin consumption test* and it evaluates the combined effectiveness of the intrinsic pathway together with platelets. Abnormality here is registered by prothrombin not being sufficiently con-

sumed and therefore remaining in the serum. There are two more tests routinely made on anticoagulated whole blood. One is to make a blood film for microscopic evaluation of cells and platelets and the other is to count the number of cells and platelets present. The latter is most often done in an automated cell counter.

For coagulation work, trisodium citrate is the usual anticoagulant. Blood would be collected by venepuncture and transferred to tubes containing anticoagulant and made up to a specific volume mark. EDTA is employed for certain platelet tests but not for coagulation samples as several clotting factors are inactivated by chelating agents such as EDTA, owing to removal of essential metals such as calcium.

Preliminary Tests on Plasma

Most tests of clotting factors are made on plasma separated from citrated blood by centrifugation. Normally, this would be high spun to remove platelets as well as the other cells. If a platelet-rich material is required, then gentle centrifugation can be employed or the blood can be left to settle under gravity.

There are two procedures that are initially done on plasma. One is the *activated partial thromboplastin time test* (APTT), which is also known as the kaolin-cephalin clotting time test. It evaluates the intrinsic pathway using kaolin to provide the initial surface activation plus cephalin to mimic the lipid from aggregating platelets. The second procedure is the *one-stage prothrombin time test*, which examines the extrinsic route using a tissue extract to simulate the product of wounded tissue. In principle, there is a wide choice of possible extracts but a saline extract of brain is the most convenient. At one time, human material would be used but safety considerations now demand an alternative and currently rabbit is the most usual source.

Typical procedures for these two methods are given next.

One-stage Prothrombin Time
Plasma sample	0.1 mL
Tissue extract	0.1 mL
0.025M-calcium chloride solution	0.1 mL—start stopwatch
Record clotting time	

Activated Partial Thromboplastin Time
Plasma sample	0.1 mL
Cephalin solution	0.1 mL
Kaolin suspension	0.1 mL
Incubate at 37°C for 2–5 min	
0.025M-calcium chloride solution	0.1 mL—start stopwatch
Record clotting time	

Upon completion of these two tests, it should be possible to locate a deficiency as being either in the intrinsic or extrinsic chain or else in the route which is common to both (*see* Fig. 29.1). However, it is necessary to exercise some caution because the procedures can be slightly insensitive to prothrombin deficiency as well as to deficiencies of factors VIII or IX around the level of 20–30%.

A third preliminary investigation done on plasma is the *thrombin time*, which is simply a measure of the time it takes for a sample to clot when thrombin is added to it. It is an indicator of fibrinogen content but it can also reflect the presence of an abnormal fibrinogen or of an inhibitory substance such as fibrin degradation products.

One-stage Assays

A simple one-stage form of assay is available for all the factors displayed in Fig. 29.1 with the exception of fibrinogen, prothrombin and factor XIII. Most are basically modifications of the preliminary tests given in the previous section, the difference being that the plasma sample is diluted and there is one additional reagent introduced, which is a plasma deficient in the factor being assayed. By these means, the test plasma is made to be the major source of the factor being tested, in the reaction mixture. Hence that factor is in the rate-determining step of the assay and clotting time varies with its concentration. Factors of the intrinsic chain, from factor XII through to factor VIII and IX are assayed by a modification of the APTT. A typical procedure in a factor XI assay would be as follows:

Diluted test plasma	0.1 mL
Plasma deficient in factor XI	0.1 mL
Cephalin solution	0.1 mL
Kaolin suspension	0.1 mL
Incubate at 37°C for 5 min	
0.025M-calcium chloride solution	0.1 mL—start stopwatch
Record clotting time	

The diluted plasma referred to above would probably be tested in a range of dilutions, for example at 1 in 10, 1 in 30 and 1 in 100, so that the final result could be computed graphically. If a factor other than factor XI were being assayed, then the appropriate deficient plasma would be substituted in the formula above. Factor V could, in principle, be tested in the same way but in practice it is better to use a modification of the one-stage prothrombin time as is used for factor VII. The latter is typically as follows:

Diluted test plasma	0.1 mL
Plasma deficient in factor VII	0.1 mL
Tissue extract	0.1 mL
0.025M-calcium solution	0.1 mL—start stopwatch
Record clotting time	

Factor X could be measured in a manner similar to the two procedures above but there is a complication in that factor X-deficient plasma is rare. However, venom from the Russell's viper will activate factor X directly, which permits another assay to be used. In this factor X assay, venom replaces tissue extract in the method above and an artificially made, deficient plasma is employed. The latter is incidentally deficient in factor VII as well as factor X but this is not a problem since the venom activates factor X directly without involving factor VII. Prothrombin (factor II) can also be measured by a snake-venom assay but this is referred to later.

Two-stage Assays

Factors VII[39] and IX can be measured very satisfactorily by the one-stage assays above but for these two factors an alternative is possible. This is the two-stage assay, which is organized so that diluted test sample and starting reagents are devoid of prothrombin. As a result, the reaction in its first stage fails to reach completion and instead the sequential steps terminate with the activation of factor X (*see* Fig. 29.1). Reagents are adjusted such that the factor VIII or IX in the diluted plasma occupy the rate-determining step in the reaction and hence the amount of activated factor X formed is proportional to the amount of factor VIII or IX originally present. After an appropriate incubation period the reaction is allowed to complete itself by adding a source of prothrombin and fibrinogen (usually normal plasma) and the clotting time of this second stage is recorded. As mentioned above, the test plasma needs to be devoid of prothrombin when used in this assay. For the factor VIII assay this is achieved by adsorbing it with aluminium hydroxide suspension while for the factor IX assay the plasma is clotted to form a serum (factor IX would be adsorbed by aluminium hydroxide).

The two-stage assay enjoyed a period of popularity that now appears to be waning. For measurement of factor IX it is seldom used. For measurement of factor VIII the two-stage assay is still very good but it does require more sophisticated reagents and more finely controlled conditions. As a result it is more prone to 'off days' than its one-stage counterpart. An area in which the two-stage assay is staging a modest revival is in the colorimetric assay for factor VIII. The available colorimetric substrates seem to have improved and it is now possible to introduce into the second stage of the factor VIII assay a substrate that changes colour with activated factor X and thus the degree of colour is a measure of the factor VIII content.

Assay of von Willebrand Factor and its Antigen

The levels of both von Willebrand factor and its antigen can be measured. Assay of the active factor is based on the finding that ristocetin (a redundant antibiotic) at an experimentally determined concentration will aggregate normal platelets if von Willebrand factor is present. Therefore, ristocetin and normal platelets are mixed with the sample and the degree of platelet aggregation determined. For a semiquantitative result the aggregation could be visually observed but otherwise special apparatus is required. One method[40] uses an aggregometer that recognizes aggregation by light transmission or scattering and provides a plot of it changing with time. Time taken to reach a particular level of aggregation is recorded for each sample and compared to those of a standard. The second method[41] involves mixing the reagents, allowing aggregated platelets to settle and then counting the number that remain unaggregated, using an electronic particle counter. Knowing the number of unaggregated platelets at the beginning allows a calculation of the percentage aggregation and this can be compared to the results for a standard sample.

The von Willebrand factor antigen is measured by conventional techniques of immunology using a specific antibody. Most usual is the Laurell method in which antibody is included in an agarose gel and samples are introduced into small holes in this gel. These traverse the gel under the influence of an applied electric field and peaks of antibody–antigen complex, whose heights are proportional to the amounts of antigen in each sample, appear after staining. Radioactive and colorimetric assays are also possible (IRMA and ELISA tests) where the antibody is adsorbed on to a plastic tube or well, reacted with test sample and then further reacted with a labelled antibody. The amount of label picked up is a measure of antigen level.

A two-dimensional Laurell technique is also very useful to detect certain abnormalities in the von Willebrand factor molecule that are manifested by an alteration in electrophoretic mobility.[42] Here the sample is run in an electrophoretic gel that does not contain antibody. After an appropriate period of time the run is stopped and the electrophoretic path in the gel is cut out. This is recast in another gel that, this time, does contain antibody. Electrophoresis continues now at right angles to the first dimension and when the run is complete the antibody–antigen complex is revealed by staining. Position and shape of these peaks of complex reveal the mobility of the sample in the first dimension and are compared with those for normal samples.

There is another method of detecting abnormalities in the von Willebrand molecule that involves electro-

phoresis.[42] In this, the sample is placed in a chemically dissociating medium and then run on a dissociating polyacrylamide gel. Using a labelled antibody, a pattern of multimers is seen on the electrophoretic track and this pattern varies according to the particular abnormality in the antigen.

Assay of Prothrombin

It might be thought that a simple one-stage assay based upon the one-stage prothrombin time test, as described for factor VII, would also be suitable for the assay of prothrombin. In practice this is a rather insensitive assay. A better method is to use the venom of the Taipan snake, which activates prothrombin directly.

A typical assay would be:

Diluted plasma	0.1 mL
Cephalin	0.1 mL
Fibrinogen solution	0.1 mL
Venom/0.025M-calcium chloride	0.1 mL—start stopwatch
Record time taken to clot	

Venom of the Tiger snake can also be used but this additionally requires factor V.

An alternative assay for prothrombin is the *two-stage prothrombin time test*. It involves clotting plasma using tissue extract and subsampling from the mixture at intervals into fibrinogen. Clotting times are converted into equivalent thrombin concentrations using a calibration curve. Then a graph is constructed of thrombin generation with time. The area under this graph is a measure of total thrombin generation and can be compared to that of a normal sample. It is a tedious and time-consuming assay and does not work well on stored samples. As a result it is usually only done where it is required to demonstrate thrombin generation in the patient's own plasma with his or her own antithrombin.

Assay of Fibrinogen

In the coagulation laboratory, fibrinogen measurement usually starts by clotting the sample with thrombin. For a rapid screening test, the clotting time alone can be taken as an indicator of fibrinogen content or, for a more quantitative test, a range of dilutions of the sample can be clotted and the dilution recorded when the clot just fails to appear. To improve the assay further, a series of dilutions of the sample and a standard can be tested, and by plotting clotting times against dilution a numerical answer can be obtained.

In the chemical laboratory, a true quantitative measure of fibrinogen is obtained by clotting the sample, washing the clot and then determining the amount of protein in it. It is even possible to weigh the dried clot and compare the result with that of a standard sample.

Assay of Factor XIII

The basis of the factor XIII test is to clot the plasma and suspend it in a solution of urea or acetic acid, when an abnormality would be indicated by the clot dissolving. Parallel tests would be run on a normal and known abnormal sample. With this type of test it is important to make sure that the patient has not been given a transfusion of blood or a plasma fraction that contains factor XIII. The half-life of the factor is relatively long and only 2% of the normal level is required for clot stability, which means that the effects of such a transfusion could persist for a long time. It would be easy to convert the above procedure into a quantitative assay by serially diluting the sample, using plasma deficient in factor XIII, and observing the clot stability of the dilutions. Usually this modification is avoided because of the rarity of deficient plasma.

Quantitative assays are also possible, based on measuring transglutaminase activity. However, results obtained are not a strict measure of biological activity and therefore they are not usually the first choice in a coagulation laboratory. On the other hand, plasma fractionators find them very useful. A transglutaminase assay is usually based on the ability of the sample to cross-link casein with labelled putrecine or cadaverine. A radioactive (usually ^{14}C) or a fluorescent label are the most common.

Assay of Antithrombin III

Antithrombin content is determined, in principle, by incubating a sample with a known amount of thrombin and assessing the amount of thrombin that remains.[43] Measuring this residual thrombin usually involves adding fibrinogen and comparing the clotting times with those of a standard (using a range of dilutions of both samples and standard). Alternatively, a colorimetric substrate can be employed, which produces colour in response to the proteolytic action of thrombin. Heparin markedly accelerates the action of antithrombin and as a result is often included in assay procedures. By the same token, antithrombin assays can be converted into procedures to measure heparin.

A variation of the above method is based on diffusion in an agarose gel. The gel contains thrombin and samples are placed in small holes in it. As the samples diffuse, thrombin is consumed by the antithrombin they contain until all of the latter is depleted. Fibrinogen in molten agarose is poured on top to reveal thrombin and hence the area of thrombin consumption. Results are computed by comparing this area with corresponding ones for standards. Immunoelectrophoretic assays as well as IRMA and ELISA techniques are also applicable to anti-

thrombin measurement when true biological activity is not needed.

Assay of Inhibitors and Antibodies

Naturally occurring inhibitors are essential as part of the control mechanisms in coagulation reactions but there are other inhibitors that can develop in the blood, usually as the result of an underlying clinical condition. In addition, antibodies can develop in response to replacement therapy, or on rare occasions they can arise in a person who had previously normal haemostasis. Antibodies to factor VIII and IX are those most commonly encountered in the coagulation laboratory.

Antibodies and inhibitors reveal themselves initially by a prolongation of the clotting time in one of the preliminary tests. Following this, their inhibitory nature can be confirmed by mixing patient's plasma with that of a normal subject and repeating the test. If inhibitors are in the test sample the clotting time will be much longer than would have been predicted from the proportions of the two plasmas in the mix.

With antibodies a quantitative assay is possible, which consists basically of mixing patients' plasma with a source of the factor in question and measuring how much of the factor remains. For most antibodies this is a fairly rapid reaction and the procedure is straightforward. However, with factor VIII antibodies, the process is more time consuming and the actual procedure adopted can influence the results obtained. Initially, this gave rise to a variety of methods and it was necessary to find a standard procedure. As a result, the Bethesda antibody assay was developed in committee.[44] It has its shortcomings but it is used almost universally.

Assay of Protein C, Protein S and Thrombomodulin

Protein C can be assayed by clotting methods as well as by colorimetric techniques that detect amidolytic activity.[45] Amidolytic activity is not necessarily the same as biological activity but at least it is one stage better than an immunological assay of antigen. Clotting methods call for great attention to detail. They are tedious and as a result the colorimetric procedures are quite popular. The original clotting methods involve adsorbing protein C out of the plasma sample, adding thrombin to activate the protein C and then antithrombin to remove excess thrombin. Anticoagulant activity of the mixture is a measure of the protein C content and is assessed by prolongation of clotting time in the APTT test. A very useful development is seen with the introduction of the venom from the copperhead snake, which directly activates protein C.[46] After activation by venom, anticoagulant action of protein C can be measured using the APTT tests or, alternatively, amidolytic action can be assayed by means of a colorimetric substrate, with the same reservations as recorded above.

Thrombomodulin greatly enhances the thrombin activation of protein C and protein S catalyses its proteolytic action. Therefore the protein C assay can be modified to convert it into a thrombomodulin[34] or a protein S[47] assay. Immunological tests for protein C, protein S and thrombomodulin are also available and these can be based on the ELISA, IRMA or the immunoelectrophoretic methods.

Test on Platelets

An initial indicator of a platelet disorder is seen in the preliminary tests referred to earlier, when the bleeding time is seen to be prolonged and the tourniquet test is found to be abnormal. The prothrombin consumption index may also be abnormal. A count of platelet numbers will also be made to identify thrombocytopenia if present.

After this the *aggregation tests* of platelet function are made. Platelet aggregation can be observed visually but machines give much more information. An aggregometer is used, which detects aggregation with time. The procedure is then simply to mix platelet-rich plasma with the reagent and allow the machine to plot out its curve. Each reagent is used at a series of dilutions so that a family of curves can be built up and compared to a similar set obtained using a normal plasma. For the normal subject, it is usually possible to observe the complete aggregation process at one or more of the intermediate dilutions. Typically, an initial aggregation is followed by disaggregation and then a second phase of aggregation occurs as a result of ADP release from the platelets. Failure to aggregate or an absence of the second wave of aggregation are the indicators of an abnormality.

The main divisions of abnormality likely to be encountered are as follows:

- *Thrombocytopenia.* Reduction in the number of platelets, which are otherwise normal.
- *Thrombasthenia.* Platelets fail to aggregate with ADP, adrenaline or collagen but aggregate normally with ristocetin. *In vivo* they would adhere normally to subendothelium but would fail to aggregate beyond a monolayer.
- *Release reaction defects.* Platelets aggregate with ADP, adrenaline, or ristocetin but fail to aggregate with collagen. In addition, they fail to show a second phase of aggregation with ADP or adrenaline. These defects can be subdivided into storage-pool deficiency, cyclo-oxygenase deficiency and defective nucleotide metabolism.
- *Defective adhesion.* Bernard–Soulier syndrome is the inherited disorder of this type. Platelets are abnormally large and fail to aggregate with ristocetin. Aggregation with ADP or collagen is normal.
- α-Granule deficiency. In 'gray platelet' syndrome, platelets show a marked reduction in the number of α-granules they contain and hence there is a

corresponding reduction in the amount of essential chemicals available for release. Platelets are variable and of slightly increased size and numbers may be reduced. As well as showing a poverty of α-granules, the platelets have a peculiar grey appearance. Aggregation with ADP or collagen is somewhat reduced.

Tests of Fibrinolysis[48]

Plasmin can be assayed by means of its lytic action on fibrin or by its caseinolytic, esterolytic or amidolytic activity. Measurements would be made with a range of sample dilutions and results compared with those for standard samples. At the moment, assays of amidolytic action using colorimetric substrates are quite popular. Plasminogen levels are determined by first activating the plasminogen with, for example, streptokinase and then measuring the resultant plasmin. Immunological assays are also available to detect the presence of the plasminogen molecule.

Blood samples for tests of existing fibrinolytic function should be taken with minimum venous stasis and immediately processed at 4°C. The following four tests are the most common.

1. Clot Lysis Time

The sample is clotted and incubated at 37°C. Time taken for the clot to dissolve is recorded and compared with results for normal samples. This is a non-specific test that only provides a rough guide to diagnosis. The initial sample can be blood, diluted blood or plasma but of the three, plasma provides the most sensitive method.

2. Euglobulin Lysis Time

The principle here is to remove fibrinolytic inhibitors by adding an acidic solution to plasma and collecting the euglobulin that precipitates. This is redissolved and made to clot by introducing thrombin or calcium or both. Clotted samples are incubated at 37°C and the times taken for clots to lyse are recorded and compared with values for normal samples.

3. Fibrin Plate Method

Fibrinogen solution is clotted in a Petri dish using thrombin. Drops of each sample are placed on the plate and left overnight at 37°C. Areas of lysis caused by samples dissolving the fibrin are a measure of fibrinolytic activity. Using plasma here results in a test that is too insensitive and it is usually a euglobin (referred to above) that is applied to the plate. Results obtained will be a measure of plasminogen activator since plasminogen itself will already be present, bound to the fibrin. It is possible to modify the test to measure plasmin content by initially heating the plate to 80°C to destroy adherent plasminogen. Similarly a heated plate can be used to measure plasminogen by activating the sample with streptokinase to convert it to plasmin before applying it to the plate.

4. Fibrin Degradation Products

These are usually detected by an immunological method involving red cells or latex particles that have been coated with antiserum. When a sample is added the degree of aggregation is a measure of the amount of fibrin degradation products present. A variation of the test also exists in which a sample is mixed with antiserum and residual antiserum is then assessed by adding cells or latex that have been coated with fibrinogen (this antiserum reacts with both fibrinogen and the degradation products).

Carrier Detection

Female relatives of patients with haemophilia A or B frequently request investigations to determine whether they are carriers of the disease. Both complaints are inherited by an X-linked recessive mechanism and often the female carrier will exhibit no signs of excessive bleeding. As discussed in the section on factor VIII above, carriers of either of these two diseases will have, on average, 50% of the normal factor level but variation between individuals is large. Therefore, a simple measurement of factor concentration detects a proportion of carriers but by no means all of them. Variation of factor IX concentration in the general population is somewhat less than that for factor VIII and, accordingly, the prediction rate for haemophilia B is slightly better. In the case of haemophilia A a significant improvement is obtained by using a ratio of the levels of factor VIII to von Willebrand factor as the predictor of carrier status. As the latter is normal in haemophilia A the expected value for the average carrier would be 1:2. Probably the reason why this ratio affords an improvement is that both factors are affected if the patient is stressed or has been exercising and therefore a ratio cancels out the effect of these conditions.

An alternative and powerful technique is now possible however, using DNA analysis, which is capable of detecting the majority of carriers.[49] Eventually it should be possible to analyse the exact mutation that causes haemophilia in any particular family and as a result any female in this family could be assessed by determining whether she possesses that mutation or not. It will be some time before all families can be characterized in this way and so, in the meantime, an alternative method is being employed. This alternative is not as good as direct sequencing of the precise mutation but is nevertheless extremely powerful. It is called restriction fragment length polymorphism (RFLP) analysis and depends on the fact that DNA in a given gene can vary from individual to individual without causing any clinical problem. Such variations usually occur in relatively unimportant parts of the gene that do not code for protein (introns). The way in which the differences are detected is to employ enzymes (restriction endonucleases) that cut the DNA only at a specific site. If this site has been changed in any way (an inherited variation), the enzyme will fail to cut at that point. This must be reflected in the fragment sizes being different from those obtained with the unchanged DNA. Fragment size is revealed by running the reaction mixture on an electrophoresis gel causing fragments to separate according to their mobility. After this the gel is overlaid with a nitrocellulose or nylon membrane and a high ionic-strength buffer is passed through the pair so as to transfer fragments still in position on to the membrane (Southern blotting method). A radioactive probe applied to the membrane reveals the position of the fragments by autoradiography.

Carrier detection then depends on using this technique on DNA from the person enquiring about her carrier status and on DNA from other members of her family. With each enzyme being used, there are only two results that can be obtained for a given gene. Either the cutting site has an attenuation or else it has not. The altered site results in a certain fragment size being obtained while the unaltered site gives a different size. The deductions then made are best illustrated by an example. Assume the results are as follows (**NB**. Females have two genes and males have one if inheritance is X-linked):

Family member	Fragment size (kb)
Female enquiring	1.8 and 1.3
Her mother	1.8 and 1.3
Her father	1.8
Her affected brother	1.8

The deduction then proceeds as follows. The mother has two different genes and the one which corresponds to a 1.8-kb fragment is the abnormal one because this is the same as that possessed by her affected son (brother of the female enquiring). The enquiring female also has two different genes and she took the one corresponding to a 1.8-kb fragment from her father. Therefore, she took her gene corresponding to a 1.3-kb fragment from her mother. However, from the deduction above, that corresponds to the unaffected one of her mother's genes. Therefore, the female is not a carrier. It should be noted that analysis is not necessary for a female whose father is a haemophiliac. She must, of necessity, receive an affected gene from her father and therefore she will definitely be a carrier.

REFERENCES

1. Rizza C.R. (1981). Management of patients with inherited blood coagulation defects. In *Haemostasis and Thrombosis* (Bloom A.L., Thomas D.P. eds.) Edinburgh: Churchill Livingstone, pp. 371–388.
2. Crossley M. et al. (1990). A less severe form of haemophilia B Leyden. *Nucleic Acids Res.*, **18**, 4633.
3. Bloom A.L. (1980). The von Willebrand syndrome. *Semin. Hematol.*, **12**, 215.
4. Kattlove H.E., Shapiro S.S., Spivack M. (1970). Hereditary prothrombin deficiency. *N. Engl. J. Med.*, **282**, 57.

5. Greipp P.R., Kyle R.A., Bowie E.J.W. (1981). Factor X deficiency in amyloidosis. *Am. J. Haematol.*, **11**, 443.
6. Beck E.A. (1979). Congenital abnormalities of fibrinogen. *Clin. Haematol.*, **8**, 169.
7. Saito H. et al. (1979). Molecular heterogeneity of Hageman trait (factor XII deficiency). *J. Lab. Clin. Med.*, **94**, 256.
8. Lorand L., Losowsky M.S., Miloszewski K.J.M. (1980). Fibrin stabilising factor. *Prog. Hemost. Thromb.*, **5**, 245.
9. Bick R.L. (1982). Clinical relevance of antithrombin III. *Semin. Thromb. Hemost.*, **8**, 276.
10. Bertina R.M. (1987). Congenital deficiencies of protein C and protein S. In *Biotechnology in Clinical Medicine* (Albertini A., Lenfant C., Paoletti R., eds.) New York: Raven Press, pp. 175–181.
11. Hardisty R.M., Caen J.P. (1981). Disorders of platelet function. In *Haemostasis and Thrombosis* (Bloom A.L., Thomas D.P. eds.) Edinburgh: Churchill Livingstone, pp. 301–320.
12. Stump D.C. et al. (1990). Pathologic fibrinolysis as a cause of clinical bleeding. *Semin. Thromb. Hemost.*, **16**, 260.
13. Tans G., Rosling J. (1987) Structural and functional characteristics of factor XII. *Semin. Thromb. Hemost.*, **13**, 1.
14. Mannhalter C.H. (1987). Biochemical and functional properties of factor XI and prekallikrein. *Semin. Thromb. Hemost.*, **13**, 25.
15. van Iwaarden F. (1987). The role of high molecular weight kininogen in contact activation. *Semin. Thromb. Hemost.*, **13**, 15.
16. Osterud B., Bouma B.N., Griffin J.H. (1978) Human blood coagulation factor IX. Purification, properties and mechanism of activation by activated factor XI. *J. Biol. Chem.*, **253**, 5946.
17. Anson D.S. et al. (1984). Gene structure of human anti-haemophilic factor IX. *EMBO J.*, **3**, 1053.
18. Leyte A. et al. (1989). The interaction between blood coagulation factor VIII and von Willebrand factor. *Biochem J.*, **257**, 679.
19. Austen D.E.G. (1979). The chromatographic separation of factor VIII on aminohexyl sepharose. *Br. J. Haematol.* **43**, 669.
20. Pittman D.D., Kaufmann R.J. (1989). Structure–function relationship of factor VIII elucidated through recombinant DNA technology. *Thromb. Haemost.*, **61**, 161.
21. Chopek M.W. et al. (1986). Human von Willebrand factor: a multivalent protein composed of subunits. *Biochemistry*, **25**, 3146.
22. Seligsohn U. et al. (1979). Activation of human factor VII in plasma and in a purified system. *J. Clin. Invest.*, **64**, 1056.
23. Mertens K., Briet E., Giles A.R. (1990). The role of factor VIII in haemostasis: infusion studies of factor VII in a canine model of factor VII deficiency. *Thromb. Haemost.*, **64**, 138.
24. Lindhout M.J., Kop-Klaassen B.H.M., Hemker H.C. (1978). The effect of γ-carboxyglutamic acid residues on the enzymatic properties of activated blood clotting X. *Biochem. Biophys. Acta*, **533**, 342.
25. Mann K.G., Nesheim M.E., Tracy P.B., (1986). Nonenzymatic cofactors: factor V. In *Blood Coagulation* (Zwaal R.F.A., Hemkar H.C. eds.) Amsterdam: Elsevier, pp. 15–34.
26. Baltlett S., Latson P., Hanahan D.J. (1980). High molecular weight factor V of bovine and human plasma. *Biochemistry*, **19**, 273.
27. Kristnaswamy S. et al. (1987). Activation of human prothrombin by human prothrombinase. *J. Biol. Chem.*, **262**, 3291.
28. Suttie J.W., Jackson C.M. (1977). Prothrombin structure activation and biosynthesis. *Physiol. Rev.*, **57**, 1.
29. Doolittle R.F. (1981). Fibrinogen and fibrin. In *Haemostasis and Thrombosis* (Bloom A.L., Thomas D.P. eds.) Edinburgh: Churchill Livingstone, pp. 163–199.
30. Lorand L., Losowsky M.S., Miloszewski Z.J.M. (1980). Human factor XIII: fibrin stabilising factor. *Prog. Hemost. Thromb.*, **5**, 245.
31. Griffith M.J. (1986). Inhibitors: antithrombin III and heparin. In *Blood Coagulation* (Zwaal R.F.A., Hemker H.C. eds.) Amsterdam: Elsevier, pp. 259–282.
32. Dahlback B., Fernlund P., Stenflo J. (1986). Inhibitors: protein C. In *Blood Coagulation* (Zwaal R.F.A., Hemker H.C. eds.) Amsterdam: Elsevier, pp.285–305.
33. Esmon C.T., Comp P.C., D'Angelo A. (1987). Protein C and protein S: physiological aspects. In *Biotechnology in Clinical Medicine* (Albertini A., Lenfant C., Paoletti R. eds.) New York: Raven Press, pp.143–152.
34. Esmon N.L., Esmon C.J. (1988). Protein C and the endothelium. *Semin. Thromb. Hemost.*, **14**, 210.
35. Mayer M. (1990). Biochemical and biological aspects of the plasminogen activation system. *Clin. Biochem.*, **23**, 197.
36. Mills D.C.B. (1981). The basic biochemistry of the platelet. In *Haemostasis and Thrombosis* (Bloom A.L., Thomas D.P., eds.) Edinburgh: Churchill Livingstone, pp.50–60.
37. Nurden A.T., Caen J.P. (1975). Specific role of platelet glycoproteins in platelet function. *Nature*, **255**, 720.
38. Rodgers R.P.C., Levin J. (1990). A critical appraisal of the bleeding time. *Semin. Thromb. Hemost.* **16**, 1.
39. Parquet-Gernez A., Mazurier C., Goudemand M. (1988). Functional and immunological assays of factor VIII in 133 haemophiliacs. *Thromb. Haemost.*, **59**, 202.
40. Macfarlane D.E. et al. (1975). A method for assaying von Willebrand factor (ristocetin co-factor). *Thromb. Diathesis Haemorrhagica*, **34**, 306.
41. Evans R.J., Austen D.E.G. (1977). Assay of ristocetin co-factor using fixing platelets and a platelet counting technique. *Br. J. Haematol*, **37**, 289.
42. Howard M.A., Oates A., Firkin B.G. (1988). Comparison of two-dimensional immunoelectrophoresis and multimer analysis in the study of von Willebrand factor. *J. Clin. Pathol.*, **41**, 346.
43. Tollefson D.M. (1990). Laboratory diagnosis of antithrombin and heparin cofactor II deficiency. *Semin. Thromb. Hemost.*, **16**, 162.
44. Kasper C.K. et al. (1975). A more uniform measurement of factor VIII inhibitor. *Thromb. Diathesis Haemorrhagica*, **34**, 869.
45. Miletich J.P. (1990). Laboratory diagnosis of protein C. deficiency. *Semin. Thromb. Hemost.*, **16**, 169.
46. Franchi F., Tripodi C., Valsechi C. (1988). Functional assay of protein C: comparison of two snake venom assays with two thrombin assays. *Thromb. Haemost.*, **60**, 145.
47. Comp P.C. (1990). Laboratory evaluation of protein S status. *Semin. Thromb. Hemost.*, **16**, 177.
48. Davidson J.F., Walker I.D. (1981). Assessment of the fibrinolytic system. In *Haemostasis and Thrombosis*

(Bloom A.L., Thomas D.P. eds.) Edinburgh: Churchill Livingstone, pp.796–808.

49. White G.C., Shoemaker C.B. (1989). Factor VIII gene and hemophilia A. *Blood*, **73**, 1–12.

FURTHER READING

Austen D.E.G., Rhymes I.L. (1975). *A Laboratory Manual of Blood Coagulation*, Oxford: Blackwell Scientific.

Bloom A.L., Thomas D.P. (1981). *Haemostasis and Thrombosis*, Edinburgh: Churchill Livingstone.

Brownlee G.G. (1986). The molecular genetics of haemophilia A and B. *J. Cell. Sci.*, Suppl. 4, 445.

Davies K.E. (1988). *Genome Analysis, a Practical Approach*, Oxford: IRL Press.

Kwaan H.C., Kazama M. (1990). Clinical aspects of fibrinolysis. *Semin. Thromb. Hemost.*, **16**(3).

Zwaal R.F.A., Hemker H.C. (1986). *Blood Coagulation*, Amsterdam: Elsevier.

30. Calcium Metabolism and Disorders of Bone

J. A. Kanis

Introduction
Physiological aspects
  Distribution and function of calcium
  Calcium balance
  Major regulating hormones
  The influencing hormones
  Calcium transport to and from the
    extracellular fluid
  Bone
  Integration of organ responses
Disorders of calcium homeostasis
  Disorders of parathyroid secretion
  Disorders of vitamin D metabolism
  Disorders of calcitonin secretion
  Hypercalcaemia
  Hypocalcaemia
  Disorders of bone turnover

TABLE 30.1
DISTRIBUTION OF CALCIUM AND PHOSPHATE IN NORMAL
HUMAN ADULTS

	Calcium	Phosphate
Total body content (for 70-kg adult)	1000–1500 g	700–1000 g (of phosphorus)
Skeleton	98.0%	85%
Skeletal muscle	0.3%	6%
Skin	0.08%	1%
Liver	0.02%	1%
Central nervous system	0.01%	1%
Other tissues	0.6%	5%
Extracellular fluid	1.0%	1%

PHYSIOLOGICAL ASPECTS

Distribution and Function of Calcium

Function of Calcium

Calcium and phosphate are widely distributed throughout living tissues. However, the great majority of calcium and phosphate is found in bone (Table 30.1) and the ability of the skeleton to turn over this calcium and phosphate is essential for growth, the prevention and healing of fractures, and the remodelling of the skeleton in response to physiological and pathological stresses. During skeletal growth and remodelling, calcium is transported to bone across the extracellular fluid compartment.

Fifty per cent of the extraskeletal calcium is found in the extracellular fluid (ECF). The ECF concentration of calcium is critical to maintain normal neuromuscular activity, and a fall in plasma calcium concentration results in tetany and convulsions. Conversely, a rise in the concentration of calcium in ECF has many adverse effects (*see* Hypercalcaemia below) including delayed neuromuscular conduction and muscle paralysis.

These two functions of calcium, the maintenance of the skeleton and of the ECF calcium concentration, are closely related and suggest that disorders of the one may induce disorders of the other. This is commonly but not invariably the case. Thus in primary hyperparathyroidism, skeletal disease and disturbed plasma calcium homeostasis commonly coexist. In contrast, in Paget's disease, bone turnover is characteristically increased but plasma calcium is usually normal.

The concentration of calcium within cells is considerably lower than in the ECF. Cytosol calcium concentrations are generally 100–1000 times lower than extracellular. Within cells, however, mitochondria are capable of accumulating large amounts of calcium against electrochemical gradients, to an extent that mitochondrial deposits of insoluble calcium phosphate can form. The activation of many different types of cells by hormones or pharmacological agents depends on increases in intracellular calcium concentrations derived from the ECF or from mitochondria.

INTRODUCTION

The past 20 years have witnessed a rapid growth in knowledge about calcium metabolism, particularly in our understanding of the biochemistry, metabolism, and actions of the calcium-regulating hormones. Not only has this clarified physiological control mechanisms, it has also resulted in a better understanding of the pathophysiology of several clinical disorders. This in turn has led to a more rational approach to investigating patients with disorders of mineral metabolism.

The purpose of this chapter is to review the pathophysiology of the common disorders of plasma calcium and skeletal homeostasis. The approach is one of applied physiology and therefore a substantial proportion of the chapter deals with normal physiology. This provides a basis for interpreting the many biochemical, histological and other investigations available to the clinician interested in metabolic bone disease. Of the many tests available, an attempt has been made to distinguish those primarily of physiological and pathophysiological interest from those of diagnostic value.

TABLE 30.2
DISTRIBUTION OF PLASMA CALCIUM

Ultrafilterable calcium (53%)	
Ionized calcium	47.0
Complexed calcium (6%):	
phosphate	1.5
citrate	1.5
HCO₃ etc.	3.0
Protein-bound calcium (47%)	
Albumin	37.0
Globulin	10.0
Total plasma calcium (2.12–2.6 mmol/L)	100%

Many intracellular processes including enzyme activity, cell division and exocytosis are controlled by intracellular calcium, and in particular the calcium-dependent regulatory protein, *calmodulin*.

Disorders of intracellular calcium homeostasis have not been recognized, perhaps partly because of the difficulties of measuring subcellular calcium concentrations. Hormonal activation is commonly associated with a stimulation of adenylate cyclases specific to the target tissue. This in turn changes the levels of cyclic AMP (cAMP) and intracellular calcium, producing further responses within the cell. In some disorders this sequence is lost and the ability of parathyroid hormone (PTH) to stimulate adenylate cyclase and other metabolic events can be used clinically to distinguish various disorders of parathyroid function.

Plasma Calcium

The concentration of plasma calcium in health is maintained within a narrow range (Table 30.2) despite the large movements of calcium across gut, bone, kidney and cells. Several hormones, including parathyroid hormone and 1,25-dihydroxy vitamin D_3 (1,25(OH)$_2$D$_3$ or calcitriol) appear to regulate the ionized fraction of plasma calcium (approx. 50% of total plasma calcium) by modulating calcium fluxes to and from the ECF. In turn the secretion rates for these hormones are regulated by the calcium concentration in the ECF.

Changes in the concentration of plasma ionized calcium are usually accompanied by changes in the total amount of calcium in the ECF since there is a passive distribution of ionized calcium throughout the ECF compartment. Within the plasma compartment, however, approximately 40% of the calcium is bound to proteins, mainly albumin, and the binding is pH dependent. Major changes in plasma protein concentration, the presence of abnormal proteins, and large shifts in extracellular hydrogen ion concentration may therefore affect the proportion of total plasma calcium that is bound. A further 5–10% of total plasma calcium is bound to small anions such as citrate, phosphate and bicarbonate, and the extent of binding may vary as the concentrations of these anions change. For these reasons the estimation of total plasma calcium may not accurately reflect the ionized calcium concentration.

Changes in the binding of calcium in plasma have some important clinical consequences. Thus, the paraesthesiae found in patients with the hyperventilation syndrome are due to a decrease in ionized calcium concentration because of alkalosis; but the total plasma calcium level is normal. Also, the infusion of alkali into patients with metabolic acidosis (e.g. in diabetes mellitus and chronic renal failure) may precipitate hypocalcaemic convulsions due to a decrease in ionized calcium without changing total plasma calcium.

In the absence of severe acidosis or alkalosis, the major factor influencing the amount of calcium bound is the quantity of albumin present, since the proportion of calcium that is bound varies little. Failure to account for protein binding may result in the erroneous diagnosis of hypercalcaemia in conditions where there is an increased level or an abnormality of plasma proteins (e.g. dehydration, prolonged venous stasis, myeloma). Also, in hypoproteinaemic states, such as disseminated carcinoma or chronic renal disease, total plasma calcium may be low, though ionized calcium is normal. Similarly, in such disorders the concentration of total plasma calcium may be normal and may mask true hypercalcaemia.

The ionized or free plasma calcium concentration should ideally be measured, since it is the physiologically relevant fraction; methods are available, based on colorimetric reaction with dyes (tetramethyl murexide) or by the use of ion-selective electrodes. They are, however, tedious to do, and require rapid and anaerobic handling of the sample. Moreover, until recently, the errors of the methods used often exceeded the errors incurred from making appropriate corrections to measured concentrations of total plasma calcium.

Many formulae have been proposed for predicting the ionized calcium from the total plasma calcium, or 'correcting' the total plasma calcium to a normal protein value. These methods depend on the concurrent measurement of total proteins, albumin or specific gravity of plasma. None of these is entirely satisfactory but a simple correction factor for plasma calcium that is widely used is to subtract from (or add to) total plasma calcium 0.02 mmol/L (0.08 mg/dL) for every 1 g/L that the plasma albumin exceeds (or is less than) 40 g/L, provided that the sample is drawn without venous stasis. Many laboratories now report 'corrected' plasma calcium, but it should be realized that these are at best a guide to the ionized calcium concentration.

The small proportion of total plasma calcium (Table 30.2) that is complexed with cations such as phosphate, citrate, and bicarbonate should not be ignored. The calcium that is normally filtered by the kidney includes this complexed calcium as well as ionized calcium, and can be measured by passing

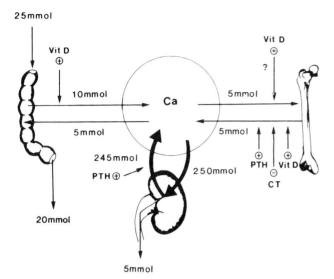

Figure 30.1 Major fluxes of calcium (mmol/day) in a healthy adult. Exchange of calcium in the extracellular fluid occurs with bone, gut and kidney. The net balance for calcium equals the net absorption minus the losses of calcium in faeces and urine, which in a healthy adult is zero. The major fluxes of calcium are regulated by the regulating hormones. PTH increases renal tubular reabsorption of calcium and bone resorption. Calcitonin (CT) inhibits bone resorption and vitamin D augments intestinal absorption for calcium. The precise role of vitamin D in augmenting bone resorption and mineralization *in vivo* is not clear.

plasma through membrane filters, which retain the protein-bound calcium. The measurement of ultrafilterable calcium may be of value when assessing the renal handling of calcium, particularly in those disorders associated with abnormalities in the complexed fraction of calcium, disorders of acid–base, phosphate or citrate metabolism for example. In normal subjects the ultrafilterable fraction of plasma calcium lies between 50 and 60% of the total plasma calcium.

Distribution of Calcium and Phosphate
Most of the body's calcium and phosphate resides in bone (98 and 85%, respectively), which is thus a major reservoir for both. Unlike calcium, the concentration of which is low in most soft tissues, about 15% of the body's phosphorus lies outside the skeleton as organic phosphate compounds such as nucleic acids, nucleotides, phospholipids and phosphorylated metabolites (*see* Table 30.1). Extracellular concentrations of phosphate vary much more than those of calcium, particularly in response to circadian rhythms and to meals. The measurement of plasma phosphate alone therefore affords less precise information than the measurement of plasma calcium, particularly when taken in the non-fasting state, and is best interpreted alongside additional investigations such as estimates of tubular reabsorption for phosphate.

Studies with radioisotopes (of calcium and strontium) have shown that in normal human adults the exchangeable pool of calcium is approximately 1–2% of the total body calcium, in the region of 2 mmol (80 mg)/kg during the first few days after injection. This nevertheless represents approximately 125 mmol, which is a substantial amount considering that the ECF contains somewhat less than 20 mmol (0.8 g) as ionized calcium. This exchangeable pool of calcium is therefore very important in plasma calcium homeostasis, and movements of calcium between body fluids, cells and surfaces of bone occur continuously.

These large and rapid fluxes of exchangeable calcium should be distinguished from the movements of calcium that occur in bone as a result of mineralization and resorption. *Resorption* is defined as the complete removal of bone mineral and matrix that occurs during physiological remodelling and is a result of osteoclast activity. This accounts for only a fraction of the total calcium exchange between ECF and bone, the remainder occurring across the large surface area of osteocytes and their canaliculi without synthesis or destruction of bone matrix. Between 1% and 4% of the adult skeleton is thought to be renewed each year. This process is not uniformly distributed throughout the skeleton, as trabecular bone has a faster turnover than cortical bone. This means that disturbances of bone-cell turnover commonly have greater effects in trabecular than cortical bone.

The body is not a closed system with respect to calcium, in the sense that calcium is lost by urinary and intestinal secretion and to a lesser extent in sweat, and enters by intestinal absorption and renal tubular reabsorption. The way in which the ECF concentration for calcium is maintained, and the way in which the body gains and loses calcium from the external environment, can be simplified by considering the roles of the major organs responsible for movements of calcium to and from the ECF, namely gut, kidney and bone.

Calcium Balance

Major Sites of Calcium Flux
The major movements (fluxes) of calcium through gut, bone and kidney in adults are shown in Fig. 30.1. Calcium enters the body by intestinal absorption. The true absorption of calcium is greater than the net absorption because some calcium is returned to the gut lumen in biliary, pancreatic and intestinal secretions. Thus, from an average daily dietary intake of 25 mmol (1 g), approximately 10 mmol are absorbed. This is offset by intestinal secretions amounting to approximately 5 mmol (0.2 g) daily, leaving a net transport into the ECF pool of 5 mmol. True and net fluxes across the gut can be measured by tracer and balance techniques, some of which are now used regularly in clinical practice.

The kidney is a major site for calcium excretion

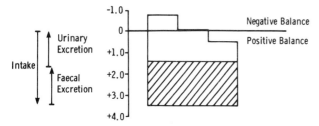

Figure 30.2 Metabolic diagram showing conventional method of calculating net balance. The daily intake of the dietary constituent (e.g. calcium) is plotted below the 0 line. From this value the faecal excretion (hatched areas) and the urinary excretion (unshaded areas) are subtracted to give the balance. The figure shows three balance periods. In the left-hand period the daily faecal output and urinary excretion exceed the dietary intake and the patient is in negative balance. In contrast, during the balance period on the right of the figure the patient is in positive balance where total excretion is less than dietary intake.

from the body. A large amount of calcium is filtered (Fig. 30.1) but most of this is reabsorbed so that only 1–3% is excreted into urine. These large fluxes through the kidney to and from the ECF compartment mean that small changes in renal tubular reabsorption may have profound effects on the ECF concentration of calcium. Since reabsorption is under hormonal control, principally by PTH, this has led to the view that the kidney is a major organ in the regulation of calcium.

Calcium is also lost from the body in sweat. This is commonly ignored in metabolic studies because the loss is small and cannot be measured easily. However, losses can be as high as 8 mmol (c. 300 mg) daily under extreme conditions.

In the mature adult who is neither gaining nor losing calcium, bone and soft tissues contribute neither a net gain nor loss of calcium from the ECF. Thus, the amount of bone resorbed (accounting for approximately 5 mmol (200 mg) of calcium daily) exactly matches the amount formed.

Calcium Balance

In the healthy adult who is neither gaining nor losing bone, the amount of calcium lost in urine is balanced by an equivalent amount of calcium absorbed by the gut (Fig. 30.1). A change in the calcium content of the skeleton must clearly result from changes in the net flux of calcium between the ECF and the skeleton. Because plasma calcium is controlled within a close range, and the bulk of calcium is in the skeleton, changes in bone mass are reflected in changes in the external balance for calcium (Fig. 30.2) rather than in changes in plasma calcium. For example, during growth, where there is a net daily gain of calcium into the skeleton, plasma and intracellular concentrations of calcium are normal. In the long term, therefore, the total body balance for calcium reflects

exactly the skeletal balance for calcium (in this case positive balance). Mineral losses begin in middle age (negative balance), particularly in women. Between the age of 25–45 years the body is for practical purposes neither gaining nor losing calcium, so that the inflow and outflow of calcium are matched.

Calcium balance is measured by the difference between the dietary intake of calcium and the combined faecal and urinary losses. In practice this is time consuming to do and needs the facilities of a metabolic unit.

Over the past few years a variety of techniques has been developed that measure skeletal mass or density. These include *in vivo* neutron activation analysis, computerized axial tomography, single- and dual-energy photon absorptiometry and dual-energy X-ray absorptiometry. These variously provide estimates of bone mineral at regional sites (appendicular or axial) or the whole body. There have been significant advances in the precision of these techniques so that balance can be measured by sequential determinations. The techniques most commonly used are single-photon absorptiometry at the wrist or mid-radius or dual-energy X-ray absorptiometry (at the spine, hip or whole body). Both have an *in vivo* reproducibility error of 1–2%. The performance characteristics of other techniques are shown in Table 30.3. These have largely replaced the traditional metabolic balance.

Calcium balance is a function of the integrated fluxes across bone, gut and kidney. These fluxes are continually changing and are affected by a variety of factors including several hormones. Thus, the concentration of calcium in the ECF is set by the relative size of the various fluxes and by the influence of these controlling agents. These hormones can be subdivided into 'controlling' and 'influencing' hormones. The *controlling hormones* are the major regulating hormones, PTH, calcitonin and the vitamin D metabolites, the secretion of each of which is altered in response to changes in plasma ionized calcium concentrations. The *influencing hormones* are those other hormones, such as thyroid hormones, growth hormone, and adrenal and gonadal steroids that have effects on calcium metabolism, but whose secretion is determined primarily by factors other than changes in plasma calcium.

Major Regulating Hormones

Parathyroid Hormone (PTH)

In the circulation, PTH consists of several polypeptide fragments, which are degraded in the liver and kidney. The major stimulus to the secretion of PTH is a fall in the ionized fraction of plasma calcium. The biological actions of PTH at a variety of target organs serve to increase plasma calcium concentration, which in turn suppresses the secretion of PTH, so that there exists an efficient negative-feedback hormonal loop.

Mammalian PTH consists of a single peptide chain,

TABLE 30.3

TECHNIQUES USED IN THE ASSESSMENT OF BONE MASS OR BALANCE

Technique	Site	Reproducibility (CV%)
Metabolic balance		5–15
Neutron activation	Hand	2–4
	Spine	2–10
	Whole body	5–10
Single-photon absorptiometry	Radius (cortical)	1–2
	Ultradistal radius	3–5
Dual-photon absorptiometry	Spine	3–5
	Hip	4–6
Dual-energy X-ray absorptiometry	Spine	1–2
	Hip	2–4
	Whole body	2–4
Bone histology	Ilium	20–30
Ultrasound attenuation	Heel	3–5
Ultrasound velocity	Patella	2–3

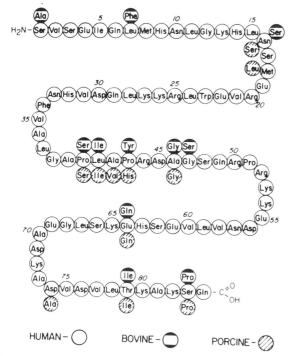

Figure 30.3 Amino acid structure of human parathyroid hormone and differences in amino acid sequence in the bovine and porcine hormone.

containing 84 amino acids. There are small differences in amino acid sequences between those so far characterized (bovine, porcine and the human hormones; Fig. 30.3). In common with several other peptide hormones, PTH is synthesized as a prohormone that contains an additional six amino acids on its N-terminal end. A further precursor form, preproPTH, containing a total of 115 amino acids, has been identified in studies *in vitro*. These precursor forms are probably converted to the 84 amino-acid peptide before secretion from the gland.

Synthesis of the different segments of the polypeptide chain has shown that only the first 32–34 amino acids (reading from the N-terminal end) are necessary for biological activity. There is evidence that cleavage occurs naturally, partly in the liver, to produce a short, N-terminal, biologically active fragment and a larger, inactive, C-terminal fragment. This cleavage may be necessary for PTH to act on bone. There are also many, less well-characterized, circulating fragments of PTH. The liver and kidney are important sites of degradation and, for example, the C-terminal fragment normally cleared by the kidney may be increased in chronic renal failure, though the circulating biological activity of PTH may be normal. This causes some problems in the interpretation of radioimmunoassay in patients with renal impairment since the C-terminal fragment is the major component measured in many assay systems. Several assays developed to detect specific sequences such as the aminoterminal portion of the molecule (the biologically active fragment) or mid-molecule sequence have been partially successful in resolving this problem (Fig. 30.4). The assay least affected by uraemia detects intact (1–84) parathyroid hormone utilizing a double antibody. Nevertheless, the characteristics of all immunoassays for PTH depend critically upon the immunoreactivity of the antibody, so that each assay system with each antiserum must be well characterized at a clinical level before full interpretation of PTH concentrations is possible.

The major physiological stimulus to secretion of PTH is a fall in the plasma ionized calcium concentration; conversely, a rise above normal suppresses PTH secretion. A host of other factors is known to influence PTH secretion including β-adrenergic agonists, vitamin D metabolites, growth hormone and somatostatin, vitamin A, prostaglandins, prolactin, dopamine and other cations such as magnesium, aluminium and strontium. With the exception of aluminium and magnesium, the physiological or

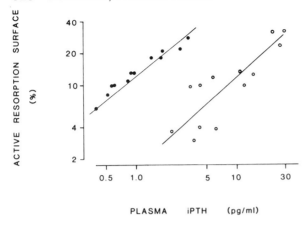

Figure 30.4 Plasma immunoreactive levels of parathyroid hormone (iPTH) in patients with end-stage chronic renal failure. Two antiserum preparations have been used and values using either assay correlate significantly with known biological effects of PTH (in this case increased bone resorption). However, the values using the 'amino-terminal' assay (closed symbols; left) are 6–10 times lower than those using a 'carboxyterminal' assay (open symbols; right).

clinical relevance of these factors is uncertain. In the presence of low levels of magnesium, the secretion of PTH is impaired and this, together with an impaired target-organ response to PTH, probably accounts for the hypocalcaemia occasionally seen in severe magnesium deficiency in man. Conversely, aluminium retention caused by uraemia inhibits the secretion of PTH. This, coupled by direct effects of aluminium on bone turnover, give rise to adynamic bone disease of chronic renal failure.

The target-organ actions of PTH include effects on bone, kidney and indirectly on gut. PTH acts on the kidney to increase the tubular reabsorption of calcium and to depress the tubular reabsorption of phosphate. This leads to a rise in plasma calcium and a fall in plasma phosphate. PTH also decreases the proximal renal tubular reabsorption for bicarbonate, which leads to a hyperchloraemic acidosis (analogous to a proximal renal tubular acidosis). A mild metabolic acidosis is often seen in primary and in secondary hyperparathyroidism. Conversely, a metabolic alkalosis is commonly observed in hypoparathyroidism and in hypercalcaemia due to malignant disease affecting the skeleton. In this latter disorder the alkalosis is partly due to suppression of PTH secretion, but the release of buffer from bone may also contribute. PTH has a further important effect on the kidney in stimulating the 1α-hydroxylase enzyme responsible for the production of calcitriol, leading to increased intestinal absorption of calcium and possibly to release of calcium from bone. Thus, many of the actions of PTH on the kidney appear either directly or indirectly to increase the concentration of calcium in the ECF.

The major effect of PTH on bone is to increase bone resorption, an effect that is readily demonstrated *in vitro*. Both primary and secondary hyperparathyroidism can be associated with obvious radiographic and histological evidence of increased bone resorption. For reasons discussed later, the increase in bone resorption is followed normally by an increase in bone formation so that the net efflux of calcium from bone is not markedly changed. Thus, in kinetic studies, the rate of mineral accretion often matches the rate of bone resorption in primary hyperparathyroidism.

There is a great deal of controversy as to whether PTH (and indeed calcitonin) can influence the rapid exchange of calcium that occurs between the ECF and bone and soft tissue, but this is likely to be so. This rapid transfer may be very important in the minute-to-minute maintenance of plasma calcium, and determines the set-point for plasma calcium.

Calcitonin

Calcitonin is produced from the C-cells of the thyroid in man. It is a peptide hormone containing 32 amino-acid residues with a disulphide bridge between cysteine residues in positions 1 and 7. The entire sequence is essential for biological activity and the gene structure of the human hormone has been elaborated. There are several differences in amino acid composition of the calcitonins from different species and these are associated with different potencies (Fig. 30.5). Surprisingly, the salmon hormone resembles the human more than other mammalian calcitonins and it is interesting that the salmon hormone is more potent on a molar basis in man than the human hormone itself.

The site of calcitonin secretion in man may not be only from thyroid tissue. The C-cells themselves are derived embryologically from the APUD-cell series, which itself is derived from the neural crest. Non-thyroidal sites for production of calcitonin include the thymus, adrenal, and possibly the pars intermedia of the pituitary gland.

Many agents are known to affect the secretion of calcitonin. These include calcium, gastrointestinal hormones such as cholecystokinin, enteroglucagon and gastrin, β-adrenergic agents, and alcohol. Since an obvious action of calcitonin is to inhibit bone resorption and thereby lower plasma calcium, it is widely believed that calcitonin is a calcium-regulating hormone with a negative feedback mechanism. Thus the secretion of calcitonin, stimulated by an increase in ECF concentration of calcium, inhibits bone resorption and lowers plasma calcium. Conversely, a decrease in plasma calcium concentration reduces the secretion of calcitonin and in turn leads to an increase in calcium release from bone. The actions of calcitonin could, therefore, complement those of parathyroid hormone in reversing changes in the ECF concentration of calcium.

The physiological role for calcitonin in man is not

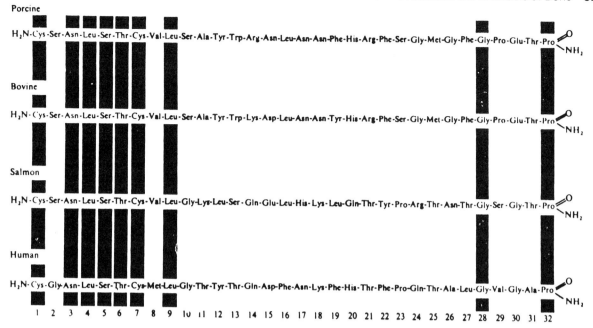

Figure 30.5 Amino acid structures of calcitonin from various species; nine of the 32 amino acids are common to all these species.

known. Although the most obvious action of calcitonin in mammals is to inhibit bone resorption, it also has effects at other sites. In the kidney it decreases renal tubular reabsorption of calcium, phosphate, magnesium, potassium and a variety of other ions, and is a powerful diuretic, but many of these effects are pharmacological. Calcitonin also inhibits the secretion of several gastrointestinal hormones including gastrin, insulin, and glucagons. Once again, the physiological importance of these effects is not clear. One difficulty of ascribing a physiological role to calcitonin is that a deficiency (total thyroidectomy) or excess (medullary carcinoma of the thyroid) of calcitonin are associated with only minor disturbances in skeletal or mineral homeostasis. Athyroidal subjects given thyroid hormones exhibit minor impairments in their ability to handle an oral calcium load in that they excrete more calcium in the urine than do normal controls. This may mean that calcitonin has some role in preventing postprandial rises in plasma calcium.

A further difficulty in assessing the role of calcitonin metabolism in man arises from the problems of its radioimmunoassay. Like PTH, calcitonin circulates in heterogeneous form and is degraded in part by the kidney. Many of the immunoreactive fragments are not biologically active and many assays measure some of these fragments. The development of assays that measure authentic 1–32 calcitonin has not resolved these problems, and there is much conflicting evidence as to how calcitonin secretion responds to various 'physiological' stresses. Despite these difficulties, however, the assay for calcitonin is useful in the diagnosis of medullary carcinoma of the thyroid and for the detection of family members with the disease in a presymptomatic form. A major clinical interest in calcitonin is its use as an inhibitor of bone resorption and turnover in Paget's disease of bone and in hypercalcaemia associated with increased bone resorption.

Vitamin D

Man derives vitamin D_3 (*cholecalciferol*) from the diet, and from the skin by ultraviolet irradiation of 7-dehydrocholesterol. Vitamin D_2 (*ergocalciferol*) is a product originally derived from the ultraviolet irradiation of plant sterols and is used to supplement the diet, particularly in margarines. In many respects vitamins D_2 and D_3 are comparable in their metabolism and in their actions.

The photochemical conversion of 7-dehydrocholesterol to vitamin D in skin is a chemical reaction not under metabolic control but there is some evidence that the conversion occurs more readily in white- than dark-skinned races. Both vitamin D and its metabolites are transported in plasma bound to a specific α-globulin. Vitamin D is fat soluble and absorbed primarily from the duodenum and jejunum into the lymphatic circulation. The vitamin is distributed in fat and muscle.

Before exerting biological effects, vitamin D undergoes a series of further metabolic conversions (Fig. 30.6). The first step involves its conversion in the liver to a 25-hydroxylated derivative (25-OHD; *calcifediol*). This is the major, circulating vitamin D metabolite and is the metabolite most commonly

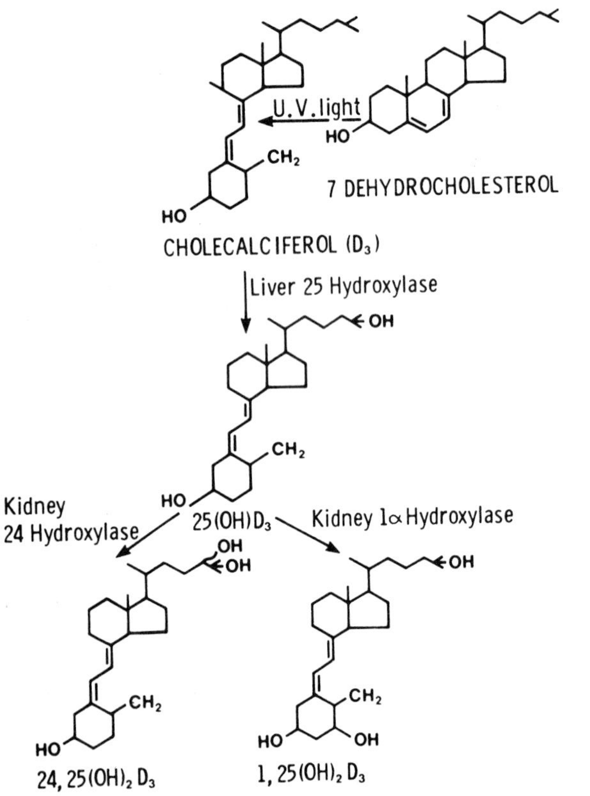

Figure 30.6 Steps in the conversion of 7-dehydrocholesterol to vitamin D and its metabolites. The site of synthesis of 25-hydroxy vitamin D_3 (calcifediol; 25 $(OH)D_3$) is in the liver. The active form of vitamin D (calcitriol; $1,25(OH)_2D_3$) is made in the kidney and placenta. Secalciferol ($24,25(OH)_2D_3$ is synthesized in several tissues, but the kidney is probably the major site.

measured clinically to provide an index of vitamin D nutritional status. There is a marked seasonal variation in plasma 25-OHD concentrations, with a peak in late summer and a trough in late winter. In winter, plasma levels may commonly approach those associated with vitamin D-deficiency states, suggesting that in northern Europe both sunlight and dietary intake may be of crucial importance in maintaining vitamin D status.

The second step in the metabolism of vitamin D is its further hydroxylation, mainly in the kidney, to either 1,25-dihydroxy vitamin D_3 (*calcitriol*) or to 24,25 $(OH)_2D_3$ (*secalciferol*). Apart from the human placenta and decidua, the kidney is the major, if not the sole site for 1α-hydroxylation, a factor that is of considerable importance in the pathophysiology of renal bone disease. The renal metabolism of calcitriol is closely regulated, and its production is favoured under conditions of deficiency of vitamin D, calcium or phosphate. Production of calcitriol is also augmented by a variety of hormones, including oestradiol, prolactin and growth hormone, but it is not clear if this is a direct effect of the hormones on the kidney or if it is mediated by changes in calcium or phosphate concentration.

In many experimental systems studied, calcitriol has the greatest biological potency. Its principal effects are to increase intestinal absorption of calcium and phosphate and to increase the resorption of calcium from bone. Although lack of vitamin D in man is associated with defective mineralization of cartilage and bone, it is still not known whether vitamin D and its metabolites act directly on bone to promote its mineralization. Despite the presence of calcitriol receptors on osteoblasts, and the production of bone-specific proteins in response to vitamin D, it is possible that the effects of vitamin D on bone mineralization are secondary to changes in ECF concentrations of calcium and phosphate. Unfortunately there are few experimental systems for studying skeletal mineralization *in vitro* and the major demonstrable effect of calcitriol on bone *in vitro* is to increase resorption. Apart from vitamin D toxicity, in which increased bone resorption is well documented, there is surprisingly little evidence that physiological doses of calcitriol, or indeed of any other metabolite of vitamin D, increase bone resorption in man.

From a teleological viewpoint, the action of calcitriol can be thought of as increasing the availability of calcium and phosphate for mineralization, or as maintaining plasma concentrations of calcium and phosphate. Calcitriol can therefore be considered to be the hormonal form of vitamin D in the sense that its secretion from endocrine tissue (the kidney) is controlled by the calcium and phosphate status of the individual, and that the action of this hormone reverses the stimulus to its secretion. The interval between stimulation of the 1α-hydroxylase and the synthesis of calcitriol is several hours so that the role of vitamin D in calcium homeostasis is to provide regulation over a longer term than the minute-to-minute regulation of plasma calcium that is achieved with PTH or calcitonin.

Receptors for calcitriol have been found in very many other tissues apart from bone and gut. A notable exception is skeletal muscle. In many tissues the vitamin promotes the differentiation of cells and has led to the use of vitamin D derivatives in proliferative disorders (some haematological malignancies, psoriasis). There is some evidence that calcitriol inhibits the secretion of PTH but the physiological significance of this genomic action is not known.

A striking weakness of skeletal muscles, particularly of the pelvic and shoulder girdles, is a well-described feature of vitamin D deficiency. Moreover, myopathy improves rapidly following treatment with vitamin D of one of its metabolites. The mechanisms whereby vitamin D produces an effect on muscle function are unknown but they may involve non-receptor membrane effects mediating calcium transfer across the sarcoplasmic reticulum or modifications in the metabolism of troponin C. It is notable that severe phosphate deficiency induced by dietary deprivation or by hyperparathyroidism is associated with muscle weakness, suggesting that the effects of vitamin D could be mediated by hypophosphataemia. However, in the inherited tubular disorder, hypophosphataemic osteomalacia, muscle weakness is characteristically absent even though profound hypophosphataemia is found. There are several other poorly understood trophic effects of vitamin D, particularly on growth, on the maintenance of intestinal mucosa and on the maturation of collagen and cartilage.

The function of secalciferol in man is unknown. In many experimental systems its production is favoured under conditions that inhibit synthesis of calcitriol such that a reciprocal relation is commonly observed between their respective production rates. Thus, under conditions of repletion of vitamin D, calcium or phosphate, secalciferol is the major circulating dihydroxy metabolite. Various observations in experimental animals and man suggest that this metabolite may have a physiological role in regulating the metabolism of cartilage or bone.

Assays for vitamin D metabolites are not generally available with the exception of the competitive protein-binding assay for calcifediol (*see* Appendix for normal ranges). These assays do not generally distinguish between $25(OH)D_2$ and $25(OH)D_3$. Plasma measurements provide a useful index of the adequacy of vitamin D nutrition in the investigation of rickets or osteomalacia. Thus, plasma concentrations of calcifediol are low in simple vitamin D-deficient states and in disorders associated with increased destruction or elimination of calcifediol. In rarer forms of rickets (discussed later), in which the metabolic defect is a failure of production of calcitriol, or is a metabolic error unrelated to vitamin D metabolism, plasma calcifediol is normal. The finding of high levels may be helpful in an occasional patient presenting with acute hypercalcaemia who withholds a history of excessive dietary intake of vitamin D. Several other vitamin D metabolites have been isolated from plasma and identified, such as 25,26-dihydroxycholecalciferol and a 23,26-lactone derivative. Some of these metabolites appear to have some biological activity but their tissue of origin and metabolic functions are not clear.

Calcitriol has a biological half-life measured in hours and a normal plasma concentration of approximately 30 pg/mL in adults. Higher concentrations are observed in growing children. Plasma concentrations of calcifediol and secalciferol are 1000-fold and 100-fold greater, respectively, than those of calcitriol; both compounds have a long biological half-life in the circulation, perhaps related to their greater affinity for the vitamin D-binding protein. Despite these differences in plasma levels, calcitriol is considered the active form of vitamin D because it is so much more potent than other derivatives in exerting actions on the target organs.

The discovery that vitamin D must be metabolized to more polar products has led to considerable advances in our understanding of the pathophysiology of a number of disorders. Nevertheless, there is a limited place for its assay in clinical practice. Methods include competitive binding assays using the cytosol or nuclear-receptor protein for calcitriol and, more recently, radioimmunoassays using antibodies raised against calcitriol. Both the receptor assays and immunoassays cross-react with other vitamin D compounds; to overcome this problem it is necessary to undertake prior extraction of the plasma followed by chromatographic separation of the metabolites, processes that are time consuming and laborious. Assay of calcitriol has a place in the investigation of several disorders of mineral metabolism including sarcoidosis, and in rare forms of osteomalacia.

The Influencing Hormones

From the preceding section, it is clear that the major regulating hormones appear to operate by increasing or decreasing plasma concentrations of calcium or phosphate in response to changes. The hormones PTH, calcitonin, and calcitriol are all present in the circulation under normal physiological conditions and their secretion might be expected to exert a continuous influence on calcium metabolism and on the rate of bone remodelling. But, as these hormones are regulated by changes in plasma concentrations of calcium, their physiological role may be less important for skeletal homeostasis than for extracellular calcium homeostasis. Other factors, some of which are at present poorly characterized, influence skeletal metabolism and maintain the integrity of the skeleton in health and under various conditions of stress. Their secretion rate is not primarily governed by ECF concentrations of calcium or phosphate.

Growth Hormone

Growth hormone is best known for its effect on growth of cartilage, an effect brought about directly and indirectly by growth hormone-dependent production of insulin-like growth factor 1 (*somatomedins*). There are several known growth factors called somatomedins, but only some are dependent on growth hormone. Growth hormone also causes an elevation in plasma phosphate by increasing the tubular reabsorption of phosphate in the kidney, and may contribute to the high plasma phosphate found in growing children and in acromegaly. Excess or deficiency of growth hormone is associated with obvious abnormalities in skeletal growth. In acromegaly there is increased periosteal apposition of bone, but, contrary to popular belief, there is no convincing evidence that acromegaly causes osteoporosis.

Thyroid Hormones

Deficiency of thyroid hormones early in life produces the well-known skeletal deformities of cretinism. Before skeletal maturity, thyrotoxicosis may increase longitudinal skeletal growth. In the adult, thyrotoxicosis may be associated with increased bone resorption, hypercalciuria, a raised alkaline phosphatase and

occasionally hypercalcaemia. These effects, probably due to direct actions of the thyroid hormones on bone, lead to a tendency for plasma calcium to rise, which in turn decreases the secretion of PTH and synthesis of calcitriol to offset this calcium challenge.

Adrenal Steroids

The most important effect of glucocorticoids on the skeleton is to regulate growth. Their actions on calcium metabolism are complex and probably involve effects on many target tissues in addition to their effects on metabolism, transport and action of other hormones. In the adult, adrenal insufficiency is not associated with marked skeletal abnormalities but is occasionally accompanied by hypercalcaemia. This is probably due to haemoconcentration (increased albumin concentration) and also to increased renal tubular reabsorption for calcium because of volume depletion.

The effect of glucocorticoid excess in inducing osteoporosis is well established. The pathogenesis is far from clear and the relative contributions of diminished intestinal absorption of calcium, diminished bone formation, and increased resorption of bone are not well defined. The ability of corticosteroids to decrease plasma calcium in hypercalcaemia other than that due to primary hyperparathyroidism has been used for many years as a diagnostic aid (*see* Hyperparathyroidism), but once again the precise mechanism of action is uncertain. However, glucocorticoids are known to inhibit the biosynthesis of prostaglandins and of some osteoclast-activating factors, which may be mediators of bone resorption and hypercalcaemia in several haematological malignancies.

Sex Steroids

Characteristic growth abnormalities are associated with deficiencies of either male or female sex hormones. They appear to play a crucial part in epiphyseal closure and in the so-called adolescent growth spurt that precedes this event. They may also influence the amount of calcium present in the skeleton in adult life. In adults the effects of oestrogens are of particular interest because of the loss of bone that occurs in women after the menopause (*see* Osteoporosis). Administration of exogenous oestrogen prevents this loss and lowers plasma calcium slightly, an effect more noticeable in postmenopausal women with hyperparathyroidism or hypercalcaemic women with carcinoma of the breast. The mechanism of action of oestrogens on bone is not known, though receptors for oestrogen have been found (by some investigators) on osteoblasts. They appear to decrease the rate of bone remodelling and increase the functional competence of bone cells, but it is not known whether these are direct or indirect effects.

Gastrointestinal Hormones

There are many interactions between calcium-regulating hormones and gastrointestinal hormones. The relations between gastrin and calcitonin secretion have been mentioned earlier. Calcium and PTH are also involved, and in hyperparathyroidism, gastrin levels are increased, owing to the ability of calcium to stimulate gastrin secretion. Of the other gastrointestinal hormones, glucagon and amylin are hypocalcaemic due to inhibition of bone resorption, either directly or by stimulating the secretion of calcitonin. Secretin may cause hypercalcaemia, possibly by stimulating release of PTH. Insulin is an important hormone for skeletal growth and insulin-dependent diabetics often have diminished skeletal mass. Insulin is one of the few hormones that has been shown to stimulate collagen synthesis *in vitro*.

Parathyroid Hormone-related Peptide

This peptide (PTHrP) shares several homologies with PTH. Its physiological role is not yet known, but one of its functions may be the placental transport of calcium. It is produced by a number of solid tumours and is responsible at least in part of the humoral hypercalcaemia of malignancy. Its activity is similar if not identical to that of PTH.

Cytokines and Growth Factors

A myriad of factors has been identified that can be shown to affect various aspects of skeletal metabolism. These include the interleukins (IL). IL-1 is a potent inducer of bone resorption and may have a role in local bone resorption in inflammatory bone disease. IL-6 and lymphotoxin (tumour necrosis factor-β; TNF-β) also activate osteoclasts and are thought to be responsible for the hypercalcaemia and bone loss seen in myeloma, which is characteristically sensitive to treatment with corticosteroids.

Several of the colony-stimulating factors (e.g. GM-CSF and M-CSF) also stimulate bone resorption. The interferons, particularly IFN-, inhibit bone resorption where this is mediated by cytokines. There are a large number of growth factors that may stimulate bone formation. These include epidermal growth factor, the transforming growth factors, and insulin-like growth factors. In most instances their physiological role is uncertain, but the TGF-βs are of great interest because they are present in bone, exposed by bone resorption and appear to stimulate the mitogenesis of osteoblasts. TGF-β may, therefore, play a part in the coupling of resorption and formation in bone remodelling.

Prostaglandins

A number of prostaglandins, particularly of the E series, resorb bone by directly stimulating osteoclastic activity. There is good experimental evidence that prostaglandins cause the increased bone resorption mediated by certain tumours *in vitro* and in experimental animals. The evidence that prostaglandins are involved in tumour-mediated bone resorption and hypercalcaemia in man is, however, circumstantial.

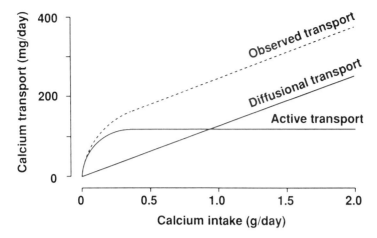

Figure 30.7 The relation between calcium intake and the amount of calcium absorbed throughout the gastrointestinal tract. The active and passive components of intestinal or calcium transport are distinguished. The observed relation between absorption and dietary intake (––––) is resolved into active and diffusional transport components. The active transport mechanism is responsible for most of the flux at low intakes, whereas diffusion assumes greater quantitative significance at high intake. In the presence of vitamin D deficiency, the active transport component is lost and absorption is linearly related to dietary intake.

Prostaglandin-synthetase inhibitors have been advocated in the treatment of hypercalcaemia due to metastases in bone, but the general experience is that very few patients respond. Prostaglandins also have anabolic effects. High doses of PGE_1 stimulate periosteal growth, which is sometimes observed as a side-effect of prostaglandin infusion in neonates (for patent ductus arteriosus). Whether or not prostaglandins have a physiological role in skeletal metabolism is not clear.

Summary
From the preceding comments it is clear that the effects of many of these hormones on the skeleton are incompletely understood. The judicious use of assays for these hormones or their metabolites is nevertheless important in investigating certain growth abnormalities, the occasional patient with hypercalcaemia, and in excluding the rare but treatable causes of osteoporosis.

Calcium Transport to and from the Extracellular Fluid

With the exception of the pregnant or lactating female, the major fluxes of calcium to and from the ECF occur across the intestinal mucosa, bone and kidney (*see* Fig. 30.1). This section describes the extent to which these fluxes are controlled by the major regulating hormones and some of the investigations available to examine these movements of calcium.

Intestine
Unlike the fluxes of calcium between the ECF and bone and kidney, intestinal absorption of calcium is episodic and dependent on an adequate supply of calcium delivered in an available form to the intestinal mucosa. The availability of calcium for absorption depends upon many dietary factors, including the presence of phosphate, oxalates, fatty acids and phytates, which bind calcium and render it unavailable for absorption. The influx of calcium depends both on active transport and diffusion processes. Absorption occurs throughout the length of the small intestine and to a lesser extent in the colon. The major sites for active transport are in the duodenum and upper part of the jejunum. However, because the duodenum is shorter than the rest of the gastrointestinal tract, more calcium is probably absorbed at sites distal to the duodenum than within the duodenum itself, at least with normal dietary intakes.

The relation between the dietary intake and the net calcium absorbed is not linear (Fig. 30.7). Net absorption of calcium increases steeply as the calcium intake rises from very low amounts, but thereafter flattens off, though does not reach a plateau. This relation is explicable on the basis of the two known transport systems; the one being an active system that is saturable and important at low concentrations of calcium, and the other being a passive diffusion process that is concentration dependent and is more important at high calcium concentrations in the bowel. This means that the net percentage of dietary calcium absorbed decreases with increasing intake, a fact that is important to take into account when assessing different types of calcium absorption tests (Fig. 30.8). A clinical consequence of this is that the use of calcium supplements alone is a relatively inefficient way of increasing net intestinal absorption unless the dietary intake of calcium is very low.

At very low intakes of calcium, net absorption may be negative. Calcium delivered into the gut

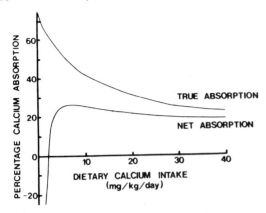

Figure 30.8 The relation between dietary calcium intake and the net and true absorption of calcium expressed as a percentage of the intake. (From Nordin B.E.C. (1976). *Calcium, Phosphate and Magnesium Metabolism*, Edinburgh: Churchill Livingstone.)

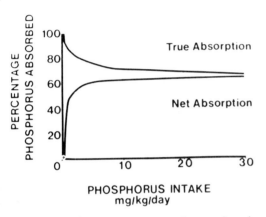

Figure 30.9 The relation between dietary phosphorus intake and the net and true absorption of phosphorus expressed as a percentage of the dietary intake. (From Nordin B.E.C. (1976). *Calcium, Phosphate and Magnesium Metabolism*, Edinburgh: Churchill Livingstone.)

weeks or months rather than hours or minutes. It is now thought that it is due to changes induced in the synthesis of calcitriol, so that the rate of net intestinal absorption of calcium returns to its original value.

The biochemical mechanisms involved in active calcium transport through the intestinal mucosa are not understood in detail, though several features of the system have been identified. Calcitriol stimulates the synthesis of a calcium-binding protein in addition to an intestinal alkaline phosphatase, by a mechanism similar to that described for many other steroid hormones. This involves the translocation of vitamin D plus its receptor protein to the intestinal-cell nucleus to increase the synthesis of mRNA and new protein synthesis. The exact function of these proteins is not clear but they could either be involved in the transmucosal transport of calcium or act as buffer to large intracellular shifts in calcium concentration.

There is now good evidence that calcium and phosphate can be absorbed separately from each other, and that calcitriol has independent effects to enhance the absorption of each. Unlike the absorption of calcium, which appears to be closely regulated, the proportion of the dietary phosphate absorbed does not decrease appreciably with increasing intake, but remains fixed at approximately 70% (Fig. 30.9). This explains in large part the increases in plasma phosphate that occur after a meal and underlines the need to study patients under controlled conditions (e.g. fasting) when assessing phosphate homeostasis.

A variety of tests is available to study calcium absorption. Calcium balance provides an index of net calcium transport (*see* Fig. 30.2). Accurate assessment of unidirectional fluxes of calcium across the gut is dependent upon tracer techniques. A standard method is to compare the plasma appearance and disappearance of an orally administered calcium isotope with the disappearance of an intravenously given calcium isotope. Absorption is calculated from the difference between the specific activities of the two isotopes in plasma. A simpler technique, but subject to more assumptions, is to follow the appearance and disappearance of a single calcium radioisotope given by mouth. The fractional absorption of calcium will depend on several factors including the availability of the calcium for absorption and the site of absorption. Of great importance is the amount of calcium carrier given with the radioisotope, since a low total calcium dose will present itself for absorption high in the gastrointestinal tract and be more clearly a function of the active transport mechanism. A higher dose of carrier (e.g. 200–300 mg) more closely approximates the calcium provided by a meal and will in addition be available for absorption at sites distal to the duodenum. Clearly the amount of calcium in the diet must also be taken into consideration when assessing the results of calcium absorption tests since, for example, a high fractional absorption of calcium does not necessarily mean that the total amount of calcium absorbed in the diet is high if the

lumen in intestinal secretions may exceed the calcium absorbed. Calcium delivered from intestinal secretions contributes to the so-called endogenous faecal calcium and can be monitored by radioisotope methods in which parenterally administered radiolabelled calcium is recovered in the faeces. In malabsorption syndromes, the endogenous faecal calcium may appear to rise, but this does not always mean that the amount of calcium secreted in the digestive juices is increased, since the rise is probably due to malabsorption of this digestive-juice calcium. Nevertheless, increased calcium secretion has been described in steatorrhoea and adult coeliac disease (gluten-sensitive enteropathy).

Man is able to adapt to variations in dietary calcium so that net absorption remains relatively constant over a fairly wide range of intakes (Fig. 30.8). This adaptation is slow and occurs over a period of diet is severely deficient in calcium, or if calcium is rendered unavailable for absorption by phosphates, phytates, fats or drugs.

A 24-h urine collection for calcium or phosphate provides an indirect index of intestinal absorption, provided that it is assumed or known that the net flux of these ions across bone and other tissues is zero. The expression of excretion as a ratio to creatinine helps to adjust for differences in body weight and for incomplete urine collections.

Increased intestinal absorption of calcium is found in several disease states such as hyperparathyroidism, sarcoidosis and idiopathic hypercalciuria, and is thought to be due to increased production of calcitriol. Conversely, malabsorption of calcium is often associated with low levels of calcitriol, for example in hypoparathyroidism, vitamin D-deficiency states and in chronic renal failure. Malabsorption of calcium also occurs in disorders in which the target tissue for calcitriol is defective. A good example of this is in untreated coeliac disease, where the flat intestinal mucosa lacks the villi and enterocytes through which calcium is normally absorbed.

Kidney
The fluxes of calcium across the kidney are much greater than those of the gut (*see* Fig. 30.1). Renal tubular reabsorption of calcium in the kidney is a complex process, and takes place at several different sites in the nephron. The total amount of calcium reabsorbed can, however, be estimated by subtracting the filtered load of calcium from the renal excretion. The filterable calcium is approximately 60% of total plasma calcium (*see* Table 30.2), and the filtered load represents the product of the glomerular filtration rate (GFR) and the filterable calcium (approx. 250 mmol (10 g) daily).

Provided that the serum calcium is stable, the total excretion of calcium reflects the net input of calcium to the ECF, largely from gut and skeletal sources. If patients are fasted (usually overnight) and urine collected thereafter in the postabsorptive state, the urinary excretion more closely reflects net efflux of calcium from bone. A 2-h urine collection is commonly used, but the timing is not critical if the urinary excretion is expressed as the calcium: creatinine ratio.

In health there is a curvilinear relation between

---

* Calcium clearance as a proportion of GFR can be derived from the urine concentration of calcium (U_{Ca}) and creatinine (U_{Cr}) and plasma concentrations of ultrafilterable calcium (P_{Ca}) and creatinine (P_{Cr}):

$$\frac{U_{Ca} \times P_{Cr}}{U_{Cr} \times P_{Ca}}.$$

The urinary excretion of calcium per unit of GFR is therefore calculated:

$$\frac{U_{Ca} \times P_{Cr}}{U_{Cr}}.$$

plasma calcium concentration (an index of filtered load, assuming no change in GFR) and renal excretion of calcium, so that tubular reabsorption cannot be assessed simply from the calcium clearance.* To take account of variations in GFR the renal excretion is commonly expressed per litre of GFR (Fig. 30.10). Any value below the lines depicting the normal relationship indicates an increase in the net tubular reabsorption of calcium and values above the lines denote decreased net reabsorption. Any value for renal excretion above normal but within the normal range for the relation between plasma and urine calcium would indicate an increase in filtered load (gut or bone derived) or a low GFR, but with normal net tubular reabsorption of calcium. Calcium excretion, measured in the fasting state, will reflect more closely calcium derived from bone resorption.

The assessment of renal tubular reabsorption in this way has several limitations, particularly in clinical disorders. Thus, the proportion of total plasma calcium that is filtered is often uncertain in the presence of alkalosis, acidosis or abnormal plasma proteins. Moreover, a change in the relation normally found between plasma calcium and its renal excretion might be expected in patients with intrinsic renal disease or during saline infusion, dehydration, or treatment with diuretics.

Despite these difficulties, the measurement of calcium excretion together with plasma calcium can help provide information about tubular reabsorption in a steady state, whereas the measurement of calcium excretion alone does not.

Whenever a steady state for plasma calcium exists, either in health or disease, calcium must be eliminated from the circulation at the same rate as it enters, whatever the GFR or tubular reabsorption. It follows that hypo- or hypercalciuria do not in themselves indicate disturbances in renal tubular reabsorption, but denote increased or decreased net input into the ECF due to changes in bone resorption or intestinal absorption. Furthermore, *under steady-state conditions*, changes in tubular reabsorption alone will not be reflected by changes in renal excretion rate, but by changes in the plasma calcium concentration.

In health, approximately 97% of the calcium filtered by the kidney is reabsorbed. Many factors influence renal tubular reabsorption, but of the various hormones mentioned PTH is probably the most important under physiological conditions. In mild primary hyperparathyroidism the hypercalcaemia is due mainly to increased renal tubular reabsorption since the fasting calcium excretion is often normal (Fig. 30.10), whereas an increase would be expected if the net flux of calcium from bone to ECF were increased. As many patients with primary hyperparathyroidism have increased bone resorption, the normal calcium excretion rate implies an increase in bone formation to match the change in bone resorption. Similarly, in hypoparathyroidism the fasting renal excretion of calcium is commonly normal (Fig.

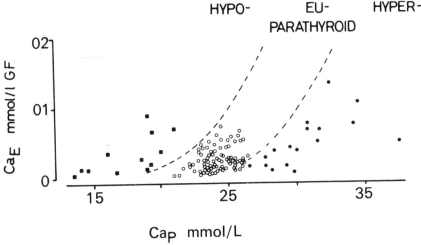

Figure 30.10 Relation between fasting urinary calcium excretion (Ca_E; expressed as mmol/L of glomerular filtrate) and plasma calcium (Ca_p) in health and disorders of parathyroid function. The broken lines denote the range ($\pm$ SD) obtained in normal subjects during calcium infusions. Patients with primary hyperparathyroidism lie on the right of the line describing normal subjects, indicating increased renal tubular reabsorption for calcium. In contrast, patients with hypoparathyroidism lie to the left of the normal line, indicating decreased renal tubular reabsorption for calcium. Note that the determination of calcium excretion alone (without concurrent measurement of plasma calcium) does not give information concerning renal tubular reabsorption for calcium. Note also that hypoparathyroid patients, and many hyperparathyroid patients have calcium excretion values that are normal. (From Kanis J.A. (1980). Etiology and medical management of hypercalcaemia. *Metab. Bone Dis. Related Res.*, **2** (3).)

30.10), though plasma calcium is low. PTH-mediated changes in plasma calcium are therefore often due to changes in renal tubular reabsorption of calcium.

Plasma phosphate concentration varies more than that of plasma calcium, particularly in response to circadian rhythms and to meals. The level of fasting plasma phosphate is set mainly by the kidney and the measurement of the renal tubular reabsorption of phosphate is often used in clinical diagnosis, such as in hyperparathyroidism. Of the several methods available to calculate phosphate reabsorption, the most appropriate from a physiological point of view is the estimation of Tm_p/GFR (the tubular maximum for phosphate reabsorption per unit of GFR). This examines the relation between filtered load and renal excretion, which, like that for calcium reabsorption, is curvilinear. A nomogram is available for deriving this measurement (Fig. 30.11).

Phosphate reabsorption is increased by growth hormone, in hypoparathyroid conditions and by phosphate deprivation. It is diminished by calcitonin, in hyperparathyroidism and in several inherited or acquired renal tubular disorders that may also be associated with defects in the reabsorption of glucose, amino acids, or bicarbonate. The calcium and phosphate ions themselves may also influence renal phosphate transport, which makes it difficult to dissociate the direct effects of hormones on tubular resorption from the other metabolic consequences of their secretion.

Both calcium and phosphate excretion are influenced by other factors, notably sodium excretion, ECF volume, and by the administration of diuretics.

There is evidence for both proximal and distal sites of tubular reabsorption, and both can be influenced by PTH. Experimental studies show that receptors for PTH exist at multiple locations in the nephron. However, in physiological terms PTH induces changes in phosphate reabsorption that occur predominantly at the proximal convoluted tubule whereas the action of PTH on calcium is mainly distal. Infusion of sodium chloride increases the excretion of both calcium and phosphate, an effect that probably contributes to its value in the acute treatment of hypercalcaemia.

The biochemical mechanisms involved in renal transport of calcium and phosphate are not elucidated but the action of PTH on the kidney is known to produce an increase in cortical adenylate cyclase activity, which increases tubular cell and urinary concentrations of 3', 5'-cyclic adenosine monophosphate (cAMP). It is not known whether this increase in cAMP is the cause of the subsequent changes in phosphate and calcium transport. However, in the clinical disorder, pseudohypoparathyroidism, there is a defective receptor mechanism for PTH in kidney (and sometimes bone) so that the administration of PTH does not always produce the normal response of an increased excretion of phosphate and cAMP. This is somewhat analogous to the failure of patients with nephrogenic diabetes insipidus to respond to arginine vasopressin (antidiuretic hormone). The estimation of urinary cAMP is also used in the investigation of hypercalcaemia. Thus, increased excretion of cAMP is seen in primary hyperparathyroidism, but depressed in most conditions where hypercalcaemia

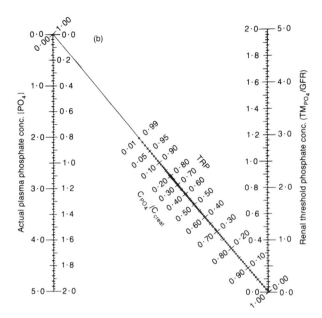

Figure 30.11 Nomogram for the derivation of $Tm_P/$ GFR (estimate of phosphate reabsorption) from simultaneous measurements of tubular reabsorption (TRP) or the ratio of clearance of phosphate to clearance of creatinine (C_{PO_4}/C_{creat}) and plasma phosphate [PO_4]. TRP can be calculated from the concentrations of phosphate and creatinine in plasma and creatinine; and urine volume is not required:

$$\frac{C_{PO_4}}{C_{creat}} = \frac{\text{urine phosphate} \times \text{plasma creatinine}}{\text{plasma phosphate} \times \text{urine creatinine}}.$$

A straight line through the appropriate values of plasma phosphate and TRP or phosphate/creatinine clearance passes through the corresponding value of Tm_P/GFR. Both Tm_P/GFR and phosphate are expressed in the same units. The scale in units of the figure are arbitrary. (From Walton R.J., Bijvoet O.L.M. (1975). *Lancet*, **ii**, 309.)

is not mediated by PTH or PTHrP. By expressing cAMP excretion so that only the nephrogenous (parathyroid-hormone dependent) component of nucleotide excretion is taken into account, the discriminatory value of the test may be considerably improved. However, a proportion of patients with hypercalcaemia associated with malignant disease, particularly squamous-cell carcinoma, but without obvious skeletal metastases may show increased production of nephrogenous cAMP. This was once thought to be due to ectopic production of PTH (so-called pseudohyperparathyroidism) but in the majority of cases there are additional circulating factor(s) such as PTHrP that stimulate both renal tubular reabsorption of calcium and the production of cAMP.

It is worth noting that the kidney is the site of degradation for many hormones including PTH and calcitonin. Renal function therefore needs to be taken

into account when assessing the results of radioimmunoassay, particularly in the case of PTH, where the C-terminal fragment normally degraded by the kidney persists in the circulation (*see* Fig. 30.4).

Bone

In the adult skeleton, in balance with respect to calcium, the amount of bone resorbed is balanced by an equivalent amount of bone formed (*see* Fig. 30.1). The processes of mineral accretion and resorption are closely coupled but do not occur in the same anatomical site at the same time.

The transfer of calcium to and from bone depends on cellular activity. In mature bone three main cell types occur. *Osteoblasts*, which form matrix, *osteoclasts* responsible for bone destruction, and *osteocytes*, themselves derived from osteoblasts, which become trapped within the bone matrix as maturation proceeds. The osteocytes are interconnected by an extensive canalicular network. This network has a large surface area (one acre (approx. 4050 m²) in man) and may be responsible for many of the rapid ion fluxes that occur in bone. The origin, life-span, and fate of the various cells in bone are only partially understood, but it is thought that osteoclasts are derived from the monocyte–macrophage lineage of haemopoetic cells, whereas the osteoblasts and osteocytes are derived from mesenchymal cells of the bone marrow stroma. The derivation of bone cells is of clinical interest in the disorder of *osteopetrosis*, which is characterized by defective bone resorption and the accretion of excessive amounts of calcium in the skeleton. A major abnormality is thought to be the defective production of osteoclasts, which is corrected by bone marrow transplantation.

The mineral component of bone is predominantly calcium and phosphate in the form of hydroxyapatite with multiple ionic substitutions. The major constituents of bone matrix are type I collagen, which is largely responsible for the tensile strength of bone, and proteoglycans. Many other proteins are found in bone. Of clinical interest is osteocalcin, a vitamin K-dependent, γ-carboxyglutamate (GLA)-containing protein (sometimes called bone gla protein; BGP). This is synthesized exclusively by osteoblasts and is laid down in bone matrix at sites of mineralization. It also appears in the circulation and its radioimmunoassay provides an index of osteoblast numbers in some skeletal disorders. Its greatest value is in the assessment of osteoporosis. The mechanisms controlling matrix production are uncertain, though the importance of normal matrix production is apparent from disorders in which it is defective, for example in osteogenesis imperfecta or in vitamin C deficiency in which synthesis of defective collagen and other bone proteins results in disturbed bone formation.

Calcification of the collagen matrix is an important step in the transition between matrix production and the formation of mineralized bone. In the skeleton, calcification takes place in two main sites—in epiphyseal cartilage during the growth of long bones, and in bone matrix during intramembranous ossification—and in the remodelling and growth of existing bone. The concentrations of calcium and phosphate in the ECF are insufficient to initiate the deposition of calcium and phosphate, but can sustain crystal growth once it has started. The first steps in calcification are now thought to take place in or around small membrane-bound vesicles found in the matrix derived from hypertrophic chondrocytes during the maturation of epiphyseal cartilage and possibly from osteoblasts in adult bone.

These vesicles are rich in alkaline phosphatase, an enyzme that has been known for many years to be associated with calcification. Alkaline phosphatase may function in calcification as a component of a membrane pump for calcium and phosphate, or it may be involved in the removal of potential inhibitors of calcification such as inorganic pyrophosphate. The possible importance of alkaline phosphatase in mineralization is illustrated in *hypophosphatasia* (a rare and recessively inherited disorder of mineralization), characterized by low or absent levels of bone-derived alkaline phosphatase. Hypophosphatasia is also characterized by increased concentrations of plasma pyrophosphate. As pyrophosphate is an inhibitor of the crystal growth of calcium phosphate, it may be responsible for the defective calcification of cartilage and bones in this condition.

Defective mineralization of adult bone results in increased amounts of osteoid. It is important to remember that the amount of osteoid present is dependent not only upon the rate of mineralization but also upon the rate of matrix formation. Increased osteoid due to an increased rate of formation occurs in hyperparathyroidism, Paget's disease, fracture repair, and the term *osteomalacia* is restricted to those conditions that result in a delay between formation of matrix and its subsequent mineralization. This occurs in vitamin D deficiency but is also found in other disorders such as hypophosphataemia, severe acidosis, and aluminium intoxication.

Phosphate plays a critical part in skeletal mineralization. Low plasma phosphate concentrations are often associated with osteomalacia and increased concentrations with the ectopic (extraskeletal) deposition of calcium phosphate. Phosphate may have specific effects on cells to enhance the uptake of calcium in calcified tissues.

It is widely held that vitamin D or its metabolites are required for normal mineralization, though there is little direct evidence for such an effect. It is therefore interesting that in many clinical disorders there is a stronger relation between levels of plasma phosphate and mineralization of bone than between levels of the active metabolites of vitamin D and mineralization. For example, in hypoparathyroidism, levels of calcitriol are classically low though mineralization of osteoid is usually normal. Conversely, in hypophosphataemic rickets, levels of plasma phosphate are low but levels of calcitriol are normal. In many of these conditions, administration of phosphate alone can improve skeletal calcification. This suggests that calcitriol may act on mineralization, predominantly by making calcium and phosphate available for mineralization. It is possible that the osteomalacia seen in simple vitamin D deficiency is partly due to the low plasma phosphate found in this disorder (in part an effect of secondary hyperparathyroidism to reduce Tm_P/GFR).

The biochemical events occurring during bone resorption are poorly understood. Some resorbing agents such as PTH and prostaglandins can stimulate the production of cAMP in bone but others such as calcitriol do not. It is interesting that in studies of isolated bone cells *in vitro*, osteoblast-like cells appear to have receptors for calcitriol and a PTH and prostaglandin-sensitive adenylate cyclase, though these cells themselves are not capable of resorbing bone. It seems likely that there is a complex humoral system of communication between various populations of bone cells, which may form the basis of the close coupling between the rates of bone formation and bone resorption. Bone resorption is accompanied by a release of acid and lysosomal enzymes capable of degrading matrix. Osteoclasts, viewed by electron microscopy, possess a ruffled border that is closely applied to the bone surface, and is the site at which removal of bone mineral and matrix occurs. The dissolution of bone matrix is associated with the release of calcium and degradation products of collagen. Proline is a major constituent of the collagen molecule, which is hydroxylated to form hydroxyproline in the post-translational stage of collagen biosynthesis. The liberation of hydroxyproline-containing peptides by osteoclasts is therefore an index of collagen degradation and of bone resorption, which can be used clinically in the assessment of metabolic bone disease. The maturation of collagen includes the formation of pyrodinolene cross-links. These, too, are liberated during bone resorption and their urinary excretion rate provides a more specific index of bone resorption than hydroxyproline excretion.

A number of agents are known to inhibit the rate of bone resorption. Administration of calcitonin inhibits bone resorption and decreases the activity and numbers of osteoclasts. Oestrogens also inhibit the rate of bone resorption, though receptors for oestrogens have not yet been convincingly demonstrated in bone cells. Other inhibitors of bone resorption include mithramycin and the diphosphonates. All these agents have been used therapeutically as inhibitors of bone resorption. Under physiological conditions, resorption of bone is probably under the control of PTH, vitamin D, thyroid hormones, and steroids, but will occur at a basal rate even in the absence of these hormones.

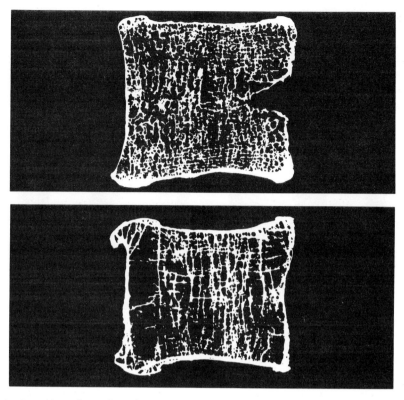

Figure 30.12 Sagittal section through a lumbar vertebra in a healthy individual (top) and in a patient with postmenopausal osteoporosis (bottom). Note the cortical shell enclosing a network of trabecular bone. In the case of postmenopausal osteoporosis the reduction in bone density is associated with a loss of trabecular elements rather than their thinning.

Organization and Turnover of Bone

Most bones comprise a compact cortical shell which surrounds a lattice work of spongy or trabecular bone tissue that houses the bone marrow (Fig. 30.12). The shape of the skeleton, its microanatomy, balance and mechanical competence are dependent upon the turnover of bone. In the adult who is neither increasing nor decreasing in skeletal mass the vast majority (95%) of movements of calcium to and from the skeleton are accounted for by the process of *bone remodelling*, which in turn is governed by the activity of bone cells. Bone remodelling represents an organized sequence of focal events on the surfaces of bone. These comprise the resorption of old bone by a team of osteoclasts that creates an erosion cavity, and the subsequent attraction of bone-forming cells or osteoblasts to sites of prior resorption (termed *coupling*). Osteoblasts thereafter synthesize an organic matrix, which, several days later after a period of osteoid maturation, undergoes mineralization. This sequence of events is particularly prominent in trabecular bone tissue (Fig. 30.13), largely because bone remodelling is a surface-based event and the surface to volume ratio is much higher (by a factor of 10) in trabecular than in cortical tissue.

In contrast to bone remodelling, *modelling* implies the continued apposition or destruction of bone, and is an important phenomenon in growth. In the adult, however, the vast majority of bone turnover is ac-

counted for by the remodelling process. For skeletal balance to be maintained, the requirement is that each erosion cavity created will be infilled with an equal volume of new bone. The remodelling process is, therefore, a very important component for the maintenance of skeletal balance and mechanical competence. Remodelling is also the major mechanism whereby bone can repair fatigue damage. Like all solid structures, bone undergoes damage by repeated stresses, but unlike inert materials can self-repair. If the remodelling activity of bone is impaired, this can give rise to fractures without necessarily altering the amount of bone. This is probably an important component of fractures that occur in the aluminium intoxication of patients with end-stage renal failure.

A number of disorders are associated with increases in remodelling activity. These include thyrotoxicosis, hyperparathyroidism and particularly Paget's disease, where focal rates of bone remodelling may be very high indeed. Increases in bone remodelling are generally associated with an increase in the number of bone remodelling units present on the bone surface at any one time. This has some implications for skeletal mass (Fig. 30.14), even when the amount of bone removed is equal to the total amount that is replaced in erosion cavities. A further consequence of increased bone remodelling is that progressively more and more of the surfaces of bone are

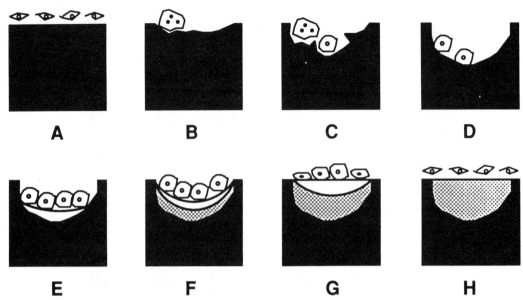

Figure 30.13 Schematic diagram to show the steps in the process of remodelling on trabecular bone surfaces. (A) the quiescent bone surface; (B) the activation of bone resorption by the focal attraction of osteoclasts; (C) the creation by osteoclasts of an erosion cavity; (D) smoothing of erosion cavities by mononuclear cells (reversal); (E) the differentiation of osteoblasts within resorption cavities (coupling); (F) the onset of matrix synthesis in mineralization; (G) the completion of matrix synthesis; (H) the completion of the remodelling sequence where the bone surface is covered by lining cells once more.

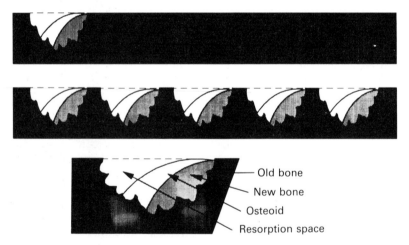

— Old bone
— New bone
— Osteoid
— Resorption space

Figure 30.14 The effect of skeletal turnover on bone and calcium balance. The upper panel depicts the normal trabecular surface where bone remodelling activity occurs on 15% of the bone surface. The resorption space occupies 2% of the bone volume and a somewhat smaller amount is occupied by osteoid. When turnover is increased fivefold without affecting the balance between the formation and resorption, the resorption and osteoid space increase proportionately. Conversely, when bone turnover is decreased, the accession of new osteoclasts to the bone surface is inhibited and bone mass will increase until the resorption space is infilled, a process that may take 1 or 2 years to be complete.

occupied by active events, either of formation or destruction. Thus, the surface coverage of bone by osteoclasts, osteoblasts and osteoid increases in proportion to the increment in remodelling. In practice, it is important to distinguish the increase in osteoid due to an increase in bone turnover from that due to defective mineralization of bone. In the latter, the thickness of osteoid is generally increased whereas in the former its surface extent is increased without inducing marked changes in the width of osteoid seam.

Bone Loss and Gain

The amount of bone deposited within erosion cavities may not equal the amount resorbed. For example, in postmenopausal osteoporosis it is clear that, although the coupling mechanism is preserved in that osteoblasts are attracted to sites of previous resorption, their numbers or competence are insufficient and the portion of new bone formed is less than that resorbed. This results in a finite deficit of bone for each remodelling sequence (Fig. 30.15). If bone turnover is ampli-

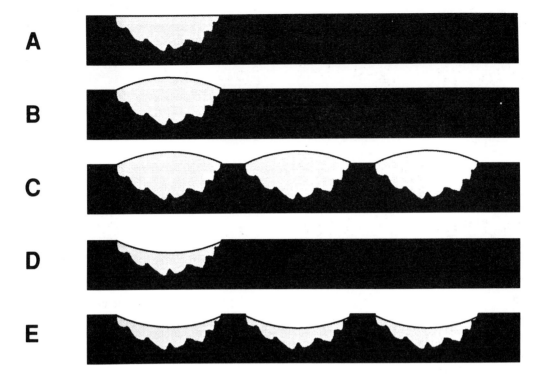

Figure 30.15 Mechanism for the production of trabecular osteoporosis and osteosclerosis. The upper panel shows a schematic representation of a normal trabecular bone surface and the infilling of a resorption bay with an equal volume of new bone. In osteoporosis, less bone is deposited in resorption cavities (D). If bone turnover is increased without altering this balance (E), the rate of trabecular bone loss will increase in proportion to the increment in bone turnover. Conversely, a decrease in bone turnover will delay the rate of bone loss. If the amount of bone deposited within resorption bays is greater than that removed each remodelling sequence will result in an increment in trabecular bone mass (B), a process that can be accelerated in proportion to the rate of bone remodelling (C).

fied, as indeed occurs immediately after the menopause, these skeletal losses will be amplified. Conversely, the amount of bone formed within erosion cavities may exceed that removed resulting in skeletal gains. Again, if bone remodelling is increased, these skeletal gains will be amplified. In the case of cortical bone, erosion cavities are tunnels within the solid geometric constraints of the cortex and cannot be overfilled. This is one of the reasons why anabolic agents such as sodium fluoride induce substantial gains in trabecular bone tissue but have little, if any, anabolic effect at cortical sites.

Bone losses and gains may also occur from uncoupled resorption and formation. In the case of uncoupled resorption, bone resorption is never subsequently followed by bone formation. This is an important component of osteolytic bone disease. It is also a component of some forms of osteoporosis, particularly that associated with immobilization and gonadal deficiency. In these disorders there is not only a decrease in trabecular width but also a marked loss of trabecular elements themselves. Indeed, there is little evidence of trabecular thinning in the case of postmenopausal osteoporosis, so that loss of trabecular elements must be partly a result of the generation of resorption cavities that transect or perforate trabecular structures. The disruption of trabecular architecture characteristic of hypogonadal states has important implications for structural strength. Selective destruction of cross-bracing elements leads to failure of the structure out of proportion to the amount of material removed. Even though remaining trabeculae in postmenopausal osteoporosis can thicken, evident even radiographically, this cannot compensate adequately and prevent skeletal failure. Similarly, therapeutic manipulation of the remodelling process might be expected to thicken remnant structures without necessarily restoring trabecular continuity. Indeed, the restoration of skeletal mass with sodium fluoride thickens remnant structures but does not increase their connectivity and probably explains why the effects on fracture frequency are less than might have been predicted from the changes in bone density.

In a variety both of physiological and of pathological states it is clear that there is a remarkably close correlation between the rates of mineral deposition, or bone formation, and mineral resorption. Even though these individual rates may be altered across a wide range, the net gains or losses of skeletal mass

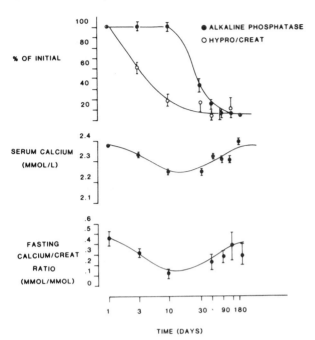

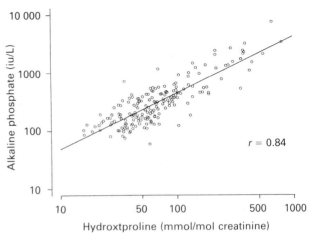

Figure 30.17 Relation between plasma alkaline phosphatase and urinary excretion of hydroxyproline in patients with Paget's disease of bone. Note the logarithmic scales indicating the close relation between these two measurements over a very wide range of values.

Figure 30.16 Biochemical responses to treatment with clodronate (3200 mg/day), an inhibitor of bone resorption, in three patients with Paget's disease (mean ± SEM). Despite the rapid bone turnover before treatment, plasma calcium and fasting calcium excretion were normal. During the early phase of treatment suppression of bone formation as judged by plasma alkaline phosphatase lagged behind inhibition of bone resorption (urinary hydroxyproline (hypro)/creatinine (creat) ratio). During this transient phase when bone formation exceeded resorption, fasting plasma and urinary calcium levels fell until a new steady-state was attained when formation matched resorption.

are minimized by the tight coupling between these rates. This is an important feature in skeletal physiology and therapeutics that is often overlooked. Thus, it is difficult to induce a sustained difference between the rates of mineralization and resorption, since a decrease in bone resorption will inevitably lead to a decrease in formation (Fig. 30.16). The process may take several years before a new steady state arises. This is one reason why treatments should be studied for long periods, since it is unwise to extrapolate long-term consequences from short-term changes.

Clinical evidence for coupling is readily seen in Paget's disease from the concurrent measurement of alkaline phosphatase and urinary excretion of hydroxyproline. There is a close correlation between these two measurements over a wide range of values (Fig. 30.17). During treatment of Paget's disease with inhibitors of bone resorption, the earliest response to treatment is a decrease in the urinary excretion of hydroxyproline. This is followed later by a diminution in plasma alkaline phosphatase activity, an index of bone formation. If treatment is sustained, the fall in alkaline phosphatase activity matches the fall in hydroxyproline excretion so that the relation between

the two measurements remains the same as before treatment.

There are important differences between the control of skeletal turnover and the regulation of the plasma calcium concentration. In disorders characterized by increased but coupled bone turnover (for example, Paget's disease), the rate of bone resorption is high. This, however, is matched by an increased rate of bone formation so that the net contribution of calcium to the ECF from the skeleton is normal. Thus under steady-state conditions there is no marked disturbance in plasma calcium unless remodelling is temporarily disturbed, during treatment for example (*see* Fig. 30.16).

It is also important to note that, whereas bone cells are intimately related to the accretion and resorption of bone mineral (approx. 5 mmol (200 mg) of calcium per day), this turnover underestimates the true exchange between plasma and bone because exchange of calcium occurs at other sites such as the osteocytic and canalicular surfaces. In the adult, these surfaces have been estimated to constitute an area of more than 1000 m² which is 100-fold greater than that of the total trabecular bone surface. This vast exchange area may act as a buffer to calcium stresses imposed on the ECF and is probably under the influence of hormones such as PTH. Indeed, this 'bone blood' membrane probably contributes to the long-term setting of the plasma calcium concentration.

Assessment of Skeletal Turnover. Skeletal turnover (bone formation, mineralization, and resorption) can be deduced from kinetic, histological or biochemical tests. Metabolic balance studies give an approximation of the net fluxes of calcium occurring across the skeleton (*see* Fig. 30.2). They do not, however, indi-

TABLE 30.4
BIOCHEMICAL INDICES OF SKELETAL METABOLISM

Measurement	Source	Changes in high bone turnover
Formation		
Alkaline phosphatase	Liver/bone/gut	Increased
Skeletal alkaline phosphatase	Bone: osteoblasts	Increased
Osteocalcin	Bone: osteoblasts	Increased
Non-dialysable hydroxyproline	Post-translational maturation of collagen	Increased
Procollagen type I	Bone: osteoblasts	Increased
Procollagen type III	? Fibrous tissue	Increased
α_2HS glycoprotein	Liver: incorporated into bone	Decreased
Resorption		
Hydroxyproline (dialysable)	Collagen degradation	Increased
Hydroxylysine and its glycosides	Collagen degradation	Increased
Glucosylgalactosyl/galactosyl hydroxylysine	Skin/bone collagen	Decreased
Acid phosphatase	? Osteoclasts	Increased
3-hydroxy-lysyl-pyridinolone	Collagen cross-links	Increased
Proline iminopeptidase	? Osteoclasts, ? osteoblasts	Increased
Urinary or serum free GLA	Osteocalcin degradation	Increased

cate the sizes of the unidirectional fluxes. This can be overcome to some extent by the use of tracer kinetic studies. For example, the rate of bone resorption can be calculated by the release of strontium or calcium isotopes from the skeleton, and together with the balance studies, resorption and formation rates can be calculated separately.

Less direct but more readily measured indices of bone turnover are the estimation in plasma of alkaline phosphatase and the urinary excretion of hydroxyproline (*see* Figs. 30.16 and 30.17). Alkaline phosphatase is derived in part from osteoblasts and contributes to the total plasma alkaline phosphatase. It is important to note that plasma alkaline phosphatase is also derived from liver and gut, and that hyperphosphatasia may also be caused by diseases of these systems. Alkaline phosphatase derived from bone has a greater heat stability and somewhat different electrophoretic mobility than that from gut or liver. The concurrent measurement of liver enzymes in plasma (e.g. 5'-nucleotidase) or isoenzyme studies of phosphatase may help to clarify the causes of hyperphosphatasia.

Hydroxyproline in small peptides derived from collagen degradation can be measured in plasma or urine. As in the case of plasma alkaline phosphatase, there are several limitations that impair interpretation of the results of these estimations. Unless the ingestion of foods rich in hydroxyproline is avoided, high urinary excretion rates may spuriously suggest increased bone resorption. Also a large proportion of the total hydroxyproline in plasma is found in the first component of complement (C1q) and collagen is present in many other structures than bone.

There are a number of other indirect indices of skeletal metabolism, variously derived from bone cells or bone matrix (Table 30.4). Many are not widely available but are utilized in specialist centres.

Bone formation, mineralization, and resorption can also be assessed from histological studies; methods exist for estimating the amount of bone undergoing these processes. For practical purposes these techniques are confined to a limited number of centres with an interest in metabolic bone disease. They are nevertheless extremely useful in understanding the pathophysiology of skeletal disorders and their response to therapeutic intervention. They depend heavily on static measurements, for example the proportion of trabecular surfaces occupied by active-looking osteoclasts, but dynamic measurements can also be obtained. The administration of tetracycline before bone biopsy results in its deposition at the calcification front. If two courses of tetracycline are given with a known time interval between them (usually 10–14 days), then the two markers can be seen on sections of the bone biopsy by their fluorescence under ultraviolet light (Fig. 30.18). In this way the extent and the rates of bone deposition and mineralization can be measured, and from these the bone formation rate. It is also possible to quantitate the activity of both osteoblasts and osteoclasts, and indeed to calculate the turnover time for bone. Bone biopsy must be necessarily confined to available skeletal sites, usually the ilium, and a major limitation of the technique is that inferences made from the biopsy may not reflect events occurring at other skeletal sites, particularly in disorders in which the skeleton is not uniformly disturbed.

Despite the many limitations in the assessment of these biochemical indices of bone turnover, there is a surprisingly good correlation between kinetic, histological and biochemical measurements in metabolic bone disease.

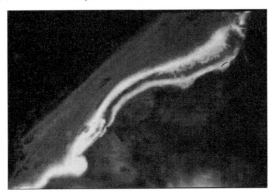

Figure 30.18 Section through trabecular bone, photographed under ultraviolet light, that has been prelabelled with tetracycline. The light bands indicate the two courses of tetracycline given, which are separated by a known time interval. This allows the rate and extent of bone formation to be calculated.

Measurement of Skeletal Mass and Loss. A variety of techniques are available for measuring bone loss. With the exception of balance and radioisotope studies, they depend on indirect determinations of skeletal mass at repeated intervals. Conventional balance studies are too insensitive to measure small losses reliably because the magnitude of daily losses of calcium, for example in osteoporosis (say 30 mg/day, equivalent to approximately 1% of bone mass per year), is beyond the detection limits of the technique. Moreover, a measurement of skeletal balance over a short period of time may not reflect long-term changes, since bone losses or gains may not occur uniformly with time.

Assessment of skeletal mass can be made from radiographs, but this method is relatively insensitive. Subjective evaluation can be improved by comparing the radiodensity of bone with standards such as aluminium step wedges and with the use of industrial film. In the hip, the loss of femoral trabecular markings on X-rays can give a semiquantitative index of bone loss (Singh score), and discriminates fairly well between patients with and without femoral-neck fracture due to osteoporosis. More precise measurements ($\pm 2\%$) can be made by measuring cortical thickness of long bones. This technique has been widely used in the metacarpal, particularly in the evaluation of osteoporosis. Cortical thickness clearly does not reflect trabecular bone density, which may be important, for example, in spinal osteoporosis. These measurements also do not take account of cortical porosity, which is a feature, for example, of primary hyperparathyroidism.

Bone mineral density can be readily measured by photon absorptiometry at peripheral sites. More recently, techniques have been developed to examine central sites such as the hip or spine by dual-energy photon or X-ray absorptiometry, and these are becoming widely available. The measurement of bone mineral density has some advantages over cortical thickness in that, for the same degree of precision, it provides an index both of cortical and trabecular density. The importance of this is that bone loss is not usually distributed uniformly between cortical and cancellous bone.

Various techniques and their characteristics are summarized in Table 30.3 above. It is important to recognize that all have their limitations, and indeed none of them measures true density. Other problems relate to the type of information obtained, the sites of measurement and their relevance to clinical endpoints such as fracture risk. They are, however, becoming a very important tool for measuring the amount of bone at a skeletal site and thus giving an estimate of fracture risk in osteoporosis, and for assessing rates of bone loss by their repeated measurement over intervals.

With respect to the use of bone mineral density as a diagnostic tool, a number of studies have examined the sensitivity and specificity of bone mass measurements. The use of these measurements for screening depends upon their ability to measure what they intend (accuracy) and the relation of this to the population variance. With the possible exception of single-photon absorptiometry the methods do not have the required accuracy, and even in the case of single-photon absorptiometry the sensitivity and specificity of the method to detect future fracture risk may not be sufficiently robust for wide-scale screening. The ability of sequential measurements to detect bone loss depends much more on the precision of the techniques (*see* Table 30.3). The more precise a technique the more certain one can be in a given period of time that a change in apparent density reflects a true change. With the more precise techniques it is, nevertheless, necessary to measure bone density at infrequent intervals, usually after at least a year or two. Rates of bone loss can also be assessed by the indirect biochemical estimates of skeletal turnover, particularly in osteoporosis where accelerated losses are associated with accelerated turnover (*see* Fig. 30.15). Thus, the combined use of physical and biochemical techniques on one occasion may improve the estimate of fracture risk compared with single physical measurement alone.

Quality of Bone. The quality of bone can be directly estimated by the use of bone biopsy. Reference has been previously made to quantitative histological techniques that are available, but it is also possible to determine the composition of bone directly (e.g. the calcium:phosphate ratio or the aluminium content by appropriate methods, including chemical analysis or physical methods such as energy-dispersive X-ray analysis under the electron microscope.

The bone biopsy can also be used to provide indices of trabecular connectivity. Skeletal radiographs have, for many years, provided an important clinical tool for the investigation of skeletal disorders. The radiographic changes that occur in various dis-

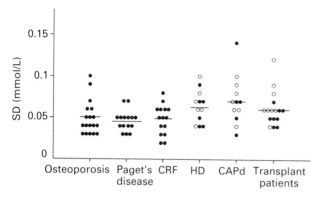

Figure 30.19 The deviation around the mean values (SD) for serum calcium concentration in patients with various disorders of calcium and skeletal metabolism. Fluctuations in serum calcium were assessed in each individual from repeated measurements over several months. Open circles denote hypercalcaemic patients. Note the relative efficiency of maintaining the set-point in disease states. CAPd, continuous ambulatory peritoneal dialysis; CRF, chronic renal failure; HD, haemodialysis.

eases are beyond the scope of this review but it is important to note that in many disorders, radiography is a relatively insensitive technique. For example, in osteomalacia occurring in the adult skeleton, radiographic appearances may be quite normal unless also associated with Looser's zones. The architectural detail on radiographs can be improved by the use of fine-grain industrial film, which is particularly important in assessing trabecular porosity and the presence of subperiosteal bone resorption.

Isotopes such as ^{89}Sr and ^{18}F have been used clinically as scintigraphic agents for detecting regions of increased bone turnover, such as in metastatic tumour deposits. Pyrophosphate, polyphosphates, and diphosphonates, all of which have a high affinity for crystals of hydroxyapatite, are widely used as bone-scanning agents by linking them to the γ-emitting isotope technetium-99m (^{99m}Tc) in the presence of stannous ions. The whole-body retention of ^{99m}Tc-labelled diphosphonates in the skeleton can be used as an integrated index of bone-cell activity.

Integration of Organ Responses

It is useful to draw some distinction between the way in which the plasma calcium is set at a particular concentration, and the way in which movements of calcium in and out of ECF are adjusted (error correction). The plasma calcium concentration is set close to a particular value in different individuals in normal and disease states. The set-point can be defined as the mean plasma calcium of an individual and the standard deviation, the efficiency with which the set-point is maintained. This efficiency is not markedly disturbed in disorders of skeletal turnover (e.g.

Paget's disease) or disorders of the major calcium-regulating hormones (e.g. hypo- or hyperparathyroidism), indicating that other factors than bone turnover or hormones are important for maintaining this efficiency (Fig. 30.19). It is likely, however, that the value of the set-point is determined by hormones, particularly PTH and its effects at the ECF–bone interface.

Deviations from this value are, however, corrected by hormone-induced changes in all the fluxes of calcium to and from the ECF compartment. Alterations in flux rates are monitored and adjusted by the changes in plasma calcium or phosphate concentration they induce. This homeostatic error correction can operate with the plasma calcium set at any number of different values, with the relative rates of entry and exit of calcium to and from the ECF being altered as drift occurs from this set-point. Thus, in hypo- or hyperparathyroidism the fluxes of calcium across the gut and in and out of bone may not be greatly different from normal, and external calcium balance can be maintained even though the plasma calcium is set at a markedly abnormal level.

When the system is disturbed, a steady state no longer exists, and the response which occurs adjusts the system so that a new steady state comes into existence. Deviations of plasma calcium away from its normal value are rapidly corrected by alterations in the secretion of the regulating hormones. PTH and possibly calcitonin can be considered the fast-acting components of the regulatory system, whereas vitamin D is responsible for adaptation in the longer term. In experimental animals, removal of sources of PTH and calcitonin (for example, thyroparathyroidectomy in dogs or rats) results in hypocalcaemia (lower set-point for plasma calcium) and in a slower than normal return of plasma calcium to starting values in response to acute changes in concentration.

In considering plasma calcium homeostasis it is useful to consider the steady-state and transient changes separately. In man, the most important regulator of acute changes in the concentration of calcium is PTH, the secretion of which increases within seconds of a fall in plasma calcium, and decreases as the ionized concentration of calcium rises. The rapid control of plasma calcium by PTH is mainly due to its ability to regulate renal tubular reabsorption of calcium and possibly by its effects on calcium exchange between ECF and bone. After parathyroidectomy, the fall in plasma calcium can be largely accounted for by a continued loss of calcium into urine, until a new steady state is achieved in which calcium excretion is the same as its starting value but takes place at a much reduced filtered load of calcium. Thus, the acute effect of PTH is to increase calcium excretion by decreasing renal tubular reabsorption of calcium, but when the steady state exists urinary calcium decreases once more, but at the expense of a lower serum calcium.

A further example of a disruption of the steady

TABLE 30.5

CAUSES OF HIGH LEVELS OF PARATHYROID HORMONE (PTH) IN PLASMA

Primary hyperparathyroidism
Single or multiple adenoma (common)
Parathyroid hyperplasia (less common)
Parathyroid carcinoma (rare)

Secondary hyperparathyroidism
Vitamin D-deficiency states
Drugs causing hypocalcaemia (e.g. phosphate, diphosphonates)
Renal failure (reduced clearance of PTH fragments, increased secretion or both)
Medullary carcinoma of thyroid
Pseudohypoparathyroidism (target-organ insensitivity to PTH)

Tertiary hyperparathyroidism
Prolonged secondary hyperparathyroidism (e.g. chronic bowel or renal disease)
Transplantation (slow parathyroid involution following restoration of renal function)

Pseudohyperparathyroidism (humoral hypercalcaemia of malignancy)
Carcinoma, e.g. squamous-cell carcinoma of bronchus, lymphomas

state is seen during an infusion of calcium, where the plasma calcium concentration will begin to rise. If the rate of calcium infusion is constant, the concentration of plasma calcium will not rise indefinitely but only until the rate of efflux of calcium from the extracellular pool (to bone, kidney, and gut and other tissues) matches the rate of influx. At this point, plasma calcium levels will not rise further, despite continuing the infusion, and a new steady state prevails. In practice, the infusion of calcium will result in the suppression of PTH secretion and a decrease in the renal tubular reabsorption for calcium. This will tend to increase the rate at which a new steady state is achieved. It is notable that the rise in plasma calcium during a calcium infusion is to some extent buffered by the exchange of calcium in bone. Thus, rises or falls in plasma calcium are partially compensated by increased net movements of calcium into or out of bone.

The response to prolonged perturbations brings in contributions from changes in vitamin D metabolism, and from the intestine and bone. An example is the adaptation that occurs to a change in dietary intake of calcium. If intake is reduced, this will tend to cause a gradual fall in plasma calcium, which will increase the secretion of PTH. Apart from its effects on the kidney, a sustained increase in PTH will lead both to enhanced turnover of bone and to an increase in synthesis of calcitriol. This in turn will enhance intestinal absorption of calcium and resorption of calcium from bone. If the reduction in dietary calcium continues, these changes will act to restore the plasma

calcium towards its previous value, and bone formation rate will increase to match the rate of increased bone resorption by the coupling mechanism. The new steady state will consist of a greater efficiency of intestinal absorption of calcium and an increased rate of entry and removal of calcium from bone, so that net balance can be maintained.

DISORDERS OF CALCIUM HOMEOSTASIS

The purpose of this section is not to give a detailed clinical description of disorders of calcium metabolism but to illustrate some of the principles of calcium homeostasis and their application to the investigation of various diseases.

Disorders of Parathyroid Secretion

Hyperparathyroidism

The term hyperparathyroidism is applied to those clinical disorders characterized by an increase in the circulating concentration of PTH (Table 30.5). These can be conveniently classified into primary, secondary and tertiary hyperparathyroidism.

Secondary hyperparathyroidism is due to a rise in PTH because of sustained hypocalcaemia, as seen for example in vitamin D deficiency or chronic renal failure. Hypocalcaemia results in the increased secretion of PTH and, if sustained, to hyperplasia of the parathyroid glands. The skeletal lesions that result are therefore a reflection of the underlying disorder (e.g. vitamin D deficiency) and the high circulating levels of PTH. Secondary hyperparathyroidism can be cured by appropriate treatment that restores the plasma calcium concentration to normal (for example, vitamin D in simple nutritional deficiency of vitamin D). This, therefore, removes the stimulus to parathyroid overactivity.

Tertiary hyperparathyroidism is a term used to denote those patients with long-standing secondary hyperparathyroidism who develop 'autonomous' gland function and hypercalcaemia. Nowadays this is most commonly seen after renal transplantation, but may also be observed in patients with long-standing malabsorption or chronic renal failure. The parathyroid glands are hypertrophied and may show histological evidence of adenomatous transformation. As in the case of many endocrine disorders, the term 'autonomous' secretion is probably a misnomer since PTH levels can be suppressed by calcium infusion or further augmented by manoeuvres that lower the plasma calcium (e.g. infusion of EDTA). Tertiary hyperparathyroidism therefore implies a change in the set-point with respect to PTH secretion for the control of plasma calcium. In contrast to secondary hyperparathyroidism, plasma calcium and PTH are both raised.

Primary hyperparathyroidism is due to the presence of multiple or single adenomata or to hyperplasia of the parathyroid glands. The causes are unknown and

TABLE 30.6
MAJOR CAUSES OF HYPOPARATHYROIDISM

Inadequate secretion of PTH
Surgical-thyroid, parathyroid and radical neck surgery
Familial
Sporadic
Di Giorge syndrome
Parathyroid disease, e.g. neoplasia, amyloid

Suppression of PTH secretion (normal parathyroid glands)
Neonatal—from maternal hypercalcaemia
Severe magnesium depletion
Non-parathyroid induced hypercalcaemia

Defective end-organ response to PTH
Pseudohypoparathyroidism types I and II

it is assumed that the abnormality is intrinsic to the parathyroid glands themselves. Primary hyperparathyroidism is rarely due to carcinoma. As in the case of tertiary hyperparathyroidism, the main biochemical abnormality is an increase in the circulating concentration of both PTH and calcium. There are, however, instances when such patients have normal total plasma calcium and intermittently high PTH levels, sometimes associated with concurrent vitamin D deficiency. Thus, primary hyperparathyroidism can be defined as a disturbance of the parathyroid glands where the circulating level of PTH is inappropriately high for the prevailing concentration of plasma calcium.

Both plasma calcium and PTH should be interpreted with caution. Thus, total plasma calcium comprises the ionized, complexed and protein-bound fraction and account should taken of possible abnormalities in protein concentration, pH and in protein binding. Hypercalcaemia itself may impair renal function, and since the kidney is an important site for degradation of PTH, increased levels of PTH in the presence of renal failure may not reflect an increase in the biologically active moiety of PTH (*see* Fig. 30.4).

In primary hyperparathyroidism, the hypercalcaemia is maintained partly by a resetting of the renal tubular reabsorption for calcium, so that reabsorption is enhanced for any given filtered load (*see* Fig. 30.10). Frequently, increased bone resorption and increased intestinal absorption of calcium (due to stimulation of production of calcitriol) are also found, and these will increase urinary calcium excretion (24-h excretion). Although resorption of bone is commonly enhanced, so too is bone formation. Thus the balance for calcium may be normal, but at the expense of an increased bone turnover so that the fasting urinary excretion of calcium is usually normal. Radiographic abnormalities (subperiosteal erosions) are more commonly seen in secondary and tertiary hyperparathyroidism and are due to abnormalities in bone architecture because of increased bone turnover. Calcium balance may be negative, particularly in patients with severe bone disease, and osteoporosis is

occasionally the major radiographic feature. Renal stones are also a common complication of primary hyperparathyroidism. The aetiology of renal stones in hyperparathyroidism is discussed elsewhere (*see* Chapter 20) but is related in part to an increase in the daily amount of calcium excreted.

Hypercalcaemia is commonly seen in patients with malignant disease. This may be variously caused (discussed later), but in some instances may be due to the production of PTHrP by the tumour itself. This syndrome has been described as ectopic hyperparathyroidism or pseudohyperparathyroidism but is now termed the *humoral hypercalcaemia of malignancy*. True ectopic hyperparathyroidism is exceedingly rare.

The majority of patients with hypercalcaemia have either primary hyperparathyroidism, without overt radiographic evidence of bone disease, or non-parathyroid malignant tumours. In the vast majority the distinction is straightforward but, in a few, diagnostic difficulties are encountered in distinguishing between these two groups. A variety of tests has been devised to distinguish these disorders, partly because of the lack, until recently, of suitable assays for PTH. The hydrocortisone suppression test was widely used. Hydrocortisone (usually 40 mg thrice daily for 10 days) fails to lower plasma calcium in primary hyperparathyroidism but usually does so in hypercalcaemia due to other causes. With the advent of radioimmunoassay for PTH, this test is becoming redundant but it still has its advocates. It is important to realize that a proportion of patients with primary hyperparathyroidism will show suppression of their plasma calcium with hydrocortisone, particularly those patients with bone disease. Furthermore, hypercalcaemia in patients with other disorders does not invariably respond to corticosteroids, particularly in patients with secondary skeletal neoplasia.

Various other tests have been devised to distinguish hypercalcaemia due to hyperparathyroidism from that from other causes. PTH has an effect on the renal handling of phosphorus and this has led to the measurement of indices of tubular reabsorption for phosphate. Many tests are available, though the estimation of Tm_P/GFR is based on sounder physiological principles than many others. In the absence of renal impairment, the plasma bicarbonate alone may be helpful. Thus in hyperparathyroidism a metabolic acidosis is commonly found, reflected as a low plasma bicarbonate, whereas in disorders where PTH secretion is depressed, a metabolic alkalosis is to be expected and frequently observed. Moreover, in hypercalcaemia due to rapid bone destruction, an alkalosis may be accentuated by the release of bicarbonate from bone. Another test is the urinary excretion of cAMP, an index of parathyroid function.

Hypoparathyroidism

Decreased secretion of PTH may arise in hypercalcaemic conditions that suppress the secretion of PTH.

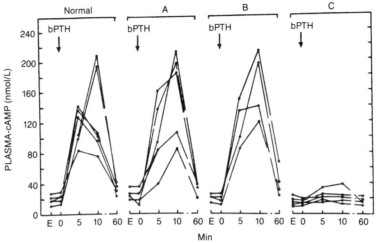

Figure 30.20 Plasma cAMP before and up to 60 min after an injection of 200 units of bovine PTH (bPTH) in normal subjects and in patients with surgical (A) and idiopathic hypoparathyroidism (B) and with pseudohypoparathyroidism (C). (From Tomlinson S., Hendy G.N., O'Riordan J.L.H. (1976). *Lancet*, **i**, 62.)

The term hypoparathyroidism is usually confined, however, to those disorders (Table 30.6) associated with defective secretion or action of PTH (the latter termed pseudohypoparathyroidism).

Many of the biochemical and metabolic abnormalities seen in hypoparathyroidism can be understood from an appreciation of the physiology of PTH. Plasma phosphate is raised due to an increase in Tm_p/GFR. Hypocalcaemia is due in part to a decrease in tubular reabsorption for calcium. PTH stimulates the synthesis of calcitriol from its precursor, calcifediol, and in hypoparathyroidism circulating concentrations of calcitriol may be low and account for decreased intestinal absorption of calcium. Hyperphosphataemia may be another reason for low levels of calcitriol because phosphate suppresses its renal production. It is also thought that hypocalcaemia is due to impaired osteocytic calcium transfer from bone because of the deficiency of PTH or calcitriol or both.

Many of the signs and symptoms of hypoparathyroidism (tetany, calcification of basal ganglia, cataract, etc.) are attributable to hypocalcaemia and hyperphosphataemia.

There exists a group of disorders termed *pseudohypoparathyroidism* in which the secretion of PTH is normal or even increased but some or all of the biochemical features of hypoparathyroidism are present. This is due to a resistance of one or more of the target-organ tissues to PTH. There is an association between pseudohypoparathyroidism and characteristic somatic features, including short stature, round face, short neck, shortening of metacarpals and metatarsals. These are not invariably found in pseudohypoparathyroidism and indeed may be present occasionally in idiopathic hypoparathyroidism when present in childhood. Rarely the somatic features of pseudohypoparathyroidism may be found in patients

with no impairment of secretion or action of PTH, a condition termed *pseudopseudohypoparathyroidism*.

Simple hypoparathyroidism most commonly results from inadvertent removal of parathyroid glands during thyroid, parathyroid or laryngeal surgery. Idiopathic hypoparathyroidism is much rarer and may be familial, sporadic or be found in combination with other disorders such as pernicious anaemia, Addison's disease or candidiasis. Rarely, hypoparathyroidism may result from infiltration of the parathyroid gland by malignant disease, haemochromatosis or amyloid. Di Giorge syndrome refers to a congenital absence of thymic and parathyroid tissue and is associated with immunological deficiencies, cardiovascular anomalies and unusual facies. Hypoparathyroidism has been reported following ^{131}I therapy, but irradiation of the neck appears to be one of the factors predisposing to hyperparathyroidism.

Apart from low or absent levels of PTH, hypocalcaemia and hyperphosphataemia in the presence of normal renal function, a biochemical characteristic of hypoparathyroidism is that patients are responsive to the action of PTH (Fig. 30.20). The renal excretion of cAMP is low and is augmented by the administration of PTH. Similarly, renal tubular reabsorption for phosphate is acutely decreased following PTH. This forms the basis of the Chase–Aurbach (Ellsworth–Howard) test.

In contrast, pseudohypoparathyroidism (also called PTH-resistant hypoparathyroidism) results from a resistance of target tissues to the action of PTH. Indeed, PTH levels are commonly high, although appropriate for the hypocalcaemia. The resistance to PTH may be partial or complete. Thus during the infusion of PTH, cyclic AMP production is not stimulated (*see* Fig. 30.16) and in many patients neither is the renal tubular reabsorption of phosphate decreased (pseudohypoparathyroidism type I). Other

TABLE 30.7
VITAMIN D-DEFICIENCY STATES

TABLE 30.7
VITAMIN D-DEFICIENCY STATES

Reduced availability of vitamin D
Inadequate sunlight or diet
Intestinal malabsorption of vitamin D, e.g. malabsorption
   syndromes, subtotal gastrectomy, ileal bypass surgery

Reduced availability of calcifediol
Liver disease
Drugs, e.g. phenobarbitone, phenytoin, glutethimide
Decreased enterohepatic circulation, e.g. malabsorption
   syndromes and liver disease
Nephrotic syndrome (urinary losses)

Reduced availability of calcitriol
Enzyme deficiency (1α-hydroxylase), e.g. vitamin
   D-dependent rickets (type I)
Enzyme destruction, e.g. chronic renal failure
Enzyme suppression, e.g. hypoparathyroidism,
   pseudohypoparathyroidism
Fanconi syndrome and acidosis
Tumour-associated osteomalacia (mesenchymal tumours)
Itai-itai disease (cadmium toxicity)

Reduced end-organ response
Vitamin D-dependent rickets type II
Anticonvulsants
? Steroid-induced osteoporosis
Coeliac disease and chronic renal failure (tissue damage to
   gut)

Uncertain or little relation to vitamin D
X-linked hypophosphataemia
Diabetes mellitus
Neonatal hypocalcaemia
Treatment with corticosteroids
Osteoporosis

patients may show a normal cAMP response but the absence of phosphaturia (type II), whereas in others responsiveness to PTH may be completely restored by calcium infusion. Not all target tissues need be affected and pseudohypoparathyroidism may be associated with osteitis fibrosa, indicating that the skeleton is sensitive to PTH.

There is a great deal of confusion concerning the definition of pseudopseudohypoparathyroidism, since affected patients may have relatives with pseudohypoparathyroidism and may indeed undergo transition from hypocalcaemia to normocalcaemia and vice versa.

Mention has been previously made of the hypocalcaemia seen in magnesium deficiency. This may be due to impaired secretion of PTH as well as diminished responsiveness of target tissue to PTH.

Disorders of Vitamin D Metabolism

Excessive Amounts of Vitamin D
Vitamin D toxicity is a common finding in clinical practice and is usually iatrogenic. Since vitamin D increases calcium absorption and in high doses aug-ments bone resorption, these patients characteristically have hypercalcaemia. Plasma phosphate concentration is commonly also high, owing to similar effects on phosphate transport. If overdosage is prolonged, increased bone resorption causes progressive loss of bone.

Under physiological conditions, the major actions of vitamin D are thought to be due to its conversion to the dihydroxylated metabolites, particularly calcitriol. However, large doses of vitamin D and calcifediol also induce toxicity, even in patients who are incapable of forming calcitriol (e.g. anephric patients). Furthermore, in patients with normal renal function and vitamin D toxicity, plasma levels of calcitriol are not increased.

The factors that augment the synthesis of calcitriol include hypophosphataemia, hypocalcaemia and increased secretion of PTH. High levels of calcitriol are found in patients with primary hyperparathyroidism and in idiopathic renal calculi and account for the increased calcium absorption found in these disorders. Increased calcium absorption is also seen in acromegaly and may be due to increased secretion of calcitriol. Sarcoidosis and other granulomatous disorders are occasionally associated with hypercalcaemia but more commonly with hypercalciuria. This is due to increased intestinal absorption of calcium associated with increased production of calcitriol by the sarcoid tissue itself. This explains the so-called vitamin D sensitivity seen in this disorder.

Defective Production of Vitamin D Metabolites
The hallmarks of vitamin D deficiency include defective mineralization of bone and retardation of growth. Simple vitamin D deficiency causes hypocalcaemia and hypophosphataemia. The hypophosphataemia results from secondary hyperparathyroidism (decreased Tm_P/GFR) and malabsorption of phosphate. Indeed it is possible that the defective mineralization of bone is due in part to the phosphate depletion associated with secondary hyperparathyroidism.

Vitamin D deficiency may be present despite adequate supplies of vitamin D because of a disturbance in its metabolism. This gives rise to vitamin D resistance in the sense that the doses of vitamin D necessary to achieve therapeutic effects are greater than the normal physiological requirements. As in the case of osteomalacia, not all vitamin D-resistant disorders are due to defective metabolism of vitamin D. Defective action or production of vitamin D metabolites may arise in a number of ways (Table 30.7), by impaired conversion of vitamin D to its natural metabolites or by its impaired target-organ responses.

Chronic renal failure, pseudohypoparathyroidism and hypoparathyroidism are disorders in which conversion of calcifidiol to calcitriol is impaired. Plasma levels of calcitriol are low and physiological quantities of calcitriol may reverse some of the biochemical abnormalities, whereas pharmacological amounts of vitamin D_3 or calcifidiol are required to achieve the

TABLE 30.8
SOME CAUSES OF OSTEOMALACIA

Vitamin D deficiency of defective metabolism (*see* also
  Table 30.6)
Nutritional deficiency of vitamin D
Lack of sunlight
Malabsorption of vitamin D
Chronic renal failure
Vitamin D-dependent rickets

Low plasma phosphate
Phosphate deficiency (diet, phosphate-binding agents)
Renal tubular disorders (vitamin D-resistant rickets)

Chronic acidosis
Ureterosigmoidostomy
Renal tubular acidosis (proximal or distal)

Drugs
Anticonvulsants
Diphosphonates
Fluoride

Inherited or unexplained
Fibrogenesis imperfecta ossium
Hypophosphatasia
Axial osteomalacia

same response. Perhaps a better example of defective conversion of vitamin D_3 to calcitriol is seen in vitamin D-dependent rickets in which many of the clinical and biochemical features are compatible with a deficient renal 1α-hydroxylase enzyme system (pseudo-deficiency rickets). There are patients with similar biochemical characteristics who have normal or high levels of calcitriol, the vitamin D equivalent of pseudo-hypoparathyroidism. This rare condition is described as vitamin D-dependent rickets type II.

The cause of osteomalacia associated with the use of anticonvulsant drugs may be the increased metabolic degradation of vitamin D to inactive metabolites because of induction of hepatic microsomal enzymes (including the cytochrome-P450 system). A more firmly established role for impaired metabolism of calcifediol is seen in the nephrotic syndrome, which may be associated with excessive urinary losses of this metabolite bound to proteins. Impairment of target-organ response to vitamin D probably occurs in coeliac disease (gluten-sensitive enteropathy) where intestinal absorption of calcium is not increased by relatively large doses of calcitriol, even when given intravenously. After effective treatment with a gluten-free diet, a normal sensitivity to calcitriol is restored. This suggests that the lack of response in the untreated disease is due to damage to the intestinal villi, which are the site of action of vitamin D metabolites on intestinal calcium transport. Impaired target-organ responses, in both the intestine and bone, may also be responsible for the disorders of mineral metabolism found in anticonvulsant use and corticosteroid treatment.

Low levels of calcitriol have also been reported in postmenopausal osteoporosis but the importance of this in its pathophysiology is controversial. It is important to recognize that osteomalacia in adults or rickets in children is not always due to deficiency of vitamin D or its metabolites (Table 30.8). A common example is X-linked or sporadic hypophosphataemia (vitamin D-resistant rickets) where defective mineralization of bone is probably due to abnormalities in phosphate transport. Hypophosphataemic causes of osteomalacia are not usually associated with changes in serum calcium. For this reason, secondary hyperparathyroidism is not observed and the turnover of bone, and hence bone-cell numbers, and the activity of alkaline phosphatase are not markedly increased.

Plasma calcifediol is the most commonly used test that is useful for assessing nutritional status with respect to vitamin D. Assays for calcitriol aid in the precise diagnosis of patients with and without vitamin D-related osteomalacia.

Disorders of Calcitonin Secretion

Increased secretion of calcitonin occurs in medullary carcinoma of the thyroid, a familial and malignant disorder of the C-cells. This may be associated with other endocrine abnormalities such as phaeochromocytoma, Cushing's syndrome and hyperparathyroidism, the so-called multiple endocrine abnormality (MEA) syndrome. Medullary carcinoma may become evident clinically by the detection of a mass in the thyroid or be suspected from the family history or the presence of associated endocrinopathies. Severe diarrhoea may occur, which is probably related to the synthesis of prostaglandins or serotonin. The lack of apparent effect of excessive amounts of calcitonin itself is one of the reasons why the physiological role of calcitonin is uncertain. The diagnosis is established by the presence of high plasma levels of calcitonin and augmented responses to provocative tests of calcitonin secretion (e.g. pentagastrin and calcium infusion).

Few metabolic abnormalities appear to be associated with calcitonin deficiency. Thus, in athyroidal man given thyroid supplements, calcium metabolism is not markedly disturbed. Defective secretion of calcitonin has been implicated in the pathophysiology of hyperparathyroid bone disease in chronic renal disease, and it is possible that osteitis fibrosa in chronic renal failure is in part due to hyperparathyroidism and in part to deficient production of calcitonin.

Hypercalcaemia

Many of the causes of hypercalcaemia have been reviewed above and are summarized in Table 30.9. Of clinical importance is the ability of hypercalcaemia to alter renal function adversely. Not only may hypercalcaemia cause intrinsic renal damage due to the

TABLE 30.9
CAUSES OF HYPERCALCAEMIA

Common
Artefactual hyperproteinaemia due to venous stasis, hyper-
    albuminaemia (dehydration, i.v. nutrition), hypergamma-
    globulinaemia (myeloma, sarcoidosis)
Carcinoma with skeletal metastases (e.g. breast, lung)
Carcinoma without skeletal metastases (humoral hypercal-
    caemia of malignancy)
Haematological tumours (myeloma, lymphoma)
Primary hyperparathyroidism

Rare
'Tertiary' hyperparathyroidism—transplantation, chronic
    renal failure, malabsorption
Vitamin D toxicity
Vitamin D 'sensitivity' sarcoidosis, hypercalcaemia of
infancy, berylliosis, etc.
Immobility—Paget's disease
Milk alkali syndrome
Thyrotoxicosis
Thiazide diuretics
Adrenal failure
Phaeochromocytoma
Familial hypocalciuric hypercalcaemia
Haemodialysis—high dialysate calcium
Pseudohypercalcaemia

TABLE 30.10
CAUSES OF HYPOCALCAEMIA

Low plasma albumin or haemodilution
    malnutrition, liver disease, etc.
Vitamin D deficiency or resistance
Acute and chronic renal failure
Hypoparathyroidism and pseudohypoparathyroidism
Hypomagnesaemia
Acute pancreatitis
Drugs, e.g. calcitonin, phosphate, diphosphonates, citrate
Carcinoma, particularly of the prostate

intrarenal deposition of calcium phosphate, but it
also decreases the renal sensitivity to arginine vasopressin and may therefore result in profound dehydration. Because there is a link between the tubular
reabsorption of sodium and of calcium, dehydration
and salt depletion increase renal tubular reabsorption
of calcium. All these factors tend to aggravate
hypercalcaemia.

The hypercalcaemia associated with malignant disease is complex and arises by several mechanisms.
Most commonly this is due to the focal skeletal
destruction of bone associated with widespread metastases. Under such circumstances the secretion of
PTH is suppressed and the decreased renal tubular
reabsorption for calcium thereby induced has a sparing effect on hypercalcaemia. This may be one reason
why patients presenting with hypercalcaemia and skeletal metastases are usually far advanced in the course
of the disease. Certain humoral agents have been

associated with osteolytic bone disease due to malignant disorders. These include the PTHrP in the case
of solid tumours and the osteoclast-activating factors
in the case of myeloma.

The investigation of patients with hypercalcaemia
is usually straightforward, and the diagnosis is commonly reached by clinical assessment and simple biochemical investigations. The majority of patients can
be accurately diagnosed by a good history including
a full drug history and the simple measurement of
plasma calcium, phosphate, creatinine, and an estimate of tubular reabsorption for phosphate such as
Tm_p/GFR. Radiographs or bone scans are also most
helpful in detecting malignant disease or hyperparathyroid bone disease. The major difficulties arise in
those patients without overt skeletal disease and hypercalcaemia. Mention has been previously made of
the investigation of such cases. These investigations,
together with a search for sarcoidosis, myeloma or a
drug history, usually yield a diagnosis.

Hypocalcaemia

The more common causes of hypocalcaemia are
shown in Table 30.10. The investigation of hypoparathyroidism has been previously discussed, but it is
important to emphasize that the distinction between
hypoparathyroid and pseudohypoparathyroid states
is academic rather than of practical clinical interest
since the treatment is the same. The measurement of
plasma calcium, phosphate and creatinine, together
with a measurement of plasma albumin will distinguish most patients with hypoproteinaemia, vitamin
D deficiency, chronic renal failure, and the hypoparathyroid states.

Disorders of Bone Turnover

There are a number of disorders associated with
abnormal bone turnover. Several are inherited diseases such as osteogenesis imperfecta, hyperphosphatasia, fibrogenesis imperfecta ossium, various
epiphyseal, metaphyseal and diaphyseal dysplasias,
and neurofibromatosis. In most of these cases there
is no apparent systemic disturbance in calcium metabolism and they are beyond the scope of this
chapter.

Paget's Disease of Bone
In Paget's disease of bone there is enhanced resorption and formation of bone but the two processes
remain coupled so that there is no marked systemic
disturbance in calcium metabolism unless the balance
between resorption and formation is temporarily disturbed. This may occur during immobilization, when
hypercalciuria or hypercalcaemia can develop. There
is probably a true association between primary hyperparathyroidism and Paget's disease, and this should
be suspected in hypercalcaemic patients. Most of the
other complications of Paget's disease arise because

TABLE 30.11
SOME CAUSES OF OSTEOPOROSIS

Primary
Old age
Natural or surgical menopause
Idiopathic juvenile osteoporosis

Secondary
Dietary deficiency of calcium or malabsorption:
   steatorrhoea
   partial gastrectomy
   chronic liver disease
Endocrine:
   hyperparathyroidism
   hyperthyroidism
   Cushing's syndrome
   hypogonadism
Metabolic:
   vitamin C deficiency
   pregnancy
   osteogenesis imperfecta
Drugs:
   corticosteroids
   heparin
Immobilization
   generalized, e.g. space flight
   localized, e.g. after fracture, paraplegia
Rheumatoid arthritis
Chronic renal failure or dialysis

and the fractures that arise. They may occur at any site but the spine, wrist and hip are characteristic.

The most common cause for osteoporosis is that associated with the menopause. The mechanism of this bone loss has been previously described. The risk of fractures increases with age, and in the case of hip and vertebral fracture this increase is exponential. The incidence of fractured neck of femur is twice as high in women than in men, but because women live longer than men the prevalence is even greater.

There are no distinctive biochemical abnormalities found in osteoporosis that are useful in clinical investigation. For example, plasma calcium, phosphate and alkaline phosphatase are usually normal. Alkaline phosphatase may, however, rise for several months after fracture. Abnormalities in PTH secretion and in vitamin D-metabolite production have been described but are of no value in making the diagnosis of osteoporosis in individuals. The evaluation of patients includes the assessment of future fracture risk (e.g. bone-density measurements), the rate of bone loss, and any secondary causes. It is important to distinguish patients with senile osteoporosis from those with more treatable forms of the syndrome, particularly endocrine disorders such as Cushing's disease and hyperthyroidism (Table 30.11). Of particular importance is the association of osteomalacia with osteoporosis in the elderly population. The manifestations of osteomalacia are often subtle in the elderly but the clinical consequences are readily treated, unlike the osteoporosis itself.

the affected bone is structurally abnormal. Bones may be painful, increase in size, become highly vascular, and more liable to deformity and fracture.

The diagnosis is made by the characteristic radiographic findings and the biochemical indices of augmented bone turnover (plasma alkaline phosphatase, urinary hydroxyproline, etc.), without disturbances in plasma calcium or phosphate. Occasionally it may be difficult to distinguish monostotic Paget's disease from fibrous dysplasia or osteoblastic secondary deposits, when bone biopsy may be helpful.

Osteoporosis
Another important group of disorders of bone turnover include the osteoporoses. Osteoporosis is the diminution of bone mass, without detectable changes in the ratio of mineral to non-mineralized matrix. This distinguishes the condition from osteomalacia, where the proportion of osteoid to calcified bone is increased. A variety of disorders causes osteoporosis, including liver disease, various endocrinopathies and chronic renal failure (Table 30.11), but it is most commonly associated with ageing (senile and postmenopausal osteoporosis). The clinical significance of osteoporosis lies in the greater skeletal fragility

FURTHER READING

Avioli L.V., Krane S.M. eds. (1977). *Metabolic Bone Disease and Clinically Related Disorders*, 2nd edn, Philadelphia: Saunders/New York: Academic Press.

Heersche J., Kanis J.A. eds. (1991) *Bone and Mineral Research Annual*, vol. 7, Amsterdam: Elsevier.

Kanis J.A. eds. (1980). Etiology and medical management of hypercalcaemia. *Metab. Bone Dis. Related Res.* **2** (3).

Kanis J.A. (1991). *Pathophysiology and Treatment of Paget's Disease of Bone*, London: Dunitz.

Lawson D.E.M. ed. (1978). *Vitamin D*, New York: Academic Press.

Nordin B.E.C. ed. (1976). *Calcium, Phosphate and Magnesium Metabolism*, Edinburgh: Churchill Livingstone.

Norman A.W., Schaefer K., Grigoleit H.G., von Herrath D. eds. (1988). Vitamin D. In *Molecular Cellular and Clinical Endocrinology*, Berlin: De Gruyter.

Smith R. (1979). *Biochemical Disorders of the Skeleton*, London: Butterworths.

Smith R. ed. (1990). *Osteoporosis 1990*, London: Royal College of Physicians.

Vaughan J.M. (1981). *The Physiology of Bone*, Oxford University Press.

APPENDIX

TABLE 30.12

TYPICAL NORMAL ADULT RANGES FOR SOME SIMPLE BIOCHEMICAL MEASURE-
MENTS USED IN THE INVESTIGATION OF PATIENTS WITH DISORDERS OF CALCIUM
HOMEOSTASIS (M OR F DENOTES SEX)

Measurement	Units	Normal range
Plasma		
Total calcium	mmol/L	2.12–2.60
Ionized calcium	mmol/L	1.10–1.35
Fasting inorganic phosphate	mmol/L	0.6–1.5
Urine		
Calcium	mmol/24 h	M: 2.5–10
		F: 2.5–9.0
Phosphate	mmol/24 h	16–32
Total hydroxyproline	μmol/24 h	M: 55–250
		F: 75–430
Fasting urine		
Calcium/creatinine ratio	mmol/mmol	0.10–0.32
Calcium excretion	mmol/L GF	<0.04
Tm_P/GFR	mmol/L GF	0.8–1.35
Total hydroxyproline/creatinine	μmol/mmol	<40
Vitamin D metabolites		
25-OHD (calcifediol)	ng/mL	5–50
$1,25(OH)_2D_3$ (calcitriol)	pg/mL	20–40
$24,25(OH)_2D_3$ (secalciferol)	ng/mL	1–5

31. Rheumatoid arthritis and connective tissue diseases

A. L. Parke

Rheumatoid arthritis
  Introduction
  Pathology
  Laboratory tests
  Therapy
  Conclusion
Connective tissue diseases
  Introduction
  Pathology
  Laboratory tests
  Therapy
  Conclusion

RHEUMATOID ARTHRITIS

Introduction

Rheumatoid arthritis (RA) is a common disease, found worldwide. It is estimated to affect about 1–2% of the population (prevalence) in the temperate zones, with a female to male ratio of 3:1. The condition occurs in families, with 11% of probands having at least one affected first-degree relative.[1] A genetic predisposition is further emphasized by the association with HLA (class II)–DR4 that has been demonstrated in numerous studies,[2,3] and it has recently been suggested that adult RA could be reclassified according to the patient's HLA genotype as some studies have shown an association between the presence of certain HLA and disease severity.[4]

Environmental associations with this disease are not so well defined, and numerous bacterial and viral agents have been implicated as inciting agents. Chronic synovitis is a consequence of injecting bacterial products into rodents.[5,6] Recent work has demonstrated resistance to the induction of adjuvant arthritis by the prior administration of specific T-cell clones and mycobacterial heat-shock protein (HSP) 65.[7] This finding, as well as the demonstration of increased levels of antibodies to mycobacterial HSP 65 and 70 in patients with RA,[8] has renewed enthusiasm for the concept that microbes may play a part in the pathogenesis.

The association with a preceding bacterial infection *is* well established in Reiter's syndrome.[9] Recent studies showing subclinical inflammatory bowel disease in patients with 'reactive arthritis'[10] and the fact that arthritis is the most common extraintestinal manifestation of inflammatory bowel disease suggests that it may be a consequence of increased bowel permeability[11] and abnormal exposure to bacterial antigens.[12] Twenty-five per cent of patients who had gastrointestinal bypass operations in the 1970s for marked obesity developed an arthritis/dermatitis syndrome. They improved after being treated with antibiotics or after having their bypass operations reversed.[13,14]

The associations between preceding infection and classical RA are, however, not so well substantiated. The drug sulphasalazine was originally designed for use in RA, as this disease was considered to be a consequence of infection and sulphonamides were the only antibiotics available at that time. Sulphasalazine *has* been shown to benefit patients with RA as well as those with spondarthropathies, suggesting that an infectious aetiology in these diseases deserves serious consideration.

RA is a systemic disease. The most common extra-articular manifestation is anaemia, but patients may present with pathology in any organ (Table 31.1). The brunt of the disease is, however, in the diarthrodial joint, although some joints are comparatively spared (Fig. 31.1). The classical presentation is that of persistent arthritis (joint swelling) in a symmetrical pattern involving large and small joints. In typical disease the patient produces antibodies directed against autologous immunoglobulin (rheumatoid factor) and shows joint destruction with the erosion of juxta-articular cartilage and subchondral bone. These patients frequently have numerous extra-articular manifestations of their disease, and additional laboratory abnormalities including antinuclear anti-

TABLE 31.1
EXTRA-ARTICULAR MANIFESTATIONS OF RHEUMATOID
ARTHRITIS

Laboratory features
Anaemia (normochromic normocytic)
Thrombocytosis
Sometimes leucopenia ± thrombocytopenia associated
  with splenomegaly (Felty's syndrome)
Rheumatoid factor
Antinuclear antibody
Cryoglobulins

Clinical features
Weight loss
Subcutaneous nodules
Eye disease: scleritis; episcleritis
Pulmonary disease: nodules, fibrosis, pleural effusions
Cardiac disease: pericarditis
Splenomegaly
Hepatic inflammation
Nephritis (associated with vasculitis)
Neurological disease: nerve entrapment (i.e. carpal tunnel),
  mononeuritis multiplex (associated with vasculitis)
Vasculitis
Amyloidosis
Sjögren's syndrome
Recurrent sepsis

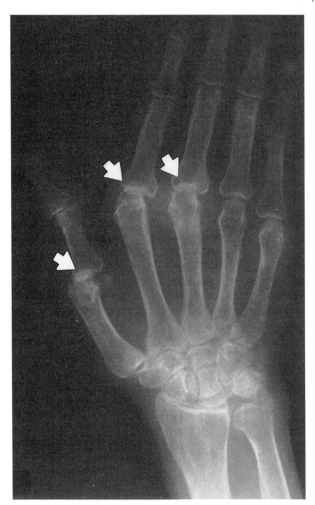

Figure 31.1 Radiograph of the hand showing preferential destruction of some joints, i.e. first, second and third metacarpal phalangeal joints (arrows) with comparative sparing of the fourth and fifth metacarpal phalangeal joints.

dous influx of PMNs. The consequences of this intra-articular production of oxygen radicals include the destruction of cartilage,[19] membrane damage and cell death.[20]

Nature of the Cellular Infiltrate

The cellular infiltrate in rheumatoid synovium is of mononuclear cells comprising macrophages, B cells and predominantly T-helper cells. Many of these intra-articular T cells are activated and there is evidence that this is due to local activation rather than the transport of activated T cells to a site of inflammation.[21] These activated T cells do contribute to the pathogenesis of RA,[22] but the inciting factors responsible for initiating this T-cell invasion and activation are as yet unknown. Studies designed to determine if specific clones of T cells are abundant in rheumatoid synovium have failed to reveal clonality.[23,24]

The B cells found in rheumatoid synovium respond to autologous immunoglobulin and collagen type II.[17,25] The local production of antibody is abundant, and results in the formation of intra-articular immune complexes and activation of complement. Some activated components of complement are chemotactic and a consequence of this is the massive infiltration of PMNs into the synovial fluid.

Mechanisms of Cartilage and Bone Destruction

The mechanisms resulting in the destruction of cartilage and bone in RA are not completely understood. Invasion by the proliferating synovium (pannus) in juxta-articular locations has been well demonstrated and it is in these sites that cartilage erosion is initially seen. The local production of numerous mediators of inflammation, cytokines, proteases, collagenases, antibodies and the formation of immune complexes with activation of complement, chemotaxis of PMNs and the generation of oxygen radicals all contribute to the articular damage.

Laboratory Tests

Diagnosis should not be made solely on the basis of laboratory tests. A competent history and physical examination are essential for determining the best laboratory tests to help confirm the diagnosis. It is apparent, however, that many patients presenting with bilateral, symmetrical, chronic polyarthritis have different diseases, although they may all fulfil criteria for RA.

Rheumatoid Factors

Rheumatoid factors (RhF) were first identified in the 1930s[26] and are now known to be antibodies directed primarily against the Fc portion of autologous or heterologous IgG. The basic tests for RhF involve coating particles or sheep red-blood cells with IgG antibody. RhF in the serum to be tested results in agglutination of the coated particles. The quantity of RhF is determined by serial dilutions of the serum to be tested, and the result is expressed as the highest

bodies and cryoglobulins. These classical patients carry a worse prognosis than others with RA who do not have these features.[15]

Pathology

Changes in the Synovium

Normal synovium is one to three cells thick and is fine and lacey (Fig. 31.2). In RA the synovium proliferates (Fig. 31.3), becomes infiltrated with monocytes and plasma cells,[16] and is the site of local antibody production.[17] Rheumatoid synovium is comparatively avascular and it has been suggested that the comparative hypoxia of this proliferating tissue may result in depletion of ATP, calcium imbalance, impaired mitochondrial function and the generation of free oxygen radicals.[18] Oxygen radicals are also a product of polymorphonuclear leucocytes (PMNs), and in the rheumatoid synovial fluid there is a tremen-

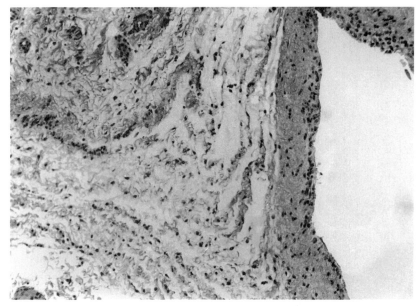

Figure 31.2 Normal synovium, which is thin, lacy and usually 1–3 cells thick.

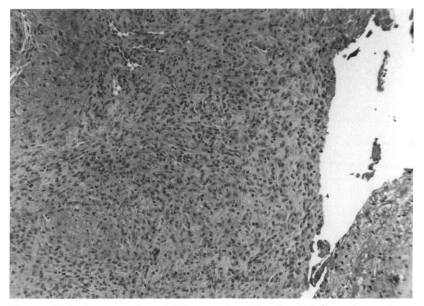

Figure 31.3 Intense cellular infiltrate and proliferation in inflamed synovium.

dilution of serum still capable of producing agglutination. These agglutination tests primarily detect 19*s* IgM RhF and may miss RhFs belonging to other immunoglobulin classes. Radioimmunoassays and enzyme-linked immunosorbent (ELISA) assays can detect IgM, IgG and IgA RhFs.

False-negative results can sometimes be produced by the failure of IgM RhF to dissociate from its autologous IgG antigen. These 'hidden' RhFs can be detected by a variety of procedures designed to dissociate the RhF from its autologous antigen.[27] The presence of RhF is not specific for RA and absence of RhF does not rule out RA as a diagnosis.

Haemotological Abnormalities

Normochromic normocytic anaemia is the most common extra-articular manifestation of RA. The precise mechanism of this anaemia is not known. These patients are not iron deficient and bone marrow studies have shown adequate iron stores. Giving iron to rheumatoid patients has been reported to be associated with a flare of synovitis in some cases.[28] An inability to utilize iron appropriately seems to be a consequence of this inflammatory disease and controlling the inflammation results in an improvement in the anaemia. True iron deficiency, however, can occur in some patients, particularly

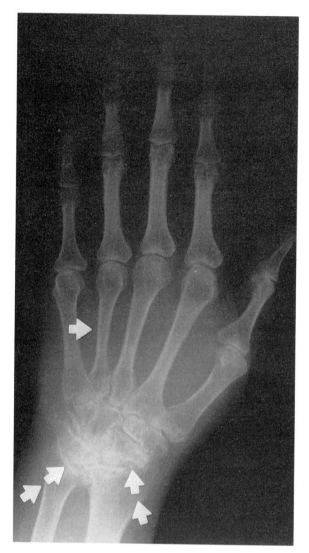

Figure 31.4 Radiograph of the hand showing preferential destruction of the carpal joints (double arrows) with sparing of other joints in the hand, i.e. the metacarpal phalangeal joints (compare with Fig. 31.1). The film also shows abnormal development of the metacarpal bones with thin tapering shafts (single arrow) and bulbous heads. These changes in the metacarpals show that the onset of disease was in childhood. This patient is a full-time medical secretary, a mother and a wife. She has had rheumatoid arthritis since the age of 2 years.

those treated with non-steroidal anti-inflammatory drugs as gastrointestinal bleeding is a common side-effect of these.

Patients with RA may have very high platelet counts. Less commonly, thrombocytopenia may be found and this may be accompanied by leucopenia and splenomegaly (Felty's syndrome). Leucopenia, of course, predisposes to infection, but even rheumatoid patients with normal white-cell counts may have impaired leucocyte function.[29] Infection is a real hazard because seeding to arthritic and prosthetic joints may occur.

Synovial Fluid

Normal synovial fluid is golden and viscous like egg white. In inflammatory disease the viscosity is reduced and the cellular content increased, replacing the golden colour with an opaque white fluid that may ultimately appear to be frank pus. Simple bedside procedures can be done to determine if the joint fluid is inflammatory. Colour and clarity give some indication of cellular content. Viscosity can be assessed by the 'string' sign where a drop of synovial fluid is dropped from the syringe into the sink, and the 'string' between the drop and the syringe measured. A normal 'string' should be close to 10 cm; a reduction in the content of hyaluronate in inflammatory fluids reduces the length of the string produced. Synovial fluid should also be examined for:

- cells (number and type present),
- crystals,
- biochemical factors (including glucose),
- complement.

The most important tests of joint fluid are, however, Gram stain and culture. It is absolutely vital to ensure that a joint is not infected as some bacterial infections can destroy cartilage within a matter of hours. This is particularly important when assessing the rheumatoid patient who has one joint that is worse than all the rest, or who states that this is 'the worst joint pain they have ever had'. This is an infected joint until proved otherwise.

Radiographic Changes

Radiological studies are essential for assessing extent of disease, progression and response. Radiographic examination must be included in the evaluation of a new patient and should include views of both hands and wrists and both feet, with oblique or 'ball catcher' views to show the metatarsal and metacarpal heads more clearly, as these often show the earliest erosive changes.

Some children presenting with chronic polyarthritis do not produce RhF, and their pattern of joint destruction is different from that seen with more classical RA (Fig. 31.4). The reason for this selective joint destruction is not understood, and it has been suggested that different patterns of joint destruction may even be seen in adults, depending on whether or not they produce RhF, although it appears that there are numerous exceptions to this. However, even patients with the most aggressive, classical RA are spared the distal interphalangeal (DIP) joints and often the fourth metacarpal phalangeal (MCP) joint on each hand (*see Fig. 31.1*).

Early radiographic changes include soft-tissue swelling and juxta-articular osteoporosis. Serial studies (at least annually) are useful in assessing progression of the disease. Aggressive therapy should be initiated early with the hope of delaying erosive changes.

Other necessary radiographs include a chest X-ray as both RA and many of its therapies can cause

TABLE 31.2
DRUG THERAPY IN RHEUMATOID ARTHRITIS

First line
Low-dose aspirin or simple analgesics
High-dose aspirin or non-steroidal anti-inflammatory
  drugs
Cyclo-oxygenase inhibitors
Leucotriene inhibitors

Second line
Hydroxychloroquine
'Disease-remittive agents', i.e.:
  Injectable gold
  Oral gold
  Methotrexate
  Sulphasalazine
  Combination therapy, i.e. hydroxychloroquine
    (combined with gold or methotrexate when these start
    to fail)
  Low-dose steroids

Third line
Immunosuppressive or cytotoxics:
  Azathioprine
  Pulse i.v. cyclophosphamide
  p.o. Cyclophosphamide
  Chlorambucil
  Cyclosporin A
High-dose steroids (pulse i.v. 1–3 g)

pulmonary problems. It is therefore essential that a chest X-ray is taken before starting treatment. Annual flexion and extension views of the cervical spine must be done to assess instability at the atlanto-axial joint and the patient must be educated about the cervical instability, even if surgery is not indicated. Failure to be aware of this problem can result in devastating spinal-cord compression.

Therapy

Table 31.2 lists the therapies currently used in RA. The term 'disease-remittive agents' is a misnomer: the disease will progress and is life-long. Whether it would progress at the same rate with or without treatment is difficult to determine. Clinically there is no doubt that the quality of life is improved by therapy; however, long-term studies show a dismal picture,[30,31] but many included patients with the most severe disease. Recent new ideas about therapy include the development of immunotherapy directed specifically at T-cell infiltrates[32] and the bombardment with multiple toxic therapies similar to the regimens used to control cancer.[33,34] Both of these ideas are distasteful, especially when it is apparent that rheumatologists are second only to oncologists in producing significant iatrogenic disease.

Conclusion

RA is a chronic life-long inflammatory disease that results in increasing disability and morbidity. Current therapies are inadequate and toxic, and our efforts should be directed towards obtaining a better understanding of the factors that appear to 'cure' or prevent RA. Some of these factors include jaundice, exogenous oestrogens[35,36] and pregnancy.[37] Exactly how these pathological and physiological states improve the clinical expression of RA is unknown.

CONNECTIVE TISSUE DISEASES

Introduction

These diseases are a consequence of a systemic inflammation in blood vessels that results in multiple end-organ damage. In systemic lupus erythematosus (SLE) the presence of non-organ-specific autoantibodies results in the formation of circulating immune complexes, activation of complement and inflammatory vessel-wall damage. The lack of control that permits the production of these autoantibodies in SLE is not well understood, but certain factors that influence their production are known and these include female sex,[38] age,[39] exposure to chemicals,[40] and certain HLA associations.[41]

Our understanding of the pathogenesis of these connective tissue diseases is minimal. This section will include three concepts relevant to the current understanding of the pathogenesis of autoimmune rheumatological disease:

1. the role of xenobiotic agents;
2. specific autoantibodies associated with distinct clinical syndromes;
3. subclinical autoimmune disease.

Xenobiotic Agents and Autoimmune Disease

The original dictum that drug-induced and idiopathic SLE are different diseases must now be questioned. Admittedly, there are some differences between them, including the nature of the autoantibodies produced; these are usually distinct, with histone antibodies being a feature of drug-induced disease[42] and antibodies to native double-stranded DNA (dsDNA) a feature of idiopathic disease.[43] Histone antibodies may also be found in idiopathic disease but antibodies to native dsDNA are very rare in drug-induced disease. It has been suggested that the different antibodies produced are responsible for the different clinical expressions, as renal disease is uncommon in drug-induced SLE.

Drug metabolism plays a large part in the development of xenobiotic-induced autoimmune disease. Slow acetylators are more likely to develop drug-induced SLE if they are exposed to hydralazine or procainamide and patients treated with *N*-acetylated procainamide develop antinuclear antibodies less frequently than those treated with the parent compound.[44]

The cytochromes P_{450} are a family of haemoproteins that are located in the endoplasmic reticulum of a variety of tissues and are concerned with the oxygenation of numerous endogenous and exogenous substrates. These enzymes play a vital part in the detoxification of exogenous agents and metabolism by certain members of this family (i.e. P_{4501} or P_{45011E}) can result in the formation of reactive intermediates that damage proteins, enzymes and DNA.[45,46] This damage can lead to mutations, malignancy, the production of neoantigens, and eventually cell damage and death.[20] Recent studies have demonstrated the presence of antibodies to various members of the cytochrome P_{450} family, and have suggested that these antibodies, by interfering with the normal function of the P_{450} cytochromes, may lead to aberrant drug metabolism resulting in drug-induced disease.[47,48]

The concept that removal of the offending chemical abrogates autoimmune disease is wrong. This has been clearly demonstrated by patients with the toxic oil syndrome,[49] and most recently, by those with the L-tryptophan-associated eosinophilia–myalgia syndrome,[50] although the exact pathogenesis of this syndrome remains unclear. A better understanding of the inciting factors that precipitate flares of SLE may show that a variety of xenobiotic agents has this potential. Sulphonamides[51] and exogenous oestrogens[52] precipitate flares of SLE in susceptible patients with idiopathic disease, demonstrating the susceptibility of so-called idiopathic disease to environment influences.

Exposure to silica, polyvinyl chloride or organic solvents may lead to the development of scleroderma or its associated syndromes, and the majority of these patients do not improve clinically when the inciting chemical is removed. Only a small proportion of people exposed to these chemicals develop disease. Recent studies have shown that patients with scleroderma do metabolize certain drugs differently, suggesting that this aberrant metabolism may contribute to the development of the disease.[53]

Autoantibodies and Specific Clinical Syndromes
The correlation of disease expression with specific autoantibody production is not a new concept. In this subsection, three syndromes will be described that have been defined by the presence of specific autoantibodies and a specific group of clinical complaints. Additional clinical and laboratory associations are defined in the section below on Laboratory Tests.

1. Mixed Connective Tissue Disease and Overlap Syndromes. In the 1970s, mixed connective tissue disease (MCTD) was defined as a separate entity based on the presence of antibodies to ribonucleoprotein (RNP).[54] It was suggested at the time that patients with MCTD should be categorized separately because:

(i) they did not develop renal disease, and therefore had a better prognosis;

(ii) they reportedly responded more dramatically to corticosteroids than patients with diffuse scleroderma.

MCTD has since declared itself to be a non-entity, and patients with this RNP antibody may express complaints compatible with dermatomyositis, scleroderma or SLE.

Some patients do not fulfil established criteria for specific diseases, and we prefer to call these examples of 'overlap syndrome'. Some of these patients are eventually found to have SLE or scleroderma, whereas others remain ill defined. Nonsense terms such as 'rupus' or 'lupatoid' have been coined for those patients with features suggestive of both RA and SLE, a testament to our lack of knowledge.

2. Phospholipid Antibody Syndrome. The (anti-) phospholipid (APL) antibody syndrome defines a group of clinical complaints associated with antibodies to negatively charged phospholipids. These antibodies are measured by three tests:

(i) the lupus anticoagulant test;
(ii) a biologically false-positive test for syphilis (VDRL);
(iii) cardiolipin antibodies, usually measured by ELISA.

The clinical syndrome associated with the presence of these antibodies has various features; most are considered to be a consequence of a thrombotic diathesis.[55,56] This diathesis may be expressed in both the arterial and venous systems, and there may be recurrent thromboses in a variety of vessels, including the cerebral vasculature. The components of the syndrome continue to expand and recent clinical associations have included the presence of mitral valve disease, Addison's disease and pulmonary hypertension.[57,58]

Patients with APLs also complain of fetal wastage.[59] It has been suggested that this is due to placental insufficiency, a consequence of thrombosis in the placental bed. Women who complain of habitual abortion (three fetal losses) do have an increased prevalence of APLs. Our recent studies have demonstrated that habitual aborters are more likely to have a biologically false-positive VDRL or IgG cardiolipin antibodies when compared with two control groups, normal mothers and women who have never been pregnant.[60] Women with habitual abortion and APL experience less fetal wastage if they are treated with anticoagulants, and/or other agents with the potential for lowering the levels of these antibodies. However, there is no good randomized controlled study; optimal therapy for these patients will not be defined until there is.

How APLs predispose patients to thrombosis or fetal wastage is not well understood. Recent evidence has suggested that abnormalities of the natural anticoagulants protein C and protein S may be associated with APLs.[61,62] Other theories are that APLs interfere with production of prostacyclin,[63] but attempts to demonstrate that they are endothelial antibodies have failed.

Some patients with APLs do not meet criteria for well-defined connective tissue diseases (such as SLE). However, they may have close family members who *do* fulfil criteria for SLE,[64] and this is not surprising as a biologically false-positive VDRL is one of the revised American Rheumatism Association criteria for SLE. This familial relationship emphasizes the close association between SLE and the APL syndrome.

Some patients with APLs (complaining primarily of habitual abortion) may be clinically healthy and yet have numerous laboratory markers for underlying autoimmune disease, including:

- antinuclear antibodies,
- antibodies to native dsDNA (Farr test),
- complement abnormalities,
- a positive Coombs' test,
- thrombocytopenia.

This has led to the concept of 'subclinical' autoimmune disease and our own experience is that follow-up of some of these 'subclinical' patients (for up to 6 years) failed to show any progression to overt clinical disease.

3. The Neonatal Lupus Syndrome. This syndrome may occur in infants born to mothers who have circulating autoantibodies predominantly directed against the Ro and La nuclear particles. The neonatal lupus (NNL) syndrome is most commonly identified by the presence of

(i) a transient photosensitive rash,
(ii) primary congenital complete heart block,[65,66]

although most affected infants do not have both of these features. Other children are less fortunate as associated features of this syndrome include the presence of myocarditis, aseptic meningitis and hepatitis.[67]

The mothers of these infants are usually clinically healthy; however, they do have autoantibodies,[66,68] and these contribute to the pathogenesis of this syndrome, although exactly how is not understood. The photosensitive rash disappears at approximately 6 months of age, and this is about the time that maternal antibody would be completely cleared from the fetal system. Unfortunately, the primary congenital complete heart block is a permanent feature, and approximately 50% of affected children will require permanent pacemakers.[67]

Certain unknown fetal determinants predict infants at risk. Mothers have been described that have had one or more affected children with normal pregnancies intervening between these affected children.[69] Fraternal twins have been born to a mother with these antibodies where one twin was affected by the syndrome and the other perfectly healthy.[70] The

nature of the fetal factors that determine disease expression is unclear.

Long-term follow-up of these clinically healthy mothers has shown that some ultimately develop a connective tissue disease, most frequently Sjögren's syndrome.[71] The abnormal pregnancy is frequently the first sign of underlying autoimmunity and may predate any overt clinical complaints by years.

Subclinical Autoimmune Disease
The APL syndrome and the NNL syndrome have both shown that the effects of autoimmunity may be expressed by clinically healthy mother's years before the individual develops clinical complaints. These syndromes have broadened our knowledge of autoimmune disease and demonstrate the limitations of criteria for defining diseases.

Pathology

Vasculitis
Vasculitis is most easily classified by identifying:

(i) the size of the vessels involved;
(ii) the nature of the histopathological changes (i.e. the presence or absence of granulomas);
(iii) deposition of immunoglobulin and/or complement at the pathological site.

SLE most frequently affects small and medium-sized vessels; less frequently large vessels may be involved. Characteristically, immunoglobulin and/or complement are deposited at the site of injury (Fig. 31.5).

The Role of Complement
The complement system is a cascade of serum proteins that interact to result in the lysis and destruction of invading organisms. Complement deficiency, therefore, results in an abnormal susceptibility to infections. Complement activation also promotes inflammation and assists in the removal of circulating immune complexes. Factors that interfere with the removal of these complexes can be expected to promote the development of immune complex-mediated disease, and congenital complement deficiency, especially of the early components of complement (C2), is associated with an increased prevalence of autoimmune diseases, particularly SLE.[72] A deficiency of one or more components of the complement cascade can be detected by a CH50 test.[73] This functional test uses antibody-coated sheep red-blood cells as targets, with their lysis being an end-point of the test, and a consequence of the complement proteins present in the test serum.

The fourth component of complement has two isotypes, C4A and C4B. C4A is particularly good at binding and precipitating immune complexes,[74] and C4A deficiency confers an increased risk for SLE.[75,76] Deficiencies of complement receptors also promote the development of these diseases. CR_1 is a receptor predominantly found on erythrocytes that

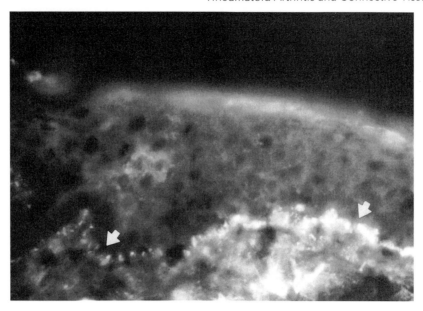

Figure 31.5 Immunofluorescence micrograph of a section from a skin biopsy with the epidermis at the top and the dermis at the bottom. The arrows show linear immunofluorescence at the dermal–epidermal junction, signifying the deposition of complement and/or immunoglobulin there, which is a characteristic finding in patients with systemic lupus erythematosus, who frequently present with a rash.

binds C3b, C4b and immune complexes. Numerous studies have demonstrated a deficiency of the CR_1 receptor in patients with SLE.[77,78]

Activation of complement both via the classical and alternate pathways occurs as part of the pathological process of SLE; the deposition of complement and immunoglobulin at the site of disease is one of its hallmarks. Such deposition may even be found in normal tissues;[79] however, the lytic and chemotactic properties of the turned-on complement system frequently result in tissue damage, leading to ischaemia and eventually necrosis (Fig. 31.6).

The activation of complement results in a fall of the serum levels of certain components of the complement system, in particular C3 and C4.[80] This fall may precede the development of clinical disease and can be used to predict flares of disease.[80-82] More recently, increased levels of activated components of complement have been found to be valuable markers of disease activity.[83,84]

Laboratory Tests

Non-organ-specific Autoantibodies
1. Antinuclear Antibodies. Antinuclear antibodies (ANAs) are the hallmark of SLE, although this test is not specific for SLE as there are numerous nuclear antigens. The most widely used screening test for ANAs is the indirect immunofluorescent (FANA) test using cellular substrate (most frequently mouse liver cells or HEp2 cells) and a fluorescein-labelled antibody to human gammaglobulin. This test is sensitive, but not specific.

Newer, more specific tests have been developed that have allowed the identification of antibodies to specific nuclear constituents, and this in turn has led to the recognition of certain patterns of immunofluoresence that indicate the presence of antibodies to specific nuclear constituents. These specific patterns include the centromere and the peripheral or 'rim' pattern. The rim pattern appears with immunofluorescence around the edge of the nucleus. This is associated with antibodies to native dsDNA and is found in patients with SLE.[85] Other, less specific patterns of fluorescent nuclear antibody (i.e. diffuse, homogeneous or speckled patterns) may be associated with numerous antibodies to different nuclear antigens, and may be found in a variety of different diseases.[86,87]

Antibodies to native dsDNA in SLE are associated with the development of renal disease.[88] These antibodies are measured by a variety of tests. The Farr test is a radioimmunoassay using labelled native dsDNA. The result is expressed as a percentage of the DNA bound by the test serum. The Crithidia test uses a flagellated organism with an organelle that contains native dsDNA.[89] This test is very specific. The Farr and the newer ELISA tests are dependent on the purity of the DNA used.

Antibodies to centromere are predominantly found in patients with CREST (**C**alcinosis, **R**aynaud's phenomenon, **E**sophageal abnormalities, **S**clerodactaly, and **T**elangectasia) syndrome.[90,91] This syndrome is a variant of scleroderma, and CREST patients classically do not develop proximal scleroderma or renal disease but may develop pulmonary hypertension.

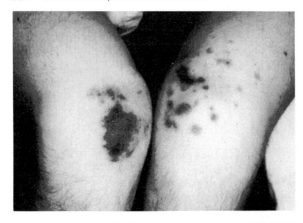

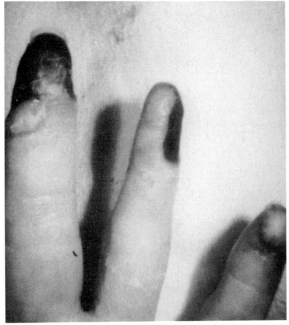

Figure 31.6 Necrosis of: (a) the skin over the knees and (b) the fingers, occurring secondarily to vasculitis.

Patients with true systemic sclerosis (scleroderma) are more likely to have antibody to Scl-70 (topoisomerase I).[92] Our laboratory experience is that patients rarely have both centromere and Scl-70 antibodies, and that presence of these antibodies is a good predictor for the pattern and extent of disease that can be expected in patients complaining of Raynaud's phenomenon.[93]

The Smith (Sm), Ro, La and RNP (ribonucleoprotein) antigens are components of extractable nuclear antigen (ENA). Antibodies to Sm antigen are most commonly found in SLE.[94] Antibodies to RNP are a requirement for the diagnosis of MCTD.[54] Antibodies to the Ro and La RNP complex are found in numerous diseases including SLE, Sjögren's syndrome, and RA. The Ro particle consists of a 60- and a 52-kDa polypeptide, and each of these fractions is associated with four RNA species.[95] The 48-kDa La polypeptide is a transcription factor, and probably

a cofactor for RNA polymerase.[96] Antibodies to the La polypeptide are usually found in patients with Ro antibodies and rarely occur alone. Antibodies to Ro and La particles are those most commonly associated with the NNL syndrome.[65,68]

A variety of the immunological techniques has been developed to detect antibodies. Some of the techniques are more sensitive (i.e. ELISA and Western blotting) than others (i.e. immunodiffusion or counter-immunoelectrophoresis (CIE). Most have been applied to detecting nuclear antibodies and the prevalence of these antibodies in specific diseases and in a normal population is obviously dependent on the sensitivity of the test used.

2. Phospholipid Antibodies. This is a family of antibodies that can be detected by a variety of tests including:

(i) a lupus anticoagulant test,
(ii) biologically false-positive test for syphilis (VDRL),
(iii) a cardiolipin assay.

(*a*) *Lupus Anticoagulant.* There are numerous tests for detecting the presence of lupus anticoagulants (LAC). A LAC results in a prolongation of the normal coagulation tests, most frequently the partial thromboplastin test. This prolongation is not corrected by adding equal volumes of normal, platelet-poor plasma, but can be shortened by the addition of lysed platelets,[97] a source of phospholipid. LACs are antibodies directed to the prothrombin activator complex, which consists of activated clotting factor Xa, factor V, calcium and phospholipid. Although the presence of these antibodies appears to prolong the normal coagulation tests, they are, in fact, associated with a thrombotic diathesis rather than haemorrhage.[55,56] The Russell viper venom test and the kaolin clotting time are the most sensitive tests for LACs.[98,99]

(*b*) *The VDRL Test.* This is a flocculation test using an alcohol-soluble lipid obtained from bovine heart. The lipid contains phospholipid, in addition to lecithin and cholesterol. Originally designed for the detection of antibody (reagin) in syphilitics, it was soon realized that some patients produced a falsely positive reaction. A biologically false-positive reaction (BFP) can now be determined by a positive VDRL test and a negative fluorescent treponemal antibody test. Some patients with BFP eventually developed SLE, and the clinical expression of the SLE sometimes occurs years after the BFP reaction had first been noted.[100,101]

(*c*) *Cardiolipin Test.* Cardiolipin assays were designed in an attempt to be more specific in detecting antibody to phospholipid (phosphatidyl diglycerol). We use an ELISA to detect cardiolipin antibodies, an assay that has only recently been standardized.[102] Lack of standardization and recent claims for the requirement of a cofactor[103,104] have caused innumerable problems, which have contributed to some of the confusion that surrounds this syndrome.

3. Other Antibodies. Antibodies to a whole variety of cellular organelles have been described. An association between antibodies to neutrophilic cytoplasm (ANCA) and Wegener's granulomatosis has now been identified.[104,105] Wegener's granulomatosis is a large-vessel vasculitis characterized by the presence of granulomas, and unlike SLE, this disease does not result in the consumption of complement. It has been suggested that ANCA levels can be used to monitor flares and to assess response to treatment.[106] If this proves to be true, the ANCA test will be a useful marker for monitoring this very serious and frequently fatal disease.

Haematological Abnormalities
Antibodies directed at various blood-cell components can result in a variety of haematological abnormalities—haemolytic anaemia (Coombs' test),[107] thrombocytopenia and neutropenia. Antibodies directed at haematopoietic stem cells may result in aplasia of all or any of these components.

Clotting abnormalities may also be found, including elevated levels of fibrinopeptide A.[108] LAC, VDRL, and cardiolipin assays should be done on all new patients as a normal prothrombin and partial thromboplastin time do not rule out the presence of LAC. Because these phospholipid antibodies are a 'family',[109] patients may have various combinations of antibody present.

Markers of Disease Activity
As mentioned above, some laboratory markers may preceded clinical signs of disease activity. A fall in serum complement levels (especially C3 or C4) or a rise in the levels of activated components of complement may herald a flare of disease.

A rise in the level of antibody to native DNA (Farr test) and a change in the pattern of immunofluorescence to a rim or peripheral ANA pattern are ominous signs.

An active urine sediment with urinary cells or casts may indicate the need for a renal biopsy. Proteinuria can be chronic and a long-term consequence of previous glomerulonephritis. The haematological markers mentioned in the previous section all signify disease activity. Lymphopenia is also found in active disease and is probably a consequence of T-cell antibodies.[110]

Markers of End-Organ Damage
The major causes of mortality in SLE are renal and central nervous pathology. Recurrent, immunologically mediated inflammation in these tissues results in permanent damage, and staging of renal lesions now includes not only the presence of acute active lesions, but also of scarring and loss of glomeruli.[111]

Persistent proteinuria and rising serum creatinine signify permanent renal damage. These patients can expect to develop renal failure, although the progression to renal insufficiency varies tremendously. Lupus patients are candidates for renal transplantation; the disease does not recur in the transplanted kidney[112] and very frequently, when the patient is in renal failure, becomes dormant. Neurological involvement, both peripheral and central, may result in permanent damage. The newer imaging techniques are currently being evaluated for use in SLE as it is really quite difficult to find a lupus patient with a normal cerebral magnetic-resonance image.

Therapy
The art of managing SLE lies in the fact that each patient must be treated differently. Frequently the patient knows that the disease is active long before there are any obvious clinical signs, and even non-specific complaints such as fatigue or aches, without true arthritis, may be markers of disease activity. When SLE patients flare they often manifest their disease in the same way; therefore the patient who has previously had renal disease may expect to develop renal disease with subsequent SLE activity if they are not treated promptly. A change in ANA pattern to a rim pattern, a rise in antibodies to native dsDNA and a fall in complement levels indicate that an immediate increase of therapy is necessary, especially in patients who have had previous major organ involvement.

Corticosteroids remain the mainstay of treatment for the lupus patient; we rarely use non-steroidal therapy because of potential renal toxicity. Antimalarial drugs with the 4-aminoquinoline radicals have been shown to be beneficial in lupus patients with arthritis and cutaneous disease, and these drugs can be used as steroid-sparing agents. It has also been shown that discontinuing antimalarial therapy can precipitate a flare of disease,[113] and therefore we frequently continue to use antimalarials (i.e. chloroquine or hydroxychloroquine) in lupus patients who have become pregnant unexpectedly.[114]

The aim is to manage the patient with the smallest amount of corticosteroid possible. Patients taking corticosteroids only once a day will get fewer side-effects, but frequently patients require massive doses of these drugs, and the long-term consequences of corticosteroids are almost as bad as the disease itself. The patient requiring high doses of corticosteroids may need immunosuppressive therapy (i.e. azathioprine or cyclophosphamide) as steroid-sparing agents. Cyclophosphamide used intermittently as an intravenous bolus every 3–4 weeks is preferable to daily therapy, especially in young women, as not only is there a potential for neoplastic change (particularly in the bladder),[115] but cyclophosphamide therapy can lead to premature ovarian failure.[116]

Recent work has suggested that methotrexate may be beneficial in managing this disease,[117,118] and methotrexate has *not* been shown to be a neoplastic agent in man. Methotrexate, therefore, would seem to be a better therapy for young SLE patients than long-term azathioprine or cyclophosphamide.

Conclusion

Several important questions relevant to this group of diseases include:

1. What is the basic deficit in the control of B-cell reactivity that leads to autoantibody production?
2. What are the factors that determine the pathological potential of antibodies? Ability to bind complement,[119,120] and ionic charge[121] are known to be important predictors of pathogenicity, but are far from the whole story.
3. Do specific antibodies dictate a set of specific clinical complaints, and if so, are these antibodies directly responsible for the pathological consequences observed?
4. What is the role of oestrogens? The female:male ratio for SLE is 9:1. Studies have shown that lupus patients metabolize oestrogens abnormally[122,123] and the incidence of SLE is increased in patients with Klinefelter syndrome.[124]
5. What is the role of xenobiotic agents in the development of autoimmunity?[125]
6. How can we treat these diseases without producing iatrogenic disease?

The SLE of the 1990s is a far cry from the devastating, frequently fatal disease of earlier decades. Subclinical disease is real, and long-term follow-up of these subclinical patients will allow the observation of a disease in evolution. We hope that time will provide a better understanding of the factors that influence the development of these diseases and some answers to the questions posed above.

REFERENCES

1. Wolfe F., Klainheksel S.M., Khan M.A. (1988). Prevalence of familial occurrence in patients with rheumatoid arthritis. *Br. J. Rheumatol.*, **27** (suppl. 11), 150.
2. Martell R.W., Du Toit E.D., Kalla A.A., Myeres O.L. (1989). Association of rheumatoid arthritis with HLA in three South African populations—whites, blacks and a population of mixed ancestry. *S. Afr. Med. J.*, **76**, 189.
3. Jajic Z., Jajic J. (1988). Antigens of HLA-DR locus in rheumatoid arthritis. *Br. J. Rheumatol.*, 27 (suppl.), 139.
4. Buchanan W.W., Singal D.P. (1990). Is there a need to reclassify adult rheumatoid arthritis? *Br. J. Rheumatol.*, **29**, 377.
5. Pearson C.M. (1964). Experimental models in rheumatoid disease. *Arthritis Rheum.*, **7**, 80.
6. Cromartie W.J. et al. (1977). Arthritis in rats after systemic injection of streptococcal cells or cell walls. *J. Exp. Med.*, **146**, 1585.
7. van den Broek M.F. et al. (1989). Protection against streptococcal cell wall-induced arthritis by pretreatment with the 65-kD mycobacterial heat shock protein. *J. Exp. Med.*, **170**, 449.
8. Tsoulfa G. et al. (1989). Raised serum IgG and IgA antibodies in mycobacterial antigens in rheumatoid arthritis. *Ann. Rheum. Dis.*, **48**, 118.
9. Reiter H. (1916). Uber eien bisher unerkannte Spirochaetenin-fektion (spirochaetosis arthritica). *Dtsch. Med. Wochenschr.*, **42**, 1535.
10. Mielants H., Veys E.M., Cuvelier C., De Vos M. (1989). Subclinical involvement of the gut in undifferentiated spondylarthropathies. *Clin. Exp. Rheumatol.*, **7**, 499.
11. Rooney P.J., Jenkins R.T., Buchanan W.W. (1990). A short review of the relationship between intestinal permeability and inflammatory joint disease. *Clin. Exp. Rheumatol.*, **8**, 75.
12. Granfors K. et al. (1989). Yersinia antigens in synovial-fluid cells from patients with reactive arthritis. *N. Engl. J. Med.*, **320**, 216.
13. Stein H.B. et al. (1981). The intestinal bypass arthritis-dermatitis syndrome. *Arthritis Rheum.*, **24**, 684.
14. Leff R.D., Aldo-Benson M.A., Madura J.A. (1983). The effect of revision of the intestinal bypass on post intestinal bypass arthritis. *Arthritis Rheum.*, **26**, 678.
15. Erhardt C.C., Mumford P.A. Venables P.J.W., Maini R.N. (1989). Factors predicting a poor life prognosis in rheumatoid arthritis: an eight year prospective study. *Ann. Rheum. Dis.*, **48**, 7.
16. Ishikawa H., Ziff M. (1976). Electron microscopic observations of immunoreactive cells in the rheumatoid synovial membrane. *Arthritis Rheum.*, **19**, 1.
17. Natvig J.B., Munthe E. (1975). Self associating IgG rheumatoid factor represents a major response of plasma cells in rheumatoid inflammatory tissue. *Ann. NY Acad. Sci.*, **256**, 88.
18. Stevens C.R., Williams R.B., Farrell A.J., Blake D.R. (1991). Hypoxia and inflammatory synovitis: observations and speculation. *Ann. Rheum. Dis.*, **50**, 124.
19. Burkhardt H. et al. (1986). Oxygen radicals as effectors of cartilage destruction. *Arthritis Rheum.*, **29**, 379.
20. Cross C.E. et al. (1987). Oxygen-radicals and human disease. *Ann. Int. Med.*, **107**, 526.
21. Burmester G.R. et al. (1984). Activated T-cells *in vivo* and *in vitro*: divergence in expression of Tac and Ia antigens in the non-blastoid small T-cells of inflammation and normal T-cells activated *in vitro*. *J. Immunol.*, **133**, 1230.
22. Maini R.N. (1989). Exploring immune pathways in rheumatoid arthritis. *Br. J. Rheumatol.*, **28**, 466.
23. Savill C.M. et al. (1987). A minority of patients with rheumatoid arthritis show a dominant rearrangement of T-cell receptor beta chain genes in synovial lymphocytes. *Scand. J. Immunol.*, **25**, 629.
24. Brennan F.M. et al. (1988). Heterogeneity of T cell receptor idiotypes in rheumatoid arthritis. *Clin. Exp. Immunol.*, **73**, 417.
25. Tarkowski A. et al. (1989). Secretion of antibodies to types I and II collagen by synovial tissue cells in patients with rheumatoid arthritis. *Arthritis Rheum.*, **32**, 1087.

26. Waaler E. (1940). On the occurrence of a factor in human serum activating the specific agglutination of sheep blood corpuscles. *Acta Pathol. Microbiol. Scand.*, **17**, 172.

27. Allen J.C., Kunkel H.G. (1966). Hidden rheumatoid factors with specificity for native globulins. *Arthritis Rheum.*, **9**, 758.

28. Wynyard P.G. et al. (1987). Mechanism of exacerbation of rheumatoid synovitis by total-dose iron-dextran infusion: *in vivo* demonstration of iron-promoted oxidant stress. *Lancet*, **i**, 69.

29. Ruderman M., Miller L.M., Pinals R.S. (1968). Clinical and serologic observations on 27 patients with Felty's syndrome. *Arthritis Rheum.*, **11**, 377.

30. Rasker J.J., Cosh J.A. (1984). The natural history of rheumatoid arthritis: a fifteen year follow-up study. *Clin. Rheumatol.*, **3**, 11.

31. Scott D.L., Coulton B.L., Symmons D.P.M., Popert A.J. (1987). Long-term outcome of treating rheumatoid arthritis: results after 20 years. *Lancet*, **ii**, 1108.

32. Herzog C. et al. (1987). Monoclonal anti-CD4 in arthritis. *Lancet*, **ii**, 1461.

33. Paulus H.E. (1990). Current controversies in rheumatology: the use of disease-modifying antirheumatic agents in rheumatoid arthritis. *Arthritis Rheum.*, **33**, 113.

34. Jaffe I.A. (1990). Combination therapy of RA—rationale and overview. *J. Rheumatol.*, **17**(suppl. 25), 24.

35. Wingrave S.J., Kay C.R. (1978). Reduction in incidence of rheumatoid arthritis associated with oral contraceptives. *Lancet*, **i**, 569.

36. Hernandez-Avila M. et al. (1990). Exogenous sex hormones and the risk of rheumatoid arthritis. *Arthritis Rheum.*, **33**, 947.

37. Hench P.S. (1938). The ameliorating effect of pregnancy on chronic atrophic (infectious rheumatoid) arthritis, fibrosis, and intermittent hydrarthrosis. *Proc. Mayo. Clin.*, **13**, 161.

38. Schurs A.H.W.M., Verheul H.A.M. (1990). Effects of gender and sex steroids on the immune response. *J. Steroid Biochem.*, **35**, 157.

39. Ruffati A. et al. (1990). Autoantibodies of systemic rheumatic diseases in the healthy elderly. *Gerontologica*, **36**, 104.

40. Uetrecht J.P., Woosley R.L. (1981). Acetylator phenotype and lupus erythematosus. *Clin. Pharmacokinet.*, **6**, 118.

41. Batchelor J.R. et al. (1980). Hydralazine-induced systemic lupus erythematosus influence of HLA-DR and sex on susceptibility. *Lancet*, **i**, 1107.

42. Tan E.N., Portanova J.P. (1981). The role of histones as nuclear antigens in drug related lupus erythematosus. *Arthritis Rheum.*, **24**, 1064.

43. Tan E.M., Schur P.H., Carr R.I., Kunkel H.G. (1966). Deoxyribonucleic acid (DNA) and antibodies to DNA in the serum of patients with systemic lupus erythematosus. *J. Clin. Invest.*, **45**, 1732.

44. Lahita R., Kluger J., Drayer D.E. (1978). Antibodies to nuclear antigens in patients treated with procainamide or acetyl procainamide. *N. Engl. J. Med.*, **301**, 1382.

45. Ioannides C., Parke D.V. (1987). The cytochrome P-488—a unique family of enzymes involved in chemical toxicity and carcinogenesis. *Biochem. Pharmacol.*, **36**, 4197.

46. Ioannides C., Parke D.V. (1990) The cytochrome P450 I gene family of microsomal haemoproteins and their role the metabolic activation of chemicals. *Drug Metab. Rev.*, **22**, 1.

47. Beaune P.H. et al. (1987). Human anti-endoplasmic reticulum autoantibodies appearing in a drug-induced hepatitis are directed against a human liver cytochrome P–450 that hydroxylates the drug. *Med. Sci.*, **84**, 551.

48. Manns M.P. et al. (1990). Identification of cytochrome P450 IA2 as a human autoantigen. *Arch. Biochem. Biophys.*, **280**, 229.

49. Noriega A.R. et al. (1981). Toxic epidemic syndrome Spain. *Lancet*, **ii**, 697.

50. Winkelmann R.K. et al. (1991). Histopathologic features of the L-tryptophan-related eosinophilia–myalgia (fasciitis) syndrome. *Mayo Clin. Proc.*, **66**, 457.

51. Hoffman B.J. (1945). Sensitivity to sulfadiazine resembling acute disseminated lupus erythematosus. *Arch. Dermatol. Syph.*, **51**, 190.

52. Jungers P. et al. (1982). Influence of oral contraceptive therapy on the activity of systemic lupus erythematosus. *Arthritis Rheum.*, **25**, 618.

53. May D.G. et al. (1990). Scleroderma is associated with differences in individual routes of drug metabolism: a study with dapsone, debrisoquin and mephenytoin. *Clin. Pharmacol. Ther.*, **48**, 286.

54. Sharp G.C. et al. (1972). Mixed connective tissue disease: an apparently distinct rheumatic disease syndrome associated with a specific antibody to an extractable nuclear antigen (ENA). *Am. J. Med.*, **52**, 148.

55. Bowie E.J., Thompson J.H., Pascussi C.A., Owen C.A. (1963). Thrombosis in systemic lupus erythematosus despite circulating anticoagulants. *J. Lab. Clin. Med.*, **62**, 416.

56. Boey M.L. et al. (1983). Thrombosis in systemic lupus erythematosus: striking association with the presence of circulating lupus anticoagulant. *Br. Med. J.*, **287**, 1021.

57. Asherson R.A., Hughes G.R.V. (1991). Hypoadrenalism, Addison's disease and antiphospholipid antibodies. *J. Rheumatol.*, **18**, 1.

58. Asherson R.A., Oakley C.M. (1986). Pulmonary hypertension in SLE. *J. Rheumatol*, **13**, 1–5.

59. Cowchock S., Smith J.B., Gocial B. (1986). Antibodies to phospholipids and nuclear antigens in patients with repeated abortions. *Am. J. Obstet. Gynecol.*, **155**, 1002.

60. Parke A.L., Wilson D., Maier D. (1994). The prevalence of antiphospholipid antibodies in habitual aborters, normal mothers and in women who have never been pregnant. *Arthritis Rheum.* (in press).

61. Malia R.G., Kitchen S., Greaves M., Preston F.E. (1990). Inhibition of activated protein C and its cofactor protein S by antiphospholipid antibodies. *Br. J. Haematol.*, **76**, 101.

62. Parke A.L. et al. (1990). The thrombotic diathesis associated with antiphospholipid antibodies may be due to low levels of free protein S. *Clin. Exp. Rheumatol.*, **8**, 210 (abstr. 51b).

63. Carreras L.O. et al. (1981). Arterial thrombosis, intrauterine death and 'lupus' anticoagulant: detection of immunoglobulin interfering with prostacyclin formation. *Lancet*, **i**, 244.

64. Parke A.L. (1989). Antiphospholipid antibody syndromes. *Rheum. Dis. Clin. N. Am.*, **15**, 275.

65. McCue C.M. et al. (1977). Congenital heart block in

newborns of mothers with connective tissue disease. *Circulation*, **56**, 82–90.

66. Scott J.S. et al. (1983). Connective-tissue disease, antibodies to ribonucleoprotein, and congenital heart block. *N. Engl. J. Med.*, **309**, 209.

67. Lee L.A. (1990). Maternal autoantibodies and pregnancy—II: The neonatal lupus syndrome. In *Pregnancy and the Rheumatic Diseases* (Parke A.L., ed.) *Baillière's Clinical Rheumatology*, vol. 4, London: Baillière, p.69.

68. Weston W.L. et al. (1982). A serological marker for neonatal lupus erythematosus. *Br. J. Dermatol.*, **107**, 377.

69. Aylward R.D. (1928). Congenital heart block. *Br. Med. J.*, **1**, 943.

70. Harley J.B. et al. (1985). (SS-A) antibody and antigen in a patient with congenital complete heart block. *Arthritis Rheum.*, 28, 1321.

71. McCune A.B., Weston W.L., Lee L.A. (1987). Maternal and fetal outcome in neonatal lupus erythematosus. *Ann. Int. Med.*, **106**, 518.

72. Agnello V. (1978). Complement deficiency states. *Medicine*, **57**, 1.

73. Rynes R.I. (1982). Inherited complement deficiency states and SLE. *Clin. Rheum. Dis.*, **8**, 29.

74. Law S.K.A., Dodds A.W., Porter R.R. (1984). A comparison of the properties of two classes, C4A and C4B, of the human complement component C4. *EMBO J.*, **3**, 1819.

75. Fielder A.H.L. et al. (1983). Family study of the major histocompatibility complex in patients with systemic lupus erythematosus: importance of null alleles of C4A and C4B in determining disease susceptibility. *Br. Med. J.*, **286**, 425.

76. Reveille J.D. et al. (1985). Null alleles of the fourth component of complement and HLA haplotypes in familial systemic lupus erythematosus. *Immunogenetics*, **21**, 299.

77. Iida K., Mornaghi R., Nussenzweig V. (1982). Complement receptor (CRI) deficiency in erythrocytes from patients with systemic lupus erythematosus. *J. Exp. Med.*, **155**, 1427.

78. Ross G.D. et al. (1985). Disease-associated loss of erythrocyte complement receptors (CR$_1$, C3b receptors) in patients with systemic lupus erythematosus and other diseases involving autoantibodies and/or complement activation. *J. Immunol.*, **135**, 2005.

79. Gilliam J.N. et al. (1975). Immunoglobulin in clinical uninvolved skin in systemic lupus erythematosus: association with renal disease. *J. Clin. Invest.*, **53**, 1434.

80. Schur P.H., Austen K.F. (1968). Complement in human disease. *Ann. Rev. Med.*, **19**, 1.

81. Lloyd W., Schur P.H. (1981). Immune complexes, complement and anti-DNA in exacerbations of systemic lupus erythematosus. *Medicine*, **60**, 208.

82. Weinstein A. et al. (1983). Antibodies to native DNA and serum complement (C3) levels. Application to the diagnosis and classification of systemic lupus erythematosus. *Am. J. Med.*, **74**, 206.

83. Belmont H.M. et al. (1986). Complement activation during systemic lupus erythematosus: C3a and C5a anaphylatoxins circulate during exacerbations of disease. *Arthritis Rheum.*, 29, 1085.

84. Abramson S. (1987). Complement activation and vascular injury in systemic lupus erythematosus. *J. Rheumatol.*, **14** (suppl. 13), 43.

85. Rothfield N.F., Stollar B.D. (1967). The relation of immunoglobulin class, pattern of antinuclear antibody, and complement-fixing antibodies to DNA in sera from patients with systemic lupus erythematosus. *J. Clin. Invest.*, **46**, 1785.

86. Harley J.B., Gaither K.K. (1988). Autoantibodies. *Rheum. Dis. Clin. N. Am.*, **14**, 43.

87. McCarty G.A. (1986). Autoantibodies and their relation to rheumatic diseases. *Med. Clin. N. Am.*, **70**, 237.

88. Koffler D., Sabur P.H., Kunkel H.G. (1967). Immunological studies concerning the nephritis of systemic lupus erythematosus. *J. Exp. Med.*, **126**, 607.

89. Aarden L.A., DeGroot E.R., Feltkamp T.E.W. (1975). Immunology of DNA. III. *Crithidia lucilliae*, a simple substrate for the determination of anti-dsDNA with the immunofluorescence technique. *Ann. N Y Acad. Sci.*, **254**, 505.

90. Fritzler M.J., Kinsella T.D., Garbutt E. (1980). The CREST syndrome: a distinct serologic entity with anticentromere antibodies. *Am. J. Med.*, **69**, 520.

91. Earnshaw W. et al. (1986). Three human chromosomal autoantigens are recognized by sera from patient's with anti-centromere antibodies. *J. Clin. Invest.*, **77**, 426.

92. Shero J.H., Bordwell B., Rothfield N.F., Earnshaw W.C. (1986). High titers of autoantibodies to topoisomerase I (Scl-70) in sera from scleroderma patients. *Science*, **231**, 737.

93. Weiner E.S. et al. (1991). Prognostic significance of anticentromere antibodies and anti-topoisomerase I antibodies in Raynaud's disease. *Arthritis Rheum.*, **34**, 68.

94. Hamburger M., Hodes S., Barland P. (1977). The incidence and clinical significance of antibodies to extractable nuclear antigens. *Am. J. Med. Sci.*, **273**, 21.

95. Wolin S.L., Stietz J.A. (1984). The Ro small cytoplasmic ribonucleoproteins: identification of the antigenic protein and its binding site on the Ro RNAs. *Proc. Natl. Acad. Sci. USA*, 81, 1996.

96. Rinke J., Steitz J.A. (1982). Precursor molecules of both human 5s ribosomal RNA and transfer RNAs are bound by a cellular protein reactive with anti-La lupus antibodies. *Cell*, **29**, 149.

97. Triplett D.A., Brandt J.T., Kaczor D., Schaefer J. (1983). Laboratory diagnosis of lupus inhibitors: a comparison of the tissue thromboplastin inhibition procedure with a new platelet neutralization procedure. *Am. J. Clin. Pathol.*, **79**, 678.

98. Rosove M.H. et al. (1986). Lupus anticoagulants: improved diagnosis with a kaolin clotting time using rabbit brain phospholipid in standard and high concentrations. *Blood*, **68**, 472.

99. Exner T. (1985). Similar mechanism of various lupus anticoagulants. *Thromb. Haemostasis*, **53**, 15.

100. Moore J.E., Shulman L.E., Scott J.T. (1957). The natural history of systemic lupus erythematosus: an approach to its study through chronic biologic false positive reactors. *J. Chronic Dis.*, **5**, 282.

101. Haserick J.R., Loreg R. (1951). Systemic lupus erythematosus preceded by false positive tests for syphilis: presentation of 5 cases. *Ann. Int. Med.*, **37**, 559.

102. Harris E.N. (1990). The Second International Anti-Cardiolipin Standardization Workshop/Kingston

Anti-Phospholipid Antibody Study (KAPS) Group. *Am. J. Clin. Pathol.*, **94**, 476.

103. Galli M. et al. (1990). Anticardiolipin antibodies (ACA) directed not to cardiolipin but to a plasma protein cofactor. *Lancet*, **335**, 1544.

104. McNeil H.P., Simpson R.J., Chesterman C.N., Krilis S.A. (1990). Anti-phospholipid antibodies are directed against a complex antigen that includes a lipid binding inhibitor of coagulation: β_2-glycoprotein I (apolipoprotein H). *Proc. Natl. Acad. Sci. USA*, **87**, 4120.

105. van der Woude F.J. et al. (1985). Autoantibodies against neutrophil and monocytes: tool for diagnosis and marker of disease activity in Wegener's granulomatosis. *Lancet*, **i**, 425.

106. Cohen Tervaert J.W. et al. (1989). Association between active Wegener's granulomatosis and anticytoplasmic antibodies. *Arch. Intern. Med.*, **149**, 2461.

107. Coombs R.R.A., Mourant A.E., Race R.R. (1945). A new test for the detection of weak and 'incomplete' Rh agglutinins. *Br. J. Exp. Pathol.*, **26**, 255.

108. Hardin J.A. et al. (1978). Activation of blood clotting in patients with systemic lupus erythematosus: relationship to disease activity. *Am. J. Med.*, **65**, 430.

109. Exner T., Sahman N., Trudinger B. (1988). Separation of anticardiolipin antibodies from lupus anticoagulant on a phospholipid-coated polystyrene column. *Biochem. Biophys. Res. Comm.*, **155**, 1001.

110. Winfield J.B., Cohen P.L., Litvin D.A. (1982). Antibodies to activated T cells and their soluble products in systemic lupus erythematosus. *Arthritis Rheum.*, **25**, 814.

111. Austin H.A. et al. (1984). Diffuse proliferative lupus nephritis: Identification of specific pathologic features affecting renal outcome. *Kidney Int.*, **25**, 689.

112. Nossent H.C. et al. (1991). Systemic lupus erythematosus after renal transplantation: patient and graft survival and disease activity. *Ann. Int. Med.*, **114**, 183.

113. Rudnicki R.D., Gresham G.E., Rothfield N.F. (1975). The efficacy of antimalarials in systemic lupus erythematosus. *J. Rheumatol.*, **2**, 323.

114. Parke A.L. (1988). Antimalarial drugs, systemic lupus erythematosus and pregnancy. *J. Rheumatol.*, **15**, 607.

115. Worth T.L.H. (1971). Cyclophosphamide and the bladder. *Br. Med. J.*, **2**, 182.

116. Kumar R. et al. (1972). Cyclophosphamide and reproductive function. *Lancet*, **ii**, 1212.

117. Rothenberg R.J. et al. (1988). The use of methotrexate in steroid-resistant systemic lupus erythematosus. *Arthritis Rheum.*, **31**, 612.

118. Wilson K., Katz J., Abeles M. (1991). The use of methotrexate in systemic lupus erythematosus. *Arthritis Rheum.*, **34** (suppl.), R39.

119. Abramson N. et al. (1970). The interaction between human monocytes and red cells: specificity for IgG subclasses and IgG fragments. *J. Exp. Med.*, **132**, 1207.

120. Huber H., Fundenberg H.H. (1968). Receptor sites of human monocytes for IgG. *Int. Arch. Allergy*. **34**, 18.

121. Ebling F., Hahn B.H. (1980). Restricted subpopulations of DNA antibodies in kidneys of mice with systemic lupus: comparison of antibodies in serum and renal eluates. *Arthritis Rheum.*, **23**, 392.

122. Lahita R.G., Bradlow H.L., Kunkel H.G., Fishman J. (1979). Alterations of estrogen metabolism in SLE. *Arthritis Rheum.*, **22**, 1195.

123. Lahita R.G., Bradlow H.L., Fishman J., Kunkel H.G. (1982). Estrogen metabolism in systemic lupus erythematosus: patients and family members. *Arthritis Rheum.*, **25**, 843.

124. Stern R., Fishman J., Brusman H., Kunkel H.G. (1977). Systemic lupus erythematosus associated with Klinefelter's syndrome. *Arthritis Rheum.*, **20**, 18.

125. Parke A.L., Ioannides C., Lewis D.F.V., Parke D.V. (1991). Molecular pathology of drug-disease interactions in chronic autoimmune inflammatory diseases. *Inflammopharm.*, **1**, 1007.

32. ClinicalBiochemistry of the Central Nervous System

G. B. Firth, G. N. Cowdrey and S. J. Frost

Introduction
Cerebrospinal fluid
  Formation and physiology
  Composition
  Lumbar puncture
  Routine examination of the CSF
The blood–brain barrier
The investigation of proteins in CSF
  Origin of proteins in normal CSF
  Origin of proteins in pathological CSF
  Other CSF proteins
Enzymology and the CNS
Cerebrovascular disorders
  Cerebral infarction
  Haemorrhage
CNS infections
Demyelinating diseases
  Multiple sclerosis
  Examination of CSF in demyelinating
    diseases
Epilepsy
Dementia
Tumours of the CNS
*Nutritional and systemic disorders affecting
  the CNS*
*The role of the laboratory in investigating CNS
  disease*
Conclusion and future prospects

INTRODUCTION

The provision of a clinical biochemistry service for investigation and management of diseases of the central nervous system (CNS) offers several interesting challenges over and above those found in other branches of the speciality. The CNS requires a highly stable internal environment in order to function normally, which results in a relative isolation of the brain and spinal cord from other parts of the body. Paul Ehrlich, over 100 years ago, first demonstrated that the injection of a dye into animals resulted in the staining of all parts of the body apart from the brain. Conversely, injection of dye directly into the subarachnoid space results in intense staining of the brain, giving rise to the concept of the blood–brain barrier. This relative segregation of the brain imposes limitation on the usefulness of investigations of blood and urine in attempting to understand and analyse changes occurring within the CNS. Furthermore, many diseases of the CNS can be localized to very small specific regions of the brain or spinal cord, leading to changes that may be difficult or impossible to detect, even within the cerebrospinal fluid (CSF).

Although there is a vast wealth of literature on the biochemistry of the CNS, only a small proportion of this knowledge can be applied directly to the investigation of neurological disease; this knowledge is, however, invaluable in helping to understand many of the subtle changes occurring within the brain. The reasons for this are numerous; in particular, many such studies have been made at the tissue or cellular level in animal models, primarily mammals and amphibians. For reasons outlined above, few of these biochemical changes at the cellular level can be detected in the biological fluids and samples generally available to the clinical biochemist. Although the composition of the CSF is the best guide available to the probable interstitial fluid composition in the brain, it is nevertheless a poor index of brain composition and metabolism. The concentration of many analytes in the CSF is also very low, resulting in analytical limitations on their precise and accurate quantitation (although the advent of techniques such as capillary gas chromatography and possibly capillary electrophoresis may help to resolve some of these difficulties). Finally, many of the biochemical changes described in man and in animals are not disease specific, limiting their usefulness in clinical diagnosis.

The introduction of computerized tomography (CT) and more recently nuclear magnetic resonance (NMR) in the neurosciences has, more so than in any other branch of medicine, revolutionized the diagnosis of neurological disease, rendering many previous diagnostic techniques in clinical biochemistry, radiology and electrophysiology virtually obsolete. Nevertheless, the pathological investigation of body fluids still has an important part to play in diagnosing and treating many neurological diseases:

1. As in other fields of medicine the appropriate use of so-called routine investigations of blood and urine can provide important information, although certain of these such as for sodium, glucose, creatine kinase, and the pituitary hormones, can be of particular significance in the investigation of neurological disease.
2. A limited range of investigations of specific value in neurological disease can be made on serum; for example, various antibody studies (e.g. acetylcholine-receptor antibodies) and investigation of certain inborn errors with neurological implications (e.g. phytanic acid in Refsum's disease). However, these are primarily diseases of the peripheral rather than the central nervous system. Measurement of heavy metals

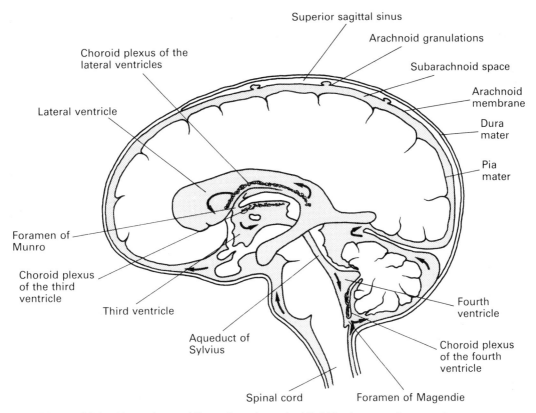

Figure 32.1 Formation and flow of cerebrospinal fluid in the central nervous system.

and catecholamines in the serum and urine can also be of value. Assay of arylsulphatase and detection of metachromatic staining deposits in the urine can be of diagnostic value in the detection of metachromatic leucodystrophy.

3. The analysis of CSF is of particular value in a number of diseases, particularly: CNS infections, suspected intracranial bleeding, multiple sclerosis and peripheral neuropathy. It is now generally contraindicated in the investigation of the unconscious patient, headaches (with the exception of those likely to be secondary to infections or haemorrhage) and in most types of suspected cerebral tumours.

4. Therapeutic drug monitoring is of particular value in neurology, primarily in serum but occasionally in the CSF. This is dealt with adequately elsewhere and will not be considered further here.

5. Very small biopsy specimens may be obtained during many neurological procedures for investigation or removal of intracerebral lesions. Examination is generally limited to routine staining of a biopsy smear in order to obtain a provisional diagnosis before debulking a tumour and only very rarely, in the more specialized neurological unit, might any biochemical investigations be called for.

CEREBROSPINAL FLUID

CSF bathes the surface of the brain and spinal cord. It is confined between the arachnoid and pia membranes and acts as a physical and biochemical buffer between the organs of the CNS and the rest of the body. It buoys up the brain, effectively reducing its weight, and is a barrier to physical injury. It provides a chemically stable fluid environment without which the brain cannot function normally and also serves as a means for removal of products of metabolism and inflammatory exudates.

Removal of wastes may be by bulk flow, diffusion or active transport. Thus, weak organic acids such as hydroxymethoxymandelic and vanillylmandelic acid can be cleared in this way.

Most nutrients that are rapidly metabolized by the brain, such as glucose, amino acids and ribonucleosides, are directly transported to the CNS across the blood–brain barrier of the cerebral capillaries. However certain micronutrients, including vitamins B_6, C, folate and deoxyribonucleosides, are transported to the brain via the CSF. The CSF–brain interface may also play a part in the regulation of respiration.

Formation and Physiology (Fig. 32.1)

The major site of CSF formation is in the choroid plexus of the lateral ventricles in the left and right cerebral hemispheres and in the fourth ventricle situated near the base of the brain. CSF formed in the lateral ventricles passes to the third ventricle through the foramen of Monro and thence to the fourth ventricle via the aqueduct of Sylvius. It then passes through two lateral apertures, the foramina of Luschka and Magendie, to the subarachnoid space surrounding the brain and spinal cord. As it flows there is a continuous exchange of nutrients and waste products between the CSF and the interstitial fluid of the brain cells. Adsorption and drainage of CSF is primarily through arachnoid granulations into the intracranial venous sinuses. These villi or granulations act as 'valves' permitting one-way flow of CSF from the subarachnoid space into the sinuses, opening or closing in response to changes in CSF pressure. This, together with the constant formation of CSF by the choroid plexus at the rate of approximately 0.4 mL/min gives direction to the flow of CSF.

The choroid plexus constitutes approximately 0.25% of the total weight of the human brain (2 or 3 g) and consists of a network of densely branched fronds, each containing capillaries surrounded by a single layer of epithelial cells. Each epithelial cell is firmly bound to its neighbour, forming 'tight junctions' that are impermeable to virtually all solutes. This creates the physical basis of the blood–CSF barrier. Blood plasma filters through the capillaries of the choroid plexus to bathe the basolateral surfaces of the epithelial cells. The plexus actively secretes water from the plasma into the ventricular space by a process involving ion transfer. Water molecules within the cell dissociate into hydrogen and hydroxyl ions, the latter combining with carbon dioxide from cell metabolism in the presence of carbonic anhydrase to form bicarbonate ions. Hydrogen ions are exchanged at the basolateral surface of the cell for sodium ions, which are pumped across the cell and into the ventricular space by an active transport system involving an Na^+, K^+-dependent, ouabain-sensitive ATPase. The resultant increase in positive charge in the ventricles is countered by the movement of chloride and bicarbonate ions from the cells into the ventricular space. Water passes from the epithelial cell into the ventricles in order to maintain an osmotic balance.

Other small molecules, including vitamins and nucleosides, are actively transported from the plasma to the ventricles. Most of the active transport processes can be shown to be rate limited if the concentration of constituents in the blood rises owing to saturation of the transport system. The epithelial cell layer acts as a virtual barrier to most blood proteins. However, certain proteins that appear to be carriers, prealbumin for example, are in higher concentration in the CSF than plasma and must be synthesized within the choroid plexus and transferred to the CSF.

A number of CNS diseases may be associated with alterations in the composition or pressure of the CSF. A variety of space-occupying lesions may obstruct the flow of CSF, leading to dilation of the ventricular system and resulting in a rapid increase in pressure. Damage to the choroid plexus by tumours, bacterial inflammation or other agents may also result in changes in CSF pressure and composition.

For a more detailed description of the role of the choroid plexus in the production of CSF and maintenance of its composition, see Spector and Johanson.[1]

Composition

In the normal healthy individual, CSF is a clear, colourless fluid of total volume approximately 140 mL, which, although it has a very low protein content similar to a plasma ultrafiltrate, differs in the concentration of various ions and other small molecules because of the active mechanisms involved in their transport into and from the CSF. These mechanisms serve to maintain the CSF concentration of most ions at remarkably constant levels despite any short-term variation in blood levels. Although sodium ion concentrations in the CSF are similar to or marginally higher than the plasma concentration, CSF levels of potassium and calcium are approximately half those found in the plasma. Lactate and phosphate concentrations in CSF are approximately a third to a quarter of plasma levels. Chloride is the dominant anion in the CSF and its concentration is rather higher than that of plasma because of the low protein concentration, in partial compliance with the Gibbs–Donnan equilibrium.

Because various constituents are either removed from or secreted into the CSF during its flow from the ventricles to the arachnoid villi its composition varies according to the site at which the fluid is sampled. The approximate concentration of constituents from normal adult CSF obtained at different sites is given in Table 32.1, although ranges will vary according to the analytical method, particularly for total protein.

Lumbar Puncture

There are four main indications for puncture:

1. For injection of radiopaque media in neuro-radiological investigation.
2. For therapeutic administration of drugs, including antibiotics, antitumour agents and local anaesthetics.
3. For therapeutic removal of CSF in patients with benign raised intracranial pressure.
4. In order to measure pressure and collect CSF for biochemical and cytological analysis in a number of neurological diseases. Examination of CSF is generally helpful in the investigation of peripheral neuropathy, particularly suspected Guillain–Barré syndrome; diagnosis of bacterial, fungal or viral infection of the CNS and in patients with suspected multiple sclerosis.

CSF is most frequently collected by lumbar punc-

TABLE 32.1
COMPOSITION OF LUMBAR, CISTERNAL, AND VENTRICULAR CSF

	Lumbar CSF	Cisternal CSF	Ventricular CSF
Total protein	0.2–0.4 g/L	0.15–0.25 g/L	0.05–0.15 g/L
Glucose	2.8–4.4 mmol/L	2.8–5.0 mmol/L	2.8–5.0 mmol/L
Cells	0–5 per 10^{-9} L	0–4 per 10^{-9} L	0–1 per 10^{-9} L
pH	7.33–7.37	7.33–7.37	
Sodium	130–155 mmol/L		
Potassium	2.3–3.5 mmol/L		

ture. However, the procedure is not without its risks and at best is uncomfortable and unpleasant for the patient. Consequently, lumbar puncture for biochemical analysis of CSF should not be undertaken lightly, particularly in hospitals that lack neurological facilities. The development of non-invasive techniques such as CT and NMR scanning has rendered 'routine' CSF examination superfluous in many diseases in which it was previously useful.[2] It is seldom indicated in patients suffering from stroke or in suspected cases of cord compression. It is generally contraindicated in any patient with a headache and definite signs of an intracerebral tumour and in the unconscious patient unless a careful neurological assessment has first been made. Although analysis of CSF can provide valuable confirmatory evidence in practically all cases of suspected subarachnoid haemorrhage, the procedure results in a dramatic deterioration in the level of consciousness with the possibility of cerebral dislocation or tonsillar coning in a small percentage of patients (see below). It is, therefore, generally considered that in most cases of suspected haemorrhage, CT scanning should be the primary investigation and only where this is negative should lumbar puncture be considered. In order to lessen the risk of a 'bloody tap' and to reduce the trauma, it is essential that the patient is correctly positioned for the puncture. For a clear account of the correct procedure the reader is referred to Patten.[3] Normally, from 4 to 6 mL of CSF is collected by lumbar puncture from the interspace between lumbar spines 3 and 4 whilst the patient is lying in the lateral position. The fluid should be allowed to flow under its own pressure and to drip directly from the puncture needle into three small, clean, sterile containers and into a paediatric fluoride tube for estimation of blood glucose. A syringe must never be used for aspiration of CSF because of the danger of damaging a nerve root or causing tonsillar impaction in cases of low CSF pressure. The containers should preferably be of plastic since glass can adsorb proteins on to its surface, and it is essential that they are labelled in the correct order of collection. Small containers are preferable for collection of CSF; a considerable amount of sample can be lost in the rubberized cap of the 20 mL glass containers that were conventionally used by many for collection of CSF.

Specimens should be sent to the laboratory as soon as possible after collection because degenerative changes in cell morphology can occur within a few hours. If there is likely to be any delay in analysing the samples they should be stored at 4°C until processed. The site of collection of the CSF, together with full relevant drug information, must be provided as this can influence the interpretation of results.

Routine Examination of the CSF

Although CSF specimens sent to the laboratory are frequently required for examination by more than one discipline, all samples should in the first instance be sent to one department for visual examination and should not be split and distributed by reception staff unless they are fully trained to do so. Apart from the necessity of identifying a 'bloody tap', the sample received is frequently insufficient for all the analyses requested and a decision may need to be taken on the order of priority of investigation.

The analysis of CSF is often one of the least well performed of any investigation in the clinical laboratory. A recent informal survey of a number of laboratories in two different Health Regions in England found that in over 50% of cases the biochemical analysis of CSF was carried out a department other than clinical biochemistry. The only examination for pigmentation was visual and in no case was scanning spectrophotometry of the specimen undertaken. In some cases where the biochemical analysis occured in other departments, the clinical biochemistry department was unsure of the methods currently being used for assay of CSF glucose or protein. Although these assays are no doubt done to acceptable standards in most cases, one would not necessarily expect other disciplines to be fully conversant with current standards of quality control and methodology in clinical biochemistry, any more than one would expect most clinical biochemists to be aware of the state of the art in other disciplines. Although in many patients undergoing a CSF examination in a general hospital, biochemical analysis may be of secondary importance to examination for the presence of leucocytes and infective agents, this is not invariably the case. The patient may require to be transferred to a neurological unit and a poorly done CSF examination at the hospital of origin may delay or confound the final diagnosis. This may necessitate the patient having to undergo a second lumbar puncture, although at that stage it may be impossible to distinguish a subarachnoid haemorrhage from an earlier 'bloody tap'.

A number of CSF investigations that were previously useful or thought to be useful have now been superseded by more specific techniques. Assay of CSF chloride rarely yields any clinically useful information and has been discontinued by most laboratories. Various indirect tests for abnormalities in gamma-globulin concentration, in particular the Pandy test and the Lange colloidal gold test, have long since been superseded by more specific electrophoretic and immunological techniques and will not be considered further here.

Inspection

Normal CSF is completely clear and colourless. Cloudiness may be caused by the presence of blood, bacteria, white cells or occasionally by radiopaque material following myelography. A traumatic tap will normally be indicated by the presence of a reducing amount of blood in each of the three successively obtained specimens that on centrifugation demonstrate a completely colourless supernatant. Similar concentrations of blood in all three specimen containers and the presence of xanthochromia are indicative of a subarachnoid haemorrhage. There are occasional exceptions to these general observations, however. Pigmentation of the CSF may be due to the presence of oxyhaemoglobin, methaemoglobin, bilirubin or bilirubin derivatives and the presence of xanthochromia must be assessed by scanning spectrophotometry, since visual inspection alone will miss many minor but nevertheless important changes and can rarely distinguish the type of pigment present. A small fibrin clot is characteristically seen in cases of tuberculous meningitis but may very occasionally occur in CSF samples having a high protein content.

Glucose

Measurement of glucose is still regarded by many as one of the most important biochemical investigations in CSF, although an accurate, precise and rapid enzymatic assay must be used and it must be properly controlled, using appropriate CSF controls, both during normal working hours and in particular out-of-hours. The specimen must have been collected into sodium fluoride preservative because glucose is rapidly metabolized in the presence of bacterial infection or a raised leucocyte count. As the CSF glucose concentration is markedly affected by the serum glucose concentration it is important that this be measured at the same time. Although a classical bacterial infection with elevated neutrophil count will give rise to little diagnostic confusion, estimation of glucose is valuable in atypical cases, particularly where there is a lymphocytic cell response. The CSF glucose is also

the first to return to normal after appropriate antibiotic therapy. Whereas the CSF leucocyte count will increase during the first 24 h after therapy in many patients before decreasing rapidly thereafter, the glucose level has returned to normal in most patients by that time.[4]

The extent of reduction of the glucose level also correlates with a poor outcome in cases of pneumococcal meningitis but not in other bacterial causes of meningitis.

Protein

There is no ideal method for the assay of total protein in CSF. Each technique will give different results, dependent upon the ratio of albumin to globulin and other proteins present in the specimen and on the type of standard material used in the assay. There is as yet no national quality assessment scheme for CSF protein assays in the UK, although various local schemes have shown that the assay has very poor accuracy that can only be partially improved by use of a common standard. Turbidimetric techniques based upon precipitation by sulphasalicylic acid or trichloracetic acid are particularly inaccurate due to variation in particle size and should no longer be used. Several methods are available based upon dye-binding techniques or on the formation of copper complexes with protein. The Coomassie blue technique is probably the most commonly used of these methods; however, it suffers the serious disadvantage of producing a lower colour intensity with globulin than with albumin and can, therefore, underestimate the total protein content of CSF samples with abnormally elevated γ-globulin levels. The recently introduced pyrogallol method largely overcomes this problem. It exhibits a more linear response over a wide range with less dye binding to the cuvette. It can be automated.

Many of the difficulties of attempting to measure total protein can be overcome by specific immunochemical assay of individual proteins and there is a good case at least for the routine measurement of IgG, particularly in inflammatory diseases and in suspected multiple sclerosis. Specific measurement of prealbumin, transferrin and β_2-microglobulin may also be useful in certain circumstances. Nevertheless, assay of total protein remains a rapid, simple, albeit insensitive marker of changes in CSF protein content and composition.

Other Routine Investigations

In addition to 'routine' biochemical investigations many CSF specimens will also undergo cell count, microbiological culture and Gram stain, and cytological examination of a fixed film preparation. Although 'cytospin' preparation of most patients' CSF for cytological investigation is routinely done in some neurological units, few unsuspected abnormalities are picked up and the investigation is more often restricted to cases of suspected carcinomatous meningitis. White blood-cell count is valuable in the identification and differentiation of bacterial, viral and fungal meningitis and will be discussed later in this chapter. Small increases in the lymphocyte cell count in the CSF are also encountered in diseases with an immunological basis, for example multiple sclerosis.

THE BLOOD–BRAIN BARRIER

Observations that led to the concept of the blood–brain barrier and the analogous blood–CSF barrier were described above. There is, in fact, no single barrier but a series of regulatory interfaces that determine the rate at which certain substances are able to pass into the brain.

The main function of the blood–brain barrier is to protect the brain from the blood *milieu* but it also controls the selective transport of certain substances from the blood to the brain. In this way, the homeostasis of the brain environment is maintained, which is necessary for normal brain function.

Similarly, the blood–CSF barrier maintains the biochemical composition of the CSF.

The impermeability of the blood–brain barrier to most substances is effected by the tight junctions between endothelial cells. However, in certain areas of the brain, the endothelial cells do not form tight junctions but allow free exchange of molecules between the blood and adjacent neurons. This means, for example, that neuroendocrine hormones released from specialized nerve terminals can freely enter the blood and influence distant target organs.

THE INVESTIGATION OF PROTEINS IN CSF

Origin of Proteins in Normal CSF

Normal CSF has a total protein concentration of between 200 and 400 mg/L, which is approximately a 1 in 200 dilution of that found in the serum. Nearly all the CSF proteins originate from the blood and are introduced into the CSF by filtration at the choroid plexi in the ventricles.

Molecular size is an important factor that determines the relative abundances of proteins in CSF, so that small proteins such as prealbumin predominate over large ones such as IgG.[5]

There is also evidence that some proteins, prealbumin and transferrin for example, are synthesized locally by cells within the CNS.

Origin of Proteins in Pathological CSF

In some neurological diseases, especially those of an inflammatory nature such as meningitis, the blood–CSF barrier becomes more permeable and permits relatively large protein molecules to pass directly from the blood into the CSF. Similar leakages of protein may also occur as the result of mechanical damage to the cerebral blood vessels.

Some proteins that are found only in trace amounts in CSF are specific to the CNS, such as S-100 protein, glial fibrillary acidic protein (GFAP) and myelin basic protein (MBP). The amount of S-100 protein is raised in CSF from patients with cerebral glioma tumours, GFAP is an astrocyte-specific protein and MBP is increased in the CSF of many patients suffering from multiple sclerosis.[6]

Intrathecal Synthesis of Immunoglobulin
In certain neurological diseases, especially multiple sclerosis, immunoglobulin (principally of the IgG class) is synthesized within the brain itself by lymphocytes. This is termed intrathecal synthesis. Intrathecally synthesized IgM and immunoglobulin free light chains may also be found in the CSF, especially in patients with infections of the CNS.

Intrathecally synthesized IgG differs from normal serum IgG in two different ways:

1. It separates into distinct bands in the γ-globulin region when subjected to electrophoresis. This phenomenon, *oligoclonal banding*, is not seen in the serum from the corresponding CSF, which confirms that it is produced exclusively within the CNS.
2. It is well established that at least a part of the intrathecal IgG has a much higher isoelectric point (pI) than normal serum IgG. These proteins have been described as highly alkaline fractions and give pI in excess of 8.0.[7–9]

As yet, there is no known explanation for the existence of these highly alkaline protein fractions in CSF. Furthermore, the mechanism responsible for this abnormal electric charge has not been explained. Similarly, their pathological significance and antigenic specificity have still to be determined.

Oligoclonal IgG bands are not specific for multiple sclerosis but have also been detected in CSF from patients with a variety of other neurological diseases including chronic infections of the CNS, neurosyphilis and Guillain–Barré syndrome. This topic is considered further below.

Detection of Intrathecal IgG in CSF by Quantitative Methods. These methods rely upon immunochemical means of measurement. Various corrections are then made in order to eliminate the effects of leakage at the blood–CSF barrier as a cause of any increased concentration of IgG in the CSF. The CSF IgG concentration is then expressed in relation either to the CSF albumin concentration or the CSF total protein concentration. An increase in the percentage value of CSF IgG concentration expressed in this way is suggestive of intrathecal synthesis of IgG.

The IgG index, introduced by Delpech,[10] has been widely used to detect intrathecal IgG synthesis. In this test, CSF and serum IgG concentrations and CSF and serum albumin concentrations are measured. The ratio of CSF to serum IgG is divided by that for CSF to serum albumin. An increased ratio indicates the intrathecal synthesis of IgG.

Tourtellotte[11] introduced a formula from which it is possible to detect intrathecal IgG synthesis by calculating the amount of IgG synthesized daily in the CNS. The formula is based on the concentration of IgG and albumin in CSF and serum; it also incorporates a number of mathematically derived constants to correct for any defect in the blood–CSF barrier.

Tourtellotte's formula for calculating intrathecal IgG synthesis is as follows:

$$\left[\left(IgG_{csf} - \frac{IgG_s}{369}\right) - \left(Alb_{csf} - \frac{Alb_s}{230}\right) \times \left(\frac{IgG_s}{Alb_s}\right)(0.43)\right] \times 5.$$

Detection of Intrathecal IgG in CSF by Electrophoresis. In multiple sclerosis and some infections of the CNS there is intrathecal synthesis of IgG that separates into discrete bands when subjected to electrophoresis. This phenomenon was first reported by Lowenthal in 1964,[12] who used agar-gel electrophoresis to study the proteins in CSF from patients with a variety of neurological diseases. He found that there were γ-globulin bands in some CSFs that were absent from normal CSF. Lowenthal believed this type of electrophoretic pattern characterized the essential protein in CSF of multiple sclerosis. Similar work was done by Latterre,[13] who made the original reference to 'oligoclonality'; by this he meant that an origin from serum could not explain these bands because any impairment of the blood–CSF barrier would allow a diffuse spectrum of γ-globulins to pass into the CSF, corresponding to that of normal serum γ-globulin.

Early electrophoretic methods were not sensitive enough to detect the proteins in CSF without having to concentrate it by almost 200 times to approach that of serum. Because this causes certain proteins to be lost through adhesion to the concentrating membranes, it has become essential to use unconcentrated CSF for electrophoresis. This is particularly relevant in the case of basic proteins such as the highly alkaline intrathecally synthesized IgG found in the CSF of most patients with multiple sclerosis.

The introduction of disc electrophoresis using polyacrylamide gel as the separation medium by Ornstein[14] and Davis[15] allowed modifications of this method to be used to analyse unconcentrated CSF for the investigation of alkaline CSF proteins, including oligoclonal bands.

The method of choice for the electrophoretic detection of oligoclonal IgG bands in unconcentrated CSF is now *isoelectric focusing* (IEF). This is the most sensitive method available for the detection of oligoclonal IgG bands, owing to its extremely high resolving power.

Isoelectric Focusing of CSF for the Detection of Oligoclonal IgG bands. In IEF, proteins migrate under the influence of an applied voltage to their respective pI in a pre-established pH gradient formed using chemicals known as carrier ampholytes. The potential of IEF for the separation of CSF proteins was first pointed out over 20 years ago. However, it is only during the last 10 years that it has gradually become a routine technique for the detection of oligoclonal bands in unconcentrated CSF.[16]

The incidence of oligoclonal IgG bands in CSF from patients with multiple sclerosis is high using IEF and detection rates of 90% and even 100% are reported, although the latter could include false-positive results due to the creation of artefactual bands by the carrier ampholytes.

The specificity of IEF for the demonstration of oligoclonal IgG bands in CSF is increased when used in combination with *immunoblotting* procedures. In immunoblotting, the CSF proteins are transferred to an immobilizing membrane such as nitrocellulose or polyvinylidenedifluoride (PVDF) directly after IEF. The immobilized replica-protein patterns are then visualized by treating the blots with specific antibody to human IgG. The signal can be further enhanced by treatment with a secondary, enzyme-conjugated antibody, followed by an appropriate colour reaction.

The detection of oligoclonal IgG bands in CSF is not complete proof of intrathecal synthesis; proteins must be shown to be unique to CSF rather than to originate from the blood before intrathecal synthesis can be established. This is most commonly achieved by comparing the IEF pattern of CSF and serum from the same patient. Bands present in the CSF but absent from the corresponding serum indicate intrathecal synthesis.

Isoelectric Focusing of CSF for the Detection of Oligoclonal IgG Bands Using an Immobilised pH Gradient. Conventional IEF is done with either agarose or polyacrylamide gels as support media and containing carrier ampholytes to form the pH gradient. However, the formation of gradients is not without difficulties, one of which is 'cathodic drifting', whereby the entire gradient migrates slowly towards the cathode electrode during IEF. As is to be expected, this drifting is particularly troublesome in the separation of very basic proteins such as highly alkaline oligoclonal IgG fractions; indeed, some of them may not be focused at all.

Another problem of IEF with carrier ampholytes is the uneven electrical conductivity and buffering capacity produced by focusing of the individual components of the carrier ampholyte solution into a series of ridges and troughs spread throughout the pH gradient. This in turn leads to the appearance of artefactual bands, even in the case of polyclonal antibody, which by all other electrophoresis methods separates as a continuous diffuse zone.

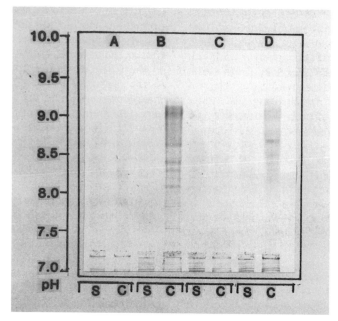

Figure 32.2 Immunoblot with a PVDF membrane from an immobilized pH gradient gel, pH 7–10, containing 0.2% V/V carrier ampholytes. Serum (S) and cerebrospinal fluid (C) from two patients without any alkaline oligoclonal IgG bands, (A) and (C), and two patients with intrathecally synthesized alkaline oligoclonal IgG bands, (B) and (D). Total amount of IgG applied in each sample is 0.1 μg. Detection is with sheep antihuman IgG, followed by donkey antisheep alkaline phosphatase conjugate and enhanced with nitroblue tetrazolium.

The recently introduced electrophoretic technique of IEF using immobilized pH gradients [17] overcomes some of these problems. Immobilized pH gradients are formed from a number of acrylamide derivatives known as immobilines. These are solutions of molecules that are bifunctional, having a buffering group at one end and a double bond at the other. The latter groups are covalently linked to polyacrylamide gel during polymerization. Hence, the buffering groups, being copolymerized within the polyacrylamide gel matrix, cannot migrate in an electric field, i.e. they are immobilized. This means that the pH gradient is stable indefinitely, unlike pH gradients formed with carrier ampholytes.

Immobilized pH gradients are capable of extremely high resolution and are stable, even at highly alkaline pH. They are therefore ideal for the investigation of the highly alkaline, intrathecally synthesized oligoclonal IgG bands associated with multiple sclerosis (Fig. 32.2).

An IEF method has now been described that uses an immobilized pH gradient extending over the pH range 7–10 for the specific detection of alkaline, intrathecally synthesized oligoclonal IgG bands in unconcentrated CSF.[18]

Detection of Oligoclonal IgM and Immunoglobulin Free Light Chains in CSF. Most of the work on oligoclonal bands in CSF has been on IgG but IgM can also have an oligoclonal distribution in CSF after IEF.

It is well recognized that an IgM antibody response occurs much earlier than an IgG. In certain condi-tions, such as when monitoring treatment of a CNS infection, it may be appropriate to examine the CSF for the presence of oligoclonal IgM bands, and then for IgG bands, which form later but remain in the CSF for many years.

Oligoclonal bands consisting of immunoglobulin free light chains are also found in the CSF of some patients. In multiple sclerosis, for example, free light chains mainly of κ class have been found in the CSF of about 85% of patients. Free light chains have also been found in the CSF of patients with viral infec-tions of the CNS and in subacute sclerosing panen-cephalitis, a rare persistent measles infection involv-ing the brain. In infection of the CNS the free light chains are mostly of the λ class.

Other CSF Proteins

Haptoglobins are a group of genetically controlled proteins with molecular sizes around 100 kDa found in the blood. Normally they are confined to the blood and excluded from entering the CSF by the cells of the blood–CSF barrier. However, in certain inflammatory neurological diseases such as menin-gitis, the barrier becomes abnormally permeable to proteins and relatively large proteins such as hapto-globins pass from the blood into the CSF. The detection of haptoglobins in the CSF, usually by disc electrophoresis with polyacrylamide gel, is an indication of an inflammatory condition within the CNS.

Transferrin exists in CSF in two distinct forms. One is the same as the one found in blood and the other, known as Tau protein, is a desialylated form of transferrin unique to CSF. Transferrin and Tau protein are immunologically identical (both react with antihuman transferrin) but have different electrophoretic mobilities (Tau protein migrates more slowly). The ratio of Tau protein to transferrin in CSF increases when tissue necrosis releases lysozomal enzymes into the CSF.

At least two other proteins that may be detected by CSF electrophoresis have been assumed to be CSF specific; these are β-trace and γ-trace proteins. In fact, both can be detected immunochemically in serum. β-Trace protein has no known physiological function and migrates in the β-region as a single band on non-sieving media or as four bands on polyacrylamide gel. The γ-trace protein has been known more recently as cystatin C and is a potent inhibitor of cysteine proteinases. It is a very alkaline protein (pI 9.2) and can therefore be mistaken for alkaline, intrathecally synthesized IgG bands unless these are specifically identified by immunofixation with antihuman IgG.

The concentration of cystatin C in CSF is reduced in many cases of multiple sclerosis and this has led to speculation that when the regulation of cysteine proteinases is lowered there is enhanced activity of these enzymes which could initiate the breakdown of myelin.[19]

Prealbumin is filtered from the blood plasma via the choroid plexi. However, prealbumin additional to the plasma variety is also synthesized by the cells of the choroid epithelium. The physiological significance of this cerebral source of prealbumin is unknown. The concentration of prealbumin is the same in ventricular and lumbar CSF, although as a proportion of the total protein content there is more prealbumin in ventricular than lumbar fluid.

ENZYMOLOGY AND THE CNS

CSF enzyme concentrations can be altered by mechanisms similar to those affecting other proteins, and they are more easily measured, which facilitated early application of their estimation. Enzymes can pass from damaged brain tissue into the CSF. Since the 1950s, it has been known that their levels are elevated as a result of brain damage. However, partly due to the advent of alternative diagnostic methods and partly because of lack of diagnostic specificity in individual clinical conditions, on the whole the procedures for enzyme assay have not become established. There is still interest, however, in their potential as an indicator of severity of damage, as prognostic indicators and as means of monitoring response to treatment. A simple marker of organic disease might also be useful in some patients in whom all other investigations are normal. Applications of enzyme assays will be described in relation to certain specific conditions, preceded by an overview of enzyme measurement in neurological cell damage.

Physiological variations in tissue enzyme levels as well as the variable spatial relations of injured tissue to the CSF circulation make relating enzyme levels to the degree of injury difficult. A correlation with injury can be found for certain enzymes such as aspartate aminotransferase (AST), lactate dehydrogenase (LDH), γ-glutamyl transpeptidase (GTT), malate dehydrogenase (MDH) and creatine kinase (CK) in the CSF.

In animal studies there is little regional variation in some enzymes such as acid phosphatases, AST, isocitrate dehydrogenase, LDH and MDH but greater variation in CK and glutamate dehydrogenase.[20] Regional variability of CK isoenzymes can also be demonstrated. Enzymes that have a more homogeneous distribution may be more useful diagnostic or prognostic indicators.

Most enzymes can probably pass from the CSF into the peripheral circulation but unless they are distinguishable from serum enzymes (e.g. unique isoenzymes) they will be masked by systemic changes in their concentration. Total AST and CK activities in serum correlate with the extent of neurological injury, although isoenzyme studies suggest this may be due to coexisting systemic trauma in severely injured patients.

An alternative approach is to measure specific isoenzymes in either CSF or blood. Although at first sight an attractive proposition, these estimations require more specific methods, such as electrophoresis or immunological assays, which increases the complexity of, and time required for, the measurements.

Neurons contain substantial amounts of the γ-isoenzyme of enolase (*neuron-specific enolase*; NSE) which is also found in neuroendocrine (APUD) cells. The β-isoenzyme is largely found in muscle and the α-isoenzyme is more widely distributed within the brain and elsewhere. Elevations of γ- and α-isoenolases in the CSF occur in a wide range of neurological conditions and lack diagnostic specificity. Despite this, measurement of isoenolases may have a role in assessing severity and monitoring treatment.

CK-BB is found in neurons and astrocytes. It is another isoenzyme that has been shown, experimentally in animals and clinically, to be increased in neurological cell damage in both CSF and serum and to be related to the degree of damage. CK-BB is found in brain tissue, which lacks significant amounts of the other isoenzymes of CK (CK-MM and CK-MB). The rise in CK-BB in the CSF reaches a maximum a few hours after events such as acute trauma and then falls exponentially with a half-life of a few hours, consistent with release from damaged cells.[21] CSF CK-BB apparently reflects prognosis in head trauma, though the value of this assay has been questioned. It may be greatly improved by either taking samples soon after the trauma or by extrapolating levels back to an estimated value for the time of injury.

Several other putative markers of neurological damage include *aldolase-C4 isoenzyme*, which is predominantly found in brain. This has been suggested as a marker for neurological damage, although there may be a lack of specificity and sensitivity.

CEREBROVASCULAR DISORDERS

The most frequently encountered forms of cerebrovascular disease are:

(i) *cerebral infarction*;
(ii) *haemorrhage*:
  - intracerebral haemorrhage,
  - subarachnoid haemorrhage,
  - subdural haematoma,
  - arteriovenous malformations or angiomas;
(iii) *miscellaneous*:
  - hypertensive encephalopathy,
  - disseminated intravascular coagulation,
  - atherosclerotic rigidity syndrome,
  - anterior spinal artery thrombosis.

Cerebral infarction occurs more commonly than cerebral haemorrhage and it may be clinically difficult to distinguish between the two. These conditions must also be distinguished from neoplastic and other space-occupying lesions as a cause of hemiparesis. It is also essential to exclude any basic disease process predisposing to intravascular thrombosis. For a detailed discussion of the pathophysiological processes and clinical presentations in the various forms of cerebrovascular disease the reader is referred to the review by Patten.[3]

Cerebral Infarction

The differential diagnosis of cerebrovascular disease is best achieved by CT, which will in most instances differentiate tumours from infarction, haematomas or angiomas. Although CSF analysis is rarely of diagnostic value in these circumstances a number of studies have shown biochemical changes in spinal fluid following cerebral infarctions, including increases in CK, AST, GTT and LDH.

Lactate dehydrogenase is said to be the most sensitive of these enzyme markers and may provide earlier evidence of stroke than may be apparent from CT scanning. It is claimed that this may be of prognostic value and also useful in differentiating strokes from transient ischaemic attacks.[22]

Although early studies suggested that CSF *ferritin* concentrations are increased in patients with strokes and transient ischaemia, more recent work has questioned the sensitivity and specificity of these associations.[23] Elevated levels are also found in viral and bacterial meningitis; furthermore, normal levels may be found in stroke victims, except where a haematoma is present.

As outlined in the preceding section, the brain is the only organ known to contain substantial amounts

of the γ-isoenzyme of *enolase* (NSE). It is elevated in the CSF in stroke and trauma but again the assay lacks diagnostic specificity as elevated levels of both the γ- and α-isoform have been demonstrated in a wide range of neurological conditions. There is a positive correlation between the volume of infarcted tissue as measured by CT and both γ- and α-enolase levels in CSF and it has been suggested that they may have a role in assessing severity of disease and monitoring treatment.[24] However, there is no evidence that the assay can provide any information over and above that obtained by CT scanning. Furthermore, repeated lumbar puncture for monitoring could not be justified. More recent studies have, however, demonstrated that the enzyme is also elevated in serum in these conditions,[25] and there may be a role for serial estimation of γ-enolase in some cases where access to CT scanning facilities is limited. Similar claims have been made for the acidic calcium-binding protein S-100, which is found in glial cells, Schwann cells and neurons, although it only appears to be elevated in patients with more severe damage.

Further studies are needed to determine whether any of these potential markers may be of diagnostic or prognostic value. On the other hand, it is essential to identify any disease process that predisposes the patient to stroke, as this is likely to be the best way of improving long-term prognosis. Diabetic patients in particular have an increased incidence of cerebral vascular disease and can suffer from a variety of cerebral vascular accidents as well as more specific, small-vessel disease affecting the internal capsule, basal ganglia and spinal cord. Biochemical, haematological and microbiological investigations should also be undertaken to eliminate other predisposing diseases including polycythaemia rubra vera, disseminated lupus erythematosus, subacute bacterial endocarditis, myocardial infarction or thyrotoxicosis.

Haemorrhage

Haemorrhages can occur into many parts of the cerebrum and cerebellum and, particularly in the case of cerebellar bleeds, can present with clinical symptoms very similar to those of subarachnoid haemorrhage. These haematomas are space-occupying lesions and the risks of lumbar puncture under these conditions can be as great as for the investigation of a tumour. CT scanning should therefore be the first line of investigation in patients presenting with a suspected subarachnoid haemorrhage, and only where the scan is normal and after a full neurological examination should lumbar puncture be done. If done within the first 48 h of the event, CT scanning will detect most cases of subarachnoid haemorrhage but after this time the probability of detecting blood on CT becomes progressively reduced. On the other hand, xanthochromia of the CSF can be detected in virtually all cases when the fluid is examined between

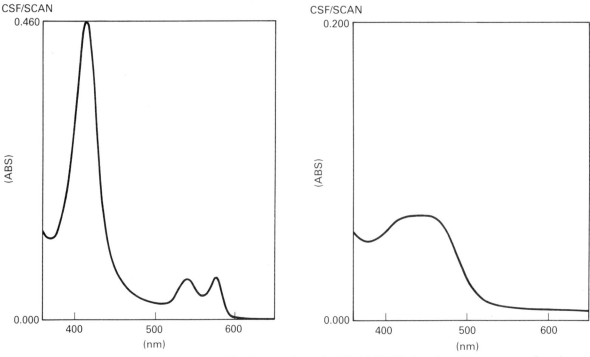

Figure 32.3 (a) Spectrophotometric scan of lumbar cerebrospinal fluid (CSF) showing the presence of oxyhaemoglobin. (b) Spectrophotometric scan of lumbar CSF showing the presence of bilirubin.

12 h and 2 weeks after the ictus, and in 70% of patients after 3 weeks and over 40% at 4 weeks.[26] This only applies, however, where the fluid is examined properly by scanning spectrophotometry.

The eye is particularly insensitive to low concentrations of haemoglobin and where the absorption due to haemoglobin at its wavelength maximum of 415 nm is less than 0.1 absorbance units, simple visual inspection will often fail to detect it. Several studies going back over 25 years and involving large numbers of samples have confirmed that whereas spectrophotometry will detect the presence of pigments in the CSF of virtually all patients with subarachnoid haemorrhage, provided the specimen is collected between 12 h and 2 weeks of the event, visual examination will fail to detect any pigmentation in nearly 50% of cases.

Three major pigments can be detected in the CSF after a subarachnoid haemorrhage or subdural haematoma—oxyhaemoglobin, methaemoglobin or bilirubin. These pigments are present in the CSF in a form that is insusceptible to ultrafiltration, and by electrophoresis it can be shown that bilirubin is bound to albumin or occasionally prealbumin. Methaemalbumin may also be detected. IEF techniques demonstrate that bilirubin can occur in the CSF in the free or conjugated form. Differences in the absorbance curves of the different bilirubin complexes can also be observed, with the conjugated bilirubinoids appearing to absorb light at a lower wavelength than the free complex.[27]

After a bleed into the subarachnoid space, free oxyhaemoglobin can be detected in the CSF superna-

tant within 4–6 h (Fig. 32.3) and this gradually breaks down to form unconjugated bilirubin over the following 2–3 weeks. After this time conjugated bilirubin can be detected. Methaemoglobin and methaemalbumin can also be detected in cases of subdural and intracerebral haematomas and some craniopharyngiomas.

On spectrophotometric analysis of a centrifuged specimen of CSF, oxyhaemoglobin can be detected by its characteristic absorption at approximately 415 nm, with lesser peaks at 540 and 575 nm. Methaemoglobin has a maximum at 406 nm with subsidiary peaks at 540, 575 and 630 nm. For methaemoglobin the absorbance at 540 nm is greater than at 575 nm, whereas for oxyhaemoglobin the two peaks are of roughly similar height. Interpretation can, however, be complicated by the presence of a background absorbance due to turbidity, which can be particularly noticeable in some abnormal fluids. Bilirubin has a wide absorbance range with a peak at about 460 nm but because of the presence of haemoglobin this can often appear as a 'shoulder' rather than a true peak. Conjugated bilirubin, on the other hand, has a maximum at 425–430 nm.

In many cases more than one pigment will be present in the fluid and care must be exercised in the interpretation of the spectrophotometric data. To simplify this the presence of xanthochromia is often defined as an extinction exceeding 0.023 absorbance units at 415 nm and/or a peak or shoulder in the absorption curve at 450–460 nm. Attempts have been made to classify further the pigmentation pattern by more detailed analysis of the form of bilirubin or methaemoglobin present, and to quantitate individually the amount of each pigment present; however, this is of doubtful clinical value. Bilirubin will cross the blood–brain barrier to some extent and increased levels will be found in the CSF of jaundiced patients. Various formulae are available to correct for this, although their validity in all cases is questionable. It must also be borne in mind that where there is an obstruction to the flow of CSF resulting in elevated protein concentrations there will also be a detectable increase in bilirubin in the CSF.

Various other changes in the composition of the CSF will follow a subarachnoid haemorrhage, although not all are well documented. An increase in total protein concentration is to be expected, owing to the presence of blood, the concentration increasing by approximately 0.01 g/L for every 1000 red cells per 10^{-9} L. Increases in various enzymes, including CK, have also been detected and there may also be changes in the level of various prostaglandins, monoamine metabolites, amino acids, somatomedins and hypoxanthine, although these appear not to be of great diagnostic value. There are also unconfirmed suggestions that the measurement of CSF lactate may be of value in distinguishing haemorrhage from a traumatic tap, although this can be achieved easily in most cases by visual and spectrophotometric examination of successively collected specimens. Changes in electrolyte homeostasis have been reported in patients with subarachnoid haemorrhage:[28] serum and CSF calcium, serum magnesium and CSF potassium concentrations were all decreased, whereas sodium levels remain unaltered. These changes cannot be explained simply in terms of damage to the blood–brain barrier. Changes in potassium concentration may be due to alteration of the active transport systems or by an increase in potassium reabsorption from the CSF; the decrease in calcium may reflect its transport into cells in a cascade of ischaemic injury. The study was, however, too small to determine whether there was any causal relation between the changes in CSF calcium and potassium and symptoms of delayed cerebral ischaemia.

Increases in neuropeptide Y have also been demonstrated in the CSF at 6–11 days after the haemorrhage. This is a potent vasoconstrictive agent that may play a part in the pathogenesis of the cerebral vasospasm which often occurs after subarachnoid haemorrhage.[29] A similar causal relation between elevated CSF endothelin and vasospasm has been suggested.[30]

CNS INFECTIONS

Infections of the CNS are responsible for considerable morbidity and mortality.[31] While investigations can usually establish the presence of infection, identification of the causative agent is often difficult, particularly after antibiotic therapy. Infections can produce biochemical effects either specific to the causative micro-organism or due to the effects of the CNS destruction and/or dysfunction. It is not surprising that in the latter case infection produces biochemical changes that are similar to those associated with other causes of tissue damage and that lack diagnostic specificity.

The most common infectious disease in neurology is *meningitis*, an inflammation of the membranes surrounding the brain and spinal cord. Biochemical tests have centred on the problem of differentiating between the various types of infecting micro-organism so that appropriate therapy can be rapidly begun. At present, probably the greatest initial weight is given to the differential white-cell count. Large numbers of polymorphs indicate the likelihood of an acute pyogenic bacterial meningitis, while viral infection produces a predominantly lymphocytic picture. Tuberculous meningitis and fungal meningitis often give modest cell counts of mixed type. Cell counts are not always unambiguous. The time taken to culture specific organisms may be prohibitive when treatment needs to be started at once.

As described above, CSF *glucose* is still a widely used test. Although insensitive, a CSF glucose below 2 mmol/L is none the less a useful, rapid indicator of a bacterial meningitis. Glucose concentration is believed to be lowered primarily by metabolism of cells in the CSF and is thus an indicator of the degree of infection. There is a role for a rapid but more sensitive and specific test to differentiate between types of meningitic micro-organism and several candidate analytes have been considered.

CSF *ferritin* is increased in viral and bacterial meningitis, the latter showing the highest values. Unfortunately it is not specific as it is also increased in some patients with strokes or transient ischaemic attacks and in some with leukaemia, particularly if there is meningeal involvement.

There has been some debate as to the source of the increased concentrations of CSF ferritin. Studies of isoforms of ferritin suggest that the increase is principally produced within the CSF or brain meninges rather than by leakage of the blood–CSF barrier. It may be an indicator of meningeal cell damage and possible release by macrophages during phagocytosis. CSF ferritin, perhaps expressed as a ratio to serum ferritin, may be of value in differentiating bacterial from viral meningitis.[32]

Lactate and *NSE* are other indicators of cellular damage that are elevated in meningitis.[21,33] NSE is increased in a range of other disorders. Lactate may be elevated by several mechanisms but the current view is that it is raised because of disordered brain metabolism and anoxia. This differs from an earlier view that it is produced by the presence of white blood cells and/or leucocyte-induced bacterial lysis.

Lactate can be raised in fungal and bacterial meningitis, including tuberculous meningitis in which levels are initially high but do not seem to correlate well with recovery or treatment. Fungal meningitis often presents non-specifically as a chronic infection. The sensitivity of fungal culture of CSF is low, and the procedure is costly and time-consuming. The presence of a high CSF lactate, although itself a non-specific finding, may alert clinicians to the possibility of unsuspected fungal meningitis.

Lysozyme is liberated from degenerating polymorphs and from monocytes and macrophages that are found in high concentration in the meninges in bacterial, fungal and granulomatous meningitis.[34] It is active against the mucopolysaccharide components of certain bacterial cell walls. Although also elevated in CSF in CNS tumours, very high concentrations are found in bacterial or fungal meningitis as compared to small elevations in viral meningitis, suggesting that lysozyme may also be valuable in differential diagnosis. Lysozyme levels seem to reflect response to treatment; however, this may be deceptive as lysozyme may be directly affected by certain drugs used in therapy.

Lactoferrin, an iron-binding protein found in the secretory granules of polymorphs and released from the cells during phagocytosis, differentiates well between bacterial and viral meningitis.[35]

Another important biochemical marker that has been advocated as differentiating bacterial from viral meningitis is *C-reactive protein* (CRP). This has a potential advantage that it can be measured in serum, the serum test giving good discrimination and being a good prognostic indicator of neurological complications. The increase in CRP seems to reflect inflammatory damage to brain tissue.[36] CRP is an acute-phase protein that can bind to cell-surface phospholipids, although its exact role is not clear. It is produced in the liver, presumably in response to toxins or metabolites produced in response to bacterial infection that escape into the circulation. CSF CRP comes from the serum and discriminates between bacterial and viral meningitis less well. CRP acts as an opsonin and the poorer discrimination of the CSF measurement may also reflect its bacterial uptake within the CSF.

Neopterin and *β_2-microglobulin* are markers of cellular immunological response and as such are relatively non-specific. CSF levels are increased (more than the increase in serum levels) in neurological illnesses including lymphoma, multiple sclerosis and a variety of infections.[37,38] They are also markedly increased in the AIDS–dementia complex. In general, levels are not related to CSF cell count or dysfunction of the blood–brain barrier, indicating that these substances are probably released locally in the CNS. Although non-specific, these markers may be a useful indicator of the presence of AIDS–dementia complex and its response to antiviral therapy; in particular, CSF neopterin levels fall dramatically after treatment with zidovudine.

Microbiological culture is at present accepted as the main means of identifying specific organisms and

establishing antibiotic susceptibility. Identification of causative agents is also possible with immunological techniques. In meningitis, specific *antigens* can be measured against the major causative organisms.[31] The detection of bacterial antigens offers potential advantages over culture in certain circumstances. There is the likelihood of increased speed of reporting. It may also be possible to detect antigens after antibiotic treatment, when cultures will be negative, and subsequently to monitor response to treatment. While this field will probably expand, at present there are methodological difficulties. Very rapid methods such as latex immunoprecipitation, which might be suitable for 'near patient testing', often suffer from lack of diagnostic specificity and non-specific reactions (e.g. to rheumatoid factor). Of several alternative analytical approaches, countercurrent immunoelectrophoresis is time-consuming. Enzyme-linked immunosorbent assay (ELISA) also suffers in this respect, though this may improve.

Immunological detection of *antibodies* against causative agents is also possible. Examples include the detection of locally produced CSF antibodies against herpes simplex virus type 1, which can be responsible for encephalitis and more rarely acute myelitis or meningitis. Antibody against neurologically active agents can also be detected in serum. For example, methods are available to detect serum antibodies to *Borrelia burgdorferi*, the causative agent of Lyme disease, a tick-borne infection that can give the symptoms of meningitis. Such biochemical and immunological investigations are increasingly likely to complement microbiological methods.

Biochemical investigations may be of value in establishing the identity of a causative organism. For example, tuberculous meningitis can be diagnosed by the detection of *tuberculostearic acid* (10-methyloctadecanoic acid), a component of the mycobacterial cell wall, in the CSF.[39] Although the equipment required at present (gas chromatography/mass spectrometry) is seldom available in routine laboratories, the test enables a relatively sensitive and specific diagnosis to be made within hours. This compares to a period of several weeks necessary to culture *Mycobacterium tuberculosis*. Tuberculostearic acid is elevated for many weeks but does not reflect the effectiveness of treatment. However, it has the diagnostic advantage that it remains in the CSF after a patient has been given antituberculous therapy on clinical grounds.

Although not completely specific, two other biochemical tests, CSF *adenosine deaminase* and the *bromide partition test*, usefully discriminate between tuberculous and other forms of meningitis.[40]

DEMYELINATING DISEASES

Multiple Sclerosis

Multiple sclerosis (MS) was first identified as a distinct neurological disease by Charcot in 1868. Since then, an enormous amount of research has sought to establish the cause of the disease, which remains unknown.

The hallmark of MS is loss of myelin, which results in the formation of lesions in the brain with characteristic toughened appearances called plaques.

MS causes a variety of neurological symptoms including visual disturbances, limb weakness and often premature death. The frequency of onset of MS begins to increase around 17 years of age, reaching a peak around 30 years of age; it is relatively rare after the age of 60.

The variable course and severity of MS is the most remarkable feature of the disease. It may be so mild as to be imperceptible and only accidentally discovered at autopsy. Alternatively, it may become progressive, or even be progressive from the onset, eventually leading to various crippling neurological symptoms. Most frequently, however, the course is a relapsing and remitting one, with new neurological symptoms developing at intervals of several months or even years between each attack. The precise nature of the neurological symptoms depends on the site of the demyelination within the CNS.

The global distribution of MS seems to be associated with particular regions rather than with any racial subgroup of people living in those regions, and is unaffected by the place(s) in which affected individuals lived during childhood.

MS is common in Europe and in North America but uncommon in northern China, northern Japan, Africa and the West Indies. The prevalence in Europe is about 40/100 000 and is particularly high in the Orkney Islands at 258/100 000 and 310/100 000 in Northern Ireland, the highest in the world.

In the CNS, nerve fibres (axons) are enclosed in a sheath of myelin laid down by specialized cells, the oligodendrocytes. The chief element of the white matter is the myelin sheath. In MS, it is not known whether the demyelination is the result of an immune attack that damages the myelin, or the oligodendrocyte or both.

Myelin is a complex combination of protein (30%) and lipid (70%), of which three major protein fractions have been investigated. Of these, myelin basic protein (MBP) has been the most extensively studied because when it is injected into an animal it elicits a cellular antibody response that produces an autoimmune disease of the brain called *experimental allergic encephalomyelitis*. This disease produces areas of inflammation and demyelination that in some respects resemble MS. MBP is, as described above, a highly alkaline protein with a pI greater than 12 and a molecular size of 18 kDa.

In MS, as demyelination in the plaques progresses the myelin sheath is broken down and fragments of MBP may be detected in the CSF. The plaques are almost always around a small vein (perivascular cuffing), which is surrounded by inflammatory cells

(lymphocytes). In the early stages of these inflammatory lesions there is a zone of oedema immediately surrounding this cuff. In active lesions, cuffing frequently infiltrates along the vein, preceding demyelination. The demyelinating plaques are frequently found in close proximity to CSF-containing areas and for that reason it has been suggested that demyelination may be due to some toxic agent in the CSF.

Demyelination is accompanied by the infiltration of brain tissue by lymphocytes, plasma cells and macrophages. The presence of T and B lymphocytes and plasma cells suggests that an antibody-dependent, cell-mediated immune response may be responsible for demyelination in MS. However, the identities of possible antigens are unknown.

There have been many attempts to identify the various specific antibodies that constitute the oligoclonal IgG bands that occur in the CSF of patients with MS. Antibodies to measles virus have been identified in the CSF of MS patients but not exclusively, as antibodies to other viruses have also been identified.

It has been suggested that the oligoclonal IgG bands may be an epiphenomenon, not related to the pathogenesis of MS, but rather that lymphocytes have penetrated the blood–brain barrier in response to an immune reaction and then secreted antibodies that they had previously been programmed to synthesize.

In MS, the proportion of κ to λ immunoglobulin light chains is frequently increased. Normally, their ratio in CSF is the same as in serum (6:4) but in MS and some other neurological diseases the two may diverge. As there is no reason to suppose that κ-chains are preferentially transported across the blood–CSF barrier, this increased ratio must be regarded as further evidence that some immunoglobulin is synthesized intrathecally.

The differential diagnosis of MS is still a difficult one because the diversity of symptoms can easily be mistaken for those of many other neurological diseases. Diagnosis is made even more difficult by the absence of a specific diagnostic test. Hence the diagnosis of MS is still primarily a clinical one.

The criteria upon which the diagnosis is made rely upon a number of schemes that classify MS into several diagnostic categories, e.g. definite, probable, possible, etc.

The latest attempt at defining rational criteria links clinical with laboratory findings. In this scheme,[41] laboratory support for diagnosis is confined to the presence of oligoclonal IgG bands in the CSF. The detection of these bands is therefore now an established and important aid in the diagnosis of MS.

Examination of CSF in Demyelinating Diseases

CSF in Multiple Sclerosis

MS is the most common demyelinating disease of the human nervous system. As outlined above, the diagnosis is still made largely by clinical criteria but is now supplemented with information from CSF in the form of the presence of intrathecally synthesized, oligoclonal IgG bands.

In MS there is an increase in the white-cell count in one-third of patients, while the remainder are normal. Two-thirds of MS patients have a normal CSF total protein concentration (0.1–0.5 g/L) and a mild elevation occurs in other patients. An elevation greater than 1 g/L is rare in MS. The total CSF IgG is usually elevated in MS, while the serum immunoglobulins are normal.

The most sensitive and useful CSF test in suspected MS is electrophoresis, preferably IEF, to identify oligoclonal IgG bands. These bands are found in over 90% of MS patients. CSF oligoclonal bands usually differ between patients with MS but they remain remarkably constant in most individual patients for years. This constancy is useful in distinguishing chronic inflammatory diseases such as MS and subacute sclerosing panencephalitis (SSPE) from acute post-infectious demyelinating diseases and Guillan–Barré syndrome, in which oligoclonal bands are transient.

In addition to helping in diagnosis of clinically definite MS, CSF studies provide more diagnostic information in cases of possible early demyelination. For example, patients with optic neuritis who also have oligoclonal bands have a significantly greater chance of developing MS than those without. Thus, the presence of oligoclonal bands in suspected early demyelination leads to a significantly greater chance of developing MS.

CSF in Guillain–Barré Syndrome

Changes in CSF in the Guillain–Barré syndrome are highly dependent on the timing of the lumbar puncture in relation to the disease course, in contrast to MS where the CSF changes are more constant over time. When the patient presents with Guillain–Barré syndrome, typically there are no excess white cells in conjunction with an elevated CSF total protein concentration, although pleocytosis does occur in about 20% of cases. An elevation of CSF total protein is characteristic, though not invariable, and in Guillain–Barré syndrome is often between 1 and 5 g/L. A raised CSF IgG concentration, IgG index and the appearance of oligoclonal bands occur in the majority of patients. These, however, are usually transient and only remain abnormal in the few patients that develop chronic disease.

CSF in Other Demyelinating Diseases

Demyelinating diseases in general all show the same CSF changes as MS. The only distinguishing features are the differing clinical presentations and the temporary nature of the CSF abnormalities in the acute demyelinating conditions. In the chronic conditions, such as SSPE, there is persistent CSF abnormality that is distinct from that in MS, except

for the characteristic elevated measles titre in SSPE.

Examination of CSF for Myelin Basic Protein

As described above, MBP is one of the major components of the myelin sheath. Increased levels of MBP or MBP fragments have been detected in the CSF in a variety of neurological demyelinating diseases, including MS.

Several radioimmunoassays have been developed but results depend upon the type of antiserum used. Not all antisera recognize the same epitopes on the MBP molecule, which may give rise to interlaboratory variations in results.

The detection of MBP in CSF is a useful research technique but is not in routine clinical use.

Examination of CSF for Antimyelin Antibodies

Antibodies to MBP are reportedly present in the CSF of all patients with clinically active MS. By contrast, patients whose disease is in remission have undetectable antimyelin antibody. Elevated levels of antimyelin antibodies are not specific for MS but they are strongly associated with disease activity and may be involved in the pathogenesis of demyelination.

EPILEPSY

The main involvement of the clinical biochemistry department in epilepsy is in the measurement of anticonvulsant drugs. Clinical biochemistry also has a role in the diagnosis of epilepsy and its differentiation from non-epileptic pseudoseizures. It is generally accepted that a certain proportion of so-called epileptics in the population fail to show evidence of organic disease on detailed examination. Furthermore, pseudoseizures can occur in a proportion of true epileptics, adding to the diagnostic confusion. This difficulty can be resolved by using electroencephalographic telemetry and closed-circuit television. However, the expense of this technique has led to considerable interest in the application of *serum prolactin* measurement to this problem.[42]

After a tonic–clonic, partial-complex seizure, plasma prolactin levels rise, reaching a peak in 15–20 min. The half-life of prolactin is approximately 20 min and levels decline to a baseline after about 60 min. Although criteria have varied, an increase in serum taken 20 min after the seizure of at least twice (sometimes three times) the baseline prolactin concentration is taken as indicating true epilepsy.

Prolactin is not elevated in CSF during the time of the test. This indicates that release of prolactin is into the peripheral circulation, presumably in response to neurophysiological disturbances.

DEMENTIA

Dementia affects approximately 5% of 65 year olds

and 20% of 80 year olds. In the elderly about 75% of cases are caused by primary brain degeneration (Alzheimer's disease). Of the rest about 15% have multi-infarct dementia but the remainder have conditions that can be treated or at least stabilized.[43] These include many biochemical causes such as hypothyroidism, vitamin B_{12} deficiency, Wilson's disease, alcohol abuse and heavy metal poisoning, as well as vascular, infectious, neoplastic, epileptic and traumatic causes. Pseudodementia in depression or after sedative or hypnotic intoxication may also mimic Alzheimer's disease.

Confirmatory diagnosis of Alzhiemer's disease requires demonstration of characteristic changes (neurofibrillary tangles and senile plaques) either at biopsy or autopsy. While clinical biochemists can shed light on some of the underlying causes (e.g. hypothyroidism), it is not surprising that there have also been attempts to develop biochemical markers for Alzheimer's disease itself.

Despite early findings that cholinergic neurons were damaged in Alzheimer's disease it was soon apparent that deficiencies in several other types of neurotransmitters and their neurons occur and that these changes may be secondary to generalized damage rather than the primary cause of the disease. Nevertheless, measurements of neurotransmitters and their metabolites in CSF show alterations in Alzheimer's disease, some of which could eventually prove diagnostically useful as well as throwing light on the pathological processes involved.

Early studies showed reductions in metabolites of CSF dopamine and serotonin but with low predictive value. Technical difficulties in measuring the low concentrations of metabolites found in lumbar CSF have tended to prevent the emergence of clinically useful tests. However, technical advances, such as improved high-performance liquid chromatographic methods may revitalize this approach. For example, in a small study, good discrimination between Alzheimer's patients and controls was found when measuring homovanillic acid and 3,4-dihydroxyphenylacetic acid in CSF.[44]

An early pathological finding in Alzheimer's disease was a decrease in the activity of *acetylcholinesterase* in the cerebral cortex. This has led to many reports of measurements of CSF acetylcholinesterase, roughly equal numbers demonstrating no change or decreased levels. These discrepancies could be partly due to sampling techniques or diagnostic inconsistency, but some variation has probably also been due to assay specificity. More recent reports of a CSF test based on the use of a monoclonal antibody specific for brain acetylcholinesterase show a reasonably good separation between patients and controls though further studies will be needed to establish the diagnostic potential of the assay.[45]

The finding of aluminium silicate deposits in the neurons containing neurofibrillary tangles has caused considerable excitement, although, as in the case of neurotransmitter changes, it has not been resolved whether they represent cause or effect. Neither is it yet clear whether aluminium intake or serum aluminium concentrations have any relation to the pathogenesis of Alzheimer's disease. High serum aluminium concentrations do occur in chronic renal failure and in patients receiving haemodialysis with aluminium-rich dialysate and are associated with a form of dementia.

Alzheimer's disease is known to have an immunological component and immunological methods seem to hold the greatest diagnostic potential. High levels of antiglial fibrillary acid protein (antiGFAP) have been found in the serum of Alzheimer patients; 80% of patients with onset before the age of 65 (presenile) but only 30% of patients with older onset (senile dementia of the Alzheimer type) had raised concentrations, as compared with raised levels in only 9% of patients with multi-infarct dementia, in no patients with stroke and in less than 2% of age-matched controls.[46] A particular application of the assay could be to distinguish Alzheimer's disease from vascular causes of dementia.

TUMOURS OF THE CNS

Primary intracranial tumours may arise from the brain and its soft tissue or bony covering or from the cranial nerves or the pituitary, while metastases may spread from virtually any other tumour to the brain, the most common primary sites being the bronchus, breast and kidney. In adults the most common neoplasms are gliomas, which are infiltrative tumours, meningiomas, which are essentially benign, or metastases, whereas in children the most common are medulloblastomas or astrocytomas, frequently arising in the posterior fossa. The CNS is the second most common site of primary tumours in children.

Most of the CNS tissues are thought to come from primitive neural epithelium, known as neuroectoderm, which subsequently differentiates through a number of stages to produce two main cell types, nerve cells and glial cells. Two main forms of glial cell can be identified—the macroglia of ectodermal origin and the smaller microglia of mesodermal origin. Macroglia develop from a common stem cell, the spongioblast, to produce three main cell types, the astrocyte, the oligodendrocyte and the ependymal cells.

All three cell types are capable of undergoing malignant transformation to produce the tumours known collectively as gliomas. A simplified classification of the major CNS primary tumours is shown in Fig. 32.4.

Pituitary adenomas are the most common pituitary tumours and are generally benign. They may be secreting or non-secreting, the non-secretory tumours being more frequently associated with compression of the optic chiasma. These tumours will be dealt with in greater detail elsewhere.

Figures provided by the World Health Organiza-

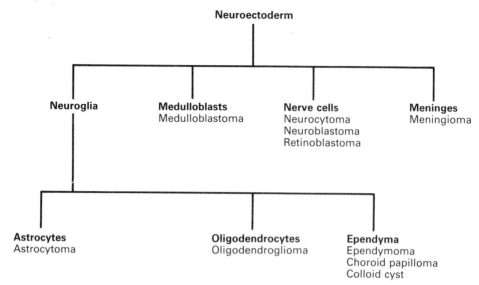

Figure 32.4 Classification of tumours of the central nervous system.

tion, based on mortality rates from malignant brain tumours from 27 countries, indicate an incidence of intracranial tumours of approximately 5 in 100 000, ranging from 1 in 100 000 in Mexico to 7 in 100 000 in Israel. However, there are a number of difficulties in interpreting these official figures and more rigorous studies, based upon defined populations, have yielded figures ranging from approximately 12 in 100 000 to as high as 46 in 100 000, the latter figure including nine cases of pituitary tumours.

The most common signs and symptoms of CNS tumours, which may occur alone or in combination, are:

- general, non-localized symptoms, e.g. epilepsy or mental symptoms;
- focal symptoms, e.g. hemiparesis or cranial nerve palsy;
- features of raised intracranial pressure, e.g. headaches.

Symptoms of raised intracranial pressure may arise as a result of a mass effect, cerebral oedema or through obstructive hydrocephalus. As well as headaches, other symptoms of raised intracranial pressure may be observed, particularly vomiting, drowsiness or visual disturbances.

The differential diagnosis of CNS tumours must include the elimination of other causes of raised intracranial pressure, including cerebral abscesses, benign intracranial hypertension and chronic subdural haematomas. Up to 95% of tumours can now be detected by CT scanning with contrast enhancement, and in most cases this would then be confirmed by biopsy.

A biopsy smear technique is generally used rather than a frozen section as this shows far more detailed cytology, although at the expense of tissue architecture. Specimens can be processed, stained and exam-

ined within 10 min with a reported accuracy of 94%, prior to surgical debulking of the tumour mass when appropriate.

Despite the high success rate of CT scanning and where necessary NMR scanning, there are still a number of advocates of the use of potential biochemical markers of malignancy in the CNS. A review cites nearly 100 papers on the use of biochemical markers of CNS tumours, including CSF cytology, human chorionic gonadotrophin, alphafetoprotein, carcinoembryonic antigen, polyamines, fibronectin and other glycoproteins, GFAP, S-100, NSE and MBP.[47] The author of this particular review went so far as to lament the fact that few of these putative markers of malignancy had found their way into clinical practice. This is despite the fact that over 70% of patients with gliomas, the most common form of CNS tumour, suffer headaches or other symptoms of raised intracranial pressure at presentation. Lumbar puncture is contraindicated, owing to the high risk of fatal herniation of the medial temporal lobe or of the cerebellar tonsils through the foramen magnum (coning). There is also the theoretical risk of promoting the spread of a metastatic tumour through the site of the lumbar puncture.

Nevertheless, lumbar puncture may occasionally be made when a tumour is not suspected, or after a careful neurological examination in some individuals when it is considered that the investigation may be of diagnostic value. This is most likely in cases of suspected medulloblastoma or pineal tumour, or carcinomatous meningitis when exfoliative cytology may be diagnostic. The detection rates are relatively low, however. CSF examination is also useful in cases of subacute meningitis of unknown aetiology for evidence of the increased protein and reduced glucose in the absence of microbial infection that is characteristic of diffuse meningeal tumours. Changes in LDH isoenzyme patterns in the CSF have been identified in cases of carcinomatous meningitis. Furthermore, considerable elevations of alkaline phosphatase have been found in cases of pulmonary carcinomatous meningitis.

Assay of serum: CSF β-HCG ratios is useful in detecting cerebral metastases of germ-cell tumours or in the diagnosis of pineal germinomas, ratios of less than 0.1 being strongly suggestive of germ-cell tumour. Increased levels of the placental alkaline phosphatase isoenzyme are also said to be diagnostic for pineal germinomas.[48] Assay of fibronectin, enolase and of β_2-microglobulin in CSF may also be of value in identifying CNS involvement in cases of acute leukaemia.

Some of these increased concentrations of biochemical markers in the CSF will 'spill over' into the blood; however, the high systemic contribution to the serum concentration of many of these markers will in most cases mask any increased contribution by the CNS. There are certain markers that are only or primarily produced by CNS tissue and in these cases, assuming that the marker is not extensively metabolized within the CNS, may appear in the serum in sufficient concentration to be detected. Although, with the exception of neuroendocrine tumours, these are unlikely to be of diagnostic value, they may be useful in monitoring therapy, whether radiotherapy or chemotherapy. Chemotherapy of CNS tumours poses particular problems, partly because of the relative impermeability of the blood–brain barrier to many of the drugs most likely to be effective. There are also difficulties in assessing the initial response to therapy because successful chemotherapy may result in cerebral oedema, resulting in an initial deterioration in the patient's condition. Several novel approaches to improve the chemotherapy of CNS tumours are being developed[49] and because of the difficulties outlined above the measurement of tumour markers in the serum could be of considerable future value in assessing the efficacy of these approaches. S-100 protein is elevated in the serum in approximately 40% of patients with CNS tumours, although there is a wide range of potential markers that have yet to be studied in detail including NSE, various growth factors and cell-surface antigens such as astrocytin and malignin. CNS tumours are immunogenic and induce an immune response; serum sample from up to 75% of patients with gliomas may contain glioma cross-reacting antibodies. Monoclonal antibody techniques to develop new tumour-specific marker assays may prove to be of value in the future.

Various non-specific changes may also be observed in the serum. The erythrocyte sedimentation rate (ESR) may be significantly increased in cases of cerebral secondaries arising from a latent systemic cancer and the non-specific acute-phase proteins, in particular haptoglobin, α_1-acid glycoprotein and α_1-antitrypsin may be elevated in a variety of primary CNS tumours, particularly gliomas. Increases in serum levels of glycoprotein associated carbohydrates including sialic acid, neutral hexose and fucose have also been demonstrated in cases of astrocytoma, meningioma and pituitary adenomas. With the possible exception of the ESR, these changes are of little diagnostic value.

Neuroblastomas affect 1 in 6000 to 1 in 10 000 children under 15 years of age in developed countries, about a quarter of cases occurring in the first year of life. It is the only childhood tumour for which a population screening test has been suggested as over 90% of clinically diagnosed cases have been shown to have elevated levels of one or more catecholamine metabolites. Most current screening assays are based on the detection of homovanillic acid or 4-hydroxy-3-methoxymandelic acid in the urine during the first 6 months of life, although various other changes have been reported in this condition including elevations in plasma levels of enolase and gangliosides. Screening programmes are already in operation in some countries, notably Japan,[50] and are likely to become more widely accepted as the techniques for detection improve.

NUTRITIONAL AND SYSTEMIC DISORDERS AFFECTING THE CNS

One would predict that virtually any systemic biochemical disorder could cause neurological symptoms if sufficiently severe. This is true of conditions affecting many common analytes such as glucose, lipids, hydrogen ions, calcium and electrolytes. Causative diseases are varied and numerous including, for example, trauma, endocrine and nutritional disorders (e.g. vitamin D deficiency). It is beyond the scope of this chapter to discuss each of these disorders, even though analyses related to systemic disease (e.g. electrolyte measurement) form a major part of the management of neurological patients.

Several vitamin deficiencies that have neurological manifestations are worthy of mention. Fifteen years ago the prevailing view was that *vitamin E* (α-tocopherol) *deficiency* had not been clearly shown to produce effects in man. Since then the consensus has changed and recent studies have implicated vitamin E deficiency as a cause of the spinocerebellar neuropathies of lipid malabsorption, including abetalipoproteinaemia.[51] Assay of vitamin E has now become an important biochemical investigation in conditions associated with lipid malabsorption and in spinocerebellar syndromes of unknown aetiology.

The mechanism by which the deficiency causes neurological damage is not clear but may be due to loss of antioxidant activity causing peroxidation of membrane phospholipids. Symptoms include progressive ataxia, nystagmus, sensory impairment, areflexia

TABLE 32.2
SUMMARY OF BIOCHEMICAL INVESTIGATIONS IN NEUROLOGY

TABLE 32.2
SUMMARY OF BIOCHEMICAL INVESTIGATIONS IN NEUROLOGY

1. *Tests probably available at the local hospital*
   Glucose, urea and electrolytes, etc.
   CSF glucose and protein (and cell count, cytology)
   Lipids, thyroid and adrenal function tests, vitamin B_{12}
   Pituitary endocrine investigations and prolactin (in epilepsy)
   Therapeutic drug measurement, alcohol
   CSF lactate
   C-reactive protein

2. *Tests that may require referral to specialist centre (for test and/or interpretation)*
   CSF electrophoresis
   Lysozyme
   Antinuclear antibody (or anticardiolipin antibody)
   Antiacetylcholine-receptor antibody
   Angiotensin-converting enzyme
   Congenital and genetic defects
   Toxic metals
   Vitamin E
   Thiamin
   Ferritin (CSF)

3. *Tests that may be performed in specialist centres (e.g. for research) but may be available only by arrangement*
   Indicators of trauma (one or more of CK-BB, B-ELI, NSE, S-100)
   Specific indicators in infection, e.g. tuberculostearic acid
   Myelin basic protein (or fragments)
   Neurotransmitters and their metabolites
   Acetylcholinesterase
   AntiGFAP
   Neopterins

and ophthalmoplegia, and sometimes generalized muscle weakness. Generalized fat malabsorption is almost always present, although a few patients have been found to have a specific defect in vitamin E absorption.

Vitamin E status can be readily assessed by measuring its concentration in serum or plasma. As levels of vitamin E reflect those of total lipid, which may be altered, for example, in cholestasis, the ratio of vitamin E to serum lipids may be measured. Alternative functional investigations have been proposed that measure the antioxidant activity of the vitamin. One example is the measurement of the formation of malondialdehyde generated by the peroxidation of erythrocyte polyunsaturated fatty acids exposed to hydrogen peroxide. It is also possible to measure breath pentane produced by peroxidation of polyunsaturated fatty acids in the body.

Of the water-soluble vitamins, nicotinic acid, thiamin and vitamin B_{12} deficiency can produce neurological symptoms. *Nicotinic acid deficiency* can produce a dementia that exhibits irritability and depression. However, laboratory investigation is unreliable.

Thiamin deficiency has both peripheral and central effects. Wernicke's encephalopathy is an acute cerebral manifestation of severe deficiency. Beriberi is a major nutritional problem in developing countries while in the West alcoholism is the major cause of deficiency, giving rise to the Wernicke–Korsakoff syndrome.[52] The most popular laboratory investigation is erythrocyte transketolase. The measurements of thiamin or its metabolites in urine or blood pyruvate levels are less helpful in establishing thiamin status.

Vitamin B_{12} deficiency can cause subacute degeneration of the spinal cord. Deficiency is established by serum measurement. True dietary deficiency is very rare. Low serum vitamin levels are caused in true pernicious anaemia by intrinsic-factor deficiency and they can also be found in generalized malabsorption states. It is important to assess folate status, usually by erythrocyte folate measurement, even though folate deficiency does not cause subacute cord degeneration. While the megaloblastic anaemia can be reversed by folate administration, in pernicious anaemia the neurological condition is not helped and may be aggravated.

THE ROLE OF THE LABORATORY IN INVESTIGATING CNS DISEASE

The average laboratory serving a range of specialities including some neurological patients will not have facilities to perform most of the investigations discussed. It may be useful to consider which investigations could be done in a routine (e.g. district general) hospital, and which should be referred to specialist centres. Table 32.2 lists some of the investigations that are likely to produce clinically meaningful results but may have to be referred to a specialist centre and some that are usually done in specialist centres but whose potential clinical role is still the subject of research. Some of the latter may nevertheless be available under certain circumstances by arrangement. Available investigations will vary depending on local facilities and as research progresses.

CONCLUSION AND FUTURE PROSPECTS

There is little doubt that clinical biochemistry will continue to have a role in the diagnosis and management of nervous disease and that research and development will continue. Improvements in existing methodology, such as high-performance chromatography, will improve understanding of the roles of neurotransmitters and metabolic abnormalities. New roles for biochemists will probably emerge, such as *in vivo* detection and monitoring of metabolic abnormalities using the technique of NMR, at present largely the province of the radiologist.

Perhaps the most far-reaching revolution in the range of available techniques lies in the fields of the 'new genetics' and in immunodiagnostics. While there are perhaps 3000 known genetic diseases, these clearly represent only a small part of the total that the 100 000 genes of the human chromosomes plays in disease. Through chromosomal mapping techniques, within the next few years a 'high-resolution' map of the human genome will become available. Once gene products are identified, complementary DNA (cDNA) can be synthesized, labelled (e.g. with phosphorus-32) and used as probes to identify abnormal genes in electrophoresed DNA of individuals. There are applications of this technique now appearing in the literature, often potentially superseding current biochemical applications.

An example of the application of recent DNA techniques is in the precise diagnosis of the rare condition, familial amyloid polyneuropathy. This is an autosomal dominant disease with insidious onset in adulthood and causes peripheral neuropathy and autonomic failure. The amyloid deposited has been identified as the product of a one-point mutation of the gene for transthyretin (more commonly known as prealbumin). The mutation can be detected using the cDNA for the transthyretin gene as a probe.[53]

Another major expansion has come about through the development of monoclonal antibodies. This has enabled a much wider range of specific antibodies to biological molecules to be produced than has been possible by polyclonal techniques. The use of monoclonal antibody to acetylcholinesterase in the diagnosis of Alzheimer's disease has been mentioned. Monoclonal antibodies are commercially exploitable and new assays such as measuring proteins from neurofibrillary tangles, also for diagnosis of Alzheimer's disease,[54] may soon be added to the diagnostic repertoire.

In the future, clinical biochemists should be actively involved in the research and development of these new techniques and their clinical applications. In addition, they are likely to be faced with a much wider choice of diagnostic tests in neurology. This will increase their responsibility for assessing which of the many investigations are likely to yield the most meaningful and beneficial clinical information and for effectively communicating this information to colleagues.

REFERENCES

1. Spector R., Johanson C.E. (1989). The mammalian choroid plexus. *Sci. Am.*, **261**, 48.
2. Pearce J.M.B. (1982). Hazards of lumbar puncture. *Br. Med. J.*, **285**, 1521.
3. Patten J. (1983). *Neurological Differential Diagnosis*, London: Harold Starke.
4. Arevalo C.E. et al. (1989). Cerebrospinal fluid cell counts and chemistries in bacterial meningitis. *South. Med. J.*, **82**, 1122.
5. Rosenthal F.D., Soothill J.F. (1962). An immunochemical study of the proteins in cerebrospinal fluid. *J. Neurol. Neurosurg. Psychiatry*, **25**, 177.
6. Wollemann M. (1974). *Biochemistry of Brain Tumours*, London: Macmillan.
7. Hosein Z.Z., Johnson K.P. (1981). Isoelectric focusing of cerebrospinal fluid proteins in the diagnosis of multiple sclerosis. *Neurology*, **31**, 70.
8. Zaffaroni M., Caputo D., Cazzullo C.L. (1983). Isotachophoresis evaluation of synthesis of intrathecal IgG subfractions in multiple sclerosis. *J. Neurol.*, **229**, 55.
9. Toutellotte W.W. et al. (1982). Isotachophoresis quantitation of subfractions of multiple sclerosis intra-blood–brain barrier IgG synthesis modulated by ACTH and/or steroids. *Neurology*, **32**, 261.
10. Delpech B., Lichtblau E. (1972). Etude quantitative des immunoglobins G et de l'albumine du liquide cephalo rachidien. *Clin. Chim. Acta*, **37**, 15.
11. Tourtellotte W.W., Ma I.B. (1978). Multiple sclerosis. The blood–brain barrier and the measurement of *de novo* central nervous system IgG synthesis. *Neurology*, **28**, 76.
12. Lowenthal A. (1984). *Agar Gel Electrophoresis in Neurology*, Amsterdam: Elsevier.
13. Latterre E.C. (1972). Protein patterns in pathological CSF. In *Multiple Sclerosis: A Reappraisal* (McAlpine D. ed.) Edinburgh: Churchill Livingstone, pp. 408–412.
14. Ornstein C. (1964). Disc electrophoresis-I. Background and theory. *Ann. N. Y. Acad. Sci.*, **121**, 321.
15. Davis B.J. (1964). Disc electrophoresis-II. Method and application to human serum proteins. *Ann. N. Y. Acad. Sci.*, **121**, 404.
16. Walker R.W.H. et al. (1983). A rapid method for detecting oligoclonal IgG in unconcentrated CSF by agarose isoelectric focusing, transfer to cellulose nitrate and immunoperoxidase staining. *J. Neuroimmunol.* **4**, 141.
17. Bjellqvist B. et al. (1982). Isoelectric focusing in immobilised pH gradients principle, methodology and some application. *J. Biochem. Biophys. Methods*, **6**, 317.
18. Cowdrey G.N. et al. (1990). The separation and detection of alkaline oligoclonal IgG bands in cerebrospinal fluid using immobilised pH gradients. *Electrophoresis*, **11**, 813.
19. Barrett A.J., Davis E.M., Grubb A. (1984). The place of human gamma-trace (cystatin C) amongst the cysteine proteinase inhibitors. *Biochem. Biophys. Res. Commun.*, **120**, 631.
20. Armbruster D.A., Greumer H. (1988). The regional variability of enzymes in the brain: relevance to CSF enzyme determinations. *Clin. Chim. Acta*, **175**, 227.
21. Rabow L. et al. (1986). CSF brain kinase levels and lactic acidosis in severe head injury. *J. Neurosurg.*, **65**, 625.
22. Lampl Y. (1990). Cerebrospinal fluid lactate dehydrogenase levels in early stroke and transient ischemic attacks. *Stroke*, **21**, 854.
23. Fehling C., Qvist I. (1985). Ferritin concentration in cerebrospinal fluid. *Acta Neurol. Scand.*, **71**, 510.
24. Hay E. et al. (1984). Cerebrospinal fluid enolase in stroke. *J. Neurol. Neurosurg. Psychiatry*, **47**, 724.
25. Persson L. et al. (1987). S-100 protein and neuron-specific enolase in cerebrospinal fluid and serum: markers of cell damage in human central nervous system. *Stroke*, **18**, 911.
26. Vermeulen M. et al. (1989). Xanthochromia after subarachnoid haemorrhage needs no revisitation. *J.Neurol. Neurosurg. Psychiatry*, **52**, 826.
27. Kjellin K.G. (1971). Bilirubin compounds in the CSF. *J. Neurol. Sci.*, **13**, 161.
28. Vonholst H., Mathiesen T. (1990). Electrolyte concentrations in serum and CSF following subarachnoid haemorrhage. *Br. J. Neurosurg.*, **4**, 123.

29. Susuki Y. et al. (1989). Increased neuropeptide Y concentrations in cerebrospinal fluid from patients with aneurysmal subarachnoid haemorrhage. *Stroke*, **20**, 1680.

30. Suzuki H. et al. (1990). Increased endothelin concentration in CSF from patients with subarachnoid haemorrhage. *Acta Neurol. Scand.*, **81**, 553.

31. Workshop conference: CSF analysis in the diagnosis of CNS inflammation (1989). *J. Clin. Chem. Clin. Biochem.*, **27**, 895.

32. Zappone E. et al. (1986). Cerebrospinal fluid ferritin in human disease. *Haematologica*, **71**, 103.

33. Royds J.A., Taylor C.B., Timperley W.R. (1985). Enolase isoenzymes as diagnostic markers. *Neuropathol. Appl. Neurobiol.*, **11**, 1.

34. Firth G., Rees J., McKeran R.O. (1985). The value of measurement of cerebrospinal fluid levels of lysozyme in the diagnosis of neurological disease. *J. Neurol. Neurosurg. Psychiatry*, **48**, 709.

35. Visakorpi T. et al. (1987). Cerebrospinal fluid lactoferrin in bacterial and viral meningitis. *Acta Paediatr. Scand.*, **76**, 987.

36. Petola H., Valmara P. (1984). C-reactive protein in meningitis. *Lancet*, **i**, 741.

37. Imercidori G. et al. (1990). Study of beta-2 microglobulin and neopterin in serum and cerebrospinal fluid of HIV-infected patients. *Acta Neurol.*, **12**, 58.

38. Brew B. et al. (1990). Cerebrospinal fluid neopterin in human immunodeficiency virus type 1 infection. *Ann. Neurol.*, **28**, 556.

39. French G.L. et al. (1987). Diagnosis of tuberculous meningitis by detection of tuberculostearic acid in cerebrospinal fluid. *Lancet*, **ii**, 117.

40. Mann M.D. et al. (1982). The bromine partition test and CSF adenosine deaminase activity in the diagnosis of tuberculous meningitis in children. *S. Afr. Med. J.*, **62**, 431.

41. Poser C.M. et al. (1983). New diagnostic criteria for multiple sclerosis: Guidelines for research protocols. *Ann. Neurol.*, **13**, 227.

42. Yerby M.S. et al. (1987). Serum prolactins in the diagnosis of epilepsy: sensitivity, specificity and predictive value. *Neurology*, **37**, 1224.

43. Davison K. (1985). Drug treatment of organic brain syndromes. *Br. J. Hosp. Med.*,

44. Koyama E., Minegishi A., Ishizaki T. (1988). Simultaneous determination of four monoamine metabolites and serotonin in cerebrospinal fluid by 'high performance' liquid chromatography with electrochemical detection; application for patients with Alzheimer's disease. *Clin. Chem.*, **34**, 680.

45. Rasmussen A.G., Adolfsson R., Karlsson T. (1988). New method specific for acetylcholinesterase in cerebrospinal fluid: application to Alzheimer's disease. *Lancet*, **ii**, 571–572.

46. Tanaka J. et al. (1988). A high level of anti-GFAP autoantibody in the serum of patients with Alzheimer's disease. *Biomed. Res.*, **9**, 209.

47. Koskiniemi M. (1988). Malignancy markers in the cerebrospinal fluid. *Eur. J. Pediatr.*, **148**, 3.

48. Milford Ward A. ed. (1990). *PRU Handbook of Clinical Immunochemistry*, Sheffield: PRU Publications.

49. Firth G.B. et al. (1988). Application of radioimmunoassay to monitor treatment of human cerebral gliomas with bleomycin entrapped within liposomes. *J. Chem. Pathol.*, **41**, 38.

50. Dale G. et al. (1988). Urinary excretion of HMMA and HVA in infants. *Ann. Clin. Biochem.*, **25**, 233.

51. Sokol R.J. (1988). Vitamin E deficiency and neurological disease. *Ann. Rev. Nutr.*, **8**, 351.

52. Haas R.H. (1988). Thiamin and the brain. *Ann. Rev. Nutr.*, **8**, 483.

53. Holt I.J., Middleton L., Harding A.E. (1989). Amyloid neuropathy. *Lancet*, **i**, 524–526.

54. Warner M. (1987). Diagnosis of Alzheimer's disease. *Anal. Chem.*, **59**, 1203.

33. The Biochemistry of Coma

J. de Belleroche and
F. Clifford Rose

Introduction
Hepatic encephalopathy
  Clinical forms
  The role of ammonia in causing hepatic
    encephalopathy
  Amino acids in cerebral metabolism
  Biochemical mechanisms involved in
    ammonia detoxification
  The role of the inhibitory neurotransmitter
    γ-aminobutyric acid (GABA)
Hypoxic encephalopathy
Hypoglycaemic encephalopathy
Ischaemia

INTRODUCTION

Coma is an altered level of consciousness where there is loss of awareness and responsiveness to intense sensory stimulation (*see* review by Plum and Posner[1]). Electroencephalographic (EEG) patterns disappear. It may be due to trauma or a disturbance in cerebral metabolism such as that caused by hypoxia, ischaemia, hypoglycaemia, hepatic encephalopathy or uraemia. The cause may be acute or chronic coma but, if coma is left unchecked there will be irreversible neuronal injury. Metabolic coma is usually characterized by normal pupillary responses, absent eye movements and generalized hypotonia. Other diagnostic features depend on the cause of the condition, whether endocrine (e.g. diabetes mellitus, hypothyroidism), or due to hepatic or liver failure, drugs (e.g. narcotics, alcohol, benzodiazepine), carbon monoxide, ethylene glycol, cardiovascular or infectious disease. Hypoglycaemia is readily treatable but may be fatal if left untreated. Opiate overdosage is a common cause of coma, which is reversed with naloxone, whilst some cases of poisoning may be reversible and only require observation and support therapy.

There is little doubt that reduced oxygen and glucose supplies and impaired liver or kidney function are primary events preceding coma but the biochemical mechanisms responsible for the subsequent events have been more elusive. Recently, the importance of altered levels of excitatory neurotransmitters such as glutamate in inducing coma has been highlighted: these are likely to contribute to many aspects of coma.

HEPATIC ENCEPHALOPATHY

Clinical Forms

There are two types of hepatic encephalopathy. An acute form, *fulminant hepatic failure*, is associated with rapid onset of liver disease; there is altered consciousness and progression to coma within a few hours or days. High blood ammonia concentrations are the main biochemical feature of this disease, especially at the height of the crisis. The second form is due to *chronic cirrhosis* of the liver, most commonly caused by alcoholism, but also by viral infections, drugs, biliary obstruction or exposure to some organic solvents. It is characterized by slowly developing episodes of neurological dysfunction followed by recovery.

The Role of Ammonia in Causing Hepatic Encephalopathy

One of the key agents implicated in the development of hepatic encephalopathy is ammonia. Elevated ammonia concentrations in blood and cerebrospinal fluid (CSF) have been reported in some cases of hepatic encephalopathy[2] and, further, treatments designed to lower blood ammonia levels are often beneficial. Ammonia is known to be a highly toxic agent, causing convulsions and death in experimental studies. The major means of ammonia removal in the body is through the urea cycle, which occurs mainly in the liver and has a large functional capacity. Infants born with a urea-cycle enzyme defect can have severe brain damage with impaired IQ scores unless the hyperammonaemia is treated at an early stage. The severity of this effect depends on the particular enzyme affected. Hyperammonaemia may also occur as a side-effect of treatment of epilepsy with valproate.

Despite these implications, acute ammonia toxicity alone is insufficient to explain hepatic encephalopathy since it is associated with convulsions rather than depressed activity. In addition, normal or only slightly elevated blood and CSF levels of ammonia occur in some cases of hepatic encephalopathy, and overall there is no clear correlation between ammonia concentrations and neurological status. Emphasis has more recently shifted to understanding the pathology of coma by concentrating on the amino acids from which the ammonia may be released. The three key amino acids involved in transferring amino groups are glutamate, glutamine and aspartate, which are important not only in the incorporation of amino groups into proteins and nucleic acids but also in the removal of excess ammonia. These amino acids also serve a fundamental role in central neurotransmission.

Amino Acids in Cerebral Metabolism

Glutamate and aspartate are abundant in the central nervous system. Both are normally present at millimolar concentrations and are potent excitatory neurotransmitters. Glutamate is metabolized by the action of glutamate dehydrogenase, a reversible enzyme, yielding ammonia and α-ketoglutarate as the products; in turn, glutamate can be synthesized from ammonia by the action of this enzyme. Ammonia can be incorporated into glutamate to yield glutamine by the action of glutamine synthetase or it can be released from glutamine by the action of glutaminase. In view of these interactions it is possible to understand how fluctuations in ammonia concentrations could have significant effects on levels of excitatory transmitters and hence levels of consciousness. Brain glutamate and aspartate concentrations are indeed consistently lowered in hyperammonaemic animals and the activity of glutaminase is regulated by levels of ammonia.

Biochemical Mechanisms Involved in Ammonia Detoxification

The body is normally well adapted for handling excess ammonia. Considerable flux in amino transfer is necessary for biosynthesis and catabolism of amino acids and products derived from them, such as proteins, nucleic acids, hormones and neurotransmitters. The liver plays a central role in these processes and in ensuring that excess nitrogen in the form of ammonia is detoxified into urea. Urea is harmless even up to millimolar concentrations; it is highly soluble and diffusible and represents an extremely efficient method for excretion of two amino groups in a single molecule, $NH_2\text{-}CO\text{-}NH_2$. The common pathway of nitrogen excretion involves transfer of amino groups from most amino acids to α-ketoglutarate forming glutamate, which, through the action of glutamate dehydrogenase in mitochondria, releases NH_3 for incorporation into carbamoyl phosphate and entry into the urea cycle. As the urea cycle occurs almost exclusively in the liver, conditions under which liver function is impaired can lead to elevated circulating levels of ammonia and resulting hepatic coma. Normally, arterial ammonia concentration is kept low at 0.02–0.03 mM but, if elevated to 0.2 mM, coma ensues. Only in the hepatic portal system are higher NH_4^+ concentrations normally found, being approximately 0.2 mM. This occurs because intestinal cells catalyse the release of NH_3 from glutamine by glutaminase in order to make NH_3 more readily available for catabolism in the liver.

Ammonia toxicity has been most markedly demonstrated by injection of urease, which hydrolyses urea to ammonia and causes rapid death. The specific mechanisms that lead to ammonia toxicity are not established but a number of hypotheses have been proposed: for example, it has been suggested that ammonia will lead to depleted levels of α-ketoglutarate and NADH, through the glutamate dehydrogenase reaction:

$$\alpha\text{-ketoglutarate} + NADH + H^+ + NH_3 \rightleftharpoons$$
$$glutamate + NAD^+ + H_2O.$$

However, a change in $NAD^+/NADH$ should be compensated by a change in ATP/ADP maintaining electron transfer flow through the respiratory chain and should not lead to a depletion of ATP. A more likely hypothesis is that elevated NH_4^+ concentration depletes glutamate levels through the glutamine synthetase reaction. Glutamine synthetase is localized in glial cells in brain and represents the major route of ammonia metabolism in brain.[3] Glial cells surround capillaries and neurons and thus are well adapted to metabolize blood-borne and neuronally derived ammonia. Experimental studies of the effect of infusion of ammonium salts show that large increases in tissue concentrations of ammonia are accompanied by increased glutamine and lactate concentrations without significant alterations in the concentrations of ATP, ADP, AMP, glutamate or α-ketoglutarate.[4] Levels of phosphocreatine and malate are decreased in some but not all studies. Glutamine levels increase with increased tissue concentrations of NH_4^+ up to a concentration of 2 μmol/g NH_4^+. Further increase in glutamine concentration does not occur with higher levels of NH_4^+, despite adequate enzyme levels, which may reflect an inhibitory effect of NH_4^+ on glutamine synthetase or an increased release of glutamine into the circulation. This detoxification method therefore appears to be operational only up to this level of saturation, which may reflect glutamate compartmentation.

After formation in the glia, glutamine is used as a source of glutamate in the neuron through the action of glutaminase. However, glutaminase is inhibited at concentrations of approximately 1 mM NH_4^+. It is likely that this concentration could be reached from normal tissue concentrations of 0.3 mM when circulating levels are increased 10-fold. Glutamate is a major excitatory neurotransmitter and is likely to mediate a large number of cognitive functions; hence a deficiency in glutamate could contribute to the neurological signs seen in liver disease before coma, such as lethargy and lack of drive. Elevated ammonia concentration could also regulate liver glycolysis through its regulatory effect to relieve ATP inhibition of phosphofructokinase. This would lead to increased glycolytic flux and lactic acidosis.

The Role of the Inhibitory Neurotransmitter γ-Aminobutyric Acid (GABA)

Recent developments suggest that increased GABA neurotransmission also plays a part in the pathogenesis of hepatic encephalopathy. There is evidence that elevated levels of endogenous benzodiazepine agonists occur in the central nervous system, which would facilitate GABA transmission. Endogenous ligands that are known to bind to the benzodiazepine site on the GABA receptor complex are inosine, hypoxanthine, nicotinamide and non-halogenated benzodiazepines. The origin of the last of these is unknown, but they could arise from fungal or bacterial sources that are able to synthesize benzodiazepines. However, non-halogenated benzodiazepine-like substances are apparently increased in individuals with hepatic failure.[5] These observations point to a rational basis for treatment of hepatic encephalopathy with benzodiazepine antagonists.

Preliminary data obtained with the benzodiazepine antagonist flumazenil indicate that this treatment rapidly reverses the symptoms of fulminant hepatic failure from cirrhosis.[6] A diazepam-binding inhibitory protein has also been characterized and may contribute to hepatic encephalopathy. This is found in high concentrations in astrocytes[7] and may affect GABA transmission through binding to the GABA receptor complex or by acting at mitochondrial benzodiazepine receptors located on the outer mitochondrial membrane of glial cells.

Hepatic encephalopathy is characterized by a marked gliosis, which indicates that this may be the principal site of energy deficit.[8] Astroglia contain the bulk of the enzyme glutamine synthetase that serves as an important mechanism for the detoxification of abnormally elevated levels of glutamate through its conversion to the inactive compound glutamine.

HYPOXIC ENCEPHALOPATHY

Hypoxic encephalopathy is a comparatively common condition that results from a reduced oxygen supply and is usually accompanied by cerebral hypoperfusion. It most commonly occurs as a result of exposure to a decreased partial pressure of oxygen (Pao_2) at high altitude or in pulmonary disease when there is impaired oxygen diffusion into the tissue.

At decreased Pao_2 values between 55 and 30 Torr (1 Torr = 1 mmHg = 133.3 Pa), impaired short-term memory results, followed by loss of judgement, euphoria, delirium, muscular incoordination and, at values below 25 Torr, loss of consciousness and coma. The latter approximates to an altitude in excess of 20 000 ft above sea level. Under these extreme conditions of hypoxia, mitochondrial respiration cannot be supported and ATP synthesis is impaired. Under conditions of moderate hypoxia, glycolysis is stimulated to maintain ATP levels, as indicated by an increased rate of glucose utilization. This is accompanied by a decrease in pH and an increase in the lactate:pyruvate ratio. With further decrease in oxygen pressure (< 40 Torr) depression in levels of phosphocreatine occurs. Loss of consciousness clearly correlates with a severe depletion of high-energy phosphates, both ATP and phosphocreatine, at lower levels of oxygen (< 25 Torr). The mechanisms affecting cognitive function during moderate hypoxia (55–40 Torr), when the cerebral metabolic rate for oxygen utilization and ATP levels are normal, are less well understood. However, the synthesis of neurotransmitters such as acetylcholine, glutamate, aspartate, GABA, dopamine, noradrenaline and 5-hydroxytryptamine (5-HT) is known to be sensitive to these levels of hypoxia. Oxygen is an obligatory component in the biosynthesis of dopamine, noradrenaline and 5-HT, whilst the synthesis of acetylcholine and amino acids is highly dependent on oxidative metabolism. Areas that are particularly vulnerable to hypoxia are the cerebral cortex, hippocampus and cerebellum. Neuronal degeneration is followed by gliosis.

HYPOGLYCAEMIC ENCEPHALOPATHY

Hypoglycaemic encephalopathy is most commonly seen in insulin-dependent diabetics and hence has a relatively high incidence. Early warning signs of hunger and anxiety can alert the patient to impending hypoglycaemia. As hypoglycaemia develops, confusion, seizures, lethargy, stupor and coma ensue. Abnormal rates of cerebral oxygen and glucose consumption are detected below 2.5 mM glucose,[9] and these are accompanied by loss of attention and confusion. Below 2 mM blood glucose, EEG abnormalities are detected and the patient falls into a stupor. At concentrations of glucose of 1 mM and below coma develops and an isoelectric EEG is obtained. At this concentration of glucose a sharp decrease in levels of both ATP and phosphocreatine is detected. Above 1 mM glucose, levels of ATP and phosphocreatine are maintained at a steady concentration.[10]

The loss of consciousness below 1 mM glucose clearly correlates with the level of high-energy phosphates. Earlier neurological signs are likely to arise through a different mechanism. They may be more dependent on localized effects on the levels of neurotransmitters such as glutamate and GABA.

ISCHAEMIA

Ischaemia due to reduced arterial blood flow, either globally through circulatory failure or locally due to narrowing or occlusion of cerebral arteries, may give rise to coma in severe cases. However, a wide range of responses is found from mild behavioural changes to severe cases leading to loss of consciousness.

The effects of ischaemia result from both hypoxia and hypoglycaemia with the accumulation of toxic metabolites such as lactate. ATP levels are maintained until a critical level is reached. Tissues such as cerebral cortex, hippocampus, basal ganglia, thalamus and cerebellum are most severely affected. In recent years, attention has focused on the role of the neurotransmitter glutamate in inducing neurotoxic damage in ischaemia. The evidence for this hypothesis comes from the fact that (i) glutamate levels are elevated in ischaemic conditions, (ii) glutamate itself is neurotoxic when tested experimentally, and (iii) agents that are antagonists at glutamate receptors have neuroprotective effects in experimental models.

Large increases in glutamate levels can be seen *in vitro* in tissue slices where a combination of hypoxic and hypoglycaemic conditions causes a substantial release of glutamate that does not occur with either condition alone and hence distinguishes the effects of ischaemia from those produced by hypoxia and hypoglycaemia.

Not only do agents preventing the effect of glutamate improve neuronal survival, but also agents that are able to reduce free-radical damage, such as free-radical scavengers, the enzyme superoxide dismutase and inhibitors of xanthine oxidase, which may contribute to free-radical production. These approaches will be important in the development of future therapeutic strategies to target drug treatments to early stages after the initial ischaemic insult where agents effective against free radicals and the action of glutamate may be most effective.

REFERENCES

1. Plum F., Posner J. B. (1980). *The Diagnosis of Stupor and Coma*. Philadelphia: Davies.
2. Caesar J. (1962). Levels of glutamine and ammonia and the pH of cerebrospinal fluid and plasma in patients with liver disease. *Clin. Sci*, **22**, 33.
3. Cooper A. J. L., Mora. S. N., Cruz. N. F., Gelbard A. S. (1985). Cerebral ammonia metabolism in hyperammonaemic rats. *J. Neurochem.*, **44**, 1716.
4. Lin S., Raabe W. (1985). Ammonia intoxication: effects on cerebral cortex and spinal cord. *J. Neurochem.*, **44**, 1252.
5. Olasmaa M. et al. (1990). Endogenous benzodiazepine receptor ligands in human and animal hepatic encephalopathy. *J. Neurochem.*, **55**, 2015.
6. Grimm G. et al. (1988). Improvement of hepatic encephalopathy on treatment with Flumazenil. *Lancet*, **ii**, 1392.
7. Alho H. et al. (1985). Diazepam binding inhibitor: a neuropeptide located in selected neuronal populations of rat brain. *Science*, **229**, 179.
8. Cavanagh J. B., Kyu M. H. (1971). Type II Alzheimer changes experimentally produced in astrocytes in the rat. *J. Neurol. Sci.*, **12**, 63.
9. Plum F., Pulsinelli W. (1986). Cerebral metabolism in hypoxic ischaemic brain injury. In *Diseases of the Nervous System* (Asbury, A. K. McKhann, G. M. & McDonald W. L. eds.) Philadelphia: Saunders, pp. 1086–1100.
10. Siesjö B. K. (1978). *Brain Energy Metabolism*. New York: Wiley.

SECTION 8
DISORDERS OF THE CARDIOVASCULAR SYSTEM

34. Hypertension
D. L. Williams and E. J. Burgess

Introduction
The control of blood pressure
   Cardiac output
   Peripheral resistance
What is high blood pressure?
   Systolic or diastolic pressure?
Causes of hypertension
   Congenital causes
   'Essential' hypertension
   Secondary hypertension
Consequences of hypertension
   'Malignant' hypertension
   Left ventricular hypertrophy and failure
   Cardiac failure
   Atherosclerosis
Biochemical diagnosis of hypertension

INTRODUCTION

Hypertension, together with hyperlipidaemia and smoking, is a major factor causing degenerative and occlusive disease of the cardiovascular system. It is thus a condition associated with significant morbidity and mortality. The diagnosis and monitoring of the majority of hypertensive patients cannot currently be assisted by biochemical tests. There is, however, a minority of hypertensive patients in whom such investigations are helpful in diagnosing the cause of the hypertension, and usually such causes are treatable. Because hypertension is a common condition, even a minority of those with the condition constitute a not insignificant number. It is for these reasons that hypertension finds a proper place in a textbook of clinical biochemistry.

THE CONTROL OF BLOOD PRESSURE

The blood volume, 4–6 L in the normal adult and comprising 6–8% of body weight, is distributed through the blood vascular system as indicated in Fig. 34.1. The vast majority is contained in the venous system at any one time. At birth, on establishing normal respiration, the parallel arrangement through the fetal pulmonary and system circulations changes so that the two circulations are in series. This chapter deals only with hypertension in the systemic circulation.

The arterial blood pressure (ABP) is determined by the cardiac output (CO) and the total peripheral resistance (TPR), such that:

$$ABP = RAP + (CO \times TPR),$$

where RAP is the right atrial pressure, often called the *central venous pressure*; it is almost identical with the ventricular end-diastolic pressure. In practice, therefore, increase in blood pressure can occur by increasing cardiac output or by increasing the peripheral resistance.

Cardiac Output

The cardiac output is determined by two factors: the volume of blood returning to the heart, *the venous return*, increase of which increases the force of ventricular contraction; and the sympathetic innervation of the heart supplemented by circulating sympathomimetic amines, which increases both the force of contraction and the heart rate.

Changes in the Venous Return

The healthy heart adjusts its output to cope with the volume of blood returning into the right atrium from the veins, the venous return. This is achieved through the Frank–Starling mechanism. The mechanism is based on the principle propounded by Starling in the Linacre Lecture of 1915, namely:

> The law of the heart is the same as the law of muscular tissue generally, that the energy of contraction, however measured, is a function of the length of the muscle fibre.

Thus, an increase in venous return increases the cardiac output not only through increase in the stroke volume, but also through the secondary effect of increasing the force of contraction by this mechanism.

The Frank–Starling mechanism is dependent upon

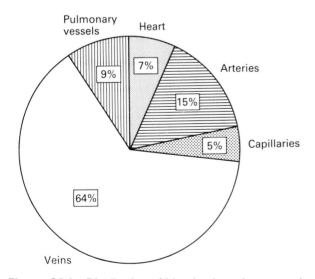

Figure 34.1 Distribution of blood volume in a normal adult.

Pulmonary vessels 9%
Heart 7%
Arteries 15%
Capillaries 5%
Veins 64%

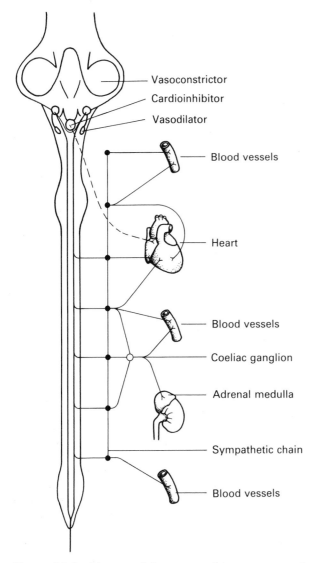

Figure 34.2 Diagram of the autonomic nervous control of the cardiovascular system (broken line, vagus nerve).

the availability of calcium ions and the sensitivity to those ions of the contractile proteins in cardiac muscle. Details of the physiology behind this principle can be found in standard physiology textbooks such as those listed at the end of this chapter.

Autonomic Nervous Control of Stroke Volume

The major nervous control of cardiac output is via the postganglionic sympathetic innervation received by all parts of the heart and reinforced by circulating catecholamines. These factors cause both *chronotropic* (increase of heart rate) and *inotropic* (increase in the force of contraction) responses.

Sympathetic stimulation causes an increase in heart rate, a more rapid rise in systolic ventricular pressure, an increase in the stroke volume and a decrease in the time required to eject the blood from the ventricle.

In contrast the vagus nerve, providing parasympathetic innervation, reduces cardiac output almost entirely by slowing the heart rate, with little effect on the contractility of ventricular muscle.

Peripheral Resistance

Peripheral resistance is under the control of three factors, the autonomic nervous system, the neuroendocrine system, and the presence of local vasoactive metabolites. These factors act on the arterioles.

Autonomic Nervous Control

In the central nervous system the medulla oblongata is the site of the vasopressor and vasodepressor centres and of the vagal nucleus. These centres respond to baroreceptors situated in the ventricular region, the aortic arch and the bifurcation of the carotid artery. They are also controlled by higher centres in the cerebral cortex and the hypothalamus (Fig. 34.2).

The direct nervous control of *vasoconstrictor* activity is mediated by sympathetic noradrenaline (norepinephrine) innervation of the arterioles. These are muscular, contractile vessels that without stimulation would dilate passively in response to increases in blood pressure. There is a constant baseline vasoconstrictor tone applied to the arterioles, which are thus in a permanent tonically active state. Further constriction and hence increase in peripheral resistance is achieved by a several-fold increase in this basal sympathetic stimulation.

Vasodilator activity is more restricted, acts more locally and does not exhibit basal tonic discharge. It is mediated both by sympathetic innervation, originating in the cerebral cortex, stimulating postganglionic cholinergic fibres and responding as part of the alert response, and by parasympathetic fibres, which act through the release of acetylcholine and various vasoactive peptides of which vasoactive intestinal polypeptide (VIP) is likely to be a major component. The role of the vasodilator nerves is mainly to redirect distribution to particular organs when they become active, rather than to oppose vasoconstrictor activity in order to decrease peripheral resistance generally.

Neuroendocrine Control

The adrenal cortex and medulla and the kidney are the main sites of hormonal control of blood pressure. The catecholamines from the adrenal medulla are released by direct sympathetic stimulation of the gland. Renin, from the kidney, causes the formation of angiotensin II. The consequence of both of these actions is to increase peripheral resistance through contraction of the arterioles. Another product of angiotensin II activity, aldosterone, released from the adrenal cortex together with some other less important mineralocorticoids, acts mainly by increasing the blood volume. In addition, vasopressin and possibly natriuretic hormones have controlling effects on

TABLE 34.1
SOME VASOACTIVE HORMONES AND OTHER SUBSTANCES

	Vasoconstrictor	Vasodilator
Hormones	Adrenaline Noradrenaline Angiotensin II Vasopressin	Adrenaline Atrial natriuretic peptide
Other vasoactive substances	Serotonin Thromboxane Prostaglandin F Endothelium-derived relaxing factor Leucotrienes	Bradykinin Histamine Prostaglandin E Endothelin Prostacyclin

blood pressure (*see* below). Table 34.1 gives a list of hormones and other vasoactive compounds.

The Renin Cascade Mechanism. The proteolytic enzyme renin is released from cytoplasmic secretory granules of the juxtaglomerular cells, which are modified myoepithelial cells of the afferent arteriolar wall. Three principal mechanisms control the secretion:

1. Renal baroreceptors, which are probably stretch receptors in the afferent arterioles; decreased stretch stimulates renin release.
2. β_1-Adrenergic stimulation (by circulating catecholamines and by sympathetic nerves).
3. The macula densa, consisting of specialized cells lining the distal convoluted tubule where it makes contact with the juxtaglomerular cells. The macula densa senses changes in the sodium (and chloride) content of the tubular fluid. Increase in the concentration of sodium ions delivered in the tubular fluid to the macula densa stimulates renin release.

All three mechanisms combine to increase renin secretion in response to salt loss, hypovolaemia, or frank hypotension. Other stimuli include stress, exercise, or standing upright. Mechanisms (1) and (3) are probably mediated by locally formed prostaglandins of the E series. There is also feedback inhibition by angiotensin II and other vasoconstrictors (e.g. vasopressin). Mechanism (2) will stimulate renin release in the absence of any change in renal blood flow or in the filtered sodium load. Increase of blood pressure as a result of increased circulating catecholamines as in phaeochromocytoma (*see* below) may thus be partly caused by stimulation of renin production. Catecholamines can therefore affect peripheral resistance both directly and indirectly through this mechanism. Although most of this stimulation is thought to act at β_1-adrenergic receptors, some α-mediated stimulation may also occur.

Renin is initially synthesized as an inactive precursor (preprorenin), then converted to a smaller inactive form, prorenin, which is processed to active renin. In plasma, levels of 'inactive renin' (probably prorenin) are considerably higher than levels of active renin. For this reason, plasma assays are made of renin activity, and not of immunoreactive renin concentration. It is not known whether circulating prorenin is a source of active renin *in vivo*.

After secretion, active renin cleaves the inert decapeptide angiotensin I from angiotensinogen, an α_2-globulin precursor produced in the liver. Subsequently angiotensin-converting enzyme (ACE) forms angiotensin II by removing a C-terminal dipeptide residue from angiotensin I. The principal site of the converting enzyme is the pulmonary vascular endothelial membrane, and the active hormone (angiotensin II) is thereby delivered to the systemic circulation.

Angiotensin II is rapidly degraded by plasma and tissue peptidases (half-life < 1 min). The initial product of action by angiotensinase A, an aspartyl aminopeptidase, is angiotensin III. This heptapeptide is equipotent with angiotensin II in its steroidogenic action (*see* below) but has only 25% of the pressor effect, and forms only a small fraction of the circulating immunoreactive angiotensin. Although probably unimportant as a circulating hormone, it has been suggested that angiotensin III may be a proximal mediator of the steroidogenic effects of angiotensin II.

Angiotensin II is the most potent known natural vasoconstrictor, causing a generalized, direct constriction of the arterioles. It also enhances sympathetic activity by both pre- and postsynaptic mechanisms. Angiotensin II causes sodium retention both by direct renal effects, and by the acute stimulation of synthesis and secretion of aldosterone by the zona glomerulosa of the adrenal cortex. Angiotensin II acts at steps both early and late in the biosynthesis of aldosterone; cortisol synthesis is unaffected.

Angiotensin II exerts central effects on the circumventricular organs (not protected by the blood–brain barrier). It has a central pressor effect, less important than the peripheral pressor effect; it also directly stimulates vasopressin secretion and the thirst response.

These various effects on blood vessels, and on sodium and water balance, combine to maintain both arterial blood pressure and adequate tissue perfusion. Angiotensin II is a major determinant of blood pressure when there is sodium depletion. In this circumstance the administration of an ACE inhibitor causes precipitous postural hypotension (leading to fainting). By contrast, in the sodium-replete state an ACE inhibitor alters neither basal plasma renin activity and aldosterone production nor blood pressure (but only inhibits the rise in aldosterone that normally occurs on standing up).

Angiotensin II is the main, but not the only, factor controlling aldosterone production. Secretion of aldosterone is very sensitive to changes in plasma potassium concentration: an increase of only 0.2 mmol/L causes the plasma concentration of aldosterone to rise by nearly 50%. Prolonged hyperkalaemia causes hypertrophy of the zona glomerulosa. Acidaemia also directly stimulates aldosterone secretion. Sodium depletion enhances the steroidogenic effects of angiotensin II.

ACTH (corticotrophin) is a minor stimulant of aldosterone synthesis (acting early in the pathway, at cholesterol cleavage and at the 11β-hydroxylation step). Acute modulation by ACTH becomes significant only in the virtual absence of renin (e.g. in primary hyperaldosteronism). Trophic effects of ACTH on the zona glomerulosa are insignificant: chronic excess of ACTH does not cause hyperaldosteronism. Similarly, electrolyte disturbance due to hypoaldosteronism is not a feature of secondary Addison's syndrome, although there may be hyponatraemia due to impaired free-water clearance. The role of other peptides of the ACTH family (derivatives of pro-opiomelanocortin) as stimulators of aldosterone secretion, and the role of dopamine, atrial natriuretic factor (ANF) and somatostatin as inhibitors, are subjects of current research. It is probable that dopamine exerts a continual inhibitory effect on aldosterone synthesis that is overcome by angiotensin stimulation; however, when this inhibition is blocked by metaclopramide, aldosterone secretion increases. ANF appears to inhibit aldosterone synthesis and block its stimulation by angiotensin II.

Vasopressin. Loss of blood, even in the absence of hypotension, triggers neurosecretion of arginine vasopressin (antidiuretic hormone, ADH) from the posterior pituitary. During hypovolaemia a loss of afferent input from stretch receptors in the atria and great veins disinhibits vasopressin secretion. In fact, hypovolaemia is a reflex stimulus to release of vasopressin considerably more potent than is a rise in plasma osmolality.

Pressor effects *in vivo* of vasopressin at ordinary physiological concentrations were first demonstrated unequivocally about two decades ago. Previously a (low-dose) pressor effect had been observed only in experimental models in which the baroreceptor reflexes were eliminated, either by anaesthesia or by neurosurgery. In recent years the view that vasopressin has a role in normal cardiovascular control, and not only in the maintenance of blood pressure during acute hypovolaemia, has gained ground.[1]

Thus vasopressin has not only a direct effect on the smooth muscle of resistance vessels, but also a central effect in which the sensitivity of the baroreceptor reflex is enhanced. Access to the brain is gained via the area postrema, a region where the blood–brain barrier is leaky and which is close to that nucleus (tractus solitarius) which receives afferent nerves from the baroreceptors. Vasopressin probably functions as a neurotransmitter in areas of the dorsal medulla and hypothalamus that exert autonomic nervous control over the cardiovascular system. This is in addition to its role as a neurosecretory hormone synthesized in the supraoptic and paraventricular nuclei of the hypothalamus.

There is also some evidence that vasopressin might have a role in the pathogenesis of hypertension. In rats with various types of induced hypertension, the plasma concentration of vasopressin is inappropriately high for the osmolality. Furthermore, injection of an antiserum specific to vasopressin temporarily lowers the blood pressure. However, the evidence against such a role in man is rather more convincing.[2] Many patients with the syndrome of inappropriate antidiuresis, due to vasopressin produced ectopically by malignant cells, remain normotensive despite very high plasma concentrations of vasopressin. These concentrations exceed the increased levels found in patients with malignant hypertension.

Atrial Natriuretic Factor (ANF). ANF can directly affect both blood volume and blood pressure: its effects broadly oppose those produced by vasopressin. The active (α) factor is a 28 amino-acid peptide released from cytoplasmic secretory granules in atrial muscle cells in response to atrial stretch by small increases in atrial pressure. ANF has little effect on vascular muscle alone, but it inhibits the vasoconstrictor effects of noradrenaline and of angiotensin II *in vitro* and their vasopressor effects *in vivo*. ANF also produces a more general inhibition of the renin axis: it reduces plasma renin activity and inhibits the release of aldosterone by angiotensin II.

Injection of anaesthetized animals with specific antiserum to ANF reduces the urinary excretion of sodium and water and sometimes raises the blood pressure. Experiments in which animals are made autoimmune to ANF suggest that it is important in off-loading the heart during acute volume expansion, but that the chronic regulation of sodium balance and of blood pressure are unaffected by a prolonged deficiency of ANF.[3] In essential hypertension the mean plasma level of immunoreactive ANF (like that of plasma renin activity) may in different individuals be the same as, or higher or lower than in normotensive subjects.

Other Vasoactive Metabolites
Various vasoactive metabolites are of importance in adjusting blood flow according to the needs of particular tissues or organs under differing physiological or pathological states. But there is little good evidence to implicate these substances in the aetiology of systemic hypertension. Acid–base changes and the release of products such as lactic acid, adenosine nucleotides, and potassium are factors causing the increase in blood flow to exercising muscle, not decrease in vasomotor tone. Hypoxia causes tissues to produce substances such as endothelium-derived relaxing factor resulting in vasodilatation, whereas a vasoconstrictor polypeptide, endothelin, also derived from the endothelium, causes contraction of smooth-muscle fibres. The flushing associated with carcinoid

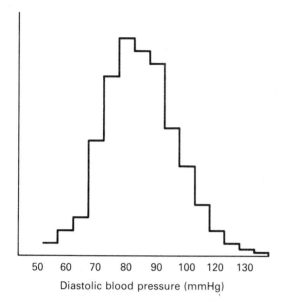

Figure 34.3 Distribution of diastolic blood pressure, men aged 45–66 years.

syndrome is probably mediated by bradykinin and other kinins rather than by serotonin, which has a vasoconstrictive action. Carcinoid syndrome is not usually associated with hypertension. There is a hypertensive variant of the similar disease, mastocytosis, probably caused by abnormal metabolism of prostaglandin D_2 (a vasodilator) to the vasoconstrictor prostaglandin F_2.

WHAT IS HIGH BLOOD PRESSURE?

Except in cases of pathological hypotension, there is an inverse relation between the blood pressure and subsequent life expectancy: this relation is continuous and shows no clear lower limit. Defining the abnormal is therefore wholly arbitrary. The best and most pragmatic approach is to set a threshold based on knowledge of the effects of treatment: that is, patients are described as hypertensive at those levels of blood pressure where therapeutic intervention confers demonstrable benefit (mainly, reduced incidence of stroke—there is little if any effect on myocardial infarction).

Systolic or Diastolic Pressure?

What is this threshold? Blood pressure is, of course, pulsatile. Systolic pressure depends particularly on the compliance of the large arteries and rises as they become more rigid with age; whereas diastolic pressure reflects the arteriolar peripheral resistance. Blood pressure rises with age. In men the rise is progressive, and in women it occurs mainly after the menopause. The increase in systolic pressure is greater than in diastolic pressure. Partly for this reason, and partly because a measure of the periph-

eral resistance was felt (perhaps unjustifiably) to have greater pathophysiological significance, clinical trials have focused almost exclusively on diastolic pressure, and most advice on treatment is based on that measure. But much of the epidemiological evidence shows that systolic pressure has a greater influence on cardiovascular risk than does diastolic pressure.

Normal ranges

The 'normal range' for blood pressure is rather like that for cholesterol; the upper limit of a statistically based normal range (containing the mean of the population ± twice the SD) overlaps with that generally considered to be the at-risk range; in other words, the normal range differs from the healthy range.

Taking blood pressure accurately and reproducibly is by no means the routine, simple, repetitive chore that it sometimes appears; it requires experience and application. Precautions must be taken to ensure that the measured blood pressure is typical of that experienced by the patient under normal conditions, and that the technique of measurement is appropriate for the physique of the patient. In order to obviate the 'alerting reaction' in which blood pressure rises during the emotional response to stress, the measurement must be repeated on at least three similar occasions and an average taken. It is important to avoid the acute pressor effects of nicotine, caffeine, or summer heat.

With regard to diastolic pressure, the consensus in the UK is that the threshold of benefit from treatment is a lower limit of about 100 mmHg for men and 110 mmHg for women (at the point of disappearance of the Korotkov sounds). Figure 34.3 shows diagrammatically the distribution of diastolic blood pressure in 1440 men chosen at random; it can be seen that a significant minority is above this limit.

As a rule of thumb, the upper acceptable limit of the normal systolic pressure is taken to be 100 plus the age in years rounded to the nearest 10 (e.g. 150 mmHg at age 50 etc.). Among the elderly, isolated systolic hypertension (without elevation of diastolic pressure) is fairly common, due probably to arteriosclerosis. A large multicentre trial of benefit from treating this form of hypertension is in progress. Other recent trial data suggest that the treatment thresholds should be set lower for the elderly, at 160/90.

CAUSES OF HYPERTENSION

Table 34.2 indicates the frequency of the main causes of hypertension. It is a summation of a number of studies that have appeared in the North American and European literature in recent years, covering some 5500 patients. Such studies vary in their classification and in the distribution of causes, but it is clear from the table that essential hypertension and disease of the kidney and its vasculature make up a very large proportion of the total cases.

TABLE 34.2
FREQUENCY OF MAJOR CAUSES OF HYPERTENSION (%)

Essential hypertension	92.9
Chronic renal disease	4.9
Renovascular disease	0.7
Coarctation of the aorta	0.1
Conn's syndrome	0.2
Cushing's syndrome	0.1
Phaeochromocytoma	0.1
Oral contraceptives	0.9
	100.0

Taken from various reports in the literature and totalling 5500 cases.

Congenital Causes

Congenital Adrenal Hyperplasia

The subject of congenital adrenal hyperplasia (the adrenogenital syndrome) is covered in detail in Chapter 41. Of the several varieties of the syndrome, the second most common variety, deficiency of 11β-hydroxylase (P-450$_{c11}$), is characterized by hypertension in addition to the androgenization typical of the syndrome in general. This is mainly due to accumulation and higher circulating levels of 11-deoxycorticosterone (DOC) (see Fig. 34.5). This mineralocorticoid is the substrate of 11β-hydroxylase in the aldosterone synthesis pathway. The depression of the equivalent enzyme activity in the cortisol synthetic pathway, responsible for the conversion of 11-deoxycortisol to cortisol, does not increase blood pressure as the accumulated substrate does not have mineralocorticoid activity. The lowered production of cortisol does, however, result in lower feedback inhibition of the pituitary ACTH-producing cells, causing increased circulating ACTH that in turn stimulates further the earlier stages of metabolism of cholesterol along the cortisol and aldosterone pathways. Consequently the build-up of DOC concentration is multiplied.

The story is, however, not entirely clear. It is thought that the same enzyme is responsible for 11-hydroxylation in both the aldosterone and the cortisol pathways; indeed it seems likely that this enzyme also catalyses the subsequent 18-hydroxylation and 18-methyl oxidase steps,[4] thus enabling the final three steps in the synthesis of aldosterone. Other work indicates that there are two closely related enzymes in the zona glomerulosa (i.e. involved in aldosterone synthesis), one of which is salt regulated; the other appears to be identical with the enzyme found in the zona fasciculata (where it is involved in cortisol synthesis). These findings may supply the explanation of the fact that not all cases of 11-hydroxylase deficiency are associated with hypertension; indeed a salt-wasting (hypotensive) state has sometimes been found.

A very rare, related condition in which hypertension is found is deficiency of 17α-hydroxylase. As can be seen from Fig. 34.4, this blocks the cortisol pathway (and also the synthesis of sex steroids) and causes increased flux through the mineralocorticoid pathway. Increased levels of DOC and its metabolites are thought to be the hypertensive factors, although aldosterone production is suppressed.

As for all cases of congenital adrenal hyperplasia, treatment is directed to reducing the high circulating levels of ACTH by replacement of the deficient cortisol. Diagnosis and monitoring of treatment are usually achieved by measurement of the blood level of 17α-hydroxyprogesterone, although this metabolite would not be a suitable indicator in cases of 17α-hydroxylase deficiency.

Coarctation of the Aorta

This condition is associated with a congenital stenosis of the aorta, usually immediately beyond the origin of the left subclavian artery and in close relation to the ductus arteriosus (or its vestigial remnant, the ligamentum arteriosum). In 40% of cases the ductus is patent and the stenosis occurs just above it. This form presents as an emergency in neonatal life as unoxygenated blood circulates through the trunk and lower limbs, making them cyanotic, whilst the upper part of the body is well perfused with oxygenated blood.

In the other 60% of cases the stenosis is below the ductus, which remains patent in only a minority of cases. The patient presents later in life with hypertension as usually measured with a sphygmomanometer on the upper arm. If the blood pressure is measured in the lower limb, however, it is found to be much lower and the pulse wave is somewhat delayed. Blood reaches the lower trunk and limbs by means of collateral blood vessels that bypass the coarctation. A typical radiological sign is 'notching' of the ribs, the notches being made by chronically enlarged intercostal arteries that are called into service to provide this collateral supply.

The condition is of limited interest in the biochemistry laboratory, but it is an important, treatable cause of hypertension. It gives rise to a high-renin, high-aldosterone hypertension, and illustrates the point that the poorly perfused kidney can, through this mechanism, overcome the inhibitory central nervous control on cardiac output that would normally be the consequence of high blood pressure in the carotid arteries.

'Essential' Hypertension

Essential hypertension is defined as hypertension stemming from a progressive rise in pressure with age *for which there is no obvious cause*. Between 90 and 95% of all hypertensive subjects will fall into this category when investigated by simple and straightforward measures. Investigations should therefore be limited to simple urinalysis, together with plasma

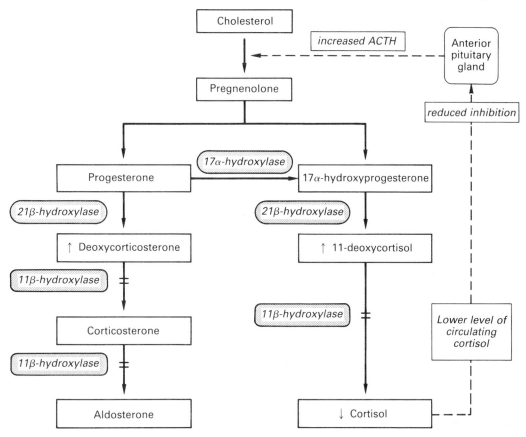

Figure 34.4 Metabolism of steroids: summary of reactions involved in synthesis of cortisol and aldosterone, and the consequences of deficiency of 11β-hydroxylase.

TABLE 34.3
CLINICAL INDICATORS OF THE NEED FOR MORE DETAILED
INVESTIGATION OF HYPERTENSIVE PATIENTS

1. The patient is young (under 30)
2. The hypertension is severe, resistant, or accelerated (malignant)
3. There are suspicious clinical features, such as the paroxysms, postural hypotension or glycosuria which may occur in phaeochromocytoma
4. There is unexplained hypokalaemia suggesting primary hyperaldosteronism
5. There is sudden deterioration of renal function when the blood pressure is lowered (particularly after ACE inhibition), suggesting renovascular hypertension
6. There is a family history of renal or endocrine disease associated with hypertension
7. The response to usually effective treatment is poor

electrolytes, glucose, urea and lipids, except in those cases in which there is one or more indicators that justify more detailed work-up.

Table 34.3 lists the features which suggest the possibility that the hypertension may not fall into the 'essential' category. In the absence of any of these features and with no evidence of pre-existing renal disease a presumptive diagnosis is made of 'essential hypertension'. Even the most diligent further search will fail to identify a secondary cause for hypertension in 99% of these cases.

Essential hypertension is now viewed as a disease with multifactorial causes, in which several genes influence the response of the physiological mechanisms outlined above to various contributory environmental and behavioural factors. The key risk factors are a positive family history, obesity, and alcohol. Not only the grossly obese or the problem drinker have excess risk of hypertension: there are continuous linear relations between the prevalence of hypertension and both excess body weight, and daily ethanol consumption. Smoking is not a risk factor for hypertension.

Causes of Essential Hypertension

Two main components of essential hypertension are apparent. Firstly, decreased compliance of the large arteries, either as part of the ageing process (arteriosclerosis) or from atherosclerosis: this elevates systolic pressure. Secondly, increased peripheral resistance, due primarily to increased tone of the vascular smooth muscle in peripheral arterioles: this elevates diastolic pressure. A further, secondary cause of increased peripheral resistance is thickening of the arteriolar walls; this is a rapid, adaptive change that occurs in response to elevated pressure.

The tone of vascular smooth muscle is governed by the sarcoplasmic concentration of ionized calcium, which is maintained always above the contraction threshold (about 10^{-7}M). A rise in calcium concentration in the vascular sarcoplasm is therefore the final common path by which all diastolic hypertension is produced.[5] A sodium–calcium exchange transporter operates across the membrane of the vascular smooth-muscle cell. Increases or decreases in the intracellular concentration of sodium drive this exchange, to produce parallel changes in intracellular calcium.

Sodium in Essential Hypertension

The role of sodium in the aetiology of essential hypertension has received a great deal of attention, and remains controversial.

Patients with essential hypertension respond to increased salt ingestion with a further increase in pressure (normotensive subjects are unaffected unless at very low intake of sodium). The pressor effect of a salt load develops relatively slowly and is mediated by a humoral agent, produced in response to volume expansion, which increases directly the contractility of the heart, arterioles, and veins, and thereby multiply accentuates venous return, cardiac output and peripheral resistance. There is a large body of evidence *in vitro* and *in vivo* that the humoral agent exerts its effect by inhibiting cardiovascular sarcolemmal Na-K-ATPase.[6]

The humoral agent in question may well be the natriuretic hormone of de Wardener.[7] This has not been identified but appears structurally similar to the cardiac glycosides, acting at the same receptors as these drugs but with far greater potency. *Natriuretic hormone is quite distinct from ANF, which does not inhibit Na-K-ATPase activity.*

De Wardener and MacGregor[8] have proposed that essential hypertension is due to an inherited variation in the ability of the kidney to eliminate sodium. The difficulty in eliminating sodium causes an increase in the concentration of natriuretic hormone, which adjusts urinary sodium excretion to normalize sodium balance. In the arteriole, this hormonal inhibitor of Na-K-ATPase causes a rise in intracellular sodium concentration, which in turn raises the intracellular calcium concentration and thus increases vascular tone, as indicated in the previous section. There is consequently a gradual rise in arterial pressure to a degree dependent on the severity of the inherited defect in eliminating sodium, and on the sodium intake.

A huge international study of the role of salt in hypertension has now been completed,[9] having included data from 52 centres in 32 countries. The median sodium excretion measured in 10 079 subjects ranged very widely between 0.2 and 242 mmol/day. Sodium excretion (equivalent to sodium intake) was related to the rate of increase of both systolic and diastolic pressure with age, but was not related either to median blood pressure or to the prevalence of hypertension. There was, however, a significant tendency for sodium intake and systolic pressure to be correlated when the data from individual centres were tested separately.

The data predict that for a reduction of 100 mmol/day in habitual sodium intake (as great as might be achieved in Western society), the increase in systolic pressure from age 25 to age 55 in a population would be less by 9 mmHg. Randomized controlled trials of the effects of restricting sodium (to 70–90 mmol/day) show reductions of about 3–5 mmHg systolic pressure in hypertensive subjects, particularly in older subjects and in severe hypertension.

In summary there is little doubt that salt contributes to essential hypertension, but it is only one of several factors and is not an overriding cause. Nevertheless, it is the only well-elucidated cause after many decades of very wide-ranging research into the aetiology of hypertension. Work on other electrolytes (K^+, Ca^{2+}, Mg^{2+}, PO_4^{3-} and Cl^-), and on possible interactions between them, is in progress.

Secondary Hypertension

Various causes of secondary hypertension are listed in Table 34.4. Many of these are important topics in their own right and are discussed elsewhere in this volume. Here we shall focus on the renal causes of hypertension, and also on two conditions where hypertension is itself the principal presenting feature: Conn's syndrome and phaeochromocytoma.

Renal Causes of Hypertension

When a renal artery is occluded, the reduction in pulse pressure stimulates renin release from the juxtaglomerular apparatus: the direct or indirect effects of angiotensin II are likely to initiate renovascular hypertension. However, the mechanisms whereby chronic hypertension associated with renovascular pathology is maintained have not been elucidated. Only about 50% of the patients in whom vascular surgery normalizes blood pressure have elevated renin in peripheral blood samples. Recent studies show that even the comparison of renin concentrations between samples from the right and left renal veins has little or no predictive value.

In many cases of unilateral renal disease, surgery or angioplasty has no effect on the blood pressure. Probably the hypertension has produced irreversible vascular changes in the contralateral kidney. A favourable outcome is most likely in young patients with a fibrous dysplasia of the renal arteries.

The mechanisms by which *bilateral* renal disease causes hypertension are still less certain. The prevalence and severity of hypertension tend to increase as the glomerular filtration rate declines: about 90% of patients with end-stage renal failure are hypertensive. These patients usually retain salt and water, and their hypertension can often be controlled without

TABLE 34.4
CAUSES OF SECONDARY HYPERTENSION

CONGENITAL
Congenital adrenal hyperplasia with deoxycorticosterone
    excess:
    11-β-hydroxylase deficiency
    17-α-hydroxylase deficiency
    11-β-hydroxysteroid dehydrogenase deficiency
Renal abnormalities:
    Dysplasia
    Liddle's syndrome
Coarctation of the aorta

ACQUIRED
RENAL
Unilateral renal disease:
    Renovascular
    Parenchymal
Chronic renal failure of any cause, e.g.:
    Urolithiasis
    Analgesic abuse
    Diabetic nephrosclerosis
    Amyloidosis
    Acute and chronic glomerulonephritis
Perirenal compression
Hypernephroma and other renin-secreting tumours of
    kidney
ENDOCRINE
Consistently hypertensive
Adrenal disorders
Cushing's syndrome
    ACTH dependent:
        pituitary
        ectopic
        pseudo (ethanol, depression)
    ACTH independent:
        adenoma
        carcinoma
        iatrogenic
Primary aldosteronism):
    Conn's syndrome
    Idiopathic
    Glucocorticoid-suppressible
    Carcinoma
Other tumours
Catecholamine-secreting tumours
Extrarenal renin-secreting tumours
May be hypertensive
Diabetes mellitus
Hyperthyroidism
Hypercalcaemia:
    Primary hyperparathyroidism
    Hypervitaminosis D
Acromegaly
DRUGS
Oestrogen/progestogen contraceptive pill
Glucocorticoids and mineralocorticoids
Liquorice and carbenoxolone
Sympathomimetics and MAO inhibitors
MISCELLANEOUS
Gestational hypertension
Raised intracranial pressure
Acute intermittent porphyria
Acute lead poisoning
Tetanus
Poliomyelitis

drugs if they are salt restricted and the excess extracellular fluid removed by short periods of ultrafiltration after haemodialysis. Occasionally, in either salt-losing chronic renal failure (which is particularly associated with obstructive uropathy) or in tight occlusion of a renal artery, there is by contrast a *contraction* of the extracellular fluid volume, sometimes with very gross hyper-reninaemia and secondary hyperaldosteronism. The cardinal features of this 'hyponatraemic hypertensive' syndrome are thirst, polydypsia, polyuria, weight loss, kaliuresis, alkalosis, and hypokalaemia.

The mechanism whereby perirenal compression (such as by a haematoma) causes hypertension is quite unknown.

Endocrine Causes
Primary Aldosteronism.
1. *Conn's Syndrome.* This syndrome when first described by Conn[10] in 1955 consisted of asymptomatic hypertension, hypokalaemia and a single adrenal adenoma. He called the condition *primary aldosteronism*. This name is now used to describe a somewhat wider syndrome of primary mineralocorticoid excess comprising hypertension, hypokalaemia with renal potassium wasting, metabolic alkalosis, and low plasma renin activity, but not necessarily associated with an adrenal adenoma. It is preferable to confine the term Conn's syndrome to those cases in whom the hyperaldosteronism is due to an adrenal adenoma to differentiate them from cases of idiopathic hyperaldosteronism, as the pathology and treatment are different between the two conditions. Occasionally there are symptoms of severe hypokalaemia: these include thirst and polyuria (due to nephrogenic diabetes insipidus), constipation, paresis, and less commonly, cramps, paraesthesiae, and tetany. The most common cause is a unilateral adenoma of the zona glomerulosa as initially described. The adenoma produces principally an excess of aldosterone. Adrenocortical carcinoma is a rare cause.

Aldosterone acts on the kidney with the following effects:

1. *Stimulates sodium reabsorption*, an action confined to the cortical collecting ducts and to the cortical connecting tubules (which link the collecting ducts to the distal convoluted tubules). Aldosterone increases the permeability of the apical (luminal) membrane to sodium and increases the mitochondrial production of ATP. The consequent rise in intracellular sodium and in ATP stimulates the activity of Na-K-ATPase in the basolateral (antiluminal) membrane. Aldosterone also causes synthesis *de novo* of these sodium pumps and their incorporation into the membrane.
2. *Stimulates potassium secretion* in the cortical collecting ducts. The increased sodium reabsorption in this nephron segment, described above (1), is electrogenic, and results in an increase in

intraluminal electronegativity. Aldosterone also increases the permeability to potassium of the apical (luminal) membrane. Both effects favour the secretion of potassium into the tubular lumen, a passive process that is ultimately driven by the basolateral Na-K pumps.

3. *Stimulates proton secretion.* Some of this effect is due to the passive movement of protons with potassium ions, in the mechanism described above (2). A more important process, which can create large pH gradients, occurs in the medullary collecting duct: aldosterone stimulates a sodium-independent, proton-secreting ATPase.

If aldosterone (or another mineralocorticoid) is administered continuously, an 'escape phenomenon' occurs after about 5–20 days (quicker when sodium intake is higher). Sodium retention then ceases, there is a natriuresis and a fall from peak levels in total body sodium and in extracellular fluid volume: the result is a new equilibrium in which both remain slightly elevated. Because of this phenomenon, oedema is no part of Conn's syndrome. By contrast, kaliuresis and proton secretion are not subject to mineralocorticoid escape, but continue unabated: therefore hypokalaemic alkalosis is characteristic of Conn's syndrome.

Sodium retention by aldosterone causes secondary expansion of the extracellular fluid volume, mediated by the arginine vasopressin system, to preserve normal plasma osmolality (a mild hypernatraemia sometimes persists). Why should this volume expansion cause hypertension? If the plasma volume is expanded by a rapid intravenous infusion of saline, there is no acute pressor effect: increase in cardiac output is merely compensated by vasodilatation and reduced peripheral resistance. Fairly prolonged hypervolaemia is required to produce any hypertension.

Hypertension in response to treatment with exogenous mineralocorticoid develops slowly, progressing long after the development of maximal sodium retention. There is initially a phase of high cardiac output, and subsequently a progressive rise in peripheral resistance. Almost certainly, a single mechanism explains both mineralocorticoid escape and any variety of volume-expanded hypertension, including that induced by salt (in patients with essential hypertension), or by mineralocorticoid.[6] This mechanism was described above (*see* Sodium in essential hypertension), the hypertensive agent being probably the natriuretic hormone of de Wardener.[7]

2. *Idiopathic Hyperaldosteronism.* It was recognized a few years after Conn's original reprt that a proportion of patients with primary hyperaldosteronism did not have a single adrenal adenoma. In particular, a group that was thought to account for 10–20% of patients with primary aldosteronism appeared to have bilateral adrenal hyperplasia, the cause for

which was unknown and which was thus called idiopathic hyperaldosteronism. Probably as a result of more thorough investigation of hypertensive patients, reports now indicate that idiopathic hyperaldosteronism accounts for some 30–50% of primary hyperaldosteronism. The zona glomerulosa may be bilaterally hyperplastic, with or without adrenocortical nodules; but the adrenals may appear completely normal, both microscopically and macroscopically. Nodules are usually multiple and bilateral, and vary in size from the microscopic up to about 2 cm in diameter. Occasionally there is a large unilateral nodule, closely resembling an adenoma; but in contrast to classic Conn's syndrome, *the nodules do not produce aldosterone*.

Against all expectation, aldosterone is not the principal mediator of hypertension in idiopathic hyperaldosteronism. The hypertension is usually not corrected by spironolactone nor even by bilateral adrenalectomy! One possibility is that the disorder is merely a type of low-renin essential hypertension. Both conditions are characterized by an enhanced sensitivity of aldosterone secretion to angiotensin II. By contrast the sensitivity to angiotensin II is diminished in adenoma, and this is useful in differential diagnosis (*see* below). Another possibility is that an aldosterone stimulating factor, first isolated by Sen et al.,[11] may be responsible. This is an anterior pituitary glycoprotein of 26 kDa: basal levels are elevated two-fold in the plasma of patients with idiopathic hyperaldosteronism, and are normal in patients with excised aldosterone-producing adenoma.[12]

3. *Glucocorticoid-suppressible Hyperaldosteronism.* This rare cause of primary aldosteronism is familial with autosomal dominant transmission. There is a bilateral hyperplasia of the zona glomerulosa, and all abnormalities are reversed by treatment with a glucocorticoid such as dexamethasone. The apparent ACTH dependence is remarkable, since ACTH has no trophic effect on the zona glomerulosa, and in any case the cortisol and ACTH levels are normal. Perhaps another derivative of pro-opiomelanocortin is responsible.[13] An alternative hypothesis is of enzymatic derangements in the zona fasciculata that permit ectopic aldosterone synthesis (normally confined to the zona glomerulosa).[14]

4. *Other Causes of Primary Aldosteronism.* Primary adrenal tumours (especially carcinomas) very occasionally secrete large amounts of deoxycorticosterone or other precursors of aldosterone. Liquorice and carbenoxolone probably act *indirectly*, by inhibition of renal 11β-hydroxysteroid dehydrogenase.[15] This enzyme converts active cortisol to inactive cortisone: when inhibited, the consequent rise in intrarenal glucocorticoid concentrations may saturate renal extravascular cortisol-binding globulin, and markedly increase free cortisol levels for action at the mineralocorticoid (or type 1) receptor. Congenital deficiency

of the same enzyme produces a syndrome of 'apparent mineralocorticoid excess'. Liddle's syndrome resembles primary hyperaldosteronism, but aldosterone levels are very low. There is probably an inherited defect accelerating sodium transport within the nephron distal to the site of action of aldosterone.

Differential Diagnosis of Primary Aldosteronism. The hypokalaemia of primary aldosteronism may well be intermittent, particularly in idiopathic hyperaldosteronism. A mild metabolic alkalosis may still be detectable; hypokalaemia can often be 'unmasked' by raising the sodium intake. Conversely, one should not be misled by the hypokalaemia of uncontrolled malignant hypertension, which merely reflects severe secondary hyperaldosteronism.

Investigation proceeds by measuring plasma renin activity and aldosterone after strict overnight recumbency while on an adequate intake of sodium (>100 mmol/day), and so far as possible after potassium repletion. Many drugs suppress renin (e.g. β-blockers, non-steroidal anti-inflammatory drugs) or stimulate aldosterone (e.g. diuretics) and all must be discontinued for 2–4 weeks before sampling; prazosin can be substituted in the interim. After the basal sample, simple tests are made of response to posture and of circadian rhythm. The measurement of plasma renin activity is repeated after 30 minutes' mobility, and of aldosterone, at midday. Diagnosis rests on a high basal aldosterone relative to renin, with negligible increase in renin after 30 minutes' upright posture. It must be appreciated that the concentrations of renin and aldosterone may not actually be outwith the respective reference ranges. Conversely, 25% of patients with essential hypertension have renin levels as low as those in patients with Conn's syndrome.

Other dynamic test manoeuvres, such as with salt depletion, salt loading (oral or intravenous), frusemide or captopril, appear to have little advantage in sensitivity and specificity over the simple procedures outlined above.

It is most important to distinguish Conn's adenoma, requiring surgical treatment, from other forms of primary aldosteronism, which require medical treatment. The investigation usually combines computerized tomographic (CT) or iodocholesterol scanning with biochemical differentiation, the latter resting on comparison of the basal and midday aldosterone levels. With renin suppressed, the control of aldosterone secretion by ACTH assumes significance: a circadian rhythm (paralleling that of cortisol) is manifest, and a remarkable fall in plasma aldosterone concentration by 50% or more occurs between 0800 h and 1200 h in cases of Conn's adenoma (or of glucocorticoid-suppressible hyperaldosteronism). This circadian fall in aldosterone would occur in the normal individual only if he were kept recumbent.

By contrast, in idiopathic hyperaldosteronism, the secretion of aldosterone is extremely sensitive to angiotensin II. In this condition, therefore, even the small postural rise in renin activity that residually occurs when renin secretion is suppressed by hypervolaemia and hypertension is nevertheless sufficient to abolish the effect of a circadian fall in ACTH. Hence the levels of aldosterone at 0800 h and at 1200 h are comparable. It is important to measure plasma cortisol concurrently with aldosterone for this test; any stress-induced rise in ACTH and cortisol will invalidate the results.

Difficult cases may justify adrenal venous sampling for aldosterone (and cortisol, as a marker), but there is often a failure to cannulate the right adrenal vein (which drains directly into the inferior vena cava).

Cushing's Syndrome. Hypertension is a common feature of Cushing's syndrome, although not always one of the major symptoms. The degree of hypertension can, however, be severe with significant consequences upon the cardiovascular system. The raised blood pressure may be caused by high renin activity, mineralocorticoid activity of cortisol or other metabolites, or increased sensitivity to the actions of catecholamines.

The topic is further discussed in Chapter 41.

Phaeochromocytoma. Phaeochromocytomas are tumours arising from chromaffin cells of the sympathetic nervous system, which release catecholamines into the circulation. Most arise in the adrenal medulla (preferentially in the right adrenal); 10% are outside the adrenals and may occur anywhere within the sympathetic paraganglia from the neck to the urinary bladder (mostly within the abdomen or pelvis). The most common extra-adrenal site is the organ of Zuckerkandl, a major source of circulating catecholamines during the first year of life (adjacent to the bifurcation of the aorta). Ten per cent of adrenal phaeochromocytomas are bilateral, and these particularly are sometimes familial forming part of the syndrome of multiple endocrine neoplasia (MEN) type II (in which phaeochromocytoma is usually preceded by the development of medullary thyroid carcinoma, C-cell carcinoma). In these syndromes there is also an association either with hyperparathyroidism (MEN type IIA); or with multiple mucosal neuromas, intestinal ganglioneuromatosis, and Marfanoid skeletal deformities (MEN type IIB). There is a separate association of phaeochromocytoma with neurofibromatosis; and also with a parathyroid hormone-*independent* form of hypercalcaemia. C-cell carcinoma sometimes causes carcinoid syndrome.

Most phaeochromocytomas are benign and curable by surgery; 10% are malignant, but even when metastasized, medical management is successful for long periods. Left undiagnosed, the patient will die from a complication of the hypertension (notably stroke and myocarditis) or, still worse, from an arrhythmia precipitated by unprepared anaesthesia, surgery, or parturition. Occasionally the tumour infarcts and may then present as an acute abdominal emergency and,

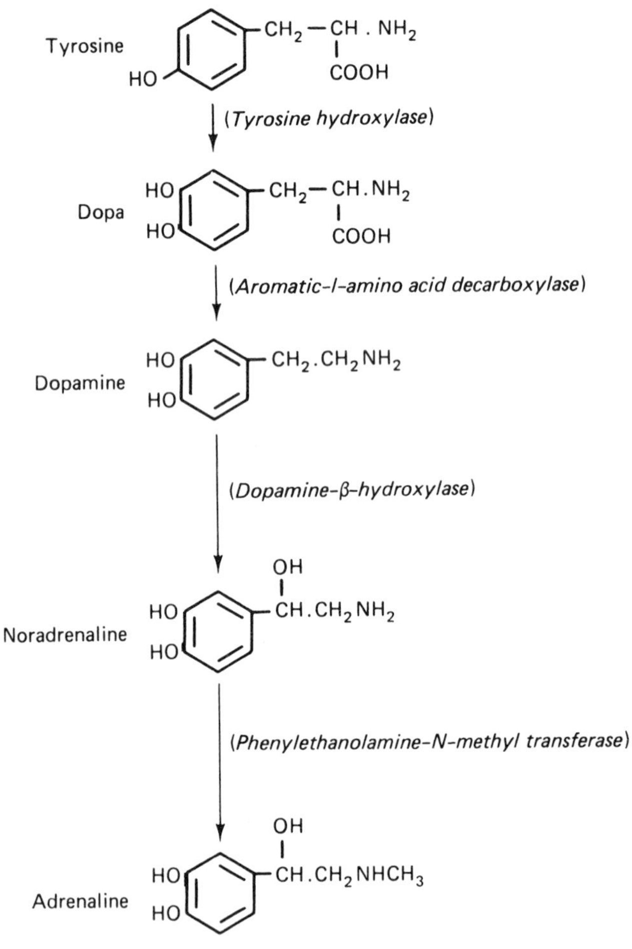

Figure 34.5 Catecholamine synthesis.

paradoxically, shock. Postural hypotension occurs commonly in phaeochromocytoma, due to blunting of the autonomic reflexes by the chronic oversecretion of catecholamines (causing for example, downregulation of receptors).

Synthesis and Secretion of Catecholamines. The synthesis of catecholamines from tyrosine is outlined in Fig. 34.5. Phenylalanine hydroxylase is absent from chromaffin tissue. Tyrosine hydroxylation is therefore the initial step and is also rate-limiting, regulating noradrenaline synthesis, which is closely matched to the rate of release: there is a preferential release of newly synthesized catecholamine. Short-term variations in the rate of release govern the activity of tyrosine hydroxylase via both end-product inhibition by catecholamines (which compete with the tetrahydrobiopterin cofactor) and protein phosphorylation, the latter through two separate mechanisms. A cyclic AMP-dependent phosphorylation of tyrosine hydroxylase increases the affinity of the enzyme for its pterin cofactor. A calcium–calmodulin-dependent phosphorylation of tyrosine hydroxylase (at a different locus) permits stimulation by an activator protein.

Long-term increases in the rate of catecholamine release will also increase the quantity of tyrosine hydroxylase by enzyme induction. In phaeochromocytoma these and other control mechanisms are impaired so that there is uncontrolled secretion of excess dopamine, noradrenaline or adrenaline.

Dopamine β-hydroxylase (DBH) is confined to the catecholamine storage vesicles and is coreleased during exocytosis, together with several vasoconstrictor and vasodilator peptides; these might contribute to a disjunction frequently observed between catecholamine levels and the degree of hypertension. Phenylethanolamine N-methyl transferase (PNMT) is rate-limiting, and is induced by glucocorticoids. These perfuse the adrenal medulla at a hundred times their systemic concentration, in blood supplied through a portal system (draining directly from the cortex). Because of this inductive mechanism, small adrenal tumours secrete mainly adrenaline (epinephrin); but larger adrenal tumours (which outstrip the normal supply of blood and cortisol), and extra-adrenal tumours, secrete mainly noradrenaline norepinephrine), and this is the most common pattern. Exceptions occur, however (due to breakdown of normal

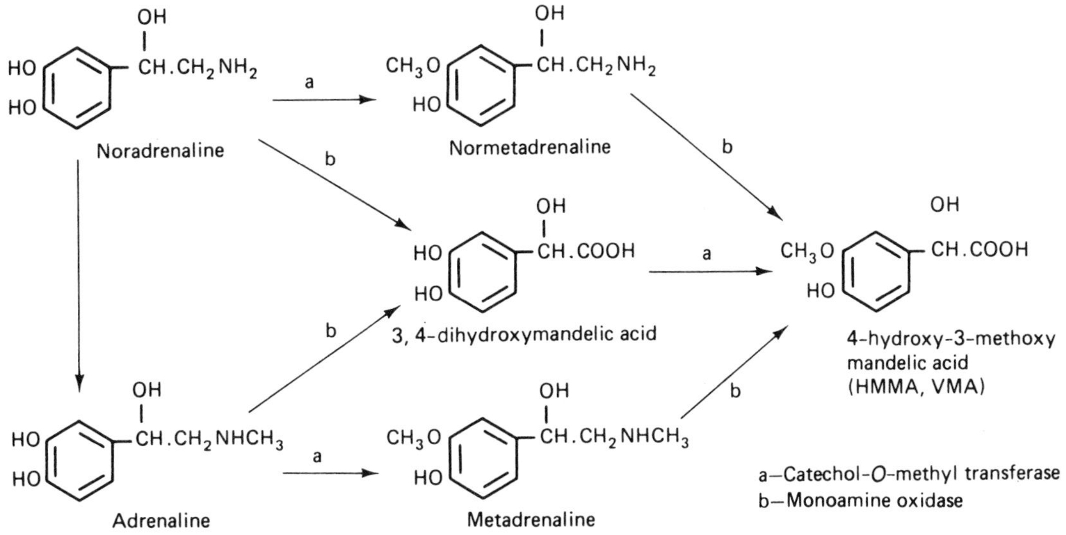

Figure 34.6 Metabolism of adrenalines (epinephrins).

control mechanisms within the neoplastic tissue). Malignant phaeochromocytomas are deficient in DBH, as well as in PNMT, and secretion predominantly of dopamine (with low levels of adrenaline) is suggestive of malignancy.

Secretion of catecholamines from normal chromaffin cells is stimulated by simple depolarization (without action potentials), and is governed chiefly by nicotinic receptors activated by cholinergic fibres within the splanchnic nerves. Adrenaline and noradrenaline are secreted from distinct cell types of their own. Secretion of adrenaline normally predominates over noradrenaline from the adrenals (except during the carotid-sinus reflex response to hypotension). In fact, 95% of the normally circulating noradrenaline originates in spill-over from sympathetic nerve terminals, and most of the circulating dopamine originates in the kidney.

Vascular Effects of Catecholamines. These are mediated variously by α-receptors, causing constriction of arterioles (and veins); β_2-receptors, causing vasodilatation; and β_1-receptors, causing positive inotropic and chronotropic effects in the heart. α-Receptors predominate in skin and splanchnic vascular beds, and β_2-receptors predominate in skeletal muscle vessels. Specific dilatory dopamine receptors (resembling α-receptors in their binding characteristics) occur in the renal arteries.

Adrenaline is an unselective α- and β-agonist; noradrenaline a selective α-agonist; and dopamine mainly β_1 (with some β_1- and α-agonist activity). Therefore, noradrenaline causes generalized vasoconstriction; adrenaline dilates skeletal muscle vessels and constricts vessels to skin and viscera; dopamine dilates the renal arteries. Noradrenaline increases both systolic and diastolic pressure. Adrenaline in-

creases systolic pressure, due to increased cardiac output; but decreases diastolic pressure, due to skeletal muscle vasodilatation. Dopamine causes hypertension only at high concentrations.

When tumours predominantly secrete noradrenaline, therefore, there is usually paroxysmal or sustained hypertension (often with reflex *bradycardia*). By contrast, predominant adrenaline secretion may cause attacks of hypotension and tachycardia; whereas dopamine secretion may cause no cardiovascular symptoms.

Metabolism of Catecholamines. The main pathways of metabolism of noradrenaline and adrenaline are outlined in Fig. 34.6, and are of key importance in diagnosis (*see* below). Perisynaptic or circulating catecholamines are taken up by two distinct carrier-mediated processes, designated uptake 1 and uptake 2. These, respectively, are neuronal and with high affinity; and extraneuronal, with low affinity but high capacity. After uptake 1, catecholamines not recaptured by neuronal storage vesicles are deaminated by mitochondrial monoamine oxidase (MAO), and the metabolites released. After uptake 2, catecholamines are metabolized (mainly in the liver and kidneys) by catechol O-methyl transferase (COMT) within the cytoplasm; the products may then become substrates of mitochondrial MAO in the same or different cells. The initial products of one route of metabolism, therefore, subsequently become free to enter the other route; circulating catecholamines are mainly initial substrates of COMT.

MAO forms aldehyde intermediates, which are oxidized by mitochondrial aldehyde dehydrogenase to form the products shown in Fig. 34.6. These intermediates are as follows. If MAO acts before COMT: 3,4-dihydroxy mandelic aldehyde (DHM aldehyde);

if COMT acts before MAO: 3-methoxy-4-hydroxy mandelic aldehyde (MHM aldehyde). Reduction of these intermediates (by aldehyde reductase) may also occur, yielding dihydroxyphenyl glycol (DOPEG) and finally methoxyhydroxyphenyl glycol (MHPG). The two principal end-products of metabolism are therefore HMMA (VMA) and MHPG; the former predominates overall, while the latter is the major metabolite of cerebral catecholamines. The metabolism of dopamine proceeds similarly via 3,4-dihydroxy phenylacetic acid (DOPAC) or 3-methoxy tyramine, to yield homovanillic acid (HVA).

The catecholamines (except dopamine), and their metabolites, are also conjugated at the phenolic hydroxy groups with the sulphate ion or with glucuronic acid. Minor quantities of catecholamines are excreted by the kidney, unchanged.

Diagnosis of Phaeochromocytoma. Current screening methods, based on high-performance liquid chromatography (HPLC–fluorimetric or HPLC–electrochemical assays) are: plasma free catecholamines; urinary total (including conjugated), or free, catecholamines; urinary metanephrines; and also, requiring less-sensitive methods of assay, urinary HMMA (and HVA). Small tumours secrete proportionately more free catecholamines, which are therefore a little more sensitive than measurements of the metabolites. Metanephrines are slightly more sensitive (and less specific) than HMMA.

Secretion may be episodic, so sampling is usually repeated. Misleading elevation of the plasma catecholamines may occur unless sampled from a supine, rested patient with a venous cannula in place for at least 30 min beforehand. Results of any of the screening tests are often borderline (less than twice the upper reference limit) in hypertensive patients, particularly if there is concomitant illness, or if the patient is on β-blockers or diuretics. When repeated (if possible off medication and free of stress), a consistent borderline elevation (3 out of 3) necessitates further investigation by a suppression test, such as with clonidine. Provocation tests are dangerous and obsolete.

The antihypertensive clonidine is a centrally acting α-agonist that inhibits central sympathetic nervous outflow, but is without suppressive effect on plasma free catecholamines elevated by phaeochromocytoma. The assay for this test must not detect conjugated plasma catecholamines as these have a longer half-life and persist after administration of clonidine to yield false-positive test results.

After diagnosis the tumour may be localized by CT scanning, or more sensitively, by scintigraphy with [^{131}I] meta-iodobenzylguanidine (MIBG), a noradrenaline structural analogue taken up by chromaffin tissue. Selective venous sampling may still be required, particularly for small or extra-adrenal tumours. Variation in adrenal blood flow (according to the vascularity of the tumour) may confound the results unless concentrations of cortisol are used as a correction factor (catecholamine : cortisol).

The patient with phaeochromocytoma must also be screened by provocative testing for medullary thyroid carcinoma, and other features of MEN type II must be looked for; if a relevant abnormality is found, family screening becomes mandatory. Annual follow-up screening is essential after phaeochromocytoma has been excised, since malignancy cannot be excluded with certainty by histological examination of the tumour.

Other Endocrine Causes. Although the above are the main endocrine diseases in which hypertension is an almost constant and important feature, a number of other endocrine diseases can also occasionally exhibit hypertension. These include:

- *Thyroid disease*: hypertension is found more frequently in hypothyroid than in euthyroid subjects. Patients with hypertension should therefore have their thyroid status assessed. Treatment with thyroid hormone usually cures the hypothyroidism and the hypertension. Hyperthyroidism is often associated with increase of systolic blood pressure, probably as a consequence of the high cardiac output in these patients; the diastolic pressure is not usually elevated.

- *Therapy with gonadal steroids*: androgenic steroids increase blood volume and hence blood pressure. Oestrogen/progestogen oral contraceptive preparations also increase blood pressure, a side-effect not observed with postmenopausal hormone replacement therapy.

- *Hypercalcaemia*: hypercalcaemic states are commonly associated with increase in blood pressure. Thus, up to half of patients with primary hyperparathyroidism also exhibit hypertension; it may not be relieved after successful treatment of the hyperparathyroidism.

- Hypertension in *pregnancy*: mothers who were hypertensive before their pregnancy are likely to experience an exacerbation of the problem during the third trimester and in subsequent pregnancy. The occurrence of hypertension in mothers who were previously normotensive is not uncommon; it is now termed *gestational hypertension*. It may be caused by disturbance of the metabolism of prostaglandins and prostacyclins. In contrast with pre-existing disease, gestational hypertension is usually self-limiting and may not recur in subsequent pregnancies. Both forms, however, can during the later stages of the pregnancy give rise to the serious complication of eclampsia.

Further information on the role of endocrine factors in the causation of hypertension can be found in reviews by Wilson and Foster and by Harris (*see* Further Reading).

CONSEQUENCES OF HYPERTENSION

'Malignant' Hypertension

This is a syndrome that can occur *in any form of hypertension* (*essential* or *secondary*), provided the pressure is high enough (diastolic usually more than 120 mmHg) or has risen abruptly. The syndrome is particularly common, however, in renovascular hypertension. The cardinal features are:

- retinopathy with haemorrhages, exudates, or papilloedema;
- proteinuria and haematuria;
- renal impairment, which progresses rapidly to end-stage failure.

The patient will certainly die within 6–12 months unless treated, and the diagnosis constitutes a medical emergency. In this accelerated phase of hypertension there is a characteristic lesion, fibrinoid necrosis, of the resistance vessels, which is manifest in the retina and kidneys. The severe small-vessel disease provokes bilateral hypersecretion of renin and this provides an element of positive feedback in the development of the disease.

Left Ventricular Hypertrophy and Failure

Hypertension causes adaptive and then degenerative changes in the heart and in the arterial tree. The heart initially undergoes hypertrophy in response to the extra work required at higher arterial pressure. But in contrast to the physiological hypertrophy associated with, for instance, a trained athlete, the blood vessels do not develop to a corresponding extent. Thus the vascular supply to the enlarged left ventricle becomes more tenuous and, together with coronary atheroma, provokes an ischaemic fibrosis leading to hypertensive heart failure, angina, or frank myocardial infarction.

Cardiac Failure

The cardiac failure associated with prolonged hypertension is initially a left ventricular failure; the hypertrophic left ventricle with its barely adequate blood supply reaches the stage when it cannot cope with an sudden increase in venous return. Typically, symptoms are initially experienced soon after retiring to bed; the increase in blood returning to the heart on adopting the recumbent position passes into the pulmonary circulation but overwhelms the failing left ventricle. The result is a sudden onset of pulmonary oedema causing acute respiratory difficulty sometimes termed cardiac asthma. Later, the right ventricle is no longer capable of responding to the increased resistance to flow of blood through the congested pulmonary circulation and in its turn, it too fails leading to a generalized failure of the heart.

Atherosclerosis

Arteries undergo adaptive medial and intimal thickening together with accelerated arteriosclerosis and accelerated atheroma. Hypertension is thought to be an important factor in the development of both of these subdivisions of atherosclerosis. Increased turbulence causes deposition of lipid-rich material from the circulating blood on to the vessel walls, especially at arterial branching points. The increased filtration pressure leads to the ingress of this material into the subepithelial space, where it causes inflammatory and necrotic changes. The increased pressure in the lumen of the vessel also jeopardizes the microcirculation in the vessel wall, possibly leading to the characteristic arteriosclerotic changes. These changes may lead to myocardial infarction and to stroke from cerebral infarction.

Resistance vessels (small arteries and arterioles) undergo degenerative change more specific to hypertension, leading to the breakdown of autoregulation, exudation, haemorrhage, and microinfarction.

In the cerebral circulation, microaneurysms form or may already be present as a congenital defect ('berry' aneurysms); increased blood pressure can cause rupture of these thin-walled parts of the vessel. These changes lead to stroke from cerebral haemorrhage, to hypertensive encephalopathy. Similar changes in the kidney can lead to impaired renal function and, if associated with impairment of the renal vascular supply, will aggravate the hypertension by stimulating the renin–angiotensin cascade.

BIOCHEMICAL DIAGNOSIS OF HYPERTENSION

Hypertension is a common disease in which it is important to distinguish those patients in whom there is a definitive cause from those who have essential hypertension. Biochemical investigations play an important part in making this distinction.

All hypertensive patients should have screening plasma urea, electrolytes, glucose and cholesterol and simple urinalysis tests. This will indicate those in whom there is a renal or diabetic cause, and if further investigation for primary aldosteronism or Cushing's syndrome is required. There is some benefit in screening for hypothyroidism in elderly hypertensive patients (both because each disease is more common in the elderly and because of an apparent association between the two).

Screening for phaeochromocytoma should certainly be done in those whose symptoms indicate the possibility. In the authors' laboratory a simple thin-layer chromatography method is in use for the semi-quantitative assessment of catecholamines; this is suitable as an initial screen and has the advantage of indicating increased concentrations of catecholamines other than the adrenalines. Other more specific but more expensive and time-consuming tests for urine catecholamines are reviewed by Weinkove.[116]

As indicated earlier (*see* Table 34.3), more detailed investigations are unlikely to be fruitful unless there are specific indications to the contrary. Then the nature of the subsequent investigation is determined by those indications.

REFERENCES

1. Harris M.C. (1988). The endocrinology of cardiovascular control. *J. Endocrinol.*, **117**, 325.
2. Padfield P.L., Brown J.J., Lever A.F., Morton J.J., Robertson J.I.S. (1981). Blood pressure in acute and chronic vasopressin excess. Studies of malignant hypertension and the syndrome of inappropriate antidiuretic hormone secretion. *N. Engl. J. Med.*, **304**, 1067.
3. Wilkins M.R., Stott R.A.W., Lewis H.M. (1989). Atrial natriuretic factor. *Ann. Clin. Biochem*, **26**, 115.
4. Yanigabashi K. et al. (1986). The synthesis of aldosterone by the adrenal cortex. *J. Biol. Chem.* **261**, 3556.
5. Blaustein M.P. (1977). Sodium ions, calcium ions, blood pressure regulation, and hypertension: a reassessment and a hypothesis. *Am. J. Physiol.*, **232**, C165.
6. Haddy F.J., Overbeck H.W. (1976). The role of humoral agents in volume expanded hypertension. *Life Sci.*, **19**, 935.
7. de Wardener H.E. (1982). The atrial natriuretic peptide. *Ann. Clin. Biochem.*, **19**, 137.
8. de Wardener H.E., Macgregor G.A. (1980). Dahl's hypothesis that a saluretic substance may be responsible for a sustained rise in arterial pressure: its possible role in essential hypertension. *Kidney Int.* **18**, 1.
9. Intersalt Cooperative Research Group (1988). Intersalt: an international study of electrolyte excretion and blood pressure. Results for 24 hour urinary sodium and potassium excretion. *Br. Med. J.*, **297**, 319.
10. Conn J.W. (1955). Primary aldosteronism, a new clinical entity. *J. Lab. Clin. Med.*, **45**, 6.
11. Sen S., Valenzuela R., Sweby R., Bravo E.L., Bumpus F.H. (1981). Localisation, purification and biological activity of a new aldosterone-stimulating factor. *Hypertension*, **3**, 81.
12. Carey R.M., Sen S., Dolan L.M., Malchoff C.D., Bumpus F.M. (1984). Idiopathic hyperaldosteronism: a possible role for aldosterone-stimulating factor. *N. Engl. J. Med.*, **311**, 94.
13. Mulrow P.J. (1981). Glucocorticoid-suppressible hyperaldosteronism? a clue to the missing hormone? (Editorial.) *N. Engl. J. Med.*, **305**, 1012.
14. Ulick S. et al. (1990). Defective fasciculata zone function as a mechanism of glucocorticoid-remediable aldosteronism. *J. Clin. Endocrinol. Metab.*, **70**, 1151.
15. Stewart P.M., Wallace A.M., Valentino R., Burt D., Shackleton C.H.L., Edwards C.R.W. (1987). Mineralocorticoid activity of liquorice: 11-beta-hydroxysteroid dehydrogenase deficiency comes of age. *Lancet*, **ii.**, 821.
16. Weinkove C. (1991) Methods for catecholamines and their metabolites in urine. *J. Clin. Pathol.*, **44**, 269.

FURTHER READING

Benowitz N.L. (1990). Diagnosis and management of phaeochromocytoma. *Hosp. Pract.*, June 15, 163.
Fraser R., Davies D.L., Connell J.M.C. (1989). Hormones and hypertension. *Clin. Endocrinol.*, **31**, 701.
Harvey J.M., Beevers D.G. (1990). Biochemical investigation of hypertension. *Ann. Clin. Biochem.*, **27**, 287.
Mitchell K.D., Navar L.G. (1989). The renin–angiotensin–aldosterone system in volume control. *Baillière's Clin. Endocrinol. Metab.*, **3**, 393.
Padfield P.L. (1989). Disturbances of salt and water metabolism in hypertension. *Baillière's Clin. Endocrinol. Metab.*, **3**, 531.
Wilson J.D., Foster D.W. eds. (1992). *Williams Textbook of Endocrinology*, 8th edn, Philadelphia: Saunders. (Especially Ch. 9, The adrenal cortex (North D.O., Kovacs W.J., DeBold C.R; Ch. 10, Catecholamines and the adrenal medulla (Landsberg L., Young J.B.); Ch. 11, Endocrine Hypertension (Kaplan N.M.)).

35. Hyperlipidaemia
A. J. Winder

The plasma lipoproteins
The central pathways of lipoprotein
  metabolism
  Chylomicrons and the exogenous dietary
    pathway
  Liver and the lipoprotein cascade
  Intracellular control of cholesterol
    metabolism
  High-density lipoproteins and reverse
    cholesterol transport
The development and progression of
  atherosclerosis
  The atheromatous plaque
  Atheroma and lipoproteins
  Hypertriglyceridaemia
  Other risk associations
  Regression of atheroma
The definition of hyperlipidaemia
  What is normal?
  Why are patients lipaemic?

THE PLASMA LIPOPROTEINS

Most lipids in plasma other than non-esterified fatty acids are transported in water-soluble form as lipoproteins. These macromolecules are in a state of flux with transfer of components between cells, tissues and other lipoproteins, but underlying component types can be defined, most readily in the fasting state.[1]

Criteria for lipoprotein classification have developed from the analytical methods that have been useful in displaying component variation. Differences of interest include the type and extent of lipid content, molecular size, charge and the pattern of apoproteins present, factors thus affecting flotation density, sedimentation velocity and mobility in various electrophoretic and separation systems. The apolipoproteins are not simply inert transport carriers of lipid but have various established and proposed active functions in lipoprotein metabolism, particularly involving interaction with cell receptors and activation of enzymes. Variation in apoprotein structure also contributes to genetic control and modulation of lipoprotein metabolism.[2]

Initial classifications based mainly on density and mobility led to that for apolipoproteins, as summarized in Table 35.1. Thus the main protein in high-density lipoprotein (α; HDL) was defined as apo A, that for low-density (β; LDL) was apo B and for very low-density (pre-β; VLDL) as apo C. VLDL actually contains all the apoproteins of major clinical interest and is thus good starting material for studies of genetic variation, but components that were both present in VLDL and not characteristic of any other group could be defined, hence apo C. This classification approach is analogous to that with vitamins, the original A,B,C, etc., being overtaken by further variation. Thus we now recognize apo A-I, A-II, etc. and components not specific for any major lipoprotein class, for example the apo E series.

The exact criteria used to define lipoproteins in laboratory studies and resulting publications are important as material described elsewhere by the same title but using different criteria may be of overlapping but different composition.[3] Thus components classified by density, such as HDL-2/HDL-3 fractions, can

TABLE 35.1
CHARACTERISTICS OF THE MAJOR LIPOPROTEINS IN PLASMA

Chylomicrons
Large particles over range up to 1×10^x mol. wt., then visible by light microscopy
Density 0.93, float up on standing or refrigeration
Mobility on agarose zero
1–2% protein, mainly A-I, A-IV, C, E, B-48
Lipid mainly triglycerides

Very low-density lipoprotein (VLDL)
Range of particles up to 1×10^x mol. wt.
Density d < 1.006 g/L
Mobility pre-β
10% protein, mainly B-100, C, E
Lipid mainly triglyceride, plus some cholesterol + ester, and phospholipid

Low density lipoprotein (LDL)
Mol. wt. 2.3×10^x
Density varies with maturity and composition in range d. 1.019–1.063
Mobility β
20–25% protein, B-100
Lipid mainly cholesterol ester plus some cholesterol, phospholipid and triglyceride

High-density lipoprotein (HDL)
Range of particles within range d. 1.063–1.210
Lipid mainly phospholipid, cholesterol ester
On the basis of density can classify as:
  HDL-2 d. 1.063–1.125. 40% protein, mainly A-I, plus A-II, C, E, trace others; mol. wt. 360 000
  HDL-3 d. 1.125–1.210, mainly A-I, A-II; mol. wt. c. 175 000
  HDL-1 is a trace fraction, enriched with apo E
HDL can also be subdivided on other criteria e.g. size, mobility, apoprotein composition

β-VLDL
Material with d < 1.006 but β-mobility
Chylomicron remnants, or released directly from small intestine

Lipoprotein Lp(a)
LDL, to which apo(a) is attached by sulphydryl links
Mobility pre-β; released directly from liver
Wide interindividual polymorphism affecting kringle 4, thus affecting apo(a) mol. wt. range 280–700 000, and density of Lp(a) at d. 1.047–1.1 g/mL

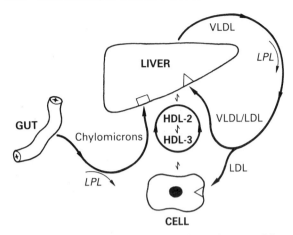

Figure 35.1 An outline of the main pathways of lipoprotein metabolism. HDL, LDL, VLDL, high-, low-, very low-density lipoproteins; LPL, lipoprotein lipase.

contain other material in the appropriate density range that has quite different structural and biological features (e.g. lipoprotein Lp(a)) and the various macromolecular precipitants—heparin, dextran, etc.—applied in the separation of HDL-2 and HDL-3 within the HDL fraction do not precipitate exactly the same material. Also, the density nomenclature (HDL, VLDL, etc.) is now preferred over earlier systems (e.g. pre-β lipoprotein), irrespective of the separation methods actually used.

THE CENTRAL PATHWAYS OF LIPOPROTEIN METABOLISM

Three essential pathways are involved, summarized in Fig. 35.2. First, exogenous dietary lipid is processed mainly as chylomicrons, which are progressively broken down in the circulation to remnants that are taken up by liver. In the VLDL second pathway, the liver then secretes newly assembled VLDL, containing mainly triglycerides, which are modified intravascularly by removal and exchange of lipid and protein to the smaller, denser and relatively cholesterol-enriched LDL. This LDL, or the definable components of intermediate density (IDL), can be recycled to liver, or taken up via specific receptors by peripheral (i.e. extrahepatic) cells as a delivery system for sterols. Finally, there are components containing as much or more protein than lipid, such as HDL, which are derived from precursors released from liver or intestine and from the spare protein/phospholipid surface coat left over as large chylomicron/VLDL particles are broken down. HDL components are involved in exchange of protein and lipid between lipoproteins and with tissues, and may contribute to a return to liver as reverse cholesterol transport. This return is important because significant degradation of cholesterol, or its excretion from the body, can only be effected by the liver.

Chylomicrons and the Exogenous Dietary Pathway

Dietary lipid is hydrolysed and then processed in the wall of the small intestine, with release into the systemic circulation as chylomicrons via the thoracic duct. Chylomicrons are large particles containing more than 99% by weight of lipid. Various apoproteins are present or transferred, mainly from HDL, the major fraction being the N-terminal sequence comprising 48% of that of apo B-100, hence apo B-48. A post-transcriptional stop codon is apparently introduced into intestinal mRNA: apo B-100 can be released by the small intestine but, in an unknown manner, this process is at least very substantially suppressed.

When fasting, or when fat intake is low, the intestine releases smaller and denser chylomicron-like apo B-48-containing lipoproteins, intestinal VLDL. Some low molecular-weight fatty acids can pass direct to liver via the portal vein and this route allows intake of medium-chain length triglyceride and fat-soluble vitamins when chylomicron formation is impaired, as in forms of abetalipoproteinaemia for which expression of the apo B gene and thus chylomicron structure or release are defective.

Chylomicrons contain triglycerides, phospholipids, and cholesterol and cholesterol esters derived from the diet and from bile. Some luminal cholesterol is esterified by intestinal acyl CoA:cholesterol O-acyltransferase (ACAT). Inhibitors of this enzyme are under review in the treatment of hyperlipidaemia, as they have the potential to reduce sterol absorption and release by intestine, and thus levels of cholesterol in serum.

Processing of chylomicrons and intestinal VLDL involves progressive hydrolysis of acyl residues in triglycerides and phospholipids, with liberation of redundant apoprotein-rich surface coat and free cholesterol. This involves lipoprotein lipase (LPL), an enzyme bound to endothelium, particularly in striated muscle and adipose tissue, which is activated by apo C-II also present in chylomicrons.

Fatty acids thus released may be transported bound to albumin, and then transferred to liver, muscle or adipose tissue for oxidation or for storage in adipose tissue after re-esterification. Subsequent lipolysis in adipose tissue, with fatty acid release into the circulation, some going to liver for assembly into lipoprotein, is suppressed by nicotinic acid and derivatives, and this effect is the basic for their use in management of lipaemic patients. Cholesterol and its esters, and spare apoprotein, are redistributed to other lipoproteins, and redundant surface coat is particularly important in the provision of precursor material for the development of mature HDL.

Patients with impaired processing of triglyceride-rich lipoproteins thus generally also show impaired generation of HDL, particularly the HDL-2 fraction, as shown in Fig. 35.2, and the benefits of exercise on lipoprotein profiles may relate to increased skeletal-

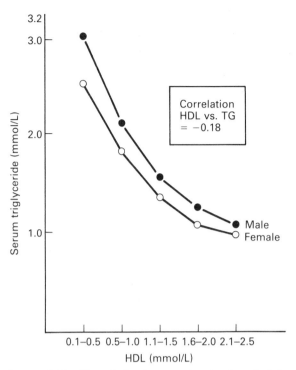

Figure 35.2 The relation between levels of total triglyceride (TG) and high-density lipoprotein (HDL) in fasting plasma for a British population; data from the National Lipid Screening Project.[14]

muscle blood flow and thus exposure of plasma lipids to LPL. This processing via LPL is also enhanced by drugs related to fibric acid. Proteoglycans are involved in linking LPL to endothelium. Intravenous heparin can be used to release this and other lipases, and postheparin lipolytic activity can then be determined in plasma.

Complete deficiency of LPL can arise through various rare, autosomal recessive, structural defects or similar deficiency of apo C-II. A circulating inhibitor of LPL with autosomal dominant transmission is also described, and in the autoimmune hyperchylomicronaemia syndrome, LPL activity may be impaired through immunoglobulin binding to LPL, apo C-II or heparin.[4] Most cases of hyperchylomicronaemia seem to be acquired, usually through diabetes and/or alcoholism; underlying genetic defects could also contribute, although this prospect is generally hard to define, or even consider, until the primary problem is controlled.

Severe deficiency of LPL activity or clearance overload as above are associated with major excess of chylomicrons and other triglyceride-rich particles; clinical features can include lipaemia retinalis, eruptive xanthomas, and a risk of abdominal pain and chemical pancreatitis. This well-known but actually quite rare association with hyperchylomicronaemia of any cause presumably arises through passive extravasation of excess lipid-rich particles into lipase-rich pancreatic tissue, with hydrolysis, fatty acid release, tissue damage, permeability change and escalating chemical pancreatitis.

Primary LPL deficiency can best be controlled by diets low in total fat: and cardiovascular risk is small, as is that of pancreatitis if total triglyceride levels are controlled below around 8 mmol/L. LPL assay precision is not high but some patients with endogenous hypertriglyceridaemia do seem to show reduced activity, as is reported for some cases with the rather loosely defined and apparently autosomal dominant disorder, familial combined hyperlipoproteinaemia, with excess of cholesterol and triglyceride in plasma. Heterozygous deficiency or variants of LPL could perhaps occasionally be involved.

Final clearance of the substantially lipid-depleted remnants of chylomicrons and intestinal VLDL involves uptake by liver in a manner strongly suggestive of a receptor-based mechanism interacting with apo E forms on the remnant particle surface, although details are not yet resolved.

An expressing apo E allele is inherited from each parent and there are three common variants E-2, E-3 and E-4. Regarding E-3 as the base form (E-3/E-3 is the most common pattern), substitutions of cystine for arginine or vice versa at positions 112 or 158 give the single charge-shift forms E-2 and E-4. In combination, these three forms encompass most, perhaps 99%, of the known variation. Additional rare variants occur for which substitutions at different sites are involved: when they also give the same charge shifts as the main variants they may be defined as E-2*, E-2**, E-4**, etc.[2] Some of this range of variants affects remnant structure, notably the E-2/E-2 combination found in 1–2% of the population, and remnants can show delayed clearance, rarely severe, however, unless a further cause of overload and/or delayed clearance such as diabetes, alcohol excess or hypothyroidism is also involved. The clinical syndrome is autosomal recessive, familial (type III) dysbetalipoproteinaemia with soft tissue and tendon xanthomas, coronary and particularly peripheral atherosclerosis, and in about half of severely lipaemic cases the striking linear palmar xanthomas. Plasma contains excess chylomicron remnants—material with VLDL density and present in the VLDL d < 1.006 density fraction, but with β-mobility on electrophoresis because apo B-48 is present. Hence these remnants are colloquially described as floating β-lipoprotein, and their identification in fasting plasma is still a benchmark diagnostic procedure for the familial disorder, as specific methodology for structural variants using electric iso focusing, immunoblotting or oligonucleotide gene probes may be confounded by the occasional rare variant form. Some of these rare variants, and occasionally the E-2 form (usually in the presence of a second defect such as heterozygous familial hypercholesterolaemia), can express with remnant delay and clinical features in heterozygous form, with a single abnormal transmitted gene. The struc tural changes induced in the remnants by the one variant protein and lipid overload restrict interaction with the proposed receptor process to such an extent that dominant expression of the defect can result. Presumably the same principle—delayed clearance as a result of variant protein plus overload-induced conformational change—explains why most apo E-2 homozygotes are not grossly lipaemic or clinically affected unless a second disorder and overload are also present.

Liver and the Lipoprotein Cascade

The liver releases VLDL, which contains some 90% by weight of endogenously synthesized lipid, mainly triglyceride with some cholesterol and phospholipid, and 10% protein, mainly apo C with some apo B-100, apo E and other trace components. VLDL is modified intravascularly through the action of LDL and component exchange, as for chylomicrons, potentially to LDL through a loosely definable, IDL stage. Thus in fasting samples, which normally contain insignificant chylomicron-related material, VLDL is the main vehicle for transport of triglyceride and LDL is that for cholesterol. LDL subclasses can also be defined. Some 70% of the cholesterol and 95% of the apo B-100 in plasma is associated with LDL: levels of cholesterol are a reasonable, and levels of apo B-100 are a close, guide to levels of LDL in plasma. Apo B-100 may therefore indicate the number of LDL particles, and thus colligative processes more related to particle number than to their composition: the development of atheroma could be such a process. Disappointingly however, in most studies levels of apo B-100 have not been obviously superior to LDL-cholesterol as markers of clinical outcome.

Modulation in the so-called lipoprotein cascade is a continuous process, with a range of material only readily compressed into apparently specific components by discontinuous separation methods such as ultracentrifugation on step gradients, further sharpened by analysis in the fasting state. A large and individually variable proportion of VLDL remnants (average around 60%) returns to liver by receptor-mediated uptake, and the exact composition of components in the VLDL/IDL/LDL cascade depends on the extent and rate of the various exchange steps. Hepatic triglyceride lipase may be involved in the conversion of some VLDL remnants to the final product, LDL. This is enriched with cholesterol and cholesterol esters, through inward transfer of cholesterol and removal mainly of triglyceride; also because of transfer, the 20–25% of protein present in LDL is essentially all apo B-100. LDL is an end-of-line component, taken up by cells and not recycled, about two-thirds returning to liver, the rest entering extrahepatic cells.

This final clearance of LDL mainly involves receptor-mediated uptake into cells, particularly by the high-affinity receptors located in coated pits on the surface of all cell types studied to date.[5] Ligand-binding regions of the receptors expressed on the cell surface bind to specific regions of apo B-100, resulting in endocytosis, fusion of the vesicles with lysosomes, hydrolysis of LDL with degradation of protein and incorporation of released lipid. Cholesterol is then esterified or re-esterified and stored in ester form through the action of the intracellular enzyme ACAT. Receptors are substantially conserved and recycled to the cell surface. Receptor expression and intracellular cholesterol synthesis are subject to feedback controls via the rate of synthesis and/or degradation of hydroxymethyl glutaryl coenzme A reductase (HMG CoA reductase), the enzyme controlling the rate-limiting step of cholesterol synthesis. These controls can stabilize levels of available intracellular cholesterol, although protection is incomplete as discussed below: some of the interlocking processes involved are summarized in Fig. 35.3. Further receptor expression on some cells promotes the uncontrolled uptake of LDL that has been modified by minor oxidative or other chemical change.[6]

This scavenger pathway has considerable implications for atherosclerosis, as discussed below. Sterol requirements of extrahepatic cells are substantially met by cholesterol delivery in LDL. Significant, although still minor, endogenous production arises in tissues with specific requirements for sterols, adrenal cortex and gonads for example. Competitive inhibitors of HMG CoA reductase—the statins—are powerful cholesterol-lowering agents. Squalene synthetase, further down the pathway, controls the committed step beyond which all components are hydrophobic and directed solely to sterol synthesis. Inhibition at this step could give a more targeted control of cholesterol synthesis without potential restriction of other non-sterol processes that are also dependent on mevalonate and HMG CoA reductase, such as synthesis of ubiquinones and dolichols.[7]

Lipoprotein(a) (Lp(a))

This is a complex directly secreted by liver, in which apo B-100 within LDL is linked through sulphydryl groups to apo(a).[8] This apo(a) has substantial structural homology with plasminogen, with a large and variable number of repeats of a mid-section (kringle four) of that structure. Apo(a) is codominantly expressed and each of the two parental alleles may involve the same or a different number of repeats, a range of 10–44 being currently reported. Thus Lp(a) may be present in a very wide range of isoforms. It is determined immunochemically with standards calibrated by weight, and by further sodium dodecyl sulphate electrophoresis, which allows some discrimination into different sized isoforms, larger isoforms associating with lower levels of Lp(a) in plasma.[8] It is not yet established whether calibration to give molar values is clinically useful. There is an association between above-mean levels of

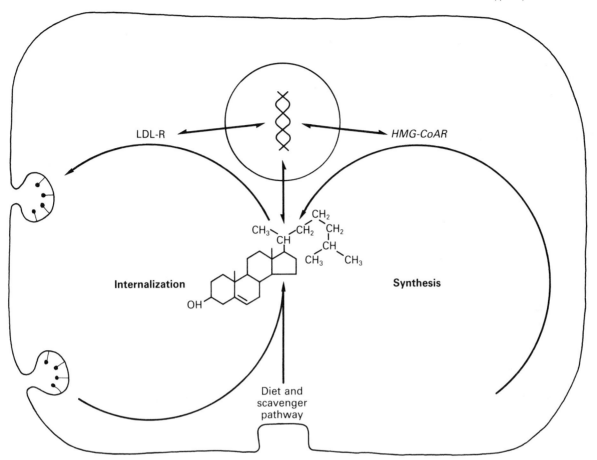

Figure 35.3 Cholesterol availability within cells: HMG-CoAR, hydroxymethyl glutaryl coenzyme A reductase; LDL-R, low-density lipoprotein receptor.

Lp(a) and premature coronary heart disease with familial hypercholesterolaemia, and also with British families with premature coronary heart disease but with generally average levels of total lipids in plasma. Such an association is not obvious in groups with high Lp(a) but low levels of LDL—black Americans and native Sudanese for example: very low levels are seen in China. Adverse relations probably arise through interference with plasminogen, and perhaps other structurally related agents affecting clot formation and dissolution and the thrombotic/thrombolytic balance in plasma. From the interpopulation data, high levels may be a conditional rather than an absolute risk and dependent on levels of LDL.

Familial Hypercholesterolaemia (FH)
Various defects in the high-affinity receptor arise in forms of FH. These are most severe in homozygotes who on family studies can be double heterozygotes for two different defects transmitted from each parent.[5] For FH homozygotes, the combined receptor defect can be substantial but not complete, and such receptor-defective homozygotes suffer slightly less severe clinical expression than with receptor-negative forms. In heterozygous FH, affecting about 0.2%

of North Europeans, the clinical expression of accelerated coronary heart disease and of tissue lipid deposits as corneal arcus and xanthomas, particularly of tendons, seems generally similar whichever molecular defect has contributed to the 50% shortfall in effective receptors. This also applies in the clinically similar disorder familial defective hyperapobetalipoproteinaemia, where the defect is in the receptor-binding domains of apo B-100. This variant arises through a point mutation affecting amino acid 3500 in the receptor sequence, hence colloquially defined as apo B-3500 FH. The two parental alleles express two populations of circulating LDL with and without the defective sequence, the defective form being predominant through delayed catabolism.

The substantial molecular heterogeneity of clinical FH, with defined genetic abnormalities in some 18% of heterozygotes only, and with the complication that functionally adequate receptor variants are also found in the normolipaemic population, means that approaches applying molecular biological screening to this clinically clear-cut but biologically very heterogeneous disorder are not yet secure. Molecular biology can be helpful in families in which the defect is known or in communities (such as French Canadians) where, through a founder effect, most cases have the same molecular defect and for which diagnostic techniques are developed. The defect in FH is also associated with enrichment of platelets with free cholesterol and their increased sensitivity to aggregating agents with increased binding of fibrinogen. Clinical outcome among patients with FH is also related to levels of Lp(a).

Lipid treatment of FH is directed at enhancing sterol excretion with oral bile-acid sequestrants—non-absorbed ion-exchange resins that complex bile acid in the intestine, preventing reabsorption and also impairing lipid absorption—plus other agents, either nicotinates or statins, to restrict endogenous sterol production. Plasma exchange, or selective plasmapheresis to remove apo B-100 lipoproteins but not HDL and other proteins, are also available.

Some patients apparently with familial hypertriglyceridaemia and VLDL excess are overproducing VLDL. Overproduction of apo B-100 lipoproteins can be involved in familial combined hyperlipidaemia, a poorly defined and almost certainly heterogeneous disorder in which LDL receptor function is normal. Accelerated coronary heart disease can also be associated with hyperapobetalipoproteinaemia, in which levels of apo B-100 are greater than expected from levels of VLDL/IDL, and of LDL, which can be small and dense. Animal studies have also shown that trivially modified LDL, such as by minor oxidation of surface LDL lipid by endothelium, is potentially atherogenic because entry into cells via specific scavenger receptors is uncontrolled,[6] as discussed below. Natural antioxidants such as vitamins C and E, and the drug probucol, may restrict this oxidative change, affecting both lipid and protein.

Intracellular Control of Cholesterol Metabolism

Homeostatic mechanisms have the potential to stabilize intracellular cholesterol levels and to protect cells from cholesterol overload, with some control of cholesterol entry and production, storage and removal.[5,7] Sterol regulatory elements within the promoter regions of the high-affinity LDL cell-surface receptor, and of HMG CoA reductase, control transcription either directly or through derived oxysterols complexed to protein, in response to the availability of intracellular cholesterol. The rate of degradation of HMG CoA reductase may also be responsive to feedback control. Control of ACAT activity is not well defined, although some oxysterols enhance activity. Mobilization of stored pools involves cholesterol ester hydrolase, modulated by phosphorylation. Extracellular cholesterol transfer probably involves receptor-based transfer to HDL fractions as discussed below. Thus, potential cell overload directs down-regulation of expression of the LDL receptor and of HMG CoA reductase, possibly with enhanced degradation, and up-regulation of the proposed HDL cell-surface receptor. Intracellular hydrolysis of stored cholesterol esters may be enhanced by new membrane synthesis as is required for cell division.

Regulation may be confounded by unregulated entry of cholesterol, as may arise for liver through high-fat diets and entry as chylomicron remnants, and more generally through the delivery of LDL-like material via the scavenger receptor, entry being driven by the level of available ligand with no feedback control. Diets rich in saturated fats seem particularly effective at down-regulating LDL receptor expression and thus reducing removal of LDL from plasma. A further complication concerns the freedom of exchange between cholesterol pools and the intracellular mechanisms for sensing and then responding to any potential deficiency or overload. These controls are not yet well understood, and specific defects could also perhaps arise, as exemplified by cell-culture studies in Niemann–Pick C disease.[9] Cells continue to express LDL receptors and internalize LDL even when overloaded with cholesterol esters compartmentalized within intracellular vesicles.

High-density Lipoproteins and Reverse Cholesterol Transport

Further lipoproteins can be defined in plasma within the density range 1.063–1.21 and containing down to some 40% lipid. This HDL is heterogeneous and a minor plasma lipoprotein fraction by weight, but as molecular weights are also relatively low, HDL components can be the most plentiful molecular lipoprotein species in plasma.

For isolation, density methods are commonly replaced by selective precipitation of non-HDL, i.e. apo B-100-rich components by polyelectrolytes, commonly using Mn^{++}/heparin or Mo^{++}/phosphotungstate systems, sometimes dextran sulphate or polyethylene glycol.[3] There are points in favour of all these methods, although as the Mn^{++}/heparin method is widely used it is now preferred, so as to render results between centres more readily comparable. The difficulty is that the various methods may not precipitate or measure exactly the same mix of HDL components, and as for the subclasses discussed below, choice of best method will depend on a clearer understanding of the metabolic role of the various HDL components in the mix.

HDL in plasma originates in precursor apoprotein/phospholipid material released from liver and intestine, and in the form of spare surface coat and lipid released during the metabolism of large triglyceride-rich particles. Nascent discoid precursor material is rapidly converted in plasma to mature HDL through fusion with mature particles and through component transfer, particularly of cholesterol, then esterified on the particle surface by lecithin–cholesterol acyltransferase (LCAT) (Fig. 35.4). This enzyme is associated with HDL in plasma and is activated by apo A–I: the cholesterol esters then formed contribute to the core of HDL fractions.

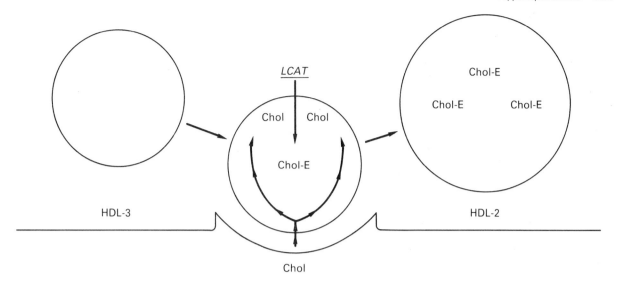

HDL cell-surface receptor

Figure 35.4 The proposed mechanism of receptor-based and high-density lipoprotein (HDL)-mediated reverse cholesterol (chol) transport: Chol-E, cholesterol esters; LCAT, lecithin–cholesterol acyltransferase.

HDL should be seen as a system complex, the exact mix and composition reflecting interactions with tissues and other plasma components at the time.[1] The HDL fraction defined by a density cut as above is not homogeneous and many techniques have been applied in further analysis, notably on the basis of density, size, apoprotein composition, electrophoretic mobility by various methods, and selective precipitation with polyelectrolytes such as dextran sulphate.

The separation by density into two major components HDL-2 and HDL-3, has been the benchmark for other approaches because of the clinical association of this approach (HDL-1 is a further, minor, apoE-rich component more evident after lipid feeding; a further dense apo A-I component has pre-β mobility and is hence called pre-β HDL). HDL-3 is smaller and denser than HDL-2 with less lipid but more apo A-I and A-II. The HDL-2 density cut contains mainly apo A-I and more lipid, particularly cholesterol ester and comprises about one-third of total HDL. It is mainly responsible for the inverse relation between levels of triglyceride and HDL shown in Fig. 35.2, the higher levels of HDL in women, and the interindividual differences in total HDL that are associated in most but not all studies with the general inverse relation within populations between HDL and coronary heart disease.

As with total HDL, the inconvenience of gradient methods has led to alternative approaches, and the HDL-2/HDL-3 cut can be more or less reproduced by selective precipitation, most commonly with specific preparations of dextran sulphate. Alternatives include a division into large and small HDL, or apo A-I-only particles and apo(A-I + A-II) particles, ap-proaches almost but not quite the same as separation by density into HDL-2 and HDL-3 subclasses.[1] Considerable additional particle subfraction heterogeneity of HDL is evident on gradient gel electrophoresis, for example.

In clinical practice the place for assays of HDL and its fractions depends on the value of the information so obtained in the diagnosis and management of patients. That requires some understanding of the interconversions affecting HDL fractions and particularly their possible contribution to reverse cholesterol transport, with implications for prevention or regression of atheroma.

HDL Metabolism

Precursor HDL material is directly released from liver and intestine, and also generated through hydrolysis of triglyceride-rich lipoproteins by LPL in capillary beds. Maturation to HDL-3 and then HDL-2 involves the development of a cholesterol ester-enriched core, through the action of LCAT on cholesterol at the hydrophilic surface of HDL-3. Further interactions probably involve a cell surface receptor-based mechanism, and cholesterol ester transfer protein (CETP: also known as lipid transfer protein 1, LTP-1) and hepatic triglyceride lipase (HTGL); outline pathways were summarized in Figs. 35.1 and 35.4. There is growing evidence of a cell-surface receptor that is specific for HDL-3 and inhibited by HDL-2 and up-regulated by cellular cholesterol loading. Interaction facilitates transfer of cholesterol to the HDL-3 surface with esterification via LCAT and its transfer to the core of the particle, thus generating the enlarged and cholesterol ester-enriched HDL-2. Transfer appears to require apo A-I. The rate-limiting step may be the intracellular mobilization of cholesterol to the cell surface for transfer, a step facilitated intracellularly by apo A-I in an as yet unknown manner.[10]

Levels of apo A-I-only HDL particles have provided the best discrimination between patients with and without angiographically proven coronary artery disease in some surveys. The glycoprotein CETP circulates in association with HDL components, and probably acts by forming an intermediary complex, to transfer cholesterol ester from HDL to VLDL/IDL/LDL in exchange for triglyceride, with regeneration of HDL-3 from HDL-2. This process is thus linked to maturation within the VLDL/IDL/LDL cascade. As these cascade lipoproteins may then proceed to hepatic degradation, this represents a potential route of reverse cholesterol transport, advantageous unless clearance of these potentially atherogenic lipoproteins is delayed. Such delay also allows further transfer of cholesterol esters into triglyceride-rich lipoproteins (probably increasing their atherogenicity unless they are themselves rapidly cleared) and triglyceride enrichment of HDL-2, via CETP. A probably lesser contribution to reverse transport may also derive from hydrolysis of HDL-2 lipid by HTGL, with transfer of cholesterol ester to liver and reconstitution of an apo A–phospholipid surface precursor of HDL-3. The drug probucol enhances CETP activity.

Genetic and Other Disorders Affecting HDL Metabolism. Several disorders affect the structure and processing of HDL and illuminate the processes of normal HDL metabolism.[11] Complete absence of circulating normal HDL arises in homozygotes for inversions and base insertions affecting the A-I/C-III/A-IV gene complex. These major defects are generally associated with premature coronary heart disease, and with tissue lipid accumulation including corneal clouding, also arising in a Fish-eye-like syndrome (*see* below) with a further defect in the A-I gene and circulating trace amounts of a truncated gene product. Substantial deficiency of circulating HDL and apo A-I is also associated with (to date) over 20 structural variants of the apo A-I gene: collectively, prevalence is at least 1/1000, probably much higher as the screening methodology primarily detects charge-shift mutations only. There is also evidence from restriction enzyme studies around the apo A-I gene of further disorders affecting gene expression.

Marked deficiency of HDL is also seen in Tangier disease, familial LCAT deficiency and the related disorder, Fish-eye disease. The primary defect in *Tangier disease* is not yet clearly defined, but involves structurally normal apo A–I and rapid turnover and catabolism of immature precursor forms of HDL include massive lipid accumulation in tissues including cornea, and a slight bias towards premature coronary heart disease in homozygotes only, perhaps

slight because levels of LDL are also low: heterozygotes have levels of HDL around the 50th percentile for their reference population.

LCAT deficiency encompasses several defects with absent or defective circulating gene product. HDL deficiency is marked, although effects on other lipoproteins are variable, tissues accumulate lipid enriched with free cholesterol, and renal involvement is commonly severe. Corneal opacification with stromal accumulation of free cholesterol and phospholipid is marked, also a feature of the so far clinically benign *Fish-eye disease*. The name was applied because the first families described had the ocular appearances of boiled fish, but at later corneal grafting to improve vision the fish-eye appearance was found to arise mainly from underlying cataracts, unrelated to the lipid disorder. Corneal appearance and biochemistry exactly resembled that of LCAT deficiency, consistent with apparent 'partial' LCAT deficiency, as was later confirmed. The defective esterification of cholesterol on HDL but not on other lipoproteins may involve structural changes at a non-catalytic site of LCAT, which, through conformational change, alter substrate specificity and impair interaction with HDL: a variant apo A–I form noted above may have a similar conformational effect.

There is a general association between levels of circulating HDL and LDL activity, and an inverse relation with activity of HDL for which genetic deficiency is associated with broadly normal levels of HDL but which is enriched with triglyceride and of HDL–2 type, and some suggestion of premature atherosclerosis.

Genetic CETP deficiency with elevated levels of cholesterol ester-enriched HDL–2 is also reported, with corneal clouding but a suggestion of longevity rather than premature atherosclerosis. There may be other forms of genetic hyperalphalipoproteinaemia of as yet uncertain basis, also associated with longevity. This may depend on plasma levels of the VLDL/IDL components into which the cholesterol ester is transferred, excess levels being adverse.

Finally, HDL deficiency can be secondary—to obesity, smoking, inactivity, some drugs (anabolic steroids, non-selective β-blockers, thiazide diuretics) for example—and a range of systemic disorders. HDL excess can also be secondary, through ethanol abuse (mainly HDL–3) and poisoning with some pesticides (e.g. DDT) for example.

THE DEVELOPMENT AND PROGRESSION OF ATHEROSCLEROSIS

Extensive and largely epidemiological observations have defined many associations with these processes, and particularly with their expression as coronary heart disease.[12] In industrialized countries the big four are hypercholesterolaemia, hypertension, cigarette smoking, and to a lesser extent, diabetes melli-

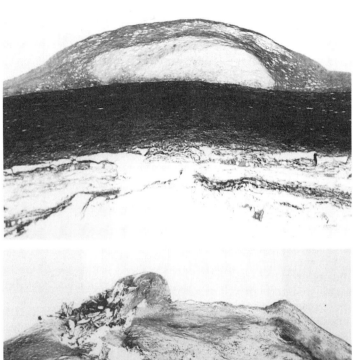

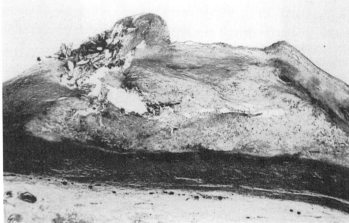

Figure 35.5 Structure and progression of atherosclerotic plaques: (a) general organization, with a central, soft, gruel-like area of lipid, cells and necrotic material, an overlying fibrous cap, and the underlying muscle coat of the arterial wall; (b) the plaque shows fissuring, rupture and thrombus formation at the exposed surface.

tus, with many other less powerful and sometimes curious and thought-provoking associations including, for example, the hardness of water, and homocystinaemia in both genetic and lesser forms. Atherosclerosis and its fundamental lesion as the atheromatous plaque is strongly associated with the clinical expression of occlusive vascular disease but the importance of other processes and particularly thrombosis must be recognized.

The Atheromatous Plaque

The essential features are a fibrous cap of connective tissue covering a gruel of lipid-enriched material present both within cells and as extracellular necrotic debris (Fig. 35.5). The proportions of these components and the complexity of plaque development can vary widely, even for plaques from the same arterial tree of the same patient. Additional features can include calcification, haemorrhage and thrombosis within the plaque, overlying thrombus, and some fibrous, vascular and lymphocytic cellular reaction in the surrounding arterial wall. Fibromuscular plaques probably arise from fatty streaks, representing superficial endothelial and subendothelial cells laden with lipid and forming at sites that suggest a relation with patterns of local blood flow and turbulence.

The uncertainty of progression arises because expression of fatty streaks and atheroma within populations is not obviously related, and if streaks are the necessary precursor lesions they do not necessarily progress. For the coronary tree, streaks and plaques have a very similar distribution, indeed suggesting at least some linked development and a moderating haemodynamic contribution. The requirements and stages of plaque development are not certain, but the idea that endothelial cell injury is involved—the reaction to injury hypothesis—is persuasive, although injury does not have to be physical.[13]

Atheroma and Lipoproteins

Permeability changes could facilitate entry of macromolecules including LDL and related lipoproteins, of cells, particularly monocyte-macrophages, and attachment of platelets at the sites of injury, particularly if endothelial denudation occurs. Progression involves accumulation of lipoprotein-derived lipid within cells. These macrophages and smooth-muscle cells are stimulated both to divide and to enhance expression of LDL-type receptors by growth factors (e.g. platelet-derived growth factor and epidermal growth factor) from platelets and other cells in arterial wall. Further recruitment and necrosis of cells follows.[13] Accumulation could involve LDL incorporating lipid and protein that has been structurally modified through oxidative interaction with endothelial cells in the extracellular space. Further oxidative and other modification (e.g. glycosylation) could also arise. Such modified material, internalized through scavenger receptors expressed on macrophages but not smooth-muscle cells, and derived lipid as ceroid, can be shown in plaques. Extravascular conversion could explain the awkward difficulty for the modified LDL proposal that such material is so hard to demonstrate in the circulation.[6] Trapping reactions through binding of LDL to vessel-wall glycosaminoglycans (GAGs) could also facilitate internalization of native or modified lipoprotein, and growth-factor effects on receptor expression could explain why accumulation of lipoprotein-lipid within smooth-muscle cells does not effectively protect against further overload by down-regulating receptor expression. HDL may compete with LDL for GAG binding and mitigate any initial trapping process. HDL also seems to be able to protect LDL from endothelial cell-mediated oxidative damage, a potential benefit independent of any effects on reverse cholesterol transport, which is discussed above.

The idea that atherosclerosis is driven by excess but trace levels of malignant 'kamikaze' lipoproteins is attractive as it would explain why levels of major plasma components such as total cholesterol, LDL or apo B-100 do not closely relate to individual clinical outcome. However, in population studies, levels of LDL do associate with outcome. Derived components in plasma, such as oxidized LDL and Lp(a), may be conditional risks, enhancing progression directly or through formation from LDL, only when levels of LDL are also excessive. These various components may also affect different steps in the process of plaque initiation and development, Lp(a) can be detected in artery wall but the key pathological effect is probably impaired dissolution of thrombus,[8] and thus simple comparisons of atherogenicity in a multistage process may be inappropriate. Arguments on the importance of trace components continue, and the outcome will be important in defining targets in the treatment of dyslipidaemic patients in general, and in defining those at particular risk of accelerated atherosclerosis and rupture of unstable plaques, probably the key process in precipitating clinical events.

Hypertriglyceridaemia

There is a general association between hypertriglyceridaemia and cardiovascular disease, and particularly with extracoronary disease where cigarette smoking, hypertriglyceridaemia and low HDL are commonly associated. When the data are analysed the association depends, in different surveys, largely or entirely on the precursor–product relation (shown in Fig. 35.2 above) between triglyceride-rich particle clearance and the generation of HDL,[14] levels of which can be estimated instead.[15] However, triglyceride levels can show some residual association with cardiovascular disease independent of HDL, notably in men with below-average levels of cholesterol and in older women, in whom levels of HDL exceed those in men.[15]

Further resolution of the value of triglyceride measurement in defining cardiovascular risk will depend on the identification of mechanisms involved. Current possibilities include associations with plasma levels of factor VII, plasminogen activator inhibitor and hypercoagulability—which could reflect incidental effects through binding and cotransport in plasma rather than specific pathological effects of triglyceride-rich lipoproteins.[16] The prospect that some triglyceride lipoproteins are readily taken up into cells and are thus highly atherogenic is also attractive, the excess levels of partially metabolized, small VLDL found in some individuals being of special interest. Compositional changes in LDL and VLDL are also common features of non-insulin dependent diabetes mellitus, the changes suggesting delayed maturation down the lipoprotein cascade, with further effects on HDL fractions.[1] From clinical associations, chylomicron remnants as β-VLDL are also plainly atherogenic, and these various associations suggest that useful information may arise from detailed analysis of triglyceride-rich lipoproteins in patients with atherosclerosis. There is also a general association between hypertriglyceridaemia and cerebral infarction, although specific mechanisms (e.g. hypercoagulability) have not been defined.

Other Risk Associations

Cigarette smoking may promote atherosclerosis through vasoconstriction, hypoxia through binding of carbon monoxide to haemoglobin, and through endothelial injury and permeability change, as may homocystine through sulphydryl-group effects on protein cross-linkage and structure,[13] effects confirmed at other sites such as lens zonule and hair keratin. Smokers may also consume less vegetable and fruit and thus particularly antioxidant vitamins, perhaps because of changed appreciation of taste. Coronary arterial segments removed at bypass surgery from heavy smokers tend to be more fibrous than fibrofatty, consistent with further growth-factor effects.

In Western populations, plaque composition is not obviously affected by coexisting hypertension, perhaps because plasma lipid levels are generally high: in animals with naturally low lipids, fibrous lesions arise if hypertension is then induced.

Regression of Atheroma

There is growing evidence that established coronary atherosclerosis can be induced to regress by extreme attention to hypercholesterolaemia and all other major risk factors, although stabilization, or a retarded rate, of progression is more commonly achieved. Prospects for regression may depend on retrieval of plaque lipid into general tissue and circulating pools,[13,17] with improved luminal diameter. This also depends on the proportions of lipid and fibromuscular obstruction. Any clinical benefit may come from this effect on the lumen, but is more likely to arise from stabilization of the increasingly lipid-depleted and fibromuscular plaque, with less risk of rupture, thrombosis and occlusion, processes strongly associated with clinical coronary events. Younger plaques seem more prone to rupture.

The question arises: is HDL good for you, and if so, how? The observations on a wide spectrum of genetic defects affecting circulating levels of HDL show that some but not all are associated with premature atherosclerosis;[11] levels alone are not a close indicator of outcome and more information is required of the processes involved.[18] Ratios of HDL/LDL or HDL/total cholesterol compound errors in both primary determinations, and are not obviously helpful when, as in Britain, LDL levels are also high.

The idea that apo A-I is acting intracellularly as a transducer, mobilizing lipid to the cell surface for transfer, fits in well with clinical observations on the apparent protective effect of apo A-I-only particles against atherosclerosis. From what is known of the processes of reverse cholesterol transport,[18] it may be that flux of lipid through HDL fractions and the lipid cascade is the essential process, of which this receptor-based step may be an important part. It probably also matters where any flux is directed, to liver directly, or through other lipoproteins that become cholesterol enriched and could enhance atherosclerosis unless their flux is also proceeding well.

Laboratory assessment of overall lipid flux in plasma is difficult *in vivo*, involving the use of stable isotopes and speculative computer modelling, and there is a real need for a practical procedure to assess this process. For the moment, levels of HDL offer a general guide to outcome within populations, perhaps because they generally reflect dietary and lifestyle habits. Except at extreme levels suggesting the presence of specific defects, attempts to raise those levels as a primary aim will not be well founded until the processes involved and their potential and specific benefits are more closely defined.

THE DEFINITION OF HYPERLIPIDAEMIA

What is Normal?

Community studies, and particularly the seven countries study of Keys, the Multiple Risk Factor Intervention Trial (MRFIT) in the USA, and recent major studies on diet, lifestyle and mortality from China all show that there is no level of serum/plasma cholesterol at which coronary heart disease does not occur, and that the relationship progressively strengthens as levels increase. The J-shaped curve relating total mortality to cholesterol seen in the MRFIT study suggested that optimal outcome arose at levels of 200 mg/dL, 5.2 mmol/L. Further analysis of outcome in that very large study strongly suggested that screenees with lower levels and premature death had pre-existing disease, mainly large-bowel carcinomas, causing the low cholesterol rather than the low level being the primary determinant of outcome. Some aspects of the risk associations of low cholesterol levels remain to be clarified and extremely low levels may be associated with an increased risk of haemorrhagic stroke (but a very low risk of the much more common coronary heart disease).

Essentially there is no absolutely safe or dangerous level of cholesterol. All recommendations on target values represent compromise, and must also be interpreted flexibly in the light of other risks also present and wide intraindividual variation in levels of cholesterol.[3]

The 5.2 mmol/L target arose through an incomplete assessment of the MRFIT data and because it was a nice round number—200 mg/dL then converted to SI units—but it has been widely endorsed internationally and certainly the risk of premature coronary heart disease at or below that value is low. It is, however, an awkward target for the UK, as some 80% of the adult population have levels above 5.2 mmol/L, that percentage differing slightly between studies depending on the age/sex mix of the adults involved.[14] For industrialized societies, levels of cholesterol increase with age (not so in native rural populations, suggesting environmental effects) and with male/female differences. Levels in men increase until a plateau around at the age of 42 years, those in women start lower but increase throughout life, as in the National Lipid Screening Project[14] for adults aged 25–59 years shown in Fig. 35.6. For both sexes, levels fall at the extremes of life and from the Framingham cohort studies this appears to be a survivor effect resulting from the death of those with higher values. For the UK, a level of 6.8 mmol/L in a 69-year-old woman may not be ideal by international epidemiological standards but it is average for her population.

Fasting triglyceride levels are also age related and slightly higher in men.[14,15] Triglyceride-rich particles are rapidly cleared from the circulation. Some postprandial hypertriglyceridaemia is normal but excess

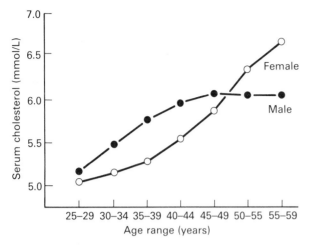

Figure 35.6 The relation between levels of total serum cholesterol and age in a British population; data from the National Lipid Screening Project.[14]

after an overnight fast is not, the difficulty being that fasting excess only reveals severe abnormalities of production or turnover. As most of us are postprandial most of the time there is growing interest in postprandial responses, triglyceride loading tests and rates of turnover rather than fixed measurements in the fasting state.[1] Levels of total cholesterol and HDL-cholesterol are rarely significantly affected by food and random samples are acceptable, although the consequent triglyceride particle-related turbidity may be inconvenient: preprandial sampling is a useful compromise.

Levels of HDL-cholesterol are similar in both sexes until puberty; the fall of about 0.3 mmol/L then seen in men and the difference persisting after the menopause in women suggesting that testosterone is more important than oestrogens in this difference. For adults, levels of HDL change little with age, and, for the manganese–heparin method, the 5th and 50th percentile values for adult British men and women are 0.9/1.3 and 1.0/1.6 mmol/L.[14] Generally similar trends for the three major lipid analytes are reported for North America.[15,19]

In clinical management the high levels of cholesterol in the UK are seen as a problem requiring political attention, and most clinical attention is directed at patients defined as hyperlipidaemic by national standards:[20,21] as a guideline, for adults of both sexes combined the 95th percentile limit for the UK is about 7.8 mmol/L.[14] Priority is also given to patients with lower levels but established or increased risk of lipid-related disease. Determination of HDL is worthwhile when that result may influence clinical management, rarely so if total cholesterol is low or very high, but helpful in borderline cases as low HDL favours more active treatment.[20] Low levels of HDL may also be familial and associated with premature coronary heart disease. HDL-cholesterol (HDLC) and a fasting sample is, however, necessary

to calculate LDL-cholesterol (LDLC), using values for total cholesterol (TC) and total triglyceride (TG), and the Friedewald calculation,[22] which in SI units is:

$$LDLC = TC - (HDLC + TG/2.2).$$

This correction assumes that triglyceride-rich lipoproteins and essentially VLDL are at average concentration and of predictable composition; the correction is not valid otherwise, for example when total triglycerides are elevated, empirically beyond 5 mmol/L.

Why are Patients Lipaemic?

In the clinical and laboratory assessment of patients it is important to note that in most studies at least 50% of patients defined as lipaemic by various criteria are lipaemic through other metabolic disorders, treatment resolving the associated lipaemia. The original classification of hyperlipidaemia into types I–V by Fredrickson and colleagues was important but based on the pattern of abnormality in the sample sent to the laboratory. The primary cause of that abnormality can often now be defined and used, thus 'mixed lipaemia secondary to diabetes' is more informative than 'type IIb disorder'. In the laboratory the terms hypertriglyceridaemia, hypercholesterolaemia and mixed lipaemia are useful shorthand.

When considering cause, golden rules are that hypercholesterolaemia in the older woman is due to hypothyroidism, and mixed lipaemia in the male executive is due to alcoholism—until proved otherwise. Autogeneration of laboratory thyroid and alcohol screens is appropriate to save a further specimen. Fasting hypertriglyceridaemia is often secondary to obesity, alcoholism, diabetes and impaired glucose tolerance, and chronic liver or renal disease.

Mechanisms for many of these associations are now defined, as for autoimmune hyperchylomicronaemia noted above,[4] and for hypothyroidism, which involves effects on LDL receptor cycling and reduced expression at the cell surface. Gene probe and linkage analysis directed at apoprotein, lipid enzyme and insulin genes and their expression suggests that partial and variably expressed underlying faults could also be involved, although the specific practical mechanisms remain ill defined. In this way the nature of polygenic disorders, with variable moderate lipid abnormalities clustering within families may be clarified, the contribution of the apo E variants to lipid levels and drug responsiveness being one such defined influence.

These 'polygenic' lipoprotein abnormalities can often be suppressed by diet, weight loss and lifestyle change.[23] It is hoped that normalization of gross plasma lipids will reduce any clinical expression, although the underlying disorder presumably remains. Some feel for why a patient is lipaemic is the most important part of management and laboratory support here is invaluable: from previous experience, associated risk, best options for treatment if appropriate, and wider genetic family implications can then be considered.

REFERENCES

1. Fruchart J-C., Shepherd J. eds. (1989). *Human Plasma Lipoproteins*, Berlin: de Gruyter, pp. 1–398.
2. Breslow J.L. (1988). Apolipoprotein genetic variation in human disease. *Physiol. Rev.*, **68**, 85.
3. 2nd Bergmeyer Conference (1989). Laboratory measurements in lipid disorders. Scand. J. Clin. Lab. Invest., **50** (suppl. 198).
4. Kihara S. et al. (1989). Auto-immune hyperchylomicronaemia. *N. Engl. J. Med.*, **320**, 1255.
5. Brown M.S., Goldstein J.L. (1986). A receptor-mediated pathway for cholesterol homoeostasis. *Science*, **232**, 34.
6. Steinberg D. et al. (1989). Beyond cholesterol: modifications of low-density lipoproteins that increase its atherogenicity. *N. Engl. J. Med.*, **320**, 915.
7. Goldstein J.L., Brown M.S. (1990). Regulation of the mevalonate pathway. *Nature*, **343**, 425.
8. Utermann G. (1989). The mysteries of lipoprotein(a). *Science*, **246**, 904.
9. Liscum L., Ruggiero R.M., Faust J.R. (1989). The intracellular transport of low density lipoprotein-derived cholesterol is defective in Niemann–Pick type C fibroblasts. *J. Cell Biol.*, **108**, 1625.
10. Oram J.F. (1990). Cholesterol trafficking in cells. *Curr. Opinion Lipidol.*, **1**, 416.
11. Schaefer E.J. (1984). Clinical, biochemical and genetic features in familiar disorders of high density lipoprotein deficiency. *Arteriosclerosis*, **4**, 303.
12. Hopkins P.N., Williams R.R. (1981). A survey of 246 suggested coronary risk factors. *Atherosclerosis*, **40**, 1.
13. Ross R. (1986). The pathogenesis of atherosclerosis — an update. *N. Engl. J. Med.*, **314**, 485.
14. Mann J.I. et al. (1988). Blood lipid and other cardiovascular risk factors: distribution, prevalence and detection in Britain. *Br. Med. J.*, **296**, 1702.
15. Stein E.A., Steiner P.M. (1989). Triglyceride measurement and its relationship to heart disease. *Clin. Lab. Med.*, **9**, 169.
16. Mann K.G. (1989). Factor VII assays, plasma triglyceride levels and cardiovascular disease risk. *Arteriosclerosis*, **9**, 783.
17. Small D.M. (1988). Progression and regression of atherosclerotic lesions. Insights from lipid physical biochemistry. *Arteriosclerosis*, **8**, 103.
18. Reichl R., Miller N.E. (1989). Pathophysiology of reverse cholesterol transport: insights from disorders of lipoprotein metabolism. *Arteriosclerosis*, **9**, 785.
19. Rifkind B.M., Lippel K. eds. (1989) Cholesterol screening. *Clin. Lab. Med.* **9**(1).
20. Betteridge D.J. et al. (1993). Management of hyperlipidaemia—guidelines of the British Hyperlipidaemia Association. *Postgrad. Med. J.,* **69**, 359.
21. O'Brien B.J. (1991). *Cholesterol and Coronary Heart Disease: Consensus or Controversy?* London: Office of Health Economics, pp. 1–100.
22. Friedewald W.T., Levy R.I., Fredrickson D.S. (1972). Estimation of the concentration of low-density lipoprotein in plasma without use of the preparative ultracentrifuge. *Clin. Chem.*, **18**, 499.
23. Shekelle R.B., Stamler J. (1989). Dietary cholesterol and ischaemic heart disease. *Lancet*, **i**, 1177.

36. Chest Pain

V. Marks

Causes of chest pain
Coronary thrombosis
   ECG
   Cardiac enzymes
   Myoglobin
   Troponin T
   Myosin
   Endothelin
   Breath pentane and reperfusion injury
   Aminoterminal type III procollagen peptide
   Thrombolytic therapy
   Other tests of myocardial infarction
Other causes of chest pain
Oesophageal pain

Chest pain is a common complaint and may be either acute, with sudden and unexpected onset, or chronic, with exacerbation. It has many causes, the most important—both numerically and clinically—being cardiac ischaemia due to narrowing or occlusion of the coronary arteries. With the greater availability of selective coronary angiography it has become apparent that up to one-third of patients complaining of angina-like chest pain have normal coronary arteries or exhibit at most only minimal main coronary artery disease.

CAUSES OF CHEST PAIN

Common causes of acute chest pain include damage to myocardium, pericardium, aorta and great vessels, pleura, rib cage and mediastinum—especially the oesophagus, the pain from which may be indistinguishable in site, character and radiation from that caused by myocardial ischaemia. Pain arising from the stomach and gallbladder may also present as acute chest pain, as may hyperventilation and other psychologically determined ailments. The differential diagnosis of acute chest pain depends, as always, upon the clinical history supplemented by a physical examination and appropriate radiological/electrophysiological and laboratory tests.

The acute chest pain that typically follows a coronary thrombosis and is caused by myocardial ischaemia, may—if sufficiently severe and/or prolonged—be accompanied by irreversible myocardial damage (myocardial infarction or necrosis) from which recovery is possible by a process of repair but leaves a scar in which cardiac muscle is replaced by fibrous tissue.

The enormous developments that have taken place within recent years in both the early and later management of myocardial ischaemia due to coronary thrombosis have put a premium on early diagnosis as there is overwhelming evidence that the sooner thrombolytic therapy is begun after the onset of a thrombotic episode—which is the almost invariable antecedent of acute myocardial infarction—the better are the chances of complete recovery.

CORONARY THROMBOSIS

Thrombosis of one of the major three, or rarely four, coronary arteries, and through which blood flow has already been restricted as a consequence of atheroma, is far and away the most common cause of acute myocardial infarction. It is the most common cause of death in middle-aged men in most of the developed countries of the world. In between 30 and 50% of people, angiography reveals that chest pain and electrocardiographic changes which respond to glycerol trinitrate can occur in the absence of occlusive coronary artery disease; these are thought to be caused by coronary artery spasm. Whether this is an important cause of actual infarction is a moot point. In most cases of acute myocardial infarction the patient has experienced the symptoms of angina for some considerable time before onset of the coronary thrombosis that precipitates the acute emergency. Nevertheless, as a result of more prolonged monitoring of ambulatory electrocardiograms (ECG), it has become abundantly clear that silent (i.e. asymptomatic) ischaemic episodes are far more common than symptomatic ones.

Typically, coronary thrombosis presents with excruciating pain in the centre of the chest, which may extend into the neck and jaw, to either or both arms, or downwards into the epigastrium. It is commonly associated with sweating and faintness, and the patient may be aware of disturbances in heartbeat and shortness of breath. Temperature is often raised, though only slightly unless the patient is also in cardiac failure, and there is often an added heart sound. The blood pressure is often below the patient's normal level, though not necessarily low in absolute terms. Very early in the onset of an attack, there may be feelings of extreme weakness and nausea, and a desire to evacuate the bowels of such intensity that the patient is unwilling to move from the lavatory.

A number of patients who experience a coronary thrombosis die instantly, presumably from ventricular fibrillation. A large number die within the first hour of onset, probably from the same cause, but are potentially susceptible to resuscitation. Experience has shown that when a patient's collapse from coronary thrombosis is witnessed and defibrillation performed within 6 min, survival is possible and achieved in upwards of 15% of all cases. The risk of imminent death diminishes rapidly the longer the patient survives an acute attack, but still remains higher than normal for a year or more following recovery.

Diagnosis of coronary thrombosis is usually made on clinical grounds, but increasingly these have been recognized as providing an incomplete picture and more and more reliance is placed upon rapid diagnostic tests, since these may determine whether thrombolytic therapy should be instituted or not. There is now very clear evidence that the earlier thrombolytic therapy is instituted the better the chance, not only of survival, but of a more or less complete recovery, with little or no myocardial scarring. Consequently there is a premium on rapid and accurate diagnosis. Just as there is much to be gained by early diagnosis and treatment of true coronary thrombosis, so there are enormous economic and clinical reasons for being able to exclude myocardial infarction as a diagnosis as rapidly and completely as possible in those patients in whom coronary thrombosis is suspected but eventually shown to be incorrect.

Because of the lack of sensitivity and specificity of the investigative procedures available it was, until very recently, widely held that a period of 24 h was required to exclude myocardial infarction in patients admitted to coronary care units for the evaluation of acute chest pain. The situation is changing rapidly, however, and it is now possible virtually to exclude a diagnosis of coronary thrombosis, even in the absence of ECG changes, within 12 h of the onset of pain.

ECG

Characteristic alterations in the ECG have long been the yardstick by which a clinical diagnosis of myocardial infarction has been substantiated. They are, however, an insensitive indicator and in a large proportion of patients the appearance of ECG changes may be delayed for up to 24 h, or may not appear at all. Consequently, whilst the test is diagnostic in something in the region of 75% of cases within the first 24 h, in the remainder a negative test result is obtained. The ECG is consequently of limited use in excluding the diagnosis of myocardial infarction. The most common and characteristic changes are an elevation of the ST segment in leads recorded over the infarcted area and of depression in leads from other areas. Q waves are seen if the infarct extends through the full thickness of the myocardium. Serial ECGs should always be taken whenever possible, especially as an abnormal ECG may be difficult to interpret in someone who has already had a myocardial infarction from which they have fully recovered.

Because of these reservations about the ECG, biochemical tests have come to play an increasingly important part in confirming the diagnosis of coronary thrombosis, and many procedures that were still under development less than 10 years ago are now in regular use. Before discussing them and their role in the early diagnosis and assessment of severity of myocardial infarction, two of the older enzyme tests, which are still nevertheless widely used, will be briefly outlined, even though their clinical usefulness is now seriously suspect.

Cardiac Enzymes

Aspartate Aminotransferase (AST)

Plasma AST (previously called serum glutamic-oxaloacetic transaminase (SGOT)) activity typically exceeds the normal range within 8–12 h of the onset of a myocardial infarction, and returns to normal within 3–4 days. As with all serum enzyme measurements, the duration of raised activity depends in part on the highest level attained. In a review of 1962 cases of myocardial infarction diagnosed clinically, an elevation of serum AST was found in 97% of them at some time or another.

Raised AST levels are, however, far from specific for myocardial infarction and are also found in hepatic congestion, primary liver disease, skeletal muscle disorders and shock, as well as in pulmonary infarction. Congestive heart failure is associated with high AST level when the liver is distended; active myocarditis tends to be associated with a modest rise in AST. Pericarditis causes an elevation in perhaps 50% of cases, and 25% of patients with pulmonary embolism show a rise in AST activity. Of patients who have undergone surgery or have suffered major trauma, 95% show a rise in AST levels—as do a high proportion of those given DC countershock for cardiac arrhythmias. Patients with diseases of the liver or biliary tract who have received intramuscular injections may also have raised AST levels.

Lactic Dehydrogenase (LDH)

Plasma LDH activity typically exceeds the normal range within 24 to 48 h of the onset of infarction, and peaks in 3–6 days. Thereafter it gradually declines to reach normal values within 10 to 14 days of the onset of the illness. True positive elevations are found in about 90% of patients with myocardial infarction, and are caused mainly, if not exclusively, by the LDH isoenzymes I and II. These isoenzymes, which have equal activity against both pyruvate and α-hydroxybutyrate when used as a substrate, were, for some time, referred to as α-hydroxybutyrate dehydrogenase (HBD) and were thought to be specific for myocardial infarction. High values are, however, found in many disorders apart from myocardial infarction, especially those associated with increased erythropoietic activity. HBD measurements have, therefore, virtually dropped into obsolescence as an aid to the diagnosis of heart disease, although electrophoretic separation and quantitation of the LDH isoenzymes continue to enjoy some popularity.

The specificity of plasma LDH assays depends on the population under test. Rises in LDH activity occur in perhaps 30% of patients with congestive cardiac failure. A number of other conditions, including haemolysis, megaloblastic anaemia, leukaemia, acute and chronic liver disease, are also associated with raised plasma LDH levels. Coronary embolism and neoplastic disease may also cause raised levels, resulting in difficulty in interpretation. Cardiac catheterization, myocarditis and shock may also cause confusion.

The practice of making serial AST and LDH measurements on patients suspected of, or actually having had, a myocardial infarction was once very popular, though never very informative except as a retrospective aid to diagnosis, and possibly therefore to prognosis. It has now been made completely obsolete by the introduction of newer, more sensitive and specific laboratory tests, except as part of a research programme for the assessment of outcomes.

The difficulty in making a firm but very early diagnosis of myocardial damage (from coronary thrombosis), which has been alluded to, was of relatively little importance whilst supportive therapy was virtually all that could be offered to the patient. The advent of thrombolytic therapy has changed all that and there is now a very real advantage in making a positive diagnosis of coronary thrombosis as soon as possible since thrombolytic treatment is more effective the earlier it is commenced.

Creatine Kinase (CK)

Among the enzymes that have been used as markers of myocardial infarction the most useful is undoubtedly creatine kinase (CK). It catalyses the reversible phosphorylation of creatine and occurs in greatest concentration in brain, heart and skeletal muscle. Creatine kinase is a dimeric protein made up of two distinct subunits known as the M and B subunits because of their association with skeletal muscle (MM) and brain (BB) creatine kinases, respectively. The main heart creatine kinase dimer consists of one M and one B subunit and is consequently known as the CK-MB isoenzyme. The heart also contains the MM dimer but it ordinarily has little diagnostic significance except to contribute to confusion.

The three CK isoenzymes can be separated electrophoretically as well as immunologically, which is the way they are now generally distinguished from one another, especially in clinical situations. A further distinction can however be made between various isoforms of the various CK isoenzymes. These different isoforms are the result of postsynthetic changes that occur in the M subunit if, and when, the enzyme gains access to the circulation. A lysine residue is cleaved from the M subunit, yielding a product with slightly different electrophoretic mobility from the parent compound. Consequently it is possible to distinguish five isoforms of CK in the circulation; the tissue form of CK-MB (referred to as $CK-MB_2$) and its transformation product (CK-MB). Similarly there are three isoforms of CK-MM, namely: the tissue form ($CK-MM_3$) and its mono- and di-delysinated products—$CK-MM_2$ and $CK-MM_1$, respectively.

Although clinical cardiological interest centres mainly upon changes in the plasma concentration of CK-MB, both it, and CK-MM, are released into the circulation following myocardial damage and much of the work on the various isoform changes that

occur, especially during reperfusion, has been done on the MM isoenzyme. The techniques currently available for distinguishing the various isoforms are too time-consuming to make their use practicable as diagnostic tools but they are enabling light to be thrown on some aspects of the reperfusion process that might otherwise have been difficult to obtain.

Plasma total CK activity (tCK) and CK-MB both tend to peak within 24 h of a myocardial infarction and to return to normal within 72 h. The specificity, and even more the sensitivity, of CK measurements in the diagnosis of myocardial infarction, however, depends on the method of assay used. Whereas in the past the methods used relied mainly on measurement of enzyme activity and its inhibition by antibodies raised against the specific CK isozymes (CK-MB), it is now possible to measure the individual isoenzymes by mass, as proteins, using direct reading immunoassays, some of which are available as rapid, one-off, bedside tests. Immunological assay techniques can be expected, within a comparatively short time, completely to replace both activity inhibition and electrophoretic separation of the CK isozymes and expression of their individual contribution to CK activity as a percentage of the total.

It has recently been shown that something approaching 100% sensitivity and 95% specificity for the diagnosis of myocardial infarction can be achieved if, instead of making just a single measurement of plasma CK or plasma CK-MB, at least three measurements are made within 12 h of the onset of pain. The results can be logarithmically transformed, plotted against time and expressed as a number reflecting the slope of the change. A slope of less than 0.015 virtually excludes myocardial infarction as the cause of the patient's illness, and a slope of more than 0.015 is virtually diagnostic of it—provided that at least one of the three measurements of tCK (or preferably, CK-MB) is above the reference range for the method used. A program developed for use with a microcomputer or programmable calculator makes calculation of the slope both feasible and practicable.

Plasma tCK and even CK-MB measurements can now be made sufficiently rapidly, precisely and accurately in the Emergency Laboratory or even in the side-room of a Coronary Care Unit to make them practicable for the specific diagnosis of myocardial infarction.

The value of single random measurement of CK-MB, though better than for most other single tests, is neither absolutely specific for the diagnosis of myocardial infarction, nor will it detect all of the cases, especially during the critical first 6 h following the onset of thrombosis, when up to 30% may still have CK-MB levels below the discriminant level. CK-MB measurements do, however, still have an important place in the decision-making process and may well sway the decision as to whether to institute thrombolytic or other invasive therapy in a probable but not absolutely certain case of myocardial infarction. The result may also delay the institution of therapy for an hour or two during which time it can be ascertained whether the plasma level of CK-MB is rising or remaining the same.

One of the main reasons for the lack of discrimination of a single measurement of plasma tCK or CK-MB is that it is not yet possible to distinguish, under clinical conditions, the MB_2 isoform (the form in which the enzyme is released from damaged myocardial tissue after myocardial infarction and whose concentration is generally below the limit of sensitivity of the assay) from that ordinarily present in the circulation (i.e. MB_1). Though generally considered very specific for myocardial infarction, a rising plasma concentration of CK-MB is not absolutely so. High and rising levels are also seen in patients with intestinal necrosis caused, for example, by mesenteric artery thrombosis. In exceptional cases this can cause confusion with myocardial infarction, especially if too much reliance is placed upon CK-MB measurements as an aid to differential diagnosis in patients in whom ECG changes are unhelpful.

Myoglobin

The cardiac enzymes enjoy their special place in the diagnosis of myocardial infarction, not primarily because of their specificity for myocardial damage, but because of the comparative ease with which they could be measured (and at a time when the measurement of other non-enzymatically active proteins was more difficult). The rise in plasma concentration of 'cardiac enzymes' is caused by their leakage out of the damaged cells and this can be monitored by means of their enzymic activity. Other cardiospecific proteins that are released into the circulation in equal or greater amounts following myocardial damage were, until recently, not so easily measured. The situation has, however, completely changed with the greater availability of rapid immunoassay techniques.

Cardiospecific myoglobin is one of the proteins that is found exclusively in the myocardium and is released into the circulation where it can be measured after damage to heart muscle. Although it has been known for a decade or more that changes in serum myoglobin are as sensitive and specific for myocardial infarction as CK-MB, it was not popular as a test because of the difficulty of measuring it rapidly and reliably. As tests designed for emergency use in the Accident and Emergency department, or even at the bedside, have become available, the measurement of plasma myoglobin levels is gaining in popularity. The main advantage of serum myoglobin measurements over CK-MB is their earlier rise above the reference range in cases of proven myocardial infarction. This facilitates even earlier definitive diagnosis than might otherwise be possible. With the rapid but still only semiquantitative assays currently available it is possible to achieve an 85% sensitivity for myocar-

dial infarction within 7 [...] likely to improve with [...] near-patient testing.

T[...]

Troponin T is a car[...] myofibril complex, wh[...] into the circulation du[...] ture is sufficiently diff[...] troponin to make its id[...] comparatively simple by an immunoassay technique that takes only 90 min to do. Its concentration in blood rises significantly above background within 3 h (i.e. quicker even than myoglobin and CK-MB) and remains elevated for longer, making it an even better marker of myocardial infarction than either of them. In one large series of 388 patients with chest pain, a plasma troponin-T measurement was 100% sensitive in detecting myocardial infarction and its overall diagnostic efficiency (number of true-positive and true-negative test results expressed as a percentage of all the positive and negative results obtained) was 98%. Experience with troponin T as a diagnostic aid is still limited but if its cardiospecificity, sensitivity for early disease and usefulness for prospective as well as for retrospective diagnosis are borne out by further experience, it is likely to become the chemical test of first choice for the diagnosis of myocardial infarction.

Myosin

Myosin heavy chains are released into the blood after a myocardial infarct and can be measured by immunoassay. The plasma concentration of myosin correlates well with infarct size in experimental animals and its use has been advocated as a guide to infarct size in man. So far, reports of its clinical usefulness for this purpose are limited. Somewhat surprisingly they do not support the contention that thrombolytic therapy limits the size of a myocardial infarct once the coronary thrombosis producing it has occurred.

Endothelin

An endothelium-derived peptide with a sustained constrictive effect on a variety of blood vessels has been isolated, characterized and called endothelin. It has been shown, using radioimmunoassay, that its concentration in blood rises in response to vascular damage and that in patients with coronary thrombosis, for example, values up to four times the upper limit of normal are common during the acute phase of the illness, falling slowly thereafter. No rises in plasma endothelin concentration are seen in patients with angina unaccompanied by cardiac ischaemia. High levels of plasma endothelin may, however, be found in other forms of intravascular damage. Its

618   Biochemistry [...]
measurement i[...]
necessarily f[...]
infarction [...]
ready e[...]
as de[...]
for [...]

blood plasma may, therefore, not
d a place in the diagnosis of myocardial
—for which many laboratory methods al-
ist—but more likely for other diseases, such
ep-vein thrombosis and the various arteritides
which such diagnostic aids are not yet available.

Breath Pentane and Reperfusion Injury

Reperfusion injury, which occurs when the blood
supply is restored to ischaemic tissue, is thought to
be mediated largely by 'free radicals', which interact
with vital structures and substances within the tissues.
Pentane is thought to be a sensitive and direct index
of lipid peroxidation *in vivo* and has been identified
as a substance whose measurement might be of use
for determining the presence and extent of tissue
damage. It could conceivably, therefore, be a useful
and early indicator of myocardial infaction and (perhaps even more important) of the rate and extent of
reperfusion as and when repair begins. The best
method currently available for the measurement of
pentane in breath, gas–liquid chromatography, is
too cumbersome for clinical use but, if further work
establishs its value as a diagnostic procedure, the
introduction of instruments, comparable in size and
simplicity of use with those employed for the roadside
measurement of breath alcohol, will surely not long
be delayed.

Aminoterminal Type III Procollagen Peptide

The speed and extent of repair after myocardial
damage are important determinants of prognosis.
Most of the biochemical markers used in the investigation of patients who have undergone myocardial
infarctions relate solely to the damage done to
the muscle tissue itself and reflected in the quantity
of intracellular enzymes and proteins leaked into the
extracellular fluid. The healing process, on the other
hand, is associated with the replacement of the infarcted material by collagen. This is accompanied by
a rise in the plasma concentration of an aminoterminal type III procollagen peptide (PIIINP), which can
be measured immunologically. As would be expected,
plasma levels of PIIINP rise slowly after a myocardial
infarct compared with the markers of acute myocardial damage, such as CK, LDH, AST, myoglobin
and troponin T, and do not reach peak levels until
about the fifth post-infarct day where they remain
for more than 3 months. How rapidly they fall thereafter is unknown but they have generally returned to
basal levels within 2 years of the infarction.

Experience with the measurement of PIIINP in
patients with myocardial infarcts and other causes of
tissue damage is still limited. But, if the early findings
are substantiated in larger and more prolonged studies, there will undoubtedly be a role for them in
assessing both the extent of the tissue damage and
completeness of healing, following a myocardial in-

farct. Both are important determinants of long-term
prognosis.

Thrombolytic Therapy

The advent of almost universal thrombolytic therapy
for acute myocardial damage due to coronary thrombosis owes much to the introduction of bioengineered
tissue plasminogen activators (TPA) and the excitement they engendered. Current evidence suggests,
however, that despite several theoretical advantages
over the older thrombolytic agents such as strep-
tolysin and urokinase, TPA is, in practice, no more
clinically efficacious. All of the thrombolytic agents
work by accelerating the destruction of the blood
clot that obstructs the coronary artery lumen and
produces the myocardial ischaemia and infarction. If
thrombolysis can be achieved quickly enough for
blood flow to be established before actual necrosis
has taken place, recovery of the damaged—but not
yet dead—muscle fibres may occur, with more or less
complete restoration of the prethrombotic situation.

All of the thrombolytic agents currently in use
work as plasminogen activators. Plasminogen—a protein that is normally present in plasma—is converted
by plasminogen activators into the enzyme, plasmin.
This degrades the insoluble fibrin that constitutes the
clot into soluble fibrin degradation products, thereby
permitting the clot to disintegrate. The speed and
effectiveness of plasmin generated by plasminogen
activators in dissolving fibrin clots are determined by
a number of modulators of plasmin action. Amongst
the most important of these is α-antiplasmin, a serine
protease inhibitor normally present in the plasma,
which rapidly deactivates plasmin by forming an
inactive complex with it. The clinical effectiveness of
thrombolytic agents might be enhanced, therefore,
by agents that delay or otherwise interfere with plasmin degradation, and there is already some evidence
that this can be achieved by a suitable combination
of a plasminogen activator, such as streptokinase,
with heparin.

The possibility that clinical laboratory measurement of some of the regulators of thrombotic and
thrombolytic activity in the plasma might predict the
propensity to myocardial infarction has aroused considerable interest. It might provide a method of screening for predisposition to coronary thrombosis that is
more sensitive than existing methods, none of which
is very satisfactory. Individuals with low plasminogen
activator activity and raised plasminogen activator
inhibitor levels, for example, are seemingly at increased risk from recurrent coronary thromboses,
though whether this is causal or consequential is still
not clear.

Use of thrombolytic agents for the treatment of
coronary thrombosis is associated with both short-
and long-term benefits, but like all therapeutic inter-
ventions is not completely without danger. Consequently it is widely believed that they should be

reserved for use in patients in whom the diagnosis of myocardial infarction is established beyond reasonable doubt, which puts a premium not only on early, but also on accurate, diagnosis.

Other Tests of Myocardial Infarction

Conventional radiology plays little part in the diagnosis of myocardial infarction except in helping to exclude other conditions such as dissection of the aorta and disease of the mediastinum, which may cause similar symptoms. Radionuclide imaging, especially with thallium, may provide independent confirmation of the diagnosis of myocardial infarction as well as information about its size and exact location.

OTHER CAUSES OF CHEST PAIN

The most common problem in acute chest pain is to distinguish myocardial infarction from other conditions with which it may be confused, and has already been addressed. Almost as important, however, is the differentiation of long-standing, or chronic, chest pain due to angina pectoris from other causes of recurrent pain.

Diagnosis of angina pectoris is still entirely clinical and relies exclusively upon obtaining a good clinical history. Provided that the clinician is satisfied that the symptoms are genuine and the history reliable, the diagnosis stands, even when the physical examination and special investigations are negative.

Many factors combine to conceal the fact that a patient has angina, and there is no completely reliable method of confirming the diagnosis. A simple question, namely 'Do you experience any discomfort in the chest on climbing hills or stairs?' frequently reveals that the pain of which a patient is complaining is really angina and not due to a skeletal, oesophageal, muscular or other cause. Myocardial ischaemia may occur in the absence of occlusive disease of the coronary arteries; indeed left ventricular dysfunction occurs in up to 35% of patients with angina and a normal angiogram. The cause of the ischaemia in such cases is postulated to be a reduction in the reserve capacity of the small arteries of the heart to expand in response to exercise. These patients cannot, therefore, increase their blood flow through the myocardium when they exercise, and they experience angina. They do not, however, exhibit any characteristic radiological or biochemical abnormalities by which they can be identified.

Another type of angina is that in which chest pain occurs at rest rather than on exertion. It characteristically develops early in the morning and may be associated with abnormalities in the ECG. Both the pain and ECG respond to glyceryl trinitrate and are thought to be due to coronary artery spasm.

OESOPHAGEAL PAIN

Regurgitation of gastric fluid from the stomach into the oesophagus may give rise to pain recognized as typical 'heart burn' or misinterpreted as chest pain indistinguishable in site, severity, character and distribution from that of myocardial infarction. Over 40% of patients with angina-like pain, but who have normal coronary arteriograms, turn out to have oesophageal reflux. This can readily be demonstrated by radiological studies but clinical biochemistry has little contribution to make unless the oesophageal ulceration, which is sometimes present, is itself a consequence of the Zollinger–Ellison syndrome, and revealed by a plasma gastrin assay.

In a substantial proportion of people investigated for severe but chronic chest pain, no physical cause can be found. In almost 60% there is some evidence of psychopathology, which is a much higher proportion than in people with coronary heart disease and left ventricular dysfunction. Hyperventilation is also often present and may itself be a cause of chronic chest pain. In this condition there are characteristic changes in blood gases, which, if the condition is sufficiently chronic and severe, may become manifest as a respiratory alkalosis.

FURTHER READING

Collen D., Stump. D.C., Gold. H.K. (1988). Thrombolytic therapy. *Ann. Rev. Med.*, **39**, 405.

Collinson. P.O. et al. (1989). Diagnosis of acute myocardial infarction from sequential enzyme measurements obtained within 12 hours of admission to hospital. *J. Clin. Pathol.*, **42**, 1126.

Eagle K.A. (1991). Medical decision making in patients with chest pain. *N. Eng. J. Med.*, **324**, 1282.

Editorial (1991). Troponin T and myocardial damage. *Br. Med. J.*, **338**, 23.

Jensen L.T. et al. (1990). Serum aminoterminal type III procollagen peptide reflects repair after acute myocardial infarction. *Circulation*, **81**, 52.

Lee T.H. et al. (1991). *N. Eng. J. Med.*, **324**, 1239.

Leger X.X. et al. (1990). Assay of serum cardiac myosin heavy chain fragments in patients with acute myocardial infarction; determination of infarct size and long-term follow up. *Am. Heart J.*, **120**, 781.

Moss A.J., Benhorin. J. (1990). Prognosis and management after a first myocardial infarction. *N. Eng. J. Med.*, **322**, 743.

Ohman E.M., Casey C., Bengtson J.R., Pryor D., Tormey W., Horgan J.H. (1990). Early detection of acute myocardial infarction: additional diagnostic information from serum concentrations of myoglobin in patients without ST elevation. *Br. Heart J.*, **63**, 335.

Schofield P.M., Brooks H.N., Bennett D.H. (1986). Left ventricular dysfunction in patients with angina pectoris and normal coronary angiograms. *Br. Heart J.*, **56**, 327.

Sherry S., Marder V.J. (1991). Streptokinase and recombinant tissue plasminogen activator (rt-PA) are equally effective in treating acute myocardial infarction. *Ann. Intern. Med.*, **114**, 417.

Weitz Z.W., Birnbaum A.J., Sobotka P.A., Zarling E.J.,

Skosey J.L. (1991). High breath pentane concentrations during acute myocardial infarction. *Lancet*, **337**, 933.

Wiman B., Hamsten A. (1990). Correlations between fibri-nolytic function and acute myocardial infarction. *Am. J. Cardiol.*, **66**, 54G.

Wu A.H.B. (1989). Creatine kinase isoforms in ischaemic heart disease. *Clin. Chem.*, **35**, 7.

37. The Hypothalamus and Pituitary and Tests of Their Functions

J.W. Wright

Introduction
Anatomy
  The hypothalamus
  The pituitary gland
The hormones of the anterior pituitary
  Growth hormone and prolactin
  Glycoprotein hormones
  ACTH and related peptides
  Measurement of anterior pituitary hormones
*Hypothalamic control of anterior pituitary
    secretion*
*Physiological control of hypothalamic–
    pituitary function*
Tests of anterior pituitary function
Growth hormone
  Regulation of GH secretion
  Actions of GH
  Tests of GH secretion
  Disorders of GH secretion

INTRODUCTION

The close functional interrelations between the hypothalamus and the pituitary gland are now well established. The concept of regulation of the anterior pituitary by releasing hormones synthesized and secreted by neuroendocrine cells in the hypothalamus and transported to the anterior pituitary via the hypothalamic–pituitary portal system has led to major advances in the understanding of anterior pituitary function in recent years. Further similar advances can be expected when the complex nature of the neurotransmitter interactions that control the synthesis and release of the hypothalamic hormones is better understood.

Releasing hormones are secreted in response to a multiplicity of stimuli, with acute responses to physiological events such as feeding and stress superimposed on underlying rhythmic variations. Two of the hypothalamic hormones (oxytocin and vasopressin) are secreted directly into the systemic circulation from the posterior part of the pituitary gland (which is, in reality, no more than a direct extension of the neural tissue of the hypothalamus) and an understanding of the physiological effects of these peptides has been obtained from study of the responses of remote, accessible structures and systems. The remaining hypothalamic hormones, however, act directly upon the anterior pituitary gland, and the inaccessibility of this system has made direct physiological study difficult. Much valuable information has been obtained from clinical research that has been driven by the anticipation of improved diagnostic and therapeutic tools. As these become available, elucidation of their place in clinical practice and the ethical issues that arise from their use and misuse will continue to stimulate research and debate.

ANATOMY

The Hypothalamus

The hypothalamus lies at the base of the brain, beneath the thalamus, between the optic chiasma and the lamina terminalis anteriorly and the mamillary bodies posteriorly. It forms the floor and part of the lateral wall of the third ventricle up to the level of the hypothalamic sulcus. In the adult human, the hypothalamus weighs less than 2.5 g. The stem of the pituitary gland arises from the infundibulum, which projects from the undersurface of the hypothalamus between the tuber cinereum and the optic chiasma. Within the hypothalamus is a number of aggregations of cell bodies—the hypothalamic nuclei—which, with the exception of the supraoptic nucleus, are poorly defined and anatomically indistinct. The cells within certain of these, particularly the supraoptic, paraventricular, infundibular and ventromedial nuclei, give rise to axons that either terminate in the median eminence or infundibulum, or pass through to the posterior lobe of the pituitary. These are neurosecretory cells and are the source not only of the posterior pituitary hormones (vasopressin and oxytocin), but also the releasing or inhibiting factors that control anterior pituitary function.

The hypothalamus is richly supplied by nerve fibres from all parts of the nervous system. In particular, there are major connections with the limbic system (hippocampus and amygdyla), the globus pallidus, the reticular formation and parts of the midbrain. These centres are among the oldest areas of the brain and are concerned with physiological homeostasis, autonomic function and arousal. The hypothalamus also receives visceral and somatic sensory impulses from spinal nerves via the mamillary bodies, an important olfactory pathway, and inputs from the newest area of the brain, the prefrontal cortex, via the corticohypothalamic tracts.

The Pituitary Gland

The pituitary gland (the *hypophysis cerebri*) comprises two distinct parts. The anterior pituitary or *adenohypophysis* consists of the anterior lobe (*pars distalis*), which constitutes about 80% of the gland, and the

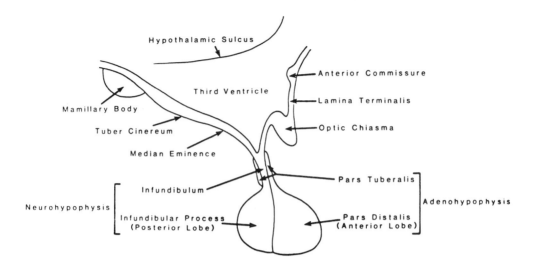

Figure 37.1 Sagittal section through the hypothalamus and pituitary (diagrammatic).

pars tuberalis, an upward extension that forms a thin cuff of cells around the front and sides of the infundibular stem (pituitary stalk). The posterior pituitary or *neurohypophysis* consists of the infundibular process (posterior or neural lobe) and the infundibulum. The area that forms the junction between the uppermost part of the infundibulum and the tuber cinereum is frequently referred to as the median eminence.

In man, a distinct intermediate lobe (*pars intermedia*) is found only during fetal life. Functionally and developmentally, the intermediate lobe should be considered as part of the adenohypophysis.

The anterior and posterior parts of the pituitary have quite different embryological origins. The adenohypophysis develops from Rathke's pouch, a midline diverticulum arising from the ectoderm of the primitive buccal cavity that migrates upwards, to fuse with a down growth of neuroectoderm from the hypothalamic part of the midbrain that becomes the posterior lobe of the pituitary. All connection between the anterior lobe and the roof of the pharynx is usually lost but the posterior lobe remains continuous with the ventral hypothalamus via the infundibular stem. The intermediate lobe develops from that portion of the adenohypophysis in contact with the posterior lobe and is separated from the anterior lobe by a cleft that represents the remnant of the lumen of Rathke's pouch.

In the adult, the pituitary measures approximately 12 mm in its transverse diameter and 8 mm anteroposteriorly. The whole gland weighs about 500 mg, slightly more in women than men, and increasing considerably during pregnancy largely due to expansion of the anterior lobe.

The pituitary gland occupies the pituitary fossa (*sella turcica*) within the sphenoid bone, which surrounds and protects it bilaterally and inferiorly. The

fossa is lined with dura mater, which envelops the gland and forms an incomplete covering over the fossa (the *diaphragma sellae*) through which the pituitary stalk passes. Beneath the pituitary fossa are the sphenoid air spaces and on each side are the cavernous sinuses, each containing the internal carotid artery and the IIIrd, IVth, Vth and VIth cranial nerves. The optic chiasma lies on the *diaphragma sellae*, immediately above the anterior part of the pituitary, where it is vulnerable to compression by suprasellar expansion of pituitary tumours.

The pituitary gland receives 80–90% of its blood supply from the superior and inferior hypophyseal branches of the internal carotid arteries. The superior hypophyseal artery supplies branches to the ventral hypothalamus and infundibulum, and a trabecular artery, which supplies the lower pituitary stalk. The neural lobe is supplied by the anterior and posterior branches of the inferior hypophyseal artery.

The arteries which supply the upper stalk and median eminence are peculiar in emptying into a system of sinusoids that are in intimate contact with the axon terminals from the hypothalamic nuclei. From these sinusoids arise the hypophyseal portal vessels, which pass down the pituitary stalk and which otherwise receives very little direct arterial blood supply. The venous drainage of the pituitary is via short veins that empty into the surrounding dural venous sinuses and, from there, into the internal jugular veins.

Histology

In practical terms, histological study of the anterior pituitary is largely confined to the identification of pituitary tumours. This should now be based upon immunological techniques (immunocytochemistry and immunofluorescence), which permit a functional rather than a purely descriptive classification of cell

TABLE 37.1

TRADITIONAL CLASSIFICATION OF ANTERIOR PITUITARY CELLS ACCORDING TO HORMONE
PRODUCTION

	Staining reactions			
Hormone	*Haemotoxylin and eosin*	*Mallory's trichrome*	*PAS–OG PAS–AB**	*Cytoplasmic granule size (nm)*
GH	Eosinophil	Acidophil	Yellow	300–450
PRL	Eosinophil	Adidophil	Yellow	500–750
ACTH and β-LPH	Cyanophil	Basophil	Red	200–400
FSH and LH	Cyanophil	Basophil	Blue	150–300
TSH	Cyanophil	Basophil	Blue	100–200

* PFA–AB, performic acid–Alcian blue; PAS–OG, periodic acid-Schiff–orange G.

TABLE 37.2

THE HORMONES OF THE ANTERIOR PITUITARY GLAND

Classification	Hormone	Chain length		Mol. wt.	Other features
Simple proteins	Growth hormone	191		21 700	Two intramolecular S–S bridges
	Prolactin	198		22 500	Three intramolecular S–S bridges
		α	β		
Glycoproteins	Thyrotrophin (TSH)	96	113	28 000	Carbohydrate substituents account for 10–20% of mol. wt.
	Luteinizing hormone (LH)	96	114	29 000	
	Follicle-stimulating hormone (FSH)	96	115	32 000	
Polypeptides	Adrenocorticotrophin (ACTH)	39		4507	See text
	β-lipoprotein (LPH)	91		9500	

types and tumours. For the most part, immunological methods have confirmed the relations between cell types and secretory products that were established by the conventional staining techniques summarized in Table 37.1. These techniques depended on the reactions of cytoplasmic secretory granules. Cells that contain few or no granules take up conventional stains poorly and are termed 'chromophobe'; these are commonly seen in both prolactin- and growth hormone-secreting pituitary adenomas, in which very little hormone is stored prior to discharge.

THE HORMONES OF THE ANTERIOR PITUITARY

The anterior pituitary hormones fall into three groups: the somatomammotrophic proteins (growth hormone and prolactin); the glycoproteins—thyroid-stimulating hormone (TSH), follicle-stimulating hormone (FSH) and luteinizing hormone (LH), which is identical to interstitial cell-stimulating hormone (ICSH); and adrenocorticotrophic hormone (ACTH) and related peptides. The major structural characteristics of these hormones are summarized in Table 37.2.

Growth Hormone and Prolactin

Growth hormone (GH) and prolactin are closely related peptides and share a common ancestral gene (along with placental lactogen). The gene for prolactin is present on chromosome 6, that for GH on chromosome 17. The genes exhibit considerable greater nucleotide homology than the 16% amino-acid sequence homology shared by the peptides for which they encode. In addition, the two hormones are secreted by similar cells of the pituitary (*see* Table 37.1) and there is some overlap in physiological effects.

There are several forms of GH in the circulation. About three-quarters are in the 22-kDa form; over half is monomeric and around one-quarter in dimeric form. A proportion of circulating GH is protein bound, mainly to a high-affinity binding protein that is identical to the extracellular domain of the GH receptor and absent in Laron dwarfism (*see* later). A second, low-affinity binding protein also exists. The biological significance of protein binding is uncertain but it clearly has an effect on metabolic clearance and may influence the binding characteristics of different monoclonal antiserum preparations. The mean half-life of exogenously administered GH in normal subjects is between 9 and 27 min. GH is largely metabolized in the liver, only a small amount appearing unchanged in the urine. It is largely for this reason that attempts to assess GH status by means of urinary GH measurements have met with limited success.

Circulating prolactin is largely in the monomeric form, although dimeric, polymeric and glycated forms also exist. The presence of different forms may account not only for variations in binding of antiserum but also for the discrepancies between bio- and immunoassayable prolactin that have been reported.

Glycoprotein Hormones

The glycoprotein hormones each comprise two separate, non-covalently bound peptide chains, the α- and β-subunits. The amino acid sequence of the α-chain is identical in all three hormones (and in chorionic gonadotrophin), although there are some differences in their carbohydrate content. The β-subunit is different for each hormone and confers biological specificity. Free α- and β-subunits both exist in the circulation. Specific assays for free β-subunits are of use in a number of clinical situations.

ACTH and Related Peptides

ACTH is one of a family of peptides that includes α-MSH (melanocyte-stimulating hormone), β-MSH, β-LPH (lipotropic pituitary hormone), γ-LPH and β-endorphin, all of which are derived from a common precursor, pro-opiomelanocorticotrophin (POMC). This large (241 amino acid) peptide undergoes extensive post-translational processing. The precise pattern of enzymatic cleavage is tissue specific, and a different pattern of smaller peptides is produced from the anterior and the intermediate lobes of the pituitary. The major hormonal products of the anterior pituitary are ACTH (1–39) and β-LPH. The products of the intermediate lobe include ACTH (1–14), corticotrophin-like intermediate-lobe peptide (CLIP or ACTH 18–39), γ-LPH and β-endorphin. A number of these peptides share not only a common heptapeptide, which confers melanocyte-stimulating properties (found in α-MSH, ACTH, β-LPH, γ-LPH and β-MSH), but also the structure of met-enkephalin (in β-LPH and β-endorphin), which confers opioid properties. ACTH is cosecreted in equimolar amounts with β-LPH. The initial enthusiasm for β-LPH assays as a more robust alternative for ACTH assays has not endured. In man, the intermediate lobe is present and functional only during fetal life; it has been suggested that the transition from intermediate to anterior lobe function and the switch to ACTH (1–39) production may play a part in the development of fetal maturity and the initiation of labour.

Measurement of Anterior Pituitary Hormones

Reliable and specific radioimmunoassay methods are available for the six major anterior pituitary hormones and these have largely replaced bioassay procedures. Problems of cross-reactivity still exist, particularly with assays for the glycoproteins. These have been partly overcome by antiserum directed against β-subunits. Variations in specificity of antiserum preparations make comparison of different assays difficult and for this reason results are related to established reference preparations.

HYPOTHALAMIC CONTROL OF ANTERIOR PITUITARY SECRETION

The synthesis and secretion of the anterior pituitary hormones are under the control of individual inhibiting or releasing factors (or hormones) produced in the hypothalamus. The structure and function of the principal hypothalamic releasing hormones have now been elucidated (Table 37.3). In common with oxytocin and vasopressin, they are synthesized within neurosecretory cells in hypothalamic nuclei and transported down the axon processes of these cells to the infundibulum. Whereas the majority of axons transporting vasopressin and oxytocin pass directly to the neurohypophysis, the anterior pituitary regulatory factors are secreted into the sinusoids of the hypophyseal portal vessels in the median eminence and pituitary stalk, from where they are carried the short distance to the adenohypophysis in the portal capillaries. Some vasopressin also follows this route, but it is not clear whether this plays a significant role in the regulation of anterior pituitary secretion.

The releasing hormones (together with vasopressin, oxytocin and a host of other neuropeptides whose regulatory function remains largely unknown) are synthesized in the supraoptic and paraventricular nuclei of the hypothalamus. High concentrations are demonstrable within the median eminence but this reflects an accumulation in and around the axon terminals rather than a site of synthesis.

Although there may be both releasing and release-inhibiting factors for several or all of the anterior pituitary hormones, all of these, with the notable exception of prolactin, are under tonic stimulatory control; it is therefore the releasing factor that is the dominant influence under normal conditions. In contrast, the major influence on prolactin secretion is an inhibitory factor (PIF) and, consequently, hypothalamic damage or pituitary-stalk section results in uninhibited hypersecretion of prolactin in association with impaired secretion of the other anterior pituitary hormones. Evidence suggests that PIF is not a peptide but the neurotransmitter dopamine.

It is clear that the hypothalamic regulatory factors are not specific in either their anatomical localization or their action on pituitary secretion. Neither is there a single factor that controls the synthesis and release of each of the pituitary hormones. Thus, GH release-inhibiting hormone (GHRIH or somatostatin) is widely distributed not only throughout the central nervous system but also the gastrointestinal tract and

TABLE 37.3
PRIMARY STRUCTURE OF THE PRINCIPAL HYPOTHALAMIC RELEASING HORMONES

pGlu-His-Pro-NH$_2$
Thyrotrophin-releasing hormone (TRH)

pGlu-His-Trp-Ser-Try-Gly-Leu-Arg-Pro-Gly-NH$_2$
Gonadotrophin-releasing hormone (GnRH)

Ala-Gly-Cys-Lys-Asn-Phe-Phe-Trp-Lys-Thr-Phe-Thr-Ser-Cys
Somatostatin

Ser-Glu-Glu-Pro-Pro-Ile-Ser-Leu-Asp-Leu-Thr-Phe-His-Leu-Leu-Arg-Leu-Arg-Glu-Val-Leu-Glu-Met-Ala-Arg-Ala-Glu-
Gln-Leu-Ala-Gln-Gln-Ala-His-Ser-Asn-Arg-Lys-Leu-Met-Glu-Ile-Ile-NH$_2$
Corticotrophin-releasing hormone (CRH)

Tyr-Ala-Asp-Ala-Ile-Phe-Thr-Asn-Ser-Tyr-Arg-Lys-Val-Leu-Gly-Gln-Leu-Ser-Ala-Arg-Lys-Leu-Leu-Gln-Asp-Ile-Met-
Ser-Arg-Gln-Gln-Gly-Glu-Ser-Asn-Gln-Glu-Arg-Gly-Ala(-Arg-Ala-Arg-Leu-NH$_2$)
Growth hormone-releasing hormone (GHRH)

the islets of Langerhans in the pancreas. In addition to its action in inhibiting synthesis and release of GH, GHRIH inhibits a variety of pituitary and extra-pituitary endocrine secretions including TSH, insulin, glucagon and renin. Similarly, thyroid-stimulating hormone-releasing hormone (TRH) is not entirely specific in its action as it stimulates the release of prolactin in addition to TSH, although the physiological significance of this is uncertain: the hypersecretion of TSH in hypothyroidism is only occasionally associated with hyperprolactinaemia, and the surge of prolactin secretion in response to suckling is not accompanied by an increase in TSH secretion. In some circumstances, TRH also stimulates the release of ACTH and GH. Dopamine, in addition to being the major (inhibitory) influence on prolactin secretion can also inhibit the release of TSH, gonadotrophins and, occasionally, GH.

The synthesis of both gonadotrophins (LH and FSH) appears to be regulated by a single gonadotrophin-releasing hormone (GnRH). The relative responses of LH and FSH to stimulation by GnRH in women of reproductive age probably depend upon the rate of stimulation and on the circulating levels of ovarian steroids.

As well as providing for translation of a neurological impulse into an endocrine response, the hypothalamic–pituitary unit provides amplification of the neuronal signal by means of a cascade system. One inevitable consequence of such a cascade is the pulsatile nature of the secretion both of regulatory factors and pituitary hormones, the rate of hormone secretion being largely determined by the frequency of the pulses of releasing factor passing down the hypophyseal portal capillaries.

A number of diseases previously believed to be due to primary excess or deficiency of pituitary hormones (e.g. Cushing's syndrome and acromegaly; isolated deficiencies of GH and gonadotrophins) may sometimes be due to over- or under-production of the corresponding hypothalamic releasing factor. As yet, this has only limited therapeutic implications.

PHYSIOLOGICAL CONTROL OF HYPOTHALAMIC–PITUITARY FUNCTION

The major factors influencing hypothalamic–pituitary activity are:

(i) neural influences from other areas of the nervous system;
(ii) hypothalamic chemoreceptors;
(iii) feedback control by target-organ hormones.

The precise origin of the neural signals concerned in the regulation of hypothalamic–pituitary secretion is unknown but they probably come from many areas of the brain and spinal cord, and are perhaps the most important of the regulatory mechanisms. Basal levels and cyclical variations in secretion rates, as well as the responses to a number of stimuli (e.g. stress, sleep) appear to be under neural control but this area of neuroendocrinology is, as yet, poorly understood.

The hypothalamus contains specific areas sensitive to certain physiological stimuli (e.g. blood glucose concentration, osmolality) that are capable of mediating acute changes in both anterior and posterior pituitary secretions. The precise anatomical localization of many of these areas is unknown but they are probably closely related or identical to the nuclei that produce the releasing factor in response to the particular stimulus.

With the exception of the positive feedback stimulation of gonadotrophin by high levels of oestrogen, secretion of anterior pituitary trophic hormones (TSH, ACTH, LH and FSH) is inhibited by the corresponding target-organ hormone. This negative feedback system is clearly seen to operate both in the presence of primary target-organ failure or hypersecretion, which result in high or low levels, respec-

TABLE 37.4

ASSESSMENT OF HYPOTHALAMIC–PITUITARY FUNCTION: SUMMARY OF INVESTIGATIONAL PROCEDURES

Axis	Tests of target-organ function	Tests of pituitary function		Tests of hypothalamic–pituitary function	
		Stimulation	Suppression	Stimulation	Suppression
HPT	Thyroid hormones (total and free T3, T4)	TRH			T3
HPA	Cortisol and other adrenal steroids	CRH		Hypoglycaemia Metyrapone	Dexamethasone
HPG	Oestradiol Progesterone HCG stimulation	GnRH		Clomiphene Oestradiol benzoate	
Prolactin	—	TRH Metoclopramide	L-dopa Bromocriptine	Hypoglycaemia	
GH	IGF-1	GHRH	Somatostatin	See Table 37.5	Hyperglycaemia

HCG, human chorionic gonadotrophin; HPA, hypothalamic–pituitary–adrenal; HPG, hypothalamic–pituitary–gonadal; HPT, hypothalamic–pituitary–thyroid; all other abbreviations in text.

tively, of trophic hormones, and also when target-organ hormones are given exogenously. Although there are a number of situations in which feedback control of hypothalamic–pituitary secretion is overridden, this mechanism is probably largely responsible for minute-to-minute control, with the background level of secretion set by suprahypothalamic influences. In the absence of assays of sufficient sensitivity to measure hypothalamic releasing factors in peripheral blood, it is difficult to tell whether feedback effects are exerted upon the hypothalamus, the pituitary or both, although it seems likely that, as with other influences, the major effect is upon the hypothalamus. Feedback control may be exerted by target-organ hormones (long loop), anterior pituitary hormones (short loop) and possibly by a very short loop system whereby hypothalamic releasing factors act to regulate their own secretion. Neither GH nor prolactin stimulate hormone production by a single target organ. Neither appears to be controlled by a simple system of feedback inhibition, although the insulin-like growth factors (particularly IGF-1) may exert some influence on GH secretion. Interestingly, these are the only two anterior pituitary hormones for which there is good evidence for the existence of a hypothalamic release-inhibiting factor.

The role of the pineal gland in the control of hypothalamic–pituitary function is largely unproven, although there is evidence that changes in melatonin secretion may be important in regulating the changes in gonadotrophin secretion that occur at puberty, and in the establishment of secretory rhythms.

TESTS OF ANTERIOR PITUITARY FUNCTION

Anterior pituitary function can be assessed indirectly by measurement of circulating target-organ hormones, or directly by measurement of pituitary hormones either in the basal state or following stimulation with synthetic releasing hormones (e.g. TRH, GnRH, corticotrophin-releasing hormone (CRH)). Additionally, the function of the hypothalamic–anterior pituitary unit can be assessed by measuring the pituitary response (either directly or indirectly) to stimuli acting at the level of the hypothalamus, such as insulin-induced hypoglycaemia. In practice, a combination of all these three approaches is generally used. Table 37.4 summarizes those tests in current clinical use.

Measurement of circulating levels of target-organ hormones is frequently adequate to exclude absolute pituitary insufficiency but gives little indication of pituitary reserve and is generally of limited value when pituitary hypersecretion is suspected.

Measurement of basal concentrations of anterior pituitary hormones is of value in confirming primary target-organ failure when high levels of the corresponding trophic hormone are found. Stimulation tests generally show an exaggerated, delayed response in these circumstances and add little further information. In contrast, in suspected hypothalamic–pituitary dysfunction, stimulation or suppression tests are usually necessary but the expectation that direct pituitary stimulation tests using synthetic releasing hormones would provide distinction between hypothalamic and anterior pituitary insufficiency has not been entirely fulfilled because the absence of endogenous tonic stimulation of the pituitary resulting from long-term hypothalamic insufficiency results in a flat response to exogenous tonic stimulation which is frequently indistinguishable from that seen in primary pituitary disease. More prolonged pituitary stimulation tests may help to resolve this problem.

Individual hypothalamic–pituitary axes may be tested separately but overall pituitary reserve is conventionally tested by means of a combined stimulation test using TRH, GnRH and insulin-induced hypoglycaemia as outlined next.

Patient fasted overnight

Time

0 min:
   In-dwelling intravenous cannula inserted

   Blood withdrawn for measurement of glucose, GH, cortisol (ACTH), TSH, prolactin, LH and FSH

   TRH 200 μg
   GnRH 100 ug $\Big\}$ given intravenously
   Insulin 0.1 u/kg
   (*see* Tests of GH secretion below)

20, 60 min:
   Blood withdrawn for measurement of TSH, LH, FSH and prolactin

30, 60, 90, 120 min:
   Blood withdrawn for measurement of glucose, GH, cortisol (ACTH)

Prolactin secretion is stimulated by both TRH and hypoglycaemia. In order to distinguish between these responses, insulin can be given at 60 min after completion of the combined TRH/LHRH test but this does not usually provide additional useful information.

Interpretation of the GH response is discussed in detail below. It is essential to achieve adequate hypoglycaemia (blood glucose falling to less than 2.2 mmol/L accompanied by clinical symptoms) in order to interpret the cortisol response; plasma cortisol should normally rise by at least 160 μmol/L (6 μg/dL) with a peak level of at least 540 μmol/L (20 μg/dL).

Normal basal TSH values are less than 6 mu/L and, with a traditional TSH assay, may be indistinguishable from zero. Using a sensitive, two-point immunoradiometric assay for TSH, it is possible to distinguish between low-normal and suppressed levels of TSH. The TSH response to TRH shows wide variations in normal subjects. The peak response occurs between 20 and 30 min and may be up to 20 mu/L. Much lower responses are also seen and using a sensitive TSH assay, a significant rise in TSH above the basal level may be considered normal. In hypothalamic or pituitary insufficiency, the TSH response to TRH is impaired, and an absent response is also seen in primary hyperthyroidism. In primary hypothyroidism, the basal TSH level is raised and the response to TRH is both augmented and prolonged.

The gonadotrophic responses to GnRH are generally proportional to the basal values. Prepubertally, the rise in FSH exceeds the rise in LH; this ratio is reversed midway through puberty. In adults, there should be a three-fold rise in gonadotrophins following GnRH. Absent or impaired values are seen with pituitary or hypothalamic disease, including many women with 'functional' or weight loss-associated amenorrhoea. Exaggerated and delayed responses are seen in patients with primary gonadal failure.

Further discussion of the hypothalamic–pituitary–adrenal,–thyroid and–gonadal axes is found in Chapters 38, 41 and 42.

GROWTH HORMONE

Regulation of GH Secretion

The major factors that influence GH secretion are summarized in Table 37.5. In the absence of specific stimuli, circulating levels of GH are low during the day, with only minor fluctuations. However, there is a marked surge of GH secretion at night, particularly in children, with one or more peaks occurring during early, deep slow-wave sleep.

GH secretion is stimulated by an increase in the circulating level of arginine and a number of other amino acids following either oral ingestion or intravenous infusion. The GH response to a fall in blood glucose concentration is related to the rate and magnitude of the fall rather than the development of a set degree of hypoglycaemia. However, the GH response to hypoglycaemia is reliable and quantifiable and remains the reference method for assessment of GH reserve.

The response of GH to neurotransmitters is complex. Acetylcholine, serotonin (5-hydroxytryptamine), α-adrenergic and dopaminergic agonists have all been shown to stimulate GH secretion. These substances probably act by modifying secretion of GH-releasing factor from the hypothalamus. There is increasing evidence to indicate that serotonin may act as the final common pathway for a number of neurotransmitters, and that a serotoninergic mechanism may be involved in the GH response to hypoglycaemia, exercise, amino acids and slow-wave sleep.

Actions of GH

GH possesses both anabolic and catabolic properties; these may be summarized as:

1. *Anabolic effects*
   - Stimulation of cellular uptake of amino acids
   - Stimulation of RNA and protein synthesis
   - Inhibition of protein catabolism and urea synthesis

2. *Catabolic effects*
   - Stimulation of lipolysis
   - Inhibition of cellular uptake and phosphorylation of glucose.

The effects on protein metabolism and tissue

TABLE 37.5

(A) FACTORS ASSOCIATED WITH STIMULATION OF GROWTH
HORMONE SECRETION

*Sleep**

Stress
Physical (e.g. surgery, exercise*)
Psychological

Metabolic factors
Fall in concentration of glucose* and free fatty acids
Rise in concentration of amino acids*
Fasting
Uncontrolled diabetes mellitus
Uraemia

Biogenic amines
Dopaminergic agonists (e.g. L-dopa*, bromocriptine, apo-
morphine)
α-adrenergic agonists (e.g. noradrenaline, clonidine*)
β-adrenergic antagonists (e.g. propranalol*)
Serotonin precursors (e.g. 5-hydroxytryptophan)
Acetylcholine agonists

Hormonal factors
GHRH, vasopressin, glucagon*, pentagastrin
Low circulating IGF-1
Oestrogens

Opiates
Morphine, enkephalin

(B) FACTORS ASSOCIATED WITH SUPPRESSION OF GROWTH
HORMONE SECRETION

Psychogenic
Emotional deprivation

Metabolic factors
Rise in concentration of glucose* and free fatty acids
Obesity

Biogenic amines
α-adrenergic antagonists (e.g. phentolamine)
β-adrenergic agonists
Serotonin antagonists (e.g. cyproheptadine, methysergide)

Hormonal
Somatostatin*
High IGF-1 level
Corticosteroid excess
Hypothyroidism

* Have been used in the clinical assessment of GH secretion.

growth are the most important physiologically; GH
deficiency in childhood results in severe impairment
of skeletal growth but in only mild metabolic effects.
In cartilage and bone, GH stimulates the synthesis of
RNA, collagen, chondroitin sulphate (proteoglycan)
and other proteins, resulting in skeletal growth. There
is also an increase in protein synthesis in muscle and
other tissues. *In vitro*, GH itself is ineffective in
stimulating anabolic processes. These effects are mediated *in vivo* by the insulin-like growth factors (IGFs),
particularly IGF-1. Initially termed 'sulfation factor'

(sic), and also known as the somatomedins because
of their growth-promoting properties, these peptides
share not only considerable sequence homology with
proinsulin but also share a number of physiological
properties with insulin (including the ability to induce
hypoglycaemia), and account for around 60% of the
bioassayable insulin activity in fasting plasma. Unlike
insulin, they are tightly bound in plasma to specific
binding proteins, the most important of which are
IGFBP-1 and IGFBP-3. The level of IGFBP-1 (quantitatively the major binding protein) and IGF-1 itself
is under the control of GH which regulates the rate
of synthesis in the liver. In contrast to IGFBP-3, the
level of IGFBP-1 shows a marked diurnal variation,
with suppression by carbohydrate feeding, and is
reciprocally related to the level of plasma insulin.

In view of the strong protein binding of IGF-1 in
plasma, the level (unlike that of GH itself) is relatively
constant and gives an intergrated measure of GH
secretion. Protein binding also results in a longer
half-life in plasma which accounts for the discrepancy
between the short half-life of GH and the duration of
its physiological actions many of which are attributable to IGF-1 rather than GH itself. Circulating
levels of IGF-1 and IGFBP-3 are also influenced by
a number of other factors, particularly nutrition;
some studies have shown a close relationship between
IGF-1 and urine nitrogen secretion in surgical patients, and it has been suggested that IGF-1 may be a
useful marker of nutritional status. It remains to be
proven that IGF-1 is sufficiently specific to fulfil this
role and that it is not simply another indicator of
disease severity. The molar concentration of IGF-1
in plasma is around 100 times that of insulin; the
precise physiological function of this large pool of
predominantly bound peptide is unknown but IGF-1
is released at sites of tissue injury and may play a
major role in the process of repair.

In contrast, tissue levels of IGF-1 may be independent of, and unrelated to, circulating GH levels. In a
number of endocrine tissues (ovary and testis for
example), IGF-1 is under the control of the corresponding trophic hormone and acts as an important
paracrine or autocrine mediator of hormone synthesis
and secretion.

The physiological effects of GH are closely interre-
lated with those of insulin. The anabolic action of
GH is synergistic with that of insulin and this action
predominates in the postprandial state following
stimulation of the release of insulin and GH by
carbohydrate and protein, respectively. The demonstration that gastrin can stimulate GH secretion indicates that the GH response to feeding may be mediated by a gut–hypothalamic–pituitary axis. However,
the majority of GH secretion occurs at night and,
although circulating insulin levels are relatively low
at this time, they may be sufficient to facilitate the
anabolic action of GH or, alternatively, the IGFs
may fulfil this role. The peak nocturnal secretion of
GH coincides with the nadir in the secretion of

cortisol, which has a catabolic effect on protein metabolism, antagonistic to that of GH.

In contrast, the catabolic actions of GH are seen in the fasting state when insulin levels are low. Lipolysis is stimulated, providing free fatty acids, which are the major energy source during fasting; insulin-dependent phosphorylation and utilization of glucose are impaired, resulting in carbohydrate intolerance in states of GH excess.

Tests of GH Secretion

Measurement of basal levels of GH are of limited value in the assessment of patients with suspected hypothalamic–pituitary disease. In normal subjects, resting levels may be low and indistinguishable from those found in in hypopituitarism; conversely, the stress of a visit to hospital and venepuncture may be sufficient to raise levels into the acromegalic range. For these reasons, the appropriate stimulation or suppression tests should be used in the investigation of patients with suspected under- or over-production of GH.

1. Stimulation Tests

In view of the discomfort and potential risk attached to many of the tests of GH secretion, a preliminary screening test should be done in all subjects (especially children) in whom deficiency is suspected. Measurement of GH after exercise and during sleep are both simple and satisfactory screening tests.

Exercise test. A single blood sample is taken 30 min after the start of a 15-min period of vigorous, preferably standardized, exercise. A serum GH value of 20 mu/L or above at this time indicates adequate GH secretion.

Sleep. A single blood sample is taken after the onset of deep sleep. Interpretation as above.

Insulin-induced hypoglycaemia (insulin stress test, IST). The test must be made with the patient resting in bed following an overnight fast. An indwelling intravenous cannula is inserted and specimens taken for basal GH and glucose assay. A single dose of soluble human insulin is then given by intravenous injection. The standard dose is 0.1–0.15 u/kg; if there is a strong possibility of hypopituitarism, a smaller dose is used, and in patients with insulin resistance (e.g. obesity, diabetes, acromegaly, Cushing's syndrome) the dose is increased to 0.2 u/kg. Blood specimens are taken at 15, 30, 60, 90 and 120 min for measurement of glucose and GH. For the test to be considered satisfactory, the blood glucose should fall to less than half the basal level or, preferably, symptomatic hypoglycaemia should be produced.

Until recently, this has been the standard provocative test for the assessment of pituitary GH reserve and the principal biochemical criterion in the selection of growth-retarded children for treatment with GH. However, the procedure is unpleasant and potentially dangerous, especially in children and in patients with pituitary or adrenal insufficiency. The IST has the advantage that it can also be used as a test for the hypothalamic–pituitary–adrenal axis, but in the majority of children with GH deficiency this is an isolated defect and formal testing of the remainder of pituitary function is not required. In these situations, an alternative to the IST (glucagon stimulation) should be used.

The IST must be done in hospital by experienced staff. The patient should not be left alone during the test and a physician should be close at hand. A patent intravenous cannula must be maintained, and the test should be terminated immediately if severe hypoglycaemia develops or if the patient loses consciousness, or if any other untoward event occurs. In the case of children, glucose should be given orally if possible (25–50 g as Hycal®); if the child is unable to swallow, glucose should be given intravenously at the rate of 2 mL/kg of 10% dextrose (200 mg/kg) over a period of 3 min, followed by an infusion at the rate of 10 mg/kg per minute to maintain the blood glucose level (measured by 'stick' test at the bedside) at between 5 and 8 mmol/L *and no higher*. Hydrocortisone (100 mg) should be given if hypopituitarism is suspected. Glucagon should not be given unless venous access is lost and, even then, no reliance should be placed upon a satisfactory response to glucagon. If there is no improvement in the state of consciousness after restoration of a normal blood glucose level, an alternative explanation for the coma should be sought. Great care must be taken not to overtreat hypoglycaemia as this can lead to severe hyperglycaemia, cerebral damage and death. *Excessive amounts of intravenous glucose must not be given.*

Caution should also be observed in patients with epilepsy and ischaemic heart disease, in whom an alternative stimulation test should be used.

Interpretation of the results is based upon the peak GH concentration reached, assuming that adequate biochemical and symptomatic hypoglycaemia was achieved. A peak value of less than 4 mu/L indicates severe GH deficiency; values between 4 and 10 mu/L represent severe partial GH deficiency, and between 10 and 20 mu/L, partial deficiency. A peak value of 20 mu/L or greater indicates adequate GH reserve.

Hypoglycaemia also stimulates secretion of ACTH and prolactin and, if required, specimens for ACTH, cortisol and prolactin should be collected at the same time as specimens for GH.

Glucagon Test. Blood samples are taken via an indwelling venous cannula at 30-min intervals before and for a total of 4 h after a subcutaneous injection of glucagon 0.03 mg/kg body weight (maximum 1 mg) in children or 1 mg in adults. Nausea may occur after the injection. At the end of the test, the child should eat lunch and should not be allowed home unless the blood glucose level is above 4 mmol/L 1 h after lunch. The GH response is enhanced by simultaneous administration of propranolol.

Clonidine. The GH response to a single oral dose of clonidine, 0.15 mg/m² surface area, may be used as an alternative to insulin–hypoglycaemia or glucagon stimulation in children as a test of GH reserve. Peak values similar to those following insulin occur between 60 and 120 min after clonidine administration. However, the dose of clonidine used may result in severe arterial hypotension.

Prolonged Oral Glucose Tolerance Test (OGTT). In normal subjects, blood GH concentration is suppressed during an OGTT, but following the rise in blood glucose concentration, the fall back towards normal provokes a rebound rise in GH occurring between 2 and 4 h after the glucose load. The GH response is less consistent than that provoked by hypoglycaemia but in normal children the serum GH usually exceeds 20 mu/L in at least one sample. The test has the advantage of safety but the disadvantage of being prolonged and requiring multiple sampling.

Arginine Infusion and Bovril Tests. Infusion of arginine stimulates GH secretion in normal subjects. After an overnight fast, arginine is given by intravenous infusion in a dose of 0.5 g/kg body weight up to a total dose of 30 g in a total volume of 100 mL. Blood samples are collected before and at 30-min intervals for measurement of GH, which usually reaches a peak value between 30 and 60 min after the start of the infusion. The test is free of side-effects, but the GH response is less consistent than the response to hypoglycaemia, particularly in adult men, who may require pretreatment with oestrogen (e.g. stilboestrol 0.5–1.0 mg every 12 h for 48 h) in order to elicit a maximal response.

In children, the amino acid content of Bovril® may elicit a GH response. Blood specimens are taken at 30-min intervals for 2 h following a drink of Bovril, 14 g/m² body surface area. Peak values are less than after insulin–hypoglycaemia and some normal children fail to respond adequately. This test has lost favour as a screening procedure.

L-Dopa. Oral (or intravenous) administration of L-dopa provokes a rise in GH and may be used as an alternative in adults in whom an insulin stress test is contraindicated. L-Dopa, 500 mg, is given after an overnight fast with blood samples before, and at 30-min intervals for a further 2 h. Concomitant administration of propranolol enhances the GH response to L-dopa. Side-effects of L-dopa include nausea, occasionally with vomiting. Peak serum GH levels usually occur between 60 and 120 min and are similar to those seen in response to hypoglycaemia.

2. Suppression Tests
Glucose Tolerance Test. In acromegaly and gigantism,

basal serum GH levels may be very high, and in the presence of characteristic clinical findings there is frequently little doubt about the diagnosis. However, in many cases basal levels are only moderately elevated but the elevation is sustained and not suppressed by physiological stimuli such as hyperglycaemia. After an overnight fast, a standard 75-g oral glucose tolerance test is performed, with specimens for GH collected at 0, 30, 60, 90 and 120 min. In normal subjects, serum GH is suppressed to less than 3 mu/L in at least one specimen, but in acromegaly and gigantism serum GH concentration remains above this level and there is frequently a paradoxical rise in response to hyperglycaemia. Similar results are obtained in response to an intravenous glucose tolerance test. In addition to abnormal GH levels, carbohydrate intolerance is found in about 25% of acromegalic patients.

Disorders of GH Secretion

Acromegaly and Gigantism

Overproduction of GH in adults results in the syndrome of acromegaly. Rarely, excessive secretion of GH occurs before puberty, before closure of the epiphyses of long bones where longitudinal growth occurs, resulting in pituitary gigantism. The causes of acromegaly are listed next:

- pituitary adenoma (common—95% of cases);
- ectopic GH-secreting tumour (very rare);
- hypothalamic GHRH-secreting tumour (very rare);
- ectopic GHRH-secreting tumour (rare);

In the vast majority of cases, the condition is believed to be due to pituitary adenoma. The annual incidence of acromegaly is around 3–4 cases per million with a prevalence in the population of about 50–60 cases per million. The condition is very insidious, usually presenting in the fourth decade but, in retrospect, often developing over many years before clinical presentation. A more aggressive course may be seen in younger patients and should arouse suspicion of an ectopic source of GHRH.

Clinical features include somatic and metabolic features (probably due largely to IGF-1 and GH, respectively), in addition to the local effects of an expanding pituitary tumour. *Somatic features* include an increase in the width of long bones and in soft-tissue thickness, giving rise to the characteristic spade-like hands and broad feet with thickened heel pad. There is also an increase in the growth of cartilaginous bone, which is not limited by epiphyseal closure, resulting in enlargement of the mandible, thickening of the skull and prominence of the supraorbital ridges that, together with coarsening of facial features due to soft tissue growth, result in the typical acromegalic appearance. Other features include cardiac enlargement, non-toxic goitre, excessive sweating, osteoarthritis, osteoporosis, pigmentation, and nasal and colonic polyps. *Metabolic features* include carbohydrate intolerance or diabetes mellitus and hypertension.

Local features are due to the pressure of an expanding pituitary adenoma causing enlargement of the pituitary fossa, which is usually evident on a lateral radiograph of the skull. Other local effects of the tumour include headache, and visual-field defects due to compression of the optic tracts by suprasellar extension. The characteristic visual-field defect is a bitemporal hemianopia (loss of the outer visual field in both eyes) resulting from compression of the optic chiasma, but any other defect may be encountered.

Other pituitary endocrine deficiencies may occur due to either compression of the hypothalamus by suprasellar extension of an adenoma, disruption of the hypothalamic–pituitary capillaries, or direct damage to pituitary tissue by an expanding tumour. Hypogonadism may result from loss of gonadotrophin secretion but some features (amenorrhoea, oligospermia, loss of libido) may be caused by hypersecretion of prolactin, which occurs in about one-third of acromegalics. If hypogonadism occurs in association with gigantism, the delayed epiphyseal fusion prolongs the period of bone growth.

Pituitary tumours occasionally undergo spontaneous infarction resulting in varying degrees of hypopituitarism. This is more common with large tumours and may produce a dramatic clinical picture (pituitary apoplexy) of severe headache, acute visual disturbance, hyperpyrexia and coma.

Rarely, acromegaly occurs as part of a syndrome of multiple endocrine adenomatosis (MEA type I; Werner's syndrome) in association with parathyroid adenomas or hyperplasia, pancreatic islet-cell adenomas (β-and non-β-cell) and carcinoid tumours of the gut.

Biochemical Investigations. Failure of serum GH concentration to suppress during a standard OGTT is characteristic of acromegaly (*see* above). Serum IGF-1 concentration is raised and, in the presence of characteristic clinical features, this may be sufficient to establish the diagnosis. The status of other hypothalamic–pituitary axes should be tested by means of appropriate provocation tests. It is particularly important to identify hyperprolactinaemia, as this may have therapeutic implications. TRH stimulation frequently produces a rise in serum GH, which is not seen in normal subjects.

Other Investigations. The diagnosis of active acromegaly depends upon biochemical criteria but other investigations are essential to determine the size of the pituitary tumour and the extent of suprasellar extension using both conventional radiography and magnetic resonance imaging. Formal plotting of visual fields is essential to document the extent of visual-field losses. Soft-tissue thickness can be assessed by a number of techniques including caliper measurement of skinfold thickness, hand volume by plethysmography or heel-pad thickness on X-ray. Such measurements, made serially, have been useful in assessing the progress of the condition and the response to treatment but have been supplanted by biochemical monitoring, particularly of IGF-1.

Treatment. The primary aim of treatment is to reduce the size of the pituitary tumour, particularly in the presence of suprasellar extension. Surgical hypophysectomy, with or without radiotherapy, remains the standard treatment in many centres. Pharmacological treatment with bromocriptine may produce some shrinkage of pituitary tumours but results have generally been disappointing. More recently, somatostatin has been shown to be effective in reducing GH secretion and tumour volume. However, this has currently to be given by frequent (thrice daily) injection and until longer-acting analogues become available, primary treatment with surgery or radiotherapy will remain the standard treatment for most patients.

Following treatment, reinvestigation is essential to assess the reduction in GH secretion and the status of other anterior pituitary hormones. After radiotherapy, GH levels may fall very slowly and may continue to decline for several years, necessitating long-term biochemical assessment.

GH Deficiency and Pituitary Dwarfism

GH deficiency in childhood results in short stature due to impaired growth of long bones. This may occur as part of a syndrome of panhypopituitarism but in the majority of cases there appears to be congenital failure of the hypothalamic stimulus to GH secretion without evidence of organic disease of either the hypothalamus or pituitary. The condition is more common in boys, is usually isolated but may be associated with deficiency of other anterior pituitary hormones, particularly gonadotrophins, TSH or ACTH. It is occasionally familial with autosomal recessive inheritance. Intrauterine growth is unaffected and birth size is usually normal, but careful plotting of height characteristically shows a reduced linear growth rate with height falling below the third percentile by the age of 4 or 5 years. There is frequently an increase in subcutaneous fat and consequently most affected children appear short and plump. Bone age as assessed radiologically is lower than chronological age but usually corresponds to height age. Puberty is often delayed, but in the absence of associated gonadotrophin deficiency, sexual development is ultimately normal and fertility may be unimpaired. Apart from a tendency to fasting hypoglycaemia and an increased sensitivity to insulin, the metabolic effects of GH deficiency are usually minimal and most adults with the condition remain asymptomatic.

GH deficiency accounts for less than 10% of cases of short stature. A summary of other causes is presented in Table 37.6. Most of those listed are not

TABLE 37.6
MAJOR CAUSES OF SHORT STATURE

Congenital
Familial short stature
Constitutional slow growth

Chromosomal abnormalities
Gonadal dysgenesis (Turner's syndrome)
Trisomies

Intrauterine growth retardation

Nutritional
Malabsorption
Protein-calorie malnutrition

Skeletal
Osteochondroplasias

Chronic systemic disease
Congenital heart disease
Chronic renal failure etc.

Emotional deprivation

Endocrine
GH deficiency
Hypothyroidism
Corticosteroid excess (endogenous or exogenous)
Congenital adrenal hyperplasia
Pseudo- and pseudopseudohypoparathyroidism
Precocious puberty
GH-receptor defect (Laron dwarfism)

TABLE 37.7
CAUSES OF HYPOPITUITARISM

Tumours
Pituitary adenoma
Craniopharyngioma
Meningioma, glioma
Pinealoma
Metastatic carcinoma

Trauma
Head injury

Infection
Basal meningitis
Tuberculosis
Syphilis

Granulomas
Sarcoidosis
Histiocytosis:
    Hand–Schüller–Christian disease
    Eosinophilic granuloma

Avascular necrosis
Post-partum (Sheehan's syndrome)
Infarction of pituitary tumour
Diabetes

Idiopathic/genetic
Isolated and multiple pituitary hormone deficiencies

Iatrogenic
Surgical hypophysectomy
External irradiation
Radioisotope implants
Suppression by prolonged endocrine therapy (corticosteroids, thyroxine)

difficult to distinguish from pituitary dwarfism and, with this exception and the probable exception of Turner's syndrome, therapy with GH plays no part in their management, but in those children in whom there is no apparent cause for short stature the possibility of GH deficiency should be investigated.

Investigation. A screening test should be done in all children in whom the diagnosis is suspected; of the tests available, exercise stimulation is the simplest and least invasive. Measurement of serum GH during the first 2 h of sleep is of value but has the disadvantage of requiring hospitalization. If the GH response to exercise or sleep is inadequate and the clinical picture is suggestive of pituitary dwarfism, a definitive test should be made. In a number of conditions, including hypothyroidism, emotional deprivation and malabsorption, the GH response to stimulation may be impaired but returns to normal on appropriate treatment.

Associated pituitary deficiencies should be excluded by means of the corresponding stimulation tests. However, it is not possible to identify gonadotrophin deficiency before the age of puberty since normal prepubertal values are low and virtually indistinguishable from those found in hypogonadotrophic hypogonadism.

In the very rare but interesting condition of Laron dwarfism, serum GH levels are normal or elevated

but levels of circulating IGF-1 are low. The defect appears to be in the gene coding for the GH receptor, resulting in low levels of tissue receptors and binding of GH, and also of the high-affinity, GH-binding protein in serum. The resultant dwarfism is resistant to GH therapy but responsive to treatment with biosynthetic IGF-1.

Hypopituitarism
The major causes of hypopituitarism are summarized in Table 37.7. In many of the conditions listed the primary defect is either hypothalamic damage or disruption of the hypothalamic–pituitary portal system. The clinical picture is very variable and depends on the underlying cause: surgical hypophysectomy is followed by rapid onset of clinical signs, with severe adrenal insufficiency developing within a few days if untreated, but in many conditions the onset is insidious and the full clinical picture may take years to develop. Surprisingly, this may be the case in hypopituitarism developing after such dramatic events as post-partum infarction or severe head injury. In these situations, GH and gonadotrophin secretion are usually lost first (failure of lactation and persistent amenorrhoea are the early symptoms of Sheehan's syndrome), with signs of thyroid and

adrenal insufficiency often developing slowly. In established hypopituitarism, the features of thyroid, adrenal and gonadal failure are combined with those of gonadotrophin and prolactin insufficiency. Symptoms and signs include growth retardation in childhood, lassitude, cold intolerance and constipation; postural hypotension, nausea and abdominal pain; and loss of libido and secondary sexual characteristics. The skin is usually pale, dry and finely wrinkled, and there is thinning of scalp and body hair. Fasting hypoglycaemia may develop and in untreated patients, coma and death may ultimately supervene.

Pituitary damage does not usually result in diabetes insipidus, although this may occur with more extensive hypothalamic involvement and occasionally latent diabetes insipidus is precipitated when treatment of hypopituitarism with steroids is instituted. The mechanism of this is not clear but may concern the relation between vasopressin and corticotrophin-releasing factor.

Biochemical Investigation. The characteristic electrolyte disturbance of adrenal insufficiency (hyponatraemia, hypokalaemia and elevated blood urea) is not usually seen in hypopituitarism, in which there is relative preservation of mineralocorticoid function. Suspicion is often raised biochemically, by the finding of target-organ failure without elevation of the corresponding trophic hormone (e.g. hypothyroidism with normal TSH concentration), but the diagnosis depends upon comprehensive testing of hypothalamic–pituitary function as outlined above. Distinction between a hypothalamic or a pituitary lesion may often be made on the basis of the prolactin concentration, which is usually raised in hypothalamic disease, due to loss of prolactin inhibitory factor, and low in pituitary disease. Additionally, prolonged or repeated stimulation with releasing factors should elicit a response in hypothalamic disease but not in primary pituitary disease.

Other Investigations. Formal visual-field testing and radiological assessment of the pituitary fossa and surrounding area should be done as in acromegaly. The choice of other investigations will be determined by the suspected nature of the underlying pathological process.

Miscellaneous

Diabetes mellitus. The GH response to a number of stimuli is increased in both insulin-dependent and non-insulin-dependent diabetes, and there is also an increase in the frequency and height of the secretory peaks of GH. The importance of this in the pathogenesis and natural history of the disease is unclear. The favourable response of diabetic retinopathy to hypophysectomy was thought to be due, in part at least, to the removal of GH but the evidence for this is inconclusive.

Liver Disease. Basal GH levels are elevated in various forms of liver disease and may show a paradoxical rise after glucose. GH is metabolized by the liver, and the elevated levels may be a reflection of decreased GH metabolism but are possibly due to increased GH secretion, which appears to occur in states of insulin resistance. Alternatively, the high levels may be due to impaired production of IGF-1 in the liver and consequent reduction in negative feedback inhibition of GH secretion.

Alcoholism. In about one-quarter of chronic alcoholics, the GH response to hypoglycaemia is either impaired or absent and in a number of cases the cortisol response is similarly affected. Abstinence from alcohol results in a return of both GH and cortisol responses. In the majority of alcoholics, this pituitary unresponsiveness to stress is asymptomatic but it is occasionally associated with the development of severe hypoglycaemia.

38. The Thyroid Gland and its Disorders

D. L. Williams and
R. Goodburn

Introduction
  Aspects of thyroid anatomy
  Functions of the gland
Physiology of the thyroid gland
  Hypothalamic–pituitary control of thyroid
    activity
  The thyroid hormones
  Metabolic and physiological effects of
    thyroid hormones
Disorders of the thyroid gland
  Pathological changes in thyroid function
  Congenital thyroid disease
  Autoimmune thyroid disease
  Goitre
Clinical aspects of thyroid dieases
  Clinical presentation
  Disorders associated with hyperthyroidism
  Disorders associated with hypothyroidism
  Thyroid disease in selected groups
Treatment of thyroid disease
  Hypothyroidism
  Hyperthyroidism
The investigation of thyroid function
  Introduction
  Thyroid function tests—indications and
    interpretation

INTRODUCTION

Disease of the thyroid gland is common and, although not usually life-threatening, it often causes major changes in the physical and mental well-being of the sufferer. Diagnosis is usually clear-cut. The available methods of treatment are straightforward, well understood and effective. The expenditure of effort and time on the part of clinicians and laboratory staff in ensuring accurate diagnosis and close monitoring of treatment is well rewarded in a noticeable general improvement in the health, both mental and physical, of their patients.

The part played by the clinical biochemistry laboratory in the diagnosis of thyroid disease varies from a relatively minor confirmatory role in the majority of patients, in whom clinical features of the disease are clear, to an important and central role in diagnosis of both adult thyroid disease, when it is mild or at an early stage, and of neonatal disease. The laboratory is also of central importance in monitoring patients during and after treatment, as changes in thyroid hormone levels inevitably precede deterioration in the patient's clinical condition. A sound understanding of the physiology and pathology of the thyroid gland will thus enable the clinical biochemist/chemical pathologist to help clinical colleagues in the interpretation of thyroid function tests, especially in those cases where the clinical features do not clearly lead to the correct diagnosis.

Aspects of Thyroid Anatomy

The thyroid gland arises during embryological development from endodermal tissue in the floor of the pharynx between the first and second pharyngeal pouches. At about the sixth week of fetal life, this area, at the rear of the developing tongue, evaginates to form a downward-growing tubular duct, the thyroglossal duct, which carries the embryonic thyroid tissue to its normal position where development of the lobes and the isthmus of the gland occurs. The duct degenerates to become a vestigial structure. Isolated nodules of thyroid glandular tissue, 'rests', can occasionally be observed at the back of the tongue or in positions along the line of the thyroglossal duct; pathological changes similar to those observed in the thyroid gland proper can occur in these. If the gland does not descend, but remains at the back of the tongue, it is termed a 'lingual thyroid' and often exhibits reduced activity.

The adult thyroid gland is a vascular structure of about 25 g in weight, formed from two conical lobes joined by an isthmus and lying anterolaterally to the trachea just below its junction with the larynx.

The gland lies invested in the cervical fascia covered by a thin, fibrous capsule. Posterior to the thyroid gland are the parathyroid glands, typically four in number and positioned two behind each lobe. There is, however, great individual variation both in the number and in the positions of the parathyroid glands, which are therefore at risk during surgical thyroidectomy. The recurrent laryngeal nerves pass on either side posteromedially to the lobes of the thyroid. These nerves innervate the vocal chords and can become damaged either by compression by an enlarged gland or during surgical operation; such damage results in hoarseness or complete loss of voice. The gland is not supplied by the recurrent laryngeal nerve but by postganglionic fibres from cervical sympathetic ganglia and also by parasympathetic fibres from the vagus. These nerves branch into plexuses on the blood vessels within the parafollicular spaces. It is not thought that any branches penetrate between the cells lining the thyroid follicle. It is likely that the thyroid nerves have a purely vasomotor function but no secretory activity.

The thyroid gland consists of follicles (Fig. 38.1), which are spheroidal groups of cells (follicular cells) forming a single layer surrounding a central core of amorphous colloid composed of thyroglobulin. The follicles range in size from 0.2 to 1 mm in diameter, the larger ones being filled with colloid and sur-

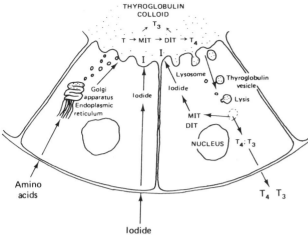

Figure 38.1 Diagrammatic representation of thyroid follicular cells. Synthesis of thyroglobulin in the endoplasmic reticulum is indicated on the left, lysis to produce T_3 and T_4 on the right. MIT, DIT: mono- and di-iodotyrosines.

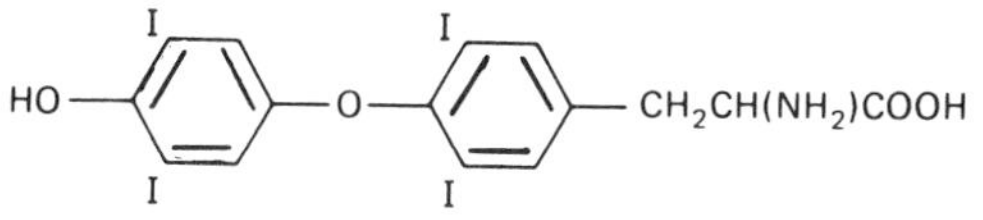

Figure 38.2 Structure of the three major thyroid hormones.

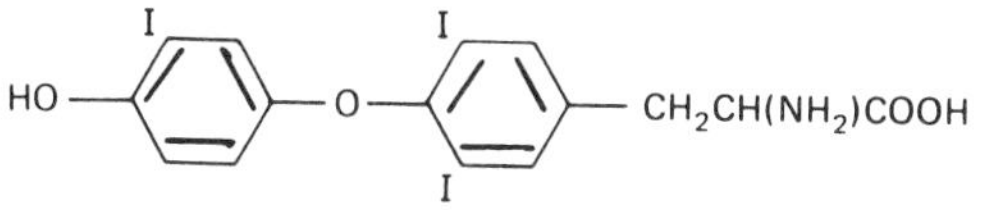

rounded by flattened follicular cells, the smaller ones being more active with less colloid and surrounded by columnar follicular cells. Between the follicles, in the 'parafollicular' region, there is a rich capillary blood supply, lymphatic vessels, and specialized parafollicular cells, which are now known to produce thyrocalcitonin. It was thought that these thyrocalcitonin-producing cells were limited to the parafollicular spaces, but it is now known that they can also occur interspersed between the thyroxine-producing cells lining the follicle. The gland is one of the most vascular organs in the body, receiving its blood supply from the superior and inferior thyroid arteries, which supply 100–125 mL of blood/min.

Functions of the Gland

The main functions of the thyroid gland are concerned with the trapping of iodine by the follicular cells, the synthesis of thyroid hormones and their storage in the follicular colloid, and their subsequent release into the bloodstream. Each of these major functions is dependent upon stimulation by thyrotrophin (thyroid-stimulating hormone, TSH) released by the anterior pituitary gland.

Thyroid Hormones

There are two major hormones produced by the thyroid gland, thyroxine (T_4), and tri-iodothyronine (T_3), together with a third compound, reverse tri-iodothyronine (r-T_3), which is endocrinologically inactive. The structures of these compounds are shown in Fig. 38.2. The thyronine molecule is formed by a condensation reaction between two molecules of tyrosine during which the amino acid side-chain of one molecule is lost and an ether (oxygen) bridge is formed between the two aromatic rings. The *in vivo* synthesis of the thyronine molecule is associated with the iodination of tyrosine, initially to form mono- and di-iodotyrosine intermediates, within the thyroid follicle.

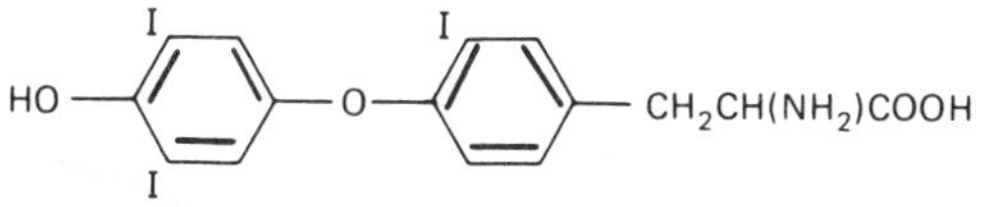

Thyroglobulin

The major source of tyrosine utilized *in vivo* for the synthesis of thyroid hormones is the protein thyroglobulin, the major component of the central colloid of the thyroid follicle. Thyroglobulin is a 19s protein with a molecular weight of about 660 000. This molecule contains some iodine and further iodination can produce 27s protein with a molecular weight of well over 10^6. Thyroglobulin is synthesized in the endoplasmic reticulum and Golgi apparatus of the follicular cell and is transported in vesicles through the apical membrane into the follicular colloid (Fig. 38.1), during which process its tyrosyl residues become iodinated. An important immunological feature, which is reflected in some forms of thyroid disease, is that thyroglobulin can act as an antigen, forming antithyroglobulin antibodies.

Thyroid-stimulating Hormone (Thyrotrophin)

The synthesis and release of thyroid hormones is under the control of TSH released from the pituitary gland. This is a glycoprotein secreted by thyrotroph cells in the anterior pituitary gland; it has a molecular weight of 2800 and is composed of two distinct polypeptide subunits. The α-subunit is very similar to the α-subunits of luteinizing hormone, follicle-stimulating hormone, and chorionic gonadotrophin. The β-subunit, however, is different and characteristic of TSH. Both subunits are required for biological activity, but it is the β-subunit that confers upon TSH its specificity. Higher molecular-weight forms of TSH ('big' TSH) have been identified in extracts of the anterior pituitary and it is likely that these larger molecules are those initially synthesized, subsequent proteolysis giving rise to the active hormone. As with most other protein and polypeptide hormones, TSH mediates its activities in the thyroid cell through cyclic AMP as a second messenger, thus increasing protein kinase activity within the cell.

PHYSIOLOGY OF THE THYROID GLAND

Hypothalamic–Pituitary Control of Thyroid Activity

The activities of the thyroid gland are stimulated by TSH from the thyrotroph cells in the anterior pituitary gland, which in turn are stimulated by thyrotrophin-releasing hormone (TRH, a tripeptide L-pyroglutamyl-L-histidyl-L-prolineamide) from the hypothalamus; TRH mediates its actions via a phospholipid second-messenger system, initiated by phospholipase C in the TRH receptor sites in the thyrotroph cell membrane. Circulating thyroid hormones inhibit this hypothalamic–pituitary drive, probably by a direct action at the anterior pituitary level; it has been postulated that this suppressive activity of the thyroid hormones is mediated through their ability to reduce the number of TRH receptor sites. The overall result is that the concentrations of circulating thyroid hormones are maintained relatively constant. Details of the hypothalamic–pituitary control mechanism are given in Chapter 37.

The Thyroid Hormones

Synthesis
The synthesis and secretion of thyroid hormones can be considered in three stages:

(i) the trapping of iodide by activation of an 'iodide pump';
(ii) the oxidation of iodide to iodine, the synthesis of thyroid hormones and their storage in thyroglobulin;
(iii) the proteolysis of thyroglobulin and the subsequent secretion of the thyroid hormones, thyroxine and tri-iodothyronine and of reverse-T_3).

Each of these stages is stimulated by TSH, which also appears to be able to increase both the size and number of thyroid follicular cells.

Trapping of Iodide. Iodide is actively transported from the blood, via the extracellular fluid, across the outer basement membrane of the thyroid follicular cell. The process is an active transport mechanism and is blocked by inhibitors of oxidation and by anoxia; ouabain also blocks the process, indicating that an ATP-ase, ionic-pump mechanism, dependent on synthesis of ATP-ase, is involved. Other negatively charged ions of similar size, such as perchlorate, thiocyanate and bromide, compete for this transport mechanism; the radioisotopic ion pertechnetate ($^{99}Tc^mO_4^-$) is also transported by this mechanism and

has proved a useful label for use in thyroid scanning.

The transport of iodine is relatively slow, equilibrium being reached at about 60 min with a concentration gradient of 40:1 in favour of the thyroid cell. In practice, however, a stable equilibrium is not achieved in view of the much faster oxidation of iodide to iodine and its subsequent incorporation into thyroglobulin. In subjects with the rare genetic defect of the iodide transport mechanism, iodide can still be transported into the cell by passive diffusion, but continuation of the process is dependent upon the intracellular utilization of the iodide; adequate uptake of iodide is achieved only if the plasma concentration of iodide is substantially higher than that normally found. Iodine is present in the environment only in limited quantities and there are geographical areas in which there is barely sufficient, even for people with normal iodide transport mechanisms. These areas would presumably provide insufficient iodide for this rare congenitally acquired deficiency.

Oxidation and Organification of Iodide. The next stage in the synthesis of thyroid hormones is a complex of three reactions, the oxidation of iodide to iodine, the iodination of tyrosine residues in the thyroglobulin molecules to mono- and di-iodotyrosines (MIT, DIT), and the joining of two iodotyrosine residues to form the complete hormones tri-iodothyronine and thyroxine.

Although the first two of these processes can take place independently *in vitro*, it seems likely that *in vivo* they are carried out sequentially on a multienzyme complex and that only small amounts of the intermediate can be identified within the thyroid cell.

The Peroxidase Reaction. At least one iodide peroxidase enzyme has been isolated from the thyroid follicular cell. It is present particularly along the apical cell border, although similar peroxidase activity can be found in membranes in other parts of the cell. The peroxidase is a haem-containing protein with an absolute requirement for hydrogen peroxide.

In cell-free systems the peroxidase can be shown to produce molecular iodine:

$$2I^- + H_2O_2 + 2H^+ = I_2 + 2H_2O.$$

In the living cell, however, it is probable that the iodination is effected by an intermediate, enzyme-bound ion (such as the iodinium ion, $E{-}I^+$) or an enzyme-bound radical ($E{-}I^\bullet$). The importance of the peroxidase located on the apical membrane of the cell is that the incorporation of iodine into the thyroglobulin molecule occurs in this part of the follicular cell, utilizing either newly synthesized thyroglobulin as it migrates into the colloid core or possibly thyroglobulin that has already reached the storage site within the follicle. These views have been confirmed by histoautoradiographic studies.

Iodination of Thyroglobulin. Thyroglobulin can be readily iodinated *in vitro* by molecular iodine. It seems likely, however, that the ionic or free-radical iodine products from the peroxidase reaction are responsible for *in vivo* iodination. The reaction also requires molecular oxygen. The products of the reaction are the iodinated tyrosines, MIT and DIT, and the iodinated thyronines, T_4, T_3 and r-T_3. The tyrosine molecules that take part in the reaction do so in their covalently bound positions within the thyroglobulin molecule and the final products are released only at a later stage when fragments of the thyroglobulin colloid are hydrolysed within the follicular cell.

The formation of the iodothyronines also takes place within the thyroglobulin molecule, by means of a reaction between two iodotyrosine residues on neighbouring polypeptide chains. Thus, tyrosine residues in peptide linkage within the thyroglobulin molecule, having initially been iodinated, participate in an intramolecular rearrangement that is associated with a conformational change of the molecule. An iodinated tyrosine residue in one part of the chain will thus gain an iodinated phenyl ring, linked via an ether bond, while the donor iodotyrosine loses a serine residue. The thyroglobulin can thus be thought of as a specialized enzyme; it has a number of active sites; it supplies two of the substrate molecules, the donor and recipient tyrosine residues; it catalyses the reaction and undergoes conformational change; but it fails to release the products of the reaction until the 'enzyme' itself is hydrolysed.

Release

Hydrolysis of thyroglobulin occurs within the thyroid follicular cell, following endocytosis of small portions of the thyroglobulin colloid by the microvilli that form the apical border of the follicular cell. The endocytosis is stimulated by TSH. Newly synthesized thyroglobulin is preferentially used for this purpose, possibly because it is sited nearest to the apical border of the cell. (A diagrammatic representation was given in Fig. 38.1.)

This process whereby small portions of the colloid are pinched off and 'ingested' by the microvilli of the follicular membrane results in small vesicles, the colloid droplets, appearing within the follicular cell. These can be seen within minutes of stimulation by TSH. The droplets migrate towards the basal membrane of the cell and merge with lysosomes. The lysosomes contain hydrolytic enzymes including peptidases, which when released into the colloid droplet cause the hydrolysis of thyroglobulin molecules into the constituent amino acids, including the iodinated tyrosines and thyronines. The iodotyrosines undergo deiodination, by active and specific deiodinases, but the iodothyronines diffuse, probably passively, through the basal membrane into the intracellular space and thence into the blood. Removal of the thyroid hormones by the bloodstream, including their binding to thyroxine-binding proteins, means that a constant gradient exists between the higher intracellular and the lower extracellular concentrations of thyroid hormones. The process of breakdown of colloid droplets and release of thyroid hormones is rapid, the colloid droplets having a half-life of about 5 min.

Circulation

On being released into the bloodstream both thyroxine and tri-iodothyronine become almost completely bound to carrier proteins. The major proteins involved in binding the thyroid hormones are thyroxine-binding globulin (TBG), which has a high affinity for the thyroid hormones but a relatively low capacity, and albumin and thyroxine-binding prealbumin (TBPA), which both have a relatively low affinity but a high capacity. TBG is a glycoprotein having a molecular weight of some 63 000 and running between the α_1- and α_2-globulin bands on electrophoresis.

Although prealbumin and particularly albumin have a much greater binding capacity than TBG, the higher affinity of TBG means that, under physiological conditions, about 75% of the circulating thyroxine and tri-iodothyronine is bound to TBG. Of the other two binding proteins, TBPA has a greater affinity for thyroxine, whereas albumin has a greater affinity for tri-iodothyronine. These two latter proteins do, however, play a much more important part in the hereditary disease, TBG deficiency.

Under normal conditions only about 1 in 3000 molecules of thyroxine is present in the free state, the remainder being bound to thyroxine-binding proteins. Tri-iodothyronine is less strongly bound so that approximately 1 in 300 molecules is free.

The role of thyroxine-binding proteins is twofold:

1. They do not pass through the renal glomerular membrane, whereas the free thyroid hormones do. Protein binding therefore conserves thyroid hormones, and particularly limits the loss of the scarce element iodine. It is interesting to note in this context that the greater binding affinity of thyroxine means that its turnover rate is only 10% per day whereas that of tri-iodothyronine is some 75% per day.
2. The large circulating pool of bound thyroid hormones is inert but in dynamic equilibrium with the small free fraction and can thus act as an available pool to replenish losses of free hormone as they are taken up into cells, metabolized and/or excreted.

Both bound and free hormones can pass relatively freely between the capillary blood and the extracellular fluid, although this ability is more pronounced in rapidly equilibrating tissues such as liver and kidney and rather less in slowly equilibrating tissues such as muscle and skin. In all tissues, however, it appears that only the free thyroid hormones can penetrate the cellular membrane and enter the cells.

TABLE 38.1
FACTORS AFFECTING THYROXINE-BINDING GLOBULIN (TBG)

Factors affecting the concentration of TBG

Rise in TBG concentration	*Fall in TBG concentration*
Physiological	
Pregnancy	
Neonatal life	
Pathological	
Chronic liver disease (sometimes)	Chronic liver disease (sometimes)
Oestrogen-secreting tumour	Androgen-secreting tumour
Acute intermittent porphyria	Active acromegaly
Acute hepatitis	Nephrotic syndrome
Hypothyroidism	Hyperthyroidism
	Protein-calorie malnutrition
	Cushing's syndrome
	Major illness
Drugs	
Oestrogens	Androgens
Contraceptive pill	Anabolic steroids
Perphenazine	Glucocorticoids (high level)

Drugs binding competitively with TBG
(causing a fall in protein-bound thyroid hormones and thus a fall in total
T_4 and T_3 concentrations, but not a fall in free hormone levels)

Salicylates
Phenytoin
Chlorpropamide
Tolbutamide
Diazepam

It is thus the free fraction that is responsible for the metabolic effects of the thyroid hormones, including the important feedback effects on the hypothalamus and pituitary gland.

In order to assess the thyroid status of the patient, knowledge of the concentration of free thyroxine and free tri-iodothyronine is more helpful than that of the total concentration of each hormone, however accurately these can be measured. This is particularly so because the concentrations of thyroxine-binding proteins, particularly TBG, can be significantly altered by physiological or pathological changes or by the effects of a wide variety of drugs. These changes result in significant alterations in the total T_4 or T_3 concentrations, but may well not affect the free fractions of these hormones. Factors affecting TBG levels are summarized in Table 38.1.

The strong binding of thyroid hormones in the blood also has a profound effect on the distribution of the hormones between the tissues. The rate of achievement of equilibrium is much slower than with substances of similar size that are not associated with binding proteins to the same extent. Several workers have suggested multicompartmental models to assess the turnover of thyroid hormones. One such model,

using four compartments namely blood, gut, fast turnover tissues (liver, kidney) and slow turnover tissues (muscle, brain and skin), has been applied in the sheep. Results suggest that a little more than 20% of thyroxine is in the plasma, a little more than 30% in the fast turnover tissues, about 45% in slow turnover tissues and about 3% in the gut.

The effect of the high degree of binding of thyroid hormones is illustrated by the fact that administration of a single dose of thyroid hormones to hypothyroid patients does not produce a maximal effect on basal metabolic rate until two days afterwards for T_3, or 10 days afterwards for T_4.

Catabolism and Excretion
The major metabolic reactions undergone by thyroid hormones are deiodination, conjugation, and deamination/decarboxylation.

Deiodination. There are at least three major deiodination reactions that iodothyronines and iodotyrosines undergo. Deiodination can occur of either the phenolic ring (3'-deiodination) or the non-phenolic ring (3-deiodination) of the iodothyronines. The deiodinases responsible for these reactions have different pH optima (pH 6–7 for the 3'-deiodinase and pH 8–9 for the 3-deiodinase). It is possible that both actions may be catalysed by the same enzyme working under different conditions. If thyroxine is the substrate, the 3'-deiodinase gives tri-iodothyronine as the initial product, whereas the 3-deiodinase produces r-T_3. The specificities of these deiodinases on T_3 and r-T_3 are such that the di-iodothyronine product has one iodine on each ring rather than both on the same ring. It should be noted that when there is reduced activity of the 3'-deiodinase there is a reduced production from thyroxine of T_3; as the same deiodinase is responsible for the breakdown of r-T_3, however, there will be an associated increase in the concentration of r-T_3. The contrary situation will occur if there is increased activity of 3'-deiodinase or a reduction of the activity of 3-deiodinase.

It has been calculated that, under normal circumstances, some 25% of thyroxine secreted by the thyroid gland is converted to T_3, this reaction being responsible for some 80% of the body's production of T_3. Some 40% of thyroxine is converted to r-T_3. It can thus be seen that the deiodination mechanism is responsible not only for initiating the catabolism and excretion of thyroxine, but also for converting it to a more active or a less active product. It is likely, therefore, that the deiodinase reaction is an important control mechanism for switching on and switching off the metabolic effects of the thyroid. It can be compared with the activation of 25-OH vitamin D.

Deiodination of MITs and DITs occurs particularly in the thyroid gland, but also in many other tissues. The tyrosine and iodine produced are then part of the general amino-acid and iodine pools, respectively.

Conjugation Reactions. Up to about 20% of the thyroid hormones undergo conjugation in the liver. T_4 preferentially forms glucuronide whereas T_3, 3,3'-di-iodothyronine and 3'-monoiodothyronine are preferentially conjugated to sulphate (it should be noted that these three compounds all have only a single iodine in the phenolic ring). The conjugates can then be excreted in the bile, although some sulphate conjugate can be found in the systemic blood. There appears to be no enterohepatic circulation of the conjugated hormones.

Deamination/decarboxylation. As might be expected from the amino-acid nature of the side chain of T_3 and T_4, deamination and decarboxylation reactions can readily occur in the liver. The immediate products are tetraiodo- or tri-iodothyroacetic acids (tetrac and triac). These compounds can be detected in the blood and have some thyroid hormone activity. Indeed it has recently been suggested that they may be the ultimate agents at the intracellular level of the activity of the thyroid hormones. At least one study has suggested that more than 40% of an injected dose of radiolabelled thyroxine was excreted as thyroacetic acid.

Thyroid Hormone—Receptor Interactions

It has been well demonstrated that the thyroid hormones interact with nuclear receptors, and that some of the effects of the hormones are mediated by this interaction. The affinity of the hormone–receptor interaction is directly related to the biological activity of the hormone. Thus the affinity for tri-iodothyronine is 10-fold that for thyroxine.

The concentration of nuclear thyroid-hormone receptors, calculated from radioligand binding studies, varies considerably from tissue to tissue. The pituitary and liver contain approximately 8000–10 000 receptors per cell, whereas the spleen and testis contain very few. In addition, differences in the interaction of the thyroid hormone with different tissue receptors may explain tissue-specific effects.

The existence of extranuclear receptors, particularly on mitochondria and cell membranes, is somewhat controversial. Stimulation of mitochondrial functions may be a result of direct T_3-mitochondrial interaction or of indirect effects. Cell membrane effects, outlined in a later section, are probably directly receptor mediated, and have been more fully established. It is likely that such extranuclear stimulations are important, but they remain to be fully characterized.

There are structural similarities between receptors for many of the hormones involved in growth and development. This has been useful in elucidating the regulation of transcriptional events, growth and development. At a more practical level, investigations on thyroid-hormone receptors may help in understanding phenomena such as thyroid-hormone resistance, and the occasional patient in whom the clinical status bears no relation to the measured hormone levels.

Metabolic and Physiological Effects of Thyroid Hormones

It is known that tri-iodothyronine has at least five times the biological activity of thyroxine. Thyroxine has virtually no activity *per se* but first requires conversion to tri-iodothyronine before it can exert its biological effects. The ratio of thyroxine:tri-iodothyronine in circulating blood, which is of the order of 50:1, is by no means constant either among normal subjects or among those undergoing thyroid investigation. Whether this is due to individual variation in the ability of tissues to convert thyroxine to tri-iodothyronine, or to individual variation in the subsequent metabolism and excretion of the hormones, is not known.

Despite much work over the last quarter of a century the precise roles played by the thyroid hormones are not fully understood. The results of excess or deficiency of the hormones on the body as a whole have been well known for many years and it has been assumed, probably correctly, that many of the pathological effects exhibited in hyper- or hypothyroidism reflect an exaggeration or a deficiency of the normal physiological function of the thyroid gland. Thus, it has been considered for many years that the thyroid hormones have a role in the control of growth, this role being reflected in the short stature of the cretin and the gigantism of the pubertal thyrotoxic. The fact that thyroid hormones have a role in controlling metabolic rate is illustrated by the extremes of basal metabolic rate (BMR) that are observed in myxoedema and thyrotoxicosis. For many years, work has been done on the cellular roles of thyroid hormones. Some of this work has tended to confuse the picture because of the use of non-physiological levels of thyroid hormones in *in vitro* studies. The cellular effects are now becoming more fully understood and it should not be long before a complete explanation of the role of thyroid hormones is available, enabling a description of the gross physiological and pathological effects in terms of the cellular biochemistry.

Generalized Effects

Effects on Growth and Development. It has been known for many years that thyroid hormones are required for the metamorphosis of amphibian animals such as the frog. In man, thyroid hormones are required for growth and development, particularly in the neonate, the child and at puberty. Part of this effect is mediated by thyroid-hormone stimulation of the hypothalamus–pituitary to produce growth hormone. Other effects seem to be independent of this ability to stimulate growth-hormone production and are probably associated with direct stimulation of protein synthesis at the cellular level. It is possible that this action also involves the production of somatomedins.

Effects on Heat Production. Thyroid hormones cause an increase in the BMR, the consumption of oxygen, and the production of heat. A long-standing and plausible theory was that thyroxine uncoupled oxidative phosphorylation, and this was shown in experiments *in vitro*. However, the level of thyroxine (or T_3) needed to elicit this response is thought to be substantially above the levels of thyroxine (or T_3) that occur physiologically. It is currently felt that if uncoupling of oxidative phosphorylation does occur, it is only in the most grossly thyrotoxic patients. It is more likely that the effects of the thyroid on heat production are a summation of a number of intracellular effects of the thyroid hormones, which are described below.

Effects on Neuromuscular Activity. Comparison of myxoedemic and thyrotoxic patients with normal subjects suggests that changes in thyroid-hormone concentrations are responsible for changes in the excitability of the central nervous system, the neuromuscular junctions, and the muscles themselves, both splanchnic and somatic. It is probable that these effects are caused by changes in membrane permeability as well as in intracellular metabolism.

Effects on Metabolic Processes

Effects on Cell Membranes. Both thyroxine and tri-iodothyronine have been shown to increase the uptake of certain amino acids and carbohydrates in isolated cell systems. This is a much more rapid effect than some of the others, occurring within minutes, and therefore probably not a consequence of the stimulation of protein synthesis. Binding sites for tri-iodothyronine have been found on cell membranes, particularly of liver, and it is probable that binding of thyroid hormones to these sites is the trigger to increased permeability.

About half of the increased oxygen consumption produced by thyroid hormones has been shown to be associated with increased activity of Na^+/K^+-ATPase. This enzyme is, of course, responsible for maintaining the extracellular–intracellular differential gradients of sodium and potassium ions. Increased ATPase activity is associated with a great increase in the utilization of energy and in the production of heat. This activity is likely to be responsible for about half of the increase in oxygen consumption produced by thyroid hormones.

Effects on Protein Synthesis. The administration of thyroid hormones increases the activity of many enzymes, including glycerol 3-phosphate dehydrogenase in mitochondria, NADPH-cytochrome C reductase, malic enzyme, α-hydroxy-α-methylglutaryl coenzyme A reductase, pyruvate carboxylase and phosphoenol pyruvate carboxylase. It is quite likely that it is by stimulating these enzymes, many of which are enzymes controlling the rate of central metabolic reactions, that some of the effects of thyroid hormones, previously described, might be affected. Similar effects on Na^+/K^+-ATPase and on growth-hormone synthesis have already been mentioned. In addition it has been known for more than 20 years that thyroid hormones cause increased albumin synthesis in man.

As these stimulatory effects of thyroid hormones are prevented by protein-synthesis inhibitors, it is now generally held that many of the actions of thyroid hormones are mediated by stimulation of the synthesis of certain proteins including enzymes and not, for instance, by direct activation of existing enzymes. Studies on the way in which this stimulation might be mediated indicate that thyroid hormones have specific effects both on the nucleus, by regulating transcription, and at the ribosome, by affecting translation. In summary, the thyroid hormones have complex effects at the subcellular level on the rate of metabolic processes.

Many of these effects may be mediated by stimulation of the synthesis of specific proteins (and possibly of the inhibition of synthesis of others), but some effects, the increased uptake of some amino acids by the plasma cell membrane for example, are likely to be independent of the protein synthesis effects.

DISORDERS OF THE THYROID GLAND

Disorders of the hypothalamic–pituitary–thyroid system can, as in most endocrine systems, result in overactivity or underactivity of the gland, or can cause no change in thyroid function. The gland can be affected by the same spectrum of disease processes that can strike other organs and tissues. Thus changes in function can be brought about by inborn errors of metabolism, congenital defects, infective disease, primary or secondary neoplastic change, toxic damage, autoimmune attack, changes in the control system, and iatrogenic factors, in addition to those ubiquitous pathologies of unknown aetiology.

Pathological Changes in Thyroid Function

The main interests of the clinical biochemistry laboratory are in distinguishing between individuals with normal thyroid function (euthyroidism) and patients with either an underactive (hypothyroidism, myxoedema) or an overactive (hyperthyroidism, thyrotoxicosis) thyroid gland. The causes of changes in thyroid activity are manifold but, as far as the management of an individual patient is concerned, once hypothyroidism, hyperthyroidism or euthyroidism has been established, there is little point in most cases in further investigation of the precise pathological cause of the disease, as the choice of treatment is limited and usually independent of the results of biochemical investigations. Thus the treatment of thyrotoxicosis, by means of surgery, radioiodine or antithyroid drugs, is decided on clinical grounds, such as the age of the patient and the appearance of the gland, and on the results of a thyroid scan, but not on either the degree of elevation of the thyroid-hormone concentrations or the detection of thyroid-stimulating antibodies.

Knowledge of the pathological cause of thyroid disease is, however, of general interest and further study of the processes involved can increase our understanding of the aetiology and may, in the long term, result in improved patient management. Also, in a small proportion of patients results of further investigations may have an immediate and direct effect on the choice of treatment. For instance, it is thought that a number of clinically hypothyroid patients, who have normal or even elevated levels of thyroxine in blood, associated with subnormal levels of tri-iodothyronine, have a reduced ability to convert T_4 to T_3 in their tissues; it would obviously be preferable to treat such patients with T_3 rather than T_4.

Specific pathological causes of thyroid disease will not be dealt with in this section, but will be mentioned when the individual diseases are discussed. Three topics, however, have more general application and these will be dealt with here; these are congenital thyroid disease, autoimmune thyroid disease and goitre.

Congenital Thyroid Disease

Congenital Hyperthyroidism

Most congenital disease of the thyroid results in diminished activity of the gland, but occasionally hyperthyroidism is observed in a neonate. Usually this is a consequence of a baby being born to a mother who is thyrotoxic and in whose blood there are high levels of thyroid-stimulating antibodies. These antibodies can pass the placental barrier into the fetal circulation and cause prolonged and inappropriate stimulation of the fetal thyroid. The condition is called neonatal Graves' disease and is usually self-limiting; in some cases, however, respiratory and cardiac involvement can lead to complications and even death. Rarely, thyrotoxicosis develops in a neonate who has a euthyroid mother and cases have been reported of babies being born with genuine hyperthyroidism, for which infection with rubella has sometimes been blamed.

Occasionally a teratoma of the ovary can contain active thyroid tissue; this congenital tumour, the 'struma ovarii', can become overactive and suppress the activity of the normal gland, thus giving rise to thyrotoxicosis in a patient with an underactive thyroid gland; the toxic manifestations do not usually present until adult life.

Congenital Hypothyroidism

The majority of congenital thyroid disease results in hypothyroidism. The incidence of congenital hypothyroidism varies to some extent from study to study, often being dependent on the population observed; it is likely to be in the order of one case per 3–4000 births. It can result from anatomical or metabolic abnormalities.

Anatomical Defects. There are a number of uncommon anatomical defects that can cause reduction of thyroid function. There can be congenital absence of the thyroid. Embryological maldevelopment of the gland can result in the whole of the gland, or part of it, being displaced from its normal position; reference has already been made to the lingual thyroid, to thyroglossal cysts, and to thyroid rests. These anatomical anomalies are often associated with reduced thyroid function; they can also be associated with normal thyroid function and it is therefore important to bear them in mind in the investigation of thyroid function in adults, as the abnormally placed tissue is capable of undergoing the same pathological changes as a normally situated gland. Surgical removal of a lingual thyroid usually demands subsequent treatment with thyroid hormone as there may be no other thyroid tissue.

Metabolic Defects. Neonatal hypothyroidism can be caused by a congenital metabolic defect. A number of such defects have been identified and include defects in the iodide concentration mechanism, defects in the iodination mechanism, and a defect in the enzyme responsible for deiodinating iodotyrosines.

The term dyshormonogenesis covers a number of specific inborn errors of thyroxine metabolism, each of which is of academic interest, but all of which are diagnosed in the same way and treated with exogenous thyroid hormones. These defects include:

1. *The inability of the thyroid gland actively to trap iodide.* Passive diffusion can, however, take place and, provided that there is a reasonable amount of iodide in the diet, this passive diffusion process can supply enough iodide to enable the gland to synthesize sufficient thyroid hormone.
2. *Deficiency in the oxidation and incorporation of iodide into thyroglobulin.* This can be associated with deafness and large, hard, multinodular goitre (Pendred's syndrome) or it may be an isolated deficiency. The only well-documented congenital defect associated with poor organification of iodide is that of the enzyme peroxidase, but it does not appear that all patients in this group have a peroxidase deficiency.
3. *Defects of thyroglobulin metabolism,* leading to deficient iodination of tyrosine, deficient conjugation of iodotyrosines to give iodothyronines and deficiencies of proteolysis, have all been postulated, in addition to the possibility of abnormal receptors for the peroxidase molecule. These defects have not yet been conclusively demonstrated, although abnormal thyroglobulin, with a high ratio of iodotyrosine: iodothyronine and increased levels of circulating iodoproteins, has been observed.

The importance of these and other causes of neonatal hypothyroidism is that, if undetected, they can cause physical and mental defects, ranging from reduced mental development to the full-blown syndrome of cretinism. Because of the relative frequency of neonatal hypothyroidism it is now the policy in the UK to screen all newborn babies 6 days after birth to indicate those which may have underactive thyroid function so that, following confirmatory investigations, treatment can be initiated at an early stage and mental retardation thereby prevented. Further details are given in Chapters 15 and 17.

Other Congenital Anomalies
Congenital Deficiency of Thyroxine-binding Globulin. Deficiency of the major thyroid hormone-binding protein in blood, TBG, is a well-known anomaly that usually has no clinical implications. The level of TBG in individuals carrying a deficient gene ranges from an immeasurably low concentration in male subjects, to detectable but lower than normal concentrations in affected female subjects. The reason for this difference is that the deficiency is inherited by an X-linked dominant trait. The fact that female carriers have intermediate levels of TBG despite the fact that one of their TBG-carrying genes is both abnormal and dominant is in accord with the Lyon hypothesis, which states that in each female somatic cell one of the two chromosomes is permanently inactivated during early fetal life. This inactivation process, however, is random so that in the single individual some somatic cells will carry a normal active X chromosome whereas others will carry an abnormal inactive X chromosome.

Congenital Thyroxine-binding Globulin Excess. In contrast to TBG deficiency, some families have been described in which there is an increased concentration of TBG. There is some doubt as to whether this anomaly is inherited by an autosomal dominant or a sex-linked dominant mode. In either case, however, it is necessary to postulate a defect a little more complicated than in most inborn errors, which results in a reduction in the level of protein and not an increase. In inherited TBG excess, it is possible that there is an inherited defect in the synthesis of a repressor gene that is normally responsible for inhibiting TBG synthesis.

Dysalbuminaemic Hyperthyroxinaemia. This is an autosomal dominant condition in which approximately half of the albumin molecules in the circulation demonstrate an increased binding affinity for T_4. The binding affinity may be as much as 50 times higher than normal, and the variant albumin becomes a major plasma binding agent of thyroxine. It is a very rare condition, and as with the previous conditions, apparently carries no pathological implications for the patient. Although this condition has been described mainly in relation to thyroxine, a few cases have been described in which a variant albumin binding tri-iodothyronine was found.

Comment. In most subjects with TBG deficiency, TBG excess or dysalbuminaemic hyperthyroxinaemia, there is no associated clinical problem. There is, however, a danger that the associated low blood total thyroxine concentration in TBG deficiency, or high total thyroxine concentration in TBG excess, may be picked up in random or screening investigations. Assays for the free hormone levels will not be affected by these genetic conditions, and should give a result appropriate to the clinical condition of the patient. In dysalbuminaemic hyperthyroxinaemia, the high-affinity albumin may interfere in assays for both total and free thyroxine, giving spuriously raised or lowered results, depending on the assay system used. Thyroxine results will usually be grossly abnormal in this case, and will not be consistent with the clinical condition of the patient. The worst case is likely to be that in which a patient has dysalbuminaemic hyperthyroxinaemia, together with a concurrent thyroid pathology. Misdiagnosis is likely if the clinician gives more attention to the test results than to clinical judgement, and a doctor unwise enough to treat patients having any of these conditions without first having assessed their clinical condition would cause iatrogenic thyroid disease.

Autoimmune Thyroid Disease

In 1956, Roitt et al. showed that antibodies capable of binding thyroglobulin existed in the plasma of patients with certain thyroid diseases. These were true autoantibodies (i.e. they were directed against normal components of the body).

Since these original observations, autoantibodies against a number of thyroid antigens have been demonstrated in association with certain thyroid diseases. These diseases have been termed autoimmune thyroid disorders and include the following:

- Graves' disease,
- Hashimoto's disease,
- primary myxoedema,
- focal lymphocytic thyroiditis.

The studies on thyroid autoantibodies led to the discovery of autoimmunity in association with other diseases (e.g. systemic lupus erythematosus, pernicious anaemia, Addison's disease) and, in a few cases, following damage to some tissues (e.g. antibodies formed to antigens released after vasectomy).

Thyroid autoimmune disease is undoubtedly the most intensively studied of the autoimmune conditions in man. These studies have been useful both as an aid to diagnostic medicine and in helping to elucidate the more widespread phenomenon of autoimmunity.

Characteristics of Autoimmune Diseases

Although many diseases have been said to have an autoimmune aetiology, very few have been shown unequivocally to conform to the strict requirements of this definition which are:

- The presence of circulating autoantibodies and / or delayed hypersensitivity reactions directed against normal body components (autoantigens) must be demonstrated in patients with the disease.
- The antigens stimulating the autoimmune reaction must be isolated and identified.
- The autoimmune reaction should be duplicated experimentally in laboratory animals.

Chronic lymphocytic thyroiditis is one of the few so-called autoimmune diseases that have been shown to meet these strict requirements.

There has been a great advance in the understanding of thyroid autoimmunity and the related abnormalities in the cellular and humoral immune systems during the last decade. Aberrant expression on the thyroid cell of molecules associated with HLA-DR class II may faciliate autoantigen presentation to helper T lymphocytes, which in turn induce B lymphocytes to generate autoantibodies. Alternatively, thyroid cell HLA-DR expression may be protective rather than pathogenetic in normal circumstances. Defective suppressor T-lymphocyte function (thyroid-antigen specific, and generalized) may also be important.

Pathological Significance of Thyroid Autoantibodies

Three major autoantibody/antigen systems are found in association with the thyroid:

(i) antibodies directed against thyroglobulin;
(ii) antibodies directed against microsomal antigen;
(iii) antibodies directed against the TSH receptor (thyroid-stimulating antibodies, and blocking-type anti-TSH receptor antibodies).

Additionally there are two systems that appear at present to have little clinical significance:

(i) antibodies directed against the second colloid antigen (CA_2);
(ii) antibodies directed against Fragraeus cell-surface antigen.

Incidence of Thyroid Autoantibodies

Before considering the significance of autoantibodies in thyroid disease, their occurrence in the blood of normal individuals must be mentioned.

The detection of thyroid autoantibodies has been facilitated by the introduction of techniques, such as haemagglutination, complement fixation, immunofluorescence, and more recently radio- and enzyme immunoassays. These techniques are generally extremely sensitive and will ostensibly detect very low levels of autoantibodies. Some of the methods, however, are prone to non-specific effects, and may show a weakly positive reaction in the absence of specific autoantibodies. Thus in one of the most commonly used techniques, haemagglutination, a titre of less than 1:20 for thyroglobulin antibodies, and 1:1600 for microsomal antibodies, is considered negative. However, positive reactions with titres well above these levels are seen in some normal individuals. The reported incidence in different studies has varied from 2% to 17.6% of the (normal) population under investigation. This wide variation may be due to regional differences or to difference in methodology. All the studies have shown that the incidence in women is substantially higher than that in men, and that, in women, the incidence increases with age and the disease is particularly prevalent in postmenopausal women.

TSH-receptor antibodies have rarely been reported in normal individuals, but this may be a reflection of the technical complexity and relative insensitivity of methods currently available for their measurement. Assay methods developed in recent years may enable a more accurate assessment of the incidence of thyroid-stimulating antibodies in the normal population. In view of the presence in a significant proportion of apparently normal subjects of antibodies against thyroglobulin and thyroid microsomes, their measurement will not give an unequivocal diagnosis of thyroid disease. However, when used in association with other thyroid function tests and other non-biochemical investigations, it will help in the differential diagnosis of simple goitre, Hashimoto's disease, de Quervain's thyroiditis, thyrotoxicosis and thyroid cancer.

Autoantibodies Directed against Thyroglobulin

Thyroglobulin is not only found in the intrafollicular colloid, but can also be identified in circulating blood. In some individuals, humoral antibodies can be found; the majority of these belong to the IgG class.

Although detection of thyroglobulin autoantibodies is relatively simple by any of the methods previously mentioned, accurate quantitation is difficult. They are most commonly found in the blood of patients with untreated Hashimoto's disease; increased sensitivity of detection allows earlier diagnosis of this disorder. Thyroglobulin haemagglutination antibody (TGHA) titres of greater than 1:640 indicate the likelihood of Hashimoto's disease (providing there is supporting clinical and biochemical evidence); much higher titres than 1:640 are commonly observed. The absence of thyroglobulin autoantibodies makes the diagnosis of Hashimoto's disease very unlikely. Positive titres are also observed in the disease described as idiopathic, or primary, myxoedema and suggest a likely aetiological link with Hashimoto's disease. Positive TGHA titres are frequently seen in patients with Graves' disease and it is possible that these patients may in the course of time revert to Hashimoto's disease. The usefulness of TGHA testing in possible thyroid cancer is dubious as the finding of a high titre will not necessarily exclude thyroid neoplasia.

In focal lymphocytic thyroiditis there is also an inconsistent appearance of TGHA. High levels are often seen in this disease, but in some cases thyroid lesions are non-progressive, produce no clinical signs, and are associated with low titres of TGHA.

There are usually moderately elevated levels of TGHA in subacute (de Quervain's) thyroiditis. This disease is also often associated with the appearance of antibodies to the second colloid antigen (CA_2), which can be shown by immunofluorescent microscopy. Thyroglobulin autoantibodies are not usually cytotoxic themselves, but are important in the induction of cell-mediated immune processes that lead indirectly to the destruction of thyroid tissue. The cell-mediated immune response is probably induced by sensitization of the thyroid cells by the IgG autoantibodies, which then allows their destruction by killer lymphocytes (K cells). Monitoring of this cell-mediated process is not easy in the laboratory.

Further complications of the autoantibody-antigen reaction include:

- the production of immune complexes in the blood of some patients with Hashimoto's disease;
- the cross-reactivity of the autoantibody with thyroxine and/or tri-iodothyronine.

This cross-reaction may give rise, when the thyroid hormones are assayed by immunoassay procedures, to results that are not in accord with the clinical condition. This characteristic of antibodies to thyroglobulin in binding thyroxine and tri-iodothyronine has been shown by autoradiography following addition of radioactive T_4 or T_3 to blood containing the antibody and also by immunofixation and radioassay techniques. It is unlikely that a similar cross-reaction also exists with other thyroid autoantibodies (although autoantibodies reacting with TSH have been reported) and it is probable that the reason for such cross-reactivity with thyroglobulin is a consequence of the fact that the thyroglobulin molecule contains thyroxine and tri-iodothyronine residues. The prevalence of titres of $antiT_4$ and $antiT_3$ antibodies sufficient to have a significant effect on the level of circulating thyroid hormones is unlikely to be high, as experience shows that even in the presence of high titres of antithyroglobulin antibodies the thyroxine and tri-iodothyronine concentrations are usually appropriate for the clinical state of the patient.

Autoantibodies Directed against Microsomal Antigens

The presence of a second thyroid autoantigen was first suspected when a positive complement-fixation reaction was observed (using a crude thyroid preparation as the antigen) in the absence of a haemagglutination reaction against thyroglobulin. Immunofluorescent studies showed that the antigen was located in the cytoplasm of the follicular cells and later studies showed it to be a lipoprotein in the membrane of the microvesicles that contain newly synthesized thyroglobulin. More recently, this group of autoantibodies has been shown to be directed against thyroid peroxidase (PO), which has been identified by Western blot and cDNA sequencing as the microsomal antigen. Thyroid peroxidase has a molecular weight of approximately 100 000. It is responsible for the iodination of tyrosine residues on thyroglobulin and the intramolecular coupling reaction of iodinated tyrosine moieties. Thyroid peroxidase is also present on the thyroid cell surface, closely associated with the TSH-receptor complex. The characterization of the antigen in this autoimmune system has prompted some workers to rename the auto antibody as antithyroid peroxidase (TPO-Ab). The traditional name of antimicrosomal antibody will, however, be used here because of its current wider acceptance.

Antimicrosomal antibodies are also found that are specific to other endocrine organs. The antibody can now be detected by complement fixation, haemagglutination, immunofluorescence, radioimmunoassay and enzyme-linked immunosorbent assay (ELISA); at best only a semiquantitative estimate of concentration can be obtained.

The thyroid microsomal antibody has a complement-mediated cytotoxic effect on thyroid tissue and a good correlation has been observed between the presence of microsomal antibody and the degree of hypothyroidism. In one study, 83% of patients with overt clinical primary hypothyroidism had antimicrosomal antibodies. The presence of antimicrosomal antibodies is also a characteristic finding in the blood of patients with Graves' disease, in which

TABLE 38.2
TSH-RECEPTOR ANTIBODY

Name of antibody	Abbreviation	Effects	Assay method
Long-acting thyroid stimulator	LATS	Present in the blood of some patients with Graves' disease; causes prolonged thyroid stimulator activity in guinea pig or mouse bioassay system	Bioassay
Long-acting thyroid stimulator protector	LATS-P	Caused anomalies in bioassays for LATS by preventing binding to the thyroid antigens; later found to have its own thyroid-stimulating activity more closely related to the severity of Graves' disease symptoms	McKenzie bioassay
Human thyroid stimulator	HTS	Increases colloid droplet formation	Bioassay
Human thyroid adenylcyclase stimulator	H-TACS	Stimulates thyroid adenylcyclase	Stimulation of adenylcyclase in human thyroid membranes
Thyroid-stimulating antibody	TSAb	In addition to being a generic name for all these substances, this term has been used for substances that increase AMP concentration in thyroid slices	Increased cyclic AMP in human thyroid slices (2-h incubation)
Thyroid growth-stimulating antibody	TGI	Increases thyroid DNA synthesis	Bioassay
Thyroid blocking antibody *and* thyroid stimulation-inhibition antibody	TSBAb TSIAb	Inhibition of TSH-mediated cAMP increase	Bioassay
Thyroid growth-blocking antibodies	TGBAb	Inhibit TSH-mediated DNA synthesis	Bioassay
Thyroid-stimulating immunoglobulin *or* thyrotrophin displacement activity *or* TSH-binding inhibitory immunoglobulin	TSI TDA TBII	Alternative name for LATS-P	Competitive receptor assay using human thyroid membrane
Fat cell-binding immunoglobulin	FBI		Radioassay using fat-cell membranes

an elevated antimicrosomal antibody titre (of greater than 1:3200) indicates severe thyrotoxicosis probably associated with concurrent cell damage.

TSH-receptor Antibodies (TR Ab)

In 1956 Adams and Purves discovered that serum taken from a patient with Graves' disease was able to mimic the action of thyroid-stimulating hormones when injected into a guinea pig; the duration of action of the serum was much more prolonged than that observed with TSH; the factor responsible for this activity was later called Long-Acting Thyroid Stimulator (LATS).

Since that time a number of investigators, using a variety of techniques, have reported several substances that have thyroid-stimulating activities. More recently, TSH-receptor antibodies have been found that inhibit rather than stimulate thyroid cell growth and metabolism. All have been shown to be G-class immunoglobulins. A rather confusing array of names has been applied to the antibodies. A list of some of the names used to describe TSH-receptor antibodies

is given in Table 38.2. The list is not entirely complete, as there is a tendency among workers in this field to invent new names for their discoveries. The major classifications are, however, included. Because they are all closely associated with the thyroid cell-surface TSH-receptor, the term TSH-receptor antibody (TR Ab) is a useful generic term for this group of autoantibodies.

TSH-receptor protein consists of two subunits, of 50 000 and 30 000 Da, linked by a disulphide bond. Similar sites have been identified on adipose tissue, testicular tissue and lymphocytes. Because TSH is required for thyroid cell growth, the interaction of TR Ab with the TSH receptor may have an agonist or antagonist effect. Thus TSH antagonistic TR Abs may be found in 5–30% of patients with autoimmune thyroiditis.

There is evidence indicating that the antibodies characteristic of Graves' disease are the *cause* of the disease, rather than a response to the pathological process. They are found in more than 90% of patients with untreated Graves' disease, and may also be found in patients with autoimmune thyroiditis, as previously mentioned. It has been suggested that autoimmune thyroid disease is a spectrum of disease states, with Hashimoto's disease and Graves' disease at the extreme ends. The pathological expression of the disease state is dictated by the predominating autoantibody, and its effects, at the time.

The TR Abs of Graves' disease are unique to the human species. Furthermore, none of the reported monoclonal antibodies propagated from animal species against the TSH-receptor has shown any stimulating activity.

It is likely that part of the TR Ab molecule has a configuration similar to that of the part of the TSH molecule that interacts with the receptor site of the thyroid follicular cell. It has been suggested that the stimulating TR Ab may bind to the epitopic region of a ganglioside component of the TSH-receptor, whereas the inhibitory antibody reacts with the glycoprotein component. An alternative explanation is that the difference between agonist and antagonist activity is dictated by affinity and specificity of the binding reaction.

Autoantibody Cross-reactions
Interactions of autoantibodies with retro-orbital tissues in classical ophthalmic Graves' disease have been postulated, and this has become somewhat controversial. There is poor evidence of tissue specificity of such antibodies, suggesting the possibility of cross-reactivities of thyroid autoantibodies with other tissues. The microsomal antigen has been observed to have similarities to the leucocyte protein myeloperoxidase of polymorphonuclear leucocytes. Such cross-reactivities may also be implicated in the links in polyendocrine disorders, and in the persistence of TR Ab after thyroid ablation treatment for thyrotoxicosis.

Methods of Measuring Thyroid Antibody Levels
A summary of methods available for the assay of thyroid antibodies other than TSH-receptor antibodies is given in Table 38.3. The wider use of more recently developed, quantitative and specific methods, such as the microELISA technique, has been a major factor in elucidating the structure, biochemistry and clinical importance of thyroid antibodies.

Incidence of Autoimmune Thyroid Disease
The clinical characteristics of autoimmune thyroid disease are diverse and not always attributable to the autoimmunity. The gland is much more prone to autoimmune disease than other endocrine glands: it also seems to be the only gland in which an autoimmune reaction can commonly cause stimulation instead of merely destruction. There is an increased incidence of other autoimmune disease in those with autoimmune thyroid disease, particularly diabetes and pernicious anaemia. Individuals with certain HLA profiles seem prone to various forms of thyroid disease. Thus there is an association between the susceptibility to subacute thyroiditis and the HLA-BW35 antigen, and a higher incidence than expected of Graves' disease in those with HLA-B8 or HLA-Dw3 antigens. Subjects with Turner's syndrome have a higher incidence of thyroid antibodies than the normal population, and it is well known that thyroid antibodies occur more frequently in women than in men.

Goitre
Goitre is the enlargement, to varying degree, of the thyroid gland. It is difficult to define accurately on the basis of thyroid size, because of the extremely large variation in size of 'normal' thyroid glands. Although the range of weight for thyroid glands is generally accepted as 25–30 g, normally functioning glands of 10–12 g may be seen in areas of high dietary iodine such as Iceland, and 50 g in areas where the intake is low, such as Switzerland before iodination of the diet was initiated.

The World Health Organization has produced a grading system for goitre (the WHO-PAHA system), which is summarized in Table 38.4.

Goitre affects at least 5% of the world population. This includes about 300 million people living in under-developed regions with iodine deficiencies, and about 100 million in areas where iodine intake is adequate.

Endemic goitre linked to iodine deficiency is an important disease economically, both because of the large numbers of people affected, and because of its effects, which may range from minor growth and mental retardation through to cretinism.

So-called simple goitre results largely from a reduced efficiency of thyroid hormone formation, resulting from a deficiency of iodine available to the thyroid gland. It may also be associated with the ingestion of goitrogens such as thiocyanate (which blocks the iodide pump), allyl thioureas (which inhibit iodination of tyrosine) and lithium (which inhibits thyroglobulin resorption)

Extreme growth stimulation by TSH as result of reduced negative feedback carries an increased risk of nodule and adenoma formation. Toxic nodular goitre is dealt with in a later section.

CLINICAL ASPECTS OF THYROID DISEASES

Clinical Presentation
Patients with thyroid disease can present with the classical symptoms of hyperthyroidism or hypothyroidism or with visible or palpable abnormality of the gland itself, which may or may not be associated with abnormality of endocrine function.

The clinical signs and symptoms of thyroid disease are well and fully presented in most general medical textbooks and in the increasing number of publications devoted to thyroid endocrinology. Description of these clinical features is therefore limited in this

TABLE 38.3
THYROID AUTOANTIBODY INVESTIGATION METHODS

Antibody	Detection system	Comments
Thyroglobulin autoantibody	Immunodiffusion	Lacks sensitivity: useful only in advanced disease Slow end-point development Non-quantitative
	Countercurrent immunoelectrophoresis	Similar to immunodiffusion, but rapid end-point development
	Latex fixation	Superseded by haemagglutination
	Haemagglutination	Commonly used assay Senstitive semiquantitative and relatively easy to do, especially in kit form
	Immunofluorescence	Requires fluorescence microscopy, and skilled interpretation Common method: non-quantitative, but very sensitive
	Radioassays (i) Competitive	Most sensitive quantitative assay; requires radiolabelled high-titre autoantibody
	(ii) Non-competitive	Relatively simple semiquantitative or quantitative system Requires radiolabelled thyroglobulin
	ELISA	Becoming very commonly used Relatively simple semiquantitative method Enzyme labels more stable than radiolabels
Microsomal autoantibody	Immunofluorescence	As for thyroglobulin autoantibody
	Complement fixation	Sensitive semiquantitative assay, giving an indication of cytotoxicity Largely superseded by haemagglutination
	Haemagglutination	As for thyroglobulin autoantibody, but subject to interference due to contamination of microsomal antigen by thyroglobulin
	Radioassay (i) Competitive	As for thyroglobulin autoantibody Requires radiolabelling of high-titre microsomal autoantibody
	(ii) Non-competitive	As for thyroglobulin Requires radiolabelling of microsomal antigen free of contamination by thyroglobulin
Second colloid autoantibody	Immunofluorescence	Seen on immunofluorescence for thyroglobulin autoantibody No other assay systems developed

TABLE 38.4
WORLD HEALTH ORGANIZATION EPIDEMIOLOGICAL GRADING
FOR GOITRE SIZE

Stage 0	No goitre visible or palpable with neck fully extended
Stage 1A	Goitre detectable only by palpation; not visible even with neck fully extended
Stage 1B	Goitre palpable, and visible only when neck is fully extended (this classification includes nodular thyroid disease)
Stage 2	Goitre visible with neck in normal position
Stage 3	Very large goitre, visible even at considerable distance

chapter to the summaries presented in Tables 38.7 and 38.10 below. Further details can be found in the excellent accounts mentioned in the Further Reading list. Clinical signs and symptoms may be less easy to recognize when the disease is mild or at an early stage, and may also be misleading when thyroid disease presents in the neonate, the child, in pregnancy or in the elderly. Attempts have been made to draw up 'score sheets', by means of which clinicians give points if certain signs or symptoms are present and subtract points if these clinical features are absent; the final sum of points indicates the probability of thyroid disease. Experience has indicated that this method is more useful in the assessment of hyperthyroidism than of hypothyroidism. Two of the most well known of the indices, the Wayne index and the Newcastle index, are compared in Table 38.5.

Disorders Associated with Hyperthyroidism

Hyperthyroidism, the clinical consequence of inappropriately high concentrations of circulating T_4 and T_3, is a relatively common condition; some authorities reserve the term for those diseases giving rise to increased activity of the thyroid gland itself, but not including increased thyroid hormone production from extrathyroidal tissues; instead they use the term

TABLE 38.5

COMPARISON OF THE WAYNE AND THE NEWCASTLE INDICES
FOR THE CLINICAL DIAGNOSIS OF HYPERTHYROIDISM

Signs	Wayne Index Score if: Present	Wayne Index Score if: Absent	Newcastle Index Score if: Present	Newcastle Index Score if: Absent
Pulse rate > 90/min	+ 3		+ 16	
Pulse rate 80/90 min	0		+ 8	
Pulse rate < 80/min	− 3		0	
Atrial fibrillation	+ 4			
Palpable thyroid	+ 3	− 3	+ 3	0
Thyroid bruit	+ 2	− 2	+ 18	0
Exophthalmos	+ 2	0	+ 9	0
Lid retraction	+ 2	0	+ 2	0
Fine finger tremor	+ 1	0	+ 7	0
Hyperkinesis	+ 4	− 2	+ 4	0
Lid lag	+ 1	0		
Hands hot	+ 2	− 2		
Hands moist	+ 1	− 1		

Symptoms	Score if present	Score if present
Increased appetite	+ 3	+ 5
Decreased appetite	− 3	
Increased weight	− 3	
Decreased weight	+ 3	
Dyspnoea of effort	+ 1	
Palpitations	+ 2	
Tiredness	+ 2	
Preference for heat	− 5	
Preference for cold	+ 5	
Excess sweating	+ 3	
Nervousness	+ 3	
Psychological precipitant		− 5
Frequent checking		− 3
Anticipatory anxiety (severe)		− 3
Age of onset (years):		
15–24		0
25–34		+ 4
35–44		+ 8
45–54		+ 12
55 and over		+ 16

TOTAL SCORES (signs + symptoms)

Euthyroid	Less than 11	− 11 to + 23
Hyperthyroid	Greater than 19	Greater than 40
Equivocal	11–19	+ 24 to + 39

TABLE 38.6

VARIETIES OF HYPERTHYROIDISM

Graves' disease (*toxic diffuse goitre*)

Toxic nodular goitre
Uninodular
Multinodular

Thyroiditis
Subacute (de Quervain's) thyroiditis
Chronic thyroiditis with transient hyperthyroidism

Nodular hyperthyroid goitre due to excess exogenous iodine (*Jod–Basedow disease*)

Excess exogenous thyroid hormone
Iatrogenic
Self-administered

Neoplasia
Follicular adenoma of thyroid
Follicular carcinoma of thyroid
TSH-secreting tumours
   Choriocarcinoma
   Hydatidiform mole
   Ectopic TSH-secreting tumours
   Pituitary TSH-secreting tumours
   (secondary hyperthyroidism)
Metastatic thyroid tumours
Thyroxine-secreting teratoma (struma ovarii)

Although the list of possible causes of hyperthyroidism is long (Table 38.6), most cases fall into the categories of Graves' disease, toxic nodular goitre and overtreatment with thyroid hormones. The more common variants of the syndrome are discussed below.

The clinical presentation of hyperthyroidism is a classical one and there is usually no difficulty in making the correct diagnosis in moderate to severe cases; mild or borderline cases are less easy to diagnose and may require a series of investigations. A summary of the major clinical features is given in Table 38.7.

Graves' Disease

Graves' disease (toxic diffuse goitre, diffuse hyperthyroidism) is the most common cause of hyperthyroidism, being especially so in women in the third and fourth decades. The clinical signs and symptoms (Table 38.7) are associated with a diffusely enlarged, non-nodular gland. In addition to the typical ophthalmic complications of hyperthyroidism (i.e. the wide-eyed stare, lid lag, and poor convergence), patients with Graves' disease may be affected by characteristic and specific ophthalmic lesions manifested by puffy, itching and inflamed eyelids associated with hyperaemic conjunctivae.

Graves' disease is known to be associated with autoimmune phenomena; in particular, thyroid-stimulating antibodies can be detected in high concentrations in the vast majority of patients with Graves' disease. These features have been mentioned earlier.

Malignant neoplastic change may rarely occur in Graves' disease. It is difficult to know whether there

thyrotoxicosis to cover the complete list of causes of increased thyroid hormone activity; in this discussion the terms are used synonymously.

It is difficult to establish the precise incidence of hyperthyroidism, but estimates suggest that it is present in about 0.3–0.4% of the population. The incidence in women of reproductive age, the group mainly affected, is substantially higher than this. There is a genetic predisposition to hyperthyroidism, particularly in that associated with Graves' disease, in which female relatives of sufferers have up to an 8% incidence of the disease.

TABLE 38.7

SIGNS AND SYMPTOMS OF HYPERTHYROIDISM (IN APPROXIMATE ORDER OF INCIDENCE)

Signs
Tachycardia (occasionally progressing to atrial fibrillation)
Enlarged, palpable thyroid gland
Warm, smooth, moist skin
Fine finger tremor
Hyperactive movements
Thyroid bruit (rushing sound of blood circulating through the thyroid heard on auscultation)
Eye signs (ranging from wide-eyed stare, mild proptosis and lid lag to gross ophthalmopathy involving damage to eyelids, cornea and extraocular muscles)
Gynaecomastia in men; breast enlargement in women

Symptoms
Nervousness and irritability
Increased sweating, especially palmar and facial
Intolerance to heat, preference for cool weather
Intermittent palpitations and an awareness of increased pulse rate
Weight loss, usually associated with increased appetite
Fatigue and weakness
Menstrual irregularity (usually oligomenorrhoea, occasionally dysfunctional uterine bleeding; reduced fertility)
Diarrhoea and hyperactive bowel

is a genuine increased incidence over the normal population, but one study has suggested evidence of malignancy in 20% of patients with toxic diffuse goitre compared with 0.5% in those with toxic nodular goitre. These figures should, however, be considered in the light of a study in Japan where carcinoma *in situ* was observed in 4% of autopsies done on subjects who had not suffered from thyroid disease, and this value rose to 28% if extensive serial sectioning of the glands was carried out. A 'cold' nodule in an otherwise 'hot', diffusely hyperplastic gland, as observed on thyroid scanning, should be taken as a warning sign that there may be an area of malignant change.

Toxic Nodular Goitre
Hyperthyroidism may be associated with one or more localized areas of the thyroid gland having increased endocrine activity; these nodules are usually palpable, exhibit increased activity on thyroid scanning, and are usually autonomous, having 'escaped' from hypothalamic–pituitary control. The increased concentrations of circulating thyroid hormones produced by the nodules are sufficient to cause negative feedback inhibition of the hypothalamic–pituitary control mechanism. This results in low circulating levels of TSH and therefore lack of stimulation of the normal thyroid tissue. Thyroid scanning will show increased activity in the nodule(s), termed 'hot nodules', with the rest of the gland showing reduced activity.

Repeat of the scan following intravenous TSH injection shows that the previously 'cold' tissue is capable of being stimulated to normal activity.

Toxic nodular goitre is observed in a somewhat older population than Graves' disease, although there is a significant overlap in the age of onset. As in Graves' disease there is a much higher incidence of toxic nodular goitre in female than in male subjects. Surveys have indicated that toxic nodular goitre is about half as common as Graves' disease, but the fact that the hyperthyroid symptoms are less severe may result in a less complete identification of subjects with toxic nodular goitre.

The clinical appearance of patients with toxic nodular goitre is variable. The symptoms are usually milder than in Graves' disease, and cardiac arrhythmias, especially atrial fibrillation, may be the only striking clinical sign, particularly in the older age group. The levels of T_4 and T_3 may be in the high-normal or borderline-high ranges, but there is suppression of TSH levels, both unstimulated, and following injection of TRH. More overtly hyperthyroid symptoms can be observed when the dietary iodine intake is increased.

Other Causes of Hyperthyroidism
Subacute Thyroiditis. This disease has a number of names, including de Quervain's thyroiditis, and it is likely that it is caused by a viral infection; mumps virus, echovirus, influenza virus and coxsackievirus have all been implicated.

The clinical features are variable, but there is usually pain and tenderness in the region of the thyroid associated with moderate pyrexia and generalized systemic symptoms such as malaise, weight loss and anorexia. Symptoms of hyperthyroidism often occur in the early stages of the disease, with increased nervousness, sweating, intolerance of heat and tachycardia being the most common. These symptoms appear to be associated with release of thyroid hormones from the thyroid gland, although during the course of the initial phase of the disease the thyroid follicles have a reduced uptake of iodine and reduced synthesis of thyroglobulin. It is obvious, if breakdown of thyroid stores is prolonged and/or severe and not accompanied by a rebuilding of the stores, hypothyroidism will follow. This is often observed, following a brief period in which the patient is euthyroid. The thyroiditis is usually self-limiting, however, and the period of the hypothyroidism, either biochemical or clinical, is usually of short duration, after which the gland returns to normal function. The amount of damage done to the gland varies from patient to patient and the average duration of the disease is from 2–5 months. In about 20% of patients, less severe recurrences delay complete recovery.

Hashimoto's Thyroiditis (Chronic lymphocytic thyroiditis) is a chronic inflammatory disease of the thyroid gland associated with a similar autoantibody picture to Graves' disease (*see* below). The aetiology is uncertain but it seems likely that it is an autoimmune disease. The similarities between the immune

TABLE 38.8
COMPARISON OF FEATURES IN GRAVES' DISEASE AND HASHIMOTO'S THYROIDITIS

Features	Graves' disease	Hashimoto's thyroiditis
Circulating thyroid antibodies	Almost always present	Almost always present
Circulating thyroid-stimulating antibodies	Almost all untreated patients	About 13%
Exophthalmos	About 50%	About 2%
Lymphadenopathy	Common	Rare
Hypergammaglobulinaemia	Uncommon	Common
Evidence of cell-mediated immunity	Yes	Yes
Association with other autoimmune diseases	Yes	Yes
Immunoglobulins in other stroma	Yes	Yes
Histocompatibility antigen link	HLA-B8, HLA-BW35, HLA-Dw3	? (conflicting evidence)

phenomena of Graves' disease and Hashimoto's disease are given in Table 38.8 .

Hashimoto's lymphocytic thyroiditis is most frequently observed in women and presents as an enlargement of the thyroid gland with relatively mild symptoms. In a minority of patients, mild to moderate symptoms of hyperthyroidism can be seen in the initial stages but more frequently the symptoms are those of hypothyroidism, and therefore the disease is described more fully in the section on hypothyroidism.

Iodine-induced Thyrotoxicosis. Increases in the incidence of hyperthyroidism have been noted in areas in which the dietary iodide level, having previously been low, has been deliberately increased, for example by iodinating bread. Subjects particularly prone to develop this complication are those in whom there is already existing thyroid pathology, particularly multinodular goitre. There have also been reports of hyperthyroidism occurring in individuals who have been given iodide-containing contrast media for radiological studies. The condition is usually mild and remits spontaneously.

Hyperthyroidism due to Excess Thyrotrophin Production (Secondary Hyperthyroidism). It is very rare for hyperthyroidism to be caused by increased production of pituitary TSH. In most of these cases a pituitary tumour is observable by radiographic methods. Occasionally, however, there is no distinct tumour, it being thought that the increased TSH secretion comes either from a microadenoma too small to observe or from general pituitary hypersecretion of TSH. Increased production of the α TSH sub-unit suggests a pituitary tumour.

Neoplastic Causes of Hyperthyroidism. It is very unusual for hyperthyroidism to be caused by over-activity of a primary thyroid carcinoma; metastases from this primary tumour may, however, produce significant amounts of thyroid hormones, not suppressed by lack of circulating TSH. Removal of such a primary tumour will not cure the hyperthyroid symptoms. Mention has already been made of the excessive production of thyroid hormones by a struma ovarii or by ectopic thyroid tissue.

Inappropriate stimulation of the thyroid resulting in hyperthyroidism can rarely occur by TSH from neoplastic tissue, which is not controlled by the high concentrations of T_3 or T_4 in the blood. Ectopic TSH-like activity can also be produced in patients with trophoblastic tumours (choriocarcinoma, hydatidiform mole) or in some forms of testicular cancer. It is probable that this TSH-like activity is associated with chorionic gonadotrophin, which is produced in large amounts by these tumours, and which has structural similarities to TSH.

Treatment-induced Hyperthyroidism. One of the most common causes of hyperthyroidism is over-enthusiastic treatment of hypothyroidism without adequate monitoring by measurement of TSH and/or thyroid hormones.

Thyrotoxic Crisis

Exceptionally, thyrotoxicosis, usually in Graves' disease or toxic nodular goitre, may become acutely exacerbated, by some precipitation cause such as infection, surgical operation or other trauma, to the severe state of thyrotoxic crisis. The symptoms and signs listed in Table 38.7 are present in an accentuated form, especially tachycardia, fever, sweating and restlessness, and sometimes delirium; later apathy, stupor and coma may occur. The condition is a medical emergency with poor prognosis, and treatment is aimed at correcting the thyrotoxicosis with anti-thyroid drugs, maintaining the cardiac output (as cardiac failure and hypotension can supervene), reducing the pyrexia and correcting body fluid, sodium and glucose levels. Despite these active measures the mortality rate is still of the order of 20%.

Disorders Associated with Hypothyroidism

Hypothyroidism is probably rather less common than hyperthyroidism, occurs most frequently in a somewhat older age group and has a sex incidence ratio of about 6:1 (F:M). There is a long list of possible

TABLE 38.9

CAUSES OF HYPOTHYROIDISM

Congenital anomalies
    Agenesis and maldevelopment
    Ectopic thyroid
    Dyshormonogenesis
    Congenital exposure to iodide or antithyroid compound
Autoimmune thyroid disease
    Autoimmune thyroiditis (Hashimoto's disease)
    End-stage Graves' disease
    Subacute thyroiditis
Iatrogenic hypothyroidism
    Post-radiation hypothyroidism
    Post-radio-iodine hypothyroidism
    Post-thyroidectomy hypothyroidism
    Excess antithyroid drugs (also some food substances)
Infiltrative disease of the thyroid
Endemic hypothyroidism
Disorders of thyroid hormone activity
    Peripheral resistance to thyroid hormones
    Antithyroid hormone antibodies
    Impared conversion T_4 to T_3
Hypothalamic†pituitary hypothyroidism
    Depressed hypothalamic function ('tertiary hypothyroidism')
    Panhypopituitarism
    Selective thyrotrophin deficiency (secondary hypothyroidism)
    Anorexia nervosa

TABLE 38.10

SIGNS AND SYMPTOMS OF ADULT-ONSET HYPOTHYROIDISM (IN APPROXIMATE ORDER OF INCIDENCE)

Dry, coarse, cool skin
Myxoedemic features (coarse skin and lips, puffy eyelids, thick tongue)
Slow, hoarse speech
Thin, dry, brittle hair
Undue sensitivity to cold (wearing warm clothes even in warm weather)
Impaired cerebration (poor memory, slow reactions both mental and physical)
Apathy, listlessness, decreased libido
Slow ankle reflex (both on contraction and especially on relaxation)
Constipation
Weight gain (often associated with decreased appetite)
Peripheral oedema
Slow pulse
Menstrual irregularity (especially menorrhagia but occasionally amenorrhoea and resulting in impaired fertility)
Deafness
Hyperlipidaemia (giving rise to xanthomata, occlusive vascular disease and its complications, cardiac enlargement and hypertension)
Myxoedema coma (rare, usually in elderly women, associated with hypothermia, poor prognosis)

aetiologies (Table 38.9) but most patients fall into one or other of the two main categories, chronic lymphocytic thyroiditis or iatrogenic hypothyroidism. The main clinical features are listed in Table 38.10.

Autoimmune Hypothyroid Disease
Autoimmune Thyroiditis (Hashimoto's disease, chronic lymphocytic thyroiditis). This category covers a group of overlapping disorders. Hashimoto's disease presents classically in middle-aged and elderly patients with the symptoms of hypothyroidism and a diffusely enlarged, horseshoe-shaped thyroid gland that has a firm, rubbery consistency. Histologically there is marked fibrosis, loss of thyroid architecture, and an infiltrate of plasma cells. It is associated with high titres of microsomal and thyroglobulin antibodies.

Also often included in the classification of Hashimoto's disease is a more common but less severe form, presenting at an earlier age and associated with low-normal or mildly subnormal thyroid-hormone concentrations. The goitre is not as firm as in the classical variant and histological examination shows predominantly lymphocytic infiltration with minimal fibrosis. There are usually high titres of microsomal antibodies, but thyroglobulin antibodies are not a common feature. The incidence of both forms of the disease is much greater in women than in men, the sex difference being more pronounced in the less severe form.

These diseases can coexist with, or follow, overt Graves' disease and it is tempting to speculate that the many similarities between these diseases (*see* Table 38.8) indicate a causal relation.

End-stage Graves' Disease. That there is a link between Graves' disease and hypothyroidism is undoubted, even if hypothyroidism resulting from radical or overenthusiastic treatment is excluded. Some patients with Graves' disease require long-term antithyroid drug therapy, or need repeat partial thyroidectomy because of recurrence of hyperthyroidism; others appear to go into remission, do not require further treatment and exhibit a reduction in antithyroid antibodies to normal levels; others, however, pass from clinically overt Graves' disease through a stage of euthyroidism to genuine hypothyroidism; this conversion frequently takes 10–15 years. It is possible that some patients with spontaneous hypothyroidism occurring in middle age have suffered from the subclinical Graves' disease. Occasionally patients presenting with hypothyroidism will admit retrospectively to symptoms suggestive of hyperthyroidism some years previously.

The ophthalmic complications of Graves' disease are increasingly being reported in patients with hypothyroidism who have not apparently suffered from hyperthyroidism previously.

In contrast some patients who develop Graves' disease do so after experiencing symptoms and showing clinical and biochemical signs of hypothyroidism that may have lasted for some years.

Subacute Thyroiditis

As mentioned previously, subacute thyroiditis, having passed through the acute inflammatory and hyperthyroid phase may revert via euthyroidism to a hypothyroid state. This is usually self-limiting but is sometimes severe enough to warrant temporary treatment with replacement thyroxine.

Endemic Hypothyroidism

Endemic hypothyroidism occurs in populations living in areas where the natural supply of iodide is suboptimal. It is associated with much greater incidence of endemic goitre, particularly in mountainous regions of the world such as the Alps, the Himalayas and the Andes. The goitre is, of course, a physiological response to the low environmental levels of iodide. Within the populations of those regions there is a spread of thyroid function from normal euthyroidism, through borderline hypothyroidism with subnormal thyroxine levels but clinical euthyroidism, to overt cretinism. Treatment is largely prophylactic, once a region has been identified as being iodine deficient. Additional iodide can be introduced into the diet, although care must be taken in initiating such measures that some individuals do not swing suddenly into a thyrotoxic phase.

Disorders of Thyroid Hormone Activity

Resistance to Thyroid Hormone Action. Results of a number of studies have implied that some patients suffer a very rare familial metabolic defect in which there is a reduced end-organ response to circulating thyroid hormones, which are usually present in such patients at substantially increased concentrations. These patients do not complain of symptoms or show signs of thyrotoxicosis; indeed they frequently appear, clinically, to be mildly hypothyroid. The reduced response is shown not only in clinical signs and symptoms, but also in a normal or reduced BMR, and in the level of TSH, which will exhibit a normal or even elevated response to intravenous injection of TRH. In past years this diagnosis has been arrived at by exclusion of other possible explanations.

Antithyroid-hormone Antibodies. The presence of high levels of circulating autoantibodies which react with thyroxine and tri-iodothyronine may give rise to clinical and biochemical findings that are totally discordant. These autoantibodies act essentially as an additional transport protein (albeit an abnormal one). It is important that this condition is differentiated from thyroid hormone resistance, since the findings may be similar. The demonstration of T_4/T_3-binding autoantibodies will differentiate the two conditions, or if this test is not available, TSH estimation may be useful. Assessment of end-organ response, such as BMR or erythrocyte sodium level, may also be helpful.

Drugs and Goitrogens Causing Hypothyroidism

In addition to those drugs that are given therapeutically with the deliberate intention of reducing thyroid activity, a number of other drugs and dietary substances are know to interfere with the production of thyroid hormones. Some of these are listed in Table 38.11.

Disorders of the Hypothalamic–Pituitary Control Mechanism

Reduced Hypothalamic Function. This is particularly noticeable in subjects who have reduced their dietary intake through personal choice or famine. Thus, in anorexia nervosa borderline-low levels of thyroid hormones, particularly tri-iodothyronine, are observed associated with low concentrations of TSH. (The findings may be complicated by a concurrent derangement of T_4–T_3 conversion; (see sick euthyroid syndrome). That the defect is not in the pituitary gland can be shown by intravenous injection of TRH when a satisfactory response, albeit somewhat delayed, can be shown. This may be associated with a similar depression of reproductive function caused by poor pituitary stimulation. The hypothyroidism has been classified as tertiary hypothyroidism.

Hypopituitarism. Secondary hypothyroidism is one of the associated symptom complexes in panhypopituitarism of whatever cause. Rarely, a condition in which there appears to be an isolated deficiency of TSH has been described. In patients with this deficiency, low levels of thyroid hormones would be associated with a low level of TSH unresponsive to TRH stimulation. The most important reason for bearing in mind the possibility of pituitary hypothyroidism is to prevent cretinism. Neonatal screening programmes that depend on the observation of a raised TSH value to diagnose neonatal hypothyroidism will miss the rare patient in whom there is associated hypopituitarism, and it may be several weeks or months before the true diagnosis is made, by which time there will have been significant delay in mental development.

Clinical Appearance of Hypothyroidism

Almost irrespective of the cause of the hypothyroidism, the clinical symptoms will fall within the classically described picture of myxoedema. These signs and symptoms are fully described in medical and endocrine text books. They were summarized in Table 38.10. There is usually no difficulty in making the clinical diagnosis of severe hypothyroidism, but it is now evident that there is a spectrum of disease ranging from mild thyroid hypofunction to gross myxoedema: patients with minimal degrees of disease often do not have clear-cut signs and symptoms. It is in these patients that biochemical, immunological and thyroid-scanning investigations are particularly helpful to the clinician. One must bear in mind, however, that borderline disease, associated with borderline clinical symptoms, is also frequently accompanied by borderline abnormal results. The possibility

TABLE 38.11
A LIST OF SOME SUBSTANCES KNOWN TO DEPRESS THYROID ACTIVITY

Substance	Mechanism of effect
Drugs	
Lithium	Possible inhibitory effect on the action of cyclic AMP
Sulphonamides	Inhibits organification of iodide (noted only in animals)
Sulphonylureas	Blocking iodide uptake (effects extremely rare in commonly used sulphonylureas, but powerful effect in carbutamide, which is now withdrawn)
Thiocyanate	Blocks uptake and binding of iodide (rarely used)
Food substances	
Soya bean flour	?Binds iodide in gastrointestinal tract and prevents absorption
Cabbage, turnip and associated vegetables	Contain thioglucosides, which are converted to thiocyanate and inhibit iodide uptake

of neoplastic change must always be considered but this diagnosis is usually made on the appearance of the thyroid gland and on the results of thyroid scanning.

If thyroid cancer has been excluded, treatment of hypothyroidism is by means of hormone replacement.

Thyroid Disease in Selected Groups

Thyroid Status in Pregnancy

Because thyroid disease is frequently experienced in women in their reproductive years, the association of thyroid disease in pregnancy is relatively common. There are a number of findings which might suggest that thyroid activity increases during pregnancy:

- There is an increased incidence of goitre and of thyroid hyperplasia during pregnancy.
- The basal metabolic rate is increased.
- The total thyroxine concentration is increased.
- The uptake of iodine by the thyroid is increased.

It is likely, however, that these are not true indicators of increased thyroid activity. The increased thyroxine concentration is associated with a substantial increase in the level of thyroxine-binding globulin (TBG). Free thyroxine concentrations indicate that there are no increases in the amount of free, active thyroid hormones, merely an increase in the protein-bound fraction. The increase in BMR is likely to be due to the increased metabolism associated with the fetoplacental unit, and the associated haemodynamic circulation of the mother. The fact that the response to injected thyrotrophin-releasing hormone, the TRH test, is exaggerated in pregnancy is also against the theory that the thyroid is overactive in normal pregnancy.

The fetal thyroid develops independently of the state of activity of the maternal thyroid gland in the normal euthyroid pregnancy. The important circulating thyroid hormones, T$_3$ and T$_4$, as well as TSH, do not pass across the placenta in significant amounts, in either direction. However, thyroid-stimulating immunoglobulins can pass from a thyrotoxic mother and cause fetal hyperthyroidism. If the maternal hyperthyroidism was not diagnosed before the onset of the pregnancy, it may be difficult to make the diagnosis as some of the symptoms of thyrotoxicosis can be confused with similar symptoms that occur in a normal pregnancy. The clinician is therefore dependent upon accurate assessment of the thyroid state of the pregnant woman, such assessment taking into account the abnormally high levels of TBG that can be expected. Often a patient with mild to moderate hyperthyroidism will cope with the pregnancy satisfactorily, but may relapse into a state of thyrotoxicosis in the post-partum period.

Hypothyroidism is rather less common than thyrotoxicosis in pregnancy, largely because it occurs mainly in a slightly older age group. Hypothyroidism is associated with subfertility, but is by no means a contraindication to pregnancy. The rate of miscarriage seems to be higher than normal in hypothyroid mothers. Biochemical diagnosis of hypothyroidism during pregnancy presents two difficulties: (i) the increased concentration of TBG may push the total thyroxine level into the normal range although the free fraction may be subnormal, and (ii) the exaggerated response to the TRH test in pregnancy may cause the misclassification of the euthyroid pregnant patient into the hypothyroid category.

Whether or not the hypothyroidism affects the development of the fetus is not clear from the literature; however, the increased rate of spontaneous abortion is sufficient indication that the hypothyroid mother should be treated during pregnancy and an attempt made to ensure that the TSH level is suppressed to normal limits.

Post-partum hypothyroidism in the mother is not uncommon. This is sometimes of temporary duration, but occasionally the pregnancy is an event that precipitates incipient hypothyroidism. The development of transient post-partum thyroid disease suggests a predisposition to thyroid disease in later life, and long-term follow-up should be recommended.

Thyroid Disease in Neonates and Children

The incidence of thyroid disease in the young is by no means as common as in the older age groups. Mention has already been made of the importance of screening for and treating hypothyroidism in neonates.

The possibility of hypothyroidism should also be considered in children with abnormally short stature, or with a reduced growth rate. It is interesting to note that the academic school performance of such children, provided the hypothyroidism was not present during the first year of life, may well appear to be better than that of their euthyroid colleagues or may appear to deteriorate somewhat when the euthyroid state is achieved through treatment; this change is particularly noticeable in children who become much more active when treated and is merely a reflection of an increased interest in activities, both mental and physical, outside the somewhat narrower school schedules.

The possibility of hyperthyroidism should always be considered in children who are excessively tall for their age, particularly when this cannot be explained on the basis of parental height, or when there is a sudden, unexpected increase in the rate of linear growth. The effect of hyperthyroidism on a child's height is particularly noticeable at puberty. Clinical examination, backed up with the measurement of thyroid hormone concentrations, can prevent excessive, but inappropriate, investigation of possible growth-hormone abnormalities.

Thyroid Function in the Elderly

Thyroid disease is more common in the elderly than in the younger population; one report has suggested that thyroid disease is present in over 5% of elderly patients. About three-quarters of thyroid disease in the elderly is hypothyroidism, the remaining quarter being associated with hyperthyroidism. Occasionally atypical presentations occur, such as 'apathetic thyrotoxicosis' and rarely myxoedema coma, a severe complication with poor prognosis, which may be associated with hypothermia, hypercapnia and hypoglycaemia.

Sick Euthyroid Syndrome

The metabolism of thyroid hormones may be significantly altered by non-thyroidal illness. Essentially, the major change is the lowering of T_3 production and r-T_3 catabolism. This results in a low plasma T_3 level, with a raised r-T_3 level. As discussed earlier, the differential deiodination of T_4 acts as a control mechanism on the metabolic effects of the thyroid hormones. It seems likely that there is a need to 'slow down' metabolic activity in illness, and that this is achieved by switching monodeiodination from active T_3 to inactive r-T_3.

Plasma T_4 and TSH levels are usually unaltered, but may become affected in severe illness. A low total thyroxine may be seen in very severe illness, but this is probably due to deranged protein binding.

The condition, known as sick euthyroid syndrome or low T_3 syndrome, is seen commonly in many illnesses. For this reason, thyroid function testing on hospital inpatients may be unwise. It is a common practice to screen elderly patients in hospital geriatric wards for thyroid disease. As many of these patients may be in hospital because of illness, this practice is likely to give rise to some misleading results. However, as genuine thyroid disease is relatively common in the elderly population, such screening may also yield useful results. Senior laboratory staff should be closely involved in interpreting and advising on thyroid function screening of the elderly and should therefore be aware of the difficulties likely to be encountered.

The syndrome is also classically seen in patients suffering from anorexia nervosa and starvation from other causes.

The use of r-T_3 assays would be useful in the investigation of sick euthyroid syndrome, but this assay is not in common use. TSH is the most reliable estimation, but postponement of thyroid function testing until the illness is resolved may be more rewarding, if clinical suspicion is not high.

TREATMENT OF THYROID DISEASE

Hypothyroidism

The aim of any treatment of hypothyroidism is simply to replace the missing thyroid hormone. Early treatment consisted of crude extracts of animal thyroid glands. Success with this encouraged the purification of the extracts to yield thyroglobulin. Modern treatment consists of chemically synthesized thyroxine or tri-iodothyronine.

In general, thyroxine is the treatment of choice, as it has a relatively long half-life, allowing stability of treatment with one daily dose once the optimum therapeutic level has been reached. Titration of the dose during initiation of therapy is easily achieved by the combined use of clinical judgement and appropriate serum hormone levels, as discussed below.

The therapeutic use of tri-iodothyronine is not very common. Unlike thyroxine, T_3 has a short half-life in serum, and maintenance of a stable treatment regimen is more difficult. Its use is generally reserved for two situations: firstly where an immediate therapeutic effect is required, such as in myxoedema coma (it is usual for the therapy to be switched to thyroxine as soon as practical in these patients), and secondly, where there is a known defect in T_4–T_3 conversion, in which the use of thyroxine would have little, if any, effect. Efficacy of treatment may be monitored clinically, but in these patients hormone investigations have an important role, because of the labile nature of the treatment and the effects of overdosage, especially on cardiac function.

Hyperthyroidism

Essentially, there are three possible courses of action in the treatment of hyperthyroidism:

(i) drug treatment to prevent the synthesis of thyroid hormones;
(ii) surgical removal of part or all of the gland;
(iii) ablation of the gland by radioactive iodine.

Drug treatment, usually by carbimazole, whose main effect is to reduce the formation of iodotyrosines, is now thought to very safe, but carries the need for a regular daily dose. Compliance may become compromised with increasing patient age, so regular outpatient supervision, backed by laboratory checks, is essential. Long-term remission is unlikely unless the therapy is prolonged (at least a year). Some clinicians may use a combined therapy of carbimazole and thyroid hormone (either thyroxine or tri-iodothyronine). Biochemical and clinical monitoring, and adjustment of dosage regimen, may be more difficult with this treatment. Carbimazole therapy is widely used to make the patient euthyroid before thyroidectomy, as the cardiac complications of thyrotoxicosis present a serious operative risk. Ten to twelve days before operation, the carbimazole is replaced with iodine, which reduces the vasculature of the gland and gives it a firm texture to assist in removal.

Partial or total *thyroidectomy* for thyrotoxicosis is a quick and effective form of treatment. In general it is a relatively simple operation, but as with any operative procedure, the patient must be assessed for risk. Early operations frequently carried the risk of removal of the parathyroid glands, as they may be variable in number and location. This is now a relatively minor risk when the operation is done by competent surgeons. Nevertheless, it is usual to monitor calcium metabolism for a short while postoperatively. After total thyroidectomy the patient will require lifelong thyroxine replacement, as outlined above for hypothyroid patients.

Thyroidectomy is also used for the treatment of thyroid carcinoma. The operative procedure may need to be more extensive than that for thyrotoxicosis, and it is essential that thyroxine replacement therapy postoperatively is sufficient fully to suppress TSH levels, in order that any metastatic tissue is not stimulated.

Iodine-131 is a very safe form of treatment, despite any initial fear of radioactivity by the patient. There may be some difficulty in accurately calculating the dose to be used, as the distribution of iodine within the thyroid is not uniform. The choice between sufficient dosage to render the patient euthyroid and complete ablation may also cause difficulties.

The use of iodine-131 for the treatment of toxic nodular goitre is effective in rendering the patient euthyroid, but will not necessarily stop growth of the goitre. The use of surgery may be preferable in these cases.

Two compounds related to thyroid hormones are also used therapeutically. The D isomer of thyroxine (dextrothyroxine) may be prescribed to assist in the lowering of cholesterol levels with minimal thyroid hormone effects. It may also be used to treat hypothyroidism when normal therapy is not tolerated. Tri-iodothyroacetic acid may rarely be prescribed for assisting in weight loss.

THE INVESTIGATION OF THYROID FUNCTION

Introduction

The assessment of thyroid function is made, first and foremost, on clinical grounds. A good history and sound examination are sufficient to make a diagnosis in patients with moderate or severe thyroid disease. Laboratory investigations in these cases are useful to give baseline information, which can be compared with the results of further investigations during the course of the treatment. Investigations also provide interesting information about the cause of the disease, although this may not be particularly important in deciding on treatment. Investigations are more important in those patients who present with an equivocal picture, although if the clinical features are borderline, results of investigations are also often borderline. In some, but not in all, studies routine screening for thyroid disease in adults has been shown to be worthwhile (most workers are agreed on the value of neonatal thyroid screening); thyroid disease is common and debilitating, there are good screening tests, and treatment is relatively simple.

The laboratory investigation of thyroid function was transformed by the advent of accurate and precise radioimmunoassay methods of measurement of the thyroid hormones and TSH, which superseded the non-specific protein-bound iodine method. The development of immunometric assays to measure polypeptide hormones such as TSH resulted in a further transformation. Assays are now commonly available with quoted sensitivities up to two orders of magnitude better than previous competitive assays, combined with a greatly enhanced precision, specificity and robustness. Additionally, the growing use of non-isotopic immunoassays and automation is beginning to have yet another impact on biochemical thyroid-function testing. Assay systems are currently available that allow the processing of large numbers of samples with almost the same ease and simplicity as that accepted for liver and renal function tests. However, it is unwise to take such simplicity for granted in immunoassays, as they are still essentially biological assays, with the inherent problems of biological systems.

The methods at present employed to measure the thyroid hormones T_4 and T_3 may measure the total (bound plus free) concentrations, or the free fraction. In recent years, practicable methods for the direct measurement of free T_4 and T_3 concentration have been developed, and both methods are now easily available.

Aims of Investigation

The aims of laboratory investigation of thyroid function are as follows:

- to use one or two well-understood and inexpensive methods for the routine investigation of patients with possible thyroid disease;
- to use the more sophisticated, difficult, time-consuming investigations in those patients in whom simpler tests have not given a satisfactory answer;
- to minimize the use of invasive techniques or those that cause discomfort or pose threats of danger to patients—in particular, as many patients with thyroid disease are women of reproductive age, the use of *in vivo* radiosotope methods should be kept to a minimum.

Thyroid Function Tests—Indications and Interpretation

Total Thyroxine

Serum total thyroxine concentration is a well-established, inexpensive, initial measurement on patients with either hypothyroidism or hyperthyroidism. It is also useful in monitoring the progress of treatment of both hypo- and hyperthyroidism. The method is practicable, relatively inexpensive, and can be automated to deal with large numbers of samples. Its major drawback is that as it is an assay of total hormone concentration a number of patients with abnormal levels of TBG, either from pathological or physiological causes, can be misdiagnosed

Our experience is that in order to avoid incorrect categorization, adequate clinical information must be given. The other drawback of total thyroxine measurements (which is also true of measurement of free thyroxine) is that they will not pick up a hyperthyroid patient who is suffering from T_3-toxicosis and in whom the thyroxine concentration is in the normal range. It is theoretically possible also that patients with hypothyroidism caused by a low T_3 concentration, but with normal T_4 level, may also be missed.

Total thyroxine results may be interpreted as follows (with some variation depending on methodology, etc.):

< 45 nmol/L (< 3.5 μg/dL)	Hypothyroid value
45–55 nmol/L (3.5–4.3 μg/dL)	Borderline hypothyroid value
56–70 nmol/L (4.4–5.5 μg/dL)	Low-normal value
71–135 nmol/L (5.6–10.5 μg/dL)	Normal value
136–145 nmol/L (10.6–11.2 μg/dL)	High-normal value
146–160 nmol/L (11.3–12.4 μg/dL)	Borderline-high value
> 160 nmol/L (> 12.4 μg/dL)	Hyperthyroid value

But these interpretations may be modified in the light of other investigations, e.g. TSH, T_3, done on the same sample, and may also be modified by the clinical appearance of the patient.

Free Thyroxine

As mentioned above, a very large percentage of thyroxine and tri-iodothyronine circulates in the plasma bound to thyroid hormone-binding proteins; it is, however, the free hormone that is likely to have biological effects at the tissue level. Thus, total thyroid-hormone measurements in blood do not give a direct estimate of the amount of the active hormones. If the amount of thyroxine-binding proteins and the degree of binding to them did not vary between individuals, the total hormone concentrations would bear a fixed relation to the free hormone concentrations. Unfortunately this is not so and various factors (*see* Table 38.1) alter the amount of binding proteins or interfere with the binding of thyroid hormones to them. Particularly important amongst these are the contraceptive pill and pregnancy, both of which cause a significant increase in the level of thyroxine-binding proteins, thereby increasing the total concentration of thyroid hormones, without necessarily influencing the concentration of the free hormones. An inappropriate diagnosis of thyrotoxicosis or T_3-toxicosis may thus be made in a euthyroid patient.

In order to overcome these difficulties a variety of methods has been investigated to make indirect estimates of the amount of free thyroid hormones. For instance, an estimate of the amount of thyroxine-binding proteins can be achieved with the T_3-uptake test, and this may be used to give an approximation to the level of free thyroxine (the *free thyroxine index*). In recent years this estimate has been superseded by direct measurement of free thyroxine, either by equilibrium dialysis or by 'analogue' methods.

The so-called analogue methods are now the most common for measuring free thyroid hormones. Since their introduction, much controversy has surrounded both their theoretical basis and practical application. However, it cannot be denied that in the vast majority of cases the methods yield clinically useful results. Essentially, the method attempts to measure the amount of free thyroxine without disrupting the T_4/TBG equilibrium, and without the TBG in the patient's serum interfering in the analytical binding reaction. This is achieved by the use of an antibody of very high avidity, together with a radiolabelled analogue of thyroxine, which will bind to the antiserum but not to TBG.

Free T_4 assays are easily available and the results are at least as useful as total T_4 in the same contexts. In many laboratories free thyroxine has replaced total thyroxine as a first line test for thyroid function (*see* Strategies below). The cost tends to be higher, especially when compared to in-house tests for total thyroxine, as free T_4 methods are more difficult to develop.

Free T_4 results may be interpreted as follows (with some variation depending on methodology etc.):

< 10 pmol/L (< 0.78 ng/dL)	Hypothyroid value
11–13 pmol/L (0.78–1.00 ng/dL)	Borderline hypothyroid value
14–24 pmol/L (1.09–1.87 ng/dL)	Normal value
25–30 pmol/L (1.94–2.33 ng/dL)	Borderline hyperthyroid value
> 30 pmol/L (> 2.33 ng/dL)	Hyperthyroid value

As with total T_4 levels, these interpretations may be modified in the light of further test results. With some free-T_4 methods, the upper part of the euthyroid range becomes extended with the age of the patient, so that in geriatric patients, results below 30 pmol/L may be considered normal.

Thyroid-stimulating Hormone
TSH measurements were excellent at confirming the majority of hypothyroid states, in which elevated levels are observed. But they were not sensitive enough to distinguish between the suppressed levels found in hyperthyroid states and the low-normal levels frequently seen in euthyroid subjects. In the last decade the development of sensitive TSH methods has enabled TSH to be used in the differentiation between these two groups. Indeed some laboratories have for some years used the sensitive TSH assay (HS-TSH) as their primary thyroid screening method for both hypo- and hyperthyroidism. A so-called third-generation TSH assay, yet more sensitive than HS-TSH, is currently being marketed; its benefits have yet to be assessed, but initial reaction suggests that its ability to distinguish between eu- and hyperthyroidism is no better than HS-TSH.

The measurement of TSH concentration is particularly useful in the following situations.

● *In patients who have clinical hypothyroidism and whose thyroxine level is significantly below the normal range.* This enables distinction to be made between patients with primary hypothyroidism, in whom the TSH value will be significantly elevated, and the very rare cases of secondary hypothyroidism, in whom the TSH concentration will be unmeasurably low (TSH measurement on its own would not identify such rare cases). It also acts as a baseline for comparison for future TSH measurements taken once treatment has been started.

● *In patients with borderline subnormal thyroxine levels, particularly if there are any clinical indications of hypothyroidism.* In these patients the TSH level may not be greatly elevated and it may be necessary to carry out a TRH test, or at least to carry out repeat investigations after 3 months in order to see if there has been any progression of the hypothyroidism. Measurement of thyroid autoantibodies may also help to confirm incipient hypothyroidism.

● *In monitoring the treatment of hypothyroidism.* TSH measurements are particularly useful in monitoring treatment with thyroxine (or tri-iodothyronine) in the early stages, when an appropriate dose is being sought, or subsequently, when it is felt that the treatment dose is not quite adequate. In these cases, when the thyroxine (or tri-iodothyronine) levels are in the lower part of the normal range, the TSH value can help to confirm the adequacy or otherwise of the treatment dose. Since the advent of sensitive TSH measurement, this estimation may now also be used, in conjunction with T_4 (or T_3) measurement, when the possibility of overdosage is being considered. Many clinicians now expect T_4 (or T_3, depending on the therapy) and TSH estimations on all patients with treated hypothyroidism, once or twice yearly, to ensure biochemical stability of the treatment regimen.

● *In patients with borderline raised T_4 and/or T_3 levels.* HS-TSH measurement may now be used in the assessment of hyperthyroidism, where the levels should be suppressed. The use of TSH in this context is discussed more fully in a later section. Secondary thyrotoxicosis, where TSH is secreted by a pituitary tumour, causing overstimulation of the thyroid, has been described, but is very rare.

● *In monitoring the treatment of thyrotoxicosis.* Patients treated with carbimazole may be biochemically assessed by measurement of the thyroid hormones. However, this group of patients tends to be slightly unstable, either because of the short half-life of carbimazole in the bloodstream, or because of their poor compliance. TSH assay in addition gives a more integrated biochemical assessment of the effectiveness of the therapy. TSH estimation is also useful in patients treated with radioiodine or thyroidectomy to monitor the effects of the treatment.

The reference euthyroid range for TSH is generally 0.4–5.0 mu/L, and for HS-TSH is 0.2–5.0 with some interlaboratory and methodological variation. The lower limit of the range of results found in hypothyroid patients is approximately 7.5 mu/L. Results falling between the euthyroid and hypothyroid ranges should be considered in conjunction with the T_4 results, and not routinely taken as indicating hypothyroidism, without careful clinical assessment and if necessary, repeat testing.

TRH Test
The TRH test has been used in the diagnosis both of hyperthyroidism and hypothyroidism. However, its necessity in the resolution of difficult and borderline cases has now been considerably reduced by the

ability of the laboratory to measure TSH with more accuracy, specificity and sensitivity. The TRH test is usually made because of borderline clinical findings followed by borderline basal thyroid-function tests. In the majority of these cases, the results of the TRH test are also borderline, and will have contributed nothing to the diagnosis. There have also been reports, though rare, that unacceptable side-effects have been observed as a consequence of TRH injection. Its role, therefore, as a test of thyroid function is doubtful, although it may still have a place in the assessment of pituitary dysfunction (*see* Chapter 37).

Tri-iodothyronine

Both total and free tri-iodothyronine may be measured in the plasma, using methods similar to those for total and free thyroxine. In the following section, references to 'T_3' may be taken to relate to either the total or free hormone levels as indicated.

The normal range for total tri-iodothyronine is 1.3–2.8 nmol/L (80–180 ng/dL), with some interlaboratory and methodological variations. Values within 0.3 nmol/L of this range may be considered borderline. The equivalent range for free T_3 is 3.0–8.6 pmol/L (185–540 pg/dL).

The major uses for the measurement of T_3 are:

- To diagnose T_3-toxicosis in patients in whom there are clinical signs or symptoms of hyperthyroidism but in whom the thyroxine concentration is within the normal range.
- To supplement thyroxine measurements in those patients who show signs of thyrotoxicosis and whose thyroxine levels are in the high-normal or border-high regions. Significantly elevated or borderline-elevated T_3 values would support the diagnosis of thyrotoxicosis, but a level well down in the normal range would contraindicate such a diagnosis.
- To monitor hypothyroid patients who are being treated with tri-iodothyronine. The T_3 measurement must be supplemented by TSH measurement as mentioned above.

The measurement of T_3 may also be of value in patients who appear to be hypothyroid but who have normal serum thyroxine concentrations. If in these patients the T_3 concentration is subnormal, it is possible that the patient is unable adequately to convert T_4 to T_3. If, as suggested, T_3 is the active metabolite of the thyroid hormones, one can see why such poor conversion may lead to signs of hypothyroidism. This situation is very rarely seen.

Reverse-T_3

Although various suggestions have been made for using the measurement of r-T_3 to assess thyroid function, it does not appear at present that a good case has been made for any particular clinical situation. Reverse-T_3 concentrations are known to rise in certain non-thyroid diseases but this knowledge is unlikely to be helpful.

Strategies for Investigating Thyroid Function

With the advent of sensitive methods for the determination of serum levels of TSH, and readily available assays for free thyroid hormones, a number of alternative strategies for biochemical thyroid-function testing have become possible. Each strategy has its proponents and merits. Currently, testing must not only be clinically efficacious, but also cost-effective. Thus, when considering which testing system to use, the laboratory must take into account financial considerations such as bed occupancy during delays in testing inpatients, and repeated outpatient or general practitioner visits for repeat of equivocal tests. Other financial factors that must be considered are the manhours required, the capital cost or lease cost of any special equipment, together with the actual reagent costs. The skill level of staff available for performance of assays (and development of in-house assays) must also be taken into account.

The major alternatives in test strategies are outlined below.

1. Perform only those tests requested by the clinician. This is an unreliable system, and is in general not cost-effective, as some hospital junior medical staff and general practitioners may not be aware of the best tests to use in any given situation. Inconclusive or misleading results may therefore be obtained, leading either to repeated testing, or to incorrect diagnosis. If this strategy is to be used, then it must be accompanied by constant and careful education programmes for the users of the service.

2. Use serum total thyroxine, an inexpensive primary test. Thereafter proceed with further, discriminatory tests on the basis of the first-line test and the clinical/therapeutic information available. In terms of laboratory costs, this system is certainly cost-effective, as in the majority of cases thyroid status will be determined with the inexpensive primary test. Further testing (free thyroxine, total or free T_3 and/or TSH) will be required where the initial result is equivocal; where differentiation between primary or secondary hypothyroidism is required, where the patient is on treatment for hyper- or hypothyroidism; or where there is a disturbance of hormone binding. This extra testing may introduce delays that make this strategy less financially attractive overall. A turn-round time for thyroid function tests, based on this system, may be as long as 9 days using in-house assays with long assay times. It is not uncommon for junior medical staff to repeat requests for thyroid function tests because of delays in receiving results, caused by batching of the second-line tests, for instance on a once-weekly basis.

3. Use a primary test that is more expensive, but partially discriminatory. Thereafter proceed with a second discriminatory test on the basis of the first-line test and the clinical/therapeutic information available. This system is identical with that described above, except that many of the equivocal results seen when using total thyroxine as first-line test are eliminated when measuring a more discriminatory primary test such as free thyroxine or HS-TSH, and there is a consequent reduction in secondary testing.

Two major strategies have been developed along these lines, using either free thyroxine or TSH as the first-line test.

(i) Free thyroxine as first line. In general, this method will not be affected by disturbances of thyroid-hormone binding. Thus the amount of secondary testing will fall, providing a faster turn round with more clinically useful results in the majority of cases. In our experience, clinical staff will often not fully inform the laboratory of treatment that the patient is receiving. Using free-thyroxine estimation as a first-line test overcomes this problem in many cases, particularly with the contraceptive pill (which is often not identified by requesters of investigations as therapy or as a drug).

Care must be exercised particularly in the interpretation of results in pregnant patients, where a lower reference range may be required, and in the elderly, where changes in albumin concentrations may give results that rise with age (depending on the particular method used), necessitating a different reference range. In addition, less common anomalies such as thyroid hormone-binding antibodies may cause misleading results. The use of secondary tests such as T_3 (total or free), or TSH will still be necessary, as with the total thyroxine-based system, but their usage will certainly be reduced.

Commercial, analogue-based methods for free thyroxine have relatively short assay times, which may help to reduce turn-round times for patient samples. The more sophisticated equilibrium dialysis assays are far more demanding and take much longer to perform. Although they are accepted as the 'gold standard' for free thyroxine methods, they have not found a place in the routine laboratory.

(ii) TSH as first line. In view of the fact that the thyroid status of the individual is reflected by the status of the thyroid/pituitary/hypothalamus feedback loop, many laboratories have used TSH as the primary indicator of thyroid function. This is based on the idea that the end-organ responses of the pituitary and the peripheral tissues are the same, or sufficiently similar, so that TSH may act as a monitor of the effects of the thyroid hormones. This strategy has only become possible with the use of sensitive, precise and specific methods based on the immunometric principle. Previous assays, based on competitive immunoassay, were too crude to allow this development.

Initially, it was thought that using TSH assays might allow the testing of thyroid function with only this single test. There were, however, a number of drawbacks to this system, and laboratories using TSH as a first-line test generally use a secondary test (total or free T_4 or T_3) as well.

The reference euthyroid range for TSH is generally 0.4–4.0 mU/L, with some inter-laboratory and methodological variation. It is important to stress that this is the range of results found in a euthyroid population. It cannot be assumed that all results below the lower limit of the range indicate thyrotoxicosis. In our experience, results obtained on clinically thyrotoxic patients are almost always undetectably low (in our assays, less tthan 0.1 mU/L), leaving an area of uncertainty between 0.1 and 0.4 mU/L. The TSH results in this area should be considered in conjunction with those of T_4 and T_3, and the patient should be carefully assessed clinically, with repeat testing if immediate treatment is considered unnecessary. Similarly, the lower limit of the range of results found in hypothyroid patients is approximately 7.5 mU/L. Results falling between the euthyroid and hypothyroid ranges should be considered in conjunction with the T_4 results, and not routinely taken as indicating hypothyroidism, without careful clinical assessment and if necessary, repeat testing. Patients treated for hypo- and hyperthyroidism may be monitered with TSH, usually with additional tests (e.g. thyroxine for treated hypothyroid patients, and T_3 for thyrotoxic patients). As with the use of free thyroxine, this strategy is not affected by patients whose hormone binding is disturbed, so the number of tests required may be reduced.

In terms of cost-effectiveness, this system is similar to that using free thyroxine as the first-line test, although TSH methods may be more expensive than those for free thyroxine, and take longer to do. Turn-round times may be slightly longer than those for the previous systems.

4. Use combined testing. The use of two or more tests concurrently (usually total or free thyroxine and TSH) has been advocated as a means of combining clinical and cost-effectiveness to the maximum. Some manufacturers have produced kits that allow the concurrent measurement of T_4 and TSH in the same tube, by the use of two different isotopic tracers. However, the testing strategy may be used just as effectively by doing two separate assays at the same time.

There can be no doubt of the advantages of assaying thyroxine and TSH at the same time in those patients who have abnormal thyroid-function tests. There is no requirement for decisions on secondary testing (usually based on inadequate clinical/therapeutic information) to be made by laboratory staff. There can be much better interpretation of borderline results, and the turn-round time is reduced dramatically. Working procedures are simplified, and reagent costs are more easily controlled. There is, however, a large wastage of reagent in testing euthyroid patients, for whom a single, inexpensive test would have been sufficient. In terms of reagent costs, this strategy may increase the expenditure significantly depending on the methodologies involved. This needs to be balanced carefully against the overall costs associated with repeat visits, waiting times, etc. outlined above.

Interpretation of Unexpected Results

It is the experience of every clinical biochemist and endocrine physician that tests of thyroid function do not always produce the expected results. Sometimes the results do not agree with the patient's presentation, sometimes the results of two tests that should complement each other turn out to be incongruous, at least at first sight. The following discussion is an attempt to explain some of the incongruity.

Erroneous Results. Errors in results can arise in a wide variety of ways. Serum samples are generally preferred, as the fibrinogen in plasma can interfere with the analytical antigen–antibody reaction in some assays, especially that for TSH. The sample must be reasonably fresh when it reaches the laboratory, so that haemolysis can be avoided, and deterioration of the thyroid hormones and the production of potentially interfering artefacts in the sample minimized.

The assay methods for thyroid function tests are more complex, involve more manipulation, demand a higher degree of technical skill and are less automated than many other tests made in the clinical biochemistry laboratory.

Tests, such as those used for urea and electrolyte determinations, have precise methodology, are fully 'automated' and are frequently linked to computerized data-handling systems. This is often not the case with the immunoassay methods used in thyroid function tests. As a result these tests are liable to greater analytical imprecision, provide more opportunity for operator error, and are subject to more likelihood of misidentification; they also produce greater interlaboratory variation.

Some unexpected results are therefore a consequence of errors made in the collection and transport of the sample or in its subsequent analysis. Because abnormal thyroid function frequently needs to be treated for the rest of the patient's life, or demands irreversible surgical or radiation treatment, it is essential that abnormal results are confirmed on a second sample before treatment, particularly if the test results are not wholly in accord with the patient's clinical condition.

In addition to genuine errors of this sort, apparently incongruous results can sometimes be obtained in which no error has occurred. These demand interpretation in the light of the patient's condition. Some apparently incongruous results that can be explained are as follows:

- *Normal T_4, low T_3.* Classically seen in the sick euthyroid syndrome: information should be sought about any non-thyroid illness that the patient may have, and advice given on whether the test should be repeated after any illness is resolved. TSH estimation may be helpful if further immediate investigation is required by clinical staff.

- *High T_4, low or normal T_3.* This can occur in thyrotoxicosis, particularly if there is an associated impaired conversion of T_4 to T_3. It could be observed in elderly thyrotoxic patients or in the sick euthyroid syndrome. TSH estimation may be helpful.

- *Low T_4, normal T_3.* These results can occur in mild or early thyroid failure, as the gland attempts to maximize the output of active hormone, in which case TSH will be at least slightly raised. They can also be an indication of iodine deficiency, as the thyroid attempts to make best use of the limited amount of iodine.

- *Normal T_4, high T_3.* This is commonly observed in T_3-toxicosis, or rarely in deliberate or accidental overdosage with T_3. It may also occur in iodine deficiency.

- *Low total T_4, low total T_3, normal TSH.* These results can be observed in subjects with congenital or acquired TBG deficiency (the use of anabolic steroids by sportsmen and as medication leads to a TBG-deficient state), and possibly in hypothermia or severe illness in patients who are usually euthyroid. Free hormone levels are usually helpful in these cases.

- *Low T_4, low T_3, low TSH.* Very low values are associated with secondary (pituitary) hypothyroidism. Moderately reduced thyroid-hormone levels with low TSH can also be associated with tertiary (hypothalamic) hypothyroidism. A TRH test would show no rise of TSH in the former case, but a normal, possibly delayed, response in the latter. It is important to bear in mind that these conditions are very rare.

- *High total T_4, high total T_3, patient not hyperthyroid.* This is a relatively common finding in patients with increased levels of TBG, as a result of oestrogen therapy, pregnancy or congenital TBG excess. The effects of the increased TBG will be negated by the use of free-hormone estimations. The possibility of antibodies to T_3 and T_4, dysalbuminaemic hyperthyroxinaemia, or a peripheral tissue resistance to thyroid hormone action should also be considered, although these are all relatively rare. The measurement of free hormones will give correct results in the case of dysalbuminaemic hyperthyroxinaemia, but not with antibodies reacting with T_4 and/or T_3. In all these patients, TSH estimation would be most helpful.

- *High T_4, high T_3, high TSH.* The comments shown in the previous section are also relevant here, but the TSH result would suggest that the patient, as well as having abnormal binding, is also suffering from some degree of hypothyroidism. This should only be used to support a clinical diagnosis, and would require considerable further investigation to determine the cause of the discordant results. The possibility of secondary hyperthyroidism, although rarer than any of the other possible explanations, must also be investigated.

Other Tests of Thyroid Function
Thyroid Antibody Studies. As mentioned earlier, a significant proportion of thyroid disease is associated with the presence of circulating antibodies to thyroid antigens. Measurement of these, both stimulatory and destructive, can help make the diagnosis when clinical appearance and hormone measurements give equivocal findings. It should be remembered that thyroid autoantibodies can be found at significant levels in subjects who are clearly euthyroid.

Thyroid Scanning. The use of thyroid scanning is a useful adjunct in the diagnosis of thyroid disease. It is particularly useful in cases of nodular goitre, and also in borderline cases. The subject is, however, beyond, the scope of this book.

The increasing use of the clinical biochemistry laboratory in the investigation of thyroid function, brought about by the development of radioimmunoassays for the hormones involved, has greatly helped in making the diagnosis and monitoring the treatment of patients with thyroid disease. These advances have also led to a greater understanding of the nature of thyroid disease.

In the long run, however, diagnosis of thyroid disease is a clinical matter and, in cases where the biochemical results and the clinical features do not completely tally, it is the latter that should determine treatment. A cautionary tale, albeit anecdotal, of one of our patients will suffice to make the point.

The patient was in her mid-fifties when she first presented to her general practitioner with symptoms and signs that he felt to be consistent with mild hypothyroidism. She was referred to a physician who requested thyroid function tests, and was surprised to find that both T_4 and T_3 (total) levels were significantly raised. Repeat tests showed the same results, and both reports stated that the requested TSH estimation was inappropriate, in view of the high levels of thyroid hormones, and was therefore not done. Following further discussion the physician persuaded us to make a TRH test. This showed, to our surprise, a TSH response a little elevated above

that normally observed, and certainly not a hyperthyroid response, despite the fact that the thyroid hormone levels continued to be significantly raised. At that time, direct measurement of free thyroxine was not available. We could not demonstrate the presence of T_3 or T_4 antibodies and therefore concluded that the patient had some peripheral resistance to thyroid hormone action. The physician agreed and advised the general practitioner that it was of no use to treat the patient with thyroxine or tri-iodothyronine as she was already producing more than enough. The practitioner argued that the patient was becoming more hypothyroid and 'needed treatment with thyroxine'; the physician's advice was unchanged. Our opinion was sought and we agreed about the uselessness of giving still more thyroxine. The general practitioner decided, in view of the patient's condition, to take no heed of the advice given and instituted thyroxine therapy. The patient recovered splendidly. It is interesting to note that we now, some years later, believe that this patient demonstrated abnormal albumin binding of thyroid hormones, and not peripheral hormone resistance. Using the more advanced biochemical testing now available, it is less likely that this apparent contradiction between biochemical and clinical assessment would arise. This does not affect the lesson, however. The general practitioner had steadfastly believed that he should treat the patient and not the biochemistry. He was absolutely correct.

SUGGESTIONS FOR FURTHER READING

Amino N. (1988). Autoimmunity and hypothyroidism. In *Clinics in Endocrinology and Metabolism: Hypothyroidism and Goitre* (Lazarus J.H., Hall R. ed.) London: Baillière Tindall.

Braverman L.E., Utiger R.D. ed. (1991). *The Thyroid*, Philadelphia: Lippincott.

Delange F. (1988). Neonatal hypothyroidism. In *Clinics in Endocrinology and Metabolism: Hypothyroidism and Goitre* (Lazarus J.H., Hall R. ed.) London: Baillière Tindall.

Larsen P.R., Ingbar S.H. (1992). The thyroid gland. In *Williams Textbook of Endocrinology*, 8th edn (Wilson J.D., Foster D.W. ed.) Philadelphia: Saunders.

Sheppard M.C. ed. (1988). Molecular biology of endocrinology. In *Clinical Endocrinology and Metabolism*, **2**(4) London: Baillière Tindall.

Thorner M.O., Vance M.L., Horvath E., Kovacs K. (1992). The anterior pituitary. In *Williams Textbook of Endocrinology*, 8th edn (Wilson J.D., Foster D.W. ed.) Philadelphia: Saunders.

39. Hypoglycaemia

V. Marks

Introduction
   Symptoms
   Pathogenesis
Fasting hypoglycaemia
   Insulinoma
   Non-insulin-secreting tumours
   Inborn errors of metabolism
   Antoimmune hypoglycaemia
Reactive hypoglycaemia
   Insulin autoimmune syndrome
   Alcohol-induced reactive hypoglycaemia
Diagnosis
   Confirmation of hypoglycaemia
   Provocative tests
   Differential diagnosis of hypoglycaemia

TABLE 39.1
CLASSIFICATIONS OF HYPOGLYCAEMIA ACCORDING TO ITS
AETIOLOGY

Pancreatic causes
Insulinoma and proinsulinoma: benign and malignant
Insular hyperplasia
MEN-1
Pancreatitis
Functional hyperinsulinism: 'nesidioblastosis'

Non-pancreatic neoplasias
IGF-II-producing tumours
Adrenal tumours
Lymphomas and leukaemias
Other tumours

Autoimmune disease
Anti-insulin-receptor antibodies
B-cell stimulatory antibodies
Anti-insulin antibodies

Endocrine disease
Pituitary insufficiency; generalized or specific
Adrenocortical insufficiency
Selective hypothalamic insufficiency

Inborn errors of metabolism
Liver glycogen disease
Galactosaemia and hereditary fructose intolerance (HFI)
Disorders of gluconeogenesis
Dicarboxylic acidurias

Liver and kidney failure
Hepatocellular disease, e.g. infective hepatitis
'End-stage' kidney
Congestive liver disease: cardiac failure

Neonatal hypoglycaemia
Temporary infantile hyperinsulinism, e.g. infants of dia-
   betic mothers and small for dates babies
'Nesidioblastosis' or 'functional hyperinsulinism'
EMG syndrome

Toxic hypoglycaemia
Iatrogenic and felonious, i.e. due to therapeutic hypoglycae-
   mic agents, e.g. insulin, sulphonylureas
Alcohol
Drugs, e.g. quinine, β-adrenergic antagonists
Poisons, e.g. *Amanita phalloides*, ackee nuts; hypoglycin

Reactive hypoglycaemia
Post-gastrectomy
'Alcohol' provoked
'Idiopathic'

Miscellaneous causes
Diseases of the nervous system
Starvation, including anorexia nervosa
Rigorous exercise (especially in combination with certain
   drugs)
Dialysis

INTRODUCTION

Hypoglycaemia is an important physical finding in a number of diseases and is the consequence of a disturbance of glucose homeostasis. It is, however, as a cause of brain dysfunction that hypoglycaemia arouses most clinical interest, especially as it may occasionally be the only pointer to the ultimately correct (i.e. aetiological) diagnosis of the patient's underlying disease.

Far and away the most common cause of hypogly-caemia encountered in clinical practice is that caused by overtreatment of diabetes with insulin, or rarely, sulphonylureas. This is usually referred to as 'iatro-genic' to distinguish it from 'spontaneous' hypoglycae-mia, which is always secondary to an underlying disease whose involvement in the causation of hy-poglycaemia is not necessarily immediately apparent. An aetiological classification listing the best recog-nized causes of hypoglycaemia is given in Table 39.1. Two clinical classifications are given in Tables 39.2 and 39.3.

Symptoms

Hypoglycaemia is arbitrarily defined as a plasma glucose concentration below 2.5 mmol/L (45 mg/100 mL) or blood glucose of 2.2 mmol/L (40 mg/100 mL). It is often associated with symptoms but not invariably. When they do occur, symptoms are always the result of activation of the nervous system, i.e. they are neuroglycopenic in origin (literally 'short-age of glucose in the neurons'), although some of the more flagrant are mediated through the sympathetic nervous system. As a result they are sometimes referred to as adrenergic rather than as neuro-glycopenic.

Three more or less distinct, but not mutually exclu-sive, neuroglycopenic syndromes can be recognized:

1. Acute neuroglycopenia is the most common of the four syndromes and results from the rapid onset of hypoglycaemia. It begins with a vague sense of ill

TABLE 39.2

CLASSIFICATION OF HYPOGLYCAEMIA ACCORDING TO THE CIRCUMSTANCES OF ITS DEVELOPMENT

A. *Fasting hypoglycaemia*

Inappropriate insulin secretion due to benign, malignant or multiple insulinomas; microadenomatosis and nesidioblastosis

Non-pancreatic IGF-II-secreting tumours

Liver and kidney failure

Endocrine diseases: pituitary, adrenal, hypothalamic, etc.

Liver glycogen disease and other inborn errors of metabolism

Starvation or substrate limitation

Autoimmunity

B. *Stimulative hypoglycaemia*

Exogenous hypoglycaemic agents; drugs and poisons

Reactive hypoglycaemias

Hereditary fructose intolerance (HFI)

Galactosaemia

Alcohol-induced (a) 'fasting' and (b) 'reactive' hypoglycaemia

TABLE 39.3

CLASSIFICATIONS OF HYPOGLYCAEMIA ACCORDING TO ITS NATURE

Fasting	v.	Stimulated
Ketotic	v.	Non-ketotic
Drug-induced	v.	'Spontaneous'
Epiphenomenon	v.	Major feature of illness
Physiological	v.	Pathological

health, often accompanied by feelings of anxiety, panic and unnaturalness. Palpitations and restlessness are common. Objectively, there may be tachycardia, facial flushing, sweating, slurring of speech and unsteadiness of gait. These signs and symptoms are transient, usually lasting only a few minutes. All except sweating, which is often exaggerated, are attenuated by pretreatment with non-selective β-adrenergic blocking agents. Untreated, the symptoms of acute neuroglycopenia usually improve as the blood glucose concentration rises spontaneously under the influence of counterregulatory homeostatic mechanisms. Rarely, however, they may progress to produce alterations of consciousness, stupor and eventually coma. These symptoms, like those that precede them, can be rapidly and completely reversed by oral and intravenous glucose. Acute neuroglycopenia is associated with an abrupt rise in the plasma concentration of many hormones such as adrenaline and noradrenaline, growth hormone, prolactin, vasopressin, glucagon, ACTH and cortisol. Measurement of the urinary cortisol:creatinine ratio may reveal a marked rise in an early morning urine sample in patients who have experienced silent nocturnal hypoglycaemia.

2. Subacute neuroglycopenia is the most common type of hypoglycaemia encountered in patients suffering from spontaneous hypoglycaemia. It results from a gradual fall in blood glucose concentration over a period of an hour or more. The florid signs and symptoms of acute neuroglycopenia are lacking. Instead there is a general reduction of spontaneous activity, and conversation and movement become minimal. Sleepiness is an early feature, but consciousness is retained until late. Behaviour patterns resembling mild alcoholic intoxication are common and even habitual tasks are performed poorly. Subjectively, discomfort is minimal for the degree of functional impairment. Most episodes abort spontaneously under the influence of counterregulatory homeostatic mechanisms; plasma hormone levels rarely rise to anything like the same extent as during acute neuroglycopenia and are often completely normal.

3. Chronic neuroglycopenia is extremely rare. It is generally only diagnosed after clinical biochemical investigations have revealed the presence of more or less unrelieved hypoglycaemia in a patient who would otherwise have been diagnosed as suffering from dementia, hysteria, depression, schizophrenia or even brain tumour.

Pathogenesis

Hypoglycaemia is the result of a greater outflow of glucose from the glucose pool than inflow from either the liver alone (during fasting) or the gut and liver combined, such as occur during, and for a variable period after, the ingestion of a meal. The constant drain put upon the glucose pool by the insulin in dependent utilization of glucose by the brain and other tissues requires release by the liver during fasting of roughly 8.5 g of glucose per hour for a typical 70-kg man. Glucose released from the liver comes partly from glycogen made from glucose taken up by the liver and stored during the absorptive phase of a meal, but mainly from new glucose molecules made by gluconeogenesis.

Interference with either glycogen breakdown or gluconeogenesis can lead to hypoglycaemia developing in the fasting state. Although increased glucose uptake by tissues such as muscle, skin and connective tissue, which do not ordinarily remove glucose from the glucose pool in the fasting state, is also a possible cause of fasting hypoglycaemia, it is rare except as a consequence of insulin overdosage and very rare cases of exercise-induced hypoglycaemia.

Under conditions of normal glucose homeostasis, insulin secretion drops almost to zero as the arterial blood glucose level falls to overnight fasting values following its temporary rise after the ingestion of a carbohydrate-containing meal. This diminution in insulin secretion has the dual effect of releasing the liver from the inhibition of glycogenolysis and gluconeogenesis that high concentrations of insulin in the portal blood impose upon it, and of reducing the peripheral glucose uptake by insulin-indendent tissues. Reduction of inhibitory effects of insulin upon lipolysis in adipocytes in the fat depots is attended by an increase in the amount of glycerol and free fatty acids (NEFA) that are released into the circulation. In the liver the glycerol is converted into glucose by the gluconeogenic pathway and the NEFA are converted into the so-called ketone bodies, that is acetoacetate and β-hydroxybutyrate, which can be utilized as fuel by most tissues of the body.

It is therefore possible to classify hypoglycaemia into a ketotic variety, in which the cause is unrelated to increased insulin, or more correctly, insulin-like action, and a non-ketotic variety in which there is an increase in insulin or insulin-like activity, and which is associated with a depression of both plasma glucose and plasma ketone levels.

The classification of hypoglycaemia into ketotic and non-ketotic varieties is clinically useful and comparatively easy now that plasma β-hydroxybutyrate measurements are so readily available. Another clinically useful classification is into fasting and stimulative (often called reactive) hypoglycaemia. The latter type of hypoglycaemia is characterized by its complete failure to develop in response to fasting no matter how long it is continued.

FASTING HYPOGLYCAEMIA

The main clinical categories of fasting hypoglycaemia are outlined in the following subsections.

Insulinoma

Inappropriate insulin release by tumours made up of typical, or sometimes atypical, β-cells of the endocrine pancreas is amongst the most important causes of hypoglycaemia, as this is usually their sole clinical manifestation. The tumours are generally small, less than 1 cm in diameter, benign, and confined to the pancreas. They occur with slightly greater frequency in women than in men, in a ratio of 6:4, and at a rate of about 1 case per million of the population per year. Symptoms of subacute neuroglycopenia typically occur in the morning before the patient rises, but they can occur at any time of the day. A careful history often reveals the occurrence, for some time before the patient requests investigation, of 'strange turns' during periods of unusually strenuous exercise, abstinence from food or in response to the ingestion of a meal. About 10% of insulin-secreting tumours are malignant, and a further 10% are either multiple, or occur as part of the multiple endocrine neoplasia I (MEN-I) syndrome. The biochemical hallmark of an insulinoma is its failure to suppress the release of insulin into the blood as the blood glucose concentration falls first to normal fasting, and then

to hypoglycaemic, levels. In other words, it is the inappropriate, rather than the excessive, secretion of insulin in the presence of hypoglycaemia—which is itself the result of continued insulin action—that is the characteristic laboratory finding by which insulinomas can be identified and diagnosed. Whilst tumorous β-cells may respond abnormally or excessively to various stimuli to insulin secretion, the results are too unpredictable to provide clinically useful information.

It is difficult, if not impossible, to distinguish the anatomical causes of hyperinsulinism resulting from abnormal β-cell function with any degree of certainty before surgical exploration. Nevertheless, because of their great numerical preponderance, insulinomas can be looked upon as being solitary, benign and present somewhere within the pancreatic substance until proven otherwise. Diagnosis is made on the basis of the demonstration of Whipple's triad—that is, the presence of a fasting blood glucose level of 2.2 mmol/L or less (plasma glucose 2.5 mmol/L) which is associated with symptoms of cerebral dysfunction that are relieved specifically by intravenous glucose; together with evidence of inappropriate insulin secretion—that is, inappropriately high plasma insulin, C-peptide and proinsulin levels in peripheral venous blood in the presence of hypoglycaemia.

Non-insulin-secreting Tumours

It has been recognized for almost as long as the history of hypoglycaemia itself that certain tumours apart from those capable of secreting insulin can, and sometimes do, produce hypoglycaemia as their most important clinical manifestation. Many of these tumours are very large but their presence may be unsuspected until hypoglycaemia makes thorough clinical investigation necessary. These tumours do not have any single histological characteristic or site of origin that distinguishes them from other tumours. Many, but not all, are malignant. The most common are fibromas and fibrosarcomas, haemangiopericytomas and primary hepatic carcinomas, but no type of tissue is exempt. The cause of the hypoglycaemia was until comparatively recently a complete mystery, but was known not to involve abnormal insulin secretion. Indeed insulin, C-peptide and proinsulin secretion is completely suppressed during hypoglycaemia. Nevertheless, clinically there is evidence of increased insulin-like action.

Advances in molecular biology have shown that many, if not all, of these tumours overproduce insulin-like growth factor II (IGF-II), which can under some circumstances exert insulin-like actions on the liver and peripheral tissues. It does this by cross-reacting with insulin receptors for which both it and IGF-I have a low affinity.

IGF-I and IGF-II ordinarily circulate in the blood at molar concentrations many hundreds of times greater than insulin itself. They are however completely and tightly bound to specific IGF-binding proteins (IGF-BP). The most important of these is, like IGF-I, produced in the liver under the influence of pituitary growth hormone. The sequence of events currently thought to account for production of hypoglycaemia by non-insulin-secreting tumours is as follows.

Overproduction of IGF-II by the tumour produces a rise in plasma IGF-II, most or all of which is bound to IGF-BP, thereby rendering it non-insulin like as far as hypoglycaemia is concerned. Nevertheless, the IGF-II does appear to inhibit growth-hormone release. As a result the hepatic production of IGF-II, and also of IGF-I itself, is reduced. When IGF-BP levels levels fall so low as to no longer be able to bind all of the IGF-II released by the tumour, an increasingly large amount of IGF-II becomes available free in the plasma to bind with insulin receptors on the liver and peripheral tissue cell surfaces. There it exerts an insulin-like action and hypoglycaemia results, probably by a combination of inhibition of hepatic glucose release and an increase in peripheral glucose uptake. Lipolysis is also inhibited as a result of the insulin-like action. Consequently plasma ketone levels are depressed, thus mimicking insulinoma. This, coupled with the finding of low plasma insulin, C-peptide and proinsulin levels, very low IGF-I and either normal or only moderately raised IGF-II levels, is virtually pathognomonic of non-islet cell tumour hypoglycaemia (NICTH).

Inborn Errors of Metabolism

Hypoglycaemia is an important feature of many inborn errors of metabolism in some of which—the liver glycogen-storage diseases, defects in gluconeogenesis and those associated with abnormalities of fatty acid metabolism for example—it may be the presenting abnormality.

Autoimmune Hypoglycaemia

This comes in three main categories. All are very rare. It is, nevertheless, said that the condition characterized by autoimmune antibodies to insulin is one of the most common causes of clinically important reactive hypoglycaemia occurring in Japan, where it was first recognized and still accounts for the majority of published cases.

Insulin-receptor Autoantibodies
The best understood type of autoimmune hypoglycaemia is that caused by stimulatory insulin-receptor autoantibodies. These react with insulin receptors, mimicking some of the biological effects of insulin itself. Thus not only are blood glucose and plasma ketone levels low, but so too are plasma insulin and C-peptide levels. Antibodies directed specifically against insulin receptors can be found if looked for, but this is still a research procedure. Hypoglycaemia

of this type is secondary to a number of different diseases, of which discoid lupus erythematosus and lymphoma are possibly the best known.

B-Cell-stimulating Autoantibodies (Pancreatic Graves' Disease)
The second type of autoimmune hypoglycaemia has been dubbed 'pancreatic Graves' disease' and is caused by stimulatory B-cell autoantibodies, which stimulate inappropriate insulin, C-peptide and proinsulin secretion just as stimulatory thyroid autoantibodies do in the thyroid. Only a very few examples of this condition have so far been described.

Insulin Autoimmune Syndrome
The third, and most common, type of autoimmune hypoglycaemia is that due to the presence of autoantibodies to insulin itself. This condition presents as a reactive rather than fasting hypoglycaemia and will be dealt with later under that heading.

REACTIVE HYPOGLYCAEMIA

Most clinically important types of hypoglycaemia, except that produced iatrogenically, develop in fasting subjects; nevertheless a temporary imbalance of glucose inflow and outflow from the glucose pool can sometimes occur. This may lead to a short-lived period of hypoglycaemia, which, in rare cases, may be sufficiently profound and prolonged to produce symptoms of acute neuroglycopenia. This situation is often referred to as 'reactive' hypoglycaemia—that is, a condition in which hypoglycaemia is a reaction to preceding hyperglycaemia. It can be produced experimentally in many perfectly normal healthy people by giving them a glucose drink on an empty stomach. In general the larger the dose (e.g. 100–150 g) the more likely reactive hypoglycaemia is to develop.

Reactive hypoglycaemia can also occur spontaneously in response to the ingestion of carbohydrate-rich meals or drinks containing large amounts of sugar, especially when these are combined with alcohol.

Reactive hypoglycaemia is a comparatively common occurrence in people with diseases that cause fasting hypoglycaemia. It also occurs, very rarely, in patients in whom the only identifiable causes are accelerated gastric emptying or increased cerebral sensitivity to a modest lowering of blood glucose concentration. Individuals in whom this occurs are often referred to as suffering from 'primary' or 'essential reactive' hypoglycaemia, which was once thought to be very common. It is now recognized, however, that this impression was a mistake and due to misunderstanding of the diagnostic limitations of the prolonged oral glucose load test. This is especially so when, as is often the case, venous rather than capillary or arterial blood was sampled.

Insulin Autoimmune Syndrome

This typically presents as a type of reactive hypoglycaemia and is caused by the gradual release of insulin from the circulating insulin autoantibody to which it is bound in the plasma. It is suggested that in this condition, insulin is released from the pancreas in response to the ingestion of food, but is prevented from exerting its full hypoglycaemic effect as a consequence of being bound to circulating autoantibodies to insulin. As a result there is a temporary hyperglycaemia following ingestion of a meal and more insulin is released from the pancreas than is strictly necessary to assimilate all of the nutrients that have been absorbed. There is, however, a residual store of insulin in the plasma in the form of antibody-bound insulin, which is released slowly into the circulation long after the stimulus to insulin secretion has gone, and at a time when insulin action would ordinarily be very low. The hallmark of this type of hypoglycaemia is high circulating levels of both insulin and insulin autoantibodies (which also interfere with insulin immunoassays, making accurate measurement extremely difficult). C-peptide levels are usually normal or high, especially if there are autoantibodies to C-peptide and/or proinsulin present as well as autoantibodies to insulin itself.

Alcohol-induced Reactive Hypoglycaemia

The ingestion of modest amounts of alcohol (e.g. 50 g) with a similarly modest amount of sugar (e.g. 50 g) on an empty stomach may stimulate more insulin secretion than ingestion of the sugar alone. The resulting hyperinsulinaemia may produce a much greater hypoglycaemic rebound than is customary and lead to marked neuroglycopenic symptoms.

DIAGNOSIS

Hypoglycaemia is merely a description of the blood glucose concentration. If it can be established as the cause of a patient's symptoms the clinician is committed to identifying the aetiology, as this determines the nature of the appropriate treatment. Conceptually, hypoglycaemia must be distinguished from neuroglycopenia, which, though usually caused by hypoglycaemia, is not necessarily so. Glucose does not pass passively from the blood into the neurons. It must first traverse the hypothetical blood–brain barrier, a major constituent of which is the specific plasma-membrane bound glucose transporter that conveys glucose from the extracellular to the intracellular fluid. There is evidence that the efficiency and capacity of this transportation can vary not only from one individual to another on a genetic basis but in the same individual from time to time depending, amongst other things, upon the normally prevailing or habitual glucose concentration in the extracellular fluid. Consequently it is possible to have genuine neuroglycopenia in the presence of normoglycaemia if transportation of glucose from outside to inside the neurons drops below the critical level, just as it is possible to have hypoglycaemia without neuroglycopenia.

Confirmation of Hypoglycaemia

There is nothing specific about the symptoms caused by hypoglycaemia except their relief by intravenous glucose. The diagnosis must, therefore, be made by establishing the presence of hypoglycaemia, defined as a blood glucose concentration of 2.2 mmol/L or less, during symptomatic episodes. In the past this often proved difficult, if not impossible, because admission to hospital for observation often produced complete remission from symptoms unless the patient was fasted for 72 h or more. It is a comparatively simple matter to teach the close family or friends, or even patients themselves, how to collect blood during spontaneous symptomatic episodes. Finger-prick blood is collected on to a properly prepared piece of filter paper or into a sodium fluoride-containing capillary tube, for accurate measurement of glucose content in a clinical laboratory. Glucose oxidase-impregnated glucose test strips designed for self-monitoring of diabetes should not be used for this purpose, as they are notoriously inaccurate in the hypoglycaemic range.

A blood glucose concentration of 4.0 mmol/L at the beginning, or early in the course of, a typical spontaneous symptomatic episode virtually rules out hypoglycaemia, and one of 2.5 mmol/L or less makes it almost certain. Intermediate values make confirmation or exclusion of hypoglycaemia as the cause of symptoms imperative before the initiation of tests designed to determine its aetiology. Most illnesses causing spontaneous hypoglycaemia do so after a comparatively short period of food deprivation, though often under these circumstances it is unaccompanied by symptoms. Blood collected after an overnight fast of 12 h or more will, provided that the test is repeated on three or more occasions, reveal hypoglycaemia in over 90% of insulinoma patients and those suffering from most other endocrine and metabolic causes of hypoglycaemia.

If clinical suspicion of hypoglycaemia is high but symptomatic episodes are infrequent—as is often the case—and overnight fasting hypoglycaemia cannot be demonstrated, it may be necessary to attempt to provoke hypoglycaemia by mimicking the conditions under which spontaneous attacks are said to occur. Clues as to precipitating causes may emerge only after a thorough history has been taken. Not only the patient, but also their relatives or friends, should be questioned as they frequently observe spontaneous attacks of which the patient has little or no recollection.

Provocative Tests

The Prolonged Fast Test

This has been considered the 'gold standard' for confirmation of fasting hypoglycaemia but is not specific for any particular disease. The patient is admitted to hospital and given nothing to eat except water, unsweetened tea or coffee (to prevent caffeine withdrawal symptoms complicating the issue) for up to 72 h. The test is continued, unless symptomatic hypoglycaemia with a recorded blood glucose concentration of 2.2 mmol/L or less (except in subjects over the age of 60, when the figure of 3.0 mmol/L is acceptable) and accompanied by characteristic electroencephalographic (EEG) changes makes earlier termination essential. The patient must not be confined to bed but should be encouraged to be moderately active whilst under supervision. Blood should be collected at frequent intervals throughout the day and night for glucose measurements, whether or not overt symptoms are present. Plasma hormone levels need only be measured if hypoglycaemia develops. Less than 1% of all patients subsequently shown to be harbouring an insulinoma fail to become hypoglycaemic under these conditions.

Asymptomatic hypoglycaemia with blood glucose levels as low as 1.5 mmol/L is said to be comparatively common in young and middle-aged women subjected to the 72-h fast, but EEG changes are not seen, plasma β-hydroxybutyrate levels rise to 1.0 mmol/L or more, and plasma insulin, proinsulin and C-peptide levels are appropriately depressed.

The Rigorous Exercise Test

The patient is brought to the Clinical Investigation Unit after an overnight fast and exercised on a treadmill or stationary bicycle until they are no longer able or willing to continue. Blood is collected and analysed for glucose, β-hydroxybutyrate and hormone content before and at 5- to 10-min intervals throughout the exercise period. Blood glucose levels can rise, fall or remain normal in healthy subjects but do not appear to influence performance. In patients with certain types of fasting hypoglycaemia, including insulinoma, blood glucose levels fall and are accompanied by neuroglycopenia symptoms and fatigue. In healthy subjects and patients with illnesses other than endogenous hyperinsulinism, plasma immunoreactive insulin (IRI) and C-peptide levels fall during rigorous exercise regardless of what happens to the blood sugar level. In patients with endogenous hyperinsulinism, plasma IRI and C-peptide levels generally do not fall below 30 and 300 pmol/L, respectively. Sufficient evidence has not yet accumulated to say with certainty how sensitive this test is, but it seems to be at least as reliable as the prolonged fast test, which requires the admission of the patient to hospital, and the intravenous tolbutamide tolerance test, whose main function is to exclude the presence of an insulinoma in a patient in whom a diagnosis of 'hypoglycaemia' had previously been made.

The C-peptide Suppression Test

Despite earlier promise, this test is of limited value because it can neither be used as a screening test for hypoglycaemia, nor as a means of excluding or confirming a diagnosis of insulinoma. It relies upon the fact that during hypoglycaemia induced by exogenous insulin (0.1 unit/kg body weight given by subcutaneous injection), plasma C-peptide levels are suppressed to below 1 μg/L (300 pmol/L) except in patients with autonomous insulin-secreting tumours. The test does, however, have an unacceptably high incidence of both false-positive and false-negative responses, such as to make it little more than an ancillary procedure. Its main use is as an early indicator of recurrence of hyperinsulinism following resection of an apparently solitary benign or malignant insulinoma.

Meal Provocation Test

Patients with the postprandial syndrome are often suspected, on the basis of an erroneous interpretation of the prolonged oral glucose load test, of suffering from meal-induced or 'essential' reactive hypoglycaemia. This diagnosis can generally be excluded by the results of ambulatory blood-glucose testing as described above. It may, however, sometimes be necessary to subject the patient to formal provocation by giving them a standard meal and observing the symptomatic, blood glucose and hormone responses to it. Only if the symptomatic disturbance (if any) is accompanied by a fall in capillary or arterial blood glucose to below 2.2 mmol/L is the first stage in the diagnosis of hypoglycaemia justified. Occasionally the coingestion of alcohol in the form of gin and tonic, with or without a starchy snack, can precipitate hypoglycaemia in susceptible subjects. It can be tested for experimentally by giving the patient 50 g of alcohol with 50 g sucrose in the form of gin and tonic on an empty stomach and collecting blood for glucose and hormone analysis for the next 4–5 h.

Other Provocative Tests

Many other tests including the 5-h oral glucose load test, intravenous tolbutamide tolerance, intravenous insulin tolerance, calcium infusion, leucine and glucagon tests, have been used in the past—either to establish hypoglycaemia as the cause of the patient's symptoms or to ascertain its aetiology—but have now largely or wholly been superseded by more clinically useful procedures. Only the extended oral glucose test will be described here, because it is so beloved by clinicians, despite having been shown to be virtually worthless for diagnostic purposes.

The Prolonged Oral Glucose Test.

This is really a research rather than a clinical tool, and has been grossly misused in the past by those who did not appreciate its limitations.

The test itself is normally made after an overnight fast. The result is markedly affected by preceding diet and the patient should have been consuming at least 200 g carbohydrate per day for 3 days or more before the test is carried out. Since many of the people in whom a diagnosis of hypoglycaemia is suspected have already made the diagnosis on themselves and begun taking a low-carbohydrate diet as advocated in many of the lay articles on this subject, attention to the dietary history is unusually important. Low-carbohydrate feeding may lead to temporary glucose intolerance and exaggerated hypoglycaemic rebound in response to oral glucose load. In this way, a self-diagnosis of 'reactive hypoglycaemia' may become a self-fulfilling prophecy.

'Arterialized' venous blood from the back of the hand (or alternatively, capillary—but not ordinarily antecubital fossa venous—blood) is collected before and at half-hourly intervals for 5–6 h. At zero time a solution containing 100 g of hydrolysed starch (glucose) is drunk over the course of about 15 min. Only if neuroglycopenic symptoms accompanied by a fall in arterialized (or capillary) blood glucose to, or below, 2.2 mmol/L are observed can the test be considered as even suggestive of genuine reactive hypoglycaemia worthy of further investigation. This must be done to determine whether reactive hypoglycaemia occurring in the course of ordinary life is the cause—or more likely not the cause—of the patient's spontaneous symptoms. In order to do this one must measure glucose in blood collected during a 'spontaneous' attack or during the performance of a 'meal provocation test'. This is a test in which a proper meal is substituted for hydrolysed starch in the prolonged oral glucose test.

Differential Diagnosis of Hypoglycaemia

The differential diagnosis of hypoglycaemia, once the first stage has been passed, is usually suggested by the circumstances under which the hypoglycaemia occurs, and the associated physical findings, if any. Knowledge of the most important causes of spontaneous hypoglycaemia, none of which is common, is essential if opportunities to carry out the most appropriate tests are not to be irrevocably lost. This is particularly true of ephemeral or non-recurrent causes of spontaneous hypoglycaemia such as septicaemia, congestive cardiac failure, alcoholic and other types of drug-induced hypoglycaemia, where collection of appropriate specimens at the time of the patient's presentation and their subsequent analysis often provides the only opportunity of making the correct aetiological diagnosis.

Plasma and Urinary Ketones

Plasma ketone measurements are easily made and are more informative than semiquantitative urinary assays. They are, like plasma pancreatic-hormone measurements, only of diagnostic value if done on samples collected whilst the subject is hypoglycaemic. In adults as in children, hypoglycaemia can usefully be subdivided into non-ketotic varieties in which, despite hypoglycaemia, plasma β-hydroxybutyrate levels are below 0.6 mmol/L, and ketotic varieties in which values of over 1.0 mmol/L are the rule. Non-ketotic hypoglycaemia is characteristic of endogenous or exogenous hyperinsulinism; hypoglycaemia secondary to IGF-1-secreting tumours, starvation or liver failure.

Plasma Pancreatic Hormone Measurements

Plasma immunoreactive insulin (IRI), C-peptide and proinsulin assays made on blood collected whilst the patient is hypoglycaemic are often of crucial importance in arriving at the correct differential diagnosis of spontaneous fasting hypoglycaemia. In all conditions causing spontaneous hypoglycaemia except endogenous hyperinsulinism due to insulinoma, nesidioblastosis or sulphonylurea overdosage, all three hormones are appropriately low in peripheral venous blood collected whilst the patient is hypoglycaemic. In most, but not all, cases of endogenous hyperinsulinism, both C-peptide and IRI are inappropriately high, though often not above the misnamed 'normal range' for fasting plasma levels. The so-called glucose/insulin ratio, expressed as a number, has in the author's view no role in the diagnosis of hypoglycaemia, any more than most derived values or ratios. In the absence of coexisting hypoglycaemia, plasma IRI and/or C-peptide measurements are extremely difficult if not impossible to interpret. High plasma proinsulin levels, on the other hand, are invariably pathological and are currently probably the single most specific and sensitive indicator of insulinoma.

Inappropriately high plasma IRI and C-peptide levels in the presence of normal or only slightly raised plasma proinsulin levels are suggestive of nesidioblastosis or sulphonylurea poisoning, whilst high plasma IRI and low or undetectable C-peptide and/or proinsulin levels are pathognomonic of exogenous insulin poisoning. Hypoketonaemic hypoglycaemia—in association with low plasma IRI, C-peptide and proinsulin levels—is highly suggestive of tumour-induced hypoglycaemia. This diagnosis can be considered established if the plasma concentration of IGF-2 is normal or high, and that of IGF-1 is low.

Other Tests

Tests designed specifically to investigate particular functions of other endocrine organs may be necessary should a definitive diagnosis not otherwise be possible. They are suggested by clinical or laboratory evidence of the various hypoglycaemia-producing endocrinopathies—hypopituitarism, Addison's disease, ACTH and/or growth-hormone deficiency for example. Neither glucagon nor adrenaline deficiencies are recognized causes of hypoglycaemia, and their measurement in plasma currently adds nothing to the diagnostic process. The analysis of plasma for alcohol and drugs (e.g. sulphonylureas) is indicated in some cases of seemingly spontaneous hypoglycaemia, but must generally be done on blood samples collected whilst the patient was spontaneously hypoglycaemic—that is, at presentation—if the results are to have any diagnostic value.

FURTHER READING

Field J.B. ed. (1989). *Hypoglycemia, Endocrinology and Metabolism Clinics of North America*, vol. 18(1), Philadelphia: Saunders.

Marks V., Rose F.C. (1981). *Hypoglycaemia*, 2nd edn, Oxford: Blackwell Scientific.

Service F.J. ed. (1983). *Hypoglycemic Disorders: Pathogenesis, Diagnosis and Treatment*, Boston, MA: G.K. Hall.

Service F.J. (1989). Hypoglycemia and the postprandial syndrome. *N. Engl. J. Med.*, **321**, 1472.

Snorgaard O., Binder C. (1990). Monitoring of blood glucose concentration in subjects with hypoglycaemic symptoms during everyday life. *Br. Med. J.*, **300**, 16.

Teale J.D., Marks V. (1990). Inappropriately elevated plasma insulin-like growth factor II in relation to suppressed insulin-like growth factor I in the diagnosis of non-islet cell tumour hypoglycaemia. *Clin. Endocrinology*, **33**, 87.

40. Gastrointestinal Hormones

V. Marks

Introduction
Physiology and pathophysiology
  Entero-insular axis
  Gastric inhibitory polypeptide
  Glucagon and glucagon-like peptides
  Gastrin
  Secretin
  Vasoactive intestinal polypeptide
  Pancreozymin–cholecystakinin (PZ–CK)
  Somatostatin
  Mixed and carcinoid tumours
  Other hormones

INTRODUCTION

The gastrointestinal (GI) tract is far from being an impassive barrier between the exterior and interior of the body with the sole function of facilitating transport of nutrients from the food into the body. It is instead the largest, and possibly the most complicated, of all the endocrine organs of the body. Indeed the term 'hormone' was coined by Bayliss and Starling in 1902 to describe the action of secretin—a product of the duodenum and small intestine—on pancreatic secretion. The study of GI hormones was, however, subsequently largely neglected and emphasis was instead given mainly to the neural regulation of intestinal secretion and mobility, its two most important physiological activities apart from the digestion and absorption of food and drink.

It has only been in the past 25 years or so that the GI tract itself, as opposed to the pancreas, has been accepted as a major endocrine organ worthy of study by endocrinologists and clinical biochemists. The upsurge of interest was largely due to the development of various techniques in peptide chemistry, in particular the introduction of immunoassay techniques, simplified procedures for isolating, sequencing and synthesizing polypeptides, and advances in DNA technology and molecular biology.

With the notable exception of 5-hydroxytryptamine (serotonin), the hormonal role of which has still not been unequivocally established, all of the gut hormones characterized (including those produced mainly or exclusively by the pancreas) are polypeptides of varying size and heterogeneity. They are produced by cells that possess a common set of cytochemical and ultrastructural characteristics, which have led to them being designated by Pearse as APUD cells from their capacity for *A*mine-*P*recursor *U*ptake and/or *D*ecarboxylation.

Many distinct endocrine-type cells have now been identified and are classified on an ultrastructural, histochemical and, increasingly, immunohistological basis. Typically, apart from those that occur clumped together in functional units in the pancreas as islets of Langerhans, they are scattered singly between the gut mucosal cells and are elongated with apical processes reaching and penetrating into the gut lumen; specific secretory granules are generally stored in the basal or serosal part of the cell.

The number of biologically active polypeptides that have either been isolated from the gut or at least partially characterized on the basis of their pharmacological effects is now very large. Only a small number have so far been shown to have clinical relevance, however, and even the physiological significance of most of them is unknown.

There is currently a widespread belief that many of the so-called GI hormones are, in effect, more akin to neurotransmitters than to traditional hormones and that they exert their influence mainly upon adjacent or nearby cells (i.e. they have a paracrine action) rather than on those at a distance. With a few notable exceptions, i.e. insulin, secretin, gastric inhibitory polypeptide (GIP), glucagon and peptide YY (PYY), most of the gut hormones are found in equal or greater concentrations in the brain. They are therefore increasingly often referred to as regulatory peptides rather than as GI hormones. Insulin, glucagon and pancreatic polypeptide are generally considered as GI hormones even though they are, at least in man, produced exclusively in the pancreas.

All of the GI hormones that have been characterized are (with the exception of insulin) single-chain polypeptides with molecular weights under 5000. All, except gastrin and cholecystokinin (CK), are basic in character. The primary and even tertiary structures of some of the GI hormones resemble each other sufficiently closely to justify grouping them together as 'families' with overlapping pharmacological and possibly even physiological functions. Members of a hormone family are thought to have evolved from a single gene or primitive precursor, which presumably had hormonal or neurotransmitter properties. The best characterized of the gut hormones and their family connections are briefly summarized in Table 40.1.

Most of the gut hormones circulate in a variety of molecular forms of different peptide-chain length and, consequently, slightly different biological, physicochemical and above all immunochemical forms. It seems probable that some of the variants represent hormone precursors and others circulating degradation products. From a diagnostic point of view this may be extremely important because, whereas the biological activities (and possibly the clinical significance) of the 'regular' hormone are generally known, the potencies of the other molecular forms are largely unknown; they may be more, equally or less biologically active than the native hormone. Nowhere is this seen more clearly than in the case of the newly discovered glucagon-like peptides.

TABLE 40.1
FAMILIES, DISTRIBUTION AND ACTIONS OF GUT HORMONES

Structural family	Members	Distribution	Main pharmacological actions
Gastrin/cholecystokinin	Gastrin	Antrum, duodenum	Stimulates gastric acid secretion; mucosal growth
	CK	Duodenum, jejunum	Stimulates pancreatic enzyme secretion
Pancreatic polypeptide	Pancreatic polypeptide	Islets of Langerhans	Inhibits pancreatic secretion
	Peptide YY	Jejunum, ileum	Inhibits gallbladder contraction
	Neuropeptide Y (NPY)	Gut/paraventricular nucleus	Stimulates appetite
Secretin	Secretin	Duodenum, jejunum	Stimulates pancreatic exocrine secretion
	GIP	Duodenum, jejunum	Stimulates insulin secretion, activates lipoprotein lipase
	VIP	Most of GI tract	Vasodilatation
Glucagon	Glucagon	Islets of Langerhans	Activates glycogenolysis
	GLP-1	Jejunum, ileum	
	GLP-1$_{(7-36)}$amide	Jejunum, ileum	Stimulates insulin secretion; lipogenesis
	GLP-2	Jejunum, ileum	
	Oxyntomodulin	Jejunum, ileum	
	Glicentin	Jejunum, ileum, pancreatic A-cells	
Endorphins	Enkephalins	Stomach, duodenum	Reduces transit time
	β-endorphin	Stomach, duodenum, jejunum	Reduces transit time
Somatostatin		Most of gut; pancreatic δ-cells	Reduces secretion of many peptide hormones and pancreatic exocrine function; portal blood flow
Motilin	Motilin	Duodenum, jejunum	Initiates interdigestive migrating motor complex
Insulin	Insulin	Islets of Langerhans	Stimulates glycogenolysis, lipolysis and glucose uptake

GIP, gastric inhibitory peptide; GLP, glucogen-like peptide; VIP, vasoactive intestinal polypeptide.

PHYSIOLOGY AND PATHOPHYSIOLOGY

Gut peptides can be divided into three functional categories: endocrine, paracrine and neural or neurocrine, reflecting their cellular relations and mode of delivery to target cells. The best recognized physiological functions are:

- regulation of gastric acid secretion;
- control of exocrine pancreatic and gallbladder function;
- control of metabolism of absorbed nutrients, either by direct or indirect action through the endocrine pancreas (the enteroinsular axis);
- control of gut motility.

The account given below includes consideration of hormone-secreting GI tumours (Table 40.2).

Enteroinsular Axis

The discovery that glucose given by mouth to healthy human subjects produces a much greater release of insulin into the circulation than an equivalent amount given intravenously has led to an intensive search for the mechanisms involved, but with only partial success. It was early concluded that the main, if not exclusive, mechanism was the release from the gut of one or more humorally active agents, which, in conjunction with the mild hyperglycaemia resulting from the absorption of glucose from the gut, stimulated the secretion of insulin by the pancreatic islet β-cells. The role of the autonomic nervous system in augmenting the insulinotropic effect of hyperglycaemia was initially considered to be insignificant, though more recent evidence suggests that this might not be the case. Indeed, current evidence suggests that demedullated nerve fibres innervating the islets via the vagus have an important role in the regulation of insulin secretion.

Many candidates have been put forward from amongst the GI polypeptide hormones as the main factor in mediating intestinal stimulation of insulin release, but none fits the bill completely. The leading contender at present is undoubtedly GIP, but glucagon-like polypeptide (GLP), secretin and vasoactive intestinal polypeptide (VIP) have all been proposed at one time or another. Pancreozymin (PZ–CK) has been considered to play an important part in the enhancement of insulin secretion consequent upon the ingestion of protein-rich meals but the case for it as an incretin remains unproven.

Dysfunction of the enteroinsular axis has been held responsible for certain abnormalities of glucose metabolism such as occur in type II diabetes (insulin-independent diabetes) and obesity, but evidence for this is still lacking. The enteroinsular axis does, however, provide a fruitful and important field of clinical biochemical research.

Gastric Inhibitory Polypeptide

The existence of a hormone with the ability to inhibit gastric acid secretion and delay gastric emptying and whose secretion was prompted by the ingestion of a fat-rich meal was postulated in 1930 by Kosaka and Lim. They named the hypothetical hormone entero-gastrone. In 1969, Brown and coworkers isolated a peptide with enterogastrone activity from a crude intestinal extract and named it gastric inhibitory polypeptide (GIP), the acronym by which it is now better known. Its amino-acid sequence has been determined and its N-terminal end bears a close resemblance to glucagon and secretin. The C-terminal amino-acid sequence, however, has no similarity to any other known intestinal polypeptide.

Regular GIP consists of 42 amino acids, and has a molecular weight of roughly 5000. There is, however, evidence of a larger variant of immunoreactive GIP of about 8000 mol. wt., whose physiology may or may not be different from that of the smaller variety and about which virtually nothing is known at the present time.

GIP-immunoreactive cells are localized mainly in the duodenum and upper jejunum, and to a much lesser extent in the lower bowel.

Interest in GIP initially centred exclusively upon its ability to affect gastric acid secretion and the rate of gastric emptying but this all changed when it was found to have extremely potent insulin-stimulatory properties that only become evident in the presence of mild to moderate hyperglycaemia. This, coupled with the fact that secretion of GIP follows the ingestion and absorption of all the major nutrients, led to its proposal as the main contender for the role of humoral mediator of enteroinsular stimulation—a position it still occupies, though less certainly than once seemed likely—and its renaming as glucose-mediated insulin-releasing polypeptide retaining the same acronym (GIP).

Whilst it seems probable, on circumstantial evidence, that abnormalities of GIP secretion are implicated in the pathogenesis of certain metabolic diseases such as obesity, no completely convincing evidence has yet been produced in support of this proposition, despite much searching. Currently, therefore, there are no clinical indications for measuring plasma GIP concentrations, even though its interest to researchers in GI and metabolic pathology is undiminished.

Glucagon and Glucagon-like Peptides

Glucagon was named for its ability to raise the blood glucose concentration when injected into fed animals. It was originally obtained as a contaminant of commercial insulin preparations and did not attract much attention from either biologists or clinicians until the mid-1950s when it was first characterized and synthesized.

Its main biological actions are the stimulation of gluconeogenesis and glycogenolysis in the liver, lipolysis in adipocytes, insulin secretion by the β-cells of the pancreas and inhibition of both gastric acid secretion and intestinal motility. Which, if any, of these actions is physiologically important in man is still unknown and there are no recognized ill consequences of glucagon deficiency such as occurs in patients who have undergone total pancreatectomy and receive adequate replacement therapy with insulin and pancreatic enzymes.

Although production of glucagon in man appears to be confined to the α-cells of the pancreas, it is produced by similar cells in the stomach in some species. A number of substances that share many of the immunological determinants of glucagon are, however, produced throughout the intestinal tract of man and other species.

The presence of glucagon-like peptides was foreseen through the ability of gut extracts to stimulate cyclic AMP in tissues in exactly the same way as pancreatic glucagon. It was soon shown that substances with similar but not identical properties to pancreatic glucagon could be found in gut extracts and that glucagon-like substances were released into the blood in response to the ingestion of some but not all nutrients.

As a result of advances in the molecular biology of the preproglucagon gene it became clear during the 1980s that whilst in the α-cells of the islets the main products of cleavage of preproglucagon are glucagon itself and a large glucagon-like fragment, this does not occur in the gut. Instead three glucagon-like peptides known as GLP-1, GLP-2 and GLP-$1_{(7-36)}$ amide are produced and secreted.

No function has yet been assigned to either GLP-I or GLP-2 though, after the discovery that GLP-$1_{(7-36)}$ amide is the most potent stimulus to insulin secretion yet, its role as an incretin has had to be considered. GLP-$1_{(7-36)}$ amide is released into the blood in response to ingestion of carbohydrate-containing meals and is therefore strongly suspected of playing an important part in the amplification of the stimulus to insulin secretion consequent upon eating a meal. The concentration in blood even after a large meal is, however, very low, especially in man. The methods of measurement are still poorly developed.

Nevertheless GLP-$1_{(7-36)}$ amide and GIP are currently considered to be the two main enteric limbs of the enteroinsular axis. It is also of some interest that these two hormones are, with insulin, almost the

TABLE 40.2
BIOLOGICAL AND CLINICAL FEATURES OF HORMONE-SECRETING TUMOURS OF THE GI TRACT

Feature	Glucagonoma	Gastrinoma	VIPoma	Somatostatinoma	Carcinoid
Signs and symptoms	Mild diabetes, skin rash, enlarged liver	Abdominal pain, diarrhoea, GI bleeding, epigastric tenderness, hepatomegaly	Profuse watery diarrhoea, flushing of skin	Hypoglycaemia or impaired glucose tolerance, hypochlorhydria, steatorrhoea, cholelithiasis	Flushing of skin, diarrhoea, oedema, heart lesions
Male:female ratio	10:90	60:40	25:75	1:2	50:50
Selective radiology	Coeliac axis arteriogram positive in < 50% of cases	Peptic ulcer, gastric mucosal hypertrophy	Coelic axis arteriogram positive in < 50% of cases	Coelic axis arteriogram positive in < 50% of cases	
Histopathology	Malignant, predominantly α-cell carcinoma	Malignant δ-cell tumour (60%), benign (20%), islet hyperplasia (20%)	'Non-β-cell' tumour (80%), islet hyperplasia (20%)	δ-cell tumour	Malignant carcinoid
Biochemistry	Mild hyperglycaemia, hyperinsulinaemia, hyperglucagonaemia	Resting gastrin hypersecretion and hyperacidity	Hypersecretion of VIP, hyperkalaemia, hypochlorhydria, hypercalcaemia (40%), impaired glucose tolerance	Hypochlorhydria, somatostatin elevated in portal or peripheral blood	Hypersecretion of 5-hydroxytryptamine (5-HT), raised urinary 5-hydroxyindoleacetic acid (5-HIAA)
Diagnosis	Inappropriately high plasma glucagon levels	Excessive gastric acid production and inappropriate hypergastrinaemia	High plasma VIP levels	Surgical exploration, raised plasma somatostatin	Raised plasma 5-HT, raised urinary 5-HIAA

VIP, vasoactive intestinal polypeptide.

only known stimulators of lipogenesis within adipocytes. GIP also stimulates lipoprotein lipase activity: thus the enteroinsular axis appears to be an important force for anabolism during times of plentiful food supplies and to have important survival value.

Glucagonoma

The syndrome of glucagon excess was first delineated in 1974. It usually presents as a dermatological problem in middle-aged or elderly women but also occurs in men. The most characteristic abnormality, apart from high fasting plasma glucagon concentrations, is a rare skin lesion known to dermatologists as necrolytic migratory erythema. Other common features of the syndrome are stomatitis, normochromic normocytic anaemia, weight loss, hypoalbuminaemia, psychiatric disturbances and a high rate of thromboembolic disease, the last named often being responsible for the patient's death. Diabetes is an inconstant feature and when present is usually mild. The disease has usually been present for a long time before the diagnosis of hyperglucagonaemia is suspected and

subsequently made by demonstrating elevated plasma glucagon concentrations in the presence of normoglycaemia or modest hyperglycaemia. This may merely reflect unfamiliarity with the syndrome and the difficulty, until recently, of obtaining confirmatory plasma glucagon assays. The causative lesion is almost invariably a malignant pancreatic endocrine tumour; this is only very occasionally resectable but, in those rare instances when it is, remission is both rapid and complete unless, and until, it recurs. Other treatments that have been tried with varying degrees of success include chemotherapy with somatostatin, streptozotocin and 5-fluorouracil, as well as thromboembolism of hepatic metastases.

No example of a GLP-1- or GLP-2-secreting tumour has yet been described but a renal carcinoma producing large amounts of a gut GLP has been reported. The most striking effect produced by this tumour was hypertrophy of intestinal mucosa, which led to the suggestion that at least one of the gut glucagon-like substances may have growth-promoting properties with respect to the intestinal mucosa.

Gastrin

An antral hormone capable of stimulating gastric acid secretion was first described by Edkins in 1905 but was not really characterized until some 60 years later when its structure was elucidated by Gregory and his coworkers in Liverpool. It was recognized from the very beginning that gastrin could exist in multiple forms. At the present time the unqualified term 'gastrin' is used to describe the 17 amino-acid polypeptide that may (gastrin II) or may not (gastrin I) be sulphated on the tyrosine in the 6-position (counting from the carboxy end); both forms are equally biologically active. Other forms in which gastrin occurs in the GI tract and circulation are referred to as 'big gastrin' (G34), 'minigastrin' (G14) and, according to some, but not all, authorities as 'microgastrin' (G4).

G17, G14 and G4 each represent the carboxyterminal of G34, which has the longest half-life in the circulation of all the gastrins and is often the most abundant form found in plasma. The various forms of gastrin share some biological and immunochemical properties but can be distinguished from each other physicochemically. The gastrins are normally produced exclusively by G-cells, which are confined to the GI tract proper and occur mainly in the gastric antrum and, to a limited extent, the upper duodenum. They may, however, be produced ectopically by any APUD-type tumour, especially those occurring in the pancreas and duodenum. Their principal physiological effects are thought to be stimulation of gastric acid and pepsin secretion, and trophic effects on the gastric and duodenal mucosa. Almost all the biological activity of gastrin is obtained with the C-terminal tetrapeptide alone and this has led to the synthesis of a 'protected' pentapeptide (Pentagastrin®), which has a longer half-life in the plasma than the tetrapeptide and has found widespread use clinically as a means of assessing gastric acid secretion.

Gastrin release is under both neural and hormonal control and is increased by eating a meal. The so-called cephalic phase of gastrin secretion is mediated via the vagus nerves and initiated by the sight, smell and taste of food. Release of gastrin during the gastric phase is caused by distension of the stomach and the presence in it of partially digested protein. All modes of release are inhibited by acidification of the antral mucosa and exaggerated by alkalinization.

Gastrin is usually present in the plasma in only very low concentrations but can be measured by radioimmunoassay with sufficient reliability to be useful clinically. However, because of the different specificities of the various antisera used against the various circulating forms of gastrin, complete agreement between assayists using different methods is not to be expected. For this reason, and because of the comparative infrequency with which it is required clinically, plasma gastrin assay is probably still best done in laboratories specializing in the technique.

Immunoassay results are usually expressed in terms of a G17 standard and overnight fasting values are generally less than 200 ng/L (100 pmol/L). Low plasma gastrin concentrations are of no diagnostic significance but elevated levels are often useful in the differential diagnosis of chronic abdominal pain, recurrent peptic ulceration and/or chronic diarrhoea, provided gastric hyperacidity can also be demonstrated to be present.

Hypergastrinaemia (Zollinger–Ellison Syndrome)

Zollinger and Ellison described the syndrome of recurrent and intractable peptic ulceration associated with hyperacidity, gastric mucosal hypertrophy and a pancreatic endocrine tumour in 1955, many years before gastrin, the causative agent, was isolated and identified; consequently it is universally known by its eponymous name rather than as hypergastrinism. The syndrome (Z-E) is rare, with a probable incidence of less than 1 per million of the population per year. This makes it almost as common as insulinoma and rather more common than most of the other tumours, apart from carcinoids, described in this chapter.

The two most important symptoms of Z-E are abdominal pain—usually due to peptic ulcer disease—and chronic diarrhoea, which, though less common, is not infrequently the presenting symptom. Men are slightly more often affected than women and most of the patients are middle aged, though no age group is completely exempt.

The illness has an insidious onset in the majority of cases and most of the patients remain undiagnosed for years, although this is changing with greater awareness of its manifestations and the greater availability of plasma gastrin assays. A family history of some form of endocrinopathy is obtained in roughly one-third of the patients, many of whom have pluriglandular disease or so-called multiple endocrine adenomatosis (MEN-I). Because of this a serum calcium measurement should always be made in patients with Z-E. In those cases in which it is due to MEN-I a high value will almost invariably be found and will influence subsequent management.

A malignant tumour of the pancreas, consisting mainly or exclusively of gastrin-secreting cells, is found in the majority of cases but it is usually slow growing and may, apart from its endocrinological manifestations exerted through secretion of gastrin, have remarkably few adverse effects. In a small percentage of cases the pancreatic tumour appears to be benign; but recent data, obtained by using plasma gastrin as a tumour marker, throw doubt on the frequency with which this is true because hypergastrinaemia often persists or recurs in cases in which complete surgical ablation was seemingly effected. In the past most Z-E tumours were large and easily palpable at operation but with improving diagnostic efficiency, tumours as small as 2–3 mm in diameter are being revealed as the cause of hypergastrinaemia, especially when preoperative localization has been possible by selective venous sampling.

In upwards of 20% of cases the pancreatic lesion causing Z-E is thought to be islet hyperplasia rather than a neoplasm but doubt has recently been cast upon this view, which was based on simple histological rather than on biochemical or immunohistochemical evidence. Islet hyperplasia is a common finding in almost all endocrine lesions of the pancreas and is often associated with an increase in pancreatic polypeptide secretion regardless of the nature of the primary endocrinopathy.

Gastrin is not a normal secretory product of pancreatic islet tissue. Its production by a pancreatic neoplasm is, therefore, an example of ectopic hormone production. Whether hyperplasia or other disease of the antral G-cells, the appropriate source of gastrin, is ever a cause of Z-E and, if so, how commonly, is highly contentious. Current evidence suggests that antral G-cell hyperfunction—with or without hyperplasia—is an even more rare clinical entity than 'classical' Z-E.

Regardless of its aetiology, Z-E is characterized clinically by gastric mucosal hypertrophy, which is readily detectable radiographically, and gastric hypersecretion and hyperacidity that persist throughout the night. These were, at one time, used as the main laboratory diagnostic criteria of the disease.

The characteristic biochemical lesion of Z-E is hypergastrinaemia in the presence of a high gastric acid secretion. Hypergastrinaemia is not of itself pathognomonic of Z-E since it occurs in a number of disorders, especially those associated with impaired gastric acid secretion—pernicious anaemia, atrophic gastritis, vagotomy and/or the excessive use of antacids and anticholinergics for examples. Modest hypergastrinaemia occurs also in a small proportion of patients with uncomplicated peptic ulcer disease, especially during treatment with cimetidine or other H_2-receptor antagonists. Hypergastrinaemia may also occur after surgical procedures that bypass the gastric antrum so that it is no longer bathed in acidic gastric juice (the retained or excluded antrum syndrome) and in pyloric stenosis with severe gastric retention.

The diagnosis of Z-E, once suspected, is seldom long in doubt as hypergastrinaemia is an invariable finding. Attention must, however, be directed towards eliciting the cause of hypergastrinaemia and establishing whether it is appropriate (i.e. high in the presence of a high antral pH) or inappropriate (i.e. high in the presence of a low antral pH). This can be achieved by measuring the hydrogen ion concentration of aspirated gastric juice and confirming that it comes into physical contact with the pyloric antrum.

Many tests have been advocated for distinguishing between the various causes of hypergastrinaemia, the two most popular depending upon the presumed

specific ability of calcium and secretin to stimulate gastrin secretion by gastrin-secreting tumours but not by normal G-cells. Neither of these presumptions has survived critical examination and currently the diagnosis of Z-E is best made by repeated measurements of plasma gastrin levels and the demonstration of *inappropriate* hypergastrinaemia. In many of the cases a tumour can be localized in the pancreas by selective arteriography or, where facilities exist, by percutaneous transhepatic pancreatic venous sampling under fluoroscopic control with measurement of plasma gastrin at various sampling points. A high success rate has been claimed for localization of gastrin-secreting tumours by this technique. This has also been applied, with slightly less success, to the localization of insulinomas, VIPomas and other endocrine tumours of the pancreas.

The recommended treatment of the Z-E syndrome has undergone several changes since the syndrome was first described. The first, and still widely practised, treatment was total gastrectomy. By removing the only known end-organ responsive to gastrin this operation completely alleviated the symptoms caused by hypergastrinaemia, though it left unaltered any subsequent ill effects caused by inexorable growth of the tumour, not to mention those secondary to total gastrectomy itself. With the advent, first, of powerful H_2-blockers such as cimetidine, ranitidine and famotidine, and then of the substituted benzimidazoles, such as omeprazole, total gastrectomy should disappear as a treatment for all but the most unusual cases.

Attempts at curative treatment by removing the pancreatic tumour were originally thought to be uniformly unsuccessful, though recent evidence suggests that this is not so and that ablation of the primary tumour might be the treatment of choice in cases in which the tumour is small and still confined to the pancreas or, even better, the duodenum, to which it has been localized by preoperative venous catheterization studies.

Follow-up studies, with regular monitoring of plasma gastrin levels, are clearly required in all cases of Z-E in which curative pancreatic surgery has been attempted, in order to detect relapse as early as possible and prevent reappearance of the full-blown syndrome.

Secretin

Bayliss and Starling demonstrated that instillation of hydrochloric acid into a denervated loop of small intestine elicited the secretion of pancreatic juice. They suggested that the humoral agent responsible for the effect should be named secretin. Half a century later the hormone was finally isolated in pure form and its amino-acid sequence determined. In spite of this and the enormous amount of work that has subsequently been done on it, little more is known about the physiology and pathology of secretin today than when it was first discovered. No diseases directly attributable to diminished, excessive or disorganized secretion of secretin have yet been discovered, although they probably do exist if only it was known what should be looked for.

Secretin is produced by the granular S-cells present in the mucosa between the crypts of villi throughout the length of the small intestine, with their greatest concentration in the duodenum. It is a strongly basic molecule containing 27 amino acids. The intact molecule is needed for complete biological activity, which appears primarily to stimulate the secretion of water and bicarbonate (but not enzymes) by the pancreas, especially in conjunction with PZ–CK. The actions of the two hormones on the pancreas are highly synergistic, at least under pharmacological conditions. Other biological actions of secretin that have been demonstrated experimentally include stimulation of water and bicarbonate secretion by the Brunner's glands of the intestinal mucosa and insulin release by the β-cells of the pancreas as well as inhibition of gastrin-induced gastric acid secretion and reduction of duodenal motility; whether any of these are physiological, or pathologically significant, is unknown.

Plasma secretin concentrations are extremely low but can be measured by immunoassay. Contradictory results have been obtained by different investigators under diverse experimental conditions. At present there are no clinical indications for measuring plasma secretin levels. The pharmacological response to secretin is sometimes used as a test of pancreatic exocrine function, especially in conjunction with PZ–CK, and occasionally in patients suspected of harbouring a gastrinoma. Its use for the latter purpose has, however, declined since it became clear that the discriminatory effect claimed for it was largely unfounded.

Vasoactive Intestinal Polypeptide

VIP is a member of the glucagon family of GI hormones and was isolated from a side fraction during purification of porcine secretin to which its structure is even more closely related than to glucagon itself. Initially characterized on the basis of its effects on blood vessels and the circulation, it was soon found to have a wide range of biological actions, many of which it shares with other members of the secretin family. Apart from its vasodilator and hypotensive effects, VIP inhibits pentagastrin and histamine-stimulated gastric acid secretion and inhibits gastrin secretion. It stimulates water and electrolyte secretion by the exocrine pancreas and colon in a manner similar to that of cholera toxin, i.e. through activation of adenylate cyclase. VIP is a stimulus to glycogenolysis in liver, lipolysis in adipose tissue and insulin secretion by the pancreas. All of these actions may be relevant to its proposed role as a neurotransmitter.

VIP contains 28 amino acids and shows consider-

able chemical homology with glucagon, secretin and GIP. Unlike the other members of the 'family' it occurs throughout the length of the GI tract and is confined to the nervous rather than to the endocrine elements. Indeed, it occurs in relatively large amounts in nerves in various other parts of the body and in the brain. Its role as a hormone has, therefore, been brought into question. Regardless of such semantics, however, VIP does occur as a natural constituent in plasma and measurement of its concentration is occasionally helpful in elucidating the cause of severe abdominal pain and/or diarrhoea.

The conditions under which VIP is released into the circulation, and its physiological role, are still poorly understood. It is apparently largely inactivated by a single passage through the liver and this may be the mechanism by which this highly biologically active substance—whose actions are normally confined to well-defined target organs innervated by peptidergic nerves—is removed and denatured when it inadvertently leaks into the general circulation.

The concentration of VIP in plasma can readily be measured by radioimmunoassay, but as measurements for clinical purposes are of limited use and only very rarely indicated, they are best made in laboratories specializing in the technique.

HyperVIPaemia (Verner–Morrison Syndrome)

Not long after the seminal description by Zollinger and Ellison of non-insulin-secreting pancreatic tumours producing abdominal disease, it was appreciated by Verner and Morrison that, in a small proportion of patients watery diarrhoea, rather than recurrent peptic ulceration, dominated the clinical picture and that gastric function tests often revealed hypochlorhydria instead of hyperacidity. This combination of symptoms is usually referred to as the Verner–Morrison or watery diarrhoea, hypokalaemia, achlorhydria (WDHA) syndrome. Differentiation from Z-E (in which diarrhoea is also often a dominant feature) cannot always be made on clinical grounds alone, but may require detailed biochemical and endocrinological examinations.

The likely cause of WDHA remained unknown for many years though recognized as being secondary, in the majority of cases, to the secretory product of a non-insulin-secreting pancreatic tumour that was neither gastrin nor glucagon. Though at first wrongly thought to be gastric inhibitory polypeptide (GIP) it was subsequently shown that VIP was the main mediator of the syndrome and that the tumours, by analogy with insulinomas, glucagonomas and gastrinomas, were VIPomas. Not all VIPomas, however, cause WDHA, nor are all cases of the latter associated with increased plasma VIP levels, although many of them are. Moreover, not all of the tumours causing WDHA, whether associated with increased plasma VIP levels or not, arise within the pancreas: some are phaeochromocytomas, ganglioneuromas or bronchial carcinomas. Many of the tumours produce more than one hormone—often three or more—and it becomes difficult to assign a causative role to any single one of them.

The WDHA syndrome is characterized by the production of copious watery stools occurring in explosive bursts with remarkably little cramping, often with long intervals, initially, between attacks. Hypochlorhydria and hypokalaemia (due to loss of potassium in the stool) are both very common and muscular weakness is usual during attacks. Skin flushes and eruptions are also common, as are psychotic episodes. Other biochemical features include hypercalcaemia and impaired glucose tolerance (probably secondary to the hypokalaemia). The condition is three times more common in women than in men and is associated with a metastatic pancreatic tumour in roughly half the cases. The others are associated with apparently benign tumours of the pancreas, simple islet hyperplasia and ectopic hormone-secreting neoplasms. The true endocrinological cause of the syndrome is not known with certainty and is probably not the same in every case. There are cogent arguments for differentiation of WDHA, caused by excessive VIP secretion, from watery diarrhoea caused by other agencies. This is justified by analogy with hyperinsulinism, which is now recognized to be only one among many causes of intractable fasting hypoglycaemia. Causes of WDHA other than VIPoma and hyper VIPaemia will undoubtedly emerge in time, possibly including increased production of prostaglandins or various combinations of gastrointestinal hormones.

Diagnosis of VIPoma is made on the basis of a high plasma VIP concentration in a patient with signs and symptoms of WDHA and confirmed radiologically and/or surgically. It must be distinguished, clinically, from the far more common conditions of surreptitious purgative-induced diarrhoea, and lesions of the bowel itself that are capable of producing intractable diarrhoea, as well as from other endocrinological causes, carcinoidosis and medullary carcinoma of the thyroid for example.

Only very rarely is total surgical ablation of a VIPoma possible although, because they are usually slow growing, removal of tumour bulk often improves symptoms and extends the patient's life.

Pancreozymin–Cholecystokinin (PZ–CK)

Pancreozymin and cholecystokinin were characterized independently on the basis of their abilities to stimulate enzyme production by the pancreas and contraction of the gallbladder, respectively. It was not until much later, during attempts at their purification and characterization in the 1960s, that they were recognized to be the same substance. It is usually referred to nowadays as cholecystokinin (CK) on the grounds of precedence or PZ–CK to emphasize its duality.

Several molecular species of CK are now recognized, the first to have been isolated and characterized being the polypeptide containing 33 amino acids (CK-33). The last five C-terminal amino acids of this and all subsequent CK variants are identical to those of gastrin with which they have some pharmacological and possibly even physiological properties in common. Most interest now focuses on CK-8, currently believed to be the most biologically important of the CK variants.

CK possesses a sulphated tyrosyl residue (C-7) similar to gastrin II but unlike the latter, sulphation is essential for full expression of the biological, though not the immunological, properties of CK. Caerulin, an amphibian skin peptide that has CK-like biological activities, shares the common gastrin–CK pentapeptide and is also sulphated at Tyr-7. Caerulin is used clinically as a stimulant of pancreatic exocrine activity in a test of pancreatic function.

In the gut, CK is found mainly in endocrine cells of the duodenum, which occur mainly in patches rather than evenly distributed. It has, however, been shown by immunohistological techniques that CK, particularly the C-8 variant, is widely distributed throughout the body, especially in the central nervous system.

The main pharmacological (biological) activities of CK, in addition to those by which it was discovered, are stimulation of intestinal motility, gastric acid secretion, secretion of Brunner's glands, pancreatic growth and possibly insulin release. In the brain CK is seemingly involved in the perception of satiety, and interest is currently more focused on this role than on its pancreas stimulatory one.

The secretion of CK into the circulation is stimulated by the presence of various amino acids and protein hydrolysates, hydrochloric acid and fatty acids in the duodenum. Its concentration in the plasma can be measured by radioimmunoassay and rises after ingestion of a mixed meal. Despite intensive efforts by investigators throughout the world, plasma CCK assays do not, at the present time, yield diagnostically useful information, though in the future they might be expected to do so in disorders of digestion and pancreatic exocrine function.

CK can be given intravenously, either as the purified porcine C-33 preparation or as caerulin, to test for pancreatic exocrine responsiveness in cases of suspected pancreatic insufficiency. It is usually administered in conjunction with natural or synthetic secretin and the rise in concentration of pancreatic enzymes (e.g. amylase, lipase and trypsin) in the plasma, or preferably in pancreatic juice obtained by endoscopic intubation, determined as a measure of pancreatic responsiveness.

Somatostatin

Somatostatin is a cyclic tetradecapeptide originally isolated from the hypothalamus by virtue of its ability to inhibit growth-hormone secretion by anterior pituitary cells in culture and subsequently found distributed in tissues throughout the body. Indeed, in the rat some 70% of total immunoassayable somatostatin occurs in the gut and a further 5% in the pancreas. In the pancreas, somatostatin is secreted by δ-cells that occur mainly in a mantle that surrounds a core of insulin-secreting β-cells and glucagon-secreting α-cells in some islets of Langerhans but also, to a limited extent throughout the exocrine pancreas.

Although the chemistry and pharmacological properties of somatostatin have been extensively studied—probably more than any other peptide hormone except insulin—its true physiological role is still enshrouded in mystery. It seems likely that somatostatin acts mainly, if not exclusively, as a paracrine regulator and/or inhibitor of nearby secretory cells whether they be in the pituitary gland, gut, endocrine or exocrine pancreas. The role of abnormalities of somatostatin secretion in the pathogenesis of disease is the subject of much speculation but there are few objective data. Even the causative role of somatostatin in the somatostatinoma syndrome described below is questionable.

Somatostatin is present in the plasma in at least two major forms, S-14 and S-28, and can be measured by radioimmunoassay. Its concentration varies in response to food and stress and at present is not attributed any diagnostic significance except in the recognition and diagnosis of somatostatinoma.

A long-acting synthetic analogue of somatostatin, octeotride, enjoys considerable popularity as a therapeutic agent for the treatment of a number of endocrine diseases resulting from overproduction of various peptide hormones. It has its greatest application in the treatment of acromegaly due to overproduction of growth hormone and hyperinsulinism due to nesidioblastosis. It is also indicated for the treatment of overproduction of peptide hormones by unresectable neoplasms.

Somatostatinoma

Tumours of the pancreas producing somatostatin as their main, or possibly sole, product were first described a little over 15 years ago but there is still not clear evidence that they are capable of producing a characteristic syndrome comparable, for example, with insulinoma, VIPoma or gastrinoma. In all of the small number of cases so far described the tumour was malignant and secreted or contained at least one other polypeptide hormone (e.g. calcitonin, corticotrophin or insulin) on immunohistological examination. Plasma somatostatin levels were many tens, or hundreds, of times higher in patients than in control subjects in all cases in which they were examined. Many either had hyperglycaemia or exhibited glucose intolerance, though one patient presented with severe and intractable hypoglycaemia. Gallbladder disease and steatorrhoea were a feature of some of the cases, but not all, and considering the pharmacological effects observed with even tiny amounts of somatosta-

tin, the mildness of the clinical and biochemical abnormalities was more remarkable than their presence.

Mixed and Carcinoid Tumours

All of the peptide-secreting tumours of the GI tract, whether they arise in the pancreas or gut itself, present common histological features, which have led to them being classed as APUDomas. Differentiation from one another may be difficult if not impossible without recourse to electron microscopy and special staining techniques. A fair proportion of all APUDomas reveal the presence of multiple hormone-containing cell types when subjected to immunohistological examination and many are classified on their histological features alone as carcinoids; indeed, many of them secrete varying amounts of 5-hydroxytryptamine (5-HT) though only a minority manifest this clinically (Table 40.2).

Assays on plasma of patients harbouring mixed tumours often reveal the presence of more than one hormone in excess, even when this is entirely unsuspected clinically. The reasons for this apparent hormonal silence are unknown.

Carcinoid tumours themselves have been recognized clinically and histologically for longer than any of the other hormone-producing tumours of the GI tract. They were first shown to be capable of producing cutaneous flushing, diarrhoea and cardiovascular disease as long ago as 1930, but it was almost a quarter of a century later that the full-blown syndrome of carcinoidosis was recognized and attributed to overproduction of 5-HT. This view is now considered somewhat simplistic insofar as 5-HT, though invariably produced in excess in carcinoidosis, is thought to be responsible for only a minority of the signs and symptoms, the majority of which are due to other hormonal products of the causative tumour. The exact nature of these secretions, and whether they are always the same, is still unknown, but the two that have been incriminated most consistently are bradykinin and the prostaglandins.

Only a tiny proportion of all tumours diagnosed histologically as carcinoids give rise to the clinical syndrome of carcinoidosis; in particular, those arising in the appendix, a favourite site, very rarely do so and consequently were, for a time, considered to be fundamentally different from those developing elsewhere, although this now seems unlikely. What causes the difference is still unknown. Carcinoid tumours developing in the pancreas are particularly likely to contain and secrete one or more polypeptide hormones of GI origin and may give rise to some very bizarre syndromes.

Men are more often affected than women and are usually middle-aged or elderly. Intermittent cutaneous flushing is the most common symptom and is present in over three-quarters of the cases. It can often be provoked by alcohol, which has been used clinically as a test for the disease. Dilation of veins on the face and the formation of venous telangiectases are common, especially over the nose, upper lip and cheek, which may give the patient a drunkard appearance. Heart lesions, especially affecting the valves, are common, as is asthma, but it is diarrhoea that is the hallmark of carcinoidosis and usually the most disabling part of the disease. It frequently accompanies or follows episodes of flushing and is characterized by borborygmi, urgency and the frequent, explosive passage of watery stools. It alone amongst the symptoms of carcinoidosis is most likely to be due to excessive 5-HT production and may occasionally be relieved by parachlorphenylalanine, an inhibitor of 5-HT synthesis. Many patients give a history of having undergone abdominal surgery previously but others have had no such premonitory signs. Enlargement of the liver due to metastases is almost invariably present by the time the patient presents with symptoms but this may be years, or even decades, after the lesion was first discovered.

Diagnosis of the carcinoid syndrome is generally made on the basis of the characteristic clinical picture and excretion in the urine of vastly increased amounts of 5-HT metabolites, especially 5-hydroxyindoleacetic acid (5-HIAA). Various provocative tests utilizing alcohol, calcium or adrenaline have been employed but do little to further the diagnosis, although they have helped to throw light on the pathogenic mechanisms involved. Plasma 5-HT levels are extremely high in patients with carcinoidosis, but great care is necessary in order to avoid confusion created by even the slightest degree of thrombolysis, as platelets contain large amounts of 5-HT that is liberated into the serum wherever they are damaged.

Treatment of carcinoidosis is essentially symptomatic and aimed at reducing tumour bulk and lessening endocrine effects on the target organs. Because they are usually so slow growing, surgical removal of carcinoid metastases from the liver, when feasible, or interruption of the arterial blood supply—by arterial thromboembolism for example—is often followed by remission of the symptoms for up to several years. Alternatively, radiotherapy or cytotoxic drugs, especially 5-fluorouracil, are worthy of trial. The diarrhoea often responds to treatment with methysergide and other 5-HT antagonists, including parachlorphenylalanine, though its side-effects so limit its usefulness that it has virtually been abandoned as a treatment for carcinoidosis. Glucocorticoids may help the asthma of carcinoidosis but so far there is little that can be done to relieve the flushing except avoidance of alcohol should this be implicated in its causation.

Other Hormones

None of the many GI hormones, apart from those already discussed, has yet been established as unequivocally involved in pathogenic mechanisms or as having diagnostic significance. Nevertheless, at least some of them are of sufficient potential importance to warrant brief discussion.

Motilin

A polypeptide capable of stimulating the contraction of the dog stomach fundus was first isolated from a crude extract of pig gut in 1971 and its structure was determined soon after. It is a single-chain polypeptide consisting of 22 amino-acid residues arranged in a sequence unlike any of the other known humorally active GI hormones. It occurs in two main forms in the plasma and tissues: a smaller one corresponding in molecular size to native motilin; a larger one of undetermined composition and behaviour.

The most clearly demonstrable properties of motilin are its ability to stimulate contraction of the gastric musculature and affect the frequency and strength of interdigestive myoelectric complexes. It has been said both to increase and to delay gastric emptying according to the circumstances of its administration and at present its physiological role in man is quite unknown, though it seems reasonable to suppose that it might be involved in regulating gastrointestinal motility. Its concentration in plasma can be measured by radioimmunoassay and shows marked interpersonal differences as well as rhythmical fluctuations, with a periodicity of roughly 90 min, throughout the day and night.

Glucose given either by mouth or intravenously produces a rapid fall in plasma motilin concentration, whereas fats and non-absorbable carbohydrates such as xylitol and lactose in lactose-intolerance subjects produce either no fall or a rise in plasma motilin concentration when they are given by mouth. Diarrhoea, regardless of its cause, is usually associated with high plasma motilin levels but whether these are causal or consequential has not yet been established.

Pancreatic Polypeptide

Polypeptides of roughly similar chemical composition, but with varied biological effects, were isolated from chicken and bovine pancreases by two groups of investigators working independently some 20 years ago. These peptides, called, for want of a better term, pancreatic polypeptides (PP), have different immunological properties according to the species from which they are isolated. Immunoassays capable of measuring PPs in man are available and have led to the accumulation of extensive knowledge of conditions under which their secretion rate is altered, the most important of which is eating. This produces a prompt and large rise in plasma PP that is abolished by vagotomy. So far, however, it has not proved possible to assign a physiological role to PP in man or to attribute any illness to abnormalities of its production. The concentration of PP in plasma is raised in many patients with pancreatic APUDomas and its measurement has been suggested as diagnostically useful in this disorder but rejected as insufficiently sensitive and/or specific. As the rise in plasma concentration of PP that occurs in response to insulin-induced hypoglycaemia is abolished by vagotomy, measurement of PP in plasma during an insulin stress test has been proposed as a test of completeness of vagal section following vagotomy for peptic ulceration. This operation has, itself, now become virtually obsolete as a result of improvements in the medical treatment of peptic ulceration and currently there are no clinical indications for measuring plasma PP levels for diagnostic purposes.

Two other peptides with sufficient similarity to PP to justify being considered as part of the same family are peptide YY and neuropeptide Y(NPY). Peptide YY and PP both inhibit pancreatic exocrine secretion, which is where their main physiological roles, if any, are thought to lie. NPY, which is found in high concentration in the hypothalamus, has the ability to stimulate appetite. Indeed it is the most potent stimulus to eating currently known and when injected directly into the paraventricular nucleus of the hypothalamus of animals may induce them to become obese, due mainly to their intense craving for carbohydrate. Whether this is of only pharmacological interest of whether it is physiologically important is unknown.

Neurotensin

Like somatostatin this 13 amino-acid polypeptide was originally isolated from extracts of hypothalamus and subsequently demonstrated by immunochemical methods to be present in the bowel where it occurs in highest concentration in the ileum. Pharmacologically, neurotensin has powerful hypotensive–vasodilatory properties and stimulates the secretion of insulin, glucagon and gastrin. Its physiological properties are unknown, but its concentration in plasma rises after ingestion of food, especially in patients who experience the dumping syndrome after partial gastrectomy. Whether neurotensin is involved in the pathogenesis of this syndrome is a matter for conjecture. At the present time there are no clear clinical indications for measuring plasma neurotensin levels.

Similar notes to the above could be written about each of the 10 or so other biologically active peptides that have been isolated from the GI tract, characterized and often sequenced, and to which a hormonal (or paracrine) role has been assigned. No good purpose would be served in doing so, however, and readers are referred to the review articles and books on this subject cited at the end of this chapter.

FURTHER READING

Buchanan K.D. ed. (1988). *Gastrointestinal APUDomas*, Proceedings of the Bayliss & Starling Society Symposium, Belfast University, 1987, London: Royal Society of Medicine.

DelValle J., Yamada T. (1990). The gut as an endocrine organ. *Annu. Rev. Med.*, **41**, 447.

Editorial (1989). Carcinoid tumours and endocrine cell hyperplasia. *Lancet*, **i**, 940.

Marks V., Morgan L. M. (1982). Gastrointestinal hormones. In *Molecular Aspects of Medicine: An Interdisciplinary Review Journal* (Baum H., Gergely J., Fanburg B.L. eds.) Oxford: Pergamon, pp 225–292.

Shuster L. T., Go V. L. W., Rizza R. A., O'Brien P. C., Service F. J. (1988). Potential incretins. *Mayo Clin. Proc.*, **63**, 794.

Turnberg L. (1991). Cellular basis of diarrhoea. The Croonian Lecture, 1989. *J. Roy. Coll. Phys. London*, **25**, 53.

Walsh J. M. (1987). Gastrointestinal hotmones. In *Physiology of the Gastrointestinal Tract*, 2nd edn (Johnson L. ed.) New York: Raven, pp. 181–253.

Wolfe M. M. and Soll, A. H. (1988). The physiology of gastric acid secretion. *N. Eng. J. Med.*, **319**, 1707.

41. Disorders of the Adrenal Cortex

P. J. Wood

Adrenal anatomy
Adrenal steroids
  Steroid nomenclature
  Steroid biosynthesis
  Inhibitors of steroid biosynthesis
  Steroid metabolism and excretion
  Actions of adrenal steroids
  Circulating steroid levels
  Corticosteroid-binding globulin
Control of adrenal steroid secretion
  Cortisol secretion
  Adrenal androgen secretion
  Aldosterone secretion
Methods for steroid measurement
  Serum corticosteroids
  Urine steroids
  Salivary and bloodspot steroids
Dynamic tests of adrenal function
  ACTH stimulation tests
  Dexamethasone suppression tests
  Insulin-induced hypoglycaemia
  The metyrapone test
  The CRH test
*Clinical investigation of adrenocortical
  dysfunction*
  Adrenocortical insufficiency
  Cushing's syndrome
  Congenital adrenal hyperplasia
  Virilizing tumours
  Hypertension

ADRENAL ANATOMY

The adrenals or 'suprarenals' are paired, triangular glands positioned just above the upper poles of the kidneys. In healthy adults, each adrenal weighs approximately 3–4 g, although at autopsy the glands are heavier (approximately 6 g) due to the effects of increased adrenocorticotrophic hormone (ACTH) resulting from terminal stress.

Each adrenal gland consists of a yellow outer cortex and an inner, pearly grey medulla, surrounded by a connective tissue capsule. The cortex and medulla have distinct embryological origins, histological appearances, and physiological and biochemical functions.

The *medulla* is derived from neuroectodermal cells and constitutes approximately 10% of the gland. It is concentrated in the head and body of the adrenal while the tail is formed almost exclusively of cortical tissue.[1] The phaeochromocyte cells of the medulla are members of the APUD (*Amine Precursor Uptake* and *Decarboxylation*) system and secrete adrenaline and smaller amounts of noradrenaline in response to sympathetic nervous stimulation.

The adrenal *cortex* is derived from cells of mesodermal origin and produces steroid hormones— a function that is exclusive to adrenal cortex and gonadal tissues. On histological examination three distinct zones of the adrenal cortex can be identified. The outermost *zona glomerulosa* is not continuous, but is present in irregular 'pockets' around the periphery of the cortex. The zona glomerulosa can synthesize and secrete the major mineralocorticoid aldosterone. The two innermost layers, the *zona fasciculata* and *zona reticularis* both have the enzyme systems necessary to produce steroids other than aldosterone. The yellow zona fasciculata consists of clear, lipid-laden cells, while the innermost zona reticularis is yellow-brown in colour and consists of compact, lipid-sparse cells. Normally the zona fasciculata is the largest zone, but increased adrenocortical secretory activity leads to depletion of lipid stores and a movement of the boundary between the zona fasciculata and zona reticularis so that the zona fasciculata narrows while the zona reticularis widens. The cells of these two zones generally function as a single unit, the clear cells of the zona fasciculata changing to the compact cells of the zona reticularis on lipid depletion following stimulation. There is evidence that the cells of the zona reticularis possess more sulphokinase activity than those of the zona fasciculata.

The adrenal glands receive their blood supply via small arteries originating in the inferior phrenic artery, aorta and renal arteries. The venous drainage differs for each adrenal gland; the right drains into the inferior vena cava while the left drains into the left renal vein. This has obvious importance when using renal vein catheterization to lateralize an adrenal lesion.

The cortical blood supply is centripetal, travelling from the subcapsular arterial plexus and perfusing the zona glomerulosa, fasciculata and reticularis in turn. ACTH stimulation increases the flow of blood through this system. Part of the blood supply to the medulla is provided by blood draining directly from the cortex. High cortisol levels in this portal blood supply perfusing the medulla induce the enzyme phenyl ethanolamine-N-methyl transferase (PENMT), which is responsible for the N-methylation of noradrenaline to form adrenaline. The capacity of the adrenal medulla to produce adrenaline therefore depends on the close association between adrenal cortical and medullary tissue.

Occasionally, accessory cortical tissue is found outside the adrenal gland proper. These accessory glands are often in the vicinity of the main glands or at retroperitoneal sites, and usually show the same three tissue zones as the cortex of the main gland, although medullary tissue is absent.

Rests of adrenal cortical tissue can occur in other endocrine organs, particularly the ovary or testis.

TABLE 41.1
TRIVIAL AND SYSTEMATIC NAMES OF SOME IMPORTANT STEROIDS

Cortisol	11β,17α,21-trihydroxypregn-4-ene-3,20-dione
Aldosterone	11β,21-dihydroxy-3,20-dioxopregn-4-ene-18-al
Deoxycorticosterone	21-hydroxypregn-4-ene-3,20-dione
Corticosterone	11β,21-dihydroxypregn-4-ene-3,20-dione
Progesterone	Pregn-4-ene-3,20-dione
Oestrone	3-hydroxyestra-1,3,5(10)-triene-17-one
Oestradiol	3,17β-dihydroxyestra-1,3,5(10)-triene
Testosterone	17β-hydroxyandrost-4-ene-3-one
17α-hydroxyprogesterone	17α-hydroxypregn-4-ene-3,20-dione
Androstenedione	Androst-4-ene-3,17-dione
Dehydroepiandrosterone	3β-hydroxyandrost-5-ene-17-one

Conversely, rests of gonadal tissue can occur in the adrenal glands. This has relevance in the investigation of steroid-secreting tumours, when tumours derived from rests of cells can show steroid patterns and responsiveness similar to those of the parent gland, leading to possible errors in conclusions as to the tumour site.

ADRENAL STEROIDS

Steroid Nomenclature

The conventional numbering and ring identification of steroids is illustrated in Fig. 41.1. Adrenal steroids can be identified in terms of systematic chemical nomenclature, main biological properties or by trivial name. Systematic names are based on the parent carbon skeletons pregnane (C_{21}), androstane (C_{19}) and oestrane (C_{18})[2]. These names are modified to indicate the presence of a double bond (-ane$\rightarrow$-ene) or triple bond (-ane$\rightarrow$-yne) with the lowest carbon number of the two adjacent carbon atoms concerned. To avoid ambiguity the second carbon number may be included in brackets. Substituents are then identified by prefixes or suffixes. Some examples are illustrated in Table 41.1.

The major steroids produced by the adrenal cortex have a planar ring structure with substituents extending above (β-configuration; extensions denoted by a solid line in Fig. 41.1) or below (α-configuration; extensions denoted by a dashed line) the plane of the rings. In the case of reduction at C5, which occurs during steroid metabolism, two distinct shapes of steroid molecule are produced depending on whether the orientation of the hydrogen atom is 5α (flat structure) or 5β (A ring at an angle to the plane of the B, C and D rings).

Adrenal steroids can also be classified by their main biological properties as glucocorticoids (main effects on carbohydrate metabolism), mineralocorticoids (electrolyte and water balance), androgens, oestrogens or progestagens. However, steroids often have effects covering more than one category—for example, cortisol has both glucocorticoid and some mineralocorticoid activity.

The shape and substituents on the steroid skeleton determine its physiological activity. The minimum requirement for glucocorticoid activity is the presence of hydroxyl substituents at 11β and 21 positions, keto (oxo) groups at C3 and C20, and a double bond between C4 and C5. The lack of hydroxyl group at C17 but presence of C21 hydroxyl group confers mineralocorticoid activity.

Aldosterone, in addition to this feature, also has an aldehyde group at C18, which through hemiacetal formation reduces the activity of the 11-hydroxyl group and therefore reduces glucocorticoid activity.

Adrenal androgens are C_{19} steroids with a 17β-keto and a 3-keto or hydroxyl group, while oestrogens are C_{18} steroids with a phenolic A ring.

Steroid Biosynthesis

The adrenal cortex secretes three main types of steroids: the glucocorticoids cortisol and corticosterone, the mineralocorticoid aldosterone and weak adrenal androgens dehydroepiandrosterone sulphate (DHAS), androstenedione and 11β-hydroxyandrostenedione. In addition, low levels of steroid intermediates (pregnenolone, 17α-hydroxypregnenolone, progesterone, 17α-hydroxyprogesterone (17-OHP), 11-deoxycortisol) and of the sex steroids testosterone and oestradiol are secreted. The steroid biosynthetic process requires cholesterol substrate and involves cleavage between C20 and C22, hydroxylation at a variety of sites, oxidation of the 3β-hydroxyl residue to a 3-keto group and isomerization of the double bond at C5–C6 to the C4–C5 position.

Steroid hydroxylation reactions are catalysed by a family of specialized cytochrome P450 enzymes, which require NADPH and molecular oxygen and which incorporate flavoproteins and non-haem proteins. These are classified as 'mixed-function oxidase' reactions because the oxygen molecule is split to yield one molecule of water and to incorporate an atom of oxygen into the steroid hydroxyl substituent.

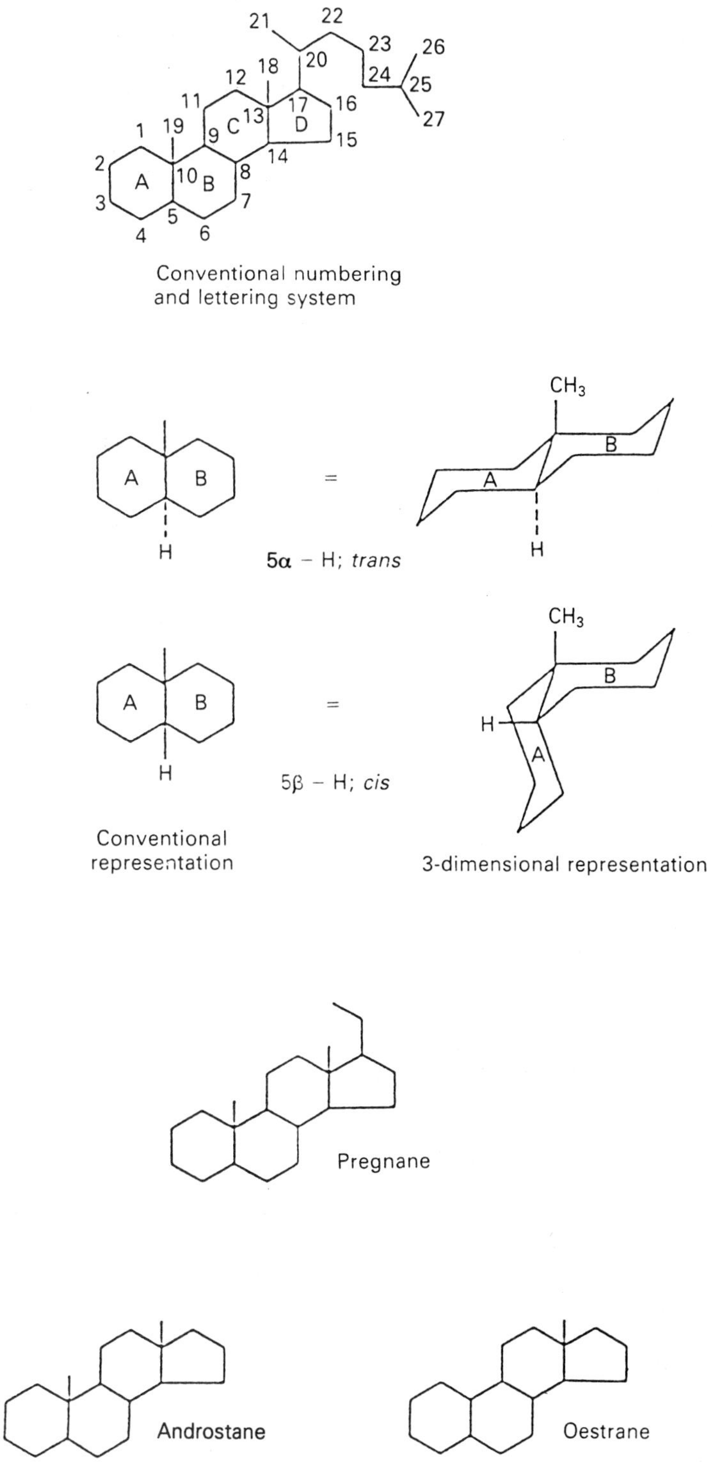

Figure 41.1 Steroid nomenclature: conventional numbering and lettering structure of 5α and 5β series of steroids and parent steroid skeletons.

An example of the mechanism for 11β-hydroxylation is given in Fig. 41.2.

Adrenocortical cells can utilize cholesterol substrate from lipid stores, from *de novo* synthesis from acetate, or from free and esterified cholesterol associated with low-density lipoprotein (LDL) in the circulation. Normally, in man, LDL-cholesterol seems to be utilized preferentially and uptake through LDL recep-

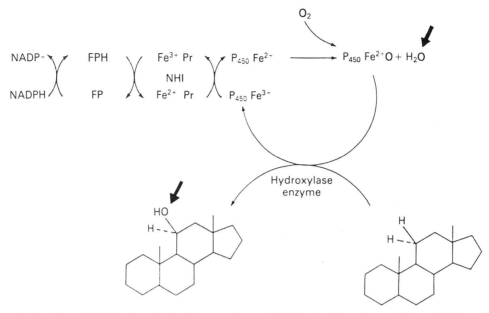

Figure 41.2 Mechanism of 11β-hydroxylation by cytochrome P450 mixed-function oxidase. FP, flavoprotein; NHI, non-haem iron protein; arrows indicate the destinations of the two oxygen atoms in the oxygen molecule.

tors on adrenocortical cells is stimulated by ACTH. At times of increased activity more stored cholesterol esters are utilized.

The main reactions leading to the production of steroids in the adrenal cortex are illustrated in Fig. 41.3.

Cholesterol substrate is cleaved by C20 and C22 hydroxylation and C20–C22 lyase reactions in the mitochondria to form pregnenolone. The lyase reaction is rate limiting in steroid synthesis and is stimulated by ACTH. Pregnenolone reaching the endoplasmic reticulum is then modified by 3β-hydroxysteroid dehydrogenase and Δ^{4-5}-isomerase, 17-hydroxylase and 21-hydroxylase reactions to produce a variety of steroids including DHAS, androstenedione, 11-deoxycorticosterone and 11-deoxycortisol. The final step involves 11-hydroxylation of 11-deoxycorticosterone and 11-deoxycortisol in the mitochondria to form corticosterone and cortisol, respectively.

There are several alternative pathways for glucocorticoid production depending on whether the 3β- hydroxysteroid dehydrogenase/isomerase reaction precedes or follows 17α- or 21-hydroxylation steps. The relative importance of these different routes is unclear, but the most likely pathways are illustrated (Fig. 41.3).

Aldosterone synthesis in the zona glomerulosa follows a similar pattern, except that the 17-hydroxylase is absent. The 11-hydroxylase and 18-hydroxysteroid dehydrogenase enzymes act on 11-deoxycorticosterone and corticosterone in the mitochondrion to produce aldosterone.

Steroid Biosynthesis by the Fetal Adrenal Cortex
The fetal adrenal cortex can be identified by the third month of gestation. Two tissue zones can be distin-

guished: a thin, outer zone of small, basophilic cells and an inner zone consisting of loosely packed, eosinophilic cells that comprises approximately 80% of the adrenal cortical tissue. The outer zone continues to develop into the adult adrenal cortex, while the inner 'fetal' zone begins to undergo involution approximately 5 days before delivery and disappears completely by 3–12 months of age. This change is accompanied by a change in emphasis from the production of 3β-hydroxy-, Δ^5-steroids and 16-hydroxylated derivatives such as DHA, DHAS and 16α-hydroxy-DHAS to the synthesis of cortisol and other Δ^4-3-keto steroids. Newborn and preterm infants in particular produce relatively large amounts of Δ^5-3β-hydroxy steroids, and caution is needed in interpreting the results of radioimmunoassay for plasma 17-OHP and other plasma steroids in these infants because of potential cross-reactivity problems.

Inhibitors of Steroid Biosynthesis

Although many inhibitors of adrenal steroid biosynthesis have been described, most are of experimental interest only.

Metyrapone competes with substrate for binding sites on the 11-hydroxylase cytochrome P450 system and therefore acts as an 11-hydroxylase inhibitor, although 20-hydroxylase inhibition has been demonstrated at high concentration. It is an effective short-term treatment for excessive cortisol production, for example in the ectopic ACTH syndrome, but its use in the investigation of disorders of the hypothalamic–pituitary–adrenal axis has little value (*see* below).

Aminoglutethimide inhibits cholesterol side-chain

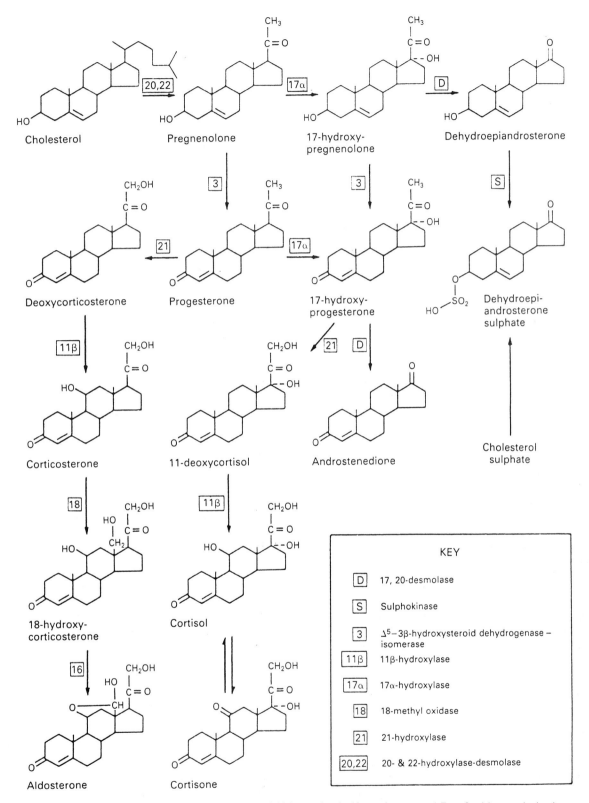

Figure 41.3 Major pathways for adrenal corticosteroid biosynthesis (from James and Few,[2] with permission).

cleavage by blocking 20-hydroxylase activity, and can also inhibit aldosterone production by blocking 18-hydroxylation. Trilostane blocks 3β-hydroxy-steroid dehydrogenase/isomerase activity; it has been evaluated for the treatment of Cushing's syndrome but is ineffective for this purpose.

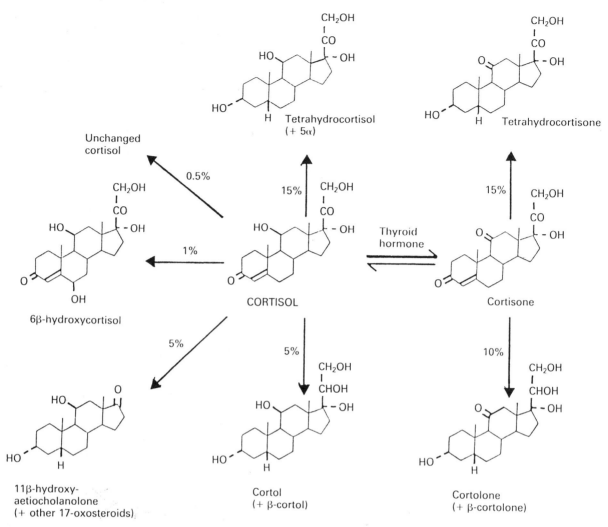

Figure 41.4 The principal metabolites of cortisol: % figures indicate the approximate percentage of cortisol converted to a particular metabolite (from Brooks,[3] with permission).

o,p'-DDD (2,2-bis(2-chlorophenyl-4-chlorophenyl)-1,1-dichloroethane) has a relatively selective cytotoxic action on adrenal fascicular and reticular cells. It has been used as a palliative in cases of unresectable adrenal carcinoma but produces extensive side-effects of anorexia, nausea, lethargy and dermatitis.

Steroid Metabolism and Excretion

The liver is the main organ responsible for adrenal steroid metabolism, although the kidneys, connective tissue and the adrenal itself have some metabolic activity. The enzyme reactions involved are reduction, hydroxylation, side-chain cleavage and esterification of products as glucuronides and sulphates. The major urinary metabolites of cortisol are shown in Fig. 41.4.

Interconversion of cortisol and cortisone is achieved by liver 11β-hydroxysteroid dehydrogenase, which catalyses the reversible oxidation of cortisol to cortisone. This reaction is influenced by thyroid hormone levels, which also modulate the rate of secretion and metabolism of cortisol. Cortisol and cortisone are reduced irreversibly at the C(4–5) double bond by at least two NADPH-requiring enzymes. One enzyme on the endoplasmic reticulum yields a 5α-oriented hydrogen atom giving rise to the 5α series of reduced steroids, while another present in the cytosol produces a 5β-hydrogen giving rise to 5β reduced steroids. The ratio of 5α to 5β metabolites depends on the particular steroid—for C_{21} steroids the 5β forms predominate while C_{19} steroids are preferentially converted to the 5α metabolites. Thyroid hormones increase the proportion of 5α reduced steroids.

A second stage involves reversible reduction of the 3-oxo group by NADPH and a 3α-hydroxysteroid dehydrogenase present in the endoplasmic reticulum and cytosol of hepatocytes. Cortisol and cortisone are transformed by these reduction reactions to a

TABLE 41.2
ACTIONS OF CORTICOSTEROIDS

GLUCOCORTICOID ACTIVITY
Intermediary metabolism
Stimulation of:
   gluconeogenesis
   hepatic glycogen storage
Breakdown of plasma and muscle protein to amino acids
Changes in lipid synthesis, storage and mobilization
Kidney
Permissive action on the ability to excrete a water load
GI tract
Permissive action on gastric acid secretion
Cardiovascular function
Positive inotropic effect on the myocardium
Permissive effect on adrenergic vasoconstriction of small
   vessels
Anti-inflammatory effects
Inhibition of synthesis and release of prostaglandins
Stabilization of intracellular lysozomes
Decreased histamine release from tissue mast cells and
   circulating basophilic leucocytes
Inhibition of capillary dilation and reduction of serum
   exudation
Inhibition of white-cell mobilization to inflamed areas
Immune system
Inhibition of interleukin-1 production by macrophages
Reduction of circulating T- and B-cell numbers
Increased antibody titre—low and moderate steroid levels
Suppression of antibody production—high steroid levels
CNS
Euphoria
Decreased seizure threshold
MINERALOCORTICOID ACTIVITY
Enhancement of renal Na^+ reabsorption
Enhancement of renal K^+, H^+, NH_4^+, Mg^{2+} excretion
Stimulation of kallikrein–kinin system

series of 5β and 5α ('allo') tetrahydrocortisol, tetrahydrocortisone, cortol and cortolone metabolites. Cortols and cortolones may be metabolized further by oxidation of the 21-hydroxyl group to a carboxyl group giving cortolic and cortolonic acids, respectively. Corticosterone is metabolized in a similar way to cortisol, with formation of tetrahydro and hexahydro products, but with approximately equal amounts of 5α and 5β derivatives.

Androstenedione is reduced to androsterone (5α) and aetiocholanolone (5β) products and similarly 11β-hydroxyandrostenedione is converted to 11β-hydroxyandrosterone and 11β-hydroxyaetiocholanolone.

The liver can hydroxylate cortisol to form 6β-hydroxycortisol, a metabolite with increased water solubility that is readily excreted by the kidney. This is a major pathway in neonates, and 6β-hydroxycortisol excretion is also increased by hepatic enzyme-inducing drugs, in liver disease, pregnancy or oestrogen therapy, and in prolonged terminal illness. Increased thyroid hormone activity diminishes 6β-hydroxycortisol output.

Approximately 5–10% of the cortisol produced undergoes side-chain cleavage at C17–20 after reduction to tetrahydro derivatives to yield the C_{19}, 17-'oxo' derivatives 11β-hydroxyandrosterone and 11β-hydroxyaetiocholanolone. This has relevance for the estimation of urinary 17-oxosteroids, as although they mainly reflect the production of C_{19} adrenal androgen metabolites, they also contain a component derived from C_{21} corticosteroid output.

Steroid metabolites are conjugated as glucuronides and/or sulphates mainly at the 3α-hydroxyl and 21-hydroxyl positions. Steroid glucuronides are produced by glucuronyl transferase, which utilizes uridine–diphosphoglucuronic acid. Steroid sulphates result from the action of steroid sulphokinase, a cytosol enzyme that requires NAD and Mg^{2+} to transfer sulphate from 5-phosphoadenosine 5'-phosphosulphate to the steroid. C_{21} steroid metabolites are mainly excreted as 3-glucuronides, as is testosterone. DHA is conjugated mainly as the 3-sulphate, while other C_{19} steroids are excreted as both sulphates (approximately 10%) and glucuronides (90%). Conjugated steroids are filtered and excreted by the kidney without reabsorption.

A small proportion (approx. 0.5%) of the cortisol produced is excreted unchanged as urinary unbound or 'free' cortisol. Unbound cortisol in the circulation is filtered at the glomerulus, and although 80–90% of this is reabsorbed, mainly in the distal tubule, the free cortisol concentration in urine represents a clinically useful indication of plasma free cortisol levels.

Actions of Adrenal Steroids

Steroid action at target cells involves combination with specific cytosol receptors and subsequent binding of the steroid receptor complex to nuclear DNA, influencing mRNA production and protein synthesis. This two-step sequence of action means that there is a delay in the effects of glucocorticoid administration because of the requirement for protein synthesis. In addition, low levels of glucocorticoids are required for the function of many biochemical and physiological systems—the so-called permissive effect.

The concept that only the 'free' fraction of a hormone in the circulation is active may be an oversimplification. There is evidence that certain tissues such as liver and placenta may mobilize some of the protein-bound steroid and therefore receive a greater proportion of the total cortisol in the circulation.[4]

Corticosteroids have widespread effects on intermediary metabolism and electrolyte balance. These actions have been classified under the broad headings of glucocorticoid or mineralocorticoid, although steroids often have both types of activity to greater or lesser extent. Table 41.2 summarizes the main physiological and pharmacological actions of corticosteroids.

Acute deficiency of corticosteroids causes increased

TABLE 41.3
NATURAL AND SYNTHETIC CORTICOSTEROID POTENCIES

Name	Anti-inflammatory relative potency (Cortisol = 1)	Mineralocorticoid relative potency (Cortisol = 1)
Hydrocortisone (cortisol)	1.0	1.0
Cortisone	0.8	1.0
Dexamethasone	30.0	(mild natriuretic)
Betamethasone	30.0	(mild natriuretic)
Prednisolone	4.0	0.5
Prednisone	4.0	0.5
Methylprednisolone	6.0	0.5
Triamcinolone	5.0	0
Fludrocortisone (9α-fluorocortisol)	10.0	125.0
Deoxycorticosterone	0	30.0
Aldosterone	0.1	600.0

sodium loss, decreased blood pressure and volume, impaired urine concentration or dilution capacity by the kidney, depletion of liver and muscle glycogen, and decreased plasma glucose levels, and a state of shock develops.

Excessive circulatory levels of corticosteroids are associated with blood volume expansion, falling plasma potassium, increased protein catabolism, increased plasma glucose, a decrease in quantity and strength of bone and other connective tissues, impairment of cell-mediated immunity and poor wound healing.

Steroid Therapy and Synthetic Corticosteroids
Corticosteroid therapy is used for a wide variety of applications including replacement in patients with deficiency, to suppress pituitary ACTH secretion, to suppress unwanted inflammatory reactions, or to reduce the immune response to antigens and organ transplants. Although both glucocorticoid and mineralocorticoid activity may be required in replacement therapy, sodium retention associated with mineralocorticoid activity is not desirable for anti-inflammatory or for immune suppression therapy.

Table 41.3 lists the major natural and synthetic corticosteroids used in steroid therapy, together with their potency relative to cortisol as anti-inflammatory agents and mineralocorticoids.

Circulating Steroid Levels

The corticosteroids present in the circulation include the glucocorticoids cortisol and lower levels of corticosterone, the weak adrenal androgens androstenedione, 11-hydroxyandrostenedione, DHA and DHAS, and the mineralocorticoids aldosterone and deoxycorticosterone. Other steroids secreted into the circulation in small amounts include testosterone, 17α-OHP and 11-deoxycortisol. Typical plasma levels and production rates for corticosteroids are set out in Table 41.4.

The cortisol present in the circulation has a half-life of approximately 66 min and exists in three forms: 70% is bound to corticosteroid-binding globulin, approximately 20% is loosely bound to albumin, and approximately 10% is unbound or free.

Corticosteroid-binding Globulin

Corticosteroid-binding globulin (CBG) or transcortin is a single-chain glycoprotein of 383 amino acids and a molecular mass of 52 000. Approximately 27% of its weight consists of carbohydrate. It is a member of the serine protease inhibitor (Serpin) family of proteins and migrates with α_1-globulins on electrophoresis. The CBG molecule contains a single steroid-binding site, which binds cortisol and corticosterone with high affinity and other corticosteroids to a lesser extent (Table 41.5).

The binding capacity of CBG in normal subjects is approximately 650 nmol/L, a level similar to the upper limit of normal for morning serum cortisol concentrations. Increases above this result in a relatively large increase in serum unbound cortisol levels. The physiological role of CBG is unclear; it has a half-life of approximately 6 days and it may serve to provide a relatively stable pool of cortisol in equilibrium with the free fraction, or to provide differential delivery of cortisol to certain tissues such as liver or placenta. Recent evidence that interaction of CBG with neutrophil elastase during inflammation results in a conformational change, with release of glucocorticoid from its binding site, suggests a possible role for CBG in targeted delivery of glucocorticoid at sites of inflammation.

CBG concentrations are increased two- to threefold in pregnancy and also are raised with oestrogen therapy; they are lower in Cushing's syndrome and in disease states associated with increased protein loss or decreased synthesis. Rare familial conditions of CBG deficiency or variants have been described.[6,7]

TABLE 41.4
SERUM CORTICOSTEROIDS

Steroid	Abbreviation	Mol. Wt.	Secretion rate mg/day (μmol/day)	Serum reference range[a]
Cortisol	Compound F	362	20.0 (55)	200–750 nmol/L (hospital inpatients)
Corticosterone	Compound B	346	3.0 (8)	2.5–60 nmol/L
11-deoxycortisol	Compound S	346	0.35 (1)	2.5–7.5 nmol/L
Deoxycorticosterone	DOC	330	0.6 (2)	1.0–3.5 nmol/L
17α-hydroxyprogesterone	17-OHP	330	1.5 (5)	Less than 14 nmol/L
Dehydroepiandrosterone	DHA	289	8.0 (30)	15–30 nmol/L
Dehydroepiandrosterone sulphate	DHAS	369	13.0 (35)	4–10 (F) μmol/L 5–13 (M) μmol/L
Androstenedione	AD	286	2.2 (8)	3–12 nmol/L
Aldosterone	Aldo	360	0.15 (0.4)	200–1000 pmol/L (ambulant) 30–400 pmol/L (supine)

[a] Morning serum or plasma levels in young adults. Reference ranges are guidelines only and will be different for different laboratory methods.

TABLE 41.5
RELATIVE BINDING AFFINITIES OF STEROIDS FOR
CORTICOSTEROID-BINDING GLOBULIN

Steroid	Relative binding affinity (expressed as a percentage relative to cortisol) (%)
Cortisol	100
Corticosterone	100
11-deoxycortisol	100
17α-hydroxyprogesterone	76
Deoxycorticosterone	63
Progesterone	36
Cortisone	12
Testosterone	8
Aldosterone	3
Androstenedione	1
Dehydroepiandrosterone	< 0.1
Oestradiol	< 0.1

Adapted from Dunn et al.[5] with permission.

CONTROL OF ADRENAL STEROID SECRETION

Cortisol Secretion

Adrenal secretion of cortisol is controlled by ACTH, a 39 amino-acid peptide that acts by receptor-mediated stimulation of cAMP production (the second messenger system) on the cells of the three zones of the adrenal cortex. The secretion of ACTH is itself stimulated by corticotrophin-releasing hormone (CRH), a 41 amino-acid peptide released from the hypothalamus under the control of the higher central nervous system, which maintains circadian rhythm and initiates emotional, pain and stress responses. The release and actions of CRH are orchestrated by the combined effects of several stimulatory or inhibitory factors. Release of CRH from the paraventricular and supraoptic nuclei in the hypothalamus is stimulated by serotonin and acetylcholine and possibly by interleukins 1 and 6, while noradrenaline, substance P, opioids, γ-aminobutyric acid and possibly atrial natriuretic peptide (99–126) are inhibitors. The action of CRH on the anterior pituitary is enhanced by vasopressin and adrenaline.

A series of negative feedback pathways also regulates the activity of the hypothalamic–pituitary–adrenal axis: decreased or increased cortisol levels stimulate or inhibit ACTH and CRH release, and ACTH may also have a negative feedback influence on CRH secretion (Fig. 41.5).

Circadian Rhythm

In a population of normal subjects, serum cortisol levels are highest at the time of waking and show a fall during the day to a nadir during the first 1–2 h of sleep; then they rise during the early morning hours to return to a maximum on waking. This pattern may vary in an individual, and is modified by changes in the sleep/wake cycle over several days, and by the pattern of light/dark. ACTH and cortisol secretion occurs in a pulsatile manner with prolonged bursts of secretory activity in the morning, intermittent activity later in the day and minimal stimulation for approximately 4 h before and 2 h after the onset of sleep.

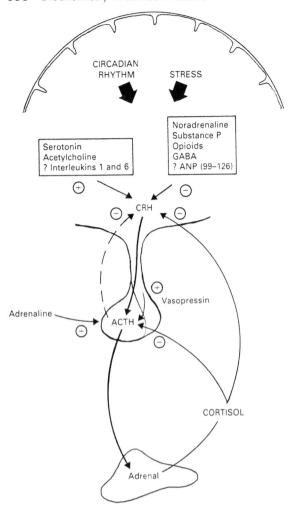

Figure 41.5 Diagram of the factors involved in the control of the hypothalamic–pituitary–adrenal axis. ACTH, adrenocorticotrophic hormone; ANP, atrial natriuretic peptide; CRH, corticotrophin-releasing hormone; GABA, γ-aminobutyric acid.

Stress

The normal circadian rhythm in serum cortisol concentrations can be overridden by the effects of psychological or physical stress, which stimulate cortisol output.

Psychological factors play a major part in determining the response to a threat. Anticipation of a stressful event can be just as potent in stimulating cortisol secretion as the event itself. Novel stimuli provoke greater responses than repeated, familiar stresses and the perception of how effectively a stress can be coped with is an important factor governing the endocrine response. The relative position of an individual in a social hierarchy also influences the stress response; this tends to be greater in those with least control over their environment.[8]

Physical stresses such as hard exercise, major surgery, burns or other major insults to the body are a potent stimulus to cortisol secretion. During major

surgery, for example, cortisol levels rise during the first 15–30 min after starting the procedure with maximum levels at approximately 1–2 h. Postsurgical complications are associated with a continuation in high plasma cortisol concentrations.

The stimulatory effects of psychological or physical stress on cortisol secretion are not overridden during dexamethasone suppression testing (*see* below).

Adrenal Androgen Secretion

In the adult, the secretion of the adrenal androgens androstenedione, DHA and DHAS follows the pattern of cortisol secretion under the influence of ACTH secretory bursts. In children the adrenal glands begin to secrete increased amounts of androgen between 6 and 8 years of age. This change in adrenal androgen secretion (the 'adrenarche') occurs before puberty and is associated with the appearance of axillary and pubic hair. ACTH and cortisol secretion do not change at adrenarche, and the factors that initiate increased adrenal androgen secretion are unknown.[9–11]

Aldosterone Secretion

Under normal circumstances ACTH has a relatively minor influence on aldosterone secretion by the zona glomerulosa, the major control being maintained by the renin–angiotensin system (*see* Chapter 34).

METHODS FOR STEROID MEASUREMENT

Older methods for assessing the hypothalamic–pituitary–adrenal axis based on colorimetric or fluorimetric assays of plasma and urine steroids with particular functional groups have been replaced by more specific radioimmunoassays (RIAs). Urine steroid profiles obtained by gas chromatography with confirmation of the identity of steroid peaks by mass spectrometry is a valuable research procedure and provides back-up to radioimmunoassay results in the investigation of possible cases of deficiency of a steroid-pathway enzyme.

Serum Corticosteroid

Cortisol concentrations can be measured by direct (non-extraction) RIA using [^{125}I] cortisol tracer with either an in-house protocol or commercially available kits.[12] Care must be taken to assess the cross-reactivity of other steroids in the assay; RIAs used to monitor the efficacy of metyrapone therapy in lowering serum (or urine) cortisol concentrations must have very low cross-reactivity with 11-deoxycortisol for example. Although most RIA methods for cortisol do not cross-react with dexamethasone, interference by prednisolone (and prednisone) is common and needs to be considered when interpreting results.

Convenient RIA methods are also available for the

measurement of 17α-hydroxyprogesterone, androstenedione, DHAS and 11-deoxycortisol. Interpretation of results is helped by a detailed knowledge of reference ranges appropriate for the method in use and for the age and population of patients studied, and by an awareness of cross-reacting and interfering factors. Most RIAs for 17-OHP will give apparently high results in preterm neonates, for example, probably because of cross-reactivity of closely related fetal steroids.[13,14]

Urine Steroid

In the past, steroids with particular substituent groupings were measured using colorimetric or fluorimetric procedures. For example, in the USA the measurement of total 17-hydroxycorticosteroids by reaction of steroids with the 17,21-dihydroxy, 20-ketone structure with phenylhydrazine (the Porter–Silber reaction) has been used. This method suffers from considerable interferences from the effects of drugs (spironolactone, phenytoin, antibiotics) and ketone-containing compounds. In the UK, urine steroid quantitation relied upon the estimation of 17-oxogenic steroids (17-hydroxyl and 20-hydroxyl or oxo group) and 17-oxosteroids using the Zimmerman reaction as an approximate guide to adrenal corticosteroid and adrenal androgen production, respectively.

A strong case has been made for the discontinuation of 17-oxogenic and 17-oxosteroid determinations on the grounds of inconvenience, poor precision, susceptibility to interference and limited diagnostic value compared with newer, more specific methods.[15] In simple obesity, for example, levels of 17-oxogenic steroids are increased because of increased rate of cortisol production and increased excretion of steroid conjugates, although serum cortisol and urine free cortisol concentrations (by solvent extraction and RIA) are unchanged. This effect severely limits the value of 17-oxogenic steroid measurements in the investigation of suspected Cushing's syndrome.

Paper chromatographic separation of 11-oxygenated from 11-deoxysteroids and estimation of an 11-oxygenation index or the measurement of urinary pregnanetriol to indentify cases of congenital adrenal hyperplasia have been superseded by RIA of 17-OHP as a screening test. Additional plasma steroid measurements can be made if necessary and a gas chromatography–mass spectroscopy urine steroid profile is helpful in confirming the site of the enzyme deficiency.

The determination of urinary free cortisol excretion by RIA is an extremely useful screen for Cushing's syndrome. Estimation of urinary 11-hydroxycorticosteroids by fluorimetric assays (Mattingly) gave considerably higher results than RIA methods and was subject to gross overestimation if urines were left to stand, owing to an increase in non-specific fluorescence.

Although direct, non-extraction RIAs are available for urine cortisol, it is important to establish that methods do not have excessive positive bias. The use of solvent extraction followed by RIA is the method of choice for urine cortisol measurement. Even with this procedure, chromatographic identification of corticosteroids has shown that only 23–70% of cortisol immunoreactivity is actually cortisol.[12]

Salivary and Bloodspot Steroids

Salivary steroid concentrations have the advantage that often they reflect the plasma free (unbound) steroid level, although this is complicated by the fact that the parotid glands may be a target for cortisol, testosterone and other steroids. Sample collection is simple and non-invasive. After freezing, thawing and centrifugation the saliva can be analysed by RIA, although assays of greater sensitivity (lower detection limits) are required to measure the lower steroid levels in saliva. The response in salivary cortisol to Synacthen (tetracosactrin) stimulation is much greater than for serum total cortisol measurements, as once the binding capacity of CBG is exceeded, a much greater proportion of cortisol secretion is unbound and is measured in the saliva.

Other steroids that can be measured in saliva include 17-OHP, androstenedione, testosterone, DHAS, progesterone, oestriol, oestradiol, aldosterone and prednisolone.[16] Potential disadvantages of salivary assays are that multiple samples may be required to give clinically useful information, and the difficulty of obtaining salivary samples in very young infants.

Bloodspot steroid assays are also valuable for the investigation of patients. Blood collection involves spotting a heel- or finger-prick sample on to filter paper, and is convenient for neonates, or for home monitoring of older children and adults. Bloodspot 17-OHP assays are useful for the diagnosis of congenital adrenal hyperplasia due to 21-hydroxylase deficiency in neonates[17] and have been used in neonatal screening trials.[18]

The assessment of a bloodspot steroid profile with sampling times of 08.00, 12.00, 18.00 and 23.00 provides additional data on the pattern of steroid levels throughout the day. Bloodspots can be taken at home by patients using an 'Autolet'® or 'Soft-Touch'® finger-prick system, and filter paper cards can be posted directly to the laboratory. 17-OHP and androstenedione profiles give useful information on the efficacy of steroid replacement therapy for congenital adrenal hyperplasia,[17,19] while bloodspot cortisol profiles help to identify those hypopituitary or hypoadrenal patients not receiving optimum corticosteroid replacement therapy.

DYNAMIC TESTS OF ADRENAL FUNCTION

The ability to test the response of the hypothalamic–pituitary–adrenal axis to challenges by agents that normally suppress or stimulate the cortisol response has provided a valuable means of improving the diagnostic efficiency of hormone measurements. The most important dynamic tests are described below.

ACTH Stimulation Tests

Synacthen (tetracosactrin) is a bioactive synthetic peptide containing the first 24 amino acids of natural (1–39) ACTH from the aminoterminal end. It is used in a short stimulation test to screen for primary or secondary adrenal deficiency, and also as a depot preparation for a 3-day stimulation test to discriminate adrenal deficiency from adrenal suppression due to hypopituitarism or long-term steroid therapy.

Short Synacthen Test

A baseline serum blood sample is taken and then 250 μg of Synacthen is injected intramuscularly. Two more blood samples are obtained at 30 and 60 min. Serum or plasma cortisol levels should rise by at least 200 nmol/L to a level greater than 550 nmol/L. Inadequate responses are seen in both primary adrenal failure (Addison's disease) and with secondary hypoadrenalism (hypopituitarism or corticosteroid therapy).

3-day Depot Synacthen Test

This test can be used to confirm a diagnosis of Addison's disease when the short Synacthen test response is impaired. Rarely, the 3-day depot test has precipitated Addisonian crisis and therefore it should only be done on hospital inpatients with medical supervision. Patients can be given low-dose dexamethasone 'cover' (0.25 mg daily) during the test if necessary. One mg of depot Synacthen is given intramuscularly at 09.00 each day for 3 days. The response is monitored by taking a baseline venous blood sample and further samples at 12.00 on the 3 days of the test. In normal subjects, plasma cortisol levels are over 1000 nmol/L at the end of the test. In Addison's there is no plasma cortisol response, whereas in cases of secondary adrenal insufficiency a delayed but significant response (at least a doubling in plasma cortisol levels) is seen.

If assays for plasma ACTH are readily available to confirm a case of Addison's disease it is not necessary to do the 3-day depot Synacthen test.

Dexamethasone Suppression Tests

Dexamethasone is a potent synthetic glucocorticoid that acts through the negative feedback system at the pituitary and hypothalamus to suppress cortisol secretion in normal subjects. It is used in a low-dose, overnight test to screen for Cushing's syndrome and in high-dose tests to help differentiate between pituitary-driven Cushing's disease and adrenal adenoma or ectopic ACTH syndrome.

Low-dose suppression test

The low-dose suppression test can be done on outpatients and involves taking 1 mg of dexamethasone by mouth at 23.00 and giving a venous blood sample for plasma cortisol at 09.00 the following day. Normally, the 09.00 plasma cortisol levels are suppressed to less than 150 nmol/L following dexamethasone administration. False-positive failure to suppress can occur in the obese, anxious or depressed patient and in those taking oestrogen or liver enzyme-inducing drugs such as phenytoin, when dexamethasone metabolism is enhanced.

High-dose Suppression Tests

The classical dexamethasone suppression test as described by Liddle[20] combines a low- and high-dose test and involves collection of 24-h urine samples for 6 days: the first 2 days are baseline collections. On the third and fourth days, dexamethasone (0.5 mg 6-hourly) is given orally and on days 5 and 6 dexamethasone (2 mg 6-hourly) is given. Responses can be monitored by urine cortisol measurements or by 09.00 plasma cortisol levels during the test. Suppression is indicated by a fall to less than 50% of basal urine cortisol or 09.00 plasma cortisol levels.

An overnight high-dose (8 mg) dexamethasone suppression test is at least as effective as the classical regimen, and is quicker and more convenient to do.[21,22] The protocol is the same as that for the low-dose overnight test, except that 8 mg dexamethasone is given at 23.00. Suppression is indicated by a fall in the 09.00 plasma cortisol level to less than 50% of previous 09.00 levels.

The use of low- and high-dose dexamethasone suppression tests to screen for Cushing's syndrome and to differentiate between pituitary, adrenal or ectopic ACTH sources is compromised by the fact that there are many exceptions to the general guidelines for interpretation. Although most patients with Cushing's syndrome fail to suppress to low-dose dexamethasone, suppression occurs in some cases of pituitary-driven Cushing's disease. The high-dose test also does not give complete discrimination, suppression sometimes occurring in cases of ectopic ACTH syndrome or adrenal tumour, and sometimes not occurring in cases of pituitary disease.

Dexamethasone Suppression Testing and Depressive Illness

Approximately 25–60% of patients with major depressive illness fail to suppress their plasma cortisol levels using a modified low-dose overnight suppression test regimen with blood sampling at 16.00 on the day after oral administration of 1 mg of dexamethasone at 23.00.[23] The test was recommended for the laboratory diagnosis of endogenous depression and for predicting the response to tricyclic antidepressants; imipramine or desimipramine were recommended for patients who did not suppress, whereas patients with normal suppression were felt to respond preferentially to amitriptyline or clomipramine.[24] Further investigation has shown that the test is of no value when used to assign patients to particular tricyclic therapy[25] and the case for dexamethasone testing in depressive illness remains unproven.

Insulin-induced Hypoglycaemia

Insulin-induced hypoglycaemia is a potent stimulus to the hypothalamic–pituitary–adrenal axis and is the only standardized test that assesses whether a patient can respond adequately to stress. The test is potentially dangerous and should be performed only under constant medical supervision with (for adults) 50 mL of 50% glucose, 100 mg hydrocortisone for intravenous injection and 1 mg glucagon for intramuscular injection available at the bedside to stop the test if necessary. It is contraindicated in patients with epilepsy, ischaemic heart disease or with known hypopituitarism. The insulin hypoglycaemia test may be combined with the thyrotrophin-releasing hormone and luteinizing hormone-releasing hormone stimulation tests when generalized pituitary hypofunction is suspected.

The test is usually done in the morning after the patient has fasted overnight, but this is not essential. In normal-weight subjects it is usually sufficient to give soluble insulin (0.1 units/kg body weight) by rapid intravenous injection through an indwelling venous cannula. Further blood samples are taken at 30, 60, 90 and 120 min for cortisol measurements. Glucose levels should be monitored frequently and preferably at the bedside to check for hypoglycemia (plasma glucose less than 2.5 mmol/L; blood glucose less than 2.2 mmol/L). If signs of neuroglycopenia or evidence of hypoglycaemia do not occur within 1 h of the initial injection, a further insulin dose of 0.1–0.2 units/kg body weight, depending on circumstances, can be given. This may occur in patients with insulin resistance—for example those with acromegaly, Cushing's syndrome or poorly controlled diabetes with high plasma glucose levels.

A normal cortisol response to insulin-induced hypoglycaemia is defined as a rise of at least 200 nmol/L to a level greater than 550 nmol/L. Plasma ACTH can be monitored at 0, 30 and 60 min, and normally shows at least a doubling in concentration. The test is used in the investigation of patients with hypopituitarism or those with possible suppression of the hypothalamic–pituitary–adrenal axis following long-term steroid therapy. Patients with Cushing's syndrome from whatever cause fail to show a rise in cortisol (or ACTH) in response to insulin-induced hypoglycaemia, a response which differs from that shown by patients with depression, where there is a further rise in cortisol output in response to hypoglycaemia. However, there is some overlap in responses to the test for patients in these two groups.

It would seem advantageous to avoid using the lengthy, sometimes uncomfortable and potentially dangerous insulin stimulation test (IST) if another simpler test could yield the same information. A strong case has been made for using the short Synacthen test rather than the IST to assess the hypothalamic–pituitary–adrenal axis.[26] Remarkable concordance between the results of the two tests was shown for the great majority of patients with hypothalamic–pituitary disorders who were investigated. Only in those patients on corticosteroid therapy or who had received a pituitary insult (post-surgery or apoplexy) within 14 days was there discordance between results for these two dynamic tests. A suitable rationale for testing therefore utilizes the short Synacthen test as a screen and reserves the IST for patients failing the short Synacthen test and those on corticosteroid therapy or who have received a pituitary trauma within 2 weeks of assessment.

The Metyrapone Test

The use of metyrapone to block cortisol secretion and to test the integrity of feedback control in the hypothalamic–pituitary–adrenal axis was first proposed by Liddle.[27] The test involves administration of 750 mg metyrapone orally every 4 h for 72 h. Plasma ACTH or 11-deoxycortisol can be measured at 0, 1, 2, 3, 4 and 24 h as an alternative to monitoring changes in urinary 17-oxogenic steroid excretion. A doubling of plasma ACTH or oxogenic steroid output or an increase of 11-deoxycortisol of greater than 300 nmol/L defines a normal response.

The metyrapone test is potentially dangerous for the investigation of hypopituitarism and should not be used for this purpose. Patients with pituitary-driven Cushing's disease show hyper-responsiveness to metyrapone in contrast to patients with adrenal tumours where there is a lack of response. However, basal plasma ACTH levels will usually distinguish these two situations and the metyrapone test is unhelpful in discriminating between Cushing's disease and the ectopic ACTH syndrome associated with slowly growing 'occult' tumours, such as bronchial carcinoids.[28,29] The metyrapone test has little to recommend it for the present-day investigation of patients with Cushing's syndrome.

The CRH Test

Although they are not widely available at present, the use of synthetic ovine or human CRH-41 can be helpful in the discrimination of Cushing's disease from 'occult' ectopic ACTH syndrome, particularly when used in conjunction with inferior petrosal sinus catheterization. Although they are equipotent, ovine CRH-41 has a prolonged effect relative to human CRH-41, possibly reflecting its longer plasma half-life (46–73 min) compared with that for human CRH-41 (25 min).

The CRH test is carried out on patients at 09.00 following an overnight fast. Thirty min after cannulating the patient, a 100-μg bolus of CRH-41 is injected and venous blood samples are taken for cortisol and ACTH measurements at 15-min intervals for 2 h.[30]

Patients with Cushing's disease generally show an exaggerated cortisol response to CRH (peak cortisol response greater than 820 nmol/L), although some may produce results that overlap with the normal range. In a recent study, for example, 14 of 18 patients with surgically proven Cushing's disease showed an increased response.[30] The use of the CRH test in combination with results of the high-dose dexamethasone test was found to give complete discrimination for Cushing's disease. Using the criteria of either enhanced cortisol response to CRH or a greater than 50% suppression of cortisol to high-dose dexamethasone a correct diagnosis was made in all 18 patients, although each test on its own gave a false-negative result in approximately 20% of patients with Cushing's disease.[30]

The exaggerated cortisol response to CRH in Cushing's disease differs from that found in depressed patients (who show a normal cortisol but subnormal ACTH response) and the obese (who have a blunted cortisol response to CRH). Patients with ectopic ACTH syndrome generally show an absent cortisol response to CRH but there is some overlap between responses for Cushing's disease and ectopic ACTH syndrome, just as there is with other tests used in the investigation of Cushing's syndrome. In a recent study the finding of a lack of ACTH response to the CRH test was associated with only a 63% chance that this was due to an ectopic source.[31]

Inferior Petrosal Sinus Catheterization
In many patients with Cushing's disease the pituitary tumour is too small to be visualized with high-resolution computerized tomography (CT), making decisions on surgery difficult. The use of inferior petrosal venous sampling in combination with the CRH test provides a valuable means of demonstrating an ACTH gradient and in confirming the diagnosis of pituitary-dependent Cushing's disease in difficult cases.

Preliminary evidence suggests that the pituitary tumour is usually found on the same side of the pituitary as the ACTH gradient, with the suggestion that if a surgeon fails to find a tumour s/he could remove half the pituitary on the side of the gradient.[30,31] The danger of causing permanent hypopituitarism associated with removal of the whole pituitary would be avoided and the procedure would give a degree of assurance that the tumour had been removed. This approach represents another potential advantage of the test but the findings require further confirmation.

The test involves taking blood samples simultaneously from catheters positioned at the left and right petrosal sinuses (which drain the pituitary gland and cavernous sinuses) or if this is not possible from left and right high internal jugular veins. Simultaneous peripheral venous blood samples are obtained for comparison. CRH-41 is injected as a bolus of 100 μg over 10 s and further bilateral samples are taken at 3, 8 and 13 min post-CRH. The finding of a plasma ACTH gradient of greater than twofold in basal or CRH-stimulated high jugular or petrosal sinus samples relative to the periphery confirms the presence of a pituitary tumour, and a gradient of more than twofold between left and right petrosal venous samples gives an indication of the position of the tumour.

In the case of ectopic ACTH syndrome no gradient is seen in petrosal sinus samples relative to peripheral ones. The results of the petrosal sampling/CRH test in two patients, one with a right-sided pituitary tumour and the other with ectopic ACTH syndrome, are shown in Fig. 41.6.

CLINICAL INVESTIGATION OF ADRENOCORTICAL DYSFUNCTION

Adrenocortical Insufficiency

Adrenocortical insufficiency is defined as primary (Addison's disease) or secondary to hypopituitarism or suppression following steroid therapy.

Primary Adrenocortical Insufficiency—Addison's Disease
Destruction of the adrenal cortex, regardless of the cause, gives rise to Addison's disease. Clinical symptoms are mainly due to cortisol and aldosterone deficiency, but they do not manifest themselves until approximately 90% of the adrenal cortex has been destroyed.

Before the mid-1950s the major cause of Addison's disease was tuberculosis, but at present autoimmune adrenal atrophy is the most common cause, accounting for approximately 80% of cases and with a higher incidence in women. Antiadrenal antibodies can be demonstrated in the serum from most patients with autoimmune adrenal atrophy but they are not present in Addison's disease due to other causes. Although in the majority of cases the adrenal glands alone are involved, autoimmune Addison's disease may be part of a polyglandular disorder with possible involvement of premature ovarian failure, hypoparathyroidism, diabetes mellitus, hypothyroidism, pernicious anaemia or vitiligo. In young male patients, adrenoleucodystrophy may present as Addison's disease in the absence of obvious neurological symptoms.

Less common causes of Addison's disease include adrenal haemorrhage, infiltration by carcinoma or fungal infection.

A rare disorder with features similar to Addison's disease, caused by lack of adrenal cortical receptors for ACTH, has been described. It gives rise to feeding problems in infancy and to stress-induced hypoglycaemia and hyperpigmentation. Secretion of aldosterone

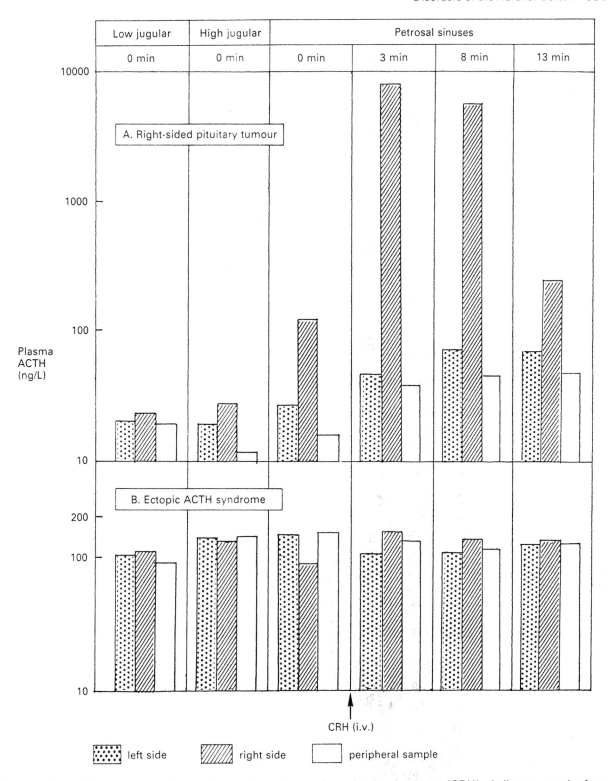

Figure 41.6 Petrosal sinus catheterization with corticotrophin-releasing hormone (CRH) challenge—results from two patients. Patient A, right-sided pituitary tumour; patient B, ectopic ACTH syndrome. (Data kindly provided by Dr S. Medbak, Department of Chemical Endocrinology, St Bartholomew's Hospital, London.)

is also decreased in this disorder, which is inherited as an autosomal or X-linked recessive trait.[32]

Another syndrome of congenital adrenal hypo-plasia with an X-linked pattern of inheritance has been reported[33] but the biochemical abnormality involved has not been identified.

Adrenoleucodystrophy. The term adrenoleucodystrophy describes two inherited disorders that affect predominantly the nervous system and adrenal gland.

The form inherited as an X-linked trait (Addison–Schilder disease) is more common and in some patients may present as primary adrenal insufficiency in childhood, adolescence, and in young adults, with neurological symptoms occurring later. To date the oldest patient to be identified with adrenal insufficiency without the neurological signs of the disorder was 34 years of age. The second 'neonatal' form is inherited as an autosomal recessive trait and presents in infants as seizures, multiple congenital malformations and psychomotor retardation with relatively minor adrenal involvement.

X-linked adrenoleucodystrophy results from a deficiency of the peroxisome enzyme lignoceroyl-CoA ligase, causing an accumulation of very long-chain fatty acids, particularly hexacosanoic, tetracosanoic and pentacosanoic acids. A significant proportion of Addison's disease in male patients may be due to adrenoleucodystropy—the incidence at the present time may be as high as 40% according to a recent study in the USA.[34] The poor prognosis associated with adrenoleucodystrophy and the potential benefits of genetic counselling and prenatal diagnosis strengthen the case for adrenoleucodystrophy screening of all male patients with Addison's disease. Conversely, patients with adrenoleucodystrophy need to be screened at regular intervals for signs of diminishing adrenocortical activity.

Clinical Presentation and Diagnostic Tests

Addison's disease may have a slow, insidious progression with gradual development of symptoms, but stress caused by an intercurrent illness may precipitate an Addisonian crisis of very sudden onset. Symptoms of Addison's disease include weakness and easy fatigability, anorexia, vomiting, diarrhoea and abdominal pain. Pigmentation of the skin, particularly in flexures such as palmar creases, in buccal mucosa, pressure points and wound scars, is seen if the adrenal insufficiency is long-standing; this results from high levels of ACTH and ACTH precursors. Amenorrhoea is common in women with Addison's disease.

Muscle weakness becomes more profound and hypotension develops as the disease progresses. Patients may be admitted in hypoglycaemic coma or they may be collapsed with hypovolaemia and acute dehydration due to water and sodium losses. In many cases of acute adrenal insufficiency the symptoms of nausea, bowel upset, muscle weakness and hypotension are similar to those of many other acute illnesses—for example, patients presenting with gastrointestinal symptoms may be mistaken for cases of severe gastroenteritis. In the absence of any obvious cause of symptoms, Addison's disease must be considered in the differential diagnosis. It is unfortunate that even in centres of excellence the majority of patients presenting in Addisonian crisis may be missed. In one series, 32 of 56 patients who died as a result of Addisonian crisis were undiagnosed or were diagnosed only in the terminal stage of the illness.[35]

If the disease shows a rapid progression, pigmentation may not be evident, and 'typical' biochemical features of a low plasma sodium and bicarbonate and raised plasma potassium and urea may be absent. A study of 20 cases of untreated Addison's disease showed that 25% of patients had normal plasma sodium, 55% normal plasma potassium, and 25% normal plasma urea concentrations.[36]

In non-acute circumstances the short Synacthen test can be used to screen for primary or secondary adrenal insufficiency, where an absent or impaired response is seen. A normal response—a rise in plasma cortisol of at least 200 nmol/L to a level greater than 550 nmol/L—excludes the diagnosis of Addison's disease but does not completely exclude insufficiency secondary to diminished ACTH secretory capacity.

If adrenal insufficiency is indicated by the results of the short Synacthen screening test, the measurement of a morning plasma ACTH level will confirm the diagnosis of Addison's disease. Plasma ACTH concentrations are very high in primary adrenal insufficiency (normally over 200 ng/L) because low cortisol levels stimulate ACTH output through negative feedback control. ACTH measurements may not be readily available, however, and in this case a 3-day depot Synacthen test can be used to discriminate between Addison's disease, where there is no plasma cortisol response, and secondary insufficiency, where plasma cortisol concentrations increase in response to depot ACTH stimulation. Low-dose dexamethasone cover can be given during the 3-day test to guard against precipitation of acute adrenal insufficiency.

Treatment with glucocorticoids and fluids should not be delayed when a patient is admitted in suspected Addisonian crisis. The minimum requirement for diagnosis is to take blood samples for cortisol and ACTH just before treatment. A short Synacthen test can be performed at a later stage, provided that the patient is switched to low-dose synthetic steroid cover (dexamethasone, 0.5 mg 8-hourly, and fludrocortisone, 0.1 mg 8-hourly) before testing. Basal plasma cortisol concentrations are usually less than 300 nmol/L in patients with Addison's disease; levels higher than this do not exclude the diagnosis, however, as they still may be inappropriately low for the stressed state of the patient. The findings of inappropriately low plasma cortisol and markedly raised ACTH results are usually sufficient to confirm the diagnosis of Addison's disease in the acutely ill patient.

Steroid-induced Suppression of the Hypothalamic–Pituitary–Adrenal Axis

Administration of large doses of glucocorticoids for short periods (1–3 days) produces only a temporary suppression of the axis, and withdrawal of corticosteroid therapy can be achieved with little difficulty. Prolonged therapy with high doses of steroids required to achieve anti-inflammatory action induces more extensive suppression of the axis. If glucocorticoid therapy is to be withdrawn, this must be done very gradually and requires a period of a year or more in some cases.

The plasma cortisol response to a short Synacthen test is usually impaired in patients on long-term steroid therapy, and although cortisol secretion can be induced by 3-day depot Synacthen stimulation this cannot be taken as evidence that the patient can respond adequately to stress, as the hypothalamus and pituitary may still be suppressed. If the patient is well enough their capacity to respond to stress can be checked by their plasma cortisol response to insulin-induced hypoglycaemia, which tests the integrity of the whole hypothalamic–pituitary–adrenal axis.

Long-term Steroid Replacement Therapy
The normal secretion of cortisol by the adrenal cortex is approximately 20 mg/day and replacement therapy is based on the administration of a similar or slightly higher dose of hydrocortisone (20–50 mg/day) or an equivalent dose of cortisone acetate, usually splitting the daily treatment 2:1 between the morning and evening doses. The doses used are often empirically chosen and it is only on detailed questioning that symptoms of under-replacement may come to light. There is a case for regular monitoring of daytime profiles of plasma or bloodspot cortisol in these patients to give additional information. Studies by Groves et al.[37] and in our laboratory have shown that patients with plasma cortisol concentrations of less than 100 nmol/L (bloodspot cortisol < 60 nmol/L) in the late afternoon have an increased incidence of tiredness and lethargy at this time. Changing the hydrocortisone dosage regimen from twice-daily doses split 2:1 to thrice-daily doses (evenly divided) resulted in a marked improvement in 'well-being' in these patients.[37]

Cushing's Syndrome

The term Cushing's syndrome refers to the features and metabolic abnormalities associated with excessive glucocorticoid activity. This may result from glucocorticoid overtreatment (the most common cause), from increased ACTH drive from hypothalamic–pituitary overactivity or pituitary tumour, from an ectopic source of ACTH, or from autonomous production of cortisol and other adrenal androgens from an adrenal adenoma, carcinoma or ACTH-independent, bilateral nodular hyperplasia. The term Cushing's disease refers specifically to the pituitary driven form of hypercortisolism, which accounts for approximately two-thirds of all cases of Cushing's syndrome; the remaining cases are approximately equally divided between primary adrenal causes and the ectopic ACTH syndrome. Cushing's disease is more common

in women (approximately 70% of cases) and although it occurs at all ages there is a peak incidence between the years of 30 and 50.[38] Cushing's disease may also present as part of the familial syndrome of multiple endocrine adenomatosis or multiple endocrine neoplasia type 1 (Wermer's syndrome), which involves primary hyperparathyroidism, pancreatic islet-cell tumours and pituitary adenomas.

Hypercortisolism can result from the production of ectopic ACTH from malignant tumours, commonly from small-cell carcinoma of the bronchus. Where there is rapid progression of the ectopic ACTH syndrome, patients may lack the typical Cushingoid features, although these may be present when the ectopic ACTH source is a slow-growing, 'occult' tumour such as a bronchial carcinoid. Rarely, hypercortisolism results from ectopic CRH production, usually with cosecretion of ectopic ACTH. In these cases, clinical presentations range from those of the rapidly progressing ectopic ACTH syndrome to features similar to those of patients with pituitary-driven Cushing's disease.[21]

Features and Investigation
The onset of Cushing's syndrome is often gradual, with symptoms of muscle weakness and tiredness occurring before other characteristic features. Weight gain is usual, but the classical feature of truncal obesity with thin arms and legs is not present in all patients. Supraclavicular and dorsal fat pads (buffalo hump), a round 'moon' face, thin, atrophic skin with purple striae over hips, lower abdomen and axillae, and signs of easy bruising may be seen. Hypertension is common but often is of only moderate severity. Impairment of glucose tolerance also is apparent but is generally mild, causing frank diabetes in approximately 25% of cases. Backache may be associated with osteoporotic changes and vertebral collapse with increased curvature of the spine may occur. Behavioural changes such as mood swings or depression often occur and may sometimes be the dominant feature on presentation. Mild hirsutism is seen in most women with Cushing's syndrome but signs of virilization such as male-pattern baldness, clitoromegaly and deepening of the voice are less common. Although Cushing's syndrome resulting from an adrenal adenoma may have features identical to those shown by patients with the pituitary-driven form, excessive androgen production together with cortisol may blunt the protein catabolic effect of cortisol; the musculature may be well preserved in these cases, although signs of virilization may be more apparent.

The investigation of patients with suspected Cushing's syndrome falls into two categories: firstly the hypercortisolism of the syndrome can be confirmed by screening tests; second-line tests can then be used for differential diagnosis. Hypothalamic–pituitary–adrenal axis testing should *not* be done in the first few days after hospital admission because stress effects are frequently observed at this time.

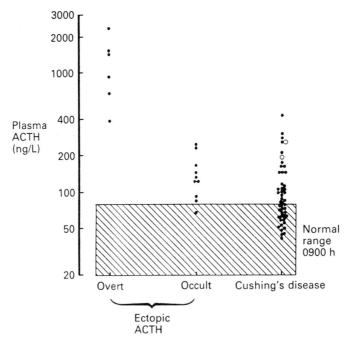

Figure 41.7 Plasma ACTH levels in patients with Cushing's disease, 'overt' or 'occult' ectopic ACTH syndrome: open circles, Cushing's disease patients on treatment with metyrapone. (From Howlett et al.,[29] with permission.)

TABLE 41.6

NEOPLASMS THAT PRODUCE BIOLOGICALLY ACTIVE ACTH

Type of neoplasm	Approx. % of cases
Carcinoma of the lung (predominantly small- or oat-cell)	50
Carcinoma of the thymus	10
Carcinoma of the pancreas (including carcinoid and islet-cell)	10
Phaeochromocytoma, neuroblastoma, ganglioma and paraganglioma	5
Medullary carcinoma of the thyroid	5
Bronchial adenoma and carcinoid	2
Miscellaneous carcinomas[a] or haematological malignancies	18

[a] For example, carcinoma of the ovary, prostate, breast, thyroid, kidney, salivary glands, testes, stomach, colon, gallbladder, oesophagus, appendix, acute myeloblastic leukaemia.
Reproduced from Odell[39] with permission.

Ectopic ACTH Syndrome

In many patients with ectopic ACTH syndrome the disease has a rapid progression and the classical signs of Cushing's syndrome may be absent, although biochemical changes are more extensive. Plasma cortisol levels can be very high (over 1000 nmol/L), with associated hypokalaemia and alkalosis. ACTH levels over 300 ng/L are strongly suggestive of ectopic ACTH syndrome, but levels for slowly growing tumours are lower and overlap completely with those found in Cushing's disease (Fig. 41.7). Pigmentation seen with ectopic ACTH syndrome results from the melanocyte-stimulating activity of ACTH, β-lipotrophin and possibly other peptide fragments of proopiomelanocortin that contain the melanocyte-stimulating hormone sequence. The types of neoplasm most frequently associated with ectopic ACTH syn-

drome are summarized in Table 41.6. Approximately 50% of patients with ectopic ACTH syndrome have carcinoma of the lung, mainly small-cell carcinoma.[39,40] However, less than 5% of patients with small-cell carcinoma of the lung have ectopic ACTH syndrome. Most normal human tissues tested contain low levels (less than 400 pg/g) of a bioinactive precursor peptide of ACTH, probably pro-opiomelanocortin (POM-C). Extracts of many different types of carcinoma contain much higher levels of ACTH precursor with average values of 22 000 pg/g,[39] although the majority of these do not cause ectopic ACTH syndrome.

The ectopic ACTH syndrome is probably associated with those tumours that are able to convert the inactive ACTH precursor into biologically active ACTH.

ACTH-independent Hyperadrenalism

In recent years a third type of adrenal lesion causing autonomous cortisol production—bilateral nodular hyperplasia—has been recognized in addition to adrenal adenoma or carcinoma.[21,38] This form of ACTH-independent adrenal hyperplasia is more common in children, and in adults it may account for approximately one-sixth of primary adrenal causes. The true incidence is difficult to determine because there are wide differences in the interpretation of whether 'microadenoma' or 'hyperplasia' are present. Bilateral adrenal nodular hyperplasia may represent the final stage in a progression from ACTH-dependent hyperplasia to ACTH-dependent nodular hyperplasia and then to ACTH-independent autonomy of cortisol production.[41] The hyperplastic appearance of the adrenal cortex suggests the possibility of stimulation by trophic factors other than ACTH, and it has been postulated that adrenal cortex-stimulating antibodies may be involved.[42]

Screening tests

Morning and midnight plasma cortisol levels, 24-h urine cortisol excretion and the plasma cortisol response to the overnight low-dose dexamethasone suppression test are all helpful in establishing the presence of hypercortisolism. For outpatients, the collection of a 24-h urine for cortisol is the most convenient screening method, but the overnight low-dose dexamethasone suppression test can also be done by taking a blood sample at clinic the following morning.

Single morning plasma cortisol concentrations are unhelpful in the diagnosis of Cushing's syndrome because in approximately 50% of cases results will lie within the morning reference range. Demonstration of a normal circadian rhythm in plasma cortisol by taking morning and midnight levels makes the diagnosis of Cushing's syndrome unlikely (although this may be seen at times in rare cases of cyclical Cushing's disease). Raised midnight plasma cortisol levels (greater than 200 nmol/L) are seen in Cushing's syndrome but are also found in seriously ill or stressed patients and in those with depressive illness.

Urinary cortisol excretion is a valuable screening test: an output of less than approximately 300 nmol/day, particularly if checked on several occasions, makes the diagnosis of Cushing's syndrome unlikely. Raised cortisol excretion is consistent with Cushing's syndrome but stress-related increases are common.

Suppression of the 09.00 plasma cortisol concentration to less than 150 nmol/L with the overnight low-dose dexamethasone test helps to exclude the diagnosis of Cushing's syndrome. Rarely, some cases of pituitary-driven Cushing's disease may suppress to low-dose dexamethasone and at times suppression may be normal in cyclical Cushing's syndrome. A lack of suppression may be seen in stressed patients, those with depressive illness or those taking enzyme-inducing drugs in addition to those with Cushing's syndrome. Paradoxical rises to low- (and high-) dose dexamethasone tests have been reported in some patients with cyclical Cushing's syndrome.

Differential Diagnosis

Once the presence of Cushing's syndrome has been established, further biochemical testing and scanning studies can be utilized to establish the aetiology of the disease. The most useful initial tests are morning plasma ACTH levels and the plasma cortisol response to high-dose dexamethasone suppression. In addition, the plasma cortisol response to insulin-induced hypoglycaemia may be helpful in confirming the lack of response seen in Cushing's syndrome and in differentiating those patients with similar endocrine results due to depressive illness. When used in combination with radiographic and CT and magnetic resonance imaging (MRI), the diagnosis can be established in the majority of cases (Fig. 41.8). The most difficult challenge lies in discriminating between pituitary-driven Cushing's disease and occult ectopic ACTH syndrome; in these circumstances a combination of the high-dose dexamethasone test and the CRH test with petrosal sinus sampling may be necessary to establish the diagnosis.

Adrenal Adenoma, Carcinoma and Primary Adrenal Hyperplasia

The finding of a suppressed plasma ACTH and the lack of plasma cortisol suppression to high-dose dexamethasone testing suggests an adrenal lesion as the cause of Cushing's syndrome. However, with some non-extraction ACTH assays, levels may not be completely suppressed, but may lie within the lowest 25% of the reference range, making interpretation difficult:[21] in these cases an extraction assay for plasma ACTH may afford better discrimination. CT scanning and, if available, MRI of the adrenal are the most sensitive means of detecting adrenal masses. Occasionally, adrenal venous sampling or iodocholesterol imaging may give additional information on tumour localization.

Cushing's Disease and Occult Ectopic ACTH Syndrome

Plasma ACTH levels lie within the upper half of the reference range in approximately 50% of cases of Cushing's disease and in the remainder of cases the levels are only moderately elevated and rarely exceed 300 ng/L. Suppression of plasma cortisol to high-dose dexamethasone testing and high-normal or moderately raised plasma ACTH are consistent with Cushing's disease. These findings can be mimicked by slow-growing tumours such as bronchial carcinoids, thymic or pancreatic tumours that produce moderate amounts of ectopic ACTH, and by some tumours in the ectopic CRH syndrome. The presence of an increased blood concentration of other markers for APUDoma tumours such as gastrointestinal hormones, carcinoembryonic antigen, calcitonin and 5-hydroxyindole acetic acid may provide additional

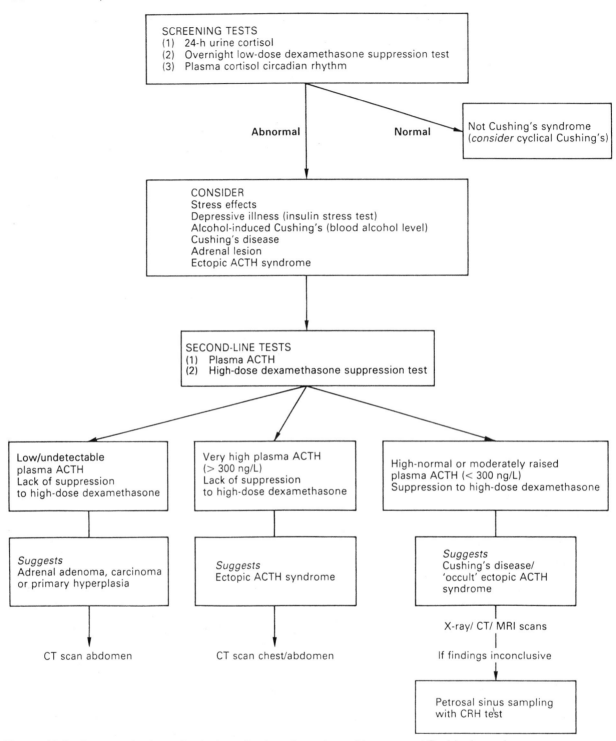

Figure 41.8 Suggested scheme for the investigation of a patient with suspected Cushing's syndrome.

evidence of ectopic hormone secretion. In many patients, small pituitary adenomas escape detection by CT scanning, although MRI may be more effective in finding these. Small occult tumours also may be difficult to identify on scanning the chest and abdomen. In the most difficult cases the use of CRH challenge with petrosal sinus venous sampling may be necessary to distinguish between ectopic or pituitary sources of high-normal or moderately elevated plasma ACTH concentrations.

Iatrogenic Cushing's Syndrome
The identification of Cushing's syndrome associated with excessive glucocorticoid treatment presents few

problems, but occasionally it may result from treatment with steroids not usually recognized as having glucocorticoid activity. Recently, several reports have identified treatment with high doses of medroxyprogesterone acetate for cancer therapy as a possible cause of Cushing's syndrome and adrenal suppression was evident on withdrawal of treatment.[43–45] Patients had suppressed plasma cortisol and ACTH levels in the presence of clinical features of Cushing's syndrome.

Cyclical Cushing's Syndrome

This term describes patients with Cushing's syndrome who show regular cycles of excess cortisol production demonstrated by at least three peaks and two troughs of cortisol production with similar time intervals between the peaks.[46] Most cases have been associated with pituitary-driven Cushing's disease, although at least two cases of cyclical ectopic ACTH-mediated Cushing's syndrome have been described. The periodicity of peaks of excess cortisol production ranges from 12 h to 85 days and, in some cases, cortisol production falls to within normal limits in the troughs. Changes in cortisol output can be monitored on an outpatient basis by measurement of cortisol in 24-h urine samples or cortisol/creatinine ratios in early-morning urine specimens; coincidence between peaks in urine cortisol, early-morning plasma cortisol and plasma ACTH levels has been demonstrated.

Clinical features also may show dramatic cyclical changes from a cushingoid appearance with facial swelling, weight gain and livid striae during a period of excessive cortisol production to a normal appearance during periods of normal cortisol output. The disorder may be more common than is generally appreciated—for example, in one study of nine patients with Cushing's syndrome, five were found to have a cyclical form of the disease.[46] A high index of suspicion is needed for patients with normal or fluctuating plasma or urine cortisol results, those showing paradoxical rises in cortisol or inconsistent responses to dexamethasone suppression, and those with a variable clinical syndrome.

Alcohol-induced Cushing's Syndrome

Acute ingestion of alcohol in amounts sufficient to cause mild to moderate intoxication stimulates adrenal cortical activity in normal subjects and in alcoholic subjects in the recovery phase.[47] Chronic alcoholism can occasionally produce a clinical appearance and biochemical pattern identical to that of fully developed Cushing's syndrome, with high plasma cortisol levels and lack of suppression to dexamethasone. The abnormal laboratory findings are corrected after as little as 1 week of abstention following hospital admission, although clandestine alcohol consumption may confuse the diagnosis. Hypercortisolism can occur in the absence of impaired hepatic function and evidence suggests that increased CRH and ACTH drive may be responsible. Blood alcohol measurements can be helpful when there is suspicion of alcohol-induced Cushing's syndrome and to confirm adherence to a regimen of alcohol abstinence before retesting the function of the hypothalamic–pituitary–adrenal axis.

Nelson's Syndrome

Small pituitary adenomas are common in Cushing's disease and treatment by bilateral adrenalectomy (more common in the past) results in the progression of the adenoma to an expanding, intrasellar tumour in up to one-third of these patients. Nelson was the first to describe a syndrome of skin pigmentation with evidence of an expanding pituitary tumour following bilateral adrenalectomy for Cushing's syndrome. Plasma levels of ACTH are very high (over 1000 ng/L) and these and high levels of other fragments of POM.C with melanocyte-stimulating hormone-like activity cause pigmentation similar to that found in Addison's disease, but of greater intensity. The tumour is often locally invasive.[48]

It is important to detect early signs of tumour growth in patients with Cushing's syndrome who have been treated by bilateral adrenalectomy. This can be achieved by monitoring for signs of increasing plasma ACTH levels that do not respond to steroid replacement therapy.

Congenital Adrenal Hyperplasia

Congenital adrenal hyperplasia describes a group of hereditary disorders of adrenocortical hormone synthesis where there is adrenal hypertrophy resulting from ACTH stimulation in response to diminished cortisol production. Reduced or absent enzyme activity at a particular stage of steroid synthesis produces a disturbance in the normal pattern of adrenal steroids and precursors; the resultant steroid hormone imbalance causes clinical effects—genital abnormalities and disturbances of electrolyte balance. Over 90% of cases are due to 21-hydroxylase deficiency, inherited as an autosomal recessive trait. Almost all of the remaining cases are accounted for by the rarer disorders 11β-hydroxylase and 3β-hydroxysteroid dehydrogenase deficiencies. Two more enzyme deficiencies, 17α-hydroxylase and cholesterol desmolase deficiency, are extremely rare. Table 41.7 sets out the clinical and laboratory findings in the three most common forms of congenital adrenal hyperplasia.

It is now clear that milder non-classical forms of 21-hydroxylase, 11β-hydroxylase and 3β-hydroxysteroid dehydrogenase deficiencies exist and that, as expected, these occur more frequently than the corresponding classical defects.[49,50]

21-hydroxylase Deficiency

Congenital adrenal hyperplasia due to 21-hydroxylase deficiency has an incidence of approximately 1 in 10 000 live births in Western Europe. Elevated levels of steroid precursors are processed in the sex

TABLE 41.7

CLINICAL AND BIOCHEMICAL FINDINGS FOR THE MOST COMMON ENZYME BLOCKS CAUSING CONGENITAL ADRENAL HYPERPLASIA

| Genital ambiguity | | Clinical features | | | | Circulating hormones | | | | | |
Female	Male	Salt wasting	Hypertension	Postnatal virilization	Enzyme deficiency	Aldo	17-OHP	AD	DHAS	Testosterone	Renin
+	0	0	0	+	21-hydroxylase: simple virilizing	N	↑↑	↑↑	N or ↑ (DHAS/AD ↓)	↑	N or ↑
++	0	+	0	+	21-hydroxylase: salt wasting	→	↑↑	↑↑	N or ↑	↑	↑↑
+	0	0	+	+	11β-hydroxylase	→	↑	↑↑	↑	↑	→↓
+	+	+	0	+	3β-hydroxysteroid dehydrogenase	→	N or ↑	N or ↑	↑↑↑	↑†	↑

N, normal; other abbreviations as in Table 41.4 and text.
†↓ or normal in male; ↑ or normal in female.
Adapted from New and Josso[49] with permission.

steroid pathway, giving rise to increased androgen production. In approximately 70% of cases the deficiency in aldosterone production is sufficiently severe to cause a salt-losing state. High levels of the precursor 17-OHP also may have a salt-losing influence caused by its antimineralocorticoid activity.[30] Female infants have varying degrees of genital ambiguity and it is now clear that there is no correlation between the degree of virilization and the severity of salt loss. Male infants have normal genitalia at birth; they may present in salt-losing crisis in the first 1–2 weeks of life or they may be unrecognized until signs of precocious puberty appear later in childhood.

Diagnosis of 21-hydroxylase deficiency can be achieved by demonstration of elevated plasma or bloodspot 17-OHP concentrations, although care is needed in the interpretation of results. Sick, preterm infants often have elevated plasma or bloodspot 17-OHP results, probably due to cross-reaction of fetal zone steroids, such as 17α-hydroxypregnenolone sulphate in the immunoassay.[14] Here it is important to observe the trend in levels and to use urine steroid profiling to check for the presence of a 21-hydroxylase block. Conversely, levels of plasma and bloodspot 17-OHP may be only moderately elevated in children with 21-hydroxylase deficiency in the first few days of life, and later blood samples and a urine steroid profile may be needed to confirm the diagnosis. Blood samples should not be taken in the first day of life as plasma 17-OHP levels remain high for the first 24 h in normal infants.

In neonates, blood samples may be taken at any time, as the circadian rhythm does not become established until approximately 10 weeks of life. After this time, morning samples should be taken, as plasma 17-OHP results may fall to levels within the reference range later in the day, even in untreated cases of 21-hydroxylase deficiency.

Monitoring of corticosteroid replacement therapy with plasma or bloodspot 17-OHP or androstenedione daytime profiles provides a convenient guide to the adequacy of replacement therapy.[17,19] Morning 17-OHP concentrations that are detectable but below 150 nmol/L (plasma) or 80 nmol/L (bloodspot) suggest reasonable control, while suppressed morning levels indicate possible over-replacement. These give a more immediate indication of control than longer-term assessments of growth rate.

The gene for the adrenal cytochrome P450 specific for 21-hydroxylation (P450 C21) has been localized to the HLA supergene on the short arm of chromosome 6. 21-hydroxylase deficiency is inherited as an autosomal recessive trait closely linked to the HLA complex. A sibling sharing both HLA haplotypes with the index case is predicted to be affected, one who shares one haplotype is predicted to be a heterozygote and one who has no HLA haplotypes in common is predicted to be unaffected.

Prenatal diagnosis of 21-hydroxylase deficiency can be achieved in the first trimester of pregnancy.[51] In families at risk for the disease, HLA serotyping and HLA genotyping using HLA class 1 and class 2 probes can be done on parents and index cases. As soon as a pregnancy is confirmed, dexamethasone therapy (1 mg/day) is instituted to provide steroid cover for the potentially affected fetus. A chorionic villus biopsy is then taken at 6–8 weeks' gestation and the karyotype and HLA genotype of cultured cells are determined. Dexamethasone therapy is discontinued if the fetus is male or an unaffected female. In cases where the risk from chorionic villus sampling is unacceptable or where results are equivocal, amniocentesis can be done from the end of the first trimester; fetal sex determination and HLA serotyping are then done to determine whether continuation of dexamethasone therapy is warranted. Levels of 17-OHP in amniotic fluid also provide useful confirmation of the deficiency where the index case was not genotyped and where dexamethasone therapy has not been started or has been discontinued before amniocentesis.

Non-classical 21-hydroxylase deficiency may produce symptoms of virilization later in childhood or in adulthood (the late-onset form) or may be asymptomatic (the cryptic form). The late-onset form may manifest itself as precocious puberty in childhood, menstrual disturbances, acne or hirsutism in adolescent women, or signs may be limited to short stature in adolescent boys and men due to early epiphyseal fusion. Non-classical 21-hydroxylase deficiency is the most common autosomal recessive disorder in man. Its HLA associations differ from those found in classical 21-hydroxylase deficiency and also differ for different ethnic groups.[50]

11β-hydroxylase Deficiency

Deficiency of the 11β-hydroxylase enzyme produces a syndrome of genital ambiguity in female infants similar to that found with 21-hydroxylase deficiency, but differs in that salt retention, hypertension and hypokalaemic alkalosis may be present, owing to the salt-retaining effects of high levels of 11-deoxycortisol and other 11-deoxysteroid precursors. The degree of salt retention varies considerably and may be mild; there is no correlation between the degree of virilization and the severity of hypertension.

Plasma or bloodspot 17-OHP concentrations may be moderately raised in 11β-hydroxylase deficiency but they are unhelpful in making the diagnosis; this is best achieved by plasma ACTH and 11-deoxycortisol measurements and by urine steroid profiling to confirm the 11β-hydroxylase block. Plasma or bloodspot androstenedione measurements can be used to assess control in terms of attenuation of adrenal androgen overproduction.

3β-hydroxysteroid Dehydrogenase Deficiency

Deficiency results in a lack of conversion of 3β-hydroxy-Δ^5 steroids to the 3-keto-Δ^4 configuration needed for all physiologically active C_{19} and C_{21}

steroids. In genetic male infants, incomplete genital development causes varying degrees of genital ambiguity at birth. Very high levels of circulating DHA, some of which may be converted in the periphery to more potent androgens, may produce clitoral enlargement in newborn female infants. Plasma levels of the Δ^5 steroids pregnenolone, 17-hydroxypregnenolone and DHA are elevated, and high Δ^5 to Δ^4 steroid metabolite ratios can be confirmed by urine steroid profiling. Salt wasting of varying degrees may be present, and there is no correlation between the degree of genital ambiguity and the severity of the enzyme defect.

17α-hydroxylase Deficiency

Approximately 40 patients have so far been identified with this disorder. Deficiency of 17α-hydroxylase blocks production of all glucocorticosteroids and sex steroids and results in pseudohermaphroditism in males and sexual infantalism in females. The 17-deoxycorticosteroids deoxycorticosterone and corticosterone are produced in large amounts and usually provide sufficient glucocorticoid activity for survival. High deoxycorticosteroid levels cause varying degrees of salt retention, hypertension and hypokalaemia, with suppression of renin.

Cholesterol Desmolase Deficiency

A total enzyme block at the stage of conversion of cholesterol to pregnenolone results in a complete absence of steroid production and would not be compatible with life. Approximately 30 patients have been described who have survived to the age of puberty or adulthood and presumably these have less severe enzyme blocks. Infants have gonadal hypogenesis or agenesis and severe fluid and electrolyte disturbances due to salt loss. Accumulation of cholesterol in the adrenal produces a yellow, foamy appearance on histological examination—hence the term lipoid adrenal hyperplasia. Serum levels of all steroids are very low.

Virilizing Tumours

Adrenal tumours that secrete androgens exclusively occur in both men and women, although they are more easily recognized in women because of associated clinical signs of virilization and menstrual disturbances. In men, suppression of gonadotrophins by excess androgens may cause infertility. Tumours may be benign or malignant and occur at any age. In women, signs of hirsutism and virilization with a rapid development over the preceding weeks or months provide useful clues. In almost all patients with virilizing adrenal tumours, plasma testosterone is markedly elevated. Often, plasma levels of the other adrenal androgens (androstenedione, DHA and DHAS) are elevated, but this is not always the case, as several reports have documented adrenal tumours that secrete testosterone only. Adrenal or ovarian

stimulation and suppression tests using oestrogen, progesterone, ACTH or human chorionic gonadotrophin (HCG) give unreliable results; some testosterone-secreting adrenal tumours respond to HCG and this may lead to incorrect conclusions as to the site of a tumour.[52]

Techniques that help with localization of such tumours include ultrasound and CT scanning, selective venous catheterization of adrenal and ovarian veins, and radiocholesterol imaging of the adrenals. Late-onset congenital adrenal hyperplasia needs to be considered as a cause of virilization in female patients. Although plasma 17-OHP levels also are raised in patients with androgen-secreting adrenal tumours, they do not suppress in response to glucocorticoid replacement therapy whereas raised levels in patients with late-onset congenital adrenal hyperplasia respond to glucocorticoid treatment.

Rare cases of adrenal tumours that secrete increased amounts of oestrogens in addition to the more usual corticosteroids have been reported. These tumours may be benign or malignant, and may cause feminization in men or interference with the ovulatory cycle in women.

Hypertension

Adrenocortical dysfunction is a rare but potentially curable cause of hypertension (*see also* Chapter 34). In many cases there is clinical and biochemical evidence of Cushing's syndrome, if this is sought. Some patients with few signs of adrenocortical dysfunction other than hypokalaemia can be shown to have some form of hyperaldosteronism (Conn's syndrome). Rarely, hypertension results from excessive production of deoxycorticosterone rather than aldosterone. Deoxycorticosterone has approximately 50% of the affinity of aldosterone for human kidney mineralocorticoid receptors, but its *in vivo* activity is attenuated by more extensive plasma-protein binding; therefore a relatively large excess of deoxycorticosterone is needed to produce the features of mineralocorticoid hypertension.

In one particular form of Conn's syndrome, glucocorticoid-suppressible hyperaldosteronism, there is an increased influence of ACTH on aldosterone production and small doses of synthetic glucocorticoids will normalize aldosterone secretion. The disorder is inherited as an autosomal dominant trait, and is also associated with increased levels of 18-hydroxycortisol and 18-oxocortisol. Measurement of these last two steroids helps to make the diagnosis in cases of partial clinical expression.[53]

The enzyme 11-hydroxysteroid dehydrogenase, which interconverts cortisol and cortisone, is thought to act as a barrier in tissues, limiting the access of cortisol to mineralocorticoid receptors. A rare syndrome of hypertension with low levels of renin, aldosterone and other mineralocorticoids, the syndrome of apparent mineralocorticoid excess, may result from impaired 11-hydroxysteroid dehydrogenase activity, allowing cortisol to act inappropriately as a mineralocorticoid.[54] The mineralocorticoid activity of liquorice derivatives is believed to involve inhibition of the same enzyme and enhancement of the mineralocorticoid activity of cortisol rather than the direct influence on mineralocorticoid receptors.

Acknowledgements

I am grateful to Drs Sammy Medbak and Keith Wakelin and to Colin Selby for their kind help with information used in this chapter.

REFERENCES

1. Neville A.M., O'Hare M.J. (1978). In *The Adrenal Gland* (James V.H.T. ed.) New York: Raven, pp.1–66.
2. James V.H.T., Few J.D. (1985). Adrenocorticosteroids: chemistry, synthesis and disturbances in disease. *Clin. Endocrinol. Metab.*, **14**, 867.
3. Brooks R.V. (1978). In *The Adrenal Gland* (James V.H.T. ed.) New York: Raven, pp.67–92.
4. Ekins R.P. (1982). In *Recent Advances in Endocrinology and Metabolism*, vol 2, Edinburgh: Churchill Livingstone, pp.287–327.
5. Dunn J.F., Nisula B.C., Rodbard D. (1981). Transport of steroid hormones: binding of 21 endogenous steroids to both testosterone-binding globulin and corticosteroid-binding globulin in human plasma. *J. Clin. Endocrinol. Metab.*, **53**, 58.
6. Lohrenz F.N., Seal U.S., Doe R.P. (1967). Adrenal function and serum protein concentration in kindred with decreased cortisol binding globulin (CBG) concentration. *J. Clin. Endocrinol. Metab.*, **27**, 966.
7. Van Baelen H., Brepoels R., De Moor P. (1982). Transcortin Leuven: a variant of human corticosteroid binding globulin with decreased cortisol binding affinity. *J. Biol. Chem.*, **257**, 3397.
8. Ur E. (1991). Psychological aspects of hypothalamo-pituitary-adrenal activity. *Baillière's Clin. Endocrinol. Metab.*, **5**, 79.
9. Meikle A.W., Daynes R.A., Araneo B.A. (1991). Adrenal androgen secretion and biologic effects. *Endocrinol. Metab. Clin. North Am.*, **20**, 381.
10. Parker L.N. (1991). Adrenarche. *Endocrinol. Metab. Clin. North Am.*, **20**, 71.
11. Parker L.N. (1991). Control of adrenal androgen secretion. *Endocrinol. Metab. Clin. North Am.*, **20**, 401.
12. Moore A. et al. (1985). Cortisol assays: guidelines for the provision of a clinical biochemistry service. *Ann. Clin. Biochem.*, **22**, 435.
13. Berry J., Betts P., Wood P.J. (1986). The interpretation of bloodspot 17α-hydroxyprogesterone levels in term and pre-term neonates. *Ann. Clin. Biochem.*, **33**, 546.
14. Wallace A.M., Beastall G.H. (1991). Direct assays for adrenal steroids in neonates. *Ann. Clin. Biochem.*, **20**, 113.
15. Rudd B.T. (1983). Urinary 17-oxogenic and 17-oxosteroids. *Ann. Clin. Biochem.*, **20**, 65.
16. Read G.F., Riad-Fahmy D., Walker R.F., Griffiths K. (eds.) (1982). *Immunoassays of Steroids in Saliva*, Cardiff: Alpha Omega.
17. Riordan F.A.I., Wakelin K., Wood P.J., Betts P., Clayton B.E. (1984). Bloodspot 17α-hydroxyprogesterone radioimmunoassay for diagnosis of congenital adrenal hyperplasia and home monitoring of corticosteroid replacement therapy. *Lancet*, **i**, 708.
18. Pang S. et al., (1982). A pilot newborn screening for congenital adrenal hyperplasia in Alaska. *J. Clin. Endocrinol. Metab.*, **55**, 413.
19. Egan S.M., Betts P., Thomson S., Wallace A.M., Wood P.J. (1989). A bloodspot androstenedione assay suitable for home-monitoring of steroid replacement therapy. *Ann. Clin. Biochem.*, **26**, 262.
20. Liddle G.W. (1960). Tests of pituitary adrenal suppressibility in the diagnosis of Cushing's syndrome. *J. Clin. Endocrinol.*, **12**, 1539.
21. Carpenter P.C. (1988). Diagnostic evaluation of Cushing's syndrome. *Endocrinol. Metab. Clin. North Am.*, **17**, 445.
22. Tyrrell J.B., Findling J.W., Aron D.C., Fitzgerald P.A., Forsham P.H. (1986). An overnight high-dose dexamethasone suppression test for rapid differential diagnosis of Cushing's syndrome. *Ann. Intern. Med.*, **104**, 180.
23. Carroll B.J. (1982). The dexamethasone test for melancholia. *Br. J. Psychiatry*, **140**, 292.
24. Brown W.A., Haser R.J., Qualls C.B. (1980). Dexamethasone suppression test identifies subtypes of depression which respond to different anti-depressants. *Lancet*, **i**, 928.
25. Peselow E.D., Fieve R.R. (1982). Dexamethasone suppression test and response to antidepressants in depressed patients. *N. Engl. J. Med.*, **19**, 1216.
26. Stewart P.M., Seckl J.R., Corrie J., Edwards C.R.W., Padfield P.L. (1988). A rational approach for assessing the hypothalamus–pituitary–adrenal axis. *Lancet*, **i**, 1208.
27. Liddle G.W. Estep H.L., Kendall J.W., Williams W.C., Townes A.W. (1959) Clinical application of a new test of pituitary reserve. *J. Clin. Endocrinol. Metab.* **19**, 875.
28. Howlett T.A., Rees L.H. (1985). Is it possible to diagnose pituitary-dependent Cushing's disease? *Ann. Clin. Biochem.*, **22**, 550.
29. Howlett T.A., Rees L.H., Besser G.M. (1985). Cushing's syndrome. *Clin. Endocrinol. Metab.*, **14**, 911.
30. Besser G.M., Ross R.J.M. (1989). In *Recent Advances in Endocrinology and Metabolism*, vol.3 (Edwards C.R.W., Lincoln D.W. eds.) Edinburgh: Churchill Livingstone, pp.135–158.
31. Loriaux D.L., Nieman L. (1991). Corticotropin-releasing hormone testing in pituitary disease. *Endocrinol. Metab. Clin. North Am.*, **20**, 363.
32. Franks R.C., Nance W.E. (1970). Hereditary adrenocortical unresponsiveness to ACTH. *Pediatrics*, **45**, 43.
33. Petersen K.E., Bille T., Jacobsen B.B., Iverson T. (1982). X-linked congenital adrenal hypoplasia. A study of five generations of a Greenlandic family. *Acta Paediatr. Scand.*, **71**, 947.
34. Moser H.W., Bergin A., Naidu S., Ladenson P.W. (1991). Adrenoleukodystrophy. *Endocrinol. Metab. Clin. North Am.*, **20**, 297.
35. Stuart-Mason A., Meade T.W., Lee J.A.H., Morris J.N. (1968). Epidemiological and clinical picture of Addison's disease. *Lancet*, **ii**, 744.
36. Irvine W.J., Barnes E.W. (1972). Adrenocortical insufficiency. *Clin. Endocrinol. Metab.*, **1**, 549.
37. Groves R.W., Toms J.C., Houghton B.J., Monson J.P.

(1988). Corticosteroid replacement therapy: twice or thrice daily? *J. R. Soc. Med.*, **81**, 514.

38. Bondy P.K. (1985). In *Williams Textbook of Endocrinology* (Wilson J.D., Foster D.W. eds.) Philadelphia: Saunders, pp.816–890.

39. Odell W.D. (1991). Ectopic ACTH secretion: a misnomer. *Endocrinol. Metab. Clin. North Am.*, **20**, 371.

40. Schteingart D.E. (1991). Ectopic secretion of peptides of the proopiomelanocortin family. *Endocrinol. Metab. Clin. North Am.*, **20**, 453.

41. Hermus A.A. et al. (1988). Transition from pituitary-dependent to adrenal-dependent Cushing's syndrome. *N. Engl. J. Med.*, **318**, 966.

42. Tedding van Berkhout F., Croughs R.J., Kater L. (1986). Familial Cushing's syndrome due to nodular adrenocortical dysplasia. A putative receptor-antibody disease? *Clin. Endocrinol.*, **24**, 299.

43. Donkier J.E., Michel L.A., Buysschaert M. (1990). Cushing syndrome and medroxyprogesterone acetate. *Lancet*, **i**, 1094.

44. Merrin P.K., Alexander W.D. (1990). Cushing's syndrome induced by medroxyprogesterone. *Br. Med. J.*, **301**, 345.

45. Siminoski K., Goss P., Drucker D.J. (1989). The Cushing syndrome induced by medroxyprogesterone acetate. *Ann. Intern. Med.*, **111**, 758.

46. Atkinson A.B., Kennedy A.L., Carson D.J., Hadden D.R., Weaver J.A., Sheridan B. (1985). Five cases of cyclical Cushing's syndrome. *Br. Med. J.*, **291**, 1453.

47. Rees L.H., Besser G.M., Jeffcoate W.J., Goldie D.J., Marks V. (1977). Alcohol-induced Cushing's syndrome. *Lancet*, **i**, 726.

48. Grua J.R., Nelson D.H. (1991). ACTH-producing pituitary tumors. *Endocrinol. Metab. Clin. North Am.*, **20**, 319.

49. New M.I., Josso N. (1988). Disorders of gonadal differentiation and congenital adrenal hyperplasia. *Endocrinol. Metab. Clin. North Am.*, **17**, 339.

50. New M.I., White P.C., Speiser P.W., Crawford C., Dupont B. (1989). In *Recent Advances in Endocrinology and Metabolism*, vol.3 (Edwards C.R.W., Lincoln D.W. eds.) Edinburgh: Churchill Livingstone, pp.29–76.

51. Speiser P.W. et al. (1990). First trimester prenatal treatment and molecular genetic diagnosis of congenital adrenal hyperplasia (21-hydroxylase deficiency) *J. Clin. Endocrinol. Metab.*, **70**, 838.

52. McKenna T.J., Cunningham S.K., Loughlin T. (1985). The adrenal cortex and virilisation. *Clin. Endocrinol. Metab.*, **14**, 997.

53. Kellie A.E. (1975). In *Biochemistry of Steroid Hormones* (Makin H.L.J. ed.) Oxford: Blackwell Scientific, pp.1–16.

54. Ulick S. (1991). Two uncommon causes of mineralocorticoid excess: syndrome of apparent mineralocorticoid excess and glucocorticoid-remediable aldosteronism. *Endocrinol. Metab. Clin. North Am.*, **20**, 269.

42. Disorders of the Reproductive System

J. W. Wright

Introduction
Normal gonadal function
    Biochemistry of gonadal steroids
    Ovarian function and its control
    Testicular function and its control
Disorders of gonadal development and sexual
        differentiation
    Chromosomal abnormalities
    Pseudohermaphroditism
Disorders of gonadal function
    Disorders in infancy and childhood
    Disorders of gonadal function in women
    Disorders of gonadal function in men
Clinical and laboratory investigation
    Measurement of gonadotrophins and
        gonadal steroids
    Subfertility: the role of the laboratory

INTRODUCTION

In both sexes, the gonads have two functions: the production of gametes and the production of steroid hormones. The ultimate purpose of these steroids is to ensure that the gametes come together at fertilization and that the fertilized ovum finds a suitable environment in which to develop and grow. In addition, they also have systemic effects on a number of tissues that are not immediately related to reproductive function. In both sexes, steroidogenesis and gametogenesis are intimately related; in the testis (but not in the ovary) these two functions are anatomically separate.

Both gonadal functions are primarily under the control of the pituitary gonadotrophins, *luteinizing hormone* (LH) and *follicle-stimulating hormone* (FSH), which are, in turn, under the control of a single *hypothalamic gonadotrophin-releasing hormone* (GnRH or LHRH). In addition, a number of other pituitary hormones (particularly prolactin and growth hormone) also influence gonadal function, albeit less directly. The gonads in turn regulate the hypothalamus and pituitary by means of a complex network of 'feedback loops'. In clinical practice, the gonads should not be considered in isolation, but as part of the hypothalamic–pituitary–gonadal axis, the components of which are closely integrated on a functional basis (*see also* Chapter 37). Furthermore, diseases of other endocrine glands, notably the adrenal, which (in the female particularly) secretes sex steroids in addition to gluco- and mineralocorticoids, can affect gonadal function. These effects may be direct, or by altering the binding of sex steroids to circulating binding protein, with clinical consequences similar to those of gonadal disorders.

NORMAL GONADAL FUNCTION

Biochemistry of Gonadal Steroids

Structure and Nomenclature
An appreciation of the chemistry of steroid hormones is undoubtedly an acquired taste, but despite the daunting appearance of what is disparagingly called 'hydroxylated chicken wire', familiarity with the structure and metabolism of the steroid hormones is repaid by a fuller understanding of the biochemical defects that occur in health and disease, and of the tests used to identify them.

The nomenclature of the ring structure is shown in Fig. 42.1. (The numbering of the ring and its three-dimensional structure are illustrated in Chapter 41.) The basic rules to remember are that:

- the saturated parent compounds are called '-anes';

- compounds with double bonds in the skeleton are called '-enes', with the positions of the double bonds identified by the number of the lower of the two carbons that they join;

- the presence of the carbonyl and hydroxyl groups is also indicated.

When multiple substituents are present, the rules are more complex.

Reduction at positions 3 and 5 is commonly involved in the metabolism of biologically active steroids and produces isomerism (Fig. 42.2). Although the 3-carbonyl group is in the plane of the ring, the hydroxyl group, following reduction, can be either on the β-side of the molecule (represented by solid bonds) or the α-side (represented by broken bonds). Similar isomerism can occur at the 5-position. These different isomers (androsterone, aetiocholanolone and their 'epi' forms) have different conformations that result in differences in biological activity. Hydroxyl groups at C20 can also be either α or β but in this case the nomenclature does not refer to the configuration of the group relative to the ring.

The trivial (i.e. commonly used) and systematic names of the major gonadal steroids and their metabolites are shown in Table 42.1.

Synthesis and Secretion
The major pathways of steroid biosynthesis in the gonads are shown in Fig. 42.3. The initial steps are identical to those involved in steroid biosynthesis in the adrenals (see Chapter 41). However, although small amounts of sex steroids may be produced in the normal adrenal (especially androstenedione in women), the gonads produce no gluco- or mineralocorticoids. All the substances shown in Fig. 42.3 have

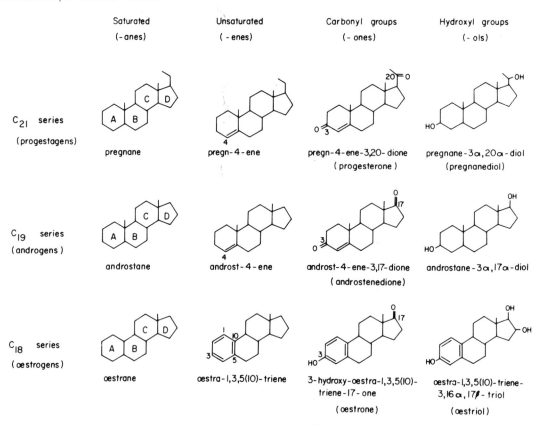

Figure 42.1 Structural nomenclature of some gonadal steroids to illustrate the principles involved.

TABLE 42.1
TRIVIAL NAMES OF THE GONADAL SEX STEROIDS AND SOME OF THEIR
METABOLITES

Trivial name	Systematic name
Aetiocholanolone	3α-hydroxy-5β androstan-17-one
Androstenedione	Androst-4-ene-3,17-dione
Androsterone	3α-hydroxy-5α androstan-17-one
Dihydrotestosterone (DHT)	17β-hydroxy-5α androstan-3-one
Oestradiol	Oestra-1,3,5(10)-triene-3,17β-diol
Oestriol	Oestra-1,3,5(10)-triene-3,16α,17β-triol
Oestrone	3-hydroxy-oestra-1,3,5(10)-trien-17-one
Pregnanediol	5β-pregnane-3α,2-α-diol
Progesterone	Pregn-4-ene-3,20-dione
Testosterone	17β-hydroxy-androst-4-en-3-one

been identified as secretory products of either the testis or the ovary or both, although those in the 5-androstene series are normally only minor products.

The total amount of a steroid entering the circulation at a given time is called the *blood production rate*. It is calculated as the concentration multiplied by the *metabolic clearance rate*. The *secretion rate* is defined as the total amount secreted from the endocrine glands. When a steroid is secreted by only one gland (e.g. progesterone in the luteal phase of the menstrual cycle), then the blood production rate is equal to the ovarian secretion rate (Table 42.2). If it is secreted by two glands (e.g. androstenedione from the ovary and the adrenal cortex), then the secretion rate will be the sum of the contributions of the two glands. Various methods of assessing these contributions in physiological and pathological states have been devised. Some hormones such as testosterone are not only secreted as such but are also produced

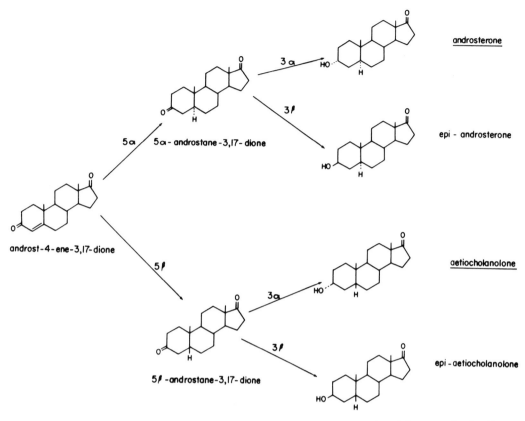

Figure 42.2 Isomerism in the C_{19} androstanes following reduction of the A-ring (also seen in the C_{21} pregnanes). Androsterone and aetiocholanolone are the two major 11-deoxy,17-oxosteroids.

in peripheral tissues (e.g. liver, skin and adipose tissue) from inactive precursors or prohormones. The total production rate is then the sum of the secretion rates from the endocrine gland *and* the contribution from peripheral non-endocrine tissues. This contribution is important in many physiological and pathological states.

Binding in Blood and Tissues

All the steroid hormones are bound to a certain extent to albumin; in addition, there are specific binding proteins for the major steroids, sex hormone-binding globulin (SHBG) and cortisol-binding globulin (CBG). The binding to these proteins is of much higher affinity than to albumin but their concentrations in plasma are very much less. For example, the binding affinity of testosterone to SHBG is 50 000 times greater than to albumin, but the concentration of albumin is 10 000 times greater than that of SHBG. The level of SHBG is increased by oestrogens and is, therefore, much greater in the female. In addition, because of the differences in binding affinities and total concentration of testosterone in males and females, about twice as much testosterone is free (unbound to *any* protein) and twice as much is albumin bound in the male as in the female (Fig. 42.4).

Because of its low binding affinity, albumin-bound testosterone is more metabolically available than the SHBG-bound hormone and may be important (along with free testosterone) not only in the male but also in hyperandrogenic states in the female.

In certain circumstances, such as hyperthyroidism, pregnancy and during oestrogen therapy, the concentrations of binding globulins and of the corresponding sex steroids are increased. The free (unbound) level remains constant and thus methods that measure this are better indicators of steroid activity than those that measure the total concentration.

Sex steroids enter their target cells by simple diffusion. In the cytosol the steroid is bound by a receptor protein of high affinity and specificity; the relative affinity of related steroids for an individual receptor is proportional to their relative biological potencies. Oestrogens and progesterone act without being further modified but in some tissues, the action of testosterone depends on prior conversion either to dihydrotestosterone (via 5α-reductase, in the skin and reproductive tract) or to oestradiol (via aromatase). Aromatization of testosterone to oestrogen occurs in the brain, and it is not clear how, following this, the steroid–receptor interaction is recognized as andro-

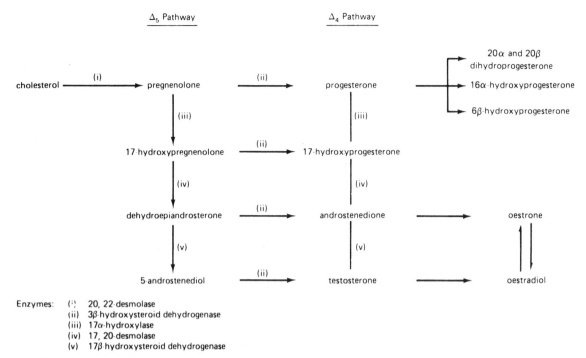

Figure 42.3 Pathways of biosynthesis of gonadal steroids.

genic, with all the psychological and physiological results that follow.

Metabolism and Excretion

Gonadal steroids undergo a complex series of reactions before eventual excretion in the urine. In part these reactions involve transformation into compounds with altered biological actions; in part they result in the formation of inactive, water-soluble conjugates that are more easily excreted.

Progesterone. The major excretory product of progesterone is pregnanediol, formed by three reduction reactions at C20, C4,5 and C3. A number of intermediary products and isomers may also appear in the urine. It should be noted that, while pregnanediol is predominantly derived from progesterone, small amounts may be derived from the metabolism of the adrenal steroids, deoxycorticosterone and 17α-hydroxyprogesterone. This latter is produced in excess in patients with congenital adrenal hyperplasia (21-hydroxylase deficiency).

Androgens. C_{19} steroids are secreted by both the adrenal cortex and the gonads. In men, the secretion of other C_{19} steroids is insignificant compared with that of testosterone from the testis. In normal women, however, only about 0.5 μmol of testosterone is secreted directly each day—part ovarian, part adrenal. A further 0.5 μmol is produced by conversion from androstenedione (Δ), the major androgen in women,

secreted both by the adrenal cortex (6 μmol/day) and the ovary (3 μmol/day). A small amount of androstenedione is also produced from dehydroepiandrosterone (DHA) and its sulphate (DHAS), which are biologically inactive steroids secreted almost exclusively from the adrenal (and, as such, useful as markers of adrenal steroid secretion). Such weak androgenicity as these steroids possess is almost certainly due to their conversion to testosterone in peripheral tissues. The term 'androgen' should thus be used with care; its use to cover all C_{19} steroids should not be taken to imply that they all possess significant biological activity.

The metabolites of all these steroids are excreted into the urine as 17-oxosteroids (also called 17-ketosteroids). This is a complex group that includes the glucuronide and sulphate conjugates of DHA, DHAS, and androstenedione, aetiocholanolone and their isomers. Testosterone and dihydrotestosterone constitute less than 1% of total urinary 17-oxosteroids, the majority being excreted as the glucuronide of testosterone itself.

Oestrogens. Most oestrogen is metabolized and excreted into the bile and thence via the faeces. A little only is excreted into the urine as a complex mixture of sulphates and glucuronides following metabolic inactivation of the oestrogen molecule at a number of sites. The major metabolite is oestriol, the measurement of which has been used as an index of fetal well-being in pregnancy.

TABLE 42.2
PRODUCTION RATES AND SECRETION RATES OF OVARIAN STEROIDS

	Phase of cycle	Plasma level (nmol/L)	Binding in plasma	Total production rate (μmol/24 h)	% from ovarian secretion (approx.)
Oestradiol	Early follicular	0.2	SHBG and	0.3	90
	Late follicular	1.2	albumin (weak)	2	100
	Mid-luteal	0.6		1	100
Oestrone	Early follicular	0.15	Albumin (weak)	0.4	70
	Late follicular	0.75		2	90
	Mid-luteal	0.3		0.8	70
Progesterone	Follicular	1	CBG	3	75
	Luteal	30		100	100
20α-dihydroprogesterone	Follicular	1	CBG	2	70
	Luteal	8		20	80
17α-hydroxyprogesterone	Early follicular	0.5	CBG	1.5	50
	Late follicular	5		12	85
	Mid-luteal	5		12	85
Androstenedione	—	5	—	10	40
Testosterone	—	1.5	SHBG Albumin (weak) CBG (weak)	1	25
Dehydro-epi-androsterone	—	15	—	30	15
Dihydrotestosterone	—	0.75	SHBG	0.2	20

CBG, cortisol-binding globulin; SHBG, sex hormone-binding globulin.

Ovarian Function and its Control

Postpubertal human ovaries are complex structures in which different cell types interact to produce sex steroids and an ovum ready for fertilization in response to cyclical stimulation by pituitary gonadotrophins.

Morphological changes

During each menstrual cycle, one (rarely more than one) follicle matures under the influence of FSH, ovulates and, if fertilization occurs, develops into a corpus luteum under the influence of LH. The corpus luteum is the major source of sex steroids, predominantly progesterone, during the postovulatory (or luteal) phase of the cycle. If fertilization does not occur, the corpus luteum regresses after about 14 days to be replaced by a corpus albicans; if fertilization does occur, the corpus luteum persists, maintained by chorionic gonadotrophin.

Sex Hormone Changes (see Table 42.2 and Fig. 42.5)

Follicular phase. During the early follicular phase, secretion of ovarian steroids is at a relatively constant and low level. As the follicle develops, ovarian secretion of oestradiol increases to reach a peak on the day before the LH peak.

Ovulatory phase. This is characterized by a sharp rise in the level of LH, which leads to final maturation of the follicle and ovulation some 24–36 h later. The LH surge is triggered by the preceding rise in oestradiol, an example of positive feedback. There is also a simultaneous but smaller peak of FSH, a reflection of the fact that the two gonadotrophins are under the control of a single hypothalamic releasing hormone.

Luteal phase. The most important biochemical feature of this phase of the cycle is the marked rise in the secretion of progesterone from the corpus luteum, which reaches a maximum about 8 days after the LH peak. It is associated with a rise in basal body temperature. If fertilization has not occurred, the FSH level starts to rise again towards the end of the luteal phase to initiate the growth of the next follicle.

In addition to a direct effect, the stimulation of ovarian steroid secretion by LH and FSH is modulated by the intraovarian production of insulin-like growth factor 1, which acts in a paracrine fashion. Similarly, high concentrations of hormones (gonadotrophins and steroids) in follicular fluid exert a local effect on follicle development.

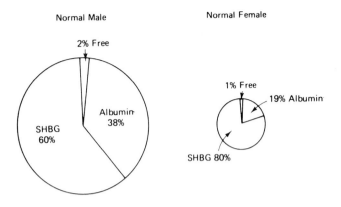

Figure 42.4 Testosterone and its binding in normal male and normal female plasma. The free and albumin-bound fractions are biologically active and available for metabolism.

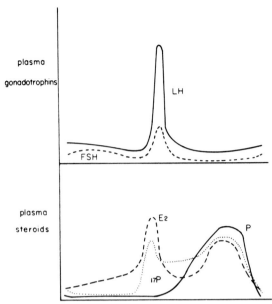

Figure 42.5 Cyclical changes in the secretion of pituitary and ovarian hormones. LH, luteinizing hormone; FSH, follicle-stimulating hormone; E₂, oestradiol-17β; P, progesterone; 17P, 17-hydroxyprogesterone.

Testicular Function and its Control

Pituitary–Leydig-cell Axis

The interstitial cells of Leydig are located in the connective tissue of the testis between the seminiferous tubules. These cells start to secrete androgens during the seventh week of fetal life; this coincides with the differentiation of secondary sexual characteristics.

In adult men, almost all circulating testosterone results from testicular secretion. Small amounts of other potent androgens such as dihydrotestosterone (DHT) are also secreted but the majority of circulating DHT is derived from peripheral reduction of testosterone. Small amounts of other steroids, including oestrogens, are also derived from peripheral conversion.

The rate of synthesis and secretion of testosterone is dependent on the rate of LH secretion. In addition to the influence of higher centres mediated by GnRH, testosterone exerts a negative feedback on LH secretion.

Pituitary–Seminiferous tubule Axis

The majority of the testis comprises a tightly coiled mass of seminiferous tubules. These are lined by specialized cells—spermatogonia—which undergo division into spermatocytes that in turn develop into spermatozoa. This process takes around 70 days. Both LH and FSH are required, LH indirectly by stimulating the production of testosterone by adjacent Leydig cells. The precise way in which FSH exerts its influence is unclear. It probably exerts a direct effect on the seminiferous tubule, and may increase testicular sensitivity to LH by increasing the number of receptors on Leydig cells.

In addition to LH and FSH, testicular (and probably ovarian) function are also influenced by *inhibin(s)* and *activin(s)*. Inhibin is a peptide produced in the Sertoli cells of the testis and the granulosa cells of the ovary. It exerts a negative feedback effect on FSH secretion and probably influences both spermatogenesis and follicular development in paracrine fashion. The activins are related peptides, also produced in the gonads; their precise action is unclear.

DISORDERS OF GONADAL DEVELOPMENT AND SEXUAL DIFFERENTIATION

The presence of the Y chromosome in the male determines testicular differentiation and development, which starts at about the fifth week of gestation. By about 8 weeks, the fetal testis starts to secrete two hormones, testosterone from Leydig cells and antiMüllerian hormone (AMH) from Sertoli cells, which are essential for the development of normal male genitalia, both internal and external, and for the suppression of female gonadal development from the Müllerian duct system.

In the female, on the other hand, the testis does not develop in the absence of the Y chromosome. Ovarian development occurs much later (not starting until about the 11th week). Neither uterus nor fallopian tubes depend upon the ovary for their development and, unlike the situation in the male, both will develop in the absence of a functioning gonad.

Congenital causes of abnormal sexual development or differentiation include chromosomal abnormalities, resulting in gonadal or seminiferous tubule dysgenesis; defects of enzymes involved in steroidogenesis; and defects in the peripheral action of testosterone (receptor defects or 5α-reductase deficiency) resulting in pseudohermaphroditism. In addition, exposure of the female fetus to androgens or synthetic progestogens may result in virilization; the male fetus is normally exposed to high levels of oestrogen and it is less clear whether additional consumption during pregnancy results in feminization.

Chromosomal Abnormalities

Gonadal dysgenesis (Turner's syndrome)
In the typical case of Turner's syndrome there is only a single sex chromosome resulting in a 45XO karyotype. A number of chromosomal errors can result in the abnormal karyotype, the most common of which is non-disjunction. The characteristic clinical features include female phenotype, short stature, sexual infantilism and a variable combination of other abnormalities of which the most frequent are webbed neck, high-arched palate, cubitus valgus, short fourth metacarpal, hypoplastic nails and coarctation of the aorta. The gonads do not develop and are present as 'streaks'. As mentioned earlier, ovarian function is not necessary for the development of the female phenotype *in utero*, but as ovarian steroids are not produced at puberty, secondary sexual development and menstruation do not occur. The diagnosis depends upon the identification of the abnormal karyotype. As expected, oestrogen levels are low and gonadotrophin levels are very high in the absence of a steroid feedback.

Many variants of the typical case are seen. Mosaicism (the development of two or more cell lines in a single individual) may be present. The most common and mildest form is the XO/XX mosaic; in these patients, additional X chromatin can be detected. These subjects are less severely affected and may be virtually normal females. More complex karyotypes also occur, including those with Y chromosomes and mixed ovarian/testicular dysgenesis.

The objectives of treatment are the achievement of maximum stature and the development and maintenance of secondary sexual characteristics. In recent years, the importance of early treatment with growth hormone has become established, with the addition of oestrogen therapy at the age of puberty.

Klinefelter's syndrome
This is the most common abnormality of testicular development in the male. The characteristic sex chromosome abnormality is 47XXY but, as with Turner's syndrome, many variants are seen. In the typical case there is a failure of pubertal development associated with small testes, azoospermia, gynaecomastia, excessive growth of the long bones, particularly the legs, giving rise to eunuchoid proportions, and some impairment of mental function and social behaviour. Testosterone levels are usually low or low-normal, while both gonadotrophins are usually elevated. The

histological appearance of the tubules and Leydig cells is characteristic but a testicular biopsy is usually unnecessary given characteristic chromosomal and endocrine findings. Treatment consists of testosterone replacement.

Pseudohermaphroditism

This term is used to cover those conditions in which the chromosomal and gonadal sex is different from the genital or phenotypic sex. Thus a male pseudohermaphrodite is an individual with a 46XY karyotype and testes, but with incomplete virilization and female appearance. A female pseudohermaphrodite is a genetic female (46XX) with ovaries, but with varying degrees of virilization, particularly of the external genitalia. True hermaphroditism is rare. These individuals possess both ovarian and testicular tissue; the karyotype may be either male or female or, in about one-third, a mosaic. The clinical picture depends on the dominant endocrine pattern.

Male pseudohermaphroditism
The causes of this are shown in Table 42.3. The most important of these are associated with either defective production or action of testosterone.

Defective Testosterone Production. This can result from a number of rare enzyme defects. Deficiencies of 3β-hydroxysteroid dehydrogenase (3β-HSD) or of 17α-hydroxylase involve the adrenal as well as the testis, and cortisol deficiency is frequently the more important feature. The diagnosis requires specialist steroid analysis, ideally coupled to mass spectrometry.

TABLE 42.3
MAJOR CAUSES OF MALE PSEUDOHERMAPHRODITISM

Defective testosterone production
Inborn errors of testosterone biosynthesis:
    3β-hydroxysteroid dehydrogenase deficiency
    17α-hydroxylase deficiency
    17,20-desmolase deficiency
Leydig-cell hypoplasia

Tissue androgen insensitivity
Androgen receptor defects:
    Complete:
        complete testicular feminization
        Reifenstein syndrome
    Post-receptor defects—defective testosterone
        metabolism:
        5α-reductase deficiency

Miscellaneous
Iatrogenic:
    Consumption of oestrogens or progestogens during
        pregnancy (?)
Persistent Müllerian duct syndrome:
    Defective synthesis or action of antiMüllerian hormone

3β-HSD Deficiency. This is characterized by ambiguous genitalia and adrenal insufficiency in a 46XY male. Levels of 17-hydroxypregnenolone and DHAS in plasma, and of pregnanetriol in urine, are high.

17α-Hydroxylase Deficiency. This results in cortisol deficiency and ambiguous genitalia in association with hypertension and hypokalaemia due to excessive production of mineralocorticoids (deoxycorticosterone and corticosterone). Diagnostically, plasma levels of progesterone and corticosterone and their urinary metabolites are high.

17,20-Desmolase Deficiency. This results in varying degrees of genital ambiguity; 17-hydroxyprogesterone and 17-hydroxypregnenolone levels in plasma are elevated.

Tissue Androgen Insensitivity. This is a more common cause of inherited male pseudohermaphroditism. This may result from either a defect in the cytosolic testosterone receptor or in the conversion of testosterone to DHT due to defective 5α-reductase deficiency. It is important to remember that DHT is not simply the active metabolite of testosterone; although the two hormones bind to the same cytosolic receptor, their activities are, to some extent at least, separate. Testosterone is largely responsible for regulating the secretion of LH from the pituitary and for the differentiation of the Wolffian duct (into seminal vesicles, vas deferens and epididymis); it is essential for spermatogenesis. The actions of DHT are important in those tissues that possess high levels of 5α-reductase, particularly the prostate, the external genitalia and the skin areas involved in secondary sexual hair growth.

Disorders of the Androgen Receptor. These may present as a number of different clinical syndromes, which are classified according to the basic sexual phenotype on the one hand and the degree of masculinization on the other.

Complete Testicular Feminization. This is the most common. It is frequently inherited as a linked recessive condition. Despite a male, 46XY genotype the patients have an obvious female body habitus and external genitalia. However, testes are present, often as masses in the groin simulating inguinal herniae, which may be the presenting feature. At puberty, breast development is usually normal but pubertal and axillary hair growth is absent or minimal. The vagina is blind-ending and there is no uterus present. Testosterone levels are in the normal male range but gonadotrophin levels may be raised due to insensitivity of the hypothalamic–pituitary androgen receptor. There is a high risk of malignancy in the ectopic testes, which should be removed surgically. Treatment is otherwise aimed at providing adequate oestrogen maintenance; no attempt should be made to reverse gender identity.

Incomplete Testicular Feminization. This is similar but with more evidence of virilization than in the complete form. Endocrine findings and treatment are similar.

Reifenstein Syndrome. This condition is similar to incomplete testicular feminization but with a predominantly male phenotype. At puberty, moderate virilization occurs but this is associated with marked gynaecomastia. Endocrine findings and treatment are similar to incomplete testicular feminization.

5α-Reductase Deficiency. This results in reduced DHT production in target tissues, particularly the external genitalia. The condition is inherited as an autosomal dominant trait. External genitalia are ambiguous with hypospadias, inguinal testes and a blind vagina, but most children are raised as females. At puberty there is marked virilization and adoption of a male gender identity, although genitalia remain poorly developed. The characteristic endocrine findings are of normal testosterone but low DHT levels, and thus a high testosterone: DHT ratio in plasma. In the urine, the aetiocholanolone: androsterone ratio is also high.

Female Pseudohermaphroditism

The major causes are shown in Table 42.4. The most important of these are associated with congenital adrenal hyperplasia due to defects in cortisol biosynthesis.

21-Hydroxylase Deficiency. This accounts for some 90% of cases. Different (but closely related) genes control the expression of the two enzymes that are involved in the cortisol pathway in the zona fasciculata and the mineralocorticoid pathway in the zona glomerulosa. More severe defects result in the 'classical' salt-wasting condition while milder defects result in simple virilization only. The condition may present

TABLE 42.4
MAJOR CAUSES OF FEMALE PSEUDOHERMAPHRODITISM

Virilization by fetal androgens
Defects of steroidogenesis (congenital adrenal hyperplasia):
  Classical 21-hydroxylase deficiency (virilization + salt wasting)
  Partial 21-hydroxylase deficiency (virilization only)
  11β-hydroxylase deficiency (virilization + hypertension)
  3β-hydroxysteroid dehydrogenase deficiency (virilization + adrenal insufficiency)

Virilization by maternal androgens
Exogenous:
  Consumption of androgens or synthetic progestogens during pregnancy
Endogenous:
  Virilizing adrenal or ovarian tumour
  Uncontrolled maternal congenital adrenal hyperplasia

as either ambiguous genitalia (females) or with salt wasting (especially males) during the first few weeks of life. The diagnosis depends on the finding of a high level of plasma 17-hydroxyprogesterone (usually well above 15 nmol/L) or its urinary metabolite, pregnanetriol. Treatment is with cortisol replacement and corrective surgery as necessary. Treatment is monitored by regular measurements of plasma 17-hydroxyprogesterone or testosterone.

11β-Hydroxylase Deficiency. This is rare (less than 5% of cases). Virilization is associated with hypertension due to increased levels of deoxycorticosterone, although aldosterone levels are low. Diagnostically, levels of 11-deoxycortisol (compound S) in plasma and of tetrahydro-S in urine are raised.

3β-HSD Deficiency. This is a rare condition, which, in addition to causing male pseudohermaphroditism, can cause virilization in females because of high levels of the weak androgen DHA.

DISORDERS OF GONADAL FUNCTION

Disorders in Infancy and Childhood

Circulating levels of gonadotrophins and sex steroids are high at birth but by 1 year of age, levels are low and non-pulsatile and remain so until the onset of puberty. Thus gonadal insufficiency is generally asymptomatic in infancy and does not present until a delay in puberty becomes apparent. On the other hand, gonadal hyperfunction gives rise to sexual precocity and therefore, by definition, becomes apparent early in childhood and occasionally at birth. Precocity may be *isosexual* (development that is premature but consistent with the genetic and phenotypic sex of the individual) or *heterosexual* (development of changes associated with the opposite sex).

Delayed Puberty

Puberty is the state of transition between childhood and full reproductive capacity. It is associated, sequentially, with maturation of the hypothalamus and pituitary, stimulation of the gonads resulting in secretion of sex steroids, and development of secondary sexual characteristics and body habitus, sexual behaviour and fertility. The trigger to puberty is unknown; body weight is important and a critical fat-cell mass may be essential for peripheral aromatization of weak adrenal androgens, a rise in the level of which is an early endocrine feature of puberty—the 'adrenarche'. This may result in 'conditioning' of the pituitary and the gonadotrophin response to GnRH stimulation. Puberty is accompanied by a decline in the level of the pineal hormone, melatonin, and high levels have been demonstrated in delayed puberty. It is not yet clear whether this is a causal relationship.

As puberty develops, the episodic secretion of FSH and LH becomes more apparent (sleep-entrained LH secretion in both sexes and, in girls, an increase in FSH secretion about 2 years earlier than that of LH). In later puberty, the LH:FSH ratio and magnitude of response to GnRH increases in favour of LH. Increased secretion of the gonadal hormones follows the rise in gonadotrophins. The development of cyclical activity in girls occurs later, with the positive feedback response to oestrogen developing after a period of anovulatory cycles.

Delayed sexual development may be due either to gonadotrophin deficiency (hypogonadotrophic hypogonadism), or to primary failure of gonadal function (hypergonadotrophic hypogonadism). The causes of hypogonadotrophic hypogonadism are similar in boys and girls, while the causes of gonadal insufficiency are generally different in the two sexes. The major causes of delayed puberty are shown in Table 42.5.

Because of the wide variation in age of onset, 'delayed puberty' is hard to define. It is important to identify those patients who will eventually undergo normal puberty (constitutional delay), those who have disorders that may be treatable, and those who have disorders that are untreatable but who require sex hormone therapy in order to achieve normal development. Early suspicion may arise because of other features or clinical conditions (e.g. following chemotherapy or radiotherapy) but early biochemical diagnosis at an age when hormone levels are normally low is difficult.

TABLE 42.5
CAUSES OF DELAYED PUBERTY

Hypergonadotrophic hypogonadism
Gonadotrophin deficiency:
    Iolated—without or with anosmia (Kallman's syndrome)
    Combined—with deficiency of other pituitary hormone(s)
CNS disorders:
    Tumours (especially craniopharyngioma)
    Cerebral trauma
    Cerebral irradiation
    Miscellaneous—infections, granulomas
Severe systemic illness
Anorexia nervosa

Hypogonadotrophic hypogonadism
Males:
    Seminiferous tubular dysgenesis (Klinefelter's syndrome)
    Testicular irradiation, trauma, infection
    Anorchia, cryptorchidism
    Chemotherapy
    Sertoli-cell only syndrome
Females:
    Gonadal dysgenesis (Turner's syndrome and variants)
    Ovarian irradiation
    Chemotherapy
    Idiopathic and autoimmune primary ovarian failure
    Resistant ovary syndrome

TABLE 42.6
CAUSES OF PRECOCIOUS PUBERTY

True precocious puberty
  Idiopathic true precocious puberty
  Tumours of the CNS (especially hypothalamic tumours)
  Other CNS disorders (e.g. infections, infiltrations,
    hydrocephalus)

Pseudo-precocious puberty
  HCG-secreting tumours (intracranial)
  HCG-secreting tumours (extracranial: e.g. teratomas,
    chorion carcinoma)
  Androgen- or oestrogen-secreting tumours
  Congenital adrenal hyperplasia
  Iatrogenic or factitious sex-steroid administration
  Miscellaneous—McCune–Albright syndrome

HCG, human chorionic gonadotrophin.

Initial biochemical classification depends upon the level of gonadotrophins. In patients with primary gonadal failure a disproportionately high level (particularly of FSH) may be detectable at a relatively early age. Chromosomal analysis should be done to exclude Klinefelter's (47XXY) and Turner's (45XO) syndromes and their variants.

Where both gonadotrophins and sex steroids are low, care must be taken to ensure that an intracranial cause requiring treatment is not present. It is important to confirm that other aspects of pituitary function are normal. Hypogonadotrophic hypogonadism (sometimes familial) may be associated with anosmia; this is believed to represent a developmental defect and is termed *Kallman's syndrome*.

Sexual Precocity
It is convenient to divide sexual precocity into *true* precocious puberty—those conditions in which there is early maturation of the hypothalamic–pituitary–gonadal axis, which is GnRH dependent and in which the gonadotrophin responses to GnRH stimulation are mature and normal—and *pseudo*-precocious puberty in which the axis is still immature but in which there is either a primary, non-pituitary source of gonadotrophins or a non-gonadal source of sex steroids, including defects in steroid production (which may result in heterosexual precocity—feminization in males or virilization in females). The conditions causing sexual precocity are listed in Table 42.6.

Idiopathic Precocious Puberty. These patients are at the youngest end of the normal distribution curve. It is more common in girls and may occasionally occur in infancy. If untreated, sexual maturation follows the normal pattern but, because of premature epiphyseal fusion, height potential is not achieved.

Tumours of the Central Nervous System. These are relatively more common in boys (in whom idiopathic precocious puberty is uncommon). Tumours that may be responsible include optic and hypothalamic gliomas, astrocytomas, hamartomas, ependymomas, pineal tumours and rarely, craniopharyngiomas.

Other Central Nervous Causes. These include hydrocephalus, encephalitis, granulomas and hypothalamic irradiation. Any of these may also cause delayed puberty and the precise anatomical localization of the lesion is clearly critical in determining the endocrine consequences.

Congenital Adrenal Hyperplasia. The virilizing forms of this condition result in androgenization in girls rather than precocious puberty. In boys they cause sexual precocity.

The McCune–Albright Syndrome. This consists of precocious puberty, polyostotic fibrous dysplasia of bone and *café-au-lait* skin pigmentation. Although there have been reports to the contrary, gonadal activation is probably independent of GnRH, and the gonadotrophin response to GnRH is characteristically prepubertal.

Disorders of Gonadal Function in Women

Disorders of gonadal function in women present clinically either as disorders of menstruation (amenorrhoea, oligomenorrhoea), or as hirsutism with or without virilization. There is frequently overlap between these. Subfertility may be a feature of either syndrome but is frequently not associated with any other apparent abnormality.

Disorders of Menstruation and Ovulation
Amenorrhoea is conventionally defined as the absence of menstrual bleeding for 6 months or more. The term 'primary amenorrhoea' is applied to women who have never menstruated and 'secondary amenorrhoea' to those who have previously menstruated. (This terminology is unfortunate and potentially confusing as it cuts across the standard endocrine classification of diseases of end-organ failure as 'primary' and those resulting from pituitary failure as 'secondary'.) Any cause of delayed puberty can result in primary amenorrhoea. In addition, any cause of secondary amenorrhoea occurring at an early age may result in primary amenorrhoea. The causes of primary and secondary amenorrhoea are shown in Tables 42.7 and 42.8.

In adult women, regular menstruation usually indicates ovulatory cycles. Confirmation of ovulation is critical in the investigation of subfertility (*see* below) but less important when fertility is not an issue.

Many of the conditions in Tables 42.7 and 42.8 are uncommon and will be suggested by particular clinical features. Thorough clinical examination is essen-

TABLE 42.7
CAUSES OF PRIMARY AMENORRHOEA

Chromosomal disorders:
  Turner's syndrome (gonadal dysgenesis)

Anatomical disorders (genital-tract dysgenesis):
  Imperforate hymen, vaginal septum, etc.

Hypothalamic–pituitary deficiency:
  Isolated gonadotrophin deficiency
  Combined pituitary hormone deficiency

Defects of steroid biosynthesis:
  17α-hydroxylase deficiency
  17,20-desmolase deficiency

Steroid-receptor defects:
  Testicular feminization

CNS disorders:
  Tumours, trauma, irradiation, etc.

Constitutional delayed puberty

Chronic systemic disease

Psychogenic:
  Anorexia nervosa, etc.

TABLE 42.8
CAUSES OF SECONDARY AMENORRHOEA

Physiological:
  Pregnancy
  Menopausal ovarian failure

Premature ovarian failure:
  Idiopathic
  Autoimmune
  Irradiation, surgery
  Infectious (mumps)
  Resistant ovary syndrome

Hypothalamic–pituitary disease:
  Hyperprolactinaemia
  Other pituitary endocrine tumours (Cushing's, acromegaly)
  Hypopituitarism (idiopathic, Sheehan's syndrome)
  Tumours, granulomas
  Infection (encephalitis, meningitis)

Polycystic ovary syndrome

Ovarian/adrenal tumours:
  Cushing's syndrome; oestrogen-, androgen-secreting

Functional disorders:
  Weight loss-associated, anorexia nervosa
  Exercise
  Severe psychological illness or stress
  Acute/chronic systemic disease

tial to determine whether secondary sexual characteristics are present and to exclude any anatomical cause of amenorrhoea. If Turner's syndrome is suspected, chromosomal analysis should be done. The presence of hirsutism is an important clinical feature.

The absence of secondary sexual hair suggests the possibility of 17α-hydroxylase deficiency or testicular feminization.

Pregnancy should always be suspected in women of child-bearing age. More usually it is of importance to exclude ovarian failure (by measurement of FSH) and hyperprolactinaemia. Functional disorders are common, and in these there is frequently no particular endocrine abnormality apart from a lack of cyclical activity.

Defects of Steroid Biosynthesis. 17α-hydroxylase deficiency and 17,20-desmolase deficiency are rare causes of sexual infantilism and primary amenorrhoea that should normally be detected during infancy or childhood.

Functional Disorders. Amenorrhoea is a common feature of emotional stress and is encountered frequently in girls moving away from home, sitting examinations or starting a new job.

Anorexia nervosa is the extreme form of weight loss-associated amenorrhoea. Endocrinologically, these patients show a regression to the prepubertal state with low, non-pulsatile levels of gonadotrophins and oestrogens. During recovery, the changes in the hypothalamic–pituitary–gonadal axis are effectively a rerun of puberty, although the positive feedback LH response to oestrogen is frequently very difficult to re-establish. Less severe but essentially similar forms of weight loss-associated amenorrhoea are seen in female athletes, models and dancers.

Polycystic Ovary Syndrome. This syndrome probably comprises a heterogeneous group of conditions that gives rise to a similar clinical picture consisting of ovulatory dysfunction, subfertility, hirsutism, obesity and polycystic ovaries in variable combination. The original description by Stein and Leventhal centred on the finding of bilateral sclerotic ovaries containing multiple follicular cysts, but it is increasingly recognized that, in many women, the diagnosis depends more upon other typical clinical and endocrine features. The aetiology of the syndrome is uncertain; the primary defect is probably abnormal secretion of androgens, which may be of either ovarian or adrenal origin or both. In as many as 40% of patients this may be due to late-onset congenital adrenal hyperplasia. Heterozygous 21-hydroxylase deficiency has recently been shown to be extremely common, with a gene frequency as high as 1 in 14 in the general caucasian population, and apparently even higher in some groups such as Ashkenazi Jews, Hispanics, Italians and Yugoslavs.

Circulating levels of both LH and androgens are raised; FSH levels are relatively low and cyclical activity is frequently absent. The sustained and acyclical LH activity may be due to resetting of the hypothalamus and/or pituitary by persistently raised levels of oestrone derived from peripheral aromatization of androstenedione. More severe hirsutism is associated with higher levels of androgens.

The prevalence of polycystic ovary syndrome in the normal population may be as high as 20%; in over 30% women with amenorrhoea; and over 80% in women with either oligomenorrhoea or idiopathic hirsutism (and regular ovulatory cycles).

Biochemical investigation is important not only in confirming the diagnosis and ruling out other causes but also in assessing the severity of the condition. The characteristic findings are a high LH:FSH ratio (the absolute level of LH is probably more important), raised levels of androgens (particularly androstenedione) and oestrone, and anovulatory progesterone levels. Androgen levels (both androstenedione and testosterone) are higher in hirsute than non-hirsute women; very high levels raise the possibility of an androgen-secreting tumour. In subfertile women a very high level of LH (> 10 mu/L) on day 8 of the cycle is associated not only with more intractable subfertility but also with a high rate of pregnancy loss if fertilization is achieved. A raised basal 17α-hydroxyprogesterone (17-OHP) level (> 6 nmol/L) suggests the possibility of late-onset congenital adrenal hyperplasia. However, basal 17-OHP levels may be normal in this condition and the diagnosis should be confirmed by demonstrating an exaggerated 17-OHP (> 15 nmol/L in heterozygotes, and > 45 nmol/L in homozygotes) in a short Synacthen test.

Recent interest has focused on the role of insulin resistance and consequent hyperinsulinaemia in the pathogenesis of polycystic ovary syndrome. This is found in both obese and non-obese women with the syndrome. In addition, levels of insulin-like growth factor 1 (1GF-1) are also raised. This may be important in view of the recently described paracrine function of IGF-1 in modulating ovarian steroid secretion. Measurement of IGF-1 in women with polycystic ovary syndrome is of interest but not, as yet, of clinical value.

Hirsutism. In the majority of women with hirsutism who do not have either polycystic ovary syndrome or late-onset congenital adrenal hyperplasia it may be difficult to detect a significant endocrine abnormality. In idiopathic hirsutism, which is characterized by a long history, the lack of virilization or menstrual irregularity and, frequently, a positive family history, there may be a modest elevation of the free androgen index, although total androgens are usually normal. Treatment in such women is usually unrewarding. In women with severe hirsutism and virilization, particularly those with a short clinical history, thorough investigation to exclude Cushing's syndrome or an androgen-producing tumour is essential. In addition to high levels of androgens, tumours frequently produce a variety of both androgen and glucocorticoid precursors. Localization of tumours may be difficult; they are frequently too small to be detected by computerized tomographic scanning, and while a high level of DHAS usually indicates an adrenal source, this can be misleading. Suppression by dexamethasone or oestrogen, or stimulation tests using human chorionic gonadotrophin have largely been abandoned, and final localization may not be made until the time of laparoscopy.

The Menopause. In a woman in her late forties suffering from hot flushes and with increasingly scant and irregular periods, biochemical confirmation of the menopause is unnecessary. In a younger woman with a less clear-cut clinical picture, the finding of a persistently raised FSH with low oestrogen levels will confirm ovarian failure. Very occasionally, this can be a transient phenomenon with the potential for at least temporary recovery.

Disorders of Gonadal Function in Men

In addition to sexual precocity and delayed puberty, disorders of gonadal function in men may present as either hypogonadism or subfertility. There is clearly considerable overlap between these clinical problems; those conditions causing delayed puberty (see Table 42.5) can also cause hypogonadism in the adult. The additional causes do not usually present until adult life.

Where appropriate, a low sperm count is the key laboratory finding. In many of the conditions listed, biochemical features may not be helpful. FSH levels will be raised only if there is significant germ-cell failure; an exaggerated response to GnRH may help to clarify the situation. With alcohol abuse, even in the absence of significant liver damage, levels of androgens and gonadotrophins may both be low and the diagnosis should be confirmed on the basis of other clinical and laboratory findings. The combination of azoospermia and a raised FSH level in an adult patient with small, soft testes indicates certain germ-cell failure. This situation is seldom, if ever, amenable to treatment and testicular biopsy rarely provides additional useful information. If the testosterone level is low, replacement therapy may be indicated.

CLINICAL AND LABORATORY INVESTIGATION

The ability to measure peptide and steroid hormones in biological fluids with increasing precision and specificity has greatly increased our understanding of the physiology and endocrine pathology of the human ovary and testis. Such measurements are of critical value in some clinical conditions but in many others they make only a very limited contribution; a careful history and clinical examination will frequently provide more information than a host of costly laboratory tests. In all instances, biochemical investigation is only one part of overall clinical assessment and an appreciation of other, non-biochemical procedures is of value.

In any case of suspected sexual differentiation, chromosome analysis should be made. A record of growth rate and timing of developmental milestones is important in elucidating abnormalities in children. Bone age, assessed by X-ray of the wrist, is an indirect measure of hormone secretion. Skeletal proportions may be altered in a number of conditions; in particular, the finding of eunuchoid measurements (arm span greater than height, an increase in lower segment:upper segment height ratio) is important in identifying hypoandrogenism. Abnormal nutritional status and body fat distribution are important not only in conditions such as anorexia nervosa but also in other disorders of puberty.

The growth and distribution of hair should be carefully assessed. Ethnic and family factors must be considered in assessing whether hair growth is clinically significant. Charts are available for semiquantitative scoring of hirsutism but these are more useful in monitoring changes than in diagnosis. Acne is a good clinical indicator of circulating androgen status (and often responds well to successful treatment). The presence of true virilization (male-pattern baldness, deepening of the voice, android muscle proportions, clitoral enlargement and, in young children, labial fusion) is a particularly important feature and suggests the presence of a significant abnormality of androgen production.

A number of criteria can be used as indirect measures of oestrogen status. Changes in vaginal epithelium and cervical mucus are useful indicators of cyclical oestrogen activity. An increase in temperature at mid-cycle provides indirect evidence of ovulation. More useful are tests that predict ovulation by detecting the mid-cycle rise in urinary LH secretion, which are widely available in kit form. Induction of a withdrawal bleed following progestogen administration indicates adequate ovarian oestrogen secretion (and, by implication, pituitary gonadotrophin secretion) and a responsive uterine endometrium. It is to some extent redundant, given the increased availability of oestrogen measurements.

Measurement of Gonadotrophins and Gonadal Steroids

Gonadotrophins

Immunoassays for the gonadotrophins are widely available and done in many laboratories. Problems have arisen in recent years, particularly with assays for LH, because of the increasing use of monoclonal antibodies, each of which is directed towards a single, precise epitope. In view of the fact that there are a number of different isoforms of LH, assays based upon different monoclonal antisera may give different results. Care must therefore be taken when comparing the results of such assays.

Gonadal Steroids

Immunoassays for the majority of gonadal steroids are now also generally available. Prior extraction procedures are frequently necessary because of the very low concentration in biological fluids of many steroids of clinical interest, for example testosterone in women and DHT in men. Appropriate selection of solvent used for extraction may, by matching the polarity of the substance measured, increase specificity as well as sensitivity. Problems of specificity are common because of the chemical similarity of many steroids measured, and the consequent cross-reactivity with many antisera.

Most measurements are made on plasma. Although urinary measurements have the theoretical advantages of ironing out circadian variations and of giving an integrated picture of overall secretion, assays of individual steroids are not used because of problems of both sensitivity and specificity; with a few exceptions the complex pathways involved in steroid metabolism make it difficult to correlate levels of steroid conjugates in the urine with circulating values. They are still used to monitor oestrogen production during ovulation induction, but plasma assays are preferable.

Steroid levels in saliva are related to *free* plasma levels and, therefore, biological activity. Despite these theoretical advantages, salivary measurements are not widely used because of assay problems (particularly matrix effects), variations in steroid levels with salivary flow rate, and public resistance to providing specimens.

Group Methods. In the past, measurements of groups of related steroids such as 17-oxosteroids in urine were the only biochemical means of assessment of gonadal function. These were frequently very blunt weapons, with compounds of particular interest often forming only a small part of the total group measured. Although such assays have largely been replaced by more specific plasma methods, measurement of urine steroids by gas or liquid chromatography, particularly if coupled to mass spectrometry, can yield useful and very detailed information but require expert interpretation.

Oestrogens. The clinical value of oestrogen measurements is limited. Total unconjugated oestradiol in plasma is the measurement of choice for most clinical purposes. Results must be interpreted in relation to gonadotrophin levels and, in menstruating women, the time of the cycle. Oestriol levels are raised in polycystic ovary syndrome but assays are not widely available.

Progestogens. Measurement of progesterone in the luteal phase is used to confirm that ovulation has occurred. In a normal, unstimulated cycle the level should be above 30 nmol/L; in stimulated cycles (clomiphene or FSH), higher values are expected. Plasma 17-OHP is used in the diagnosis of congenital adrenal hyperplasia. In the late-onset variety, the diagnosis is confirmed by measuring the 17-OHP response to Synacthen stimulation.

Androgens. Assays of different sensitivity may be required for men and women as the expected values differ greatly. Correction for binding improves the value of the assay (*see* below). Measurement of DHT is not widely used; sensitivity is a problem because levels are normally very low. In women, measurement of adrenal androgens is important. Androstenedione is of particular value in polycystic ovary syndrome and with androgen-producing tumours. DHA and its sulphate DHAS are useful markers of adrenal androgen production and response to treatment. Group methods for total 17β-hydroxy androgens based on the use of SHBG as binding protein are of limited value and have largely been replaced by more specific assays.

Free vs. Total. Although progesterone and oestradiol are protein-bound (to CBG and SHBG, respectively), it is the binding of testosterone to SHBG, and its effects on plasma levels, that is of particular clinical importance. Small variations in the biologically active free fraction cannot be distinguished if only total levels are measured. Free testosterone concentration can be measured by equilibrium dialysis but this is not suitable for routine use. A practical alternative is to measure SHBG concentration directly by immunoassay and to express the ratio of testosterone to SHBG as the free androgen index (FAI). In many women with idiopathic hirsutism, FAI is raised although total testosterone concentration is normal.

Dynamic Tests

Human Chorionic Gonadotrophin Stimulation Test. In boys with delayed puberty in whom testosterone levels are low and gonadotrophin levels are equivocal, measurement of testosterone following stimulation with chorionic gonadotrophin can be used to assess testicular potential. It can also be useful as a therapeutic trial.

GnRH Stimulation Test. Assessment of the pituitary gonadotrophin response to stimulation with the hypothalamic GnRH should theoretically give an indication of pituitary reserve. This test is less useful than had been hoped, for a number of reasons. A normal pituitary response requires priming of the pituitary with sex steroids and/or GnRH itself. Thus, in the prepubertal pituitary, the response to stimulation may be flat even though the gland is potentially normal (a similar response may be seen in women with anorexia nervosa and other functional causes of amenorrhoea). In addition, the gonadotrophin response to GnRH is, in general, proportional to the basal gonadotrophin level and the stimulation test frequently gives no additional information.

Subfertility: The Role of the Laboratory

Although subfertility is conventionally defined as failure to conceive after 12 months of unprotected intercourse, only about 90% of *fertile* couples will conceive in this time and only 95% by the end of 2 years. Overall, at least 10% of couples are relatively subfertile and this is clearly a major clinical problem. The major causes of subfertility are shown in Table 42.9. The prevalence of contributing factors varies greatly from series to series, and the figures shown are therefore, approximate. In at least 15% of couples there are both male and female factors. *Endometriosis* is a very common finding in subfertile women but it is frequently minimal and it is not clear whether this is any more than an incidental association. Conventional treatment is most successful in women with amenorrhoea; moderately successful in the presence of oligomenorrhoea and unexplained infertility; and least successful in the presence of sperm disorders or tubular damage.

Biochemical tests play a limited part in the investigation and management of male infertility. They may be useful in detecting alcohol abuse or other systemic disease but are rarely of more specific value. Hyperprolactinaemia is rare in men but should be excluded if there is marked oligospermia. The key investigation is a complete semen analysis and trial preparation of sperm for insemination or *in vitro* fertilization as appropriate.

In contrast, the laboratory plays a major part in establishing the diagnosis and in monitoring the response to treatment in the female. Documentation of regular ovulation (day 21 progesterone > 30 nmol/L) is essential. Confirmation of ovulation does not exclude such common conditions such as polycystic ovary syndrome, mild hyperprolactinaemia and hypothyroidism, in which factors other than anovulation (e.g. short or inadequate luteal phase) may contribute to subfertility. If suspected, appropriate tests (day 8 LH, androgens, prolactin, T_4 and thyroid-stimulating hormone) should be made, even in women found to be ovulating.

It is particularly important to exclude *hyperprolactinaemia* as a cause for subfertility because it can be treated so successfully in most cases. It may be associated with any menstrual pattern from complete amenorrhoea to normal, regular menstruation. There is a marked diurnal variation in prolactin secretion, with

TABLE 42.9
CAUSES OF SUBFERTILITY

Male factor	25–40%
Ovulatory dysfunction	20–30%
Tubular damage	15–20%
Cervical/immunological	5%
Endometriosis	10%
Coital failure	5%
Unexplained	20–30%

levels high overnight and declining during the first part of the day. More reliable information may be obtained from specimens taken in the afternoon. The significance of values between 500 and 1000 mu/L, particularly in women who are ovulating normally, is debatable; they should be interpreted with caution because treatment may not result in increased fertility.

In addition to biochemical tests, many other clinical and radiological investigations are essential before treatment (particularly assisted conception) is undertaken. These include a postcoital test, plus laparoscopy and dye studies, and hysterosalpingogram (both to ensure tubal patency).

It is not possible to carry out a successful programme of assisted conception without dedicated laboratory support. Although pelvic ultrasound is the major method used to follow ovulation induction, close biochemical monitoring is also considered essential to assess periovulatory oestradiol and LH levels, and oestradiol and progesterone levels in the luteal phase. The results of these assays are frequently needed for immediate decision making, and although highly sensitive assays may not be required, there *is* a need for rapid, reliable assays, made daily (including weekends).

Acknowledgement

This chapter is based upon Chapter 40 by Professor Stephen Jeffcoate in the previous edition. Some of the figures and tables are also based on those from the previous Chapter. The author and editors are grateful to Professor Jeffcoate for giving his permission.

BIOCHEMICAL ASPECTS OF TOXICOLOGY AND PHARMACOLOGY

43. The Biochemistry and Toxicology of Metals

A. P. Taylor

Introduction
Non-essential elements
  Aluminium
  Lead
  Mercury
  Cadmium
  Arsenic
  Beryllium
Essential trace elements
  Selenium
  Zinc
  Copper
  Cobalt
  Manganese
  Nickel
  Chromium
Other aspects of trace element metabolism
  Total parenteral nutrition
  Chronic renal failure and maintenance
    haemodialysis
  Trace elements as pharmacological agents
  Trace elements in the monitoring of disease
Summary

INTRODUCTION

The biological functions and properties of trace elements or heavy metals (these terms are often, but inaccurately, used synonymously) are of interest to a wide range of disciplines. While in occupational health and toxicology the consequences of gross exposure are studied, natural requirements, availability and deficiencies of the essential elements are of nutritional interest. Physiologists, biochemists and bioinorganic chemists are concerned with mechanisms, of absorption for example, and with interactions with other systems. Epidemiological research suggests that there are correlations between morbidity and environmental exposure to certain trace elements, yet a few elements can be used as pharmacological agents. The interests of clinicians and clinical chemists overlap with all of these specialities and so occupy a central position, drawing upon each of them and relating one to another.

Prior to the development of sensitive analytical techniques, particularly atomic absorption spectrophotometry, trace elements were largely ignored. Recent years have seen a radical change and measurements of concentrations in the nanogram per gram range in sample volumes of no more than 50 μL are relatively straightforward and inexpensive. As predicted in the first edition of this book, the impact of inductively coupled plasma-mass spectrometry is now evident, especially for the measurement of stable isotopes. Annual reviews,[1] which discuss recent analytical advances and also the clinical applications of these techniques, are particularly helpful. As a consequence of increased analytical activity the importance of trace elements in clinical situations other than gross toxicity is much more widely appreciated. In addition, hazards associated with environmental pollution receive considerable public attention, such that screening and monitoring programmes are established. The result is that, as never before, clinical chemists are required to be conscious of circumstances where advice and analysis are appropriate. Many of the issues discussed in this chapter were featured in a comprehensive review, which may be consulted for further information.[2]

Certain elements are *essential* to human life and well-being, but most are *non-essential* with no known function.[3] Elements present in large amounts within the body (e.g. calcium, sodium) are termed the *bulk* elements, while others are the *trace* elements. A useful definition describes the trace elements as those that constitute less than 0.01% of the dry weight of the body. Elements may be essential or non-essential but all can be toxic at certain levels of exposure. Nevertheless, because elements such as lead are usually measured when poisoning is suspected while those such as zinc are generally investigated in deficiency conditions, trace elements are often considered at the concentrations at which they usually occur within the body as either essential or toxic. This chapter will focus mainly on the effects of excessive exposures. Conditions due to deficiencies of essential elements are covered in Chapter 1 'Nutritional Disorders'.

NON-ESSENTIAL ELEMENTS

Aluminium

Aluminium is widely distributed throughout the environment. Nevertheless, incorporation into foods and beverages is generally very small so that dietary intake is usually about 5 mg/day. In many areas, aluminium is added to the drinking water derived from ground water sources as part of the treatment process to remove undesirable organic material and may be at a concentration of up to 200 μg/L, or even higher. In addition, drinking waters formed from sources derived from acidic rain can have high concentrations of aluminium due to solution of the metal from soil.

Physiology

In healthy individuals there is virtually no gastrointestinal absorption (less than 1%) of the ingested aluminium. Absorption is promoted a little by acidic food contents and considerably by formation of a citrate ligand. Other factors also influence absorption but the detailed mechanisms are not fully understood. These factors include vitamin D, parathyroid hormone, other elements (Fe, Si, F, Ca, P) and, possibly, interactions with some drugs. Absorbed aluminium is excreted in the urine so that accumulation in tissues is small (except for the lung where macrophages retain aluminium-containing particles by phagocytosis). There is an even distribution between plasma and erythrocytes, and within the plasma most aluminium is bound to transferrin.

Toxicity

Aluminium is the toxic agent responsible for the condition of *dialysis encephalopathy* (dialysis dementia). This is now rarely seen but, before the latter 1970s, patients with chronic renal failure, who were treated by haemodialysis with fluids prepared from water with high concentrations of aluminium, accumulated the metal in their tissues. As most of the plasma aluminium is protein bound, an effective concentration gradient is maintained and the metal present in the dialysis fluids readily diffuses into the blood. Dialysis dementia was characterized by the development of neurological symptoms 1–3 years after a patient started dialysis. The initial sign was speech hesitancy and an inability to articulate words at the completion of a dialysis session. This gradually extended for longer periods until it was a permanent feature. Other neurological symptoms also appeared, with myoclonus, convulsions, coma and death within about 6 months of the first onset of symptoms. Aluminium toxicity also includes osteomalacia, anaemia and, less severely, ectopic calcification and arthropathy. Treatment with desferrioxamine mobilizes accumulated aluminium, with formation of a low molecular-mass complex that is excreted into the dialysis fluid. Accumulation of aluminium has been reduced by the use of purified water for preparation of dialysis fluid and the close surveillance of patients. Plasma aluminium concentrations are typically less than $3.7\,\mu\text{mol}/\text{L}$ ($100\,\mu\text{g}/\text{L}$) and neurological symptoms are encountered only in unusual conditions. However, the osteomalacia and anaemia continue to present problems in the management of patients with chronic renal failure, mainly due to the large doses of aluminium hydroxide given orally as antihyperphosphataemic agents. In addition to patients on haemodialysis, toxicity has been reported in those treated by continuous ambulatory peritoneal dialysis, children with renal failure given aluminium-based phosphate binders and in some occupational exposures to aluminium dusts. Contamination of intravenous nutrition fluids, albumin and soya-based infant formulas may occur during preparation with tissue accumulation in those who receive these.

Aluminium may be involved with neurodegenerative disorders. It is present in the core of senile plaques found in the brains of patients with Alzheimer's disease and there is epidemiological evidence for an association between the incidence of this disease and the concentration of aluminium in drinking water. It is similarly suggested that the high water aluminium concentrations, together with low levels of calcium and magnesium, may be responsible for amyotrophic lateral sclerosis in the native population of the Pacific island of Guam. For a short time in 1988 the residents of an area in Cornwall, England received acidic drinking water with very high concentrations of aluminium and other metals after a contamination incident. Many individuals have since reported bone and joint pain and/or short-term memory loss.[4] Sensitive tests of neurocognitive function showed small, temporary deficits in some subjects but whether this can be attributed to the contamination requires further investigation. Similar tests have shown impaired performance in other groups with chronic exposure to low levels of aluminium. Subjects investigated this way are patients with chronic renal failure, who were well controlled and did not have grossly elevated serum aluminium levels, and miners deliberately exposed to aluminium dust for prophylactic purposes to prevent silicosis. Despite impaired performance in these tests the participants in these studies had no overt signs of neurological disorders.

Toxicity of aluminium is evident clinically and in experimental animals. However, the cellular mechanisms by which toxicity is produced are unclear. With *in vitro* investigations, influences on nuclear, metabolic and neurotransmitter functions, and increased reactive-oxygen activity can be demonstrated. Which of these, or other, effects are ultimately responsible for aluminium toxicity is still to be determined.

Lead

Lead occurs naturally in the environment of man—in food, drinking water, the atmosphere and in street dust. Concentrations in food have been steadily getting lower as a result of more careful preparation and packaging and more stringent statutory limits. Concentrations are generally well below $1\,\mu\text{g}/\text{g}$ and drinking water seldom contains more than $10\,\mu\text{g}/\text{L}$. The WHO provisional tolerable weekly intake of lead for adults is set at 3 mg. Recent measurements of total diets suggest the intakes are much lower, approximately $20\,\mu\text{g}/\text{day}$. Atmospheric lead is also decreasing in Britain as a consequence of the reduction in the amount added to petrol in 1986 and the increased use of unleaded fuel. These changes have contributed to significant reductions in blood lead concentrations of the general population and have also been seen in many other countries. In areas where the drinking water supply is acidic and lead plumbing is present the water is the most important source of exposure (> 100 μg/day).

Physiology

Metabolic studies and isotope absorption experiments indicate that adults normally absorb 5–10% of their daily intake. Young children, however, absorb very much more (40–50%) of the ingested lead. Availability of lead for absorption, however, is much more varied than these results suggest. In animals, absorption is inversely related to dietary calcium and phosphorus, zinc and iron. High fat and high protein diets promote absorption while the anion associated with lead also affects its uptake. Approximately 30–50% of inhaled lead is absorbed, either across alveolar membranes or, following transfer of coarse particles from the lung by ciliary action, via the alimentary tract. A typical urban atmosphere contains around 0.2 μg/m³ and is therefore relatively less important than dietary and other sources of lead.

Rabinowitch et al.[5] described the distribution of lead as approximating to a three-compartmental model. Absorbed lead rapidly associates with erythrocytes (less than 5% of lead in blood is within the plasma). From this first compartment, with a mean life of 35 days, lead passes into the urine (200 nmol/day) or is transferred into the other two compartments. From the second, represented by the soft tissues, a small amount of lead is excreted into nails, hair, and alimentary secretions, while the third—primarily the skeleton—serves as the long-term store with a very slow turnover rate and containing 99% of the total body lead.

Lead readily crosses the placenta and is a well-recognized abortifacient.

Toxicity

Industrial. That lead is an extremely versatile and important raw material in very many industries is attested by its continuous use for 6000 years.[6] Despite the well-recognized hazards associated with its use, including a number of widespread mass poisoning episodes, no suitable alternative is available and therefore many men and women continue to be occupationally exposed to lead and its compounds.

In England and Wales approximately 20 000 persons employed in a wide range of industries such as metal smelting, battery, paint, glass and ceramicware manufacture are recognized by the Health and Safety Executive (HSE) as requiring regular monitoring to safeguard against lead poisoning. There are, in addition, those who fall outside the regulations within which the HSE acts and may present through their general practitioner to the hospital without necessarily giving details of their lead exposure.

Signs and Symptoms. The characteristic clinical features of chronic inorganic lead poisoning include weakness and fatigue, anaemia, abdominal pain, gastrointestinal symptoms, chronic renal failure, deposition of lead as a blue line in the gums, and a peripheral neuropathy with tremor and weakness. Lead binds to thiol groups and is therefore an enzyme inhibitor. The activities of erythrocyte pyrimidine nucleotidase and Na⁺, K⁺ ATPase are reduced in lead poisoning, but the enzymes most studied are those of haem synthesis (Fig. 43.1), with inhibition of δ-aminolevulinic acid-ALA dehydratase, δ-ALA synthetase and ferrochelatase well documented following exposure to lead.[7]

Exposure to organic lead compounds occurs in very few occupational processes but, if severe, a syndrome quite distinct from inorganic lead poisoning ensues characterized by an encephalopathy with hallucinations, delusions and convulsions. There is moderate increase in the blood lead concentration although the proportion in the lipid fraction of blood is much higher than in inorganic lead poisoning.

Laboratory investigations. Measurement of the *blood lead concentration* in a properly collected venous blood sample is the best single test of lead absorption, although urinary lead excretion, particularly following stimulation with orally administered chelating agents, also demonstrates body lead. Blood lead concentrations in non-occupationally exposed adult men are less than 0.8 μmol/L and a little lower in women and children. Recent or prolonged exposure is indicated by increased blood lead concentrations and symptoms, which can be severe if the blood lead is greater than 4.0 μmol/L, may appear. At blood lead concentrations greater than 70 μg/dL (3.4 μmol/L), monitoring of lead workers becomes more intensive (40 μg/dL in women of child-bearing age) and they are removed from occupational exposure to lead. Provision for surveillance of lead workers in Britain is given in the Lead Regulation,[8] which requires blood lead concentrations to be measured in everyone who works with lead. Lead has been measured in the plasma of occupationally exposed subjects. The concentration is proportional to the total blood lead and, despite its availability to other tissues, plasma lead is no better indication to toxicity than total blood lead.

Tests to assess the effects of lead upon the pathway of *haem synthesis* have been used as alternatives to the measurement of lead in blood (Fig. 43.1). Because these tests, unlike the blood lead concentration, are a direct measure of the degree of biological damage wrought by lead they may better demonstrate the state of health of lead workers. Furthermore contamination of the sample during collection does not affect the result of the tests and some are sufficiently simple to be done at the collection site. Increases in urinary coproporphyrin and δALA-excretion, resulting from the effect of lead on the haem biosynthetic pathway, have been used for many years to monitor lead workers but these tests do not provide any further information than is obtained from the blood lead alone and screening by using these measurements

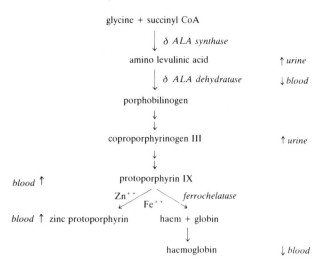

Enzymes with reduced activity due to lead are shown in italics.
Intermediates with altered concentrations are indicated together with body fluid in which assayed.

Figure 43.1 Effect of lead upon haem synthesis.

has virtually been abandoned. Measurement of zinc protoporphyrin, in addition to lead in blood, is the simplest and most common additional investigation. Three-monthly estimations of blood haemoglobin were introduced in 1964 as the first statutory test for lead workers but, as with punctate basophilia, alterations are not consistently seen in lead workers until the blood lead levels are greater than 5.5 μmol/L.

Whereas measurement of haemoglobin lacks sensitivity to the presence of lead, measurement of erythrocyte δ-ALA dehydratase is oversensitive. Inhibition of this enzyme occurs at blood lead levels below 1.0 μmol/L and has no role in monitoring occupational exposure. Inhibition by lead of the enzyme ferrochelatase causes accumulation of protoporphyrin IX in red cells. A simple procedure for fluorometric measurement of free erythrocyte protoporphyrin following ethyl acetate extraction was described by Piomelli.[9] Subsequently, it was demonstrated that protoporphyrin IX accumulating in the red cell is complexed with zinc and that this zinc–protoporphyrin complex (ZPP) can also easily be assayed. With the development of small, portable, dedicated fluorimeters, measurement of ZPP has provoked considerable interest. Piomelli[9] demonstrated a logarithmic correlation between protoporphyrin and blood lead and in the USA it was recommended that that erythrocyte protoporphyrin should be used in environmental screening surveys and only when this is increased should blood lead determination be considered. This approach was never accepted in the UK and it is now recognised that for environmental monitoring where blood lead concentrations may only be slightly increased ZPP is not a helpful investigation. While ZPP measurements have a role, as a rapid contamination check if any unexpectedly high lead result is obtained, this test cannot replace measurement of lead in blood.

To determine the test or combination of tests that best predicts or reflects morbidity, Irwig et al.[10] correlated the prevalence of various symptoms with the concentrations of blood and urine lead, urine δ-ALA and packed cell volume in 639 workers receiving considerable occupational lead exposure. The best prediction of morbidity was given by blood lead alone and the effects of lead upon porphyrin metabolism were not related to clinical findings. This work, involving a large number of subjects, 25% of whom had blood lead concentrations greater than 5 μmol/L, emphasizes the importance of the blood lead in occupational exposure and that other tests should only be considered where it is impracticable to achieve reliable blood lead results.

Non-industrial. While industrial exposure is responsible for the majority of cases of lead poisoning, there are many other sources of lead to which the population in general may be exposed (Table 43.1). Some of these, for example children with pica (where the behaviour of putting toys etc. in the mouth is prolonged) who are at risk from paint or dust in old buildings, acidic drinks stored in lead-glazed vessels, lead in petrol exhaust, are well recognized. Some are of incidental interest, being of relevance only when adding to a pre-existing problem of lead exposure. Cases of poisoning attributed to Surma, an Indian eye cosmetic containing up to 90% of lead sulphide, are now being recognized. A related problem concerns unconventional medicines that may be used by some populations. An airline pilot 'treated' in India for diabetes was diagnosed by a doctor in this country as having lead poisoning. His blood lead concentration was 4.2 μmol/L and two Ayurvedic medicines that were analysed in our laboratory contained 1.8% and 3.8% of lead. Similar episodes can be expected to occur in other groups. A surprisingly large number of cases of toxicity have been reported in persons who have been shot and where the bullet or pellets remained in the body. Variants of the Munchausen syndrome, with deliberate self-administration of lead, have been discovered.

Signs and Symptoms. Symptoms associated with lead poisoning are the same as in industrial exposure, but without the tolerance to lead found in lead workers these patients are affected earlier and more severely. This is especially so in children, where encephalopathy and death may be the eventual outcome. Acute poisoning following excessive exposure to lead is extremely uncommon. Weakness, nausea, vomiting and abdominal pain occurred in a group of drug addicts who stole lead-and-opium pills and injected a suspension of these in water. Those severely affected developed liver failure and reversible renal tubular necrosis, while neuropathy with respiratory paralysis was present in one case.

TABLE 43.1

NON-INDUSTRIAL SOURCES OF LEAD SHOWN TO CAUSE
TOXICITY OR TO BE POTENTIAL HEALTH HAZARDS

Domestic water system
Glazed jugs, bottles, glasses
Kettles and boilers
Embedded bullets
Indoor firing range
Batteries burned for fuel
Newsprint
Dust, soil
Toothpaste tubes
Sniffing petrol fumes
Herbal and Ayurvedic medicines
Surma and other cosmetics
Paints, varnish, inks
Lead-containing opium
Contaminated food
Air

Laboratory Investigations. As with lead workers the most important test is the measurement of *blood lead*; wherever a confirmed result of greater than 1.5 μmol/L is discovered, follow-up is essential. This should include an attempt to identify and if possible eliminate the source of exposure, the evaluation of the clinical effects of the lead already absorbed, and, where appropriate, initiation of treatment to reduce the body burden. While the use of chelating agents is essential when the blood lead concentration is dangerously high, this is not without risk of producing side-effects and the preferred treatment is removal from the source of exposure. Removal may be impossible in certain situations; where the patient lives close to a smelting works or where the source of exposure has not been discovered for example. Re-exposure is then inevitable and it is necessary to assess fully the clinical and biochemical effects of the lead because in these cases, too, treatment with chelating agents may be required.

The tests suggested above as alternatives to blood lead are all of value, although changes are not always due to lead. Zinc protoporphyrin is elevated in iron-deficiency anaemia to levels comparable to those in lead poisoning. Furthermore, because of the 3-month life-span of red cells a change in ZPP will inevitably lag behind absorption or elimination of lead. Inhibition of erythrocyte δ-ALA dehydratase is a very sensitive test of lead exposure and similarly a reduced haemoglobin concentration demonstrates the biochemical effects of lead. A diagnosis of lead poisoning may be suspected by the coincidental finding of low haemoglobin and punctate basophilia during routine haematological investigations of patients not known to be exposed to lead.

Lead poisoning should be considered in the differential diagnosis of unexplained encephalopathy in children. In urgent circumstances, blood lead can be measured within minutes of receipt of sample and meanwhile radiological examination for lead in the gut and for 'lead lines' in the long bones performed.

Lead excreted with the faeces represents the fraction of ingested lead that has not been absorbed, together with the very small amount present in intestinal secretions.[5] As the diet is the major source for intake of lead, measurement of faecal lead is a valuable determination in children following severe poisoning, when blood lead levels may remain high and it is necessary to discover whether this represents re-exposure or equilibration with the lead in bone.

Subclinical Lead Exposure

There is now little doubt that residents of areas with increased environmental lead have blood lead concentrations that are greater than those living in other areas. This is particularly evident around lead smelters, but is also observed in subjects living within 100 m of major roadways, or in high traffic-density areas. Children have mean blood lead concentrations that decline with increasing distance between the primary source of lead and the home. Contamination of dust, soil and vegetation, with subsequent ingestion, is probably more important than inhalation as the route of absorption. Soft acidic water is plumbosolvic and considerable lead can enter the domestic water of homes with lead pipes and/or lead-lined tanks. A positive correlation was found between blood and water lead concentrations of households studied in Glasgow. Although moderate lead exposure does not produce symptoms of classical lead toxicity, it can be recognized by abnormal biochemical findings. It has been suggested that a continuous low-level exposure to lead is responsible for subtle changes in neural function and for other effects that are summarized as subclinical lead toxicity.[11]

Several workers have measured neurocognitive development in children exposed to small amounts of lead. Results from these studies are ambiguous and only a few took thorough account of confounding variables such as age, and social and family environment.[2] However, a series of more rigorously controlled studies in recent years from different countries using different test methods has shown more or less consistent results. The investigators conclude that lead exposure is associated with a small but measurable reduction in IQ. While the effects are small and have not been found by all workers, the impact of low-level lead exposure on children cannot be dismissed. A number of reports show raised blood lead concentrations in mentally handicapped children, but this is probably a reflection of the habit of pica, which is particularly prevalent in subnormal and hyperactive children. Beattie et al.[12] retrospectively measured lead in the drinking water of the houses occupied during pregnancy by the mothers of 77 mentally retarded children and 27 non-retarded matched controls. The probability of mental retardation was significantly increased when water lead exceeded 800 μg/L. Among the deficiencies of this work was the failure to obtain controls matched for maternal age and birth order.

Notwithstanding these limitations, excess lead exposure during fetal development remains a possibility in these cases. In a subsequent investigation the same team measured the concentrations of lead in blood samples collected from the same children during the first 2 weeks of life (collected for phenylketonuria screening). The mean blood lead in the retarded group, 1.25 μmol/L, was significantly higher than in the controls, 1.0 μmol/L. These results emphasize the sensitivity of the fetus to lead and indicate that attention to household water levels is a priority in high-risk areas.

While other associations between high concentrations of lead in water and clinical or laboratory changes have been described (e.g. hypertension and chronic renal insufficiency), it is still the relation between lead and mental development that is the most emotive and most discussed aspect of subclinical lead toxicity.

Mercury

Historically, industrial exposure to mercury rivals that of lead. Pliny, the Roman historian, was aware of the practice among those working with compounds of this metal of using thin bladder skins to prevent inhalation of mercurial dust—an extremely early example of occupational hygiene.

Physiology

Exposure and Absorption. *Methyl mercury* is present in the environment as a consequence of microbial methylation of inorganic mercury. The normally very low levels are concentrated in fish and other aquatic life; thus total mercury in the range 0.05–0.5 μg/g has been measured in a variety of species including tuna fish, with 80–95% as the methyl compound. Seafood is the main source of exposure to methyl mercury and any containing more than 0.5 μg/g is not permitted to be sold. The maximum recommended intake is 200 μg/week, but is usually much less and only populations with a large fish consumption would approach this level. Discharge of industrial effluent into coastal waters around Minamata and Niigata in Japan was responsible for several hundred cases of severe methyl mercury poisoning. Large quantities of fish containing up to 50 μg/g of mercury were eaten and 115 known deaths occurred. Furthermore, at least 22 babies were born with brain damage following fetal exposure to the methyl mercury. Methyl mercury presents a minor occupational hazard. It is applied to seeds, bulbs and tubers as an antifungal agent, and persons handling these have a limited exposure. Treated seeds, however, were responsible, in Iraq, for thousands of cases of poisoning where imported seed grain was unwittingly used to prepare bread. Similar incidents occurred in Pakistan, Ghana and Guatemala.[14] Intestinal absorption of alkyl mercury compounds is virtually total in man. Organic mercury compounds included in certain soaps and creams are absorbed through the skin.

Metallic mercury is employed in a wide range of equipment, for example electrical switches, scientific instruments, solders, amalgams, and electrodes. As a consequence of its high vapour pressure, volatization and exposure is inevitable. Of the inhaled mercury vapour, 70–80% crosses the alveolar membrane and is retained. While fewer in number than 100 years ago, cases of toxicity continue to be regularly reported. Elemental mercury is not absorbed in the gut and is innocuous even following intravenous injection or aspiration into the lungs.

Other *mercury compounds* are less important. Aryl compounds are also used as fungicides on seeds, as slimicides in paper mills and in wallpaper pastes, and previously as diuretics. They are relatively non-toxic. Exposure to inorganic salts is rather more complex. Suspended as dust, inhalation occurs followed (as with lead) by absorption or removal with bronchial secretions. Gastrointestinal absorption depends upon solubility, but does not exceed 20% of the ingested material. In addition to causing considerable irritation, absorption undoubtedly occurs through the skin, although the amounts retained have not been determined. Inorganic compounds are used in pigments, for timber preservation, in photography and as antiseptics.

Distribution and Excretion. Methyl mercury is very lipid soluble and is rapidly distributed throughout the whole body. Radioactive tracer studies indicate that 10% of the dose goes to the head, with significant amounts also in the liver and kidney. Red-cell concentrations are about 10 times that of the plasma and account for 5% of the dose. Because of the low plasma concentration, little mercury is available to the kidney for filtration and urinary excretion; 90% of elimination is into the faeces via the bile. There is significant transfer across the placenta into the fetus and also into breast milk. A consequence of the mobility of methyl mercury between blood and tissue is that rates of clearance from the blood, the brain and the whole body are very similar. Following a tracer dose of methyl mercury an average half-time of 70 days has been calculated. The concentration of methyl mercury in the blood is the best assessment of both body burden and brain level and at a steady state of exposure the blood level is proportional to intake. Methyl mercury in hair correlates with blood concentration at the time of hair formation and thus a retrospective index of exposure is possible. The total mercury concentration of blood is less than 30 nmol/L except where fish consumption is considerable and may then be four to five times this level, although individual values as high as 1000 nmol/L have been reported.[13]

Elemental mercury is initially concentrated in the red cells. Subsequent to oxidation by catalase the mercuric ion transfers to the plasma so that 24 h after exposure the ratio of red-cell to plasma mercury is about 2:1. Thereafter, the concentrations decline, with half-times of around 3 days. During the first few days following exposure, faecal excretion is greater than urinary loss and a small proportion of the retained mercury is re-excreted from the lungs. There is no correlation between urinary excretion and the plasma concentration, indicating that glomerular filtration is not a predominant pathway for removal of mercury. However, mercury ions are gradually redistributed throughout the body and accumulate predominantly in the kidney, where tubular secretion into the urine then occurs. An important feature in the metabolism of elemental mercury is that while distribution following oxidation is similar to that of ingested salts, some persists for sufficient time to diffuse from the blood into other tissues. Elemental, atomic mercury is lipophilic and, therefore, crosses the blood–brain barrier and accumulates in neural tissue. Placental passage also occurs; mercury accumulates in fetal membranes and is found in cord blood at concentrations equivalent to those in maternal blood.[13] The blood mercury concentration is meaningful only after a recent exposure. With the short half-times referred to above, intermittent exposure causes considerable fluctuations in blood levels, while with a single exposure most disappears within a few days. Determination of urine mercury is the best index of chronic exposure,[14] with normal excretion being less than 50 nmol/24 h or less than 5.5 nmol/mmol of creatinine in randomly collected samples.

Distribution and toxicity of inorganic and organic mercury compounds are modified by inorganic selenium. Retardation of growth caused by oral or parenteral administration of mercury compounds is not observed when selenite is given simultaneously. Protection appears to be afforded by a novel plasma protein to which selenium binds via a sulphydryl group and which in turn traps the mercury, preventing it from leaving the vascular compartment.

Toxicity

Signs and Symptoms. Toxicity to alkyl mercury compounds has been thoroughly documented following the mass poisonings in Japan and Iraq. Amin-Zaki et al.[15] have summarized their prolonged observations of children from rural Iraq. Neurological symptoms—ataxia, dysarthria and constriction of the visual fields (the classical signs of organic mercury poisoning)—were most evident. Hyper-reflexia was noted in all cases; muscle weakness and paraesthesia, tremor and twitching were also generally present. The severity of poisoning correlated with the blood mercury concentration, which ranged from 2.5 to 25 μmol/L (normal less than 30 nmol/L), and was dependent upon the amount of methyl mercury consumed. As in previous reports there was a latent period of up to 6 weeks, with accumulation of mer-

cury, before onset of symptoms. Japanese reports of Minamata Bay incidents, where exposure continued for several years with very much higher body burdens being attained, suggested that toxicity was irreversible. In Iraq, however, consumption ceased much earlier and considerable improvement in the condition of these children has slowly taken place.

Much more common than poisoning due to alkyl mercury compounds is toxicity due to *inhalation* of metallic mercury vapour; while the hazards associated with the handling and use of this metal are ignored, cases will continue to occur. Very rarely, acute exposure to high concentrations of mercury vapour takes place, producing a diffuse interstitial pneumonitis. Fever, chills, nausea and general malaise develop rapidly, together with tightness in the chest and paroxysmal coughing. Death from lung oedema occurs within 3 days in very severe cases. Where there is chronic, moderate exposure to mercury vapour, symptoms develop insidiously over several weeks or even years. Mercurialism is characterized particularly by muscle tremor and erethism. Fine muscle tremor of the arms, interfering with writing and other delicate finger work, is an early feature. Facial muscles are often involved and therefore speech may also be affected. In prolonged cases the tremor becomes progressively generalized, involving the entire voluntary muscle system. Sudden limb jerking and muscle spasm can develop, with inability to walk or even sit. Pronounced changes in mood and behaviour with feelings of listlessness and disinterest, gradually leading to withdrawal from social life, form part of the condition of erethism. Subjects also become irritable and over-reactive, and tend to sweat or blush readily. These patterns of mood change are noticed by friends and relatives rather than by the exposed person.

Other symptoms include stomatogingivitis, headache, double vision, anorexia, diarrhoea and weight loss. Mercurialentis, a brown discoloration of the lens, is a feature of chronic exposure to mercury vapour and is not a sign of toxicity. The intensity of the colour is proportional to length of exposure, but does not interfere with vision.

Current occupational hygiene measures ensure that the full clinical picture of mercurialism is rarely encountered and where a history of exposure is known it is easily recognized. Attention is now centred upon early diagnosis where symptoms are non-specific. Also a problem is the detection of mild mercurialism in patients whose exposure is unrecognized and who present to clinicians with headache, diarrhoea or tremor. Mercurialism is readily reversed by removal from the source of exposure and, if necessary, treatment with chelating agents.

Soluble mercury salts produce intense inflammation of exposed mucous membranes. There is immediate corrosion and necrosis of the mouth, throat, oesophagus and stomach, followed by pain, vomiting and diarrhoea. In severe overwhelming cases, death from haemorrhage, shock and circulatory collapse occurs within a few hours. With less severe exposure the primary lesions begin to heal, but further inflammation to the gastrointestinal tract occurs a few days later as secretion of mercuric ions with saliva and colonic fluid commences. Stomatogingivitis, ulcerative colitis and blood loss gradually subside and recovery ensues within a few weeks. Renal tubular necrosis may also be produced, which, if not interrupted by death, gradually recovers as the epithelium regenerates, only rarely leaving residual damage. Powders containing calomel (mercurous chloride) were once used to soften the gums of young children cutting teeth and many developed a widespread erythematous rash. Increased urinary mercury excretion has been demonstrated in this condition of pink disease (acrodynia); therefore, although not proven, mercury is believed to be responsible.

Accounts of nephrotic syndrome following exposure to ammoniated mercury ointments, or to metallic mercury vapour, appear to represent idiosyncratic responses and are not general features of mercury toxicity.

Laboratory Investigations. Conclusive demonstrations of toxicity depend on measurement of mercury in blood or urine. As mentioned above, the long half-life and good correlation with body and brain burdens make the concentration of mercury in blood the best index of exposure to methyl mercury. In other situations, mercury is rapidly cleared from the blood and determinations in urine are probably more valuable. In cases of toxicity, rates of excretion are very high, with milligram amounts being recorded. Lower levels are found during occupational monitoring and there is fluctuation in excretion from day to day. Smith et al.[14] found excellent correlation between time-weighted exposure and urine mercury excretion in a study of 642 workers manufacturing chlorine, although correlation between excretion and symptoms was less good. Lauwerys and Buchet[16] also showed significant correlation between urine mercury and exposure to vapour. Experience in our laboratory is in agreement with this. It has been shown that even the very limited exposure to which dental workers are subjected can be demonstrated in the urine. In early-morning urine samples, the ratio of mercury to creatinine is up to three times that found in unexposed subjects. Furthermore, where samples were received from several persons working in a practice, one result was at least 50% higher than the others and was invariably from the person preparing amalgam and working adjacent to the amalgamator.[17]

Cadmium

Unlike lead and mercury, industrial exposure to cadmium is a recent phenomenon and involves fewer subjects.[18] Zinc and lead ores invariably contain a significant proportion of cadmium; the processes of smelting and refining therefore produce dust and vapour laden with this metal. Electroplating, soldering, brazing and the disposal of industrial waste also generate cadium-rich vapour and dust. Acute exposure can be lethal, but the effects of chronic exposure are misleadingly deceptive, with severe, irreversible morbidity suddenly appearing after many years of apparent well-being. Other than occupationally, the sources of exposure to cadmium are food (shellfish, beef and pork kidney) and tobacco. Sufficient is absorbed for the metal to accumulate throughout life, with a body burden of 20–50 mg, mostly in the kidney, being reached. Following an environmental tragedy in Japan, where wastes from a cadmium mine contaminated drinking water and growing crops, a unique syndrome with bone pain and osteomalacia was observed in postmenopausal, parous women. Hypertension can be experimentally induced by prolonged administration of low levels of cadmium to rats and rabbits. There are some data that suggest hypertension and cadmium may be related in man, but this is far from resolved.

Physiology

The UK daily dietary intake is around 15–30 μg. Retention of ingested cadmium varies from 0.7% to 15.6% and is increased at low dietary concentrations of both cadmium and calcium. The proportion of cadmium absorbed is variable, but may be as high as 50%. Within industrial locations, absorption of up to 50 μg/day takes place. By contrast, less than 1 μg/day is absorbed by non-exposed subjects, although 20 cigarettes contribute a further 2–4 μg daily.

After absorption, cadmium is transported within the plasma primarily to the liver. There it is complexed with metallothionein, an inducible protein with a molecular mass of 6000, containing a high proportion (30%) of cysteine residues. This complex is slowly redistributed to the renal cortex via glomerular filtration and tubular reabsorption. Cadmium levels in whole blood increase following exposure, and then recede as the metal is sequestered into the liver and kidney. Urinary excretion is no more than 18 nmol/day (unless renal damage has occurred), although there is a small increase with age. Combined biliary and urinary excretion is normally less than 10% of the retained cadmium. It follows from these very low rates of cadmium excretion, and from its accumulation in the kidney and liver, that overall removal rates are very slow. Few studies have been made in man but from the available data it is apparent that cadmium is virtually fixed within the kidney and only very slowly removed from the liver (half-lives of 17–33, and 7 years, respectively).[19]

Toxicity

Antagonistic interactions with certain essential elements are responsible for many of the biochemical effects of cadmium. Metals, especially zinc, can be displaced from enzymes, e.g. carbonic anhydrase.

Competition for binding sites is the presumed mechanism here and also in the interference with the metabolism and storage of copper. There is evidence of similar competition between cadmium and both iron and calcium for intestinal transport.[19] Cadmium also inhibits formation of 1,25–dihydroxycholecalciferol, thereby further interfering with calcium metabolism.

Acute exposure to cadmium oxide vapour causes profound damage to the respiratory system. After a latent period of about 2 h there is painful tightness across the chest with dyspnoea, bronchitis and pneumonitis, irritation to the throat and severe, sometimes fatal, pulmonary oedema. Ingestion of cadmium compounds is followed within minutes by gastroenteritis—nausea, vomiting, salivation, diarrhoea, abdominal pain, weakness and headaches being induced. There are few fatalities, possibly because of the emetic effect of high oral cadmium intake.

Chronic inhalation or ingestion eventually precipitates irreversible damage to the kidney, the lungs and possibly bone. Cadmium as the metallothionein complex is stored in the renal cortex. In this form it is apparently innocuous until what appears to be a critical cortical concentration of 200 $\mu g/g$ wet weight is achieved. Capacity to store the complex further is overwhelmed and renal tubular damage is manifest with low molecular-weight proteinuria, glycosuria, phosphaturia and aminoaciduria. The increase in excretion of low molecular-weight proteins is one of the earliest signs of damage, and measurements of β_2-microglobulin or retinol-binding globulin are used for the early detection of renal dysfunction. The effects on skeletal tissue are complicated. The osteomalacia of cadmium exposure is generally explained as secondary to the renal damage. Inhibition of intestinal absorption of calcium, either by a direct effect in the lumen or as a consequence of impaired vitamin D metabolism, will accentuate the calcium deficiency.

While skeletal effects are extremely uncommon in cadmium workers, osteomalacia was a consistent feature in the *itai itai* disease in Japan. In this condition the bones became so fragile that considerable pain (*itai itai* literally means 'ouch, ouch') and fractures were caused by very light pressure. In addition to the osteomalacia, renal manifestations, iron-deficiency anaemia, chronic gastritis and enteropathy were observed. The aetiology of such strikingly severe osteomalacia involves more than just contamination of crops and water by cadmium. The victims were calcium depleted by child-bearing and inadequate diet; a low fat diet together with limited exposure to sunlight caused vitamin D deficiency. The conditions existed, therefore, with low dietary calcium and protein for enhancement of absorption of cadmium into a body ill-equipped to cope with the abuses inflicted.

From various surveys the incidence of carcinoma among men chronically exposed to cadmium at work is reported to be from 0.93 to 8.1%. In 248 workers the incidence of carcinoma was not increased but four men with prostatic cancer were seen, which was considerably in excess of the expected 0.58 cases.

Hypertension can be induced in rats and rabbits by long-term, low-level, cadmium feeding experiments designed to simulate normal human exposure. Paradoxically, chronic exposure to higher amounts of cadmium does not have this effect and hypertension is not a feature of occupational exposure or of the *itai itai* disease.

Laboratory Investigations

Laboratory investigations are required if undue non-industrial exposure is suspected, to determine the level of exposure and to assess the body (or renal) burden of cadmium following long-term accumulation.

Interpretation of blood and urinary levels depends on the frequency of exposure. Where a steady state of chronic, low-level exposure obtains, both the urine excretion and blood concentrations of cadmium correlate with body burden. With exposure such as to produce urinary levels of 10 nmol/mmol creatinine, there is considerable risk of renal tubular dysfunction. However, after a recent acute exposure a surge up to 50 nmol/mmol creatinine may be achieved without associated renal damage. The urinary cadmium is not then an index of body burden. Cadmium in blood reflects recent exposure and concentrations will fluctuate considerably. A major problem in occupational monitoring is early detection of renal tubular damage, before irreversible changes occur. Sensitive laboratory tests are the measurement of retinol-binding protein and β_2-microglobulin. Excretion of these low molecular-weight proteins is correlated with the number of years of exposure.

Arsenic

Fish and shellfish concentrate arsenic as organo-arsenic compounds that are not metabolized and have very low toxicity. Exposure to the more harmful inorganic arsenic occurs at work (manufacture of glass, as a pigment, in the semiconductor industry, use as a wood preservative) or in unusual incidents such as attempts at murder. Acute exposure can give symptoms with rapid onset; headache, nausea and severe gastrointestinal irritation are accompanied by intense abdominal pain, vomiting and diarrhoea. In profound poisoning there is dehydration, oliguria and circulatory collapse with encephalopathy and death. Chronic exposure causes gastrointestinal discomfort, thick reddening areas of skin and pruritic, pinpoint dermatitis. There is also loss of hair and a peripheral neuropathy. Persons working with arsenic have a greater than expected incidence of lung cancer. Exposure to inorganic arsenic is best monitored by measurement of the urinary excretion but high total arsenic concentrations can be obtained for a few

TABLE 43.2

TRACE ELEMENT CONCENTRATIONS IN BLOOD, SERUM AND URINE[21]

Element	Reference range (serum/plasma)	Urine
Aluminium	< 0.4 μmol/L	< 0.5 μmol/24 h
Chromium	1–10 nmol/L	1–27 nmol/24 h
Cobalt	1–7 nmol/L	< 17 nmol/24 h
Copper	13–23 μmol/L	< 1.0 μmol/24 h
Manganese	6–18 nmol/L	2–3 nmol/24 h
Nickel	4–48 nmol/L	1–30 nmol/24 h
Selenium	1.1–1.9 μmol/L	0.24–0.70 μmol/24 h
Zinc	11–24 μmol/L	4.5–9.0 μmol/24 h
	Blood	
Antimony		< 8 nmol/24 h
Arsenic	< 0.53 μmol/L	< 0.67 μmol/24 h
Cadmium	< 55 nmol/L	< 10 nmol/24 h
Lead	< 1.7 μmol/L	< 400 nmol/24 h
Mercury	< 30 nmol/L	< 50 nmol/24 h

days after eating seafoods. Urine samples should be collected when no fish has been consumed for at least 3 days or the analysis should include a procedure to separate inorganic from organic arsenic before the measurement.

Beryllium

Beryllium is a hard, light metal with a high melting point. It forms high-tensile alloys that are used in space exploration vehicles and missiles, electronic components and in nuclear reactors. Beryllium is very toxic and has one of the lowest occupational exposure limits of all metals. Dust, fume or vapour is absorbed by the lung and intestine and the acute effects are inflammation of the throat and chest, dermatitis, conjunctivitis and pulmonary damage. Chronic exposure causes berylliosis, a syndrome with breathlessness, cough, chest pain, patchy shadowing on chest X-ray, tiredness, anorexia and loss of weight.

ESSENTIAL TRACE ELEMENTS

An element is defined as essential if it occurs in the natural environment, is found in physiological amounts in the diet, is present in tissues at relatively constant concentrations, is found in the newborn and/or maternal milk, if withdrawal produces similar structural and physiological abnormalities in different species that are prevented or reversed by addition of the element, and where a biological function is associated with the element. Essential elements have various functions, most of which fall into the areas of enzyme activity, hormonal activity, vitamins, structure and support, and oxygen transport.

Mechanisms exist for the regulation of body burden and blood concentrations of essential elements. For most elements intestinal control is important, while for some regulation is at the level of excretion. Further control may be achieved by immobilization either by storage or by formation of complexes with other elements, thus reducing the physiologically active fraction of the total body load. Exposures to catastrophic amounts of essential elements will overwhelm the mechanisms for regulation and precipitate toxic symptoms. The essential element to which there is the least tolerance is selenium.

Normal plasma and urinary levels[20] are summarized in Table 43.2.

Selenium

Selenium is an essential trace element, which functions as part of the antioxidant system. Animal diseases caused by deficiency and overload are widely recognized and are associated with variations in the selenium content of soils and plants. Syndromes of deficiency and toxicity are known in man, which in some situations are also associated with natural dietary intakes.

Physiology

Incorporation of selenium into plants reflects the concentration of the element in soils. Dietary intakes are dependent, therefore, on the country of origin of vegetable foods, especially grain and cereal products. Other selenium-rich foods are meat, seafood, mushroom and garlic (the characteristic garlic odour is due to dimethylselenide). The usual intakes are about 40–200 μg/day but extremes of consumption occur in some communities. Selenomethionine in plant material and yeast has a higher bioavailability (85–100%) than the forms in other foods and selenite (20–50%).

Absorbed selenium compounds are reduced in the liver to selenide, which is incorporated into dimethylselenide and the trimethylselenonium ion. The kidney excretes a large proportion of metabolized selenium but some of the element is also lost through the kidney within a few hours of absorption. Nève et al. have produced a thorough discussion of measures to assess selenium status (selenium concentrations in plasma, blood, erythrocytes, platelets, urine; glutathione peroxidase activity in plasma, erythrocytes, platelets).[2] The importance of appropriate reference intervals and the different sensitivities of these markers to depletion and repletion of selenium were noted. Plasma selenium concentrations reflect low dietary intakes and tissue concentrations. Urinary excretion correlates significantly with both low and increased dietary intakes. Glutathione peroxidase activity in plasma falls rapidly in selenium depletion but the activity in the erythrocyte responds much more slowly. In addition to intake, concentrations are influenced by age, pregnancy and illness.

Selenium (as selenocysteine) is at the active site of glutathione peroxidase, the enzyme that catalyses the reduction of hydrogen peroxide by glutathione. Glutathione peroxidase is involved with the metabolism of fatty acids but of special importance is its antioxidant function. Highest levels of activity are present in liver and erythrocytes, with less in kidney, spleen and lung. Lowest activities are found in plasma, muscle and brain.

Toxicity

Signs of selenium toxicity in animals were described by Marco Polo whilst in China. More recently, residents of an area of China developed selenosis when, for a number of years, they ate vegetables grown in seleniferous soils. The predominent symptoms were of dry, brittle hair, easily broken at the scalp and intolerable itching; brittle, streaked nails; red, swollen skin with eruptive blisters on the limbs and neck; tooth decay. Neurological signs—paraesthesia, hyper-reflexia, hemiplegia—were present in severe cases. Chronic occupational exposure (gun metal, electronics manufacture, glass manufacture, etc.) produces similar effects, with gastrointestinal symptoms and a pungent, garlic-like odour to the breath also reported. Almost identical symptoms were noted in the victim of an attempted murder who unwittingly ingested selenious acid. In a few cases of acute exposure to selenium compounds the main symptoms were of inflammation and haemorrhage of mucosal surfaces, and the garlic breath.

Zinc

Zinc is a cofactor for many enzymes including those associated with nucleic acid and protein metabolism. It is particularly important, therefore, for growth and development and for repair of damaged tissue. Deficiency can have profound effects on well-being and the body is remarkably tolerant to large amounts of the metal. However, zinc toxicity does occur in some unusual circumstances.

Ingestion of food contaminated by zinc while stored in galvanized containers causes nausea, vomiting, diarrhoea and fever. Identical symptoms were observed in a woman receiving home haemodialysis against fluids prepared from rainwater stored in a galvanized tank (she lived in a very arid area and all water needed to be preserved). Extreme lethargy, light-headedness, staggering and difficulty in writing legibly were experienced by a 16-year-old boy who ingested 12 g of metallic zinc. Inhalation of zinc oxide fumes causes a pneumonitis that may be fatal.

Measurement of zinc in a sample of serum or plasma collected to avoid contamination is the simplest laboratory test of body zinc. Urinary excretion can also be helpful to assess the level of exposure.

Copper

Copper overload can develop from increased exposure or, in Wilson's disease, as a consequence of an inability to excrete the metal.

Ingestion of copper salts, either by accident or following suicidal or homicidal intent, produces a complex clinical picture. Nausea, vomiting and diarrhoea may be followed, if toxicity is severe, by intravascular haemolysis marked by increased plasma haemoglobin and bilirubin, reticulocytosis and haemoglobinuria. Acute renal failure due to tubular obstruction by haemoglobin, deposition of copper in the kidney and dehydration occurs a few days later and may be fatal despite haemodialysis. A similar syndrome was recognized some years ago in patients receiving haemodialysis using Cuprophan as the dialysis membrane or dialysis fluid plumbed through copper tubing. Once the cause was determined, further cases were prevented.

Wilson's disease (hepatolenticular degeneration) is a rare inherited disorder of copper metabolism.[2] The main features are cirrhosis of the liver, renal tubular dysfunction and progressive degeneration of the central nervous system. A pathognomonic sign is the green-brown Kayser–Fleischer rings in the iris. Onset of symptoms is usually during the teens, although it has been reported at 6 years of age and is seen earlier in female than in male subjects. Neurological symptoms include poor coordination, a slight tremor, dysarthria, dysphagia and choreiform movements. These signs are, however, often preceded by hepatic dysfunction, which can present in a variety of ways including chronic active hepatitis, acute hepatitis and cryptogenic cirrhosis. Low ($< 9 \mu$mol/L) concentrations of copper in serum are usually evident (although normal concentrations exist in a proportion of cases where there is severe hepatocellular necrosis), while urinary excretion is considerably increased ($> 1.5 \mu$mol/24 h). These determinations, together with measurement of caeruloplasmin in serum, are the appropriate biochemical investigations for the diagnosis of Wilson's disease. Where these results are ambiguous a liver biopsy specimen can be collected and the copper measured. Grossly increased concentrations will be found.

Irreversible damage to the liver and brain can be prevented if treatment with the chelating agent penicillamine is commenced at an early stage of the disease. High oral doses of zinc are also effective and appear to work by competing with copper for absorption in the gut.

Cobalt

The only known physiological role for cobalt in man is in vitamin B_{12}. Exposure to inorganic cobalt can occur at work (e.g. production and use of tungsten carbide materials, manufacture of alloys and pigments), from corrosion of cobalt-alloy joint prostheses or as an agent to stimulate erythropoiesis (*see below*).

Cobalt cardiomyopathy was recognized after brewers added cobalt chloride to beer. (Cobalt was included to stabilize the 'head' on a glass of beer, which was otherwise discharged by traces of detergents.) Subjects developed fulminating heart failure and polycythaemia. Occupational exposure to cobalt powder or to dust associated with tungsten carbide causes interstitial changes to the lungs known as hard metal disease. This painful, debilitating condition is irreversible and exposed workers should be carefully monitored with regular lung-function tests and assessments of exposure (cobalt in air and/or cobalt in end-of-shift, end-of-week urine specimens). Animals treated with large doses of cobalt chloride developed polycythaemia and hyperlipaemia.

Manganese

Manganous ion is an activator of many enzymes including RNA polymerase and RNA-dependent DNA polymerase; thus this metal is vital for the synthesis of nucleic acids and protein. Manganese also plays a part in various endocrine systems. Manganese is relatively non-toxic, requiring considerable, long-term exposure (e.g. during mining) to evoke neurological symptoms similar to those of Parkinson's and Wilson's diseases. Chronic manganese toxicity was demonstrated in an Aboriginal community in northern Australia who lived in an area where the soil was manganese rich. Only some of the group were affected and psychiatric changes also occurred.

Nickel

Nickel toxicity is rarely seen in man. Acutely, oral administration to animals has few effects for 24 h but there is then gastrointestinal irritation, vomiting and diarrhoea. Gastritis and neurological symptoms (tremor, chorea, paralysis) occur after parenteral administration. Chronic oral exposure produces some enzyme changes in heart, liver, kidney, testis and there is thickening of lung walls after long-term inhalation. Effects in man are those of contact dermatitis and tumours of the respiratory tract (lung, nasal sinus) in workers (refining, plating, polishing). Nickel subsulphide dust is the probable carcinogenic agent.

Chromium

Occupational exposure to chromium compounds occurs during tanning of animal hides and in the electroplating industry. Dermatitis is the most usual symptom but skin contact with chromic acid sometimes occurs due to splashing or more severe accidents. In addition to the burning, dermal absorption takes place, with high plasma concentrations and accumulation of chromium in several tissues. The kidney is the most vulnerable organ.[21]

OTHER ASPECTS OF TRACE ELEMENT METABOLISM

Total Parenteral Nutrition

Subjects with intestinal incompetence following infarction, radiotherapy, surgery, etc. can be treated by prolonged or even permanent total parenteral nutrition. Technical problems associated with intravenous feeding have been superseded by those attendant on the gradual development of deficiencies of micronutrients. These conditions arise because trace element requirements, especially during physiological crises, are not known. The trace element content of intravenous fluids and supplements is not always available and the symptoms of deficiency (with the exception of zinc) are poorly described. Even where mineral supplements are deliberately included, they may be readily available for urinary excretion and not be taken into the tissues in the amounts required to maintain balance. In this important area of trace element metabolism there is an urgent requirement for methods for multi-element analyses at very low concentrations. Considerable information can also be obtained from veterinary research, which for many years has been concerned with recognition of trace element deficiencies in animals.

Chronic Renal Failure and Maintenance Haemodialysis

During a period of routine haemodialysis the body is intimately exposed to far greater volumes of dilute fluid than normally occur through drinking. The consequences of such exposure may be either losses of essential elements or acquisition of toxic elements. It appears, however, that losses probably do not occur. There are no reports of trace element deficiencies in these patients and investigations made during dialysis indicate that only small concentration changes occur, which are very soon repaired. Movement of elements from the dialysis medium into the blood does take place. Uptake of aluminium leading to dialysis dementia has already been described. In addition, copper, zinc and nickel from the dialysis equipment will contaminate the fluids and pass into the patient. Because of the continuing developments in dialysis equipment, fluids, and treatment regimens it is not inconceivable that further examples may arise; metal toxicity should therefore be considered if haemodialysis patients develop unexplained or unexpected symptoms.

Trace Elements as Pharmacological Agents

The history of deliberate administration of trace element compounds probably coexists with the history of industrial usage, with mercury (to treat syphilis), lead (to induce abortions) and arsenic (with homicidal or suicidal intent) as notable examples. More recently, chrysotherapy using soluble gold compounds like sodium aurothiomalate to treat rheuma-toid arthritis and cancer chemotherapy with *cis* complexes of platinum diamine compounds have had spectacular successes in some patients. Together with the benefit gained from such therapy there is the equally evident toxicity, which limits extensive use. Cobalt salts have been used to stimulate erythropoiesis in cases of refractory anaemia. However, like gold and platinum, the associated toxicity of cobalt limits the therapeutic usefulness. Pharmacological uses of these and other metals such as bismuth, lithium and zinc have been reviewed.[2]

Trace Elements in the Monitoring of Disease

In some pathological conditions, apparently unrelated to their normal metabolism, changes in blood concentrations of trace elements have proved valuable in predicting the clinical course or the response to treatment. Thus an increased serum copper concentration is a poor prognostic sign in Hodgkin's disease and in certain neoplasms (e.g. acute lymphoblastic leukaemia) in which concomitant hypozincaemia may also exist. Copper and caeruloplasmin concentrations in serum from patients with rheumatoid arthritis are similarly increased during the active stages of the disease, returning to normal during remission.

SUMMARY

There are several areas of the biochemistry and toxicity of trace elements that will almost certainly be prominent among future developments. Investigations of the effects of long-term exposure to elements at lower concentrations than those associated with classical toxicity; investigations with lead, cadmium and aluminium reveal some curious effects of low-level exposure that require further study. Further efforts will be made to determine the metabolism of the essential elements and to recognize clinical syndromes associated with their deficiency; widespread use of prolonged total parenteral nutrition is providing many opportunities for this work. The interactions between trace elements, now recognized as being important in intestinal absorption, will be studied at other sites. New advances in analytical techniques will undoubtedly play a major part in these developments and, to give confidence to results that are close to the detection limits of the instrumentation, greater emphasis will be placed on reference materials and quality-control procedures.

REFERENCES

1. Taylor, A., Branch S., Crews H., Wells D.J. and White M. (1994). Atomic spectrometry update—clinical and biological materials, foods and beverages. *J. Anal. Atomic Spectrom.*, **9**, 87R.
2. Taylor A. ed. (1985). Trace elements in human disease. *Clin. Endocrinol. Metab.*, **14**, 513.
3. Schwarz K. (1977). In *Clinical Chemistry and Chemical Toxicology of Metals* (Brown S.S. ed.) Amsterdam: Elsevier/North Holland.
4. Eastwood J.B., Levin G.E., Pazianas M., Taylor A., Denton J., Freemont A.J. (1990). Aluminium deposition in bone after contamination of drinking water supply. *Lancet*, **ii**, 462.
5. Rabinowitz M.B., Wetherill G.W., Kopple J.D. (1976). Kinetic analysis of lead metabolism in healthy humans. *J. Clin. Invest.*, **58**, 260.
6. Barltrop D. (1977). In *Clinical Chemistry and Chemical Toxicology of Metals* (Brown S.S. ed.) Amsterdam: Elsevier/North Holland.
7. Clayton B. (1975). Lead: The relation of environment and experimental work. *Br. Med. Bull.*, **31**, 236.
8. Health and Safety Commission (1985). *Control of Lead at Work. Approved Code of Practice*, London: HMSO.
9. Piomelli S. (1973). A micromethod for free erythrocyte porphyrins. The FEP test. *J. Lab. Clin. Med.*, **81**, 932.
10. Irwig L.M., Harrison W.O., Rocks P., Webster I., Andrew M. (1978). Lead and morbidity: a dose–response relationship. *Lancet*, **ii**, 4.
11. Waldron M.A., Stofen D. (1974). *Sub-clinical Lead Poisoning*, London/New York: Academic Press.
12. Beattie A.D. et al. (1975). Role of chronic low-level lead exposure on the aetiology of mental retardation. *Lancet*, **i**, 589.
13. Clarkson T.W. (1977). In *Clinical Chemistry and Chemical Toxicity of Metals* (Brown S.S. ed.) Amsterdam: Elsevier/North Holland.
14. Smith R.G., Vorwald A.J., Patil L.S., Mooney T.F. (1970). Effects of exposure to mercury in the manufacture of chlorine. *Am. Ind. Hyg. Assoc. J.*, **31**, 687.
15. Amin-Zaki L., Majeed M.A., Clarkson T.W., Greenwood M.R. (1978). Methylmercury poisoning in Iraqi children; clinical observations over two years. *Br. Med. J.*, **1**, 613.
16. Lauwerys R.R., Buchet J.P. (1973). Occupational exposure to mercury vapors and biological action. *Arch. Environ. Health*, **27**, 65.
17. Marks V., Taylor A. (1979). Urinary mercury excretion in dental workers. *Br. Dent. J.*, **146**, 269.
18. Piscator M., Pettersson B. (1977). In *Clinical Chemistry and Chemical Toxicity of Metals* (Brown S.S. ed.) Amsterdam: Elsevier/North Holland.
19. Webb M. (1975). Cadmium. *Br. Med. Bull.*, **31**, 246.
20. Minoia C. et al. (1990). Trace element reference values in tissues from inhabitants of the European Community I. A study of 46 elements in urine, blood and serum of Italian subjects. *Sci. Total Environ.*, **95**, 89.
21. Garstang, F.M., Day J.P., Ackrill P., Williams P. (1983). In *Chemical Toxicology and Clinical Chemistry of Metals* (Brown, S.S., Savory, J. eds.) London: Academic Press.

44. Laboratory Investigation of the Poisoned Patient

M. J. Stewart

Introduction
  Drug interactions
The role of the laboratory
  Sample collection
  Laboratory assistance
Methods of screening for drugs and poisons
  Immunoassays
  Radioimmunoassays
  Thin-layer or paper/fibre chromatography
  Extraction
  Gas–liquid chromatography (GLC)
  Gas chromatography–mass spectrometry
    (GC–MS)
  High-performance liquid chromatography
  Specific methods
  Problems with screening
Treatment
  General
  Gastric lavage and emesis
  Forced diuresis
  Haemodialysis
Interpretation of clinical chemistry tests in
    cases of poisoning
  Blood-gas analyses
  Osmolality
  Electrolytes
  Enzymes
  Myoglobin
  Interferences
Common drugs and poisons
  Aminoglycosides
  Anticonvulsant drugs
  Benzodiazepines
  Carbon monoxide
  Cardioactive drugs
  Alcohols
  Hypnotic drugs
  Inorganic anions
  Metal poisoning
  Narcotic drugs
  Organochlorides
  Organophosphorus compounds
  Paracetamol (acetaminophen)
  Paraquat
  Salicylates
  Theophylline
  Tricyclic antidepressants
Conclusions

INTRODUCTION

Poisoned patients account for approximately 10% of all acute admissions to medical wards in British hospitals and a similar pattern is seen in other developed countries. Not all of these patients are there as a result of self-poisoning attempts. Some are poisoned by accident and a minority of cases, including a significant number of children, are due to administration of drugs or poisons by others.

Many poisoning victims die before reaching hospital and many analyses are made in forensic departments. Of those who are admitted to hospital, approximately 95% are discharged well, the exceptions being those who are moribund on arrival following severe respiratory depression, or who have ingested drugs or poisons that have an irreversible action, such as paraquat.

The pattern of poisoning reflects, but lags behind, prescribing patterns; nowhere is it more of a truism that 'common drugs are taken commonly'. Despite this fact there are always single cases of poisoning with uncommon agents that may be difficult to diagnose and manage and are, unfortunately, often under-documented.

The incidence of acute self-poisoning in the UK is either static or falling. Excess of most drugs elicits side-effects that are related to the concentration of drug in the plasma. (Idiosyncratic side-effects such as agranulocytosis or haemolysis are seldom dose-related and present as acute problems of toxicity.) There is however, increasing recognition of the problem of chronic toxicity. This falls into two categories:

(i) unwitting exposure to toxins in the environment including the workplace;
(ii) chronic overdosage with prescribed drugs.

The first category will only be covered here in relation to pesticides and some heavy metals (*see* Chapter 43); the second category is familiar to the toxicologist involved in drug analysis, who will commonly find cases of overdose as a result of inappropriate use of therapeutic drugs. Common examples of chronic iatrogenic toxicity are the build-up of toxic levels of phenobarbitone and phenytoin in patients on long-term treatment and the development of high concentrations of tricyclic antidepressants or digoxin in the elderly as a result of reduced clearance. Chronic lithium toxicity also occurs, and for this reason patients on this drug for long periods should be monitored regularly, especially if there are changes in clinical state. Inappropriate dosage during intravenous therapy with agents such as theophylline, diazepam, chlormethiazole, methotrexate and aminoglycosides can also give rise to iatrogenic overdose, and in these cases quantitative, timed analyses may be required to elicit the full facts.

TABLE 44.1

BIOCHEMICAL TESTS FOR USE IN SPECIFIC CASES FOR DIAGNOSIS/PROGNOSIS

Test	Drugs/poisons
Acetone	Isopropanol
Alanine aminotransferase	Paracetamol, mushroom poisoning
Calcium	Calcium-complexing agents, theophylline
Carboxyhaemoglobin	Carbon monoxide
Cholinesterase	Organophosphorus compounds
Creatine kinase	Muscle toxins, cocaine
Glucose	Oral hypoglycaemic agents, insulin
Iron	Iron
Methaemoglobin	Oxidizing agents
Potassium	Potassium supplements, digoxin, theophylline
Sodium	Lithium

Drug Interactions

Most of the common drug interactions are known, and data should be available through hospital pharmacies. There may be occasions where an interaction is suspected in the absence of any evidence of dosing with a particular drug; in these cases a simple screen may be of use.

Knowledge of the effects of common drugs when taken in overdose is not always available on the spot and advice may have to be sought outside the receiving hospital. In the UK, rapid advice is available through the Regional Poisoning Treatment Centres in London, Cardiff, Birmingham and Edinburgh, from where advice on interpretation of laboratory results, prognosis and treatment is available 24 h a day. The 'viewdata' system, available on a telephone-linked visual display unit, is supported and maintained by the Poisons Centres and is a valuable source of up-to-date information on diagnosis and treatment in the UK and parts of Europe.

THE ROLE OF THE LABORATORY

The clinical biochemistry laboratory is involved in all serious cases of poisoning by virtue of the derangements that occur in respiratory, cardiac, renal and hepatic function and in other major homeostatic mechanisms; it is now accepted that a limited range of drug estimations should be available in all such laboratories and that a wider range of assays, for both screening and for quantitative determination, should be available in a few selected centres.

In addition, there are a few specific biochemical investigations that may contribute to diagnosis and prognosis and that require to be available on demand (Table 44.1).

The average hospital laboratory is not equipped to provide a comprehensive screening service in order to confirm or eliminate the presence of all drugs in common use, or to provide quantitative assays for the large number of drugs and poisons. However, one study has shown that in only 7% of cases did the results of a comprehensive screening procedure alter the treatment contemplated. In addition, screening procedures in laboratories where experience is limited have led to errors both of omission and commission in the 'identification' of drugs.

In an increasing number of cases the plasma or serum concentration of a drug is found to be most useful clinically; this trend will continue as methods improve in sensitivity and as information about the pharmacokinetics of more drugs at therapeutic concentrations becomes available.

While quantitative determination of drugs is increasingly possible, close liaison between the physician and the analyst is necessary if results are to be correctly interpreted.

Sample Collection

There is no ideal body fluid that can be used to answer all clinical questions related to drug ingestion and the choice of specimen is limited by clinical considerations; however, some general rules apply, as follows.

- In cases of suspected overdose, the most valuable specimen is the one taken on admission and will, in an unconscious patient, most conveniently be a *10-ml heparinized blood sample*. Follow-up specimens are valuable in some cases, but the on-admission specimen gives a baseline against which to consider both the clinical progress of the patient and the results of subsequent assays.

- Wherever possible, both a *urine* and a blood sample should be obtained. Urine can often be obtained voluntarily or by gentle compression of the bladder; catheterization should not be done unless there are clinical reasons for so doing. For quantitative analyses, *plasma* or *serum* are the fluids of choice.

- The only advantage of *gastric aspirate* is that the unchanged drug or poison may be found in the aspirate, often in much higher concentrations than in blood or urine; this may be of use for drugs that have a high volume of distribution, for example some neuroleptics. Aspirate should be obtained before and not *after* stomach wash-out or use of emetics.

Laboratory Assistance

Within limits the laboratory should be able to aid the clinician in:

- confirmation of diagnosis;
- prognosis;
- monitoring of treatment.

Confirmation of Diagnosis

The physician presented with an unconscious or semi-conscious patient has a diagnostic problem that is best solved by a thorough history and clinical examination. Only after this should requests for drug analyses be made. More important in the first instance are *glucose analyses*, because both hypo- and hyperglycaemia can and have been confused with drug overdosage. The presence of ethanol, often in addition to other drugs, should be looked for and an attempt made to obtain details of the amount ingested. The plasma osmolality can often be of use in such circumstances. With a good examination a guide will be obtained to the drugs or poisons ingested in the majority of cases, the exception being children and drug addicts (who are poor historians and may well have purchased adulterated or mixed drugs).

In such cases the priority assays, as in any acute emergency, will be blood-gas analyses, glucose, urea and electrolytes. In fitting patients, calcium analyses are mandatory.

Screening. Because treatment of overdose for the vast majority of drugs is conservative, the necessity for screening, particularly out of normal working hours, is reduced to the resolution of two problems:
(i) the differentiation of a drug overdose from some other clinical condition giving the same signs;
(ii) the positive identification of drugs or poisons for which there is a specific treatment available (Table 44.2). (This may be in the form of a quantitative analysis where such is necessary as an emergency.)

If it is proposed to use a non-specific treatment such as the instillation of charcoal slurry in order to prevent further absorption of the 'drug', then the identification of the drug in question is not necessary because the treatment carries little risk of harm to the patient. If, on the other hand, haemodialysis or charcoal haemoperfusion are contemplated, the identification of the drug should be attempted (if not known from the history) because not all drugs are dialysable and there is a certain risk attached to the procedure. Dialysis may, of course, be instituted in

patients with renal failure and in these cases there is a less urgent requirement for drug identification.

Prognosis

In most cases of drug overdose, prognosis is more related to the general state of the patient on admission and the quality of care than on the levels of drug detected in the plasma; however, there are a few drugs and poisons for which a knowledge of the plasma concentration on admission can indicate a prognosis or a need for specialized treatment (see below).

Monitoring

Plasma concentrations of other drugs obtained in cases of overdose must be interpreted with caution; the following questions should be answered:

1. *What is the accepted concentration range for this drug in patients taking a standard dose?* There is a large group of drugs for which this information is not known and only an upper limit, which may be 'undetectable' by the method in use, is quoted. A list of drugs commonly encountered in cases of self-poisoning, along with plasma concentrations above which toxic effects would be expected, is given in Table 44.3.

2. *Is the patient in the habit of taking the drug in question or is this a single exposure?* The importance of this question is often overlooked, as a naïve patient may show a different response to a given concentration of a drug than a patient who is accustomed to that drug (Fig. 44.1).

(When answering both of these questions it is pertinent to be aware that the examples given relate to concentrations in plasma and not those in urine or gastric washings.)

3. *How is the patient handling the drug?* The rate of fall of a drug concentration should approximate to the known biological half-life, some examples of which are given in Table 44.3. Much useful informa-

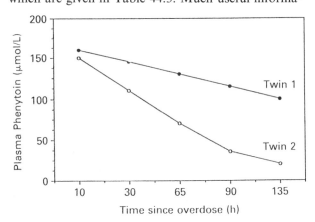

Figure 44.1 Elimination of phenytoin in identical twins who took similar overdoses of phenytoin, showing the faster half-life in twin 2, who was on regular phenytoin therapy.

TABLE 44.2
AGENTS USED FOR THE SPECIFIC TREATMENT OF INDIVIDUAL POISONS

Agent	Type of poisoning	Mode of action	Notes
N-acetylcysteine	Paracetamol	Restores glutathione Protects against hepatocellular damage	Not of use > 16 h after ingestion (given i.v.)
Ammonium chloride	Basic drugs, which are excreted unchanged	Acidifies the urine	Use with great care and continued blood-gas monitoring
Atropine	Organophosphorus poisoning	Competitive inhibitor	Titrated against clinical condition Large doses may be required
Calcium gluconate	Fluorides Hypokalaemia, hypermagnesaemia Oxalate	Binds fluoride Restores plasma Ca^{2+}	Large quantities may be required
Dicobalt edetate	Cyanide and substances metabolized to cyanide	Chelates CN^-	Dangerous if cyanide not present
Dimercaprol	Heavy metals and arsenic	Chelating agent	
Ethanol	Methanol and ethylene glycol	Inhibits metabolism to formic acid or oxalate	Maintain plasma EtOH at 20–40 mmol/L
Folinic acid	Methotrexate	Provides folate analogue	(Leucovorin)
Glucagon	β-blockers	Bypasses blockade	
Methionine	Paracetamol	Restores glutathione and protects against hepatocellular damage	Given orally Contraindicated if vomiting
Methylene blue	Nitrates, dapsone, phenols, promaquine	Reconverts methaemoglobin to haemoglobin	Patients may show blueing of skin
Naloxone	Opiates	Competitive inhibitor	Rapid action but may require repeated doses
Penicillamine	Copper, gold, lead, mercury and zinc	Chelating agent	
Propranolol	Ephedrines, theophylline (β-stimulants)	Blocks β-receptors	
Sodium bicarbonate	Salicylate Phenobarbitone Primidone	Alkalinization of urine, solubilization of ionized acids	Check urinary pH with labstix, avoid fluid overload, check electrolytes regularly and replace K^+
Sodium nitrite	Cyanides Hydrogen sulphide	Produces cyanomethaemoglobin or sulphmethaemoglobin	Use with sodium thiosulphate
Sodium thiosulphate	Cyanides	Restores conversion of CN^- to thiocyanate	Use with sodium nitrite
Vitamin C	Cresols, dapsone, primaquine, nitrates	Reducing agent—promotes conversion of methaemoglobin to haemoglobin	Large doses are non-toxic
Vitamin K	Common anticoagulants e.g. warfarin	Restores synthesis of vitamin K necessary for clotting	

tion may be obtained if more than one analysis is made, with a known time interval between the analyses. The three patterns of plasma concentration vs. time curves that may be found in the early stages following overdose are shown in Fig. 44.2.

Once equilibration between plasma and tissues has occurred, the normal sequence of events is a fall in plasma drug concentration accompanied by an improvement in the clinical condition of the patient. In cases where the clinical condition does not improve at a rate which would be expected, further analyses should be made. A fall in plasma level indicates that the detoxification mechanisms of metabolism and elimination are acting to reduce the effects of the drug; however, the possible presence of unmeasured active metabolites should not be forgotten. The principal active metabolites are given in Table 44.4.

A static or slow-falling drug concentration in

TABLE 44.3
TOXIC CONCENTRATIONS AND APPROXIMATE HALF-LIVES OF COMMONER DRUGS AND POISONS

| Drug/poison | Toxic concentrations | | $t_{\frac{1}{2}}$ |
	Mass	Molar	
Amitriptyline	1 mg/L	3.6 μmol/L	20–25 h
Amphetamine	200 μg/L	1.5 μmol/L	
Barbiturates (hypnotic)	10 mg/L	44 μmol/L	5–40 h
Carbamazepine	12 mg/L	50 μmol/L	10–20 h
Chloramphenicol	75 mg/L	232 μmol/L	2–6 h
Chlordiazepoxide	200 μg/L	600 nmol/L	7–15 h
Chlormethiazole	25 mg/L	155 μmol/L	3–7 h
Codeine	500 μg/L	1.6 nmol/L	2–4 h
Diazepam	1 mg/L	3.5 μmol/L	30–55 h
Digoxin	2.5 μg/L	3.2 nmol/L	25–50 h
Dihydrocodeine	5 mg/L	12.5 μmol/L	~4 h
Ethanol	800 mg/L	17 mmol/L	~0.25 h Dose dependent
Gentamicin	12 mg/L	—	2–4 h, less if chronic
Glutethimide	10 mg/L	46 μmol/L	5–40 h
Imipramine	1 mg/L	3.5 μmol/L	10–25 h
Lithium	—	1.7 mmol/L	16–30 h
Methadone	2.0 mg/L	6.5 μmol/L	24–45 h
Methaqualone	10 mg/L	4.5 μmol/L	20–60 h
Methotrexate	4.5 mg/L	1 μmol/L	5–10 h, depends on time of exposure
Morphine	200 μg/L	700 nmol/L	2–4 h
Nitrazepam	200 μg/L	660 nmol/L	23–30 h
Nortriptyline	1 mg/L	3.8 μmol/L	20–40 h
Paracetamol	225 mg/L	1.5 mmol/L (at 4 h)	> 4 h
Paraquat	100 μg/L (at 24 h)	530 nmol/L (at 24 h)	
Pethidine	800 μg/L	3.2 μmol/L	3–10 h
Phenobarbitone	30 mg/L	130 μmol/L	50–150 h
Phenytoin	20 mg/L	80 μmol/L	6–24 h
Primidone	10 mg/L	46 μmol/L	4–12 h
Propoxyphene	500 μg/L	1.5 μmol/L	8–24 h
Quinine	10 mg/L	25 μmol/L	4–15 h
Quinidine	6 mg/L	17 μmol/L	4–12 h
Salicylate	345 μg/L	2.5 mmol/L	Dose dependent
Theophylline	30 mg/L	166 μmol/L	3–12 h
Valproate	200 mg/L	1400 μmol/L	11–17 h

These values are ones above which toxicity will occur in the vast majority of subjects; some may show toxicity below these values.

plasma is not uncommon in the early stages after overdose and may be due to one or more of the following causes:

- reduced renal perfusion, preventing the excretion of water-soluble drugs or metabolites;
- reduced hepatic perfusion, preventing access of drug to metabolizing enzymes;
- peripheral hypoxia, reducing the activity of metabolic enzymes;
- saturation of eliminating mechanisms by high concentrations of drug;
- inhibition of metabolizing enzymes by drug interference (Fig. 44.3).

A rising plasma drug concentration is less common, but may be observed in the following cases:

- In the early stages of alkaline diuresis where plasma pH is high, plasma levels of salicylate or phenobarbitone may rise due to a shift of drug from the tissues or gut into the plasma in advance of its elimination via the kidney.
- Some drugs, notably glutethimide, undergo enterohepatic circulation giving rise to fluctuating plasma levels.
- Following periods of haemodialysis or similar active methods of elimination, the plasma drug levels, which may have been reduced to low values, may rise due to re-equilibration with drug in the tissues (rebound) (Fig. 44.4).
- Following inadequate gastric lavage, reabsorption of drugs may take place at a faster rate once blood pressure is restored in hypotensive patients.

TABLE 44.4

COMMON DRUGS OR POISONS THAT HAVE ACTIVE METABOLITES

Drug	Active metabolite	Notes
Amitriptyline	Nortriptyline	Similar action to parent Concentrations may be summed
Carbamazepine	Carbamazepine-5,10-epoxide	Similar activity to parent
Chlorpromazine	Several	
Diazepam	Desmethyldiazepam	Most benzodiazepines have active metabolites
Ethanol	Acetaldehyde	Increased if patient receiving disulfiram
Ethylene glycol	Oxalate	Complexes calcium
Glutethimide	Several	Undergoes enterohepatic reabsorption/excretion
Imipramine	Desmethyl imipramine	Similar action to parent Concentrations may be summed
Methanol	Formate	Causes severe acidosis
Morphine	Morphine-6-glucuronide	Higher activity than morphine
Paracetamol	N-acetyl quinoneimine	Binds to thiol groups Usually inactivated by GSH
Primidone	Phenobarbitone	Prolonged coma can ensue
Procainamide	N-acetyl procaineamide	Similar reaction to parent Concentrations may be summed
Quinine/quinidine	Several	
Theophylline	3-methylxanthine	50% potency of parent
	Caffeine	Only in neonates

GSH, reduced glutathione.

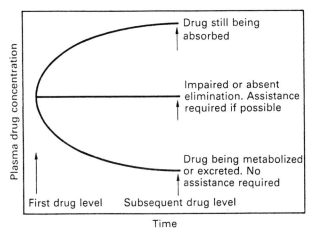

Figure 44.2 Stylized interpretation of concentration/time curves post-overdose.

Some of the most mystifying cases in which drug levels have remained high or fluctuated for many days have been traced to continued intake by the patient, replenished by friends or relatives, or from unwitting absorption of drugs hidden in the small intestine, rectum or vagina. This latter is proving much more common with the practice of smuggling drugs in the intestine (body packing). Such causes should be considered when logic fails.

Finally, a seriously poisoned patient may be treated with large volumes of intravenous fluids; it should be remembered that these may give rise to alterations in plasma drug concentrations unless care is taken in the selection of sampling sites, and time is allowed for equilibration.

METHODS OF SCREENING FOR DRUGS AND POISONS

Although provision of a comprehensive toxicology service is still a specialist activity requiring considerable experience, advances in technology now allow the general clinical chemist to provide a useful first-line screen for the most commonly encountered organic substances.

Immunoassays

These are available for those drugs that are most commonly considered for therapeutic purposes, or for those that are regularly abused. These assays can provide a rapid, qualitative answer and in some cases a full, quantitative result. They are of particular use in poisonings with theophylline, anticonvulsants, digoxin and quinidine. The analyst should know the cross-reactivity of the antiserum involved, and be aware that in overdose there may be other factors present, i.e. large amounts of metabolite or several other drugs, which may interfere with the test procedure. Immunoassays are very useful for confirmation where the drug ingested is clearly suggested, but too expensive for wide-range screening.

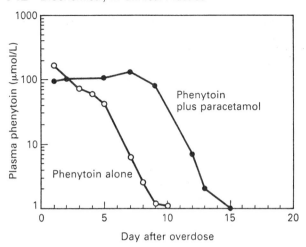

Figure 44.3 The effect of concurrent paracetamol ingestion on phenytoin metabolism. Both overdoses in the same patient, on one occasion with and on one without paracetamol. The effect of hepatocellular damage on phenytoin elimination is dramatic.

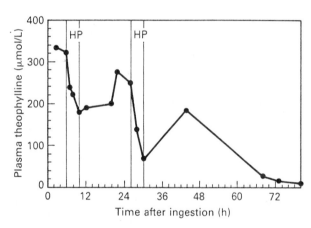

Figure 44.4 'Rebound' of plasma theophylline following periods of charcoal haemoperfusion (HP). Theophylline removed from the plasma is replenished from the tissues and/or the gastrointestinal tract (the patient was not washed out).

Radioimmunoassays

These are available for a number of less commonly encountered drugs, including paraquat and buprenorphine (Temgesic), that are difficult to estimate by other methods.

Thin-layer or Paper/Fibre Chromatography

This provides the most wide-ranging screening process and can be very economical. The system used needs to be standardized with respect to extractions, chromatography and colour development. Commercial systems such as TOXILAB™ provide such a systematic approach. The two golden rules for visual chromatography are (i) to document carefully and

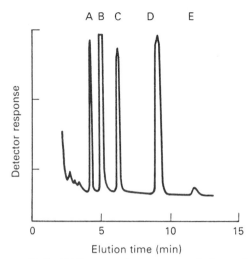

Figure 44.5 GLC trace of an extract of plasma from a patient with an overdose of amitriptyline given diazepam after admission—indicates the need for a sample *before* therapy is started. A, amitriptyline; B, nortriptyline (metabolite); C, internal standard; D, diazepam; E, diazepam metabolite.

(ii) to report only when sure of identification. Mixed overdoses and the presence of metabolites can provide confusing pictures, but despite this the procedure is highly useful and also satisfying for the analyst.

Extraction

For all chromatographic methods, the key to good results is in the extraction procedure. With the exception of the optimized commercial systems that employ ion-pairing agents, the most reproducible methods, which are applicable to most drugs, employ solid-phase extraction on reverse-phase silica columns.

Gas–Liquid Chromatography (GLC)

Capillary gas chromatography, with its high resolving power, has now been sufficiently well investigated as to provide a good, rapid, routine method for detection of the majority of drugs in plasma and urine. At least two columns are required in order to resolve most problems. A typical capillary GLC trace is given in Fig. 44.5.

Gas Chromatography–Mass Spectrometry (GC–MS)

The linking of mass spectrometry to GLC now provides, in theory, the ultimate in toxicological analysis and it is true that almost all of the substances of interest may be identified using this technique, the omissions being those substances that are non-volatile, thermolabile or inorganic. The problem with the use of GC–MS in a clinical toxicological role is that the amount of information provided may lead to much 'chasing of hares'—drugs present in trace amounts of which some have been given for therapy after admission. GC–MS should therefore be used selectively as a second-line approach where a large amount of an unidentified substance is present and the clinical picture is still unclear. Commercial libraries of drug spectra are still deficient in the data required to identify many metabolites and care must be taken to avoid wasted effort in chasing the 'last peak'.

High-performance Liquid Chromatography

This technique, which offers considerable advantages over GLC by virtue of the achievable flexibility and selectivity, and over immunoassays by virtue of its low costs, has not found a large niche in toxicology because of its limited potential as a screening tool. When specific drugs are sought, the ability to perform some analyses by direct injection of a deproteinized blood sample without extraction has been used to effect for analytes such as theophylline, paracetamol, salicylate, anticonvulsants, opiates and amphetamines. It does, at present, remain a tool for specialist rather than general interest in clinical toxicology.

Specific Methods

There are many drugs and poisons for which specific methods are required. Examples are carbon monoxide (as COHb) by oximetry; salicylate and paracetamol by specific colorimetric methods; lithium, by flame photometry (not for urine, where atomic absorption spectrometry is required); paraquat by derivative spectrophotometry; cyanide, heavy metals by atomic absorption spectrometry and a number of less common poisons. Several methods exist for alcohols, including enzymatic and electrochemical methods for both breath and head-space analysis on blood. While these are excellent for ethanol analyses, a GLC method should be used where other alcohols are suspected. The general clinical chemistry laboratory should be able to provide some of these as part of the routine repertoire. In particular, lithium, iron, salicylate and paracetamol should be available on demand in all general laboratories.

Problems with Screening

The inexperienced clinician may overestimate the ability of the laboratory to provide help in diagnosis in cases of poisoning, and a full discussion should precede analyses of all but the most straightforward of cases. Apart from the history and clinical signs, details should be obtained of therapy given on site, in the ambulance, in the casualty department and in the ward. It is not uncommon to find that a search for drugs, successfully completed, has detected only the drugs given to the patient on admission. Specimens taken *before* the instigation of therapy are far more valuable than those obtained later in which the presence of therapeutic drugs, especially those such as chlorpromazine or some antibiotics, can interfere with some screening methods.

Examples of some drugs that are used to treat poisoned patients are given in Table 44.5.

TREATMENT

General

Regardless of the availability of laboratory support, immediate clinical measures will be instituted in all cases of serious poisoning. Conservative therapy consists of the maintenance of a clear airway and adequate blood pressure.

Correction of cardiac arrhythmias may be necessary where drugs such as digoxin, trichloral or tricyclic antidepressants have been taken, and assisted ventilation in cases with respiratory depression. The use of the endotracheal tube is mandatory if gastric wash-out or emesis is to be carried out and has contributed greatly to the fall in the number of deaths in hospital caused by inhalation of vomit by patients who may have been only mildly poisoned or merely drunk.

Fluid therapy is commonly used in severe cases in order to maintain an adequate hepatic and renal blood flow, without which the elimination of drugs by physiological means cannot proceed.

As with any patient receiving intensive therapy, the regular monitoring of blood gases, urea, and electrolytes (especially potassium) is required.

With few exceptions, drugs are eliminated from the body by a combination of hepatic metabolism to more water-soluble metabolites, followed by renal or biliary excretion of the metabolites. Some drugs, notably salicylate and paraquat, are excreted by the kidneys with little delay due to metabolism. In addition, alcohol and some volatile solvents may be excreted in part via the lungs. However, the majority of drugs require to be metabolized by the liver to some extent before excretion either in the urine or bile, and it is for this reason that maintenance of adequate hepatic blood flow is necessary.

Patients who have been admitted late to hospital may already have a degree of renal impairment following a period of hypotension. Some poisons such as paraquat and heavy metals can lead to the rapid development of acute renal failure, and a similar condition occurs when the nephron is exposed to large amounts of haemoglobin or myoglobin.

Gastric Lavage and Emesis

In children, the use of emetics has always been the method of choice but, although there is a risk of damage from inhalation of gastric contents, with proper precautions this procedure is now again gaining favour over gastric wash-out in adults. Where an emetic is required, ipecacuanha is preferred. Use of

TABLE 44.5
SOME DRUGS USED TO TREAT POISONED PATIENTS

Drug	Reason for use	Notes
Adrenaline and noradrenaline	Reversal of asystole	Affects glucose and cortisol
Anexate	Antagonizes benzodiazepines	
Chlormethiazole	Anticonvulsant	Dangerous in alcohol excess
Chlorpromazine	Tranquillizer	High doses given metabolites Observe TLC
Cimetidine (ranitidine)	Prevention of ulcers in patients with endotracheal intubation	Red spot on TLC with acid development
Diazepam	Anticonvulsant	May be given in large doses
Dopamine	Reversal of hypotension	
Frusemide	Diuresis	
Glucagon	Hypoglycaemia	
Ipecacuanha	Emetic	Loss of H^+ and K^+ from stomach
Lignocaine	Antiarrhythmic	
Naloxone	Opiate antagonist	Large doses may be given
Paraldehyde	Anticonvulsant	Samples may smell of paraldehyde

TLC, thin-layer chromatography.

salt water for this purpose may give rise to severe hypernatraemia; cases of permanent brain damage as a result of this procedure have been documented. Electrolyte analyses before and after gastric lavage or use of emetics are a useful safeguard.

Gastric lavage is still regarded as a necessary procedure in cases of salicylate poisoning but is still used less commonly in other cases of severe poisoning and only where there is reasonable suspicion that the stomach contains significant quantities of the drug. Provided that a cuffed endotracheal tube is employed, the procedure is safe in skilled hands, the only common fault being insufficient volume of lavage fluid. Approximately 20 L of water are required for a thorough lavage.

In some cases, such as iron, paraquat and cyanide poisoning (*see* below), specific substances are added to the lavage fluid in order to prevent further absorption.

A considerable body of opinion now supports the use of activated charcoal in lavage fluid, not only to prevent further absorption of drugs, but also to increase the clearance of drugs that are secreted into the gastrointestinal tract via the enterohepatic or enteroenteric circulation. Whole-gut irrigation with activated charcoal is now used routinely in some centres.

Forced Diuresis

This technique is designed to increase the flow of urine and thus enhance the elimination of those drugs that are excreted unchanged by renal excretion. Large volumes of intravenous fluids are given, accompanied by diuretics, usually frusemide. Unfortunately, most drugs require hepatic metabolism as the first and often rate-limiting step, and the procedure in practice is limited to a small group of drugs. In one or two

cases, elimination may be aided by alteration of the urinary pH so as to increase the solubility of the ionized drug and reduce tubular reabsorption.

Sodium bicarbonate generates an *alkaline* urine in which phenobarbitone and salicylate are excreted at an increased rate; potassium supplements are required in order to avoid hypokalaemia and both blood gases and electrolytes should be checked during this procedure, as hypernatraemia can result from excessive use of this sodium salt.

The checking of urinary pH during alkalinization diuresis is a simple but often neglected procedure that can assist the clinician in the balance of fluid therapy. An example of the fluctuations in the excretion of phenobarbitone with urinary pH is given in Fig. 44.6.

Acid diuresis, using ammonium chloride solution, has been advocated as useful in the treatment of poisoning with basic drugs such as quinine and quinidine, amphetamine and fenfluramine. While there is no doubt that the removal of these drugs is enhanced by this procedure, there are considerable risks of the development of a severe metabolic acidosis. Regular blood-gas analyses and urinary pH checks are mandatory during this procedure. As there is now widespread experience with haemodialysis, this procedure should replace diuresis with acidification or alkalinization for all but mild cases.

Haemodialysis

Despite considerable efforts to improve the efficiency of the procedure, haemodialysis is effective in removing only a rather small number of water-soluble drugs from the body, and there is still some morbidity associated with the technique, especially when applied in an emergency.

For this reason it should not be used routinely for

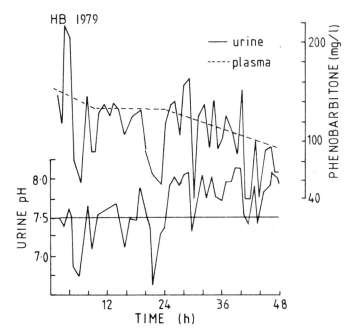

Figure 44.6 The pattern of phenobarbitone excretion in urine during alkaline diuresis with alternate 500-ml bags of 5% dextrose, 0.9% saline and 1.2% HCO₃. Only when urine pH is greater than 7.5 does phenobarbitone excretion increase significantly.

the treatment of drug overdose. Drugs that may be removed by haemodialysis are lithium, alcohols, salicylate, phenobarbitone and barbitone. Although many of these may be eliminated naturally or with the help of diuresis, on occasions the priority is to reduce the drug level rapidly and in these cases haemodialysis should be considered. It is also necessary in cases where the normal excretory mechanisms are impaired or diuresis is contraindicated, such as in patients who have developed pulmonary oedema or acute renal failure following shock or rhabdomyolysis.

The cautious approach to haemodialysis applies also in the main to charcoal haemoperfusion, although this technique is technically simpler. Studies on a wide variety of drugs show that relatively small amounts are removed by this technique, largely because most of the drug is inside the cells and plasma levels available for exchange or adsorption are low.

An example of the different effects of haemoperfusion on the plasma concentrations of phenytoin and phenobarbitone in a severe case of poisoning with these two drugs is shown in Fig. 44.7.

INTERPRETATION OF CLINICAL CHEMISTRY TESTS IN CASES OF POISONING

Blood-gas Analyses

It is sometimes difficult to place a correct interpretation on the initial results of blood-gas analyses. A variety of combinations, from pure respiratory acidosis due to acute respiratory depression to acute metabolic acidosis from methanol or ethylene glycol poisoning, is encountered. The most common finding is a mixed respiratory and metabolic abnormality, the most severe of which may be the mixed respiratory alkalosis and metabolic acidosis of salicylate poisoning. It is necessary for the clinical chemist to become expert at interpreting blood gas results and to be aware of the expected changes in the more common types of overdose. It is also useful to discuss such results with the clinician because in the acute state little notice may be given to correction of blood-gas results for temperature in patients who arrive hypothermic after a period of unconsciousness in an unheated building or outside. Correction for the hyperpyrexia observed in patients recovering from barbiturate overdose is also required. Tables or nomograms for temperature correction of blood-gas results should be available in the emergency laboratory.

Osmolality

With the advent of improved osmometers, increasing use is now being made of osmolality measurements and the question is sometimes posed as to their usefulness in drug overdose. In general, increases in osmolality due to the presence of the drugs themselves are relatively rare. The exceptions being salicylate, where a change of 5–10 mosmol/kg may be observed, or alcohols where the rise may be significantly more than 20 mosmol/kg. The concentrations of most other drugs, even in severe cases, are insufficient to have a marked effect on osmolality, although the secondary effect due to production of metabolic acids may be dramatic.

Electrolytes

Measurement of sodium concentration may provide a useful aid in the differential diagnosis of the unconscious patient, both hypo- and hypernatraemia being found on occasions. Potassium levels are almost universally raised (except in salicylate poisoning) due to underlying acidosis or interference with the Na/K pump; however, in theophylline poisoning hypokalaemia may be severe. The need for electrolyte determinations *on admission* cannot be too highly stressed, as without these the alterations observed during and after therapeutic procedures cannot be fully interpreted.

Calcium analyses, while seldom diagnostic, are mandatory in fitting patients. The author has seen several cases of patients given large amounts of diazepam for fits subsequently found to be related to hypocalcaemia. Calcium concentrations are also mandatory in the monitoring of theophylline, fluoride, and ethylene glycol poisoning (*see* bel

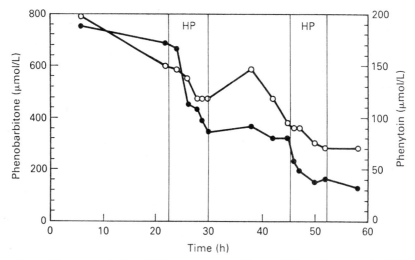

Figure 44.7 The effect of haemoperfusion (HP) on phenobarbitone (○) and phenytoin (●) in a mixed overdose. Considerable reduction in phenobarbitone concentrations contrasts with the minimal effect on the less polar phenytoin.

Enzymes

The severely poisoned patient may show a variety of non-specific enzyme abnormalities due to the metabolic changes present and also to the effect of prolonged hypothermia or immobilization before admission. Levels of aspartate aminotransferase and creatine kinase may be extremely high in patients who have lain unconscious on underperfused muscles. It is seldom therefore possible to make use of enzyme analyses in the first 24 h. The exceptions to this general statement are the use of baseline estimation of alanine aminotransferase in paracetamol overdose and of pseudocholinesterase estimations in cases of organophosphorus poisoning. The measurement of γ-glutamyl transferase may give an indication that there has been induction of the microsomal P450 system by alcohol or drugs, and may give a guide as to the likely response to the drug taken in overdose. In particular, patients who are chronic alcoholics are far more susceptible to paracetamol poisoning than abstainers.

Myoglobin

Visual examination of the urine detects myoglobinuria in the early stages; however, once renal failure ensues it may be necessary to screen the plasma for myoglobin and haemoglobin in cases where intravascular haemolysis or rhabdomyolysis have occurred.

Rhabdomyolysis, the release of myoglobin from myocytes, is much more common in cases of poisoning than is usually assumed. A mild degree is associated with hypoxic or hypothermic muscle tissue such as exists in the late-admitted, comatose patient. More severe rhabdomyolysis, which can lead to acute renal failure, is associated with major cases of poisoning with a wide variety of drugs, but is especially common in theophylline poisoning. Myoglobin may be screened for in plasma or urine but rhabdomyolysis is seldom considered before the development of renal insufficiency as evidenced by a falling creatinine clearance.

Interferences

Despite volumes written on the interaction of drugs with biochemical tests, few drugs that are commonly taken in overdose interact with the common biochemical test procedures. Interference may be by physiological means or by a direct chemical reaction of the drug (or more commonly its metabolites) with the test procedure. Literature references to interactions should be treated with some care, as a drug that interferes with one method may interact differently with another. A good example of this is oxazepam, which gives false-positive interaction with some older methods for blood glucose, although not with glucose oxidase-based assays; *N*-acetyl cysteine can give rise to false-positive hyperglycaemia and ketones if the specimen is taken from a site close to an intravenous infusion.

For this reason, reports of changes in the common variables of clinical chemistry in cases of drug overdose should be interpreted with care and the detailed method used for that analysis should be investigated.

In general, simple screening methods and side-room tests are more liable to interference from drugs than more sophisticated methods (e.g. Clinitest® tablets) will show false-positive results following ingestion of trichloral compounds or salicylate because these drugs produce metabolites that are reducing agents.

Major interferences are caused by the pharmacological effects or side-effects of the drugs on the metabolites. Thus, narcotic drugs may give rise to increased plasma amylase levels due to spasm of the sphincter of Oddi and overdose with hypoglycaemic drugs may give an expected fall of blood glucose to undetectable levels. Also predictable are the chelation of calcium by oxalate following ingestion of ethylene glycol (see below), the similar dramatic fall in calcium levels following poisoning with fluorides, and the hypokalaemia and hypercalcaemia of theophylline overdose.

Drugs can also interact with the analytical methods for other drugs. Specific methods are required wherever possible, although even the most specific can be prone to interference on occasion by high levels of metabolites of concurrently ingested drugs.

COMMON DRUGS AND POISONS

Aminoglycosides

Aminoglycoside poisoning is usually associated with over prescription, especially during intravenous therapy. There is no specific therapy, but serial plasma concentrations should be measured in order to determine re-start of therapy if required.

Anticonvulsant Drugs

This group of drugs is widely available and commonly gives rise to both chronic iatrogenic toxicity and acute overdose. Where the overdose is by a patient who is accustomed to the drug taken the effects are less severe than when they are taken by a relative who is not receiving therapy, as both phenytoin and phenobarbitone induce their own metabolism.

The salient points concerning anticonvulsant overdose are as follows:

Carbamazepine
Symptoms are more variable and may be more severe than with other anticonvulsants, and may include arrhythmias, similar to tricyclic poisoning, hyperreflexia and bizarre behaviour. Convulsions and coma occur in more severe cases. Treatment of the clinical symptoms is conservative, with caution in the use of antiarrhythmic drugs. In severe cases, where active elimination is indicated, activated charcoal or charcoal haemoperfusion has been shown to be of some use. The criteria for use are as for other drugs.

Phenytoin
Symptoms include nausea and vomiting, nystagmus and ataxia (patients may be suspected of being drunk!) and, rarely, increasing coma. Concentrations are in excess of 100 μmol/L. Treatment is purely supportive and active measures are relatively ineffective and should only be attempted (haemoperfusion) where the endogenous elimination is in absent, or where the plasma concentration is in excess of 250 μmol/L. Serial monitoring is required in order to advise on when to reintroduce therapy in known epileptics in order to avoid fits.

Primidone
Symptoms are as above, but with the added risks of renal failure due to precipitation of primidone crystals in the nephron. In severe cases the crystals may be readily identified in the urine. Primidone is metabolized to phenobarbitone, and later treatment is as for that drug. The risks of acute renal failure give a likelihood that haemodialysis rather than alkaline diuresis should be considered as first choice for elimination of phenobarbitone in cases involving primidone.

Phenobarbitone
Phenobarbitone is the only barbiturate for which self-poisoning (and iatrogenic poisoning) are still common. Symptoms are similar to those for phenytoin, but the long half-life can lead to extremely long periods of coma if the dose taken is high or if as a result of primidone overdose (see above). In mild cases, as judged clinically, conservative therapy with monitoring of blood gases is sufficient, with measurement of phenobarbitone at daily intervals in order to determine the reintroduction of therapy in epileptics. In severe cases, where elimination is impaired, or there are other reasons for requiring a more rapid return to consciousness, elimination of phenobarbitone may be assisted by alkaline diuresis, haemodialysis or charcoal haemoperfusion. Alkaline diuresis, involving the use of 1.2% $NaHCO_3$, with 0.9% saline and dextrose as required, should maintain the urine pH above pH 7.5 and not overload the circulatory system. Electrolytes should be measured frequently and potassium replaced as required. Diuretics may be needed to avoid fluid overload. Provided that intensive care is given, recovery should be uneventful.

Sodium Valproate
Valproate has gained an unenviable reputation for toxicity due to the infrequent occurrence of acute hepatocellular failure in children treated with the drug. The occurrences are not related to plasma concentration and represent an idiosyncratic reaction, possibly due to a genetically controlled metabolic defect. Plasma valproate concentrations are not of use in such cases other than to confirm compliance, nor are they particularly helpful in acute overdose with large amounts of valproate in epileptics or others in whom complete recovery is usually uneventful after conservative therapy. Haematological variables should be monitored during and for a week after treatment.

Benzodiazepines

The most commonly encountered drugs in poisonings in the UK are the benzodiazepine group of hypnotics and tranquillizers. These drugs are relatively safe when taken alone in overdose, and, provided that there is a clear history, there is seldom a requirement for drug analysis as an aid to treatment.

If untreated, coma may last for some days after a severe overdose; there is little respiratory depression and either conservative therapy, or in more serious cases, the use of the specific benzodiazepine antagonist flumazenil (Anexate) will result in full recovery. The exception is in cases where large amounts of alcohol have also been taken, where there may be respiratory depression, prognosis is poorer, and deaths do occur.

In a very few cases of long-standing coma, a request may be received to confirm that the drug in question is indeed a benzodiazepine in order to allay the fears of the clinician or to avoid other diagnostic procedures. There is a wide range of half-lives among the benzodiazepines and a knowledge of these, coupled with two serial analyses, can give some idea of the likely time of recovery of consciousness. In such cases, the estimation of benzodiazepines that have one or more active metabolites must be interpreted with care, as the half-lives of the metabolites may differ considerably from that of the parent drug.

Benzodiazepines are commonly prescribed to patients who require sedation after poisoning or overdose. A drug history should be obtained before searching for this group of drugs.

Carbon Monoxide

Carbon monoxide poisoning still presents regular problems in the UK, the cause being burning coke in unventilated rooms or deliberate self-exposure to car exhaust fumes.

Carbon monoxide (CO) has an affinity for haemoglobin that is 200–300 times that of oxygen; other haem-containing proteins, such as a cytochromes, are similarly affected.

The clinical diagnosis is seldom in doubt in severe cases and the possibility of cerebral oedema should be investigated by retinal examination. Interpretation of blood carboxyhaemoglobin (COHb) concentrations are complicated by the fact that some smokers may show concentrations in excess of 10% and that patients are frequently treated with oxygen in the ambulance before admission. Once the patient is removed from the source of CO and breathes air, the half-life for conversion of COHb to HbO_2 is approximately 320 min. The conversion of COHb to HbO_2 may be augmented by the use of pure oxygen when $t_{\frac{1}{2}}$ is reduced to 80 min. Hyperbaric oxygen at 3 atm. is no longer regarded as necessary despite the theoretical advantages.

Syncope, headaches, nausea and convulsions leading to coma are associated with levels in excess of 30% COHb. Exchange transfusion has been advocated but is not recommended unless the patient is moribund. A high proportion of patients who survive severe poisoning show late encephalopathy, which is not related to COHb concentrations.

Carboxyhaemoglobin concentrations are most easily measured using a co-oximeter. Gas chromatographic methods are also available.

Cardioactive Drugs

Digoxin, quinidine and β-blocking agents are in common use and available in many households, especially among the elderly.

Digoxin

Digoxin poisoning may occur acutely or may build up gradually during therapy. The clinical presentation is with nausea and vomiting, and severe bradycardia occurs. Patients may complain of seeing yellow. Unfortunately, the electrocardiogram is not always simple to interpret and a plasma digoxin level may be of assistance. Optical immunoassays now allow digoxin assays to be provided out of normal working hours. Consultation with the clinician in charge is mandatory.

It is important to realize that, although a digoxin level in excess of 3.0 nmol/L is indicative of toxicity, there is no good relation between toxicity and plasma level. In particular, because digoxin interferes with the Na^+/K^+ flux in the cell membrane, the potassium level should be measured in all cases. A 'normal' digoxin level may be responsible for toxicity in the presence of hypokalaemia, and as digoxin and diuretics are commonly prescribed together, hypokalaemia is not uncommon and must be excluded, because it is easily treated. Hyperkalaemia can be caused by digoxin overdose, as can hypomagnesaemia. Digoxin toxicity may, if severe, be treated with anti-digoxin antibody, which is available via the pharmacy departments of larger hospitals; however, the number of occasions on which it is warranted are few and limited to patients with renal failure or levels in excess of 7 nmol/L.

Quinine and Quinidine

These optical isomers are most commonly encountered following accidental ingestion, especially in children. Both cause severe arrhythmias when present at toxic concentrations (above 20 μmol/L) and severe intravascular haemolysis can occur at relatively low concentrations. In quinine poisoning, temporary or permanent blindness may occur. Tinnitus is a useful clinical sign. The older literature is confused in relation to levels, as earlier fluorescence methods measured not only the drugs but also their major metabolites.

Confirmation of the presence of one or other of these drugs may be rapidly made by the viewing of urine under an ultraviolet lamp at 254 nm, where a strong blue fluorescence will be seen. However, the fluorescence is so strong that a positive reaction will be obtained after the ingestion of a bottle of tonic water. Confirmation of toxicity requires quantitative estimation of plasma concentration using a method such as HPLC or optical immunoassay; at toxic concentrations there is sufficient cross-reactivity with quinine for the diagnosis to be confirmed using quinidine immunoassays.

Both quinine and quinidine are strongly protein bound and the elimination rate may be of the order of 2–3 days. The effectiveness of acid diuresis and haemoperfusion is still doubtful and these procedures should be done only under careful monitoring of acid–base status.

β-Blocking Agents

Those agents are now being encountered more frequently in cases of overdose. There are no specific laboratory-based diagnostic tests. Treatment is preferably by large (10 mg) doses of glucagon.

Alcohols

Ethanol

Ethanol is so familiar a poison that it tends to be dismissed in all but the most serious cases of overdose, being present, along with other drugs, in over 60% of all cases of self-poisoning.

The levels of alcohol found in self-poisoned patients may be grossly elevated, up to five or six times the UK legal limit for driving (16 mmol/L). In such cases the physician has to decide the relative contribution of alcohol to the patient's state of consciousness and also whether it is necessary to screen for other drugs such as paracetamol.

In many cases the procedure adopted is to wait and observe the clinical condition over a few hours, when considerable improvement in the patient's state of consciousness normally occurs. Alcohol has a short half-life and is eliminated rapidly; thus most patients will show a fall in plasma concentration of between 2 and 5 mmol/L per hour unless there is impairment of hepatic blood flow.

By far the best method for the emergency estimation of ethanol in blood is head-space analysis using an alcohol meter. The method correlates well with GLC and the instrumentation is economical, reliable and available for instant use. Analyses are simple and accurate. Enzymatic methods, employing alcohol dehydrogenase, are widely available and may be used where an alcohol meter or gas chromatograph is not available. Gas chromatography, with direct injection of blood, has the advantage that other alcohols may also be rapidly quantitated, and should be used in all cases where there is a concurrent metabolic acidosis.

Osmometry is of use where a specific method for alcohol is unavailable. A high osmolality in the absence of either hyperglycaemia or uraemia and with no acidosis is likely to correlate with ethanol concentrations. Where an acidosis is also present then methanol may be implicated, but differentiation from ketoacidosis and lactic acidosis is necessary. Hypoglycaemia may occur especially in children, and should be looked for. Some alcoholics develop a form of

ketoacidosis with low glucose levels. Fructose, which has, in the past, been given as an antidote for ethanol poisoning, can contribute to metabolic acidosis once metabolized and should not be used in treatment. Alcohol is a diuretic and aids its own elimination from the body. Haemodialysis is highly effective for removal of all alcohols and may be required in patients with blood alcohol levels in excess of 50 mmol/L.

As mentioned above, the upper legal limit in the UK for ethanol in the blood of vehicle drivers is 16 mmol/L (80 mg/100 mL). In severe cases, blood ethanol levels may reach more than 60 mmol/L (400 mg/100 mL).

Ethylene Glycol

Ethylene glycol, used commonly as antifreeze, may be ingested deliberately by alcoholics as well as accidentally by children. Most commercial preparations are brightly coloured, blue being favoured as the historical colour of poisons.

A history is very important because, in the absence of suspicion that ethylene glycol has been ingested, treatment may be delayed until too late. The initial presentation may be merely drowsiness, but this rapidly progresses to coma and eventually renal failure. Fitting is a poor prognostic sign.

Ethylene glycol is metabolized via glyoxylate to oxalic acid. The latter complexes calcium and leads to precipitation in the renal tubules with eventual renal failure. There is some delay between ingestion and the appearance of a metabolic acidosis. In severe cases, microscopic examination of the urine will reveal calcium oxalate crystals.

Treatment priorities are the maintenance of the plasma calcium concentration, prevention of further metabolism of ethylene glycol, and correction of the severe metabolic acidosis. Inhibition of further metabolism may be effected by use of competitive inhibition of the enzyme alcohol dehydrogenase by ethanol. Ethanol should be infused intravenously so as to maintain a blood alcohol level in excess of 22 mmol/L. Once this is achieved there is relatively little risk of oxalate production and therefore hypocalcaemia and renal failure may be avoided. The earlier the alcohol treatment is started the better, and on no account should the clinician wait until the appearance of a metabolic acidosis. The ethylene glycol may be removed by haemodialysis if necessary, but as some is eliminated unchanged by the kidney, maintenance of a satisfactory urine flow in conjunction with alcohol may prove sufficient.

In patients who present late and in whom metabolic acidosis has developed, the maintenance of pH in the physiological range by use of bicarbonate should be considered; however, sodium concentration tends to rise unacceptably before adequate bicarbonate can be given.

Frequent calls for blood gas, sodium, potassium and calcium measurements may well be justified in severe cases, but the prognosis is poor once renal failure has occurred. The presence of ethylene glycol and methanol (present in some brands of antifreeze) may be confirmed by GLC analysis. Quantitative analyses are not required unless dialysis is contemplated. There are now good theoretical reasons to propose 4-methylpyrazol (an alcohol dehydrogenase inhibitor) as an alternative antidote for both ethylene glycol and methanol poisoning, but to date there is little experience with this in man.

Isopropanol

Although taken uncommonly, this can give rise to difficulties in diagnosis. There is a raised osmolality, which is less than stoichiometric. Isopropanol is metabolized to acetone, which may be screened for. GLC analysis will detect both parent drug and metabolite. Metabolic acidosis is not severe in pure isopropanol poisoning.

Methanol

Methanol may be taken deliberately by alcoholics, many of whom are remarkably resistant to its effects because they also consume large quantities of ethanol. It may also be ingested accidentally. Methanol, like ethylene glycol, is metabolized by alcohol dehydrogenase but to formaldehyde and then to formic acid. It produces a severe and recalcitrant metabolic acidosis, which may require large amounts of sodium bicarbonate for correction.

The presenting features are headaches, blurring of vision, dilation of pupils and, in severe cases, coma. The diagnostic features in initial laboratory investigation are high plasma osmolality and metabolic acidosis; as this picture is similar to that obtained in other metabolic disorders, confirmation of the presence of methanol by GLC analysis may be required.

Treatment is by inhibition of metabolism using oral or intravenous ethanol and correction of the metabolic acidosis. Plasma methanol concentrations in excess of 14 mmol/L are an indication for haemodialysis, as is deepening acidosis. Dialysis should be continued until the level falls to 7 mmol/L.

Chronic methanol abuse can lead to blindness; transient and permanent blindness have been described after acute overdose.

Hypnotic Drugs

Although this group of drugs once constituted the most common cause of severe self-poisoning, changes in prescribing patterns have drastically reduced the clinical problems. Unfortunately, clinical expertise in dealing with hypnotic overdose is also now less widespread. The drugs prescribed as 'sleeping pills' include intermediate-acting barbiturates, methaqualone, glutethimide and meprobamate, chlormethiazole, trichloral compounds and a variety of benzodiazepines. With the exception of the last two groups of drugs, these are depressants of the central nervous system and can lead to severe coma with hypotension, depressed respiration and, potentially, hypothermia. Diagnosis of hypnotic poisoning is usually made from the history and on clinical grounds. Unless a rapid screening method that is at least semiqualitative is available on-call, the determination of drug levels as an emergency is of little relevance.

Treatment is conservative and only in the most severe cases (unresponsive coma with no signs of improvement in the first few hours) need effort be made to remove the drugs by external means. Cases of overdose with each of these drugs have been treated by haemodialysis and haemoperfusion and some reduction in the plasma level may be obtained, but the importance of maintaining adequate liver perfusion in order to allow detoxification of the drugs by the normal hepatic metabolic pathways must be stressed. In particular, there is no case for the use of forced alkaline diuresis or haemodialysis, which are ineffective for this group of compounds and (in the case of forced diuresis) may lead to the development of pulmonary oedema, especially in cases of *methaqualone* poisoning.

Glutethimide

Although uncommon, glutethimide is a particularly complex drug when taken in overdose because it is metabolized to an active intermediate. Some metabolites are excreted via the bile and reabsorbed from the small bowel, a cycle of events that can lead to fluctuating grades of coma. In such cases the use of activated charcoal is advised in order to prevent reabsorption.

The method of choice for the determination of the *barbiturates*, *methaqualone* and *glutethimide* is gas chromatography. The glutethimide metabolites show a characteristic pattern on some stationary phases. Hypnotic barbiturates may be rapidly screened by using enzyme immunoassay, but no reagents are readily available for the less common glutethimide and methaqualone.

If analyses are performed, the interpretation of plasma levels must be made with caution. The severity of the case should be assessed by clinical examination of the patient, as patients who are chronic users of hypnotics may have induced metabolic pathways and show reduced response to relatively high plasma drug concentration.

Chlormethiazole

This is currently in use in the UK as a hypnotic with a short half-life (3–5 h), which is of value in the elderly. The drug is also used for the treatment of delirium tremens, as an intravenous preparation for sedation of aggressive patients, and in pre-eclamptic toxaemia. The oral preparation is dangerous in overdose because it is a central depressant, and severe coma and death have been reported. Problems are also not infrequently encountered during and after continuous intravenous infusions. Although in theory chlormethiazole estimations should not be necessary, there is still no widespread clinical experience of overdosage with this drug and laboratory support may be helpful. Chlormethiazole is highly volatile and analytical methods that involve evaporation of organic solvents should be avoided. A rapid micro-method is available. The standard forensic ultraviolet method cross-reacts with inactive metabolites and should not be used for clinical purposes.

Trichloral compounds

These drugs, used as hypnotics because of their relatively short half-lives, are uncommonly seen nowadays in overdose cases. Vomiting is common but the clinical problem concerns the bizarre disturbances of cardiac function. Treatment with intravenous propanolol restores the electrocardiogram to normal and may need to be repeated until the drug is eliminated. *Chloral hydrate* and its related compounds have good and bad features as far as the analyst is concerned. The end-product is trichloroacetic acid and there is a variety of intermediates. Detection of the end-products is simple and involves heating the plasma or urine with pyridine in the presence of alkali. A red colour in the pyridine layer indicates a drug of this type. The test may be made quantitative in plasma. Care must be taken to avoid false-positive reactions from chloroform, which can cause contamination if it is being used nearby in the laboratory. Patients receiving trichloral at therapeutic doses (1 g) excrete urine that is strongly positive for reducing substances. Hepatic and renal damage subsequent to overdose have been reported.

The *hypnotic benzodiazepines* have been discussed earlier in this chapter.

Inorganic Anions

The ions most commonly encountered in cases of self-poisoning are the oxidizing agents, notably *chlorate* from weedkiller, with *bromate, iodate* and *nitrate* being encountered less commonly. *Cyanide* poisoning is also still relatively common as an accidental occurrence. *Fluoride* from rat poison has been taken, with fatal results in some cases, and there is still a small number of reports of overdosage with *bromide* used as a sedative.

Chlorate

Chlorate and related oxidizing anions exert their toxic effect by oxidation of oxyhaemoglobin to met-haemoglobin, with a similar action on the haem moieties of the cytochrome system.

Confirmation in cases of mild poisoning is best made by using the screening test on urine, which consists of the addition of diphenhydramine solution. In severe cases the test will give a blue colour, indicating a positive, in plasma, but this may be masked by the brown coloration of methaemalbumin. The use of spectral methods for the quantitation of methaemoglobin are rather unsatisfactory and provide little more information than that which may be seen with the naked eye. Derivative spectra are more useful than zero order. Modern co-oximeters will give a quantitative measurement of methaemoglobin. In severe cases the cells will lyse and the haem moiety becomes attached to plasma albumin forming methaemalbumin. In such cases the plasma is likely to be dark brown in colour and may need to be diluted before testing with diphenhydramine for the presence of oxidizing agents.

The clinical picture of patients with a muddy skin colour is due to a combination of methaemoglobinaemia and some cyanosis. In cases of nitrate poisoning, lysis of the cells is uncommon and treatment is with methylene blue, 1–2 mg/kg, repeated as necessary. Oxygen may also be required. Patients treated with methylene blue may show rapid changes of skin colour, which should not be a cause for concern. Treatment is highly effective and patients have survived methaemoglobin concentrations of 75%.

In more severe cases, where chlorate is involved, lysis of the cells occurs. In such cases methylene blue treatment is less effective and the treatment of choice is exchange transfusion because this both removes the abnormal pigments, thus protecting the renal tubules, and provides fresh red cells. In addition, the risk of a raised plasma potassium level from haemo-lysed cells is diminished. Exchange transfusion is preferable to haemodialysis, which removes the potassium and anions but does nothing to prevent the deposition of methaemoglobin and methaemalbumin in the renal tubules. In a few cases, haemolysis and methaemoglobin production are the result, not of self-poisoning, but of the idiosyncratic response to a drug at a therapeutic dose.

Bromide

The most common cause of bromism today is the prescription of the hypnotic Carbromal to elderly patients. Bromine levels may build up over weeks. Bromide poisoning is serious and the clinical picture may fluctuate due to slow, erratic absorption. Available preparations also contain amylobarbitone and a screen for barbiturates may give a lead. In severe cases a haematological screen is required in order to detect clotting abnormalities.

If high, bromide will falsely elevate plasma chloride concentrations as estimated by standard colorimetric techniques, but the interference is less than stoichio-metric. Once suspicion is aroused, estimation of plasma bromide by a colorimetric method may be necessary in order to follow the fall in concentration, which may be slow. Diuresis and peritoneal dialysis are of limited effectiveness, but activated charcoal haemoperfusion has been used with some success.

Cyanide

More cases of accidental than suicidal poisoning

occur at present, the cause often being the mixing of acid with cyanide waste in drains or waste tips. Cyanide poisoning is often implicated in cases of death by inhalation of smoke from burning plastics.

Patients exposed to cyanide require immediate treatment because there may well be a lag between exposure and development of severe symptoms. Dyspnoea with no cyanosis may be present, with vomiting and the gradual loss of consciousness. There is seldom time to confirm diagnosis before treatment.

Two forms of treatment are available. First, conversion of haemoglobin to methaemoglobin using *nitrite*. The methaemoglobin reacts with further cyanide to form cyanomethaemoglobin, which is relatively nontoxic. The cyanide is then converted to thiocyanate by injection of sodium thiosulphate. The initial nitrite administration may be enhanced by the use of amyl nitrite inhalation. Reagents must be fresh. Oxygen therapy is only effective if given with nitrite/thiosulphate.

An alternative form of treatment involves the use of the specific chelating agent 'kelocyanor' but as this compound is toxic in the absence of cyanide, it should never be used in cases where there is doubt.

Identification and estimation of cyanide in blood may be done most simply using a Conway diffusion method; however, retrospective analysis of thiocyanate in urine is a simple way of confirming cyanide intake. Blood cyanide levels in smokers can be as high as 150 μg/L but following poisoning may be considerably higher, in the mg/L range. Blood taken for cyanide estimation should be collected into fluoride/oxalate and should not be stored for long periods.

Fluoride

While uncommon, poisoning with fluoride is invariably serious. The fluoride effectively removes calcium from the plasma as may be evidenced by measurement of calcium levels. Calcium estimation is mandatory and active replacement of calcium in massive amounts may be required to control fits. Magnesium is also reduced. Diuresis should be induced to aid the elimination of the anion, and haemodialysis may be considered but there is often little time and adequate calcium replacement is seldom given rapidly enough. A bad prognostic sign is increasing hyperkalaemia and metabolic acidosis. Fluoride can be measured using an ion-specific electrode.

Nitrite

Nitrite may itself be taken as a poison, in which case methaemoglobinaemia follows, complicated by a severe hypotension that is resistant to many vasopressors.

Metal Poisoning (*see* also Chapter 43)

Aluminium

Chronic aluminium poisoning is now known to be a hazard to patients receiving haemodialysis or chronic ambulatory peritoneal dialysis. All water and reagents used in the preparation of such dialysis fluids must be checked for aluminium content before use, or certified to have an Al^{3+} concentration of less than 2 μmol/L. Aluminium encephalopathy is known to occur in patients with plasma Al^{3+} concentrations of greater than 6 μmol/L. Acute aluminium poisoning is uncommon, despite public perceptions to the contrary.

Iron

The majority of cases of iron poisoning occur accidentally in young children, although on occasion self-poisoning attempts in adults occur. The mortality in severe iron poisoning is high if untreated and urgent efforts must be made to remove the iron from the body. The clinical course of severe iron poisoning may show periods of several hours in which there are few symptoms, so the assessment of severity of iron poisoning requires emergency iron analysis and every laboratory should be equipped to make such an estimation. It is probably preferable to use in emergency the method used normally during the day. Where a single analysis is done manually, iron-free acid-washed glassware should be kept aside for this eventuality. Iron-binding capacity, if available quickly, is useful because a total iron concentration greater than the total binding capacity is diagnostic. Once treatment has started, measurement of both iron and iron-binding capacity can give clinically misleading information. Severe poisoning is indicated if the iron level exceeds 150 μmol/L in an adult or 90 μmol/L in a child.

Treatment consists of chelation of the iron both in the gut and the bloodstream using the specific chelating agent *desferrioxamine*. Some of the agent is left in the stomach. Following lavage, intravenous desferrioxamine is given with intramuscular supplement if necessary until plasma iron levels return to acceptable levels (150 μmol/L). The excretion of chelated iron requires an adequate urine flow; where this is not obtained, dialysis may be required. The urine in patients treated with desferrioxamine may appear dark orange due to the chelated iron, and inexperienced clinicians should be reassured that this is not a cause for concern.

Lead

Acute lead poisoning is uncommon but chronic cases occur both from industrial exposure to lead dust and in children who ingest some older paints. Lead analyses should be made by a specialist laboratory because the analytical procedure using atomic absorption spectroscopy is difficult to accomplish accurately without continuous practice. Lead levels above 0.07 mg/100 mL in blood or 15.3 in urine are indicative of excess exposure to lead. A rapid index of lead poisoning may be obtained in any laboratory using a kit method for δ-aminolaevulinic acid, which increases if later steps in porphyrin synthesis are blocked by lead. Lead poisoning leads to neurological signs, which are the most usual presenting symptoms, but chronic renal damage is a risk. Treatment is by the use of the chelating agents in combination. Again, an adequate urine flow is required for effective treatment. Occupational screening is now mandatory in industries where the risk is recognized.

Lithium

The use of lithium as an antidepressant has regained favour now that plasma concentrations may be readily monitored, as the drug has a narrow therapeutic index with plasma concentrations of 0.7–1.3 mmol/L necessary for effective therapy and levels in excess of 1.5 mmol/L associated with toxicity. Concentrations of greater than 3 mmol/L are potentially life-threatening. Most cases of toxicity are due to build-up over a short period following a change of dose, development of renal insufficiency or salt depletion. In patients receiving regular therapy, low concentrations are of concern because the tissue stores are already filled. In cases not previously exposed to the drug, early high levels are less worrying because distribution will cause a rapid fall, even in the absence of excretion.

The symptoms of lithium toxicity are in the main concerned with the central nervous system, but gastrointestinal problems are seen and, in some patients, a nephrogenic diabetes insipidus occurs which may be refractory to treatment.

Diagnosis and prognosis depend upon estimation of the plasma lithium concentration, the patient with high levels being treated urgently using forced alkaline diuresis or haemodialysis, both of which are effective. During either of these procedures a close watch should be kept on the concentrations of sodium, potassium, and lithium itself. Treatment should be stopped once the plasma lithium concentration falls to within the therapeutic range, as complete removal of the drug may give rise to serious effects in those on long-term therapy. A method for the emergency estimation of lithium should be available in each district general hospital. Flame emission photometry is a satisfactory and simple technique. It is not suitable for the estimation of urinary lithium levels, for which an atomic absorption spectroscopic method should be used.

Some patients receiving lithium therapy develop hypothyroidism and patients on lithium who show symptoms of myxoedema should be checked for thyroid status.

Mercury

Acute poisoning with mercury is more common than would be expected. Metallic mercury, even if ingested, is relatively low in toxicity, but ingestion of mercuric chloride or the incorrect use of mercuric chloride solutions are the major causes of mercury poisoning. Chronic poisoning may be caused by elemental mercury, which sublimes from spillages (e.g. broken thermometers or dental amalgam). Mercury vapour is toxic when inhaled. A source of this hazard in clinical chemistry laboratories is from thermometers breaking in GLC ovens. The symptoms are neurological, and renal damage may occur.

Mercury is estimated by atomic absorption spectrophotometry. Concentrations in excess of 0.5 μmol/L in urine are diagnostic of chronic poisoning.

Treatment of mercury poisoning in cases where the mercuric chloride is ingested is by gastric lavage with sodium formaldehyde sulphoxylate. This reduces the mercuric ion to the less toxic mercurous form. Chelation of the ions with dimercaprol or N-acetyl D,L-penicillamine is used to remove inorganic mercury.

Narcotic Drugs

Narcotic overdose in the UK is associated with drug abuse, with the exception of *propoxyphene* poisoning, which occurs in patients taking preparations containing paracetamol and propoxyphene (Distalgesic and co-proxamol). For this reason, paracetamol estimations should be performed on all patients diagnosed as suffering from narcotic poisoning.

Diagnosis of narcotic poisoning depends upon the clinical picture of coma with respiratory depression and pin-point pupils, both of which respond rapidly to adequate doses of the specific opiate antagonist, *naloxone*. Naloxone thus contributes to both diagnosis and treatment.

There are no specific laboratory tests required in order to diagnose narcotic poisoning; however, amylase levels may be raised due to constriction of the sphincter of Oddi. Retrospective confirmation may be made by urine analysis, which may be of use in determining the drug or drugs taken and assist in after-care; plasma concentrations of narcotics have little significance. Specimens should be obtained *before* the start of naloxone treatment. A variety of other drugs, especially barbiturates, may be present. Specimens obtained from addicts have a high chance of carrying a risk of hepatitis; therefore unnecessary blood samples should not be taken. Patients admitted late after overdose with narcotic agents may well have suffered irreversible cerebral anoxia. In such cases, requests for screening for drugs preparatory to the potential donation of organs may be requested. In such cases the analyst should consider the half-lives of the ingested drugs and those drugs (including antibiotics) given after admission to hospital, as these may obscure the picture when using methods such as thin-layer chromatography. The length of time that drugs of abuse remain positive in the urine (using National Institute for Drug Abuse guidelines) is of the order of 1–3 days, but this may be prolonged in cases of poisoning. Active elimination methods are not useful in such cases.

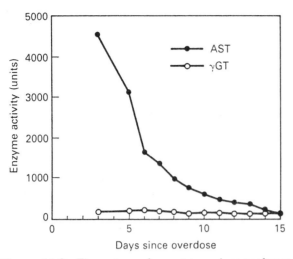

Figure 44.8 The pattern of aspartate aminotransferase (AST) and γ-glutamyl transferase (γGT) in plasma following a paracetamol overdose. Although the difference is not always so marked the use of AST rather than γGT as an index of hepatocellular damage is clear.

Organochlorides (e.g. DDT, pentachlorophenol (PCP))

Cases of poisoning are uncommon in Britain but, when encountered, may be severe with hepatic and pulmonary damage predominating. There is no specific treatment available unless convulsions are present, in which case intravenous diazepam may be used. There is, however, a tendency for low Ca^{2+} levels to be encountered. Ca^{2+} should be estimated on at least two occasions and the patient treated with calcium gluconate if necessary.

Organophosphorus Compounds

The major problem associated with this group of compounds is inhibition of cholinesterase activity by phosphorylation of the serine residues of the enzyme. Treatment is with atropine and pralidoxine (PAM). The latter competes for the organophosphorus compound, enhances its hydrolysis and regenerates the active enzyme.

Measurement of organophosphorus content of body fluids is unhelpful in diagnosis and treatment but may be required for subsequent enquiries; therefore samples, especially those obtained early, should be kept. Estimation of red-cell cholinesterase levels is the most sensitive index; if below 50% of the lower limit of the normal range, treatment should be started, even in the absence of symptoms. Most laboratories offer only plasma pseudocholinesterase estimations. These should be available at short notice, as treatment needs to be continued, in some cases for days, until levels approach the normal range.

Paracetamol (Acetaminophen)

Poisoning with paracetamol, a mild analgesic available without prescription, is common in the UK and is increasing in the USA, where the drug is known as acetaminophen.

There are few clinical signs associated with severe paracetamol overdose in the early stages and confirmation may be required by analysis. The drug is, however, commonly formulated in combination with other drugs, notably the narcotic propoxyphene (*see* above), and should be sought in cases of self-poisoning with narcotics and in other cases where the exact nature of the poison(s) is not clear.

Paracetamol is toxic via an active metabolite that actively binds to thiol groups. The metabolite is produced to a large extent in the hepatocytes and acute hepatocellular damage is caused if the concentrations of metabolite exceed the available concentrations of glutathione, which acts as a scavenger. Individuals with reduced glutathione production due to liver disease or malnourishment and those with induced microsomal oxidation enzymes, who produce relatively higher amounts of metabolite, are more at risk than healthy subjects. Patients with alcohol problems are thus doubly sensitive to paracetamol.

The clinical course of severe paracetamol overdose mirrors that of other causes of acute hepatocellular damage and may progress to hepatic failure and death.

Early death has occurred in those with oesophageal varices or piles, owing to failure in clotting mechanisms due to the fall-off in production of prothrombin.

Less severe cases may recover and in untreated cases, or those treated late, the estimation of aspartate aminotransferase and bilirubin concentration for some days may be of prognostic value but γ-glutamyl transferase concentrations are not helpful (Fig. 44.8).

Provided that diagnosis is made within 12 h of ingestion of the drug, the mode of treatment is now well established and should be available in district general hospitals in the UK. Intravenous administration of N-acetyl cysteine, which is available commercially, can provide the necessary thiol groups and protect the hepatocytes from damage. Oral therapy with methionine has been advocated, but as nausea may be present in a proportion of cases and absorption may be compromised in cases of mixed overdose (due to hypotension), the intravenous route is advisable.

The decision on treatment can be made logically only after determination of the plasma paracetamol concentration. If this lies above the 'treatment line', which relates plasma paracetamol concentration to time since ingestion on nomograms, then treatment is necessary. Patients with concentrations well below the line are not at risk. There are inevitably grey areas associated with uncertainty about drugs and the rule must be to treat if in doubt. Treatment at later than 16 h has not been shown to be effective, thus reinforcing the requirement for rapid early analysis.

There have been conflicting views of the validity of plasma paracetamol measurement arising from the use of different methods for the measurement. It is important that the method used must detect only paracetamol and not the metabolites, which may be present in high concentrations. The preferred method for routine use is the specific enzymatic colorimetric method.

Paraquat

Poisoning with paraquat and the similar compound, diquat, still gives rise to fatalities each year. Most of the fatal cases are caused by the agricultural concentrates, which are dark-brown liquids resembling the cola soft drinks. The concentrates are extremely toxic, one mouthful being sufficient to cause death, and may also be absorbed through the skin if gloves are not worn, and inhaled with spraying if a mask is not used. The garden herbicides ('Weedol' and 'Pathclear') are in granular form and require some effort to ingest; however, in some suicidal attempts up to three sachets dissolved in water have been taken.

Paraquat is toxic to the lung after a lag period of up to 3 weeks. In severe cases, renal failure is an early feature with lung pathology appearing later. Diagnosis of paraquat overdose may be made rapidly using a urine specimen. Sodium bicarbonate 10 mg is added to 2 ml of urine to render it alkaline, followed by 10 mg sodium nitrite. A strong blue colour indicates the presence of paraquat.

Paraquat is rapidly excreted via the kidney in the early stages after ingestion and even a small dose may give rise to a strong colour reaction in the urine. Prognosis is entirely dependent on the measurement of the level of paraquat in the plasma at a known time after ingestion (Fig. 44.9). Experience to date indicates that patients with plasma paraquat levels well above the line are unlikely to survive, although death may be delayed for days or weeks. Patients with levels well below the line survive with supportive therapy, which may include treatment of transient renal failure.

Current treatment consists of gastric lavage using bentonite clay or fuller's earth in order to adsorb paraquat. The procedure is cathartic, which also aids gut clearance. Prolonged haemodialysis or charcoal haemoperfusion are claimed to remove considerable amounts of paraquat but only if instituted early while the plasma level is still high. Starting dialysis at later times has not so far proved effective in improving the prognosis.

The methods of choice for the emergency measurement of paraquat are colorimetric involving derivative spectroscopy, which are adequate for prognostic purposes, it being necessary to estimate concentra-

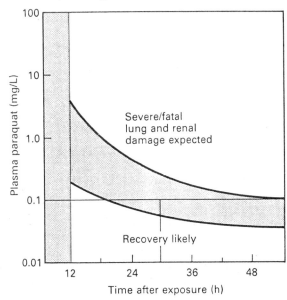

Figure 44.9 The prognostic nomogram for use in cases of poisoning with paraquat; prognosis is guarded in the shaded area.

tions down to 10 mg/L. The contribution of diquat is seldom significant, comprising some 14% of the paraquat concentration at all levels.

Salicylates

Salicylate, like paracetamol, is freely available in the UK and represents a still-common cause of severe poisoning in both adults and children with a high mortality (1–7%). The most toxic form is methyl salicylate (oil of wintergreen), which can be absorbed via the skin.

Aspirin (acetylsalicylate) is hydrolysed to salicylic acid, which is the major component in plasma. Further metabolism to salicyluric and gentisic acids, along with conjugation, occurs before excretion in the urine at therapeutic doses. In overdose the binding sites for salicylate are swamped and salicylate is excreted in the urine, largely unchanged. Excretion is related to urinary pH.

When used for long-term therapy (e.g. for rheumatoid arthritis) the plasma concentration of salicylate may be up to 2.5 mmol/L. Above this concentration, or in previously unexposed patients, salicylate can exert a stimulatory effect on the respiratory centre, leading to hyperventilation, which is commonly observed in adult patients who have taken an overdose. However, this takes some time to develop and it is not uncommon for a patient to present with no clinical signs who subsequently turns out to have a high plasma salicylate concentration. In an untreated case the hyperventilation increases in severity, leading to a loss of CO_2. Re-equilibration of the bicarbonate buffer system leads to a fall in HCO_3 to extremely low levels, and at the same time there is increasing

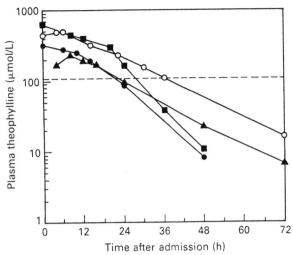

Figure 44.10 Variation in elimination in the early stages following theophylline overdose in four patients.

dehydration due to pure water loss via the lungs. At this stage the blood-gas picture in such a patient shows a simple respiratory alkalosis. If treatment is not instituted, the combination of lactic acid production from the diaphragm plus other metabolic acid production caused by the action of salicylate as an uncoupling agent for oxidative phosphorylation causes the development of an increasing metabolic acidosis.

The depleted bicarbonate buffer system is inadequate in the face of the acid load and there develops a severe metabolic acidosis in the presence of an existing respiratory alkalosis. At this stage, loss of consciousness may occur and the prognosis is increasingly poor.

In the absence of a good history the plasma salicylate concentration is necessary for confirmation of diagnosis because the combined metabolic acidosis and respiratory alkalosis presents a difficult blood-gas picture and salicylate overdose has been confused with diabetes mellitus, especially as salicylate metabolites are reducing agents that interfere with Clinitest®, but not with specific tests for glucose.

The plasma salicylate concentration should be related to the putative time of ingestion of the drug. Levels in excess of 5.0 mmol/L should be regarded as serious and levels in excess of 7.5 mmol/L as severe. The colorimetric method of Trinder is adequate and simple, but a more precise method involving enzymatic hydrolysis is now the method of choice. In these cases, gastric lavage is mandatory because there is a tendency for aspirin tablets to form a mass in the pylorus and for continued absorption to occur. In cases where gastric wash-out is not done, the plasma concentration may well increase after admission.

The aim of treatment of salicylate poisoning is to hasten the removal of the drug from the body and to replace the bicarbonate buffering capacity and thus restore the pH to normal. Both of these requirements may be met by the administration of alkali.

Alkalinization using 1.2% $NAHCO_3$ with replacement of K^+ as required should restore the plasma water and lead to the production of urine of pH > 7.5 without development of hypokalaemia.

In severe cases, monitoring of salicylate, potassium and blood gases may be required until the plasma salicylate concentration falls below 2.5 mmol/L. As with other drugs, if an inadequate flow of urine is obtained despite diuretics, then removal of the drug by haemodialysis may be required.

Theophylline

Iatrogenic theophylline poisoning is relatively common and is more properly discussed in Chapter 45. The introduction of sustained-release theophylline preparations and its monitoring has led to an increase in availability, which is reflected in increased incidence in cases of poisoning. Theophylline poisoning is one of the most serious medical emergencies, with a considerable number of deaths associated.

Theophylline acts by inhibiting phosphodiesterase and thus cAMP degradation, and by stimulating catecholamine release. The clinical effects are protean, and include nausea and vomiting progressing to severe cardiac arrhythmias, but may develop after a delay of 24–36 h, by which time tissue theophylline levels may be extremely high if untreated. The metabolic effects include hyperglycaemia, hypophosphataemia and hypercalcaemia, and hypermagnesaemia. Hypokalaemia is unusual in the early stages, but at later stages, following development of acute renal failure, hyperkalaemia ensues. Renal damage due to rhabdomyolysis, which is most common in patients who present late to hospital, makes the maintenance of electrolyte imbalance more complicated. The treatment of choice is charcoal both orally, in non-vomiting patients, and as haemoperfusion in more serious cases (plasma theophylline > 300 μmol/L at 4 h or $t_{\frac{1}{2}}$ > 24 h); however, the correction of cardiovascular and metabolic effects takes priority. Treatment should be initated as soon as possible after admission. Some centres use magnesium hydroxide in addition to charcoal, but magnesium defects are more safely corrected with intriavenous fluids. Serial monitoring of plasma theophylline concentration is mandatory in suspected overdose. Because the elimination kinetics in the early stages are non-linear (Fig. 44.10), measurements should continue until it is certain that the half-life is stable and the concentrations are returning towards the therapeutic range. Theophylline measurements should be available on call. Both optical immunoassays and rapid HPLC methods provide the means.

Tricyclic Antidepressants

Despite the fact that many less toxic antidepressants are available, this group of drugs still gives rise to a relatively high proportion of serious poisoning cases. The diagnosis is seldom in doubt since the cholinergic symptoms are well recognized. Cardiac arrhythmias are common and may persist, with a danger of cardiac arrest for some time after recovery of consciousness. For this reason, electrocardiographic monitoring should be instituted in all serious cases.

Where screening is requested it should be noted that there is a delay of up to 12 h in the excretion of tricyclic drugs and their metabolites. A urine specimen taken on admission may not show more than a trace and a plasma screen is of more assistance. A qualitative enzyme immunoassay is available, and both ultraviolet fluorescence and GLC methods are simple.

In overdose, plasma concentrations in excess of 1 mg/L may be found but they are highly variable and not prognostic. This is high enough to give an identifiable spectrum on simple ultraviolet analyses of an extract of alkalinized serum. There is a rapid screening test for the presence of *imipramine* and *desmethylimipramine* in plasma and urine, using the Forrest reagent, which may be of use diagnostically.

Amitriptyline and *imipramine* are metabolized to their pharmacologically active demethylated derivatives before excretion. It is possible to advise on the necessity for active elimination measures by measuring the concentrations of the unchanged drug and its metabolite over 12 h. The parent drug concentration should fall, accompanied by an initial rise and then a fall by the metabolite.

CONCLUSIONS

The correct laboratory investigation of the poisoned patient requires a considerable knowledge of both the clinical and analytical aspects of toxicology.

There are few drugs and poisons for which specific clinical knowledge is required, but it is in such cases that mistakes may be made because of failure both to appreciate the dangers of a specific toxic mechanism and to treat it with sufficient emergency. Time and effort may be wasted in screening for drugs or performing a qualitative assay when all that is required is an estimate of, for example, plasma calcium.

Similarly, insufficient use is made of the simple concept of half-life in order to determine the patient's ability to eliminate a drug and thus determine the likely recovery time or need for intervention with a procedure such as dialysis.

Methods for the rapid and specific determination of drugs and poisons in plasma are improving daily, with HPLC and immunoassay methods in particular providing some exciting possibilities. Clinical chemists faced with the task of assisting clinicians in treating poisoned patients have never had more at their disposal; the correct application of such methods is the greater challenge. The main problem now is to determine whether the work put into the analyses is justified by the clinical problem. Too many analyses are performed, the results of which are never discussed or acted upon.

The interpretation of the results obtained is by no means simple. A simple rule of thumb for the biochemist involved in clinical toxicology should be 'Do not carry out a quantitative analysis unless either you or the clinician making the request are able to interpret the result.' Using this guideline, over half of requests for drug analyses can be avoided and much time, effort and money saved. The exception to the rule is where the analyses are contributing to the build-up of information on uncommon or novel drugs; in such cases, research laboratories rely on clinical biochemists to forward samples to them for analysis and information on interesting cases to poisons information units.

Careful attention to the clinical problem and selection of the relevant specimen at the correct time, coupled with the choice of a specific method, are the current priorities in this fascinating field of clinical care.

SUGGESTIONS FOR FURTHER READING

Curry A.A. (1984, pt.1; 1986, pt.2). *Analytical Methods in Human Toxicology*, London: Macmillan.

Doull J., Klaasen C.D., Amdur M.O. (1991). *Cassaret and Doull's Toxicology*, 4th edn, New York: Macmillan.

Gossel T.A. and Bricker J.D. (1994) *Principles of Clinical Toxicology*, New York: Raven Press.

Gough T. ed. (1991). *The Analysis of Drugs of Abuse*, Chichester: Wiley.

Haddad L.M., Whichester J.F. (1990). *Poisoning and Drug Overdose*, 2nd edn, London: Saunders.

Henry J., Volans G. (1985). *ABC of Poisoning*: Drugs, London: British Medical Association.

Moffat A.C. ed. (1986). *Clarke's Isolation and Identification of Drugs*, 2nd edn, London: Pharmaceutical Press.

Proudfoot A. (1993). *Diagnosis and Management of Acute Poisoning*, Oxford: Butterworth-Heinemann.

Vale J.A., Meredith T.J. (1981). *Poisoning, Diagnosis and Treatment*, London: Update Books.

45. The Regulation and Monitoring of Drug Therapy

G. Mould

Introduction
Pharmacokinetic factors affecting drug
   concentrations
  Bioavailability
  Bioequivalence
  Plasma protein binding
  Elimination half-life
  Steady state
  Clearance
Pharmacodynamic factors
Uses and abuses of TDM
  Target range
  Criteria for measurement
  Drug choice
  Indications for drug measurement
  Methods of measurement
Dose individualization
  Population data
  Dose individualization techniques
Recent advances in TDM
  New drugs
  Diagnostic procedures
  Near-patient testing
Quality control in TDM
  External quality control of drug analysis
  TDM audit
Conclusion

INTRODUCTION

It is well established that there is a wide variation in clinical response following drug administration. Variation in part can be predicted by a knowledge of the clinical pharmacokinetics and pharmacology of the drug under evaluation, so that in most cases, doses can be tailored to meet the individual patient's requirements. Dose individualization, as it is often referred to, is largely done intuitively by physicians when prescribing according to the patient's characteristics or some biochemical measure. Nevertheless, it is the pharmacokinetics of the drug and alterations in the pharmacodynamics of treatment that determine efficacy. The monitoring of drug therapy is therefore important. The concept of therapeutic drug monitoring (TDM) had arisen from these principles, although TDM itself is concerned with the measurement of a relatively small number of drugs in patients, the results of which are (or should be) interpreted with the help of pharmacokinetic principles. This implies a relatively routine commitment to consulta-

tions in clinical pharmacokinetics. At the centre of these consultations it is clear that pharmacists and biochemists in particular have a major part to play, and a number of studies have highlighted in particular the pharmacist's role.[1] However, multidisciplinary approaches are required to make the most effective use of the available resources. In this chapter, the important features of the individualization of drug therapy required to ensure better patient care are considered.

PHARMACOKINETIC FACTORS AFFECTING DRUG CONCENTRATIONS

It would be inappropriate to review the complex theory of pharmacokinetics, which has been and still is the subject of many textbooks; nevertheless, it is important to appreciate that a thorough knowledge of pharmacokinetics is required successfully to interpret clinical drug concentrations. Some of the more important considerations are discussed next.

Bioavailability

Bioavailability is a measure of the amount of unmetabolized drug appearing in the general circulation, which in turn is dependent on the amount absorbed. Measurement of the concentration of drug in the body will give a measure of these differences, and the bioavailability of a drug is therefore an important consideration in evaluating response. Bioavailability should be differentiated from *bioequivalence*, which compares bioavailability values from different preparations. As a patient may need to take a different formulation for a number of reasons, it is important to be aware of any differences in response that this may cause. A comparison of the total amount of drug absorbed following intravenous dosage with that of the non-parenteral route gives an indication of the absolute bioavailability of that route. This is expressed as a ratio or percentage and can be calculated by measuring the area under the curve (AUC) from the time:drug-concentration profile.

After intravenous administration it is assumed that the drug is completely available; however, after oral administration this may not always be so. For some drugs only a percentage reaches the general systemic circulation. The physical characteristics of the drug can influence the amount of systemic absorption. Digoxin is sparingly soluble in intestinal contents so that only between 60 and 70% of the drug is absorbed from most commercially available tablet formulations.

A reduction in bioavailabilty can also be a result of *first-pass metabolism*, where a drug is metabolized significantly before reaching the general circulation after absorption. First-pass metabolism strictly assumes extensive hepatic extraction, but it can also be due to gastrointestinal-wall metabolism or microbial metabolism. For example, recent studies have shown that cyclosporin is metabolized by human gut mucosa

TABLE 45.1

LIST OF DRUGS FOR WHICH BIOAVAILABILITY PROBLEMS HAVE
BEEN IDENTIFIED

Oral preparations
  Atenolol
  Calcium carbonate
  Carbamazepine
  Chloramphenicol
  Co-proxamol
  Diazepam
  Diltiazem
  Digoxin
  Ferrous sulphate
  Glibenclamide
  Griseofulvin
  Lithium
  Mianserin
  Medroxyprogesterone acetate
  Naproxen
  Nortriptyline
  Phenytoin
  Procainamide
  Propranolol
  Theophylline
  Tamoxifen
  Thyroxine
  Valproate

Parenteral preparations
  Vancomycin

Topical preparations
  Betamethasone valerate cream and ointment
  Fluocinolone acetonide cream
  Triamcinolone acetonide cream and ointment

and it is this that probably accounts for its variable (1–89%) bioavailability.[2] Most drugs have an insignificant first-pass effect but there are a few important drugs that have either a variable or low bioavailability, or even both. For example, amiodarone has a bioavailability of between 30 and 80%. For those drugs with a low therapeutic ratio, variability in absorption is important. Felodipine, a β-adrenoreceptor agonist, has a bioavailability of approximately 30%. On the other hand, it has been reported that the bioavailability of dihydroergotamine averaged 0.5% following a 10-mg dose.

Other problems are highlighted by the effect of food, which may significantly alter bioavailability. The angiotensin-converting enzyme inhibitor captopril is a good example, where a reduction of between 35 and 55% was shown to occur after ingestion of food (breakfast). Interestingly, its antihypertensive effect does not appear to have been compromised, despite the lower concentration of drug.

Bioequivalence

Interest in bioequivalence has been stimulated by recent efforts to reduce budgets by prescribing drugs generically, not by brand name. This has led to a proliferation in the number of generic drugs available and concerns by pharmacists and clinicians alike as to whether the alternatives are equivalent in their availability and activity to their branded counterparts, the problem being that variations in bioequivalence between the formulation of one manufacturer and that of another can lead to significant changes in clinical response.

Not surprisingly, many of the recent reports on bioequivalence have arisen from outcomes in anticonvulsant treatment. Indeed one company has recently withdrawn its current brand of phenytoin because of bioequivalence problems. On the other hand, another company has issued a statement to the fact that no problems exist. Because careful monitoring is required for these and other drugs with narrow therapeutic ratios, TDM is essential whilst transferring from one preparation to another, although clinical reports rather than anecdotal ones have been few. Nevertheless, loss of seizure control and unexpected toxicity have been reported in three patients who received generic carbamazepine rather than the branded one, Tegretol.[3] One patient lost her job and insurance cover as a result. Unfortunately, drug concentrations were not determined in the reported cases and comparisons between the preparations could not be made. What comparisons have been made show little difference in the pharmacokinetics of a new, chewable preparation of carbamazepine and ordinary Tegretol tablets. Changing between these two preparations at least should present no problems.

In another example, in which drug concentrations were measured, a young woman experienced increased seizure frequency when a generic primidone was dispensed in place of Mysoline.[4] The trough phenobarbitone (the major metabolite of primidone) concentration decreased from 76 to 39 μmol/L after 10 days of generic drug, despite an increase in the primidone dose from 500 to 625 mg. In response to criticisms, the company producing the generic preparation re-evaluated their *in vitro* dissolution data and reported that the results were 'within standard specifications', although they provided no data to support their claims. Similar seizure problems have been reported following ingestion of imported tablets containing sodium valproate substituted for Epilim. Other drugs for which bioavailability problems have been reported are shown in Table 45.1.

In the main, bioequivalence data presented to regulating authorities are not readily available, because companies are reluctant to divulge their results, but data should be readily available to make value judgements. Measuring and comparing the AUC is the most convenient way of comparing different preparations *in vivo*, and the US Federal Drug Agency has found that the average difference between the observed mean AUCs of the brand name and generic product is about 3.5%.[5] As we are looking for over a 15% difference to demonstrate bioinequivalence, this represents excellent agreement. Of course, AUC comparisons are not the only measure of bioequivalence; it is assessment of clinical difference that is really required.

Those involved with TDM should be aware of possible problems and bioinequivalence should always be considered as a possible cause of unexplained changes in response to a drug, especially if the benefits and side-effects of that drug are correlated with blood concentrations. Enlightened practitioners should be able to identify this. Not only is identification needed, it is also essential that experiences of adverse effects with generic drugs are documented. Only then can we decide whether generic drugs are really as good as their branded counterparts.

Plasma Protein Binding

Many drugs are highly bound to plasma proteins. Acidic drugs are bound to albumin, whilst basic drugs are bound to lipoproteins or to α-acid glycoprotein. The intensity of action of any reversibly acting compound that reaches its site of action by diffusion rather than by active transport is determined by the unbound or free fraction rather than by the total concentration. Standard methods for determining serum concentrations do not discriminate between free and total drug. If the binding of a particular drug were constant and predictable from one subject to another, then it would be of no importance that both bound and free components were measured simultaneously, as the total concentration would accurately reflect the free, pharmacologically active, concentration. However, for some drugs, and in some specific circumstances this relation is not constant.

Diseases that elevate acid glycoprotein, such as Crohn's disease, or which reduce albumin concentrations, such as hepatic disease or malnutrition, can give rise to altered binding of drugs. The measurement of total concentrations in these circumstances may under- or overestimate a drug's therapeutic or toxic effects. Protein binding may also be reduced in the neonate.

For other drugs, for example valproic acid, the binding to plasma proteins is limited and the fraction of drug that is bound decreases as the concentration is raised. In these circumstances, serum concentrations of total drug will not provide a good indication of free drug concentration and thereby pharmacological effect. It would be desirable in theory, therefore, to measure the concentration of free drug in serum, but in practice methods currently available for measuring unbound concentrations are unsatisfactory and in the majority of cases are unlikely to lead to better patient care.

Elimination Half-life

The elimination half-life is defined as the time required to reduce the plasma concentration to one half its value. The half-life is important in determining the time to reach steady-state drug concentrations, which for all practical purposes is within three to four half-lives. Normally the half-life is dose independent, but there are important exceptions, notably phenytoin, whose half-life is concentration dependent and increases with increasing plasma concentration. A patient in the author's hospital was admitted with an elevated and toxic phenytoin serum concentration of 200 μmol/L. The drug was stopped, and the time taken for the concentration to decline to a more acceptable 80 μmol/L was 15 days. This is equivalent to a half-life of about 11 days. The quoted half-life of phenytoin at therapeutic concentrations is 15 h.

Steady State

A steady state is achieved when the amount of drug administered in a given time is equal to the amount of drug eliminated in the same time. At steady state the plasma concentration of the drug at any time during any dosing interval should be identical and the peak and trough concentrations do not change. This enables a calculation of the average steady-state concentration to be made.

For a drug with so called one-compartment characteristics, the time to reach steady state is independent of the dose, number of doses given and the dosing interval, but as indicated in the previous section, it is directly proportional to the elimination half-life.

Clearance

Metabolic clearance for some drugs shows extremely wide interindividual variation. It has been shown that a number of drugs are under pharmacogenetic control. Some of these pathways are relatively minor; nevertheless, some are important. For example, metoprolol has a variable metabolism and it has been suggested that the oxidation phenotype of the patient may influence the incidence of adverse reactions.[6] However, the therapeutic ratios of most β-adrenoceptor blocking agents are wide, so that the differences may not be clinically significant. Other drugs exhibiting similar problems include phenelzine and isoniazid. Polymorphic metabolism of drugs may be observed between races. For example, single doses of nifedipine are metabolized more slowly in patients from South Asia than from Europe.

PHARMACODYNAMIC FACTORS

A knowledge of pharmacodynamics results in an appreciation of the interpatient variability in clinical response and its modification by certain clinical conditions or by concurrent drug therapy. It goes some way to countering the arguments against TDM, for it rationalizes drug monitoring in certain conditions and explains the variability in response for a given concentration. Thus, digoxin toxicity can manifest itself in the patient who has hypokalaemia despite normal drug concentrations, and thyroid disease can alter the response of the same drug. Some patients are well controlled at drug concentrations lower than the standard target range, whereas others may require concentrations above the recommended range in order to achieve a satisfactory response.

It should be appreciated that some drugs are converted to active metabolites in the liver. In some instances, however, active metabolites may be formed in the target tissue and when this occurs, the relation between concentration and effect may be a poor one. α-Methyldopa is a good example of such a drug; its conversion into α-methylnoradrenaline and other amine metabolites in central and peripheral noradrenergic neurons is responsible for its hypotensive action. The blood-pressure reduction long outlasts measurable concentrations of the parent compound in blood.

It can be seen that apart from obvious conditions of overdose and underdose, such as non-compliance, one should report drug concentrations as subtherapeutic or toxic with caution. The clinical condition and the pharmacodynamic response of the patient must always be considered when drug concentrations are being interpreted.

USES AND ABUSES OF TDM

For the vast majority of drugs, clinical end-points are the easiest method of deciding therapeutic efficacy. There are, however, a few drugs for which drug measurement is essential, although even within this group there are drugs for which there is still controversy as to its usefulness. Furthermore, the effective use of TDM involves not only the measurement of drug concentrations in blood (or other body fluids) but more importantly the evaluation and interpretation of the results. As such, TDM is dependent on two critical assumptions. Firstly, that there is a clear relation between the blood drug concentration and the drug's therapeutic or pharmacological effect; secondly, that a so-called target range exists, consisting of a range of concentrations against which doses are adjusted. Although these criteria are well defined, the potential for abuse exists. The concept of the therapeutic range (or *target range*, which is to be preferred) is a good illustration of the potential for TDM abuse.

Target Range

The target range is a range of concentrations within which the majority of patients are known to experience maximum clinical benefit. I prefer the term target range to therapeutic range as it retains the important elements of the concept of TDM without assuming a therapeutic validity, which a single measurement cannot make. There is undoubtedly a general movement away from rigid ranges, as many inexperienced users assume that the target range for most drugs has been well defined through carefully controlled clinical trials and thereby abuse its usefulness. In reality, a target range is a range of concentrations within which the probability of the desired clinical response is relatively high and the probability of unacceptable toxicity low. Examples of some of the common drugs in TDM illustrate these considerations.

Phenytoin

The initial prospective study in 1960 of 12 hospitalized patients with severe, generalized seizures receiving phenytoin and phenobarbitone showed good control only when the phenytoin concentration was greater than 40 μmol/L.[7] The same study demonstrated good control in a series of outpatients with concentrations above 60 μmol/L, whilst others had concentrations below 56 μmol/L and experienced no side-effects. On the other hand, of those patients whose concentrations were above 120 μmol/L, 74% experienced side-effects. Subsequent studies reported phenytoin toxicity at concentrations above 80 μmol/L and the widely used target range of 40–80 μmol/L became established. In the light of current clinical thinking, there is probably insufficient evidence for the lower limit. Many patients can be controlled with serum concentrations ranging from 4 to 20 μmol/L. Certainly, phenytoin toxicity is less likely with concentrations below 100 μmol/L in adults and children, and seizures due to phenytoin are usually associated with concentrations above this figure. However, it should be remembered that some patients will require serum concentrations above 80 μmol/L to achieve satisfactory control. Due consideration should be given to the general clinical picture before a definitive recommendation on phenytoin dosage may be made.

Digoxin

A number of clinical studies have demonstrated that there is a significant difference between the mean values of digoxin concentrations in patients with and without toxicity,[8] and most workers prefer to maintain the steady-state concentration of digoxin between 1.3 and 2.6 nmol/L. Within this range there is undoubtedly a variable response. The positive inotropic effect begins at low concentrations, which increases as the digoxin concentration increases. The usual range for the inotropic effect is 1.3–2.0 nmol/L, whereas chronotropic effects are seen at concentrations greater than 2.0 nmol/L. Furthermore, some patients will tolerate higher concentrations, and may require up to 3.5 nmol/L to be adequately controlled.

In general there is therefore a reasonable relation between the digoxin concentration in plasma and its therapeutic effect. It must be appreciated that, because of the nature of the target range, some patients may develop toxic symptoms when the digoxin concentration approaches 2.0 nmol/L. Toxicity is virtually certain, however, in all patients above 3.8 nmol/L.[9]

Theophylline

The relation between the drug concentration of theophylline and its clinical effect, for example, has been studied extensively and the range of 55–110 μmol/L has been widely used as the reference range. However, recent reports suggest that definite clinical improvement may well be obtained at concentrations below 110 μmol/L. On the other hand, theophylline toxicity is closely linked with concentrations exceeding 140 μmol/L.[10]

Lithium

The target range for lithium in which optimum benefit occurs has been revised over the years. A number of recent studies reviewing long-term therapy have suggested a reference range of 0.9–1.2 mmol/L in acute mania and a lower range of 0.6–0.9 mmol/L as prophylactic therapy in other illnesses.[11] The target range should be tailored to the condition being treated.

Free-drug Measurement

It should be appreciated that the target range is calculated as total drug, that is, both protein bound and free drug. There are a number of situations where the bound fraction is displaced, leading to an increase in the free fraction. In these cases, although the concentration of total drug may not alter, the therapeutic effect may increase because of the altered ratio of bound to free drug. Some workers advocate measurements on saliva to determine the free concentration, as in most circumstances, saliva is a fair estimate of the free fraction. It is, however, a poor substitute for actual plasma free-drug measurements, although salivary measurements do have their value for difficult children, where venesection can be a particularly traumatic experience.

Criteria for Measurement

In addition to the above criteria for selecting drugs for regular measurement, others exist. The following criteria represent current thinking in the application of routine TDM:

- The drug should have a constant and reversible action at the receptor site.
- The concentration of total drug in blood should reflect the concentration of free (unbound) drug at the receptor site and the pharmacological effect should be proportional to this concentration.
- The drug should have a narrow therapeutic ratio.
- The drug should have a specific and suitable assay.
- The drug demonstrates interpatient pharmacokinetic variability.
- The drug has adequate pharmacokinetic data avail-

able from which suitable interpretation can be made regarding a given drug concentration.
- The drug has sufficient clinical data to define the target and toxic ranges.

The number of drugs that fulfil most of the criteria and as such are ideal candidates for inclusion into TDM programmes is small (Table 45.2). The selection is further hampered by the controversy that exists between those on the one extreme who question the value of TDM and those on the other extreme, notably the manufacturers of diagnostic kits, who encourage a wider drug involvement in TDM. The dilemma is undoubtedly fuelled by the lack of carefully controlled trials and well-documented evidence of correlations between concentration and therapeutic effect.

Drug Choice

The choice of drug for TDM is limited because there are only a few drugs for which unequivocable target concentrations have been established; this indicates the fairly rigorous prerequisites that determine whether the target range for a particular drug does relate to clinical effect.

The controversial drugs for inclusion in a TDM programme include sodium valproate. Certainly, there is no correlation between valproate dose and serum concentration (Fig. 45.1), even on an mg/kg basis, but its therapeutic effect is dependent on the type of epilepsy being treated, so that the value of monitoring may be restricted to the detection of patient compliance. Other controversial drugs include clonazepam and primidone; the tricyclic antidepressants such as imipramine, amitriptyline and clomipramine; amikacin; other antiarrhythmics such as verapamil and mexiletine; and caffeine. Here, measurement may or may not be useful and more studies are needed to confirm the usefulness of TDM for these drugs.

Paracetamol and salicylate estimations, although mainly requested for toxicological purposes, need also be considered, especially salicylate, which should be monitored when given to children to treat rheumatoid disease.

The actual range of drugs measured by a particular centre will vary. The range requested at the author's hospital in 1990 is illustrated in Fig. 45.2. The percentage of measurements has not changed significantly during the last 10 years of that hospital's involvement in TDM, with the exception of the emergence of carbamazepine as the major anticonvulsant and the decrease in the use of phenobarbitone. The small number of other drugs (about 2%) also constitutes a changing variety. For example, cyclosporin, amiodarone and vancomycin were measured in 1990 and methotrexate, primidone and disopyramide in 1980.

TABLE 45.2
LIST OF DRUGS AVAILABLE FOR THERAPEUTIC DRUG MONITORING TOGETHER WITH DETAILS OF THEIR TARGET RANGE AND DETAILS FOR COLLECTION

Drug	Ideal sampling time	Target range	Resampling time (days)
Anticonvulsants			
Carbamazepine	Pre-dose	17–32 μmol/L (in combination)	1–10
		34–51 μmol/L (as single drug)	1–10
Phenytoin	Any time	40–80 μmol/L	7–10
Phenobarbitone	Any time	40–130 μmol/L	14
Cardiac drugs			
Amiodarone	Pre-dose	0.8–4.6 μmol/L	14
Digoxin	At least 6 h post-dose	0.9–2.6 nmol/L	7
Bronchodilators			
Theophylline	Pre-dose or during infusion	55–110 μmol/L (children and adults)	1–2
		33–66 μmol/L (neonates)	3–4
Immunosuppressants and cytotoxics			
Cyclosporin	Pre-dose	50–250 μg/L	2–4
Methotrexate	24 h post-dose	< 2.2 μmol/L	
Antibiotics			
Gentamicin	Pre- and 1 h post-dose	4–10 mg/L (peak)	1
		< 1.5 mg/L (trough)	
Vancomycin	Pre- and 3 h post-dose	30–40 mg/L (peak)	2
		5–10 mg/L (trough)	
Central-acting drugs			
Lithium	12–18 h post dose	0.5–1.2 mmol/L	4–5
Nortriptyline	Any time	190–540 nmol/L	7

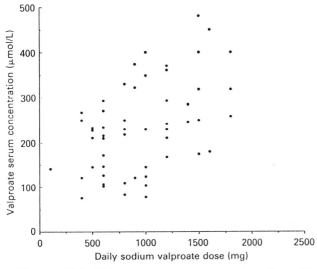

Figure 45.1 Valproate serum concentrations from 57 patients (taken at least 4 h post-dose) receiving varying doses of sodium valproate.

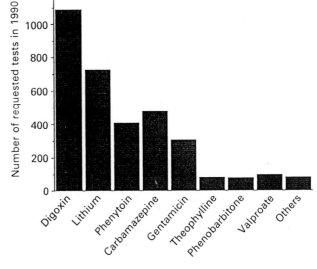

Figure 45.2 Number of requests received by a Therapeutic Drug Monitoring Service during 1990 in a district general hospital.

Indications for Drug Measurement

TDM is demanding and some of its applications are irrelevant. It is important, therefore, to be aware of indications for drug measurement, for we must not measure for the sake of measuring. However, it must be said that some levels are requested in order that the clinician may 'feel better', and who is to say that this is not a valid reason—judiciously used!

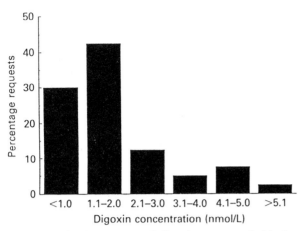

Figure 45.3 Percentage of digoxin requests (with the measured concentration) in 98 patients diagnosed as having possible digoxin toxicity.

During the auditing of TDM services, the main indications for drug measurement are those outlined below. Other reasons are of doubtful benefit.

Patient Compliance

The assessment of compliance traditionally uses close questioning of the patient or, in the case of clinical trials, some form of tablet counting. Both of these methods are inaccurate. As TDM has become more widely used, it has proved a popular way of detecting compliance. Many may feel, however, that this method is expensive; but provided that measurement is possible, it is reliable, and when the cost of the treatment itself and the costs of non-compliance are taken into account, it may prove not all that expensive ... Of particular relevance are those patients who are non-compliant whilst in the community, but, in hospital, may become toxic because of regular compliance. In these cases, a random estimation may be of value. Elderly people are particularly vulnerable to non-compliance, especially when the number of drugs prescribed is considerable.

An interesting development in this field has been the incorporation of a small quantity of an easily measurable compound into the drug being administered. Phenobarbitone, in very low doses of 2 mg, has been used extensively for this purpose, and a relation between the dose and plasma concentration can be used as a marker of non-compliance. Phenobarbitone has little variability in steady-state concentrations among individuals and minimal fluctuation throughout the day. It is suggested that this method is more sensitive than others available.

Diagnosis and Confirmation of Drug Intoxication

In some cases it is impossible to distinguish between symptoms of overdosage and those due to undertreatment. Phenytoin is particularly difficult and in many patients fitting has been observed with plasma concentrations of over 120 μmol/L. Plasma concentrations of the antidepressant nortriptyline that exceed 650 nmol/L cause increased depression. In addition, persistently high plasma concentrations of a drug may lead to a slow onset of toxic symptoms (e.g. lithium). Digoxin is another example, where an increase in the pulse rate may not necessarily reflect inadequate treatment. A survey of requests at the author's hospital for digoxin measurement where digoxin toxicity was specifically considered demonstrated a significant number (30%) of concentrations below 1.0 nmol/L (Fig. 45.3). It is assumed that these patients were not toxic. Potassium concentrations were all normal; thyroid status was not documented. The number of requests querying toxicity was approximately 11% of the total number of requests. The results demonstrate the difficulty in determining digoxin toxicity.

The only valid way to make the differential diagnosis of drug intoxication is to measure the blood concentration. If it is excessively high, the dose needs to be withheld. Too often these effects are unrecognized and the patient is treated with another drug to control the iatrogenic disease.

Multiple Drug Therapy

Many tables exist listing probable drug interactions. Most are predictable and the need for drug measurement is unnecessary. However, previously unreported drug interactions are constantly being detected, and when these involve drugs that can be measured it is essential to monitor the interaction to avoid potential toxicity.

Two recent important examples are worth mentioning. The plasma concentration of digoxin may be increased by as much as 70% in patients when large doses of erythromycin, for example 500 mg four times daily, are given concurrently. Not all patients are affected in the same way, although a similar interaction has been observed at the author's hospital, with the result that the patient became clinically toxic. The elimination half-life measured in this patient was similar to published values. It is thought that reduced intestinal metabolism in some patients may be the reason for increased digoxin concentrations. Other drugs causing more predictable increases in digoxin concentrations include amiodarone, high doses of verapamil, and quinidine.

A second case report highlighted the interaction between phenytoin and metronidazole. Again, this is an unpredictable interaction leading to significantly higher phenytoin concentrations, which in turn may result in phenytoin toxicity. It would appear that metronidazole causes enzyme inhibition of phenytoin, and that this effect may reflect the length of time the two drugs are given together. As this is an unpredictable interaction it is important to monitor phenytoin concentrations.

Altered Disease or Physiological States

It goes without saying that alterations in renal or hepatic function will affect the elimination of some drugs. Those with a narrow therapeutic index, such as digoxin or gentamicin, are particularly sensitive to changes in renal function. Drug measurement is therefore indicated in changing organ function. Pregnancy also alters drug disposition.

Inadequate Therapeutic Response

A patient may fail to respond to therapy for a number of reasons (such as delayed absorption) and a drug-concentration estimation may help to eliminate one area of doubt. An interesting case was highlighted recently with the use of intranasal feeding. The dose of phenytoin syrup had to be increased to 800 mg daily, well above the normal therapeutic dose, before reasonable amounts of phenytoin were absorbed as measured by TDM, and before the patient felt better. All prior efforts made to increase absorption, such as altering the timing of administration to avoid giving it at the same time as liquid food intake and washing the syrup through the tube with plenty of liquid, did not overcome the problem.

Methods of Measurement

The various methods involved in drug measurement have changed significantly over the last 20 years so that measurement has been greatly simplified. This is largely the result of the development of the immunoassay technique, which, because of its sensitivity and ease of use, was readily adapted for drug measurement. Development of the more traditional chromatographic techniques, such as high-pressure liquid chromatography and gas–liquid chromatography, has been less dramatic.

The early immunoassay techniques were based on phase separation, and it was not until the advent of non-isotopic homogenous assays, which became commercially available and were exploited by Syva® 'as EMIT®, that the method had a real impact. Interestingly, this initiative coincided with an accelerated interest in TDM, which enabled the discipline to become important in its own right. Because the expertise associated with the measurements tended to reside in clinical biochemistry laboratories, drug measurement, and for some this meant TDM, became established in the laboratory. As a result, many other manufacturers entered the field, presenting an array of different kits and methods to the clinical chemistry laboratory as the ultimate in TDM. This trend has continued unabated, but one hopes that cost-conscious monitoring will bring some order to the market.

DOSE INDIVIDUALIZATION

As drug effects are related to plasma concentration and are influenced by pharmacokinetic processes, it follows that the application of kinetic data to an individual patient will reduce some of the differences in drug response. The utilization of population data

in pharmacokinetics describes this variability in terms of factors that are called *fixed* or *random effects*. Fixed effects are the population average values of pharmacokinetic variables, and are a function of patient characteristics, underlying disease and pharmacological considerations. The random effects quantify the residual variability arising from the differences between patients. Both effects require consideration and a number of approaches have been described to apply population data to interpret or construct individual dose regimens.

Population Data

Population data are essential for most of the techniques to individualize drug doses and may be obtained in different ways. Most estimations are obtained from single-dose pharmacokinetic studies, and journals are replete with these. A disadvantage is that the majority of studies involve healthy volunteers and some form of extrapolation to patients is required. This may be especially so for the elderly.[12] Another method involves measurements during steady-state conditions, following multiple doses, where useful information may also be obtained provided that samples are taken at known and specific times during a dosing interval. Data may then be analysed using linear correlation or using non-linear models, such as NONMEM®, a program that needs a mainframe computer and a certain amount of expertise to run.

Dose Individualization Techniques

The methods described for dose individualization range from the manipulation of standard pharmacokinetic equations and clearance models, to predictive algorithms and nomograms, to methods that incorporate complex mathematical principles. In particular, the Bayesian technique is the most popular of the mathematical methods and requires computerized techniques to arrive at a result.

Simple Kinetic Formulae

Most drugs exhibit so-called one- or two-compartment elimination. Kinetic formulae can be constructed to predict either the steady-state concentration, the maximum concentration, or the minimum concentration following doses at steady state. Some of these calculations can be done manually and are relatively easy. Nevertheless, it may be more convenient to use computer programs to predict the concentrations. Various programs have been developed and are available. A popular one was the Sharp minicomputer, which is small enough to be carried about. It can therefore be taken on the wards, which has obvious attractions. Nevertheless, its use was limited and it is not now available.

Although population kinetic data such as elimination half-life can be used in the various formulae, the variability due to kinetic, pathophysiological and considerations and drug interactions needs to be carefully considered. A value of a plasma concentration measurement for a given dose of drug can be used in one of the above formulae and the clearance calculated and the drug concentration can be assessed. The following assumptions have been made:

- the systemic availability remains constant;
- enzyme's stimulation or (inhibition) provides different estimates of steady state;
- metabolism remains linear over the dose range employed.

In most cases, oral bioavailability remains constant in the dose ranges employed, although the new drug cisapride is a notable exception. Enzyme induction, however, may occur with increasing doses. For example, carbamazepine induces its own metabolism and drug clearance increases from a value of about 0.6 L/h per kg to 1.0 L/h per kg over an initial 3- to 4-week period. For this reason, measurement of carbamazepine plasma concentrations should not be made until at least 4 weeks after the start of therapy.

The metabolism of most drugs is linear over normal dose ranges; however, there are a number of exceptions. Phenytoin exhibits non-linear kinetics over a wide dose range and theophylline may exhibit non-variability at high doses. The consequences of these kinetics are that after discontinuing dosing, for example, the fall in phenytoin concentration is initially zero order and only later becomes first order. For a patient with concentrations above the target range and subsequent toxicity, it may take a significant time after the cessation of therapy for acceptable non-toxic levels to be reached. This may also occur with high concentrations of theophylline. Second, changing the drug input high dose for a time will lead to a disproportionate change in the average steady-state concentration. This occurs primarily with phenytoin across a wide range of concentrations and has been well documented.

Using kinetic formulae for dose prediction is valuable when interpreting results from TDM. It is limited, however, by the inaccuracies of individual pharmacokinetic variables from population data estimates of these used in the calculations.

Nomograms and Algorithms

This approach is to use nomograms based on population data and many types have been produced. For example, gentamicin interpretation can be made by at least five different published nomograms—Mawer,[13] Chan,[14] Hull–Surubbi,[15] and Dettli.[16] There are others. When these were compared as a group, dose predictions based on those nomograms produced initial gentamicin peak and trough levels that were therapeutic in a maximum of only 57% of cases.[17]

The nomogram published by Richens and Dunlop[18] is a popular one for phenytoin and has proved useful.

Another approach is to use data generated from patients taking a single dose, measuring the concentration at a fixed time-point afterwards and correlating that concentration with a subsequent concentration taken during steady-state conditions. This is termed the *single-point method* and has been used for a number of drugs. The dose of lithium was individualized using this technique in a group of 20 patients, which produced predictions of steady-state lithium concentrations within 0.2 mmol/L of the actual concentration in 85% of the cases.[19]

Feed-back Mechanisms

Most instances of population-data usage are in the interpretation of analytically generated patient data during TDM. Most practitioners would compare predicted and measured concentrations using simple kinetic formulae as above. However, the more sophisticated techniques using Bayesian feedback mechanisms are popular provided the computer hardware is readily available. These methods rely on initial population data being revised in the light of one or more subsequent blood measurements. Various computer programs are available for general use, such as OPT,[20] Abbottbase (Abbott Diagnostics, Chicago, USA), SIMKIN,[21] and MwPharm (Mediware, Groningen, Holland). However, these methods are time consuming, which is sometimes not appreciated, and are really best left for the difficult interpretations.

Methods in Practice

In spite of the availability of population data and techniques to use them, the TDM practitioner relies more on intuitive judgement and pharmacokinetic experience to make recommendations, and most patients' cases are probably solved in this way. Certainly there are many computer programs available for assessing pharmacokinetic data. However, although evaluations of the individual programs have been made, but very few comparative data are available and there is an obvious need to compare the various software packages that are available.

There has been an attempt by the newly formed Clinical Pharmacokinetics Society in the UK to assess the results obtained from artificially generated problems presented in their quarterly *Newsletter*. Unfortunately, the number of centres participating in this quality assessment scheme for interpretation has been disappointingly low. It is therefore essential that experiences gained during interpretation are communicated with other practitioners for, in spite of the variety of ways for interpretation that exist, there is a need to ensure that the final outcome is better patient care.

RECENT ADVANCES IN TDM

The number of new and developing innovative approaches for TDM has been small, but a few are worth reporting.

New Drugs

The number of new drugs offered for routine TDM is few. The two major drugs for which monitoring has been shown to be important are amiodarone and cyclosporin.

Amiodarone

Amiodarone is an antiarrhythmic drug that is effective in the treatment of a variety of broad spectrum of arrhythmias, often those that are life threatening and have proved refractory to other therapy. Its unusual pharmacokinetics and its potential to cause serious side-effects have led to attempts to relate its plasma concentrations to measures of clinical efficacy, in an effort to optimize therapy. In adults the elimination half-life is over 50 days, and this can result in a slow onset of efficacy, so that normally a loading dose is given over a period of 1 week. Furthermore, it is strongly protein bound and has a wide volume of distribution.

The data relating to clinical efficacy show a poor correlation between antiarrhythmic efficacy and plasma concentrations of the drug and its metabolite desethylamiodarone. This is probably due to the wide spectrum of arrhythmias that respond to the drug, which in turn results in a wide range of concentrations that are able to suppress the arrhythmia. In the main, few arrhythmias will respond to drug concentrations of below 1.0 mg/L and it would appear that concentrations above 3.0 mg/L are associated with an increased risk of serious adverse effects.

Assessment of the ratio of the parent drug to its metabolite is also useful, especially because the analytical method normally used measures both drug and metabolite. During chronic therapy the ratio is close to unity. If the ratio is significantly greater than unity, it can increase the confidence with which non-compliance may be suspected.

Is measurement of amiodarone an important new addition to TDM? Certainly, there are substantial between-patient differences in the amount of drug absorbed, owing to its variable bioavailability, and this indeed is most easily assessed through measurement. However, its long half-life makes dose titration difficult. Interpretation of the result must therefore reflect the extended time that must exist between dose adjustments.

Cyclosporin

This is another new drug for which measurement is clearly indicated. However, although there is a vast amount of literature describing different methods of analysis for the drug, little useful information on the correlation between efficacy and plasma concentration is available.

The establishment of a therapeutic target range for steady-state concentration has been hindered by the many different assays available for cyclosporin. Some have suggested that whole-blood cyclosporin concentrations of below 300 μg/L are infrequently associated with toxicity in renal grafts. However, healthy kidneys may be able to tolerate higher concentrations of up to 450 μg/L. The concentrations for hepatotoxicity are not clearly established. Organ rejection is less common when whole-blood concentrations are greater than 100 μg/L. Other workers have suggested a reference range for renal transplant patients of whole-blood concentrations between 350 and 400 μg/L, as measured by immunoassay techniques using a monoclonal antibody. Nevertheless, this target range needs to be adjusted when the risk of nephrotoxicity is increased and where there is an increased risk of rejection. If TDM is not to fall into disrepute through this drug, then good prospective studies are essential in defining a good target range.

Other Drugs

Indications for monitoring other drugs are limited. A number of new assays have been developed for drugs in current use, and have been used to monitor their usefulness. For example, morphine and its metabolites are the subject of a recent study, as is 6-mercaptopurine. Their usefulness, however, is limited. The same is true for vigabatrin, a recently introduced antiepileptic agent. A convenient analytical method for this drug has been developed by workers at HeathControl. It is disappointing to observe that of the requests sent in to that centre, a large proportion (greater than 95%) were incompletely documented.

Diagnostic Procedures

A recent study has established that the formation rate of the lignocaine metabolite monoethylglyinexylide in patients who are potential organ donors is correlated with the viability of the donor organ in terms of transplant survival in the recipient.[22]

Near-patient Testing

Immobilization of the key reagents on to a solid matrix has resulted in a further simplification of analytical techniques. These methods (e.g. Acculevel®, ARIS®) require only the addition of analyte in the sample to activate the whole analytical process, and have enabled pharmacists to take a more active interest in TDM analysis. The main advantage of these simpler systems is their amenability to near-patient testing and the rapid production of results. The need for rapid results from TDM is far from obvious. The desire for speed must be weighed against the reliability of results, and more importantly their cost and the ability to interpret them. Thus, in an epilepsy clinic, where it is certainly useful to have the results immediately, does the combination of a pharmacist to interpret the results, an analyst to process the sample and the clinician to act upon it, make the cost somewhat high?

QUALITY CONTROL IN TDM

Control of both the analysis and of the interpretation is necessary for proper drug monitoring procedures. Both aspects need controlling. Whereas control of drug analysis is commonplace, TDM auditing is still in its infancy.

External Quality Control of Drug Analysis

In the early days of pharmacokinetic analysis, the need for assay precision was not readily apparent and carry-over samples provided some control. When results were compared between different laboratories it was assumed that each assay was measuring equivalent values. However, on the whole this was never investigated. It was not until the advent of routine TDM, when samples from a common pool were distributed to different laboratories, that the wide variation in results was revealed. Because of the wide spread of results observed, national external quality assessment schemes for drugs were started. These schemes enabled samples to be sent to participating laboratories and the results compared by the organizers. The results of the analysis and their statistical interpretation were then returned to each laboratory. The introduction of these schemes has undoubtedly led to an improvement in the quality of the work offered by participating laboratories, together with the more rigorous control by manufacturers. All laboratories involved in pharmacokinetic monitoring should be in at least one of these external schemes, as it is important to stress that differences in results which occur are not always appreciated by those using packaged immunoassay analytical analyses.

On the whole, results from the different methods are now comparable. A recent study from Italy[23,24] concluded that the variation in digoxin measurement is less satisfactory than with theophylline and the anticonvulsants. The between-laboratory variation for the anticonvulsant drugs and theophylline was between 6.6 and 24.1% at clinically relevant concentrations and there was good agreement in the results from the Syva EMIT® and the Abbott TDX® methods. For digoxin the figures for the variation were 11.4–46.9% for concentrations between 0.3–6.7 nmol/L. These data are similar to the results obtained from the Guildford EQAS for digoxin, where the variation is between 9.0–40.0% for a mean concentration of 0.5–3.3 nmol/L (Fig. 45.4). However, if the very low digoxin values (< 0.7 nmol/L) are omitted from both ranges, the coefficient of variation is significantly reduced to under 23%, and is

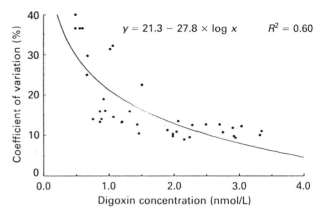

Figure 45.4 Correlation of the mean digoxin concentrations (nmol/L) from 36 samples distributed to 50 laboratories over 12 months, with the coefficient of variation of the mean (%).

then comparable with other analytes. The conclusion of these results is that the choice of a particular chromatographic method or immunoassay kit is governed by management and economic considerations and is consequently based on sample throughput, availability of equipment and of trained personnel, rather than with strict regard to the accuracy and precision of the measurements obtained.

In the UK there are external quality-assurance schemes for most of the drugs measured in TDM. Normally, samples are prepared by spiking with pure drug into human serum. Samples are sent out at intervals for assay each month (usually three samples per month). The main schemes together with their organizers and phone numbers in the UK are in Table 45.3.

TDM Audit

The quality of formalized TDM services is being widely studied in the USA. One method of monitoring has included assessing the quality of the interpretation provided by the service. This has been achieved by reviewing information records from the TDM service at monthly intervals and comparing these with a number of objective criteria that were approved by the local pharmacy and therapeutics committee. The criteria assessed volumes of service, documentation, correct use of calculations, choice of target peak and trough concentrations, renal function monitoring, incidence of drug-related toxic symptoms, and outcome data from the physician's progress notes. The results are summarized in a trend report and corrective actions may be taken. This has led to improved documentation. Another team evaluated the quality of their service by auditing dosing guidelines and the accuracy of pharmacokinetic calculations.

Very few studies have been conducted to ascertain the quality of existing TDM services in the UK.[25] A

TABLE 45.3

QUALITY ASSESSMENT SCHEMES IN THE UK FOR DRUGS USED IN TDM

Drug	Assessment scheme	Organizer(s)
Digoxin	Guildford EQAS	Dr G. Mould 0483 571122 ext. 2241
Antiepileptic drugs Respiratory drugs Antidepressant drugs	HeathControl EQAS	Cardiff Bioanalytical Services Ltd 0222 223357; 0222 372311
Gentamicin Vancomycin	National Antibiotic Scheme	Dr G. Snell 081-200 4400 ext. 3913
Cyclosporin	St George's EQAS	Dr D. Holt 081-767 9686

number of mechanisms exist for measuring the quality of service and these include quality audits, continuous assessments, surveys, peer review and feedback systems. A recent survey has shown that clinical pharmacokinetic services have increased the appropriateness of the measurement of serum digoxin concentrations from 44% where no service existed to 74% following active participation.[26] Another mechanism is that of performance indicators or measures of performance. These can be developed from continuous assessments and are usually objective measures of quality. These types of audit are necessary to demonstrate the usefulness of TDM.

CONCLUSION

It is now a number of years since the onset of TDM. The initial enthusiasm for the discipline has given way to a certain amount of pessimism regarding its future. This is probably due more to the fact that few additional drugs have been made available for monitoring. Thus, the expansion in drug measurement that was anticipated has not materialized. However, this period of stabilization may be beneficial, if only to provide time to re-emphasize the fact that proper documentation and accurate interpretation for good TDM are essential. Once this is fully appreciated, then the discipline has a stronger base from which to move forward.

REFERENCES

1. Klamerus K.J., Munger M.A. (1988). Effect of clinical pharmacy services on the appropriateness of serum digoxin concentration monitoring. *Am. J. Hosp. Pharm.*, **45**, 1887.
2. Tjia J.F., Webber I.R., Back D.J. (1991). Cyclosporin metabolism by the gastrointestinal mucosa. *Br. J. Clin. Pharmacol.*, **31**, 344.
3. Sachdeo R.C., Belendiuk G. (1987). Generic versus branded carbamazepine. *Lancet*, **ii**, 1432.
4. Wyllie E., Pippenger C.E., Rothner A.D. (1987). Increased seizure frequency with generic primidone. *J. Am. Med. Assoc.*, **258**, 1216.
5. Nightingale S.L., Morrison J.C. (1987). Generic drugs and the prescribing physician. *J. Am. Med. Assoc.*, **258**, 1200.
6. Lewis R.V., Ramsay L.E., Jackson P.R., Yeo W.W., Lennard M.S., Tucker G.T. (1991). Influence of debrisoquine oxidation phenotype on exercise tolerance and subjective fatigue after metoprolol and atenolol in healthy subjects. *Br. J. Clin. Pharmacol.*, **31**, 391.
7. Buchthal F., Svensmark O., Schiller P.J. (1960). Clinical and electroencephalographic correlations with serum levels of diphenylhydantoin. *Arch. Neurol.*, **2**, 624.
8. Aronson J.K., Grahame-Smith D.G., Wigley F.M. (1978). Monitoring digoxin therapy. *Q. J. Med.*, **186**, 111.
9. Lee T.H., Smith T.W. (1983). Serum digoxin concentration and diagnosis of digitalis toxicity. *Clin. Pharmacocokinet.*, **8**, 279.
10. Chrystyn H., Mulley B.A., Peake M.D. (1988). Dose response relation to oral theophylline in severe chronic obstructive airways diseases. *Br. Med. J.*, **297**, 1506.
11. Schou M. (1988). Serum lithium monitoring of prophylactic treatment. Critical review and updated measurements. *Clin. Pharmacokinet.*, **15**, 283.
12. Thompson A.H., Tucker G.T. (1992). Gerontokinetics—a reappraisal. *Br. J. Clin. Pharmacol.*, **33**, 1.
13. Mawer G.E., Ahmad R., Dobbs S.M., McGough J.G., Lucas S.B., Tooth J.A. (1974). Prescribing aids for gentamicin. *Br. J. Clin. Pharmacol.*, **1**, 45.
14. Chan R.A., Benner E.J., Hoeprich P.D. (1972). Gentamicin therapy in renal failure. *Ann. Intern. Med.*, **76**, 773.
15. Hull J.H., Surubbi F.A. (1976). Gentamicin serum concentrations: pharmacokinetic predictions. *Ann. Intern. Med.*, **85**, 183.
16. Dettli L.C. (1974). Drug dosage in patients with renal failure. *Clin. Pharmacol. Ther.*, **16**, 274.
17. Thomson A.H., Campbell K.C., Kelman A.W. (1990). Evaluation of six gentamicin nomograms using a Bayesian parameter estimation program. *Ther. Drug Monitoring*, **12**, 258.
18. Richens A., Dunlop A. (1975). Serum phenytoin levels in the management of epilepsy. *Lancet*, **ii**, 247.
19. Browne J.L., Huffman C.S., Golden R.N. (1989). A comparison of pharmacokinetic versus empirical

lithium dosing techniques. *Ther. Drug Monitoring*, **11**, 149.

20. Whiting B., Kelman A.W., Bryson S.W. (1982). OPT: a package of computer programs for computer optimisation in clinical pharmacokinetics. *Br. J. Clin. Pharmacol.*, **14**, 247.

21. Ginery J.W., Embil A.S., Robinson D.J., Jernigan J.A. (1987). Serum phenobarbital concentration predictions by a personal computer software system. *Ann. Pharmacother. DIC*, **21**, 895.

22. Ollerich M., Burdelski M., Lautz H.-U., Schulz M., Schmidt F.-W., Herrman H. (1990). Lidocaine metabolite formation as a measure of liver function in patients with cirrhosis. *Ther. Drug Monitoring*, **12**, 219.

23. Clinical Pharmacology and Toxicology Study Group, Italian Society for Clinical Biochemistry. (1991). Interlaboratory variability in drug assay: a comparison of quality control data with reanalysis of routine patient samples. I. Anticonvulsant drugs and theophylline. *Ther. Drug Monitoring*, **13**, 131.

24. Clinical Pharmacology and Toxicology Study Group, Italian Society for Clinical Biochemistry. (1991). Interlaboratory variability in drug assay: a comparison of quality control data with reanalysis of routine patient samples. II. Digoxin. *Ther. Drug Monitoring*, **13**, 140.

25. Hallworth M.J. (1988). Audit of therapeutic drug monitoring. *Ann. Clin. Biochem.*, **25**, 121.

26. Mould G.P., Marks V. (1987). An audit of digoxin serum concentration monitoring. *Br. J. Clin. Pharmacol.*, **23**, 138P.

Index

Abetalipoproteinaemia, 296
Abdomen, acute *See Acute abdomen*
Abdominal pain, 400
  acute, 399 *See also Acute abdomen*
  causes of, 402
  in paroxysmal nocturnal
    haemoglobinuria, 461
  in porphyrias, 416
Abortion, 552
Acanthocytosis, 297
Acetaldehyde, 136
Acetate,
  alcohol oxidation and, 136
Acetazolamide, 46
Acetoacetyl-CoA thiolase deficiency,
  282
Acetylcholine,
  in Alzheimer's disease, 148
  in depression, 148
Acetyl coenzyme A in injury, 194
Achlorydria, 351
Acid-base balance,
  after shock or trauma, 197
  potassium and, 780
Acidosis, 41–49
  causes, 39
  causing hyperkalaemia, 72
  effect of, 41
  hypoxic lactic, 42
  lactic, 43
  metabolic, 34, 41, 44
    hyperchloraemia and, 45
    inborn errors causing, 46
  renal tubular, 41
  respiratory, 46
Acidurias,
  diagnosis, 241
  mental retardation and, 254
  organic, 279
AIDS, 572,
  incidence of, 246
  malabsorption in, 374
Acrodermatitis enteropathica, 21
Acredynia, 730
Acromegaly, 523, 541, 630, 678, 693
Activated partial thromboplastin time
  test, 506
Acute abdomen,
  in children, 401
  clinical diagnosis, 399–408
  clinical examination, 401
  differential diagnosis, 402
  history taking, 400
  medical conditions simulating, 407
  palpation in, 401
  special investigations, 402
  steps in diagnosis, 400
Acute-phase reactant proteins, 479,
  480
Acute tubular necrosis, 334
  potassium loss in, 71
Acyl CoA:cholesterol -acyl-

transferase, 602
Acyl-CoA dehydrogenase deficiencies,
  258, 282, 283, 298
Acyl-CoA derivatives, 281
Addison-Schilder disease, 696
Addison's disease, 95, 158, 333, 551,
  588, 692, 694
  causes of, 694
  depression in, 145, 151
  diagnostic tests, 696
  hyperkalaemia in, 72
  presentation, 696
  treatment, 696
  water retention in, 64
Adenosine deaminase test, 572
Adenosine 3,5-phosphate, 190
Adenylsuccinate deficiency, 288
Adipsia, 96, 98, 101
Adrenal cortex,
  destruction of, 694
  disorders of, 681–706
  dynamic tests of function, 691
  fetal, 684
  function, 694
  steroids, *See Adrenal steroids*
Adrenal cytochrome P450, 703
Adrenal gland,
  adenoma, 699
  anatomy, 681
  androgen secretion, 690
  bilateral nodular hyperplasia, 699
  carcinoma, 699
  cortex *See Adrenal cortex*
  medulla, 681
  virilizing tumours, 704
Adrenal hyperplasia,
  congenital, 590, 701, 716
    screening, 250
  nodular, 699
Adrenal steroids,
  actions of, 687
  biosynthesis, 682
    in fetal cortex, 684
    inhibitors of, 684
    pathways, 685
  blood spot, 691
  in calcium metabolism, 524
  circulating levels, 688
  classification, 682
  electrolytes in colon and, 85
  long-term replacement therapy, 697
  measurement, 690
    in urine, 691
  metabolism and excretion, 68
  metabolites, 687
  nomenclature, 682, 683
  potencies, 688
  production, 684
  salivary, 691
  secretion, 689
  therapy, 688
Adrenal tumours,
  causing aldosteronism, 594
Adrenaline,
  conversion from noradrenaline, 681
  iron metabolism and, 157

metabolism, 597
  in phaeochromocytoma, 151
Adrenocortical insufficiency *See
  Addison's disease*
Adrenocorticotrophic hormone, 623,
  624, 625, 631
  in Addison's disease, 151
  aldosterone synthesis and, 588
  in Cushing's syndrome, 697, 698
  ectopic syndrome, 170, 684, 694,
    698
    in Cushing's syndrome, 687, 698,
      699
  hypoglycaemia and secretion of, 629
  in hypopituitarism, 152
  neoplasia causing, 698
  release following injury, 191
  in stress, 150
  stimulation tests, 692
Adrenoleucodystrophies, 158, 271, 696
Adult GM$_2$ gangliosidosis, 158
Adult respiratory distress syndrome,
  190
Age,
  mineral loss in, 518
Alaninaemia, 277
Alanine aminotransferase, 386
  monitoring in transplantation, 212
Albumin, 464, 483
  assessment of loss, 363
  bilirubin binding, 308, 384
  in disease, 484
  electrophoresis, 488
  excretion, 118
  following trauma, 194
  function, 483
  genetic variations, 484
  in liver disease, 390
  in protein energy malnutrition, 10
  synthesis, 390
  unconjugated bilirubin binding to,
    263
  in urine, 319
Alcohol, 121–143
  absorption, 121
  action on brain, 154
  acute intoxication, 123
  affecting plasma osmolality, 123
  breath analysis, 123
  causing brain damage, 126
  causing cell damage, 122
  clinical biochemistry of, 121
  dependency, 126
    definition, 121
  effect on liver, 130, 132
  excess, 121, 124–137 *See also
    Alcoholism*
    acute, 129
    definition, 121
    enzyme activity in, 122, 128
    factors predisposing, 124
    genetic factors, 125
    identification, 126, 128, 137
  excretion, 121
  GGT and, 128, 129
  inducing hyperlipidaemia, 133

isotransferrins, 133
liver cirrhosis and, 129, 131
MCV and, 130
macrocytosis and, 130
measurement of, 127
metabolism, 121
minor haemoglobins and, 136
oxidation, 122, 136
p-hexosaminidase and, 132
plasma glutamate dehydrogenase and, 132
plasma transaminases and, 130, 131
poisoning, 745, 749
psychiatric aspects, 153
recent intake of, 127
in saliva, 123
salsolinol and, 136
urinary dolidhols and, 136
urinary excretion, 122, 123
withdrawal, 124, 153
Alcohol abuse *See Alcohol, excess*
Alcohol dehydrogenase, 122, 154, 348
Alcohol polymorphism, 125
Alcoholic black-outs, 153
Alcoholic bone disease, 139
Alcoholic myopathy, 139
Alcoholism
    adhehyde dehydrogenase polymorphism and, 125
    biochemical test abnormalities in, 138
    cardiomyopathy in, 139
    causing Cushing's syndrome, 701
    clinical features, 127
    complications of, 138
    definition, 121
    disease complications, 127
    early signs of, 127
    enzyme ratios in, 131
    fatty liver and, 130
    glutaric acid and, 135
    growth hormone and, 633
    hepatic enzyme induction and, 136
    IgA concentrations and, 132
    ketoacidosis in, 140
    lipid abnormaslities and, 132
    liver disease in, 396
    muscle disease in, 139
    pancreatitis and, 406
    pellagra in, 17
    plasma proteins in, 132
    predisposing factors, 125
    state markers, 127
    transferrin index, 134
    treatment centres, 127
    uric acid in, 133
    vitamin B deficiency in, 16
Aldehyde dehydrogenase, 122
    polymorphism, 125
Aldolase deficiency, 309
Aldolase-C4 isoenzyme, 569
Aldosterone, 332, 682
    blood pressure and, 586
    deficiency, 73
    effect on sodium reabsorption, 56
    influencing potassium excretion, 69

potassium loss and, 71
production, 334, 587
renal effects of, 593
sodium retention from, 593
synthesis, 591, 684
tubular response to, 334
Aldosteronism, 593, 595
Alfacalcidol, 336
Alkali in ketoacidosis, 115
Alkaline Bohr effect, 424
Alkaline phosphatase, 387–389, 396, 530
    alcohol and, 130, 131
    causes of increase of, 389
    in liver disease, 387
    measurement, 387
    range in children, 293
Alkaline tide, 39
Alkalosis, 49–51
    causing hypokalaemia, 70
    effects of, 49
    metabolic, 48, 49
    post-prandial gastric secretion and, 39
    respiratory, 49, 50
Alkaptonuria, 323
Allergy, 472
Alpha fetoprotein, 486
    as marker for Down's syndrome, 234, 235
    as screening test, 232
    as tumour marker, 179
    clinical use of, 180
    low, 235
    measurement in liver disease, 392
    raised, 233
Aluminium, 723, 724
    physiology, 724
    toxicity, 335, 724 752
Alveolar dysfunction, 48
Alzheimer's disease, 288, 576
    acetylcholinesterase in, 575, 579
    biochemical aspects, 148
    depression in, 147
    immunology of, 575
Amenorrhoea, 171, 716
Amino acids,
    abnormal, in urine, 320
    activity in brain, 228, 581
    following trauma, 194
    in haemoglobin, 422
    in protein energy malnutrition, 7, 10
    RNA triplet code, 428
Aminoacidurias, 271–278
    mental retardation and, 278
    in neonates, 295
α-Amino-*n*-butyric acid:leucine ratio, 135
Aminoglutethimine, 684
Aminoglycosides,
    poisoning by, 747
5-Amino-imidazole carboxamide, 455
Aminolaevulate, 411
    formation of, 409
    toxic effects of, 416
    in urine, 409

5-Aminolaevulinate synthetase, 410
Aminopyrine removal and breath test, 393
Aminoterminal type III procollagen peptide, 618
Aminotransferases,
    in liver disease, 386
    measurement of, 385
Amiodarone, 759, 767
Amitriptyline poisoning, 740, 757
Ammonia,
    detoxification, 582
    effect on brain, 275
    in liver disease, 394
    metabolism, 275
    role in hepatic encephalopathy, 581
    toxicity, 582
    urinary,
        carbonate dehydratase and, 37
Ammonium chloride,
    metabolic acidosis and, 44
Ammonium ion,
    formation of, 37
Amniocentesis, 238
    dangers of, 233
    first trimester, 238
    problems of, 238
    second trimester, 238
    timing of, 234
Amniotic fluid cells,
    enzyme assay, 239
Amniotic fluid acetylcholinesterase, 232, 233
Amniotic fluid supernatant metabolism, 241
Amphetamine poisoning, 740
Amsterdam dwarfs, 256
Amylase, 367
    in diagnosis of pancreatitis, 368, 407
Amyloid, 487
Amyloidosis, 500
Amyotrophic lateral sclerosis, 724
Anaemias, 453–463
    aplastic, 453
        iron overload in, 451
    in blood dyscrasias, 461
    blood loss causing, 457
    in chronic renal failure, 336
    in Crohn's disease, 375
    diagnosis, 462
    Fanconi's, 288
    folate deficiency, 456
    from cancer, 179
    in G-6-P dehydrogenase deficiency, 251
    haemolytic, 457, 463
        congenital, 457
        haptoglobin in, 483
        unstable haemoglobins and, 431
    iron deficiency, 449, 450, 463, 490
        cobalt and, 22
        ferritin in, 449
    laboratory diagnosis, 463
    in malnutrition, 454
    megaloblastic, 18, 455, 463
    in myeloma, 462

oxygenation and, 424
pernicious, 155, 350, 351, 362, 456
    gastric carcinoma and, 456
in protein energy malnutrition, 11
in rheumatoid arthritis, 546, 548
sickle cell,
    simulating acute abdomen, 408
    tests for, 438
in systemic disease, 461
vitamin B_{12} deficiency, 454, 456
vitamin E and, 15
Anaesthesia,
    effect on gastric mobility, 221
Analbuminaemia, 484
Androgens, 710
    disorders of receptor, 714
    growth and, 303
    measurement of, 720
    production, 710
    secretion, 690, 712
    tissue insensitivity, 714
Androgen secreting tumours, 718
Aldosterone,
    secretion, 690
Anencephaly, 231, 232
Aneurysms,
    berry, 599
Angina pectoris, 619
Angiotensin,
    blood pressure and, 586
    conversion of, 334
Angiotensin-converting enzyme, 334
Angiotensin I, 84, 587
Angiotensin II, 84, 96, 587
Angiotensin III, 84
Angor amini, 151
Anorexia nervosa, 654, 717
Anion gap, 67
Anorexia, 221
    in marasmus, 3
Anoxia,
    mental consequences, 152
Anthropometry, 9
α_1Antichymotrypsin, 481, 482
    electrophoresis, 489
Anticonvulsant drugs,
    poisoning by, 747
    rickets and, 14
Antidiuretic hormone See Arginine
    vasopressin
Antidiuretic properties,
    drugs possessing, 90
AntiMullerian hormone, 712
Antinuclear antibodies 552
Antiplasmin, 504
Antithrombin III, 482
    assay of, 509
    biochemistry, 504
α_1Antitrypsin, 392
    clearance of, 363
    deficiency, 309
    in disease, 481
α_2Antitrypsin, 481
Anxiety, 148
Aorta, coarctation of, 590
Apgar score, 262

Aphoria, 16
Aplastic anaemia, 453
    iron overload in, 451
Apoferritin, 447
Apolipoprotein C, 483
Apotransferrin, 447
Appendicitis,
    acute, 399, 403–405
        in children, 403, 404
        differential diagnosis, 404
        investigation, 404
        radiography, 404
    investigation, 402
    perforation, 400
    ultrasonoraphy and laparoscopy,
        405
Appestat, 27
Appetite, 27, 221
APUD cells, 169, 520, 568
APUDomas, 678, 679, 699
Arachidonic acid cascade, 190
Arginase, 276
Arginine infection test, 630
Arginine vasopressin, (AVP), 54, 295,
        321, 621
    action on distal tubules, 87, 89
    amino acid sequence, 88
    blood pressure and, 588
    chemical structure, 88
        erratic release of, 174
    in syndrome of inappropriate
        antidiuresis, 172, 174
    in neonates, 306
    leak of, 174
    neurosecretion and, 89
    nicotine test, 89, 99
    origin of, 174
    production of, 88, 91, 334
    release following injury, 192
    resistance to, 96
    response to plasma osmolality, 76
    role in water balance, 88
    secretion, 76
        factors influencing, 55
        following injury, 192, 196
        inhibition of, 63, 89
        mechanism of, 89
        osmotic, 55
        posture affecting, 55
        sodium controlling, 80
        stimulation, 58, 89
    urea clearance and, 326
    in urine, 55, 100
    water absorption and, 85
    water homeostasis and, 83
Arginosuccinic aciduria, 258
Arginosuccinic aciduria, 258
Arsenic, 731
Artificial respiration, 50
Arylsulphatase deficiency, 241, 268
Ascites, 178
    cancer causing, 176
    in cirrhosis, 66
Ascorbic acid See Vitamin C
Aspartate,
    in cerebral metabolism, 581
    tests of, 385

Aspartate aminotransferase,
    in central nervous system, 568
    in coronary thrombosis, 615
    in liver disease, 387
    in neonates, 294
Aspartate transaminase, 212
Aspartylglucosaminuria, 268, 270
Asphyxia, 261
Aspirin,
    monitoring, 762
    poisoning, 739, 740, 744, 745, 754
    Reye's syndrome and, 301
Asthma, 472
Astrocytomas, 575
Ataxia telangiectasia, 258, 288
Atheroma,
    in children, 251
    in diabetes mellitus, 111, 118
Atherosclerosis,
    development of, 608
    diabetes and, 109
    hypertension and, 591, 599
    hypertriglyceridaemia and, 610
    plaques, 609
    regression of, 611
    risk associations, 610
Atransferrinaemia, 485
Atrial natriuretic factor, 588
Atrial natriuretic peptide, 56, 334
    following injury, 192
Autoerythrocyte sensitization, 500
Autoimmune disease,
    alkaline phosphatase in, 388
    Down's syndrome and, 288
    of connective tissue, 550
    subclinical, 552
Autonomic nervous system,
    in blood pressure, 586
Azathioprine, 200

B-3500 FH, 605
Barbiturate poisoning, 740, 750
Bartter's syndrome, 71
Basal metabolic rate, 224
Base excess or deficit, 40
Behavioural disturbances,
    in mental retardation, 260
Bence-Jones protein, 462, 474, 487
    electrophoresis, 490
    in urine, 321
Bence Jones proteinuria,
    fanconi syndrome and, 330
    in myeloma, 177, 178
Benzodiazepines,
    poisoning by, 747, 751
Beri-beri, 265, 578
Bernstein test, 348
Beryllium, 732
Beta blocking agents,
    poisoning by, 739, 749
Beutler method, 249
Bicarbonate,
    acid urine and, 332
    actual concentration, 40
    buffering, 32, 36
        components, 34

increased use of, 41
in children, 293
control by kidney, 35
in gastrointestinal tract, 39
generation, 34
loss of, 35,44
in metabolic alkalosis, 49
rate of production, 36
reabsorption, 36
renal production, 35,45
replacement of, 36
repletion in kidney, 38
secretion, 39
standard concentration, 40
Bicarbonaturia, 333
Biguanides, 43
in diabetes, 112, 116
Bile,
excretion of, 385
Bile acid
breath test, 360, 362
measurement, 390
Bile duct absorption, 375
Bile salts,
malabsorption, 362
Biliary atresia, 309
Biliary colic, 400
Biliary obstruction, 385
Bilirubin,
in acute pancreatitis, 407
binding to albumin, 308, 384
in brain haemorrhage, 570
conjugated, 384
direct and indirect, 383
monitoring in transplantation, 212
neonatal excretion, 307
tests of, 383, 384
types of, 383
unconjugated,
albumin binding, 263
urinary, 324
Bilirubin encephalopathy, 264
Biochemistry service,
paediatric, 314
Biological disorders,
with psychiatric component, 144
Biotidinase deficiency, 251, 283
Birthweight 304
2,33,Biphosphoglycerate, 424, 425
Blackwater fever, 460
Bladder stones, 344
Bleeding disorders, 500
see also Clotting factors etc
Bleeding times, 506
Blood,
pH, 40, 51
porphyrins, 417
in prenatal diagnosis, 238
in rheumatoid arthritis, 548
samples,
fetal, 239
in poisoning, 737
Blood-brain barrier, 560, 565
Blood-CSF barrier, 562
Blood coagulation, 467, 495–513
see also Haemostasis etc

in connective tissue disease, 555
fibrinolytic mechanism, 496
general mechanism, 495
Blood count,
in diarrhoea, 374
Blood dyscrasias, 461
Blood gases,
derived values, 40
estimations, 40
in heart transplants, 206
in liver transplants, 211
in poisoning, 745
in respiratory distress syndrome,
305
in respiratory dysfunction, 47
Blood-gas analysis, 745
Blood loss causing anaemia, 457
Blood pressure,
see also Hypertension etc
autonomic nervous control of, 586
control of, 585
height of, 59
neuroendocrine control, 586
normal ranges, 589
systolic or diastolic, 589
Blood sugar in pancreatitis, 407
Blood volume,
distribution of, 585
Blue bloaters, 48
Body composition,
in marasmus, 4
in protein-energy malnutrition, 5
Body mass index, 25
Body weight,
measurement, 219
Bone,
assessment of loss, 536
calcium in, 517
calcium transfer to, 529
defective mineralization, 530
destruction in rheumatoid arthritis,
547
disorders of, 302, 515, 529
effect of parathyroid hormone on,
520
loss and gain, 532
mass, 519
mineral content, 529
mineral density measurement, 536
oestrogens affecting, 524, 530
organization and turnover, 531
phosphate in, 517
prostaglandins affecting, 524
quality of, 536
remodelling, 531
resorption, 530, 535
hypercalcaemia and, 166, 167
stress damage, 531
turnover, 534
disorders of, 543, 544
Bone disease, 302, 515, 529
alcoholic, 139
in prematurity, 312
renal disease and, 335
Bone gla protein, 529
Bornholm disease, 408

Borrelia burgdorferi, 572
Bovril test, 630
Bradycardia,
reflex, 597
Bradykinin, 589, 678
Brain,
alcoholic damage, 126
amino acids in, 581
aneurysms, 599
cellular organization, 145
complexity of, 145
congenital abnormalities, 266
demand for glucose, 261
development of, 284
energy requirement, 146
growth spurt, 254
gut hormones in, 670
hypoglycaemia affecting, 297, 310
kernicterus damaging, 254
metabolism, 228
metastases, 577
nutrition and, 228
oxygen consumption, 146
pathogenic mechanisms, 256
peroxysmonal disorders affecting,
284
in Reye's syndrome, 301
in respiratory distress syndrome,
305
toxic effect of ammonia, 275
tumours, 60
vulnerability of, 254, 256
Brain death, 200
Brain haemorrhage, 569
Breath tests, 358, 359
bacterial overgrowth, 360
bile acid, 360, 362
for fat malabsorption, 359
hydrogen, 358, 360
lactulose hydrogen, 363
[14]C xylose 361
Bromide partition test, 572
Bromide poisoning, 751
Bromosulphthalein,
hepatic removal of, 393
Bronchitis, 47
Bronchopulmonary dysplasia, 305
Bronchospasm,
in carcinoid syndrome, 175
Bronchus,
carcinoma of, 64
Bronze baby syndrome, 309
Brucellosis, 492
Brush border oligosaccharides, 376
Buffer base, 40
Buffering, 32
bicarbonate, 33, 34, 36, 41
haemoglobin, 49
phosphate, 33
protein, 33
Burns,
anaemia in, 460
catabolic hormones and, 227
nutrition and, 227

CA 19–9,

as tumour marker, 186
Cachectin, 165
Cachexia,
  in cancer, 164, 228
Cadmium, 730–731
Caerulin, 677
Caeruloplasmin, 480, 485
  in children, 294
  in disease, 486
  in liver disease, 393
Caffeine, 394
Calcitonin, 520
  role of, 520
  secretion, 542
Calcitriol, 336
  calcium metabolism, 522
  synthesis, 541
Calcium,
  absorption, 335, 526
  balance, 517, 518
  binding, 516
  in cerebrospinal fluid, 562
  colonic absorption, 364
  concentration,
    in cells, 515
    in pancreatitis, 407
  deficiency in neonates, 311, 313
  distribution of, 515, 517
  excretion, 517, 527
  in extracellular fluid, 515, 520, 530, 537
  fluxes across kidney, 527
  function of, 515
  homeostasis, 537
    disorders of, 538
    ranges for measurement, 545
  influencing hormones, 518
  intestinal absorption, 525
  metabolism, 515–545
    adrenal steroids in, 524
    cadmium affecting, 731
    cytokines and growth factors in, 524
    following surgery, 196
    gastrointestinal hormones and, 524
    growth hormone in, 523,524
    hormones controlling, 516, 518, 523
    integration of responses, 537
    neonatal, 311
    regulation, 534
    sex steroids in, 524
    thyroid hormones and, 523
    vitamin D in, 521
  parathyroid hormone regulating, 518
  plasma, 516, 518
  in poisoning, 746
  relation of diet and absorption, 525, 526
  renal excretion, 517, 527
  renal transport, 528
  resorption, 517
  sites of flux, 517
  in sweat, 518

transfer to bone, 529
transport, 525
urinary, 322
Calcium salts,
  in renal stones, 229
Calcium stimulation test, 353
Calmodulin, 516
Campylobacter-like organisms test, 353
Canavan's disease, 158, 271
Cancer antigens, 185
Capillary blood sampling, 247
Carbamazepine, 766
  poisoning, 747
Carbaminohamoglobin, 48
Carbamyl phosphate synthetase, 301
Carbinazole in hyperthyroidism, 655
Carbohydrate,
  digestion and absorption, 355
  incomplete catabolism, 31
  tests of absorption, 358
Carbohydrate-deficient transferrin, 134
Carbohydrate metabolism,
  in cancer, 165
  in diabetes, 104
  effects of tumours on, 161
  following trauma, 193
  inherited disorders, 299
  in protein-energy malnutrition, 8
Carbamylphosphate synthetase, 276
Carbonate dehydratase,
  bicarbonate reabsorption and, 36
  potassium and, 39
  urinary phosphate and, 36
  urinary sodium and chloride and, 38
  urinary ammonia and, 37
Carbonate dehydrogenase, 34
Carbon dioxide,
  combining with globin, 424
  control of respiratory centre, 34
  generation, 31
  hydrogen ion homeostasis and, 32
  plasma total, 39,50
  removal from lungs, 34
Carbon dioxide tension,
  arterial, 51
  fall in, 50
  in respiratory distress syndrome, 306
  in respiratory dysfunction, 47
Carbon monoxide poisoning, 748
Carcinoembryonic antigen, 492
  as tumour marker, 182
  clinical use of, 183
  structure, 182
Carcinoid syndrome, 174–176, 322, 595, 679
  biochemical detection, 175
  features of, 175
  pathophysiology, 175
Carcinoid tumours, 174, 176, 353, 378, 673, 678
  classification, 175
  ectopic ACTH and, 170

Cardiac arrhythmias 74
Cardiac output, 585
  control of, 586
Cardioactive drugs, 748
Cardioeipin test, 554
Cardiomyopathy, 139
  cobalt, 734
Cardiovascular system,
  tumours of, 178
Carnitine, 313
  deficiency, 283
Carnitine acyl transferase, 194
Carnosinaemia, 277, 278
Carnosine in muscle, 139
Carotaenaemia, 13
Cataracts, 285
Catecholamines,
  depression and, 147
  insulin and, 108
  metabolism, 597
  in peripheral resistance, 587
  secretion, 597
  synthesis, 596
  trauma and, 191, 193
  vascular effects of, 597
Cells,
  electrolyte composition of, 53
Cell damage,
  from alcohol, 122
Cell membranes, 53
  effect of thyroid hormones on, 640
Cell metabolism,
  effects of hypoxia on, 190
Cellobiose/mannitol test, 358
Central nervous system,
  cellular organization, 145
  clinical biochemistry, 560–580
  complexity of, 145
  energy requirements, 146
  enzymology and, 568, 569
  infections, 571
  in nutritional disease, 577
  oxygen consumption, 146
  role of laboratory in disease, 578
  tumours of, 575, 577
    causing precocious puberty, 716
    markers for, 576
Central venous pressure, 585
Cerebral infarction, 569
  hypertriglyceridaemia and, 610
Cerebrospinal fluid, 561–565
  analysis of, 561
  antimyelin antibodies in, 574
  composition of, 560, 562, 563
  in demyelinating disease, 573
  electrophoresis, 490, 491
  formation and flow, 561
  glucose in, 564
  in Guillain-Barré syndrome, 574
  haptoglobins in, 567
  immunoglobulins in, 565
  immunoglobulin free light chains in, 567
  inspection of, 564
  lumbar puncture, 562
  myelin basic protein in, 574

physiology of, 561
pigmentation, 564
protein in, 564, 565
ranges in children, 294
routine examination, 563
transferrin in, 568
transport in, 562
xanthochromia of, 569
Cerebrotendinous xanthomatosis, 258, 271
Cerebrovascular disorders, 568–571
Chemotrypsin test, 371
Chest disease,
    simulating acute abdomen, 408
Chest pain, 614–620
Chief cells, 348
Children, 292
    see also neonates etc
    acute abdomen in, 401
    acute appendicitis in, 403
    atherosclerosis in, 251
    biochemistry service for, 314
    CSF in, 294
    disorders of gonadal function in, 715
    gallstones in, 458
    glomerular filtration rate in, 294
    hyperammonaemia in, 299
    hypoglycaemia, 297
    lead poisoning in, 727
    liver transplantation in, 213
    plasma lipids in, 296
    range of plasma constituents, 293
    renal function in, 294
    renal tubular function in, 295
    sample collecting, 292
    thyroid disease in, 654
    urine values in, 294
    with short stature, 302
Chloral hydrate poisoning, 751
Chlorate ions,
    poisoning by, 751
Chloride
    in cerebrospinal fluid, 562, 564
    in extracellular fluid, 53
    plasma concentration, 51
    urinary, 38
Chlormethiazole poisoning, 740, 750
Cholecalciferol *See Vitamin D*
Cholecystokinin, 349, 670
Cholesterol,
    in cells, 605
    control of metabolism, 606
    fetal, 296
    growth and, 303
    high levels, 612
Cholesterol desmolase deficiency, 701, 704
Cholinesterase,
    in liver disease, 391
Choriocarcinomas, 181
Chorionic gonadotrophic stimulation test, 720
Chorionic villi,
    biopsy, 239
    in Down's syndrome, 234

enzyme essay from, 240
fetal genetic material in, 241
Choroid plexus,
    cerebrospinal fluid formation in, 562
Christmas disease, 496
Chromatography in poisoning, 742
Chromium, 22, 734
Chromosomal disorders,
    causing congenital malformations, 260, 713
    mental retardation and, 288
Chylomicrons, 602
Chyme, 85
Cimetidine, 349
Citrate balance, 34
    balance, 341
    renal stones and, 341
Citrullinaemia, 280
Clonidine test, 629
Clot lysis time, 510
Clotting factors,
    assays of, 505
    basic properties, 496
    biochemistry, 500
    DNA analysis, 511
    inhibitors and antibodies, 509
    one stage assays, 507
    reactions, 495
    test's, 505, 506
    two-stage assays, 507
Clotting factor II (prothrombin), 502
    biochemistry, 503
    deficiency, 498, 500
Clotting factor V, 498, 503
    assay, 507
    biochemistry, 503
    deficiency, 498
Clotting factor VII,
    biochemistry, 502
    deficiency, 498, 500
Clotting factor VIII,
    antibodies, 500, 509
    assay, 507
    biochemistry, 501
    carrier detection, 511
    deficiency, 496, 497, 502
    treatment with, 497
Clotting factor IX, 511
    antibodies, 509
    assay, 507
    biochemistry, 501
    deficiency, 496, 500
    treatment with, 497
Clotting factor X, 507
    biochemistry, 503
    deficiency, 498, 500
Clotting factor XI,
    antibodies, 500
    assay, 507
    biochemistry, 501
    deficiency, 498
Clotting factor XII (Hageman),
    assay, 507
    biochemistry, 500, 501
    deficiency, 498, 500

Clotting factor XIII, 503
    assay, 509
    biochemistry, 504
    deficiency, 498
Clotting time, 506
Clozapine,
    dopamine and, 147
Coagulation cascade, 189
Cobalt, 733
    cardiomyopathy, 734
Coeliac disease, 357, 358, 526
    steatorrhoea in, 376
    vitamin D and, 542
Cold haemoglutinin disease, 459
Colic, 401
Collagen matrix, 529
Colon,
    absorption and secretion, 364
    decreased transit time, 365
    diminished absorption, 365
    motility, 364
    salt and water excretion, 364
    sodium absorption in, 57
    tests of function, 364–367
    water absorption in, 85
Colony-stimulating factors, 524
Colorectal tumours, 366
Coma,
    biochemistry of, 581–584
    hepatic, 581
    hypoglycaemic, 583
    hypoxic, 583
    in hypernatraemia, 62
    ischaemic, 583
Complement cascade, 190
Complement system, 467
    activation, 478
    in connective tissue disease, 552
    defence role, 477
    deficiencies, 478
    genetic deficiencies, 477
    in immune-complex disease, 478
    laboratory measurement, 479, 480
    physiology, 475
    value of measurements, 477
Computerised tomography scans, 560
Confusion with insulinoma, 145
Congenital diseases,
    preventive measures, 237
Connective tissue disorders, 550–556
    antibody detection, 553
    autoantibodies in 551
    blood abnormalities 555
    end-organ damage, 555
    laboratory tests, 553
    markers of activity, 555
    mixed, 551
    pathogenesis, 550
    pathology, 552
    therapy, 555
Conn's adenoma, 595
Conn's syndrome, 56, 71, 704
    causing hypertension, 593
    glucose tolerance in, 72
Contaminated small bowel syndrome, 377

Convulsions,
folate deficiency and, 264
pyridoxine-dependent, 278
Copper, 733
deficiency, 21
metabolism in Wilson's disease, 286, 330
transport, 287, 485
values in children, 294
Copper-containing enzymes, 287
Coproporphyria, 415
Coproporphyrin, 411
Cori cycle, 162, 298
defective, 299
Corneal opacification, 608
Coronary heart disease 605, 606, 608, 611
Coronary thrombosis, 614
cardiac enzymes in, 615
ECG in, 615
thrombolytic therapy, 618
Corticosteroids,
see also under Adrenal steroids
actions of, 687
deficiency of, 687
in serum, 689
Corticotrophin-releasing factor, 151, 626
Cortisol,
circadian rhythm, 689
depression and, 149
'free', 322, 687
urinary estimation, 691
in circulation, 688
influencing AVP, 55
interconversion, 686
measurements, 690
metabolites, 686
release following injury, 191
response to hypoglycaemia, 693
secretion, 689
stress and, 690
synthesis, 591
Cortisone-binding globulin, 709
Cortisone,
interconversion, 686
Cot death, 299
CRH test, 693
Craniopharyngioma, 303
Creatine,
in children, 293
clearance, 326, 327
daily excretion, 318
Creatine kinase, 293, 616, 617
in cerebrospinal fluid, 568
in coronary thrombosis, 616
Creatinine,
in children, 295
concentration, 328, 329
C-reactive protein, 467, 480, 483, 491, 492
alcohol and, 132
following injury, 194
in meningitis, 572
CREST, 553
Cretinism, 286

Crigler-Naijjar syndrome, 254, 308
Crithidia test, 553
Crohn's disease, 357, 358, 362, 364, 375, 686
Cryoglobulins, 475, 476
Cushing's syndrome, 28, 542, 544, 685, 693, 697–701, 704
alcohol-induced, 701
corticosteroid-binding globulin in, 688
CRH test, 693
cyclical, 701
differential diagnosis, 699
ectopic ACTH in, 172
features of, 697
hypertension in, 595
iatrogenic, 700
investigation, 697, 700
potassium loss in, 71
psychiatric factors, 151
screening, 692, 699
tests, 693, 694
with carcinoma of lung, 170
Cyanide-nitroprusside test, 320
Cyanide poisoning, 739, 744, 751
Cyanocobalamin *See Vitamin B₁₂*
Cyanosis, 433
haemoglobin M and, 434
in methaemoglobinaemia, 434
Cyclic AMP,
calcium and, 516, 528
in hypoparathyroidism, 540
Cyclosporin, 758
administration and dosage, 201, 209, 214
assay, 202
effect on fat metabolism, 164
elimination, 201
follow-up, 202
for children, 214
in heart and lung transplantation, 208
in liver transplantation, 213
metabolism, 201
monitoring, 205, 767
monotherapy, 206
nephrotoxicity, 201, 204, 208, 209
neurological defects, 214
in renal transplantation, 204
side effects, 201
in transplantation surgery, 200
Cystathiononuria, 278
Cystatin C, 568
Cystic fibrosis,
genetic counselling in, 250
lung transplant for, 209
neonatal screening, 250
sweat tests, 372
Cystinuria, 320, 330, 342
malabsorption in, 379
Cytochrome B₅, 433
Cytochrome B₅ reductase, 434
Cytokines, 524
Cytomegalovirus infection 209

Deafness, 256, 257

Dehydration,
in infants, 79
in kwashiorkor, 3
mental aspects, 154
in prematurity, 79
Dehydroepiandrosterone, 682
de Lange syndrome, 256
Delirium tremens, 124
Dementia, 574
causes, 575
Demyelinating diseases, 572–574
cerebrospinal fluid in, 573
Demyelination, 573
11-Deoxycorticosterone, 590
Deoxyhaemoglobin, 421
DNA analysis,
clotting factors, 511
fetal sexing, 243
gene tracking, 242
identifying mutations, 243
prenatal diagnosis by, 241
Depression,
in Addison's disease, 145, 151
dexamethasone suppression tests and, 692
in hypothyroidism, 151
neuroendocrinological aspects, 149
neurotransmitters and, 147
Desferroxamine, 752
in iron overload, 452
Desmethylimipramine,
poisoning by, 757
17,20-Desmolase deficiency, 714
Desmopressin acetate response test, 98
Dexamethasone suppression test, 692
for depression, 149
Diabetes insipidus, 633
cranial, 94
diagnosis, 100
head injury and, 96
nephrogenic, 92, 97, 98, 330, 333
investigation, 101
pharmacologically-induced, 90
water depletion in, 60
Diabetes mellitus, 103–120
acute abdomen and, 408, 508
aetiological classification, 107
aetiology of, 105
antigens, 105
blood glucose estimation in, 109
causing osmotic diuresis, 61
classification, 105, 107
complications, 109
see also under those complications
control and, 113
long-term, 117
control of, 113
diagnosis, 109
impaired glucose tolerance and, 110
dietary treatment, 111
encephalopathy, 583
fat metabolism in, 104
gamma glutamyltransferase in 389
glucose in urine, 319
growth hormone response, 633

in haemochromatosis, 450
hyperglycaemic emergencies, 114
hyperglycaemia in 116
hypokalaemia in, 71
incidence of, 106
insulin-dependent, 105
insulin therapy in, 112
ketosis in, 42
lactic acidosis in, 116
microalbuminuria in, 321, 330
nephrogenic, 93
non-insulin dependent, 28, 105
    insulin resistance in, 109
    oral hypoglycaemic agents in, 112
obesity and, 106, 109
oral hypoglycaemic agents in, 112, 118
in pancreatic insufficiency, 377
pancreatic transplantation for, 214
pathogenesis, 106
patient in, 110
polyuria and polydipsia in, 92, 99
pregnancy and, 110
protein glycosylation, 430
renal disease in, 330
steroid-induced, 204
transient in neonates, 311
traumatic, 193
treatment, 111
    home monitoring in, 114
    monitoring, 113, 114
    type 1,
        aetiology of, 105
        pathogenesis, 106
    type II,
        aetiology, 106
        pathogenesis, 106
viruses associated with, 106
Diabetic coma, 114
    hyperglycaemic non-ketotic, 115
Diabetic ketoacidosis, 68, 104, 114
    diagnosis and treatment, 114
    insulin resistance in, 108
    pathogenesis, 114
    role of laboratory, 115
Diabetic neuropathy, 117
Diabetic retinopathy, 117
Diagnex blue test, 351
Dialysis encephalopathy, 153, 724
Diarrhoea, 365, 366
    aetiology, 366
    in appendicitis, 404
    biliary causes, 375
    in carcinoid syndrome, 175
    clinical assessment, 372
    in Crohn's disease, 375
    definition, 365
    disorders causing, 375
    from laxative abuse, 378
    general investigations, 373
    in hypolactasia, 376
    idiopathic, 362
    investigation, 372, 373
    in malabsorption, 372
    in marasmus, 4
    mechanisms of, 365

osmotic, 366
radiology of, 374
secretory, 366
sodium depletion in, 60
spurious, 372
in ulcerative colitis, 2376
urinary sodium and, 68
water loss from, 79
Diarrhoea mortice, 366
Diazepam-binding inhibitor, 148
Dicopac test, 363
DIDMOAD, 94
Diet,
    biochemical values and, 293
    for obesity, 29
    in treatment of diabetes, 111
Di George syndrome, 312, 540
Digoxin, 764
    poisoning, 740, 748
    therapeutic monitoring, 761, 764
1,25-Dihydroxycholecalciferol, 325, 335–336
3,4,Dihydroxyphenylacetic acid, 575
1,25 Dihydroxy vitamin D, 516
DTPA clearance, 326,327
Dipsticks in urine screening, 318
Disaccharidase deficiency, 358
Disalotransferrin, 135
Disequilibrium syndrome, 153
Disseminated intravascular
    coagulation, 189, 460
Diuresis,
    alcohol causing, 124
    osmotic, 61, 94
    causing hypokalaemia, 70
    causing hyponatraemia, 65
    effects of, 95
    sodium reabsorption and, 55
Diverticular disease, 372
Dolichols, 136
Dopamine,
    alcohol and, 126
    causing polyuria, 94
    in depression, 148
    inhibiting pituitary hormones, 625
    iron metabolism and, 157
    in schizophrenia, 147
    synthesis, 583
Dopamine β-hydroxylase, 596
l-Dopa test, 630
Down's syndrome, 148, 260, 288
    prenatal screening, 233
        detection rates, 235
        maternal markers, 235
        methods, 234
    translocation type, 234
Drugs,
    bioavailability, 758
    bioequivalence, 759
    clearance, 760
    dosage, 765
    first pass metabolism, 758
    half-lives, 740, 760
    iatrogenic toxicity, 736
    immunoassays, 741
    inadequate response, 765

indications for measurement, 763
interactions, 737
intoxication, 764
mental retardation and, 267
metabolites, 741
monitoring *See Therapeutic drug
    monitoring*
multiple therapy, 764
overdose, 323, 736
    prognosis in, 738
plasma protein binding, 760
radioimmunoassays, 742
screening for, 741
    problems, 743
steady state, 760
urinary screening, 322
Drug abuse, 753
Drug concentrations,
    factors affecting, 758
Drug therapy
    psychiatric side-effects, 158
Dry mouth, 82, 96
Dubin-Johnson syndrome, 394, 411
Duchenna muscular dystrophy, 250
Dumping syndrome, 349, 378
Duodenal ulcers, 351
    H.pylori in, 353
Duodenum,
    function of, 356
Dwarfism, 631, 632
Dysalbuminaemic
    hyperthyroxinaemia, 642
Dysfibrinogenaemia, 498
Dyshormonogenesis, 641
Dysostosis multiplex, 268
Dystrophia myotonia, 109

Eclampsia, 598
Ectopic ACTH syndrome, 170, 684, 687, 694, 698, 699
Ehlers Danlos syndrome, 287, 500
Eisenmenger syndrome, 209
Elasase, 369
Elderly,
    nutritional support for, 226
Electrolytes,
    see also specific electrolytes
    absorption in intestine, 36, 354
    colonic absorption, 364
    composition of body, 53
    disturbances and mental
        retardation, 263
    in heart transplantation, 206
    in hypertension, 592
    investigation in diarrhoea, 373
    in poisoning, 745
    in renal transplantation, 203, 204
    in short bowel syndrome, 377
    sources of loss, 58
    in urine, 321
Electrophoresis, 566
ELISA test, 553
Elliptocytosis, 458
Embden-Meyerhof pathway, 460
Emesis in poisoning, 743
Emphysema, 47

Encephalopathy,
   dialysis, 724
   of environmental origin, 261
   hepatic, 581
   hypertensive, 599
   hypoglycaemia, 583
   hypoxic, 583
   ischaemic, 583
Endocrine disorders,
   causing mental retardation, 286
   psychiatric disorders and, 150
Endocrine hypofunction syndromes,
   176
Endocrine tumours,
   effects of, 168
   glucose and, 162
Endothelin, 617
Energy metabolism,
   in cancer, 164
   in malnutrition, 8
Energy nitrogen ratios, 226
Energy requirements,
   of burns patients, 227
Enolase, 569
Enteral nutrition,
   of burns patients, 227
   in cancer, 229
Enteric hyperoxaluria, 342
Enterochromaffin hyperplasia, 353
Enterocolitis,
   radiation, 378
Enzymes,
   in central nervous system, 568
   liver damage and, 130
   in poisoning, 746
   in protein energy malnutrition, 6
Enzyme assay,
   with amniotic fluid cells, 239
   with choronic villi, 240
Enzyme ratios in alcoholism, 131
Epilepsy, 264, 574
Epiphyseal dysplasias, 543
Epstein-Barr virus infection, 388
Ergocalciferol, 521
Erythroblastosis fetalis, 311
Erythrocytes,
   abnormalities in malaria, 437
   breakdown products, 457
   in carbon dioxide-bicarbonate ratio,
     34
   glucose entry, 110
   half-life, 457
   hormones in production, 454
   life-span, 455
   maturation, 453
   mean corpuscular volume, 130
   membrane defects, 457
   metabolic defects, 458
   porphyrins in, 412, 414
   producing bicarbonate, 46
   protoporphyrin, 449
   superoxide dismutase, 135
Erythrocyte-δ-aminolaevulinic acid
    dehydratase, 137
Erythropoiesis, 453
   ineffective, 447

   sites of, 453
Erythropoietin, 325, 335, 453
   action of, 454
   recombinant, 454
   mRNA, 454
ETDA clearance, 326
Ethanol,
   in body fluids, 128
   poisoning, 739, 740, 749
Ethylene glycol, 342
   poisoning, 44, 749
Euglobulin lysis time, 510
Euglycaemic clamp, 107
Experimental allergic
    encephalomyelitis, 573
Extracellular fluid, 53, 325
   calcium in, 515, 525
   chloride in, 53
   electrolyte composition of, 53
   neonatal, 306
   sodium in, 56
   thirst control and, 82
   water in, 56
Eyes in mental retardation, 256, 257

FK506, 202
Fabry's disease, 258, 269, 270
Faecal fats,
   assessment of, 359
   in diarrhoea, 374
   in pancreatic assessment, 371
Faecal isotopes test, 362
Faecal nitrogen test, 371
Faecal occult blood, 366
Faeces,
   porphyrins in, 411, 412, 417
Faecolith, 405
Familial amyloid polyneuropathy, 579
Familial periodic paralysis, 71
Fanconi's anaemia, 288
Fanconi syndrome, 331, 333
   hydrogen ion in, 332
Farber's disease, 258, 269, 270
Farr test, 553
Fasting in investigation of diarrhoea,
   375
Fat,
   assessment of, 9
   breakdown in diabetes, 111
   energy from, 27
   intestinal absorption, 356,359
   malabsorption, 359
   metabolism,
     after injury, 193
     in cancer, 164, 165
     in diabetes, 104
Fatty acids,
   absorption, 364
   dehydrogenation, 281
   incomplete metabolism, 31
   non-esterified, 104
   oxidation of, 298
   release of, 602
Feeding, 221, 222
Felty's syndrome, 549
Ferritin, 447

   amino acid sequences, 447
   as iron storage protein, 447
   in cerebral infarction, 569
   in cerebrospinal fluid, 569, 571
   in liver disease, 394
   measurement of, 449
   in meningitis, 571
   response to infection, 450
Ferrochelatase, 726
Fertility and subfertility, 720
Fetal blood sampling, 239
Fetal body water, 306
Fetal hypoxia, 263
Fetal liver,
   biopsy, 239
Fetal sexing, 243
Fetal thyroid, 653
   deficiency, 286
Fever,
   water depletion in, 60
Fibrin,
   biochemistry, 503
   degradation products, 511
   function of, 495
Fibrin plate test, 510
Fibrinogen, 483, 491
   assay, 508
   biochemistry, 503
   deficiency, 498
   electrophoresis, 490
Fibrinolysis,
   defects in, 499
   mechanism, 496
   tests of, 510
Fibrogenesis imperfecta ossium, 543
Fibronectin, 490, 577
Fish eye disease, 608
Fitzgerald factor, 501
Flaky-paint dermatosis, 3
Flatus, 365, 401
Flaujeac factor, 501
Fluid and electrolyte balance,
   disorders of, 53–75
     in neonates, 306
     psychiatric aspects, 154
    following trauma, 195
    role of kidney, 76
Flumazenil, 583
Fluoride poisoning, 752
5-Fluorouracil, 17
Flushing in carcinoid syndrome, 175
Folate, 18
   deficiency,
     anaemias in, 454, 456
     convulsions in, 264
     mental retardation and, 265
    intestinal absorption, 356
Folic acid, 455
   deficiency, 18
     mental aspects, 156
Follicle stimulating hormone, 152, 623,
     625, 707, 711, 712
   in polycystic ovary, 717
   in puberty, 715
Food,
   chemical nature of, 27

Food intake,
in cancer, 165
Formiminoglutamic acid, 19, 455
Fragile X syndrome, 254, 289
Frank-Starling mechanism, 585
Free-radical scavenging, 122
Free water clearance, 82
Free water excretion, 54
Fructose-l-6-dehydrogenase, 44
Fructose intolerance, 282, 309, 324, 331
Fucosidosis, 270

g-cell hyperplasia, 352
Galactitol, 285
Galactokinase deficiency, 285
Galactosaemia, 309
mental retardation and, 285
neonatal screening, 249
Galactose,
elimination capacity, 393
serum and urinary, 320, 359
Galactose-l-phosphate, 285
assay, 249
Galactose-l-phosphate uridyl transferase,
assay of, 249
Galactosialidosis, 271
Gallstones, 400, 406, 458
Gamma aminobutyric acid (GABA) 148, 260
disorders of metabolism, 277
role, in hepatic encephalopathy, 582
transaminase deficiency, 279
Gamma glutamyltransaminase, 131
Gamma-glutamyltransferase, 128, 388
measurement of, 137, 388
in pregnancy, 130
screening test, 396
Ganglioside metabolism,
disorders of, 268
GM$_2$ gangliosidoses, 270
Gastrectomy, 351, 376, 378
Gastric emptying and motility, 348
Gastric inhibitory peptide, 29, 349, 671
Gastric juice,
sodium depletion in, 60
Gastric lavage in poisoning, 743
Gastric metaplastic islands, 353
Gastric secretion,
assessment of, 350
diarrhoea and, 365
Gastrin, 352, 670, 674
acid inhibition of, 349
growth hormone secretion and, 628
release of, 349, 674
Gastrin-containing cells, 348
Gastrin-secreting tumours, 379
Gastrin stimulation tests, 352
Gastrinoma, 352, 353, 673
Gastritis,
H.pylori and, 353
Gastroenteritis, 62
gastrointestinal function, 347–382
see also specific organs

Gastrointestinal hormones, 670–680
calcium metabolism and, 524
distribution and activity, 671
obesity and, 29
physiology and pathophysiology, 671
Gastrointestinal protein, 363
Gastrointestinal tract,
as endocrine organ, 670
handling of bicarbonate in, 39
hormone secreting tumours, 673
hypokalaemia affecting, 72
potassium loss in, 70
in protein-energy malnutrition, 6
tumours affecting, 178
Gastrosporillium hominis, 348
Gastrotomy, 222
Gaucher's disease, 269, 270
Gene mutations,
effects of, 246
Gene therapy, 244
Gene tracking, 242
Gene transfer, 269
Genetic counselling, 246, 289
in cystic fibrosis, 250
Genetic disease, 237
Genetic heterogeneity, 255
Genetic material,
from chorionic villi, 241
Genito-urinary tract,
obstruction, 92
Gestational hypertension, 598
Gestational trophoblastic tumours, 181
Giantism, 630
Gilbert's disease, 308, 394
hyperbilirubinism in, 396
Glandular fever, 388
Glial fibrillary acidic protein, 565
Gliomas, 576
Gliosis, 583
Globin,
combining with carbon dioxide, 424
cooperativity, 422
gene structure, 426
introns, 426
structure, 422
in thalassaemia, 435
Globoid cell leucodystrophy, 158
glomerular filtration, 54
in children, 294
Glomerular filtration rate, 56, 58, 325–330
age changes, 325, 328
assessment of, 326
calcium clearance and, 527
in children, 294
monitoring changes, 329
plasma B$_2$ macroglobulin and, 329
plasma creatinine concentration and, 328, 329
plasma urea and, 328
Glomerular proteinuria, 320, 329
Glomerular ultrafiltration, 329
Glomerulonephritis,
renal failure from, 202

Glomerulo-tubular imbalance, 295
Glucagon, 108, 672
calcium and, 524
secretion in trauma, 191
Glucagon-like peptide, 671, 672
Glucagon test,
of growth hormone, 629
Glucagonoma, 673
Glucaric acid, 135
Glucocorticoids,
activity, 687
growth and, 303
production, 684
Glucocorticoid suppressible hyperaldosteronism, 594
Gluconeogenesis, 103, 281
after trauma, 195
in cancer, 162
in children, 298
impairment of, 43
in protein-energy malnutrition, 8
Glucose,
blood concentration, 666
brain and, 228, 261
in cerebrospinal fluid, 561, 564
in erythrocytes, 110
estimation in diabetes, 109
hepatic uptake, 105
homeostasis, 309
in hypoglycaemia, 116, 663
intolerance, 377
metabolism, 103, 671
chromium and, 22
in malignancy, 161
production in cancer, 163
in protein-energy malnutrition, 11
tests in diarrhoea, 374
transport, 666
uptake of, 55
in peripheral tissue, 104
in urine, 319
Glucose tolerance,
in Conn's syndrome, 72
in diabetes, 110
in protein energy malnutrition, 8
Glucose tolerance test, 111, 112
Glucose-galactose malabsorption, 356
Glucose-6-phosphate,
acidosis and, 43
Glucose-6-phosphate dehydrogenase,
deficiency, 307, 438, 458
neonatal screening, 251
Glutamate in cerebral metabolism, 581
Glutamate dehydrogenase,
alcohol and, 132
Glutamate formimimo synthase deficiency, 278
Glutamine synthetase, 582
Glutaric acid, 282
Glutathione, 277
oxidation, 458
Glutathione peroxidase, 733
Glutathione S-transferase, 391
Glutathioninuria, 277, 278
Gluten-sensitive enteropathy, 376

Glutethimide poisoning, 750
Gluttony, 27
L-Glyceric aciduria, 342
Glycine, as inhibitory
    neurotransmitter, 274
Glycogen,
  in brain, 146
  breakdown, 103
  hepatic reserves, 192
  in liver, 103
  storage in children, 298
Glycogen storage disease, 43, 302, 665
Glycolic aciduria, 342
Glycolysis, 190
  pathway, 459, 460
Glycoproteins, 479
  hormones of pituitary, 624
Glycosaminoglycans, 610
  in urine, 320
Glycosuria, 331
Goitre, 646, 647
  toxic nodular, 649, 650
Gonadal dysgenesis, 713
Gonadal function,
  disorders of,
    investigation, 718
    in men, 718
    in women, 716
Gonadal steroids,
  binding, 709
  biochemistry of, 707
  causing hypertension, 598
  effects of, 717
  dynamic tests of, 720
  excretion, 710
  isomerism, 709
  laboratory investigation, 718
  measurement of, 719
  metabolism, 710
  nomenclature, 707, 708
  structure, 707
  synthesis and secretion, 707, 710
  trivial names of, 708
Gonadotrophins,
  levels in childhood, 715
  measurement, 719
Gonadotrophin-releasing hormone,
  707
  stimulation test, 720
Gonads,
  disorders of development, 712
  functions of, 707
    disorders of, 715
Graves' disease, 641, 643, 644, 645,
    648
  end-stage, 651
  features of, 450
  ophthalmic complications, 651
  pancreatic, 665
Growth disorders,
  in mental retardation, 259
Growth hormone, 627–733
  actions of, 627
  alcoholism and, 633
  in calcium metabolism, 523
  deficiency, 303, 631

in diabetes mellitus, 633
following injury, 192
liver disease and, 633
neurotransmitters and, 627
obesity and, 29
regulation of, 627
secretion of, 628, 629
  disorders of, 630
Growth hormone release inhibiting
    hormone, 624
growth rate, 302
Guillain-Barré syndrome, 574

H_2 antagonists, 348
H_2 receptors, 349
Haem, 420
  precursors, 411
  synthesis, 409–411
    lead and, 726, 727
Haem pocket, 421
Haemochromatosis, 450–452
  clinical features, 450
  diagnosis, 451
  idiopathic, 450
  treatment, 451
Haemodialysis,
  in poisoning, 744
  psychiatric aspects, 153
  trace elements and, 734
Haemoglobins, 482
  abnormal, 420, 427
  alcohol and, 136
  amino acid abnormalities, 431
  in bicarbonate buffering, 34
  buffering, 33, 49
  chain separation, 442
  deletions and insertions, 428
  DNA analysis, 443
  embryonic, adult and fetal, 425
  expression, 425
  fetal,
    hereditary persistence, 436
    measurement, 439
  function, 420
  gene duplications, 426
  gene mapping, 443
  genetics, 425
  glycosylated, 430
  Hill equation, 423
  introns, 426
  iron content, 446
  lead and, 726
  Lepore, 436, 441
  oxygen affinity, 423, 424, 440
  oxygen transport, 446
  peptide mapping, 443
  point mutations, 428
  production, 425
  pseudogenes, 426
  sickle-cell, 430, 431, 442
    interaction with other
      haemoglobins, 431
  structure, 420
  termination, frameshift and
    nonsense errors, 49
  tetramer, 422, 423

unstable, 431, 432
in urine, 321
variants, 420, 427, 428
  distribution of, 430
  identification of, 442
  isolation of, 442
  oxygen affinity, 432
Haemoglobin A_2,
  measurement of, 439
Haemoglobin 6, 113
Haemoglobinopathies, 420–445
  definition, 420
  electrophoresis, 440
  laboratory diagnosis, 438
    interpretation, 440
  preparation of haemolysate, 438
  routine screening, 438
  specific, 431
  specimen collection, 438
  stability test, 439
Haemoglobinuria, 457
Haemoglycaemia, 263
Haemolytic anaemias, 457, 463
  acquired, 459
  cold and warm antibody types, 458
  congenital, 457
  in connective tissue disease, 555
  haptoglobin in, 483
  infection in, 459
  microangiopathic, 460
  unstable haemoglobins and, 431
Haemolytic disease of newborn, 307
Haemolytic jaundice, 396
Haemopexin, 486
Haemophilia A and B, 496
  carrier detection, 511
Haemophilia B Leyden, 497
Haemopoiesis, 454
  growth factors in, 455
Haemosiderin, 447, 450
Haemostasis, 496 *See also Blood
    coagulation, Clotting factors etc*
Hair,
  distribution of, 719
  kinky, 21, 258, 287, 393
  in kwashiorkor, 4, 9
  in vitamin A excess, 13
  morphology, 9
Hand-Christian-Schuller disease, 94
  haptoglobin, 482, 491
  in cerebrospinal fluid, 567
  electrophoresis, 489
  in liver disease, 483
  structure, 482
Hartnup disease, 258, 278, 330, 379
Hashimoto's disease, 643, 644, 645,
    649, 651
Head injury,
  cranial diabetes insipidus and, 96
  nutrition and, 228
Heart,
  hypokalaemia affecting, 72
  law of, 585
Heart and lung transplantation, 207,
    210
  domino procedure, 207

immunosuppression in, 208
preoperative assessment, 207
rejection, 208, 209
Heart disease,
cyanotic, 310
Heart failure,
in carcinoid syndrome, 175
congestive, 615
hypertension in, 599
hyponatraemia and oedema in, 65
sodium in, 56, 65
Heart rate, 586
Heart transplantation, 206
rejection, 207
*see also Heart and lung
transplantation*
Heat production, 640
Heavy chain disease, 475
Heavy metal poisoning, 333
Heinz body formation, 432
Helicobacter plyori, 348
acid-related disease and, 353
antibodies, 354
breath tests for, 354
clinical biochemistry of, 353
Henderson-Hasselbach equation, 32,
34
Henoch-Schonlein purpura, 500
Hepatitis,
alcoholic, 130
fetoprotein in, 392
cholinesterase in, 391
5'nucleotidase in, 391
viral, 386
alkaline phosphatase in, 388
gamma glutamyltransferase in,
389
Hepatitis,
aminotransferase in, 386
Hepatitis B,
transplantation and, 204
Hepatitis C,
aminotransferases in, 386
Hepatolenticular degeneration *See
Wilson's disease*
Hepatomas, 163
Hepatomegaly,
in protein-energy malnutrition, 3, 4
Hermaphroditism, 713
Hernia, 401, 405
Herpes zoster, 408
Hexoaminidase,
alcohol and, 132
Hill equation, 423
Hirsutism, 718
Histidaemia, 273, 278
Hodgkin's disease, 480
alkaline phosphatase in, 388
renal effects, 178
Hoesch tests, 412
Homocarnosinosis, 277, 278
Homocholic-tauro acid test 361, 375
Homocitrullinurias, 276
Homocystinaemia, 609
Homocystinuria, 254, 258, 274, 320
neonatal screening, 249

Homogentisic acid, 323
Homovanillic acid,
in Alzheimer's disease, 575
in central nervous system tumours,
577
Hormonal excess syndromes, 168
Hormones,
as tumour markers, 182
ectopic, 171
synthesis, 169
secretion by tumours, 170,171
in urine, 322
vasoactive, 587
see also Steroid hormones, etc
Hormone-deficiency syndromes, 176
tumours causing 176, 177
Hospitals,
incidence of malnutrition in, 218,
222
nutritional assessment of patients,
219
nutritional support team, 218
Human chorionic gonadotrophin,
as maternal marker, 235
as tumour marker, 180
structure, 180
Humeral hypercalcaemia of
malignancy, 166, 167
Hunter's syndrome, 257, 270
Hurler disease, 270
3β-HSD deficiency, 714, 715
Hyaline membrane disease,
See Respiratory distress syndrome
Hydrocephalus, 576
Hydrochloric acid, 349
Hydrogen ion,
assessment of status, 39
disturbances in balance, 40
excretion of, 332
in children, 295
overproduction, 42
physiological processes yielding, 31
secretion, 36, 37
shuttle, 38
Hydrogen ion concentration,
buffering, 32
disturbances of, 31–52
investigation of, 50
Hydrops foetalis, 307
3-Hydroxyacyl-CoA dehydrogenase
deficiency, 283
5-Hydroxyindole acetic acid, 322
3-Hydroxyisobutyryl-CoA decyclase
deficiency 282
11-Hydroxylase deficiency, 590, 703,
715
17a-Hydroxylase deficiency, 704, 714
21-Hydroxylase deficiency, 250, 714
Hydroxy-methoxymandelic acid, 322,
577
17a-Hydroxyprogesterone, 250
Hydroxyproline, 535
3β Hydroxysteroid dehydrogenase
deficiency, 703
5-Hydroxytryptamine, 505, 589
alcohol and, 126

in Alzheimer's disease, 148
breakdown products in urine, 175
in carcinoid tumours, 174
in depression, 148, 149
hormonal role of, 670
iron metabolism and, 157
overproduction of, 678
oxygen in synthesis, 583
Hyperadrenalism, 699
Hyperaldosteronism, 70, 333, 704
idiopathic, 594
Hyperammonaemias, 275, 280, 281
causes of, 300
in children, 299
encephalopathy in, 581
secondary, 276, 277
Hyperamylasaemia, 368
Hyperapobetalipoproteinaemia, 605, 606
Hyperbilirubinaemia, 384
conjugated, 398
unconjugated, 307, 308, 384
Hypercalcaemia, 15, 98, 542–543
in cancer, 165
biochemistry of, 167
mechanism, 166
cancer therapy causing, 168
causes of, 543
causing hypertension, 598
causing nephrogenic diabetes
insipidus, 93
following renal transplants, 336
hormone-dependent form, 595
in haematological malignancy, 167
idiopathic, 312
in malignant disease, 161, 539, 543
mental aspects, 156, 286
neonatal, 312
with hypercalciuria, 340
Hypercalciuria, 343, 523
calcium absorption in, 527
hypercalcaemic states with, 340
renal, 340
resorptive, 340
stone formation and 339
types of, 340
Hypercapnia, 152
Hyperchloraemia, 45
Hypercholesterolaemia, 603, 605
in children, 296
familial, 246, 605
neonatal screening, 251
Hyperchylomicronaemia, 603
autoimmune, 612
Hypercortisolism, 697
Hypergamma globulinaemia, 472
Hypergastrinaemia, *See Zollinger
Ellison syndrome*
Hyperglycaemia, 281
abdominal pain from, 403
after injury, 192
emergencies, 114
mental aspects of, 152
neonatal, 311
non-ketotic, 274
tumours causing, 161
Hyperinsulinism, 28

causing hyperglycaemia, 310
in children, 299
Hyperkalaemia, 72, 73–74
acidosis causing, 41,73
aldosterone deficiency causing, 73
effects of, 74
following renal transplantation, 336
in periodic paralysis, 74
in renal failure, 73
treatment of, 74
Hyperleucine-isoleucinaemia, 278
Hyperlipidaemia, 601–613
alcoholism causing, 133
in children, 296
classification, 612
in cyclosporin treatment, 207
definition, 611
effect on sodium concentration, 63
pancreatitis and, 369
Hypernatraemia, 60
causes, 68
causing mental retardation, 264
effects of, 62
from excessive sodium intake, 62
psychiatric aspects, 154
in trauma, 196
treatment of, 63
Hyperornithinaemia, 278
Hyperosmolality, 68
Hyperoxaluria, 343
renal stones and, 342
secondary, 342
Hyperparathyroidism, 515, 520, 524,
538–539
bone in, 527, 530, 531
calcium absorption in, 527
calcium flux in, 537
cyclic AMP in 528
in neonates, 312
pancreatitis and, 369
primary, 340, 538
renal excretion of calcium in, 527
secondary, 536
tertiary, 336, 536
in transplantation, 204
Hyperphagia, 221
Hyperphenylalaninaemia, 272
Hyperphosphataemia, 540
in cancer, 168
in tumour lysis syndrome, 168
Hyperphosphatasia, 543
Hyperphosphaturia, 343
Hyperproinsulinaemia, 108
Hyperprolactinaemia, 625
Hyperprolinaemia, 278
Hyperproteinaemia, 63
Hypertension, 585–600
in aldosteronism, 593
alcohol intake and, 121
aortic coarctation causing, 590
biochemical diagnosis, 599
cadmium and, 731
catecholamines and, 597
causes of, 589
congenital causes, 590
in Cushing's syndrome, 595

endocrine causes, 593, 598
essential 590, 591, 592
following renal transplantation, 204
gestational, 598
in heart failure, 599
hypercalcaemia causing, 598
hyponatraemic, 593
in left ventricular failure, 599
malignant, 599
phaeochromocytoma causing, 595
potassium loss and, 70
in pregnancy, 598
renal causes, 204, 592
secondary, 334, 592
Hypertensive encephalopathy, 599
Hyperthyroidism, 391, 709
causes, 648
in children, 654
congenital, 641
disorders associated with, 647
function tests, 656, 657
mood changes in, 150
neoplastic causes, 650
in pregnancy, 653
secondary, 650
symptoms, 649
treatment of, 655
treatment-induced, 650
varieties of, 648
Hypertriglyceridaemias, 610
alcohol and, 132
in cancer, 164
in children, 296
Hyperuricaemia, 341
Hyperuricosuria, 343
stone formation and, 340
Hypervalinaemia, 278
Hyperventilation syndrome, 152
HyperVIPaemia, *See Verner-Morrison
syndrome*
Hypnotic drugs,
poisoning, 750
Hypoalbuminaemia, 164, 484
Hypoaldosteronism, 73, 588
Hypoandrogenism, 719
Hypocalcaemia,
cancer and, 168
causes of, 543
mental aspects, 156
neonatal, 264, 311
Hypocalcuria, 15
Hypocitraturia, 341
Hypodipsia, 96, 98, 101
Hypogamma globulinaemia, 471
Hypogonadism, 718
Hypoglycaemia, 116–117, 662–669
ACTH secretion and, 629
affecting brain, 297
asymptomatic, 667
autoimmune, 665
causes,
Addison's disease, 696
in children, 298
inborn errors, 665
neonatal, 310
shock, 193

vitamin D deficiency, 13
causing mental retardation, 261
in children, 297, 298
classification, 662, 663
coma in, 583
confirmation of diagnosis, 666
definition of, 116, 652
diagnosis, 666
differential diagnosis, 668
fasting, 664
hypoketonaemic, 668
insulin-induced, 693
investigation in children, 299
ketones in, 68
ketotic and non-ketotic, 664
leucine-sensitive, 299
mood changes in, 152
neural function and, 146
parenteral feeding and, 313
pathogenesis, 663
plasma pancreatic hormone
measurements, 668
precipitating factors, 116
provocative tests 667
reactive, 665, 668
alcohol induced, 666
stress-induced, 694
sulphonyluria-induced, 116
symptoms of, 662, 663
treatment of, 116
tumour-associated, 162
Hypoglycaemic agents, 112
Hypogonadism, 715
Hypohaptoglobinaemia, 483
Hypokalaemia, 70–73, 98
acidosis and, 45
alkalosis causing, 49
causes of, 70
corticosteroid excess causing, 71
diabetes causing, 71
diuretics and, 70
effects of, 71
hypertension and, 593
polyuria and, 96
renal disease and, 71
in theophylline poisoning, 756
treatment of, 72
Hypolactasia, 349
diarrhoea in, 376
Hypolipidaemia, 296
Hypomagnesaemia, 311, 312
Hypomagnesuria, 343
Hypomania, 148, 149
Hyponatraemia,
after injury or surgery, 64, 192, 196
causation, 55
in congestive heart failure, 65
correction, 67
diuretics causing, 65
effects of, 66
hypo-osmolality and, 68
in hypothyroidism, 64
in nephrotic syndrome, 66
in porphyria, 416
potassium depletion causing, 65
spurious, 63

Hyponatraemic hypertension, 593
Hypoparathyroidism, 286, 539–541
  calcium flux in, 537
  causes of, 539
  in neonates, 311, 312
Hypophosphataemia, 168
Hypophosphatasia, 312, 530
Hypopituitarism, 64, 632, 692
  causing hypothyroidism, 652
  psychiatric aspects, 152
Hyporeninaemic-hypoaldosteronism
    333, 335
Hypotension,
  in carcinoid syndrome, 175
  sodium depletion and, 59,60
Hypothalamic-pituitary-adrenal axis,
    689
  steroid suppression, 696
  testing response, 691
Hypothalamic pituitary function, 626
Hypothalamus, 621
  anatomy, 621
  appetite and, 27
  AVP production in, 88
  controlling pituitary secretion, 624
  obesity and, 29
Hypothermia, 8
Hypothyroidism, 641
  autoimmune, 651
  causes of, 651
  in children, 654
  clinical appearance, 652
  congenital, 286, 641
    neonatal screening, 245, 247, 248
    prevalence, 248,249
  disorders associated with, 650
  Down's syndrome and, 288
  drugs causing, 652
  function tests in, 656,657
  hyponatraemia in, 64
  in lithium poisoning, 753
  obesity and, 28
  in pregnancy, 653
  psychiatric aspects, 150
  secondary, 652
  stature in, 303
  symptoms, 651
Hypoxaemia, 261
Hypoxia,
  causing ventricular haemorrhage,
    262
  effect on cell metabolism, 190
  encephalopathy in, 583
  fetal, 263
  mental aspects, 152, 261
Hypoxic lactic acidosis, 42

I-cell disease, 241,271
Ileocaecal valve, 356
Ileum,
  dysfunction, 361
  function, 356
Iminoglycinuria, 330
Imipramine, 740, 757
Immune-complex disease, 492
Immune response, 472

Immunoglobulins, 467
  age changes in children, 293
  antigenic heterogeneity of, 468
  biological properties, 468
  in cerebrospinal fluid, 564, 565, 567
  deficiencies, 470, 471
  in diarrhoea, 373
  electrophoresis, 490, 566
  functions of, 469
  intrathecal synthesis, 565
  in liver disease, 492
  measurements, 475
  normal ranges, 470
  sensitizing thyroid gland cells, 644
  structure, 468
  synthesis, 468
Immunoglobulin A, 403, 469, 471, 472
  alcoholic cirrhosis and, 132
Immunoglobulin D, 470
Immunoglobulin E, 470
  measurement, 472
Immunoglobulin G, 469, 471, 492
  in cerebrospinal fluid, 565
  in hepatitis, 472
Immunoglobulin M, 469, 471
  in congenital infection, 472
Immunosuppression, 200
  combination therapy, 204
  double therapy, 205
  in heart and lung transplantation,
    208
  in liver transplantation, 213
  maintenance treatment, 205
  monotherapy, 206
  quadrupal therapy, 205
  triple therapy, 204
  in renal transplantation, 204
  with renal dysfunction, 205
Inappropriate diuresis, syndrome of,
    64, 89, 97, 169, 172, 174, 588
  causes of, 83, 90
  clinical features, 172
  diagnosis, 63, 97, 174
  effects of, 59
  effect of chemotherapy on, 174
  investigation of, 101
  trauma and, 195
  treatment, 174
  tumours associated with, 172
Inborn errors of metabolism,
  acidosis and, 42, 46
  acute illness and, 303,304
  hydrogen ion disturbance in, 51
  hypoglycaemia in, 665
  mental retardation and, 254
  pathogenesis, 255, 256
Indocyanine green, 393
Infection,
  ferritin response to, 449, 450
  haemolytic anaemia in, 459
  iron metabolism in, 449
  metabolic disorders and, 260
  renal stones and, 343
  rheumatoid arthritis and, 546
  vitamin A and, 12
Infectious diseases

plasma proteins in, 492
Inferior petrosal sinus catheterization,
    694
Inflammation,
  mediators of, 189
  plasma proteins in, 479, 491
  proteins and, 467
Inflammatory response to injury, 189
Injury,
  acid base balance following, 197
  carbohydrate metabolism following,
    192
  endocrine changes after, 191
  fat metabolism following, 193
  fluid and electrolytes and, 195
  inflammatory response to, 189
  lactic acidosis in, 197
  metabolic response, 191
  plasma proteins following, 194
  potassium loss in, 70
  protein metabolism following, 194
  renal failure in, 198
Insulin, 104–105, 670
  action of GIP on, 672
  binding to receptor, 105
  categories of, 112
  counter regulatory hormones, 108
  in diabetes mellitus, 112
  effects of, 105
  immunoreactive, 668
  impaired secretion in cancer, 162
  inducing hypoglycaemia, 116
  in ketoacidosis, 115
  obesity and, 28
  potassium uptake and, 71
  in protein-energy malnutrition, 8
  release of, 671
    following injury, 192
    from pancreas, 104
  role in metabolism, 105
  secretion in hypoglycaemia, 663
  skeleton and, 524
  structure of, 104
Insulin autoimmune syndrome, 665,
    666
Insulin-like growth factor, 28, 163,
    664
Insulin receptors, 105
Insulin-receptor autoantibodies, 665
Insulin resistance, 107–109
  cancer and, 162
  causes of, 107
  Kahn model, 109
  non-esterified fatty acids and, 108
  pseudo-, 108
  theory of, 107
Insulin stress test, 629
Insulin test of acid secretion, 351
Insulinoma, 145, 163, 664, 667
Intensive care,
  clinical biochemistry in, 189–198
Interferon, 462, 524
Interleukins, 479
Interstitial cell-stimulating hormone,
    623
Interstitial fluid, 53

Intestinal absorption of calcium, 525
Intestinal obstruction, 400, 405–406
  investigations, 405
Intestinal permeability, 357
Intestines,
  see also Small intestine
  atrophy of, 225
  bacterial overgrowth in, 360
  calcium in, 55
  enzymes, 354
  water absorption in, 85
Intracranial pressure,
  causing respiratory alkalosis, 50
Intralipid, 225
Intravascular haemorrhage in RDS,
  305
Intravenous feeding,
  causing diuresis, 94
Intravenous hypertonic saline test, 99
Intraventricular haemorrhage,
  in prematurity, 263
Intrinsic factor, 356, 362
Inulin clearance, 326, 327
Iodide,
  oxidation and organization, 636,
  ·642
Iodide peroxidase defects, 286
Iodide trapping, 636
Iron,
  body content, 448
  body turnover, 447
  bound to transferrin, 448
  deficiency, 438
    diagnosis of, 448
    functional, 450
    mental aspects, 157
    in rheumatoid arthritis, 548
    transferrin and, 485
  distribution in body, 446
  in haemoglobin, 446
  intestinal absorption, 356
  losses, 448
  oxidation states, 446
  poisoning, 744, 752
  storage, 446, 448
Iron-binding capacity, 448, 449
Iron deficiency anaemia, 446, 449, 450,
  463, 490
  ferritin in, 449
  from cadmium, 731
Iron metabolism, 454
  disorders of, 446–452
  major pathways, 48
  proteins in, 447
Iron overload,
  diagnosis, 448
  ferritin, 450
  secondary, 451
Irritable bowel syndrome, 372, 376
Ischaemia causing coma, 583
Islets of Langerhans, 367
  insulin release from, 104
  toxins to cells, 106
Isoleucine, 282
Isopropanol,
  poisoning, 750

test, 439, 442
Isotransferrins, 133
Isovaleric acidaemia, 282, 283, 319
Isovaleric aciduria, 258

Jaundice,
  breast milk, 308
  creatine concentration and, 329
  in G-6-P dehydrogenase deficiency,
    251
  haemolytic, 396
  neonatal, 263, 307, 459
  obstructive, 391, 396
  neoplasia causing, 178
  with parenteral feeding, 313
Jejunostomy, 222
Jejunum,
  function, 356
  resection, 377

Kahn model, 109
Kala azar, 492
Kallikrein (Fletcher factor), 189, 501
Kasahara isoenzyme, 388
Kayser-Fleischer rings, 286, 733
Kearns-Sayre syndrome, 280
Keratomalacia, 12
Kernicterus, 308
  brain damage from, 254
  causing mental retardation, 263
  prevention of, 308
Ketoacidosis, 42
  alcoholic, 140
Ketoacids,
  longer-chain, 43
Ketoaciduria,
  branched-chain, 283
Ketogenic amino acids, 31
Ketones,
  as brain fuel, 228
  in hypoglycaemia, 668
Ketone bodies,
  production, 104
Ketonuria,
  in children, 298
Ketosis,
  in diabetic mellitus, 42
Ketotic hyperglycaemia, 274
  idiopathic, 298
Kidney,
  see also heading beginning Renal
  age changes, 325
  aldosterone action in, 593
  as endocrine organ, 325
  blood flow, 79, 878
  cadmium affecting, 731
  calcium flux, 527
  calcium leak 340
  in calcium metabolism, 519
  control of bicarbonate, 35
  counter-current mechanism in, 87,
    93
  in diabetes, 117, 321
  dysfunction
    immunosuppression and, 201,
      204, 205

  effect of tumours on, 176
  endocrine function, 334
  feedback systems, 330
  handling of potassium, 69
  handling of salt and water, 54
  hormone degradation in, 529
  hydrogen ion homeostasis and, 32
  in hypertension, 592
  hypokalaemia affecting, 72
  medullary cystic disease, 92
  myeloma affecting, 177
  non-Hodgkin's lymphoma in, 176
  parts of, 86
  potassium excretion, 72
  protein breakdown in, 467
  repleting bicarbonate, 38
  role in fluid balance, 76
  selenium in, 732
  stones in *See Renal stones*
  tests of function *See Renal function
    tests*
  transplantation *See Renal
    transplantation*
  tubular function,
    age changes, 325
    in acute renal failure,
    in children, 295
    defects, 93
    inborn errors affecting, 330
  tubular maximum, 331
  tubular necrosis, 334
  tubular phosphate handling, 331
  water reabsorption, 86
Kinins, 189
  deficiency, 498
Kininogen, 501
Klinefelter's syndrome, 713
  sex hormones in, 260
Korsakoff psychosis, 15, 16, 153, 155,
  578
Krabbe's disease, 271
Krebs cycle, 103, 104, 190
Kussmaul respiration, 41
Kwashiorkor, 1, 264, 454
  causes, 2
  cell lipid in, 6
  clinical features, 3
  marasmic, 4
  pathophysiology, 5
  prevalence, 3
  vitamin B deficiency and, 18

Lactase deficiency, 356
Lactate in meningitis, 571
Lactate dehydrogenase,
  as tumour marker, 185
  in central nervous system, 568
  in cerebral infarction, 569
  in neonates, 294
Lactate metabolism,
  disorders of, 279
Lactic acidosis, 43
  aetiology of, 281
  in cancer, 163
  causes, 43
  complicating diabetes, 116

following injury, 197
pyruvate and, 43
type A, 163
type B, 163
Lactic dehydrogenase,
    coronary heart disease and, 615
Lactoferrin, 472
Lactose absorption test, 358
Lactose tolerance,
    in protein energy malnutrition, 7
    tests, 358
Lactulose-breath-hydrogen test, 363
Laron dwarfism, 303, 632
Laurell technique, 508
Laxatives, 323, 365, 378
Lead, 724–728
    effect on fetus, 728
    industrial toxicity, 725
    intake of, 724
    non-industrial poisoning, 726
    physiology, 726
    poisoning, 156, 449, 752
        investigations, 725, 727
        mental retardation and, 267
        symptoms, 725,726
    subclinical exposure, 727
    toxicity, 725
Lecithin-cholesterol acyltransferase,
    607, 608
    familial deficiency, 297
    in liver disease,395
Leigh's encephalopathy, 279
Leprechaunism, 109
Lesch-Nyhan disease, 260, 287
Leucine, 282
    in maple syrup urine disease, 249
Leucine sensitive hypoglycaemia, 299
Leucocytosis in intestinal obstruction,
    405
Leucodystrophies, 271
Leukaemia, 461
    chronic lymphatic, 461
    chronic myeloid, 459, 462
    hairy cell, 462
    lymphoblastic, 462
    treatment, 462
Leukaemia inhibitory factor, 479
Liddle's syndrome, 595
Lignocaine,
    hepatic clearance, 394
Lingual thyroid, 634
Lipaemia retinalis, 603
Lipase,
    in diagnosis of pancreatitis, 368
Lipids,
    alcoholism and, 132
    in cancer, 164
    in children, 296
    in kwashiorkor, 6
Lipid transfer protein, 607
Lipoperoxidation, 289
Lipoproteins,
    atheroma and, 609
    characteristics, 601
    classification, 601
    high density, 602, 607

age changes in, 612
    disorders of, 605
    metabolism, 607
    reverse cholesterol transport and,
        606
    intermediate density, 602, 604
    low density, 602, 604, 609
    metabolism, 602, 607
    in Tangier disease, 297
    very low density, 602, 603, 604, 606,
        610
Lipoprotein(a), 604
Lipoprotein cascade, 604
Lipoprotein lipase, 602, 603
Lipoprotein X, 394
Lipotrophic pituitary hormone, 624
Lithium,
    poisoning, 736, 740, 745, 753
    therapeutic monitoring, 762
Lithium salts,
    effect on water balance, 93
Liver,
    ALA synthetase in, 420
    alcohol affecting, 130, 132
    alcohol metabolism in, 122
    in ammonia detoxification, 582
    bromosulphthalein and indocyanine
        removal, 393
    caffeine clearance, 394
    in calcium metabolism, 519
    cancer of, 179, 392
    clotting factors in, 503
    copper affecting, 733
    drug metabolism in, 761
    encephalopathy, 581
        GABA in, 582
        role of ammonia, 581
    enzyme induction, 135
    fetal,
        biopsy of, 239
    glucose production in, 103
    glucose uptake, 105
    glycogen stores, 298
    ketone body production in, 104
    lignocaine clearance, 394
    lipoprotein cascade and, 604
    metastatic destruction, 163
    paracetamol damaging, 754
    plasma proteins in, 389, 465
    in poisoning, 743
    in protein catabolism, 466
    protein synthesis in, 390
    selenium in, 732
    steroid metabolism in, 686, 687
Liver cirrhosis, 285, 581
    alcoholic, 120, 131
    aminotransferases in, 386
    oedema in, 66
    proteins in, 392
    transplantation and, 211
Liver disease,
    albumin in, 390
    alcohol causing, 130, 396
    alkaline phosphatase in, 387
    aminotransferases in, 386
    arterial ammonia in, 394

bile acids in, 391
caeruloplasmin in, 393, 486
clotting factor deficiency in, 498,
    500
encephalopathy in, 581, 582
GGT in, 129
glutathione-S-transferase in, 391
growth hormone in, 633
haptoglobin levels in, 483
hyperbilirubinaemia in, 385
immunoglobulin response in, 472
lecithin cholesterol acyltransferase
    in, 395
lipoprotein X in, 394
neonatal, 308
plasma proteins in, 492, 493
in porphyria, 417
protein measurement in, 392
Liver disease clinics,
    alcoholism identification by, 127
Liver failure,
    fulminant, 581
    psychiatric aspects, 153
Liver function tests, 383–398
    application of, 395
    batteries of, 395
    clearance tests, 393
    monitoring with, 397
    profiling, 395
    role in diagnosis, 396
    screening, 395
    types of, 383
    use of, 395
Liver profiles, 383
Liver transplantation, 210–214
    biochemical monitoring, 212, 213
    in children, 213
    immunosuppression, 213
    indications for, 211
    metabolic changes during, 211, 212
    neurological complications, 214
    patient selection, 211
    perioperative monitoring, 211
    postoperative monitoring, 212
    rejection, 214
Long acting thyroid stimulator, 645
Looser's zones, 537
Lowe's syndrome, 278
Lumbar puncture, 562
Lundh meal, 139, 369, 370, 371
Lungs,
    in hydrogen ion homeostasis, 32
    small cell carcinoma of, 172
    transplantation, *see Heart and lung
        transplantation*
Luteinizing hormone 152, 623, 625,
    707, 711, 712
    in polycystic ovary, 717
    in puberty, 715
Lyme disease, 572
B Lymphocytes, 573
    immunoglobulin synthesis in, 468
    malignant proliferation, 473
    in rheumatoid arthritis, 547
B Lymphocyte stimulating
        autoantibodies, 665

T Lymphocytes, 573
T helper lymphocytes, 547
Lymphomas,
    effect on kidney, 176, 178
    in transplantation, 209
Lyonization process, 497
Lysine, 282
Lysinuria protein intolerance, 276, 278
Lysosomal disorders, 268
    diagnosis, 268
    mental retardation in, 254
    treatment, 269
Lysozyme in meningitis, 572

McCune-Albright hypoplasia, 716
Macrocytosis, 130
Macroglobulin, 481, 482
    electrophoresis, 489
Magnesium, 520
    cancer and, 168
    colonic absorption, 364
    psychiatric aspects, 156
    surgery and, 196
Malabsorption, 4, 372–379
    aetiological classification, 313
    drug induced, 378
    faecal fats in, 359
    pellagra in, 17
    symptoms, 372
    zinc excretion in, 21
Malaria, 436, 437, 459
Malate dehydrogenase, 568
Maldigestion, 359
Malnutrition,
    anaemia in, 454
    consequences of, 221
    growth and, 302
    in hospital patients, 218
    incidence in hospitals, 222
    marginal, 2
    mental retardation and, 264
    metabolic rate and, 8
    protein-energy,
        see Protein-energy malnutrition
    transferrin in, 485
Manganese, 22, 156, 734
Mania, 148, 149
Mannitol, 95
Mannosidosis, 270
Maple syrup urine disease, 258, 282, 319
    neonatal screening, 249
Marasmus, 1
    anaemia in, 454
    body fat in, 5
    causes, 2
    clinical features, 3
    hair in, 9
    hypothermia in, 8
    pathophysiology, 4
    prevalence, 3
March haemoglobinuria, 321
Maroteau-Lamy disease, 268, 270
MELAS, 280
Meal provocation test for
    hypoglycaemia, 667

Meckel's diverticulum, 349
Medulloblastoma, 575
Melanogen, 323
Melanosis coli, 378
Meningioma, 575
Meningitis, 571
    fungal, 571
    tuberculous, 564, 571
    viral, 572
Menkes kinky hair syndrome, 21, 258, 287, 393
Menopause, 718
Menstruation,
    disorders of, 716
Mental handicap, *See Mental retardation*
Mental retardation,
    aetiology, 254, 255
    aminoacidurias and, 271, 278
    biochemical disturbances and, 253
    chromosomal disorders and, 288
    convulsions with, 265
    deafness in, 256, 257
    definitions, 253
    degenerative nervous disease and, 267
    detection of metabolic disorders, 256
    in Down's syndrome, 288
    endocrine disorders causing, 286
    environmental causes, 254, 261
    ethical considerations, 289
    galactosaemia causing, 249, 285
    genetic counselling, 289
    growth disorders and, 259
    histidinaemia and, 273
    homocystinuria, 274
    in homocystinuria, 249
    hypervalcaemia and, 286
    hypernatraemia causing, 264
    hypoglycaemia and, 261
    inherited and acquired, 252–291
    investigation of, 262
    laboratory investigations, 260
    lead and, 267
    in Lesch-Nyhan syndrome, 287
    in low birthweight infants, 262
    malnutrition and, 264
    metabolic disorders causing, 254
    neurological signs, 259
    ocular defects and, 256, 257
    organic acidurias and, 279
    pathogenesis, 254
    in phenylketonuria, 253
    purine and pyrimidine metabolism and, 287
    vitamin deficiency and, 265
Mercurialentis, 729
Mercurialism, 729
Mercury, 93, 728–730
    poisoning, 157, 753, 729
MERRFA, 280
Mesenteric embolism, 401, 402
Metabolic acidosis, 211
Metabolic disorders,
    inherited, 157

    peculiar odours in, 258
    see also Inborn errors of metabolism
Metabolic encephalopathies, 152
Metachromatic leucodystrophy, 158, 268, 269, 271
Metals,
    biochemistry and toxicity, 723–735
Metformin in diabetes, 112, 116
Methaemalbumin,
    in pancreatitis, 407
Methaemoglobin, 570
Methaemoglobin A, 433, 439
Methaemoglobinaemia, 433, 434, 751
Methanol poisoning, 750
Methaqualone poisoning, 740,750
Methionine, 754
Methotrexate poisoning, 739
Methoxyflurane, 342
Methylacetyl-CoA tiolase deficiency, 282
3-Methylcrotonyl-CoA carboxylase deficiency, 282
3-Methylcronyl glycinuria, 258
Methylene tetrahydrofolate reductase deficiency, 278
3-Methylglutaconic aciduria, 282
Methylmalonic acidaemia, 282
Methyl mercury, 728
Methyl salicylate poisoning, 754
Metyrapone, 684
Metyrapone test, 693
Mevalonic aciduria, 282
Microalbuminuria, 114, 118
B_2-Microglobulin, 572
Microglobulin, 329, 486
Milk alkali syndrome, 340
Minerals,
    in brain metabolism, 228
    in cancer, 165
    disorders of, 156, 311
    loss of, 518
    in total parenteral nutrition, 224
Mineralocorticoids, 687
Mitochondrial respiratory chain disorders, 280
Molybdenum cofactor deficiency, 287
Monoamine oxidase, 597
Monoclonal gammapathy, 473, 490,
    aetiology, 473
    electrophoresis, 489
    measurement, 475
    prognosis, 476
    of undetermined significance, 474
Mood, swings of, 147, 150
Morquio disease, 270
Mosaicism, 713
Motilin, 679
Mucoliposes, 268
Mucopolysaccharides, 268, 270
Mucopolysaccharidoses, 269, 320
Mucosulphatitosis, 268
Multiple carboxylase deficiency, 258
Multiple endocrine abnormality syndrome, 542
Multiple endocrine adenomatosis, 169, 631, 674, 697

Multiple endocrine neoplasia
    syndrome, 151, 169, 595, 664
Multiple sclerosis, 572
    cerebrospinal fluid in,573
Multiple sulphatase deficiency, 271
Munchausen's syndrome, 158, 408,
    726
    by proxy, 158, 159
Muscle,
    amino acids in, in trauma, 194
Muscular dystrophy, 250
Mycobacterium tuberculosis, 572
Myelin,
    antibodies, 574
    basic protein, 565, 574
    loss of, 573
    proteins in, 573
Myelodysplasia, 462
Myelofibrosis, 462
Myeloma, 340, 462, 474, 486
    hypercalcaemia in, 165, 167
    immunoglobulins in, 474, 475
    renal syndromes associated with,
    177
Myocardial disease 387, 616
Myoglobin,
    in cardiac disease, 617
    in poisoning, 746
    in urine, 321
Myopathy, 522
Myosin in myocardial infarction, 617
Myxoedema, 643
Myxoedema madness, 151

Naloxone, 739, 753
Narcotic drugs,
    poisoning by, 753
Natriuretic hormones, 592, 593
Nausea,
    stimulating AVP, 55
Necrolytic migratory erythema, 673
Neonatal biochemistry, 292–315
Neonatal screening,
    action on results, 247
    benefit to family, 246
    benefit to individual, 245
    benefit to society, 246
    collecting sample, 246
    cost of, 247
    epidemiological benefits, 246
    for biochemical disorders, 244–252
    for phenylketonuria, 27
    practical aspects, 246
    programmes, 247
    reasons for, 245
Neonates,
    blood samples from, 314
    disorders of calcium in, 311
    disorders of gonadal function, 715
    Graves' disease in, 641
    21-hydroxylase deficiency in, 703
    hypercalcaemia in, 312
    hyperglycaemia in, 311
    hypocalcaemia in, 264
    hypoglycaemia in, 310
    immunoglobulin deficiency in, 470

jaundice in, 263, 307
    monitoring, 308
    liver disease in, 308
    lupus syndrome, 552
    protein binding in, 760
    range of plasma constituents in, 293
    respiratory distress in, 304
    see also Respiratory distress
        syndrome
Neoplasia, *See Tumours*
Neopterin, 376, 572
Nephritis,
    potassium losing, 71
Nephrocalcinosis, 340
Nephrotic syndrome, 320, 482
    albumin in, 484
    calcifediol in, 542
    electrophoresis, 489
    in myeloma, 178
    oedema in, 66
Nesisioblastosis, 299, 311
Neural tube defects, 487
    screening for, 231
    vitamins and, 266
Neuroblastomas, 577
Neurofibromatosis, 543
Neurogenerative disorders, 270
Neuroglycopenia, 116, 152, 666, 668
    acute, 662
    chronic, 663
    subacute, 663, 664
Neurohormones, 146
Neurohypophysis, 622
Neurolipidoses, 270
Neurological disease,
    aluminium and, 724
    biochemical investigations in, 578
    diagnosis, 560
    degenerative, 267
Neuromediators, 146
Neurometabolic disorders, 256
    diagnosis of, 260
Neuromodulators, 146
Neuromuscular activity,
    thyroid hormones and, 640
Neuron-specific enolase, 568
    as tumour marker, 185
Neuropeptide Y, 571, 680
Neurophysins, 88
Neuroregulation, 146
Neurotensin, 680
Neurotransmitters, 146
    alcohol affecting, 124
    growth hormone and, 627
    hypoxia affecting, 261, 583
    involvement in disease, 146
    psychiatric disorders and, 147
    in schizophrenia, 147
Newborn,
    haemolytic disease of, 307
    haemorrhagic disease of, 500
Nickel, 734
Nicotinamide adenine nucleotide, 122
    reduced, 122
Nicotine test, 89, 99
Nicotinic acid, *see Vitamin B$_3$*

Niemann-Pick disease, 270, 606
Nitrate poisoning, 739, 751
Nitrite Poisoning, 752
Nitrogen balance,
    head injury and, 228
Nitrogen excretion, 61
Non-insulin-secreting tumours, 664
Non-suppressible insulin-like activity,
    163
Noradrenaline,
    alcohol and, 126
    in Alzheimer's disease, 148
    conversion to adrenaline, 681
    iron metabolism and, 157
    phaeochromocytoma and, 151, 597
    secretion following injury, 191
    synthesis, 583
Nuclear magnetic resonance scans,
    560
5′ Nucleotidase in liver disease, 391
Nutrition,
    see also Malnutrition etc
    assessment in hospital patients, 219
    biochemical indices, 220
    burns and, 227
    in cancer patients, 228
    classification in children, 3
    energy requirements, 224
    enteral, *See Enteral nutrition*
    in head injury, 228
    mental retardation and, 264
    monitoring in hospital, 226
    of surgical patient, 226
    of sick patient, 218–230
    patient monitoring, 226
    postoperative, 221
    protein requirements, 224
    providing support, 221
    requirements, 223
    support for patients, 226
    total parenteral, *see Total parenteral*
        nutrition
Nutritional disorders, 1–24
Nutritional support team, 218

Oasthouse disease, 258
Obesity, 25–30
    aetiology, 26
    assessment of, 25
    calorie theory, 26
    classification, 26
    definition, 25
    diabetes and, 105, 109
    growth hormone and, 29
    gut hormones and, 29
    hormonal aspects, 28
    insulin and, 28
    morbid, 27
    personal factors, 27
    reasons for concern, 26
    sympathetic nervous system and, 29
    treatment, 29
Obstructive uropathy, 177
Occipital horn syndrome, 287
Octeotride, 678
Odours,

metabolic disorders and, 258
Oedema,
  in beri-beri, 16
  in congestive heart failure, 65
  fluid retention with, 65
  intermittent idiopathic, 66
  in kwashiorkor, 2, 3, 9
  in liver cirrhosis, 66
  in nephrotic syndrome, 66
  in protein-energy malnutrition, 1
Oesophagus,
  acid-perfusion test, 348
  acid reflux, 347
    operative procedure, 350
  ambulant monitoring of, 347
  assessment of function, 347
  carcinoma of, 60
  pain in, 619
Oestrogens, 709
  effect on bone, 524, 530
  measurement of, 719
  production, 710
Oligoclonal banding, 565
  detection of, 566
Oncofetal proteins, 179
Opiates,
  poisoning by, 739, 753
Oral feeding, 221
Oral glucose test, 667
Oral glucose tolerance test, 630
Organic acidurias,
  in mental retardation, 279
Organochloride poisoning, 754
Organophosphorus poisoning, 739,
  748, 754
Ornithine transcarbamylase, 299
Orocaecal transit time, 363
Orosomucoid, 483, 491
Orotic aciduria, 288, 301
Osmolal clearance, 82
Osmolality, 80
  alcohol affecting, 123
  measurement of, 67
  normal, 100
  in poisoning, 745
  thirst and, 82
Osmometry, 80
Osmoreceptors, 83
Osmoregulation, 61, 83
Osmotic diuresis, 61, 91, 94
Osteitis fibrosa, 335
Osteocalcin, 529
Osteoclast activating factor, 168
Osteogenesis imperfecta, 500, 543
Osteomalacia, 13, 335, 530, 537
  acidosis causing, 41
  causes of, 542
  differential diagnosis, 14
  from cadmium, 730, 731
Osteopetrosis, 529
Osteoporosis, 529, 544
  in alcoholism, 139
  differential diagnosis, 14
  postmenopausal, 532, 533, 542, 544
Ovarian steroids, 711
Ovary,

function and control, 711
  teratoma of, 641
Overbreathing,
  alkalosis from, 50
Overlap syndromes, 551
Ovulation, 716
Oxygen,
  haemoglobin affinity, 423, 424
    measurement of, 440
  transport in haemoglobin, 446
Oxygen consumption of brain, 146
Oxygen tension,
  in respiratory dysfunction, 47
  stimulatary effect, 48
Oxygen transport,
  modification of, 424
Oxyhaemoglobin, 423
  as buffer, 49
  in brain haemorrhage, 570
Oxynotic cells, 348
Oxytocin, 88, 621

pH,
  arterial, 51
  determination, 40
  in blood, 40, 51
Paba test, 370
Paediatric biochemistry, 292–315
Paget's disease of bone, 531, 543
  bone loss and gain in, 530, 534
  calcitonin in, 521
Pancreas,
  breath tests, 371
  disease of, 367
  enzymes, 367, 371
  exocrine function,
    assessment of, 369, 370, 376
    in coeliac disease, 376
    in diarrhoea, 376
    insufficiency, 377
  function, 367–372
  indirect tests of, 371
  islet hyperplasia, 675
  metastases, 677
  proteases, 356
  in protein-energy malnutrition, 5
  regulation of secretion, 367
  transplantation, 214
  tubeless test of function, 370, 371
  tumours, 678
Pancreatic cholera, 378
Pancreatic Graves' disease, 665
Pancreatic hormone measurements,
  668
Pancreatic juice, 79, 367
Pancreatic lipase, 367
Pancreatic polypeptide, 679
Pancreatitis,
  acute, 367, 406
    assessment of severity, 369
    clinical features, 406
    in alcoholism, 138
    investigations, 407
  chemical, 603
  chronic, 369, 377
    in alcoholism, 138

diagnosis, 368
Pancreolauryl test, 370
Pancreozymin 671
Pancreozymin-cholecystokinin, 676,
  677
Panic attacks, 148, 152
Paracetamol,
  detection in urine, 323
  effect on liver, 391
  monitoring, 762
  poisoning, 739, 740, 754
Paraldehyde poisoning, 44
Paralytic ileus, 403
Paraproteins, 472, 474, 475
Paraquat poisoning, 740, 744, 754
Parathyroid function,
  in hypercalciuria, 340
Parathyroid hormone,
  amino acid structure, 519
  in calcium metabolism, 516
  effect on bone, 520
  high levels of, 538
  regulating calcium, 518
  secretion, 519
    disorders of, 538
  target-organ actions, 520
Parathyroid hormone-related peptide,
  524
Parathyroid hormone related proteins,
  167
Parenteral nutrition, 313
Parietal cells, 349
Parkinson's disease, 147
Paroxysmal cold haemoglobinuria,
  459
Paroxysmal nocturnal
  haemoglobinuria, 461
P-component, 487
Pelizaeus-Merzbacher disease, 158
Pellagra, 17, 155, 265
  in carcinoid syndrome, 175
Pendred syndrome, 257, 642
Pentgastrin test, 350
Pentane in breath, 618
Pentose phosphate pathway, 458
Pepsinigen, 352
Peptic ulcer, 400, 402, 406
Peptide YY, 670, 680
C-peptide, 668
  suppression test, 667
Pericarditis, 615
Periodic paralysis, 74
Peripheral neuropathy,
  in vitamin deficiency, 456
Peripheral resistance, 586
Peritonitis, 400, 402
Pernicious anaemia, 350, 351, 362, 456
  gastric carcinoma and, 456
Peroxidase reaction, 636
Peroxisomal disorders,
  affecting brain, 284
  biochemical assays, 285
  mental retardation and, 254
Peutz-Jegher polyp, 402
Phaeochromocytoma, 322, 587, 595
  diagnosis, 598

screening for, 599
psychiatric aspects, 151
poisoning, 739, 740, 745, 747
Phenylalanine, 271
enzyme deficiency of hydroxylation, 272
Phenylalanine hydroxylase, 248
Phenyl ethanolamine-N-methyl transferase, 681
Phenylketonuria, 241, 272–273
adult, 273
classical, 271
cofactor-deficient, 272
definition, 271
genetics, 273
hair and skin in, 258
maternal, 260
mental retardation and, 253, 261
neurological signs, 272
odour of, 258
screening, 245, 247, 248, 272
treatment, 273
Phenytoin, 759
interaction with metronidazole, 764
poisoning, 740, 747
therapeutic monitoring, 761
Phlebotomy, 451, 452
Phosphate,
in cancer, 168
deficiency, 522
depletion in neonates, 312, 313
distribution of, 515, 517
extracellular concentration, 517
following surgery, 196
plasma, 528
range in children, 293
reabsorption, 528
in skeletal mineralization, 530
tubular handling, 331
urinary,
carbonate dehydratase and, 36
Phosphate buffering, 33
Phospholipase,
in diagnosis of pancreatitis, 269
Phospholipids,
in shock, 190
in surfactant, 305
Phospholipid antibodies, 551, 554
Pigmentation,
in Addison's disease, 696
in Cushing's syndrome, 698
in precocious puberty, 716
Pigments in urine, 323
Pineal gland, 626
Pink puffers, 48
Pipe colic acidaemia, 278
Pituitary dwarfism, 631
Pituitary gland, 621–633
adenoma, 575, 700
anatomy, 621
anterior,
hypothalmic control of, 624
measurement of hormones, 624
tests of function, 626
histology, 622
hormones of, 623

tumours, 631
Pituitary-Leydig cell axis, 712
Pituitary-seminiferous tubule axis, 712
Placental alkaline phosphatase, 183
Plasma,
blood clotting tests on, 506
composition of, 54, 293
cooling, 81
osmolality, 67, 76
water content, 80
Plasma arginine vasopressin, 100
see also Arginine vasopressin
Plasma enzymes,
excess alcohol and, 128
Plasma lipids,
fasting, 297
in children, 296
Plasma proteins, 53, 54, 464–494
see also specific proteins
in alcoholism, 132
in blood clotting, 467
in cancer, 164
catabolism, 466
clinical applications, 464
distribution, 465
effect of steroids on, 465
electrophoresis, 465, 467
following injury, 194
functions of, 467
genetic variants, 465
historical aspects, 464
immune defence by, 467
in inflammation, 467, 491
in liver, 389
measurement in disease, 490
metabolism of, 465
oncofetal, 467, 486
in protein-energy malnutrition, 10
signal, 467
synthesis, 465
tissue-derived, 467
transport, 467, 483
Plasma transaminases, 130
Plasmin,
activators, 505
biochemistry, 504
formation, 496
Plasminogen,
biochemistry, 504
function, 496
measurement, 520
Plasminogen activators,
in myocardial infarction, 618
Plasminogen activator inhibitor, 610
Plasmodium falciparum, 438
Platelets,
α-granule deficiency, 510
biochemistry, 506
defective adhesion, 510
disorders, 499
function of, 495
release reaction defects, 510
tests of, 520
Platelet monoamine oxidase, 126
Plumbism, 156
Pneumonia, 47

Pneumonitis,
from mercury, 729
Poisoning,
antidotes, 739
blood-gas analysis in, 745
chromatography in, 742
clinical chemical tests, 746
diagnosis, 738
electrolyte measurements in, 745
emesis in, 743
enzyme abnormalities, 746
forced diuresis in, 744
gastric lavage in, 743
haemodialysis in, 744
laboratory investigation of, 736–757
monitoring, 738
myoglobin measurement in, 746
osmolality measurement, 745
prognosis, 738
radioimmunoassays, 742
sample collection, 737
screening, 741
self-, 736
treatment, 743, 744, 746
Pollutants,
mental retardation and, 267
Polycystic ovary syndrome, 717
Polycythaemia, 433, 454, 499
Polycythaemia rubra vera, 459
Polydipsia, 76
causes, 92
clinical aspects, 91
in diabetes, 111
hypokalaemia and, 96
investigation of, 97
primary, 95
psychogenic, 95, 98, 100
secondary, 92
Polyethylene glycols, 358
Polymerase chain reaction,
fetal sexing with, 243
in prenatal diagnosis, 241
Polyneuritis, 64
Polypeptide-secreting tumours, 378
Polyuria, 76
causes, 92
clinical aspects, 91
in diabetes, 111
genito-urinary obstruction and, 92
hypokalaemia and, 96
iatrogenic, 95
investigation of, 97
primary, 92
secondary, 95
in sepsis, 94
Pompe's disease, 270
Ponderstat, 27
Porphobilinogen,
excretion, 411, 417
formation, 409
urinary, 323, 412
Porphobilinogen deaminase, 413, 415
Porphobilinogen synthetase deficiency, 413, 414, 415, 416
Porphyria, 323, 409, 412–418
acute attacks, 415

acute intermittent, 157, 415
clinical features, 415
congenital erythropoietic, 416,417
enzyme defects in, 413, 414
from cancer, 179
gene carriers, 418
hereditary copro-, 415, 416,417
laboratory diagnosis, 417
laboratory differentiation, 414
latent, 414
main types, 409
molecular pathology, 415
PBG synthetase deficient, 413, 414,
    415,416
variegate, 415, 416, 417, 418
with skin lesions, 416, 417
Porphyria cutanea tarda, 413, 415, 416
Porphyrins,
determination of, 412
total concentration, 413
enzymes, 413
Porphyrinogens, 410
Portal hypertension, 66
Porter-Silber reaction, 691
Postoperative care, 189–198
Potassium, 69–74
see also Hypokalaemia,
    Hyperkalaemia, etc
absorption in colon, 364
in acute renal failure, 334
carbonate hydratase and, 39
in cells, 53
in cerebrospinal fluid, 562
depletion,
    bicarbonate and, 49
    in hyponatraemia, 65, 66
    in protein-energy malnutrition, 5
dietary intake, 69
distribution, 69
excretion, 593
following trauma, 195
interrelation with sodium, 69
in poisoning, 745
reabsorption, 69
renal excretion, 73
renal handling, 69
renal loss, 70
    urinary, 71, 322
Potassium-losing nephritis, 71
Prader-Willi syndrome, 260, 289
Prealbumin, 579
in cerebrospinal fluid, 568
electrophoresis, 488
measurement, 392
Prednisolone, 691
Pregnancy, 717
albumin in, 484
alcohol intake and, 121
alkaline phosphatase in, 387
corticosteroid binding globulin in,
    688
diabetes in, 110
folic acid in, 457
GGT activity, 130
hypertension in, 598
pernicious anaemia in, 456

pre-eclampsia, 460
sex steroids in, 709
tests for, 319
thyroid disease in, 653
thyroid function tests in,659
vitamin intake, 266
Prekallikrein, 501
Premature infants,
biochemistry for, 304
metabolic bone disease, 312
RDS in, 263, 305
ventricular haemorrhage, 262
Prenatal diagnosis,
by biochemistry, 239
gene therapy for, 244
inherited metabolic disease, 237–244
objectives, 237
obtaining sample, 238
polymerase chain reaction in, 241
with DNA analysis, 241
Prenatal screening,
criteria for, 231
for neural tube defects, 231
maternal biochemical markers, 235
time for, 232
Primidone poisoning, 740, 747
Progesterone, 691, 709, 710
measurement, 691, 719, 720
Proinsulin assays, 668
Prolactin, 623
in epilepsy, 574
insufficiency, 632
stimulating secretion, 627
Prolactin inhibitory factor, 624
Prolonged fast test for hypoglycaemia,
    667
Pro-opiomelanocorticotrophin, 624
Pro-opiomelanocortin, 171, 173, 698
Pripionyl CoA, 281
Propoxyphene poisoning, 753
Prostaglandins, 166, 190, 678
in brain haemorrhage, 571
effect on bone, 524
steroid hormones and, 524
Prostate specific antigen, 184
Prostatic acid phosphatase, 184
Prostatic cancer, 184
Prostatic hypertrophy, 184
Protease inhibitors, 480
Proteins,
catabolism, 466
in cerebrospinal fluid, 564, 565
colonic degradation, 365
in diarrhoea, 373
digestion and absorption, 356
electrophoresis, 392
gastrointestinal loss, 363
glycosylated, 113, 118
in iron metabolism, 447
in liver disease, 392
plasma, *see Plasma proteins*
requirements, 224
    in burns patients, 227
stone formation and, 341
synthesis, 465, 466
Protein buffering, 33

Protein-calorie malnutrition,
    see Protein-energy malnutrition
Protein-energy malnutrition, 1
amino acid metabolism in, 7
body composition in, 5
in cancer patients, 228
carbohydrate metabolism in, 8
causes, 1
in children, 1
classification, 1
clinical features, 3
investigations, 11
long-term effects, 6
metabolic disturbances, 4
pathogenesis, 2
pathophysiology, 4
plasma proteins in, 10
prevalence, 2
prognosis and mortality, 4
protein metabolism in 7
scoring system, 1, 2
urea metabolism in, 8
Protein-energy ratio, 224
Protein fiasco, 2
Protein gap, 2
Protein metabolism
in cancer, 164
following injury, 194
in protein energy malnutrition, 7
Protein synthesis, 7, 640
Protein C, 503, 551
assay, 509
biochemistry, 504
deficiency, 499
inhibitor, 499, 503, 504
Protein S, 551
assay, 509
biochemistry, 504
deficiency, 499
Protein S-100, 577
Proteinuria, 319, 320,
in connective tissue disorders, 555
in diabetes, 118
following transplantation, 336
glomerular, 320, 329
in myeloma, 178
postural, 330
tubular, 320
Proteolysis-inducing factor, 194
Prothrombin,
assay, 508
biochemistry, 503
consumption test, 506
deficiency, 498
Prothrombin time test, 506, 508
Pseudoxanthoma elasticum, 500
Pseudohermaphroditism, 713, 714
Pseudohypoaldosteronism, 73
Pseudohypoparathyroidism 286, 540,
    541
Pseudopseudohypoparathyroidism,
    540, 541
Psychiatric disorders, 144
laboratory investigations, 159
neuroendocrinological aspects, 149
of biochemical origin, 144–160

neurotransmitters and, 147
Puberty,
  delayed, 302, 715
  precocious, 716
Pulmonary embolism, 387
Pulmonary emphysema, 481
  transplantation for, 207
Pulmonary hypertension, 551
Pulmonary oedema, 47, 195
Pulmonary tuberculosis, 245
Purine metabolism,
  disorders of, 287
Purine nucleoside phosphorylase
  deficiency, 288
Purpura,
  thrombotic thrombocytopenia, 460
Pyloric stenosis,
  bicarbonate in, 49
Pyridoxine,
  See Vitamin B₅
Pyridoxine-dependent convulsions,
  278
Pyruvate,
  conversion to lactate, 44
  lactic acidosis and, 43
Pyruvate carboxylase, 44, 280
  deficiency, 282
Pyruvate dehydrogenase, 43, 279
  deficiency, 279
Pyruvate kinase, 459
Pyruvate metabolism,
  disorders of, 279

Q fever, 492
Queterlet index, 25
Quinidine poisoning, 740, 748
Quinine poisoning, 740, 748

Ranitidine, 349
Rapoport-Leubering cycle, 424, 425
Rapid urease test, 353
Reactive arthritis, 546
Rectal bleeding,
  in ulcerative colitis, 376
Rectal carcinoma, 70
Red cells, *See also under erythrocytes*
Red cell inclusions, 438
Reductase deficiency, 714
  in homocystinuria, 275
Reflex bradycardia, 597
Refsum's disease, 284
Regan isoenzyme, 388
Rehydration, 116 114
Reifenstein syndrome, 714
Reiter's syndrome, 546
Renal arterial stenosis, 204
Renal colic, 400
Renal disease,
  bone disease and, 335
  chronic, 334
  in diabetes, 321, 330
  plasma calcium in, 516
  plasma proteins in, 492
  polyuria and polydipsia in, 92
  subclinical, 320
Renal failure,

after injury, 198
calcium metabolism in, 541
chronic,
  acidosis in, 333
from myeloma, 177
hyperkalaemia in, 73
osteoporosis in, 544
sodium reabsorption in, 56
transplantation for, 202
in trauma, 195
tubular function in, 333
water and sodium retention in, 65
Renal function, 86–88
  in children, 294
  development, 294
Renal function tests, 325–327
  GFR, 325–330
  tubular function, 330
Renal osteodystrophy, 335
Renal stones, 338–345
  aetiology, 539
  age factors, 343
  causes, 344
  clinical features, 344
  composition of, 343
  dietary factors, 343
  formation of, 338
  frequency of, 339
  hypercalcaemia and, 340
  hypercalciuria and, 34
  infection causing, 343
  laboratory examination, 338
  mechanical factors, 343
  oxalate, 342
  presentation of, 339
  risk factors, 343
  sex ratios, 343
  sodium intake and, 343
  uric acid and, 340, 341
  water factors, 343
Renal transplantation, 200, 202–206
  complications, 203
  immunosuppression in, 204
  patient selection, 203
  polyuria following, 92
  postoperative monitoring, 203
  renal function after, 336
Renal tubular acidosis, 41, 177, 322,
  520
  hypercitraturia from, 341
Renal tubular damage,
  acidosis from, 45
Renal tubular function,
  in children, 295
Renin, 334
  synthesis, 587
Renin-angiotensin-aldosterone system,
  83, 84, 85, 321
  in children, 293
  following injury, 192
Renin cascade mechanism, 587
Reperfusion injury,
  breath pentane and, 618
Reproductive system, 707–721
  see also Gonads etc
Reserpine, 147

Respiration, 446
Respiratory acidosis, 46
Respiratory alkalosis, 49, 50
  causes, 50
  in liver transplantation, 211
Respiratory centre, 34
Respiratory distress, 40, 310
  blood gases in 47
Respiratory distress syndrome, 262,
  304, 305
Restriction length fragment
  polymorphism, 511
Retinol, *See Vitamin A*
Retinol-binding protein, 10
Retinopathy,
  diabetic, 117
Retinopathy of prematurity, 305
Reye's syndrome, 276, 283, 290, 299,
  300, 301
Rhabdomyolysis 139, 746, 756
Rhesus incompatibility, 307
Rheumatoid arthritis , 485, 546–550
  cellular filtrate in, 547
  drug therapy, 550
  extra-articular, 546
  haematological abnormalities, 548
  immunotherapy, 550
  laboratory tests, 547
  pathology, 547
  radiography, 549
  synovial fluid in, 549
Rheumatoid factor, 547
Riboflavin, *See Vitamin B₂*
Rickets, 13, 312
  rarer forms, 523
Rigorous exercise test, 667
Rotor's syndrome, 394

Salicylate overdosage, 43, 301
Saliva, 79
  adrenal steroids in, 691
  gonadal steroids in, 719
Salla disease, 268, 271
Salsolinol, 136
Salt in hypertension, 592
Salt wasting, 306
Sample collecting,
  ethical problems, 292
Sandoff's disease, 158, 240, 270
Sanfilippo disease, 270
Saralasin, 84
Sarcoidosis, 15, 340
Sarcosinaemia, 278
Scheie disease, 270
Schilling test, 362, 456
Schindler disease, 71
Schistosomiasis, 344
Schizophrenia, 150
  neurotransmitters and, 147
Scleroderma, 551,553
Screening programmes, 245
Scurvy, 18, 500
Secalciferol, 522
Secretin, 349, 670, 675
Secretin-cholecystokinin test, 369
Secretin stimulation test, 352

Selenium, 732–733
  deficiency, 224
  toxicity, 157
Sella turcica, 622
Sepsis, 94
Serotonin, *See 5-Hydroxytryptime*
Severe combined immunodeficiencies,
      470
Sex hormone binding globulin, 709
Sex steroids,
  in calcium metabolism,
    see also Gonadal steroids
Sexual differentiation, 712, 713, 719
Sham feeding test, 351
Sheehan's syndrome, 94, 632
Shock, 189
  bacterial, 479
  from blood loss, 457
  hypoglycaemia in, 193
Short bowel syndrome, 226, 349, 376
Sialidosis, 271
Sick cell syndrome, 64, 68, 190
Sick euthyroid syndrome, 191, 192,
      654
Sickle cell anaemia, 308, 431
  abdominal pain in, 408
  interaction with other
        haemoglobins, 431
  tests for, 438
Siderosis, 416
Singh score, 536
Sipple's syndrome, 151
Sjögren's syndrome, 552
Skeleton,
  effect of calcium on, 730, 731
  homeostasis, 523
  measurement of mass and loss, 535
  metabolism, 535
  mineralization, 522
Skin,
  in beri-beri, 16
  in kwashiorkor, 3
  water loss through, 79
  in zinc deficiency, 21
Skin disease, 258, 493
Skinfold thickness in obesity, 25
  measurement, 220
Sly disease, 270
Small intestine,
  absorption, 355, 358, 359
  assessment of function, 354
    in diarrhoea, 374
    tests of, 357
  digestion,
    carbohydrates, 355
    fats, 356
    protein, 356
  fat absorption in 358, 359
  function, 356
  mucosal damage, 357
  tumours, 378
  water and electrolytes in, 354
Sodium,
  see also Hyponatraemia,
      Hypernatraemia etc
  abnormalities of, 56

absorption in colon, 57
assessment of, 56
atrial natriuretic peptide and, 56
in cells, 53
in cerebrospinal fluid, 562
controlling AVP secretion, 80
depletion, 57
  diarrhoea and, 60
  following trauma, 195
  hypotension and, 59, 60
  in protein-energy malnutrition, 5
  water depletion and, 59, 60
  without water depletion, 58
dietary intake, 57
in essential hypertension, 592
exchangeable, 57
excessive secretion, 57
in extracellular fluid, 53, 56
following trauma, 195
homeostasis with water, 79
interrelation with potassium, 69
loss of, 59
plasma level, 61
reabsorption, 56
renal handling of, 54
renal reabsorption, 54, 56
renal stones and, 343
retention, 65
  alcohol and, 124
  aldosterone causing, 594
  angiotensin causing, 597
transport, 53
urinary, 38, 322
  measurement, 68
Sodium space, 57
Sodium valproate,
  monitoring, 762
  poisoning, 740, 747
  treatment with, 301
Somatomedins, 523, 571
Somatostatin, 348, 588, 677
  in Alzheimer's disease, 148
Somatostatinoma, 673, 678
Sperm counts, 718
Spherocytosis, 307
  hereditary, 457
Sphingomyelin, 268
Spina bifida, 231
Spleen,
  platelets in, 505
Starvation, 70
Steatorrhoea, 359, 362
  clinical assessment, 372
  disorders causing, 375
  general investigations, 373
  investigation of, 372
  in malabsorption, 372
  in pancreatitis, 377
  radiology, 374
Steatosis, 130
Stein-Leventhal syndrome, 717
Steroids,
  see also Adrenal gland, steroids etc
  blood production rate, 708
  effect on plasma proteins, 465
  in heart and lung transplants, 208

metabolic clearance rate, 708
metabolism of, 591
nomenclature, 682, 683, 707
Steroid induced diabetes, 204
Stomach,
  acid secretion, 349
  assessment of function, 348
  basal and peak acid output, 350
  carcinoma, 456
  glandular cells, 348
  motility and emptying, 348
  mucus-bicarbonate layer, 348
  secretion,
    diarrhoea and, 365
  secretory tests, 350,351
Stomatogingivitis, 730
Stools,
  microbiological analysis, 374
  osmotic gap, 376
  'silver', 373
Stress,
  cortisol and, 690
  hypoglycaemia in, 694
  neuroendocrinological aspects, 149
String sign, 549
subacute sclerosing panencephalitis,
      567, 574
Subarachnoid haemorrhage, 570, 571
Subdural haematoma, 570
Subfornical region, 84
Succinic semialdehyde dehydrogenase
      deficiency, 279
Sulfation factor, 628
Sulphasalazine/sulphapyridine test,
      363
Sulphite oxidase, 287
  deficiency, 278
Sulphonylurias, 112, 116
Superoxide,
  in RDS, 305
Superoxide dismutase, 122, 289, 584
  alcohol and, 135
Superoxide ion, 122
Surfactant, 304, 305
Surma, 726
Sweat,
  calcium in, 518
  tests, 372
Synacthen,
  in ACTH stimulation tests, 692
  for Addison's disease, 696
Synovial fluid, 549
  synovitis, 546
Synovium,
  in rheumatoid arthritis, 547
Systemic lupus erythematosus, 500,
      550, 552
  similar syndromes, 478

Tamm-Horsfall glycoprotein, 320
Tamoxifen, 168
Tangier disease, 297, 608
Tape worms, 456
Tau protein, 568
Tay Sachs' disease, 158, 268, 269, 270
^{99m}Technectium colloid scan, 351

Telangiectasia, 500
Teratogens, 266
Testicular feminization, 714
Testis,
    ectopic, 714
    function, 712
    germ cell tumours, 181
Testosterone, 688, 712
    defective production, 713
    fetal, 712
    measurement, 691
    production, 711
    in polycystic ovaries, 718
Tetany, 49
Tetrahydrobiopterin metabolism, 266
Thalassaemia, 308, 420, 436
    diagnosis, 442
    fetal haemoglobin and, 439
    haematology of, 434
    iron overload in, 452
    malaria and, 437
    molecular defects, 435
    pathology, 434
    red cell abnormalities and, 437
Thalassaemia major, 440
Thalassaemia minor, 437
α-Thalassaemias, 435, 436
    gene deletions, 443
β-Thalassaemia, 436
    diagnosis, 444
    gene deletions, 436
    iron overload, 451
β-Thalassaemia minor,
    diagnosis, 439
    red cell indices, 435
Thallium poisoning, 157
Theophylline, 766
    poisoning, 740, 756
    therapeutic monitoring, 762
Therapeutic drug monitoring, 758–770
    audit, 768
    choice of drug, 762
    drug concentrations , 758
    drug intoxication, 764
    free-drug measurements, 762
    indications for measurement,763
    methods, 766
    methods of measurement, 765
    nomograms and algorithms, 766
    patient compliance, 764
    pharmacodynamic factors, 760
    quality control, 768
    recent advances, 767
    target range, 761
    use and abuse of, 761
Thiamin, See Vitamin B₁
Thiamine pyrophosphate, 155
Thirst, 82–85
    in elderly, 82
    experimental aspects, 83
    factors causing, 82
    mechanism, 60
    osmoreceptors governing, 83
    temporary relief of, 83
Thrombasthenia, 510
Thrombin time test, 507

Thrombocythaemia, 499
Thrombocythpenia, 499, 510
    in rheumatoid arthritis, 549
Thrombolytic therapy, 618
Thrombomodulin, 504
    assay, 509
Thrombospondin, 504
Thromboxane A₂, 190
Thyrocalcitonin, 635
Thyroglobulin, 638
    antibodies, 643, 647
    iodination of, 637
Thyroglobulin haemagglutination
        antibody, 644
Thyroid gland, 634–661
    anatomy, 634
        in hypothyroidism, 641
    antibody levels, 646
    antithyroid hormone antibodies,
        652
    autoantibodies, 643, 647
    autoimmune disease, 643
        cross-reactions, 646
        incidence of, 646
    calcitonin production in, 520
    carcinoma, 635
        diarrhoea in, 379
    congenital disease, 641
    disorders of, 640
        autoimmune, 642
        clinical aspects, 646
        hypertension in, 598
        in neonates and children, 654
        in pregnancy, 653
        surgical treatment, 655
        treatment of, 654
        Wayne and Newcastle index, 648
    in elderly, 654
    fetal, 286, 653
    function of, 635
        following injury, 191
        investigation of, 655, 658
    function tests,
        in diarrhoea, 374
        erroneous results, 659, 660
    hormones, 635–40
    binding, 638
        calcitonin affecting, 521
        calcium metabolism and, 527
        circulation, 637
        conjugation, 639
        deamination, 639
        deiodination, 638
        disorders of, 652
        effect on growth, 640
        excretion, 638
        in hyperthyroidism, 649
        metabolic effects, 639
        release, 637
        synthesis, 636
    malignant changes in, 648
    microsomal antibodies, 644, 647
    pathological changes, 641
    physiology of, 636
    substances suppressing activity, 653
Thyroiditis,

de Quervain's, 644
    focal lymphocytic, 643, 644
    subacute, 649, 652
Thyroid peroxidase, 644
Thyroid stimulating hormone, 152,
        623, 625, 627, 631, 635
    deficiency of, 652
    in depression, 149
    measurement of, 657, 659
    in neonatal screening, 249
    neoplastic disease and, 650
    receptor antibodies, 643, 656
    receptor protein, 645
    releasing hormone, 625
Thyrotoxic crises, 150, 650
Thyrotoxicosis, 523, 531
    iodine-induced, 650
    treatment, 657
Thyroxine, 635, 636, 638, 639
    in children, 294
    conversion, 639
    free, 656, 659
    measurement, 656, 658
    in neonatal screening, 249
    release and circulation, 637
Thyroxine-binding globulin, 637,
    congenital deficiency, 642
    congenital excess of, 642
    factors affecting, 638
Thyroxine-binding prealbumin, 10,
        637
Tildon-Cornblath syndrome, 283
Tissue plasminogen activators, 618
Tonsils,
    yellow-orange, 297
TORCH agents, 472
Total parenteral nutrition, 218, 222–
        226
    complications, 225
    energy-nitrogen ratios, 225
    energy requirements, 224
    indications for, 222
    micronutrient requirements, 225
    minerals in, 224
    nutritional requirements, 223
    patient assessment, 220
    preparation, 224
    protein requirements, 224
    route of access, 222
    trace elements in, 734
    vitamins in, 224
Trace elements,
    see also Metals
    biological function, 723
    deficiency and excess, 21
    disease monitoring, 735
    essential, 723, 732
    haemodialysis and, 734
    metabolism, 286
    nonessential, 723
    in pharmacological agents, 734
    status determination, 220
    total parenteral nutrition and, 734
Transcellular fluid, 57
Transferase deficiency, 275
Transferrin, 447, 485

carbohydrate deficiency, 134
in cerebrospinal fluid, 568
circulation, 447
electrophoresis, 490
iron bound to, 448
iron saturation, 449
in protein energy malnutrition, 10
saturation, 451
Transferrin index, 134
Transketolase, 126
Transplantation surgery,
    see also organs concerned
    assessment of donors, 200
    biochemical detection of rejection,
        215
    biochemistry and, 199–217
    cyclosporin in, See Cyclosporin
    domino procedure, 207
    FK506 in, 202
    follow-up, 202
    immunosuppression in, 200
    multiple organs, 215
    patient survival, 199, 200
    success rate, 199, 200
Transthyretin measurement, 392
Tricyclic antidepressants 740, 756
Triglycerides 349
Triglyceride lipase, 604, 607
Tri-iodothyronine, 635, 636, 638, 639
    in children, 294
    measurement of, 658
    release and circulation, 637
    reverse, 635, 636
        measurement, 658
    therapeutic use of, 654
Trimethylaminuria, 258
Triolein breath test 360, 371
Trisomy 21, See Down's syndrome
Trometamol, 95
Tropical ataxic neuropathy, 18
Troponin, 617
Trypsin, 367
    immunoreactive, 369
Trypsin test, 371, 372
Trypsinogen, 369
Tryptophan, 176
Tryptophan-associated eosinophilia-
        myalgia syndrome, 551
Tuberculosis, 694
Tuberculostearic acid, 572
Tuberculous meningitis, 564, 571
Tuberous sclerosis, 254
Tumours,
    alkaline phosphatase in, 388
    anaemia and, 179
    ascites with, 178
    associated with SIAD, 172
    biochemistry of, 161–188
    carbohydrate effects, 161
    cardio-vascular effects, 178
    causing hormone-deficiency
            syndromes, 176
    causing nephrotic syndrome, 178
    causing obstruction, 165, 177
    ectopic hormone secretion by 171
    energy metabolism in, 164

fat metabolism in, 164
first manifestations, 161
hormonal excess in, 169
hormone-deficiency syndromes and,
        177
hormone secretion, 170
hypercalcaemia in, 165, 539, 543
jaundice and, 178
metabolic effects of, 161
mineral metabolism in, 165
nutrition and, 228
oncodevelopmental products, 161
paraneoplastic effects, 161
phosphate in, 168
plasma calcium in, 516
plasma proteins in, 493
porphyria caused by, 179
protein metabolism in, 164
renal effects of, 176
with ectopic ACTH, 170
Tumour lysis syndrome, 168, 177
Tumour markers, 179–186
Tumour necrosis factor, 165
Turner's syndrome, 302, 713, 717
Twin pregnancy,
    screening, 233
Tyrosinaemia, 258, 278, 309
    hereditary, 416

Ulcerative colitis, 376, 388
Uraemia,
    parathyroid hormone and, 519
    psychiatric aspects, 153
Urea,
    as diuretic, 96
    in children, 294
    in sodium depletion, 58
    in urine, 321
Urea breath tests, 354
Urea broth test, 353
Urea clearance, 326
Urea cycle, 582
    disorders of, 276, 277, 281, 300
    enzyme deficiencies, 276, 394
    inherited defects, 301
Urea metabolism in malnutrition, 8
Ureteric stones, 344
Ureters,
    transplantation, 45
Uric acid,
    in alcoholism, 133
    lithiasis, 341
    neuropathy, 177
Uridine diphosphate galactose, 285
Uricosuria, 340
Urinary creatine-height index, 10
Urinary retention, 184
Urinary tract, stones in, See Renal
        stones
Urine,
    acidification, 332
    in acute abdomen, 402
    alcohol excretion in, 122, 123
    amino acid excretion, 320
    5-aminolaevulinate in, 409
    analysis of, 317

in appendicitis, 404
biochemical screening 318
calcium in, 339, 518
chemical analysis, 317–324
concentration, 54
    AVP and, 55
    diurnal rhythm, 82
    in excessive sodium intake, 62
    infant ability, 81
    quantitative, 81
    renal mechanisms, 86
cortisol in, 699
dipsticks for, 318
dolichols in, 136
drug screening, 323
early morning sample, 318
electrolytes in, 321
electrophoresis, 490 , 491
enzyme activity in, 321
glucose detection in, 319
hormones in, 322
5-HT breakdown in, 175
ketone bodies in, 104
mercury in, 729
microglobulin in, 486
normal sodium concentration, 68
osmolality, 321
    measurements, 67
output in infants, 79
pigments in, 323
porphobilinogen in, 412
porphyrins in, 417
    measurement, 412
in prenatal diagnosis, 238
potassium loss in, 70
potassium measurements, 71
protein in, 319, 320, 321
random samples, 318
red, 412
reducing substances in, 319
salsolinol in, 136
samples in poisoning, 737
screening, 319
sodium measurement, 68
steroid measurement, 691
stone formation, 338
timed collection, 318
types of sample, 317
urea in, 321
Urine arginine vasopressin test, 100
Urobilinogen in urine, 324
Uroporphyrinogen decarboxylase, 415

Vagotomy, 351
Valine, 282
Vanadium toxicity, 157
Vasculitis, 552
Vasoactive intestinal polypeptide, 586,
        671, 676
Vasoconstriction, 586
Vasodilatation, 586
Vasopressin, 588
VDRL test, 554
Venous return, 585
Ventricular haemorrhage, 262
Vernier-Morrison syndrome, 676

Vigabatrin, 767
VIPoma, 378, 673
  diagnosis, 677
Virilization, 719
  fetal 714
Viruses associated with diabetes, 106
Vitamins,
  absorption, 356
  in brain metabolism, 228
  as coenzymes, 19
  deficiency, 11
    in cancer, 228
    clinical features, 12
    in hypolipidaemias, 296
    in hospital patients, 218
    mental retardation and, 265
  dependency, 266
Vitamins,
  excess, 11
  status, 19
  in total parenteral nutrition, 224
Vitamin A,
  deficiency, 12
  excess, 12
  infection and, 12
  toxicity, 156
Vitamin B,
  determination of status, 19
Vitamin B_1, 15
  cobalt and, 22
  deficiency,
    in alcoholism, 138
    psychiatric aspects, 154
  subclinical deficiency, 16
  in Wernicke's encephalopathy, 126
Vitamin B_2, 17
  deficiency, 578
Vitamin B_3, 17
  deficiency, 155
Vitamin B_5, 17
  deficiency, 342
Vitamin B_6, 126, 155
Vitamin B_{12}, 17
  cobalt and, 733
  deficiency, 18
    anaemia in, 454, 456
  in liver, 394
  malabsorption of, 362, 456
  metabolism, 455
Vitamin C, 18
  deficiency, 18
Vitamin D,
  action of, 541
  in bone mineralization, 530
  in calcium metabolism, 521
  deficiency, 11, 13, 265, 522, 530, 541,
    542
    alcoholism and, 140
    myopathy in, 522
    renal tubular acidosis in, 332
  excessive amounts of, 11, 340, 541
  metabolism, 523

toxicity, 14
  translocation, 526
Vitamin D_2, 521
Vitamin D_3, 522
Vitamin D metabolites, 523
  defective production, 541
Vitamin D resistant rickets, 14, 542
Vitamin E,
  deficiency, 15, 266
  toxicity, 15
Vitamin K,
  deficiency, 15, 498, 500
Volvulus, 406
Vomiting,
  in appendicitis, 404
  AVP and, 55
  causing hypokalaemia, 70
  in intestinal obstruction, 405
  water loss via, 79
Von Gierke's disease, 282
von Recklinghausen's disease, 181
von Willebrand factor, 497, 501
  assay of, 505, 508
  biochemistry, 502
von Willebrand's disease, 496, 497,
  502

WDHA syndrome, 676
Warburg effect, 162
Warfarin, 15
Water,
  abnormalities of, 56
  absorption, 85, 354
  assessment, 56
  balance in infancy, 79
  composition of body, 53
  compulsive drinking, 96, 154
  control of, 76
  cooling, 80
  decreased intake, 91
  depletion,
    causes, 60
    following trauma, 195
    in neonates, 306
    psychiatric aspects, 154
    with little sodium depletion, 60
  distribution in body, 77, 78
  diuresis, 82, 92
  dynamic aspects, 78, 79
  excessive intake, 90
  excessive retention, 63
  homeostasis,
    AVP and, 83
    clinical aspects, 91
    imbalance, 90
    physiological control, 80
    with sodium, 79
  inadequate intake, 60
  input and output, 77, 78
  insensible loss, 79
  intestinal transport, 85
  intoxication, 66, 154

loss of, 78
  metabolism after trauma, 196
  reabsorption,
    assessment, 333
    AVP in, 87
    factors influencing, 54
    in loop of Henle, 86
    in proximal tubule, 86
  renal handling of, 54
  renal stones and, 343
  requirement for, 77
  retention, 63, 65
    in alcohol intoxication, 124
    mechanism, 64
Water deprivation test, 98
Watson-Schwartz test, 412
Wegener's granulomatosis, 555
Weight loss,
  in cancer, 164, 165
  in carcinoid syndrome, 175
Weight norms, 25
Wermer's syndrome, 631, 697
Werner-Morrison syndrome, 378
Wernicke's encephalopathy, 15, 16,
  153, 154, 578
Whipple's triad, 664
Williams factor, 501
Wilm's tumour, 96
Wilson's disease, 21, 286, 331, 723
  alkaline phosphatase in, 388
  aminotransferases in, 386
  caeruloplasmin in, 393, 485
Woman's disease, 270

Xanthine nephropathy, 177
Xanthine oxidase, 287, 305, 584
  deficiency, 339
Xanthochromia of CSF, 569
Xanthomas, 603, 605
Xenobiotic agents, 550
Xeroderma pigmentosum, 288
Xerophthalmia, 12
X-linked adrenoleucodystrophy, 284
X-linked agammaglobulinaemia, 470
X-linked disorders, 242
X-linked Schlindler's disease, 158
Xylose absorption test, 357
^{14}C-d-Xylose breath test, 361

Zellweger syndrome, 256, 284
Zinc, 733
  colonic absorption, 364
  deficiency and excess, 21
    mental aspects, 156
  metabolism following surgery, 196
Zinc-protoporphyrina complex, 726,
  727
Zollinger-Ellison syndrome, 252, 350,
  351, 352, 619, 674
  diagnosis, 675
  diarrhoea in, 365
  treatment, 675